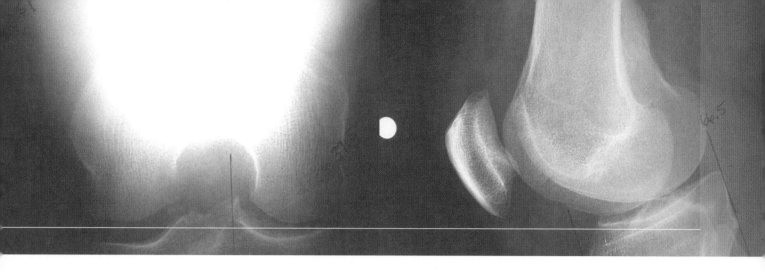

Surgical Techniques of the Shoulder, Elbow, and Knee in Sports Medicine

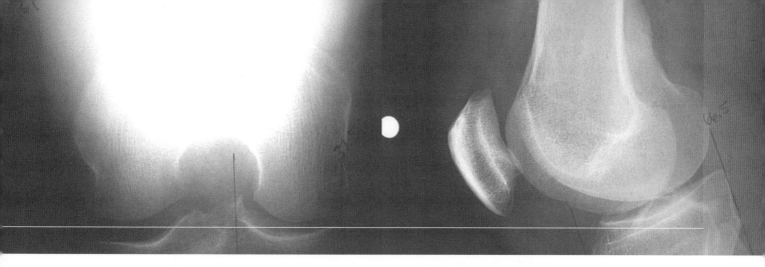

Surgical Techniques of the Shoulder, Elbow, and Knee in Sports Medicine

Associate Editors

Andreas H. Gomoll, MD
Instructor of Orthopaedic Surgery
Harvard Medical School
Cartilage Repair Center
Department of Orthopaedic Surgery
Brigham and Women's Hospital
Boston, Massachusetts

Jeffrey Rihn, MD
Fellow
Orthopaedic Spine Surgery
The Rothman Institute and
Thomas Jefferson University Hospital
Philadelphia, Pennsylvania

Edited by

Brian J. Cole, MD, MBA
Professor
Departments of
Orthopedics and Anatomy and Cell Biology
Section of Sports Medicine
Section Head, Cartilage Restoration Center at Rush
Rush University Medical Center
Chicago, Illinois

Jon K. Sekiya, MD, MC, USNR
Associate Professor
MedSport-Department of Orthopaedic Surgery
University of Michigan
Ann Arbor, Michigan

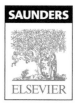

SAUNDERS

ELSEVIER

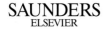

1600 John F. Kennedy Blvd.
Ste 1800
Philadelphia, PA 19103-2899

SURGICAL TECHNIQUES OF THE SHOULDER, ELBOW,
AND KNEE IN SPORTS MEDICINE

ISBN: 978-1-4160-3447-6

Copyright © 2008 by Saunders, an imprint of Elsevier Inc.

Notice

Knowledge and best practice in this field are constantly changing. As new research and experience broaden our knowledge, changes in practice, treatment and drug therapy may become necessary or appropriate. Readers are advised to check the most current information provided (i) on procedures featured or (ii) by the manufacturer of each product to be administered, to verify the recommended dose or formula, the method and duration of administration, and contraindications. It is the responsibility of the practitioner, relying on their own experience and knowledge of the patient, to make diagnoses, to determine dosages and the best treatment for each individual patient, and to take all appropriate safety precautions. To the fullest extent of the law, neither the Publisher nor the Editors assume any liability for any injury and/or damage to persons or property arising out of or related to any use of the material contained in this book.

The Publisher

Library of Congress Cataloging-in-Publication Data
Surgical techniques of the shoulder, elbow, and knee in sports medicine / edited by Brian J. Cole . . . [et al.]. – 1st ed.
    p. ; cm.
    Includes bibliographical references and index.
    ISBN 978-1-4160-3447-6
  1. Arthroscopy.   2. Shoulder–Surgery.   3. Elbow–Surgery.   4. Knee–Surgery.   5. Sports medicine.   I. Cole, Brian J.
    [DNLM: 1. Arthroscopy.   2. Elbow–surgery.   3. Knee–surgery.   4. Shoulder–surgery.
5. Sports Medicine–methods. WE 304 S961 2008]
RC932.S83 2008
617.4′720597–dc22   2007039759

Publishing Director: Kim Murphy
Developmental Editor: Ann Ruzycka Anderson
Publishing Services Manager: Tina Rebane
Design Direction: Louis Forgione
Marketing Manager: Catalina Nolte

Printed in China

Last digit is the print number: 9 8 7 6 5 4 3 2 1

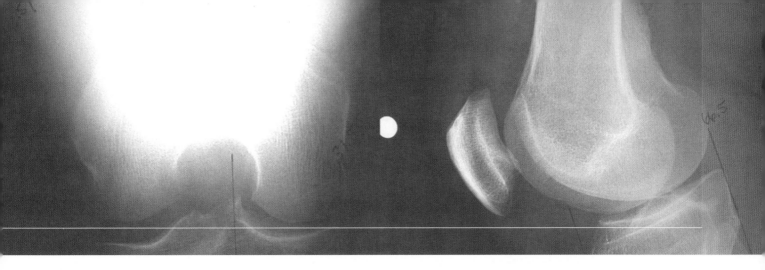

Contributors

Christopher S. Ahmad, MD

Assistant Professor of Orthopaedic Surgery, Center for Shoulder, Elbow and Sports Medicine, Columbia University, New York, New York

Joshua M. Alpert, MD

Resident, Orthopedic Surgery, Rush University Medical Center, Chicago, Illinois

Annunziato Amendola, MD

Professor, Orthopaedics and Rehabilitation, University of Iowa; Director, University of Iowa Sports Medicine Center, University of Iowa Hospitals and Clinics, Iowa City, Iowa

Ammar Anbari, MD

Attending, Orthopaedics, Sports Medicine and Cartilage Restoration, William W. Backus Hospital, Norwich, Connecticut

Kyle Anderson, MD

Director, Sports Medicine and Shoulder Fellowship, Department of Orthopaedic Surgery, William Beaumont Hospital; Team Physician, Detroit Lions, Detroit, Michigan

James R. Andrews, MD

Medical Director, American Sports Medicine Institute; Orthopaedic Surgeon, Alabama Sports Medicine and Orthopaedic Center, Birmingham, Alabama

Robert A. Arciero, MD

Professor, Orthopaedic Surgery, Department of Orthopaedics, University of Connecticut and John Dempsey Hospital, Farmington, Connecticut

Ryan A. Aukerman, MD

Orthopaedic Surgery Sports Medicine Specialist, Department of Sports Medicine, Gem City Bone and Joint; Team Physician, Department of Sports Medicine, University of Wyoming, Laramie, Wyoming

Frederick M. Azar, MD

Professor and Residency Program Director, and Sports Medicine Fellowship Director, Campbell Clinic– University of Tennessee, Memphis, Tennessee

Bernard R. Bach, Jr., MD

The Claude N. Lambert–Susan Thomson Endowed Professor of Orthopedic Surgery, and Director, Division of Sports Medicine and Sports Medicine Fellowship, Rush University Medical Center; Team Physician, Chicago White Sox and Chicago Bulls, Chicago, Illinois

Champ L. Baker, Jr., MD

Clinical Assistant Professor, Department of Orthopaedic Surgery, Tulane University School of Medicine, New Orleans, Louisiana; Clinical Assistant Professor, Department of Orthopaedics, Medical College of Georgia, Augusta; and Staff Physician, The Hughston Clinic, Columbus, Georgia

Champ L. Baker, III, MD

Resident, Department of Orthopaedic Surgery, University of Pittsburgh Medical Center, Pittsburgh, Pennsylvania

Joshua A. Baumfeld, MD

Sports Medicine, Department of Orthopaedic Surgery, Lahey Clinic, Burlington, Massachusetts

Matthew T. Boes, MD

East Bay Shoulder and Sports Medicine, Orinda, California

Kevin F. Bonner, MD

Assistant Professor of Surgery, Eastern Virginia Medical School, Norfolk; Orthopaedic Surgeon, Jordan-Young Institute, Virginia Beach, Virginia

Craig R. Bottoni, MD

Chief of Surgery, Aspetar Sports Medicine Hospital, Doha, Qatar

Mark K. Bowen, MD

Associate Professor of Clinical Orthopaedic Surgery, Northwestern University Medical School; Active Attending, Northwestern Memorial Hospital, Chicago, Illinois

Declan J. Bowler, MD, FRCSI (Tr & Orth)

Fellow in Sports Medicine, The Hughston Clinic, Columbus, Georgia

Michael B. Boyd, DO

Attending Physician, Department of Orthopaedic Surgery, St. Mary's Hospital and Deaconess Hospital, Evansville, Indiana

James P. Bradley, MD

Clinical Associate Professor of Orthopaedic Surgery, University of Pittsburgh Medical Center; Orthopaedic Surgeon, University of Pittsburgh Medical Center Shadyside and St. Margaret Hospitals; Head Orthopaedic Surgeon, Pittsburgh Steelers Football Team, Pittsburgh, Pennsylvania

Karen K. Briggs, MPH

Director of Clinical Research, Steadman Hawkins Research Foundation, Vail, Colorado

Charles H. Brown Jr., MD

Medical Director, Abu Dhabi Knee and Sports Medicine Centre, Abu Dhabi, United Arab Emirates

Shervondalonn R. Brown, MD

Department of Orthopaedic Surgery, University of Pittsburgh, Pittsburgh, Pennsylvania

Stephen S. Buckhart, MD

Director of Medical Education, The San Antonio Orthopedic Group, San Antonio, Texas

William Bugbee, MD

Associate Professor, Department of Orthopaedic Surgery, University of California, San Diego; Attending, Lower Extremity Reconstruction and Cartilage Restoration, Division of Orthopaedic Surgery, Scripps Clinic, La Jolla, California

Anthony M. Buoncristiani, MD

Sports Medicine, University of Pittsburgh Department of Orthopaedic Surgery, Pittsburgh, Pennsylvania

Charles A. Bush-Joseph, MD

Associate Professor, Department of Orthopaedic Surgery, Rush University Medical Center, Chicago, Illinois

Bradley Butkovich, MD, MS

Sports Medicine Fellow, Orthopaedic Surgery, Orthopaedic Research of Virginia and Tuckahoe Orthopaedic Associates, Ltd., Richmond, Virginia

Thomas R. Carter, MD

Emeritus Head of Orthopedic Surgery, and Consultant, Orthopedic Surgery, Arizona State University, Tempe, Arizona

Justin W. Chandler, MD

Resident Physician, Department of Orthopaedics, University of North Carolina at Chapel Hill and University of North Carolina Hospitals, Chapel Hill, North Carolina

Neal C. Chen, MD

Resident, Orthopedic Surgery, Harvard Combined Orthopedic Residency, Boston, Massachusetts

Steven B. Cohen, MD

Assistant Professor, Department of Orthopaedic Surgery, Thomas Jefferson University; Orthopaedic Surgeon, Rothman Institute; Assistant Team Physician, Philadelphia Phillies Baseball Team, Philadelphia, Pennsylvania

Brian J. Cole, MD, MBA

Professor, Departments of Orthopedics and Anatomy and Cell Biology, Section of Sports Medicine; Section Head, Cartilage Restoration at Rush, Rush University Medical Center, Chicago, Illinois

Alfred J. Cook Jr., MD

Senior Resident, Orthopaedic Surgery, Northwestern Memorial Hospital, Chicago, Illinois

Andrew J. Cosgarea, MD

Associate Professor and Director of Sports Medicine and Shoulder Surgery, Department of Orthopaedic Surgery, Johns Hopkins University, Baltimore, Maryland

Edward V. Craig, MD

Professor of Clinical Surgery (Orthopaedics), Weill Medical College of Cornell University; Attending Orthopaedic Surgeon, Hospital for Special Surgery, New York, New York

R. Alexander Creighton, MD

Assistant Professor of Orthopaedics, University of North Carolina at Chapel Hill and University of North Carolina Hospitals, Chapel Hill, North Carolina

Nader Darwich, MD

Deputy Medical Director, Abu Dhabi Knee and Sports Medicine Centre, Abu Dhabi, United Arab Emirates

James B. Day, MD, PhD

Assistant Professor and Chief of Orthopaedic Trauma Service, Department of Orthopaedic Surgery, Marshall University, Joan C. Edwards School of Medicine; Director of Orthopaedic Trauma, Department of Orthopaedic Surgery, Cabell Huntington Hospital, Huntington, West Virginia

David R. Diduch, MS, MD

Professor of Orthopaedic Surgery, University of Virginia; Head Orthopaedic Team Physician and Sports Medicine Fellowship Director, University of Virginia, Charlottesville, Virginia

Kevin M. Doulens, MD

Clinical Fellow, Sports Medicine, Orthopaedics and Rehabilitation, Vanderbilt University Medical Center, Nashville, Tennessee

Bradley D. Dresher, MD

Colorado Springs Orthopaedic Group, Penrose Community Hospital, Colorado Springs, Colorado

Jeffrey R. Dugas, MD

Affiliate Professor, College of Health and Human Services, Athletic Training Department, Troy University, Troy; Fellowship Director, American Sports Medicine Institute, Birmingham, Alabama

Craig J. Edson, MHS, PT, ATC

Sports Medicine Specialist, Sports Medicine Outpatient Rehabilitation, Geisinger/HealthSouth, Danville, Pennsylvania

Neal S. ElAttrache

Kerlan-Jobe Orthopaedic Clinic, Los Angeles, California

LCDR Christopher I. Ellingson, MD

Orthopaedic Surgeon, US Naval Hospital Sigonella, Naval Air Station Sigonella, Italy

Gregory C. Fanelli, MD

Fanelli Sports Injury Clinic, Geisinger Medical Center, Danville, Pennsylvania

Jack Farr, MD

Associate Clinical Professor of Orthopaedic Surgery, Indiana University School of Medicine; Orthopaedic Surgeon, St. Francis Hospital and Health Centers and Indiana Orthopaedic Hospital, Indianapolis, Indiana

Diego Fernandez, MD

Professor of Orthopaedic Surgery, Department of Orthopaedic Surgery, University of Bern and Lindenhof Hospital, Bern, Switzerland

Larry D. Field, MD

Clinical Instructor, Orthopaedic Surgery, University of Mississippi School of Medicine; Co-Director, Upper Extremity Service, Mississippi Sports Medicine and Orthopaedic Center, Jackson, Mississippi

Fred Flandry, MD, FACS

Clinical Associate Professor, Department of Orthopaedic Surgery, Tulane University School of Medicine, New Orleans, Louisiana; Attending Surgeon and Director of Medical Education, The Hughston Foundation, Columbus, Georgia

David C. Flanigan, MD

Assistant Professor of Orthopedics, The Ohio State University; Team Physician, The Ohio State University Athletic Department, The Ohio State University, Columbus, Ohio

Freddie H. Fu, MD, DSc (Hon), DPs (Hon)

Chairman, Orthopaedic Surgery, University of Pittsburgh Medical Center, Pittsburgh, Pennsylvania

John P. Fulkerson, MD

Clinical Professor of Orthopedic Surgery, University of Connecticut School of Medicine, Farmington, Connecticut

Raffaele Garofalo, MD

III Orthopaedic and Traumatologic Unit, University of Bari, Bari; Consultant, Shoulder Unit, Humanitas-Gavazzeni Unit, Bergamo, Italy

Scott Gillogly, MD

Medical Staff, Department of Orthopaedic Surgery, St. Joseph's Hospital, Atlanta, Georgia

Robert J. Goitz, MD

Associate Professor and Chief, Head and Upper Extremity Surgery, Department of Orthopaedic Surgery, University of Pittsburgh Medical Center, Pittsburgh, Pennsylvania

Andreas H. Gomoll, MD

Instructor of Orthopaedic Surgery, Harvard Medical School; Cartilage Repair Center, Department of Orthopaedic Surgery, Brigham and Women's Hospital, Boston, Massachusetts

Christopher D. Harner, MD

Professor, Department of Orthopaedic Surgery, University of Pittsburgh; Medical Director, Department of Orthopaedic Surgery, University of Pittsburgh Medical Center, Center for Sports Medicine, Pittsburgh, Pennsylvania

Timothy J. Henderson, MD

Orthopedic Surgery and Sports Medicine, University of California, Los Angeles, Medical Center, Los Angeles, California

Thomas F. Holovacs, MD

Instructor in Orthopaedic Surgery, Department of Orthopaedics, Harvard Medical School; Instructor in Orthopaedic Surgery, Department of Orthopaedics, Massachusetts General Hospital, Boston, Massachusetts

David P. Huberty, MD

The San Antonio Orthopedic Group, San Antonio, Texas

Mary Lloyd Ireland, MD

President/Director, Kentucky Sports Medicine Clinic, Lexington, Kentucky

Kent R. Jackson, MD

Fellow, Sports Medicine and Shoulder Service, Hospital for Special Surgery, New York, New York

Jeffrey T. Junko, MD

Clinical Instructor, Orthopaedics, Northeastern Universities College of Medicine; Director of Resident Education, Orthopaedics, Summa Health System, Akron, Ohio

Warren Ross Kadrmas, MD

Fellow, Sports Medicine and Shoulder Service, Hospital for Special Surgery, New York, New York; Staff Orthopaedic Surgeon, Wilford Hall Medical Center, Lackland Air Force Base, Texas

Christopher C. Kaeding, MD

Professor of Orthopaedics and Director of Sports Medicine, Department of Orthopaedic Surgery; Head Team Physician, Department of Athletics, The Ohio State University, Columbus, Ohio

Richard W. Kang, MD

Resident, Orthopedic Surgery, Rush University Medical Center, Chicago, Illinois

Lee D. Kaplan, MD

Assistant Professor of Orthopedics, University of Wisconsin Medical School; Attending Physician, Orthopedics, University of Wisconsin Hospital and Clinics, Madison, Wisconsin

Matthew A. Kippe, MD

Department of Orthopedic Surgery, Hawthorn Medical Associates, North Dartmouth, Massachusetts

Jason Koh, MD

Associate Professor of Orthopaedic Surgery, Northwestern University Feinberg School of Medicine, Chicago, Illinois

Pradeep Kodali, MD

Resident Physician, Department of Orthopaedic Surgery, McGraw Medical Center–Northwestern University, Chicago, Illinois

Melissa W. Koenig, MD

Instructor, Department of Orthopaedic Surgery, George Washington University and George Washington University Hospital, Washington, DC

Eric J. Kropf, MD

Resident Physician, Orthopaedic Surgery, University of Pittsburgh Medical Center, Pittsburgh, Pennsylvania

John E. Kuhn, MD

Associate Professor and Chief of Shoulder Surgery, Division of Sports Medicine, Department of Orthopaedics and Rehabilitation, Vanderbilt University Medical Center, Nashville, Tennessee

Joanne E. Labriola, MD

Clinical Instructor, Department of Orthopaedic Surgery, University Health Center of Pittsburgh, Pittsburgh, Pennsylvania

Christian Lattermann, MD

Assistant Professor for Orthopaedics and Sports Medicine, and Director, Center for Cartilage Repair and Restoration, Department of Orthopaedic Surgery, University of Kentucky, Lexington, Kentucky

Jason W. Levine, MD

Assistant Professor, Department of Orthopaedics, University of Toledo Medical Center, Toledo, Ohio

C. Benjamin Ma, MD

Assistant Professor in Residence, Orthopaedic Surgery, University of California, San Francisco, San Francisco, California

Augustus D. Mazzocca, MS, MD

Assistant Professor, Orthopaedic Surgery, University of Connecticut, Farmington, Connecticut

David R. McAllister, MD

Associate Professor and Chief, Sports Medicine Service, Department of Orthopaedic Surgery, University of California, Los Angeles, David Geffen School of Medicine; Associate Team Physician, Athletic Department, University of California, Los Angeles, Los Angeles, California

Eric McCarty, MD

Associate Professor and Chief of Sports Medicine and Shoulder Surgery, Department of Orthopaedic Surgery, University of Colorado Health Science Center; Attending, Boulder Community Hospital, Boulder, Colorado

L. Pearce McCarty, III, MD

Sports and Orthopaedic Specialists, PA, Minneapolis, Minnesota

Mark D. Miller, MD

Professor, Department of Orthopaedic Surgery, University of Virginia, Charlottesville; Team Physician, James Madison University, Harrisonburg, Virginia

Craig D. Morgan, MD

Clinical Professor, University of Pennsylvania; Associate Clinical Professor, Thomas Jefferson University, Philadelphia, Pennsylvania; Orthopaedic Surgeon, Morgan Kalman Clinic, Wilmington, Delaware

Bradley J. Nelson, MD

Associate Professor, Department of Orthopaedics, University of Minnesota, Minneapolis, Minnesota

Gregory P. Nicholson, MD

Associate Professor, Orthopaedic Surgery, Rush University Medical Center, Chicago, Illinois

Gordon Nuber, MD

Professor of Clinical Orthopaedics, Northwestern University, Chicago, Illinois

Brett D. Owens, MD

Adjunct Assistant Professor, Department of Surgery, Uniformed Services University, Bethesda, Maryland; Orthopaedic Surgeon, Keller Army Hospital, West Point, New York

Michael J. Pagnani, MD

Director, Nashville Knee and Shoulder Center; Head Team Physician, Nashville Predators Hockey Club, Nashville, Tennessee

Scott D. Pennington, MD

Assistant Clinical Instructor, Department of Orthopaedics, Harvard Medical School; Shoulder Fellow, Department of Orthopaedics, Massachusetts General Hospital, Boston, Massachusetts

R. David Rabalais, MD

Sports Medicine and Shoulder Surgery Fellow, Department of Orthopaedic Surgery, University of Colorado Health Science Center and Boulder Community Hospital, Boulder, Colorado

Christopher A. Radkowski, MD

Pittsburgh Bone and Joint Surgeons, PC, Jefferson Hills, Pennsylvania

Kristin N. Reinheimer, PA-C

Geisinger Sports Medicine, Geisinger Medical Center, Danville, Pennsylvania

Eric P. Rightmire, MD

Attending Physician, Orthopedic Surgery, Jordan Hospital, Plymouth; Orthopedic Surgeon, Plymouth Bay Orthopedic Associates, Duxbury, Massachusetts

Jeffrey A. Rihn, MD

Fellow, Orthopaedic and Spine Surgery, The Rothman Institute and Thomas Jefferson University Hospital, Philadelphia, Pennsylvania

David Ring, MD, PhD

Assistant Professor, Orthopaedic Surgery, Harvard Medical School; Medical Director and Director of Research, Orthopaedic Hand and Upper Extremity Service, Massachusetts General Hospital, Boston, Massachusetts

Anthony A. Romeo, MD

Associate Professor, Department of Orthopaedics, Rush Medical College and Rush-Presbyterian–St. Luke's Medical Center, Chicago, Illinois

Scott Alan Rodeo, MD

Associate Professor of Orthopaedic Surgery, Weill Medical College of Cornell University; Associate Attending, Sports Medicine and Shoulder Service, Hospital for Special Surgery; Associate Team Physician, New York Giants, New York, New York

William G. Rodkey, DVM (Diplomate), ACVS

Director, Basic Science Research, Steadman Hawkins Research Foundation, Vail, Colorado

Mark W. Rodosky, MD

Assistant Professor of Orthopaedic Surgery and Chief, Shoulder Service, Department of Orthopaedic Surgery, Division of Sports Medicine, University Health Center of Pittsburgh, Pittsburgh, Pennsylvania

L. Joseph Rubino, MD

Assistant Professor, Orthopaedics and Sports Medicine, Wright State University, Dayton, Ohio

Marc R. Safran, MD

Professor of Orthopaedic Surgery, Associate Director of Sports Medicine, and Fellowship Director, Department of Orthopaedic Surgery, Stanford University, Stanford, California

Brett S. Sanders, MD

Assistant Clinical Instructor, Department of Orthopaedics, Harvard Medical School; Shoulder Fellow, Department of Orthopaedics, Massachusetts General Hospital, Boston, Massachusetts

Felix H. Savoie III, MD

Professor of Orthopaedic Surgery, Tulane University School of Medicine, New Orleans, Louisiana

Jon Sekiya, MD

Associate Professor, Department of Orthopaedic Surgery, University of Michigan, Ann Arbor, Michigan

Fintan J. Shannon, FRCS (Trd Orth)

Fellow, Sports Medicine and Shoulder Service, Hospital for Special Surgery, New York, New York

James P. Sieradzki, MD

Resident, Orthopaedic Surgery, McGaw Medical Center, Northwestern University Feinberg School of Medicine, Chicago, Illinois

Adam M. Smith, MD

Kentucky Sports Medicine, Lexington, Kentucky

Stephen J. Snyder, MD

Director, Shoulder Arthroscopy Service, Southern California Orthopedic Institute, Van Nuys, California

John W. Sperling, MD, MBA

Associate Professor, Department of Orthopedic Surgery, Mayo Clinic College of Medicine; Consultant, Department of Orthopedic Surgery, Mayo Clinic, Rochester, Minnesota

Kurt P. Spindler, MD

Kenneth D. Schermerhorn Professor and Vice Chairman, Department of Orthopaedics and Rehabilitation; Director, Sports Medicine and Orthopaedic Patient Care Center; Head Team Physician, Vanderbilt Athletics, Orthopaedics and Rehabilitation, Vanderbilt University Medical Center, Nashville, Tennessee

James S. Starman, BS

Department of Orthopaedic Surgery, University of Pittsburgh Medical Center, Pittsburgh, Pennsylvania

J. Richard Steadman, MD

Orthopaedic Surgeon, Steadman Hawkins Clinic; Founder and Chairman of the Board, Steadman Hawkins Research Foundation, Vail, Colorado

Scott P. Steinmann, MD

Associate Professor, Department of Orthopedic Surgery, Mayo Clinic College of Medicine; Consultant in Shoulder, Elbow, and Hand Surgery, Department of Orthopedic Surgery, Saint Mary's Hospital, Rochester, Minnesota

Justin P. Strickland, MD

Resident, Department of Orthopedic Surgery, Mayo Clinic Graduate School of Medicine, Rochester, Minnesota

Kenneth G. Swan, Jr., MD

Sports Medicine and Shoulder Surgery Fellow, Department of Orthopaedic Surgery, University of Colorado Health Science Center and Boulder Community Hospital, Boulder, Colorado

Raymond Thal, MD

Assistant Clinical Professor of Orthopaedic Surgery, George Washington University School of Medicine, Washington, DC; Orthopaedic Surgeon, Town Center Orthopaedic Associates, Reston, Virginia

Fotios Paul Tjoumakaris, MD

Attending Physician, Cape Orthopaedics, Department of Orthopaedics, Cape Regional Medical Center, Cape May Court House, New Jersey

Albert Tom, MD

University of Connecticut Sport Medicine Fellow, Department of Orthopaedics, University of Connecticut, Farmington, Connecticut

Max Tyorkin, MD

Associate Attending, Orthopaedic Surgery, Beth Israel Medical Center and Lenox Hill Hospital, New York, New York

Nikhil N. Verma, MD

Attending Orthopedic Surgeon, Department of Orthopaedic Surgery, Rush University, Chicago, Illinois

Jon J. P. Warner, MD

Professor of Orthopaedics, Department of Orthopaedics, Harvard Medical School; Chief, Harvard Shoulder Service, Department of Orthopaedics, Massachusetts General Hospital, Boston, Massachusetts

Russel F. Warren, MD

Professor of Orthopaedic Surgery, Weill Medical College of Cornell University; Surgeon-in-Chief Emeritus and Attending Orthopaedic Surgeon, Hospital for Special Surgery; Team Physician, New York Giants, New York, New York

Robin V. West, MD

Assistant Professor, Department of Orthopaedics, University of Pittsburgh, Pittsburgh, Pennsylvania

Thomas L. Wickiewicz, MD

Chief, Sports Medicine and Shoulder Service, Department of Orthopaedic Sports Medicine, Hospital for Special Surgery, New York, New York

Riley J. Williams III, MD

Associate Professor, Department of Orthopedic Surgery, Weill Medical College of Cornell University; Attending Orthopedic Surgeon, Sports Medicine and Shoulder Service, Hospital for Special Surgery New York, New York

Vonda J. Wright, MD

Assistant Professor, Department of Orthopaedic Surgery; University of Pittsburgh Medical Center, Center for Sports Medicine, University of Pittsburgh, Pittsburgh, Pennsylvania

Shawn W. Wynn, MD

Orthopaedic Sports Medicine Fellow, Orthopaedic Surgery, University of Wisconsin Hospitals and Clinics, Madison, Wisconsin

Robert W. Wysocki, MD

Orthopaedic Surgery Resident, Department of Orthopaedic Surgery, Rush University and Rush University Medical Center, Chicago, Illinois

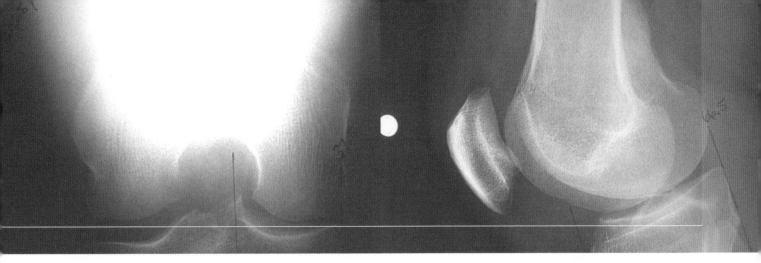

Preface

As educators, our most formidable challenge is to teach proper decision making and the techniques required to succeed in the operating room setting. As students, we are continuously pressured to compress the learning experience outside of the operating room into efficient and digestible bits of information. We all recognize the importance of having access to accurate, timely, and concise tools to supplement our knowledge base. The emergence of digital content has positively influenced our access to up-to-date information, yet falls way short of the tangible benefits derived from a manageable textbook that remains comprehensive yet not overwhelming. Simply "reading" about surgical procedures seems somewhat at odds with "doing" a series of steps that require dexterity and skill. More importantly, the act of physical repetition is what seems to propel us along the typically steep learning curve, especially when it involves the arthroscope.

Surgical Techniques of the Shoulder, Elbow, and Knee in Sports Medicine was developed with these principles in mind. The principle objective of this textbook was to maximize its value by remaining thorough in the breadth of open and arthroscopic procedures covered, yet extraordinarily concise in specific content. Authors have uniformly adhered to a template that we believe will optimize an efficient learning experience that is graphically consistent, simple, and descriptive. To this end, each chapter is crafted with a brief introduction, a thumbnail of only the most relevant pre- and postoperative considerations, a thorough and graphically supported step-by-step explicit description of the procedure, and a table with the most up-to-date results related to that specific procedure. Simply stated, it is exactly what you need to know prior to entering the operating room.

It is nearly impossible to cover every joint in a single-volume textbook. While the term "sports medicine" has broad-reaching connotations, the vast majority of the surgical armamentarium required of the orthopaedic surgeon who practices sports medicine and arthroscopy involve the shoulder, elbow, and knee. Thus, *Surgical Techniques of the Shoulder, Elbow, and Knee in Sports Medicine* intentionally limits the number of joints to those most commonly seen and treated, but covers them comprehensively without exception. Most importantly, the content is provided by authors who have largely developed and popularized the exact procedure discussed.

Part 1, The Shoulder, covers the general technical aspects of shoulder arthroscopy, including patient positioning, arthroscopic portal placement, and the instrumentation and specific steps required to pass sutures and tie knots. Then the fun begins. Because there are so many different techniques performed to address the same pathology, we include more than a dozen chapters describing the treatment of shoulder instability, including the management of bone loss with allografts and coracoid transfer. Similarly, the management of rotator cuff pathology is addressed by no less than six graphic chapters, including the role and techniques for tendon transfer. Finally, The Shoulder is complemented by chapters that address the treatment of the most common entities, including SLAP tears, shoulder stiffness, AC joint instability, biceps tendon tears and instability, and glenohumeral arthritis. Part 1 is a stand-alone compendium of the treatment of virtually every clinical problem seen by the shoulder surgeon.

Part 2, The Elbow, is also comprehensive in that it includes the requisite steps required to perform elbow arthroscopy, such as patient positioning, portal placement, and a review of normal arthroscopic anatomy. In addition to providing excellent chapters on the most common conditions that we treat arthroscopically (e.g., osteochondritis dissecans, stiffness, synovitis, athritis, and lateral epicondylitis), it is unique in that it contains an entire section on the most important open elbow procedures. Surgeons who treat athletes with ulnar and lateral collateral ligament disruption, elbow stiffness, biceps tendon tears, and epicondylitis will recognize that the section on open procedures of the elbow is thorough and completely up-to-date with surgical principles and techniques.

Part 3, The Knee, is another virtual compendium that includes the complete management of any knee-related pathology. For example, management of meniscus-related issues has led to the development of multiple techniques to excise, repair, and replace the meniscal-deficient knee. Seven chapters thoroughly review all of these techniques. Articular cartilage, the subject of stand-alone textbooks, is completely covered with the management of virtually every problem that involves cartilage and bone short of arthroplasty. Ten chapters are provided to enable the reader to perform any cartilage repair procedure in addition to realignment osteotomy. One of the most exciting sections is the management of the anterior and posterior cruciate ligaments. This section includes single- and double-bundle techniques written by the surgeons who have popularized these procedures. Finally, including the management of the multi-ligament injured knee, arthrofibrosis, and the patellofemoral joint completes a text that leaves the reader with little need to turn to any other resource.

Surgical Techniques of the Shoulder, Elbow, and Knee in Sports Medicine is the product of more than two years

of hard work by its contributors. These authors are frequently asked to further the education of others, yet never seem to wane in their enthusiasm and completeness. It is an honor to work with the contributors of this textbook, and the readers will appreciate the highly edited and consistent style that completely eliminates the noise of unnecessary information.

We would like to also thank our families, who once again have created an environment where a labor of love can result in something invaluable for our students and, more importantly, for our patients. Specifically, Dr. Cole would like to thank Emily, Ethan, Adam, and Ava for their willingness to occasionally forego a late-night story so daddy can stay awake to edit these chapters. Dr. Sekiya would like to thank his wife Jennie for her never-ending support and understanding and their son Kimo. We would like to thank our co-editors for helping complete the final details of this task, Dr. Andreas Gomoll and Dr. Jeffrey Rihn. Their diligence has definitely kept this project on time and even ahead of schedule. Finally, we would thank the Publishing Director at Elsevier, Kim Murphy, for governing the entire process until the book was released. So, read this text and prepare to challenge your mentors. *Surgical Techniques of the Shoulder, Elbow, and Knee in Sports Medicine* will allow you to do just that.

Brian J. Cole, MD, MBA
Jon K. Sekiya, MD, MC, USNR

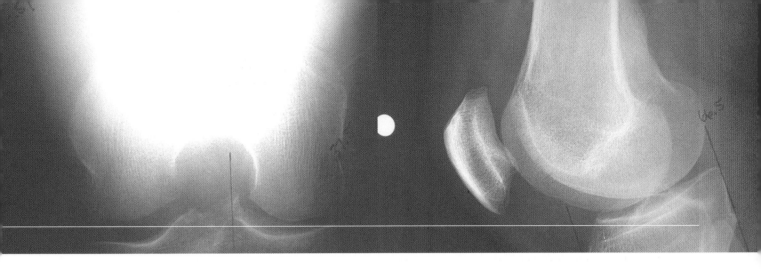

Contents

Video Supplement

PART 1

The Shoulder

Patient Positioning, Portal Placement, Normal Arthroscopic Anatomy, and Diagnostic Arthroscopy

Kevin F. Bonner, MD

Shoulder arthroscopy has become a key component in both the diagnosis and treatment of various pathologic conditions of the shoulder. Arthroscopy allows a detailed examination of the glenohumeral joint as well as of the subacromial space, with minimal patient morbidity compared with classic open procedures. As we have gained experience and arthroscopic techniques have continued to evolve, our ability to treat patients with minimally invasive arthroscopic procedures has only improved our care of patients. Adherence to the basic principles of shoulder arthroscopy, including proper patient positioning and portal placement, is essential no matter the level of the surgeon's experience. On the basis of these principles, each surgeon should develop an effective, reproducible technique that methodically examines the shoulder joint. To recognize truly pathologic conditions of the shoulder, it is paramount to have a firm understanding of normal anatomic variants that are common in the shoulder. This appreciation will prevent inaccurate diagnosis and improper treatment. Our ability to effectively and efficiently perform shoulder arthroscopy is associated with reduced patient morbidity and quicker rehabilitation.

Anesthesia

Based on the preference of the anesthesiologist, the surgeon, and the patient, shoulder arthroscopy can be performed under general anesthesia, interscalene block (i.e.,

regional), or a combination thereof. Certainly, regional anesthesia may be advantageous for many procedures performed in an outpatient setting.

Anesthetic Considerations

- Keep mean arterial pressure between 70 and 90 mm Hg (systolic blood pressure of 100 mm Hg) to maximize visualization.[10]

- Obese patients with a large abdomen may be at increased risk for superior vena cava compression (resultant hypotension) when they are placed in a beach chair position.

- Temporary ipsilateral phrenic nerve palsy routinely results from an interscalene block.[14]

- Interscalene block complications can be minimized if the block is performed before the induction of general anesthesia and when a nerve stimulator is used.[1]

Examination Under Anesthesia

An examination under anesthesia should be performed on all patients before they undergo arthroscopy. The examination under anesthesia can detect side-to-side differences in laxity and motion that may be helpful in confirming a diagnosis and developing a treatment plan (Table 1-1).

Table 1-1 Motion Abnormalities and Potential Associated Pathologic Conditions

Motion Abnormality	Potential Pathologic Condition
Increased external rotation	Subscapularis rupture
Limited forward flexion–external rotation	Adhesive capsulitis, osteoarthritis
Limited internal rotation with arm abducted 90 degrees	Isolated tight posterior capsule
Increased anterior translation	Microinstability, secondary or internal impingement

Box 1-1 Grades of Shoulder Translation and Instability (Head Relative to Glenoid)

- Grade I: Translation to the glenoid rim
- Grade II: Translation over the glenoid rim with spontaneous reduction
- Grade III: Translation over the rim of the glenoid, head remains locked

Checklist for Examination Under Anesthesia (Both Shoulders)

- Forward flexion
- Internal and external rotation—arm abducted to 90 degrees and at the side
- Anterior translation is determined and graded. Abduct the arm to 90 degrees and apply an axial load and anterior force to the proximal humerus (Fig. 1-1 and Box 1-1).
- Posterior instability is tested by flexing the shoulder to 140 degrees. The humerus is adducted to 15 degrees as a posteriorly directed axial force is applied.
- Sulcus sign

Patient Positioning

On the basis of the surgeon's preference and training and the proposed surgical procedure, the patient is placed into

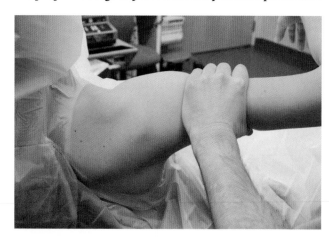

Figure 1-1 Examination of degree of anterior shoulder instability.

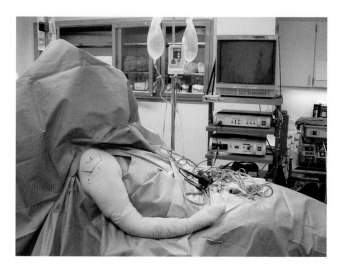

Figure 1-2 Beach chair position.

either a beach chair or lateral decubitus position. Most procedures can be performed through either position.

Beach Chair Position (Fig. 1-2)

- Place the patient on the edge of the table to optimize access to the shoulder (removable backs are optimal if the bed is equipped).
- Support the patient's head and neck in neutral position.
- Place the table into 10 to 15 degrees of Trendelenberg.
- Flex the table 45 to 60 degrees.
- Place the lower legs parallel to the floor.
- Elevate the back of the table.
- Tilt the table away from the operative side slightly.
- Firmly support the thorax on the operative side (helps diminish neck angulation).

Lateral Decubitus Position (Fig. 1-3)

- Place the patient on a beanbag or stabilizing device with bone prominences padded.

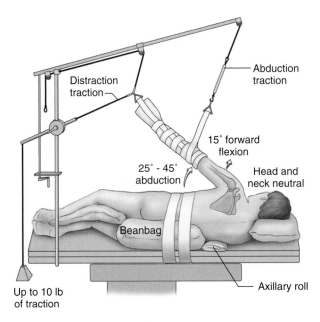

Figure 1-3 Lateral decubitus position.

Labels in figure:
Distraction traction — Abduction traction — 15° forward flexion — 25°-45° abduction — Head and neck neutral — Beanbag — Axillary roll — Up to 10 lb of traction

- Roll the torso posterior 25 degrees to position the glenoid parallel to the floor.
- Place an axillary roll.
- Secure torso.
- Suspend the arm so that it can be prepared and draped.
- Place the arm into a foam traction sleeve and connect to traction device.
- Position the arm in 25 to 45 degrees of abduction and 15 degrees of forward flexion.
- Apply traction with the arm in neutral.
- Place 10 pounds of weights for longitudinal traction and a similar or lower amount for abduction traction.
- For larger or well-muscled individuals, 15 pounds is acceptable.
- More than 20 pounds is not recommended (increased risk of neurapraxia[5,13]).
- Ensure that the head is in neutral position after traction is applied.

Skin Preparation and Draping

The shoulder is prepared and draped following established surgical principles.

- Allow access to at least the middle of the scapula posteriorly.
- Placement of a snug plastic U-drape with the U facing inferiorly tends to direct extravasating fluid away from the neck and trachea.[2,13]

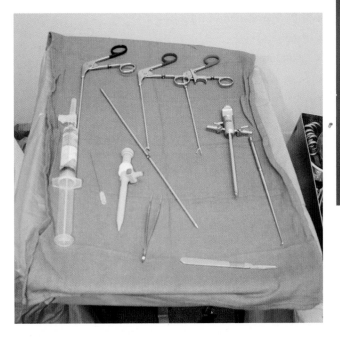

Figure 1-4 Basic shoulder arthroscopy instruments.

Equipment Set-up

After positioning of the patient, the equipment is set up. A tower containing a video monitor, control box, light source, and power shaver is set up opposite the operative side to allow optimal visualization for the surgeon and the assistant (see Fig. 1-2). The fluid pump is also placed on the opposite side of the surgeon to allow visualization of fluid pressure. Bipolar or monopolar devices may be placed adjacent to the pump system with controls placed at the surgeon's feet.

In the beach chair position, the surgeon stands slightly behind the patient's shoulder and the assistant stands at the level of the arm so that the arm can be positioned throughout the case. If the lateral decubitus position is used, the surgeon stands above the patient's shoulder and the assistant is positioned just below the surgeon toward the foot of the table. The surgical scrub technician typically stands behind the surgeon and assistant or alternatively may be just distal to the first assistant. A Mayo stand is placed just distal to the first assistant and should contain basic shoulder arthroscopy equipment or any equipment that will be used frequently for the case (Fig. 1-4).

Instrumentation for Basic Shoulder Arthroscopy

- 30-mL syringe
- 30-degree arthroscope
- Cannula

1

- Inflow and suction tubing
- Probe
- Spinal needle
- Motorized shaver
- Electrocautery (monopolar or bipolar cautery and ablation device very useful)

For more advanced reconstructive procedures, the necessary cannulas, fixation devices, and instruments must be available. It is recommended that these devices be available in the surgical suite in case of unexpected pathologic findings during the procedure.

Pumps and Fluid System

Sterile saline, which is infused with a fluid management pump, is preferred for shoulder arthroscopy. Alternatively, a gravity-driven system may be used. Either will allow the surgeon to increase or decrease the fluid pressure throughout the case, based on visualization.

Optimizing Visualization with the Fluid System

- Addition of epinephrine into the fluid bags improves hemostasis.
- Inflow is connected to the scope cannula.
- Outflow is initially through the scope cannula but is switched to the anterior or lateral cannula once it is available for optimized fluid management.
- Fluid pressure within the joint is kept below 70 to 80 mm Hg and can typically be maintained at 35 to 40 mm Hg.
- Subacromial space pressure may need to be intermittently increased until hemostasis is obtained with cautery (drive scope toward bleeding vessel— inflow clears visual field).
- Maintenance of outflow helps prevent extravasation into the tissues.

Portal Placement

Once the patient is positioned, a surgical marking pen is used to accurately outline bone landmarks of the shoulder. After the patient's anatomy is outlined, the proposed portals should be marked (Fig. 1-5). Multiple portals can be used during shoulder arthroscopy, depending on the specific procedure to be performed (Fig. 1-6).

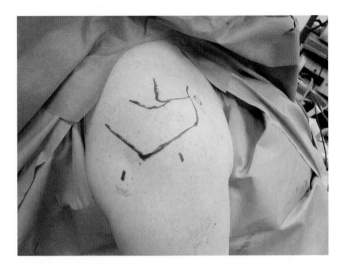

Figure 1-5 Outlined anatomy and proposed portal placement.

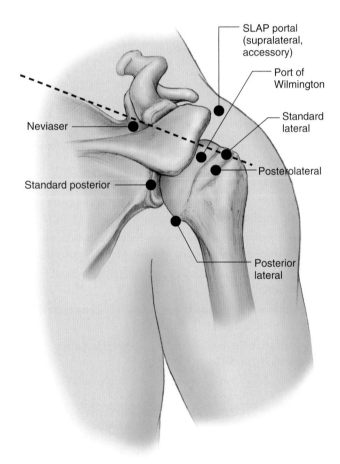

Figure 1-6 Posterior and lateral portals. (From Mazzocca AD, Cole BJ, Romeo AA. Shoulder: patient positioning, portal placement, and normal arthroscopic anatomy. In Miller MD, Cole BJ, eds. Textbook of Arthroscopy. Philadelphia, Elsevier, 2004:74.)

Posterior Portal

All arthroscopic shoulder procedures begin with placement of the arthroscope into the glenohumeral joint through the posterior portal. There are several methods to aid in determining optimal posterior portal placement. One method is to measure from the posterolateral corner of the acromion. The appropriate starting position for a posterior portal typically lies 1 to 1.5 cm medial to the lateral edge of the posterolateral acromion as well as 2 to 2.5 cm distal. Another method involves manual palpation of the posterior "soft spot," which represents the interval between the infraspinatus and teres minor muscles. In addition, the surgeon can translate the humeral head posteriorly while palpating the glenohumeral joint line (Fig. 1-7).

Posterior portal placement for the lateral decubitus position is slightly different from that for the beach chair position. In the lateral position, because of glenohumeral distraction, the posterior portal tends to be erroneously positioned too medial and proximal. It is generally recommended to place the portal 3 cm inferior and in line with the posterolateral acromion.[8]

The skin is injected with a local anesthetic with epinephrine, and a 5- to 6-mm incision is made through the dermis with a No. 11 scalpel blade. Some surgeons prefer to insufflate the joint with 20 to 30 mL of saline to facilitate safe trocar introduction. The arthroscopic cannula is introduced with a blunt trocar. While using the dominant hand to hold the cannula, the surgeon palpates the tip of the coracoid process with the nondominant hand to serve as a guide while the cannula is gently inserted through the posterior capsule and into the joint (Fig. 1-8). Alternatively, one may wish to palpate the shoulder with the same hand as the shoulder being operated on and to insert the scope with the contralateral hand. It may be helpful to aim the arthroscopic trocar toward the coracoid as an anatomic landmark because this will typically place the cannula in line with the glenohumeral joint. Gentle pressure is used to enter the posterior joint capsule. Do not use excessive pressure if the trocar does not "pop in" through the capsule. However, there may be significant variability in the pressure required to enter the shoulder joint, depending on the thickness of the posterior capsule. If there is difficulty finding the joint line, the assistant may gently rotate the humeral head to determine whether the cannula is positioned against the humeral head or the glenoid. It may also be helpful to have the assistant grab the arm distal to the axilla and create an abduction distraction force on the joint to open the joint space.

Anterior Portal

The standard anterior portal is placed in the rotator interval or triangle formed by the subscapularis, humeral head, and biceps tendon. An outside-in technique uses a spinal needle that is placed just lateral to the coracoid through the rotator interval. The spinal needle can be used to optimize portal placement and angulation (Fig. 1-9). Before an incision is made, it is helpful to determine whether more than one portal will be required (Bankart or superior labral anterior-posterior [SLAP] repair) because portals should be established as far apart as possible to aid in triangulation and to reduce crowding. A 5- to 6-mm skin incision is made with a No. 11 scalpel, and under direct visualization, a plastic cannula and trocar are advanced through the rotator interval and into the joint. Typically, this anterior cannula is connected to plastic tubing and used as outflow to gravity.

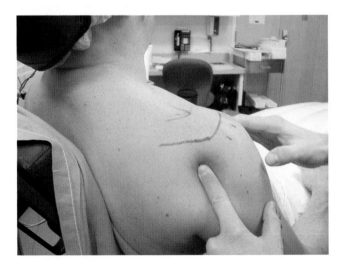

Figure 1-7 Palpation of posterior "soft spot" while translating head posterior.

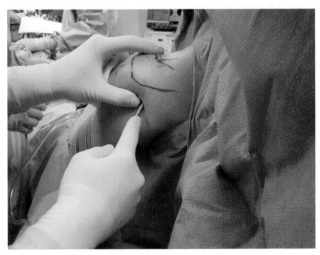

Figure 1-8 Insertion of the arthroscope into the glenohumeral joint.

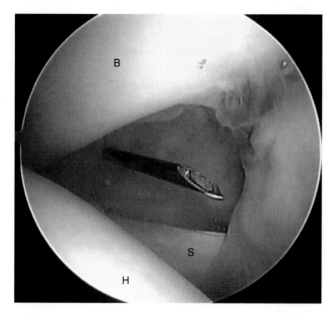

Figure 1-9 Determination of proper anterior portal placement (left shoulder). B, biceps tendon; H, humeral head; S, subscapularis.

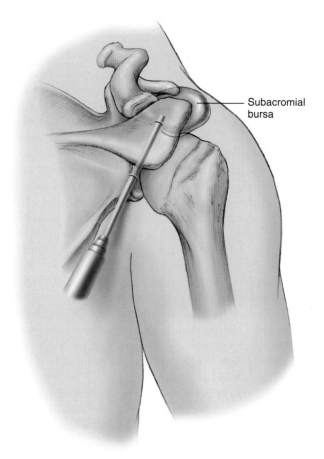

Subacromial bursa

Figure 1-10 Subacromial bursa.

An alternative technique to making the anterior portal is the inside-out method using a Wissinger rod. With this technique, the arthroscope is driven into the anterior triangle. The arthroscope is then removed and a Wissinger rod is passed through the cannula, going through the anterior capsule and tenting the skin anteriorly. A portal is made through the skin, and a plastic cannula may then be placed over the rod and delivered into the joint anteriorly.

Subacromial Space

Once the glenohumeral arthroscopy is complete, the trocar should be reinserted into the cannula to enter the subacromial space. The cannula is then pulled back outside the joint and gently slid over the rotator cuff in an anterolateral direction to enter the subacromial space. Alternatively, the trocar can be used to palpate the posterior acromion and slid directly underneath the acromion in an anterolateral direction. The trocar should be used to sweep in a medial to lateral direction to break up a portion of the bursa, which may help in the distention of this potential space. The subacromial bursa is generally located in the anterior half of the acromion (Fig. 1-10). Distal traction on the lower humerus will assist in opening a tight subacromial space.

Standard Lateral Portal

A standard lateral portal is used to access the subacromial space. The axillary nerve, the significant structure at risk,

is located 3.8 to 5.1 cm distal to the acromion.[4] The anterior posterior position of the standard lateral portal should be in line with the notch formed by the posterior aspect of the clavicle and the spine of the scapula. The portal will be approximately 2 cm distal to the acromion. Fine-tune the final portal location with the use of a spinal needle under direct visualization once the arthroscope is in the subacromial space. Do not make this portal too close to the acromion. Placement of traction on the arm will assist in opening the subacromial space. A dull trocar is used to enter the subacromial space after the incision is made in the dermis (Fig. 1-11).

Accessory Anterior Portals (Fig. 1-12)

Anterior Superior Portal

- Within the superior rotator interval just adjacent to the acromion
- Useful for labral reconstructions and SLAP repairs

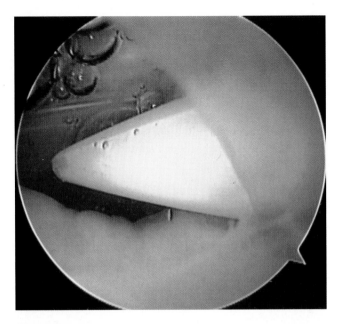

Figure 1-11 Trocar entering subacromial space.

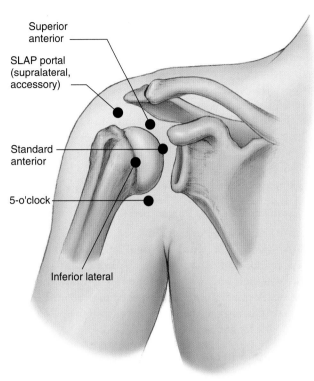

Superior anterior

SLAP portal (supralateral, accessory)

Standard anterior

5-o'clock

Inferior lateral

Figure 1-12 Anterior portals. (From Mazzocca AD, Cole BJ, Romeo AA. Shoulder: patient positioning, portal placement, and normal arthroscopic anatomy, In Miller MD, Cole BJ, eds. Textbook of Arthroscopy. Philadelphia, Elsevier, 2004:72.)

- Separate the two portals in the rotator interval as much as possible

Superior Lateral Portal

- Placed just lateral to the acromion[6]
- Spinal needle is used to enter the subacromial space or joint obliquely
- Useful for arthroscopic rotator cuff repair

Neviaser Portal

- Placed in the notch between the posterior acromioclavicular joint and the spine of the scapula
- Useful for arthroscopic rotator cuff repair, distal clavicle resection, and SLAP repairs
- Suprascapular nerve and artery approximately 3 cm medial to the portal[4]

Anterior Inferior Portal (5-o'clock)

- Useful for arthroscopic labral reconstruction
- Lateral to the conjoined tendon and in the lower third of the subscapularis muscle
- Average of 22.9 mm from the musculocutaneous nerve and 24.4 mm from the axillary nerve[3]
- Cephalic vein is the closest structure at risk (average of 9.8 mm from the portal[7])

Inferior Lateral Portal

- Over subscapularis tendon, coming from a lateral to medial direction.
- Useful for Bankart repairs.

Accessory Posterior Portals

Portal of Wilmington

- Used for posterior superior labral repairs on the glenoid
- 1 cm lateral and 1 cm inferior to the posterolateral corner of the acromion
- Goes through the infraspinatus tendon (no cannula)

Posterolateral Portal (7-o'clock)

- Useful for posterior arthroscopic stabilization procedures
- 2 cm inferior and lateral to the standard posterior portal

Diagnostic Arthroscopy and Normal Anatomy

Shoulder arthroscopy always begins with insertion of the arthroscope into the glenohumeral joint through the posterior portal. Once the posterior portal is established, the surgeon should develop a systematic approach to evaluate the glenohumeral joint and subacromial space (Box 1-2). It may be helpful to divide the joint into sectors. Rotating the 30-degree objective in conjunction with moving the arthroscope throughout the shoulder will allow a more efficient and thorough evaluation.

1. Establish Posterior Portal (See Earlier)

Once in the shoulder initially, proceed to the rotator interval to evaluate for tendinitis and inflammation of the biceps tendon and rotator interval. Also attempt to determine whether one or more anterior portals may be required. A spinal needle may be used to probe the interarticular structures at that time as well as to help establish a landmark for the anterior portal.

2. Establish Anterior Portal (See Earlier)

Once the cannula is inserted into the rotator interval under direct visualization, it can be used as a working portal as well as for outflow.

3a. Evaluate Anterior Superior Sector

Diagnostic evaluation should commence by visualizing various structures in the anterior superior sector. This includes the biceps tendon, the superior labrum, the coracohumeral ligament, and the superior glenohumeral ligament as well as the anterior superior labrum. The biceps tendon attaches to the supraglenoid tubercle on the posterior superior aspect of the glenoid rim. The biceps origin is attached to the superior labrum or to significant fibers in the anterior superior and posterior superior labrum (Fig. 1-13).

Box 1-2 Surgical Steps in Diagnostic Arthroscopy

1. Establish posterior portal 　Evaluate rotator interval
2. Establish anterior portal
3. Evaluate 　a. Anterior superior sector 　b. Anterior sector 　c. Inferior sector 　d. Rotator cuff insertion and humeral head 　e. Posterior sector
4. Establish lateral portal
5. Evaluate subacromial space

With use of a probe from the anterior portal, the labrum and biceps attachment site are evaluated. There is often a normal recess under the superior labrum where the biceps complex attaches to the glenoid, which is often diagnosed as a SLAP tear by inexperienced arthroscopists. If the hyaline cartilage of the glenoid articular surface can be followed to the base of the superior labrum, the biceps anchor is stable and should not be repaired with sutures (Fig. 1-14). Overhead athletes should be evaluated with

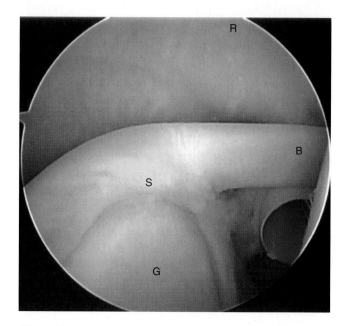

Figure 1-13 Biceps insertion into superior labrum. B, biceps; G, glenoid; R, rotator cuff; S, superior labrum.

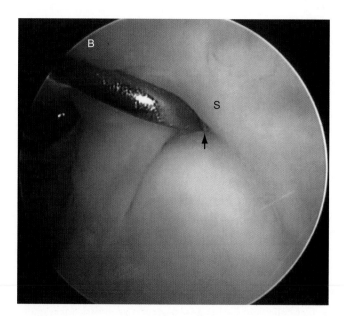

Figure 1-14 Normal recess under superior labrum (arrow). B, biceps; S, superior labrum.

the arm abducted and externally rotated in an attempt to visualize the peel-back phenomenon. When the arm is abducted and externally rotated, the superior labrum may rotate off the superior glenoid posteriorly and superiorly. This may be visualized better through the anterior cannula or portal.

The biceps should be thoroughly evaluated from the insertion point down through the intertubercular groove (Fig. 1-15). The biceps can be followed into the bicipital groove by forward flexion, elbow flexion, and slight internal rotation of the arm. The tendon can be further evaluated by use of a probe or grasper to pull the tendon farther into the joint (Fig. 1-16). The biceps tendon is bordered by the subscapularis tendon medially as well as by the supraspinatus tendon laterally. Injury or disruption of the superior glenohumeral ligament, coracohumeral ligament, or subscapularis can cause medial biceps instability. The structures surrounding the biceps tendon, including the coracohumeral ligament and superior glenohumeral ligament, should be evaluated at this time. The coracohumeral ligament encircles the biceps tendon after it originates at the base of the coracoid, sending fibers to the biceps tendon and the supraspinatus tendon as it inserts into the front of the subscapularis tendon (Fig. 1-17). The superior glenohumeral ligament runs from the anterior superior aspect of the glenoid to insert into the upper portion of the lesser tuberosity (see Figs. 1-15 and 1-17) and is considered the floor of the bicipital groove.

The anterior superior labrum is evaluated next. It is this region of the shoulder that shows a significant degree of anatomic variability. Four common anatomic variations are seen involving the anterosuperior labrum and middle glenohumeral ligament (Fig. 1-18). This variability may be physiologic detachment with a confluence of the middle glenohumeral ligament, simple detachment (sublabral hole), or complete absence.[12,15]

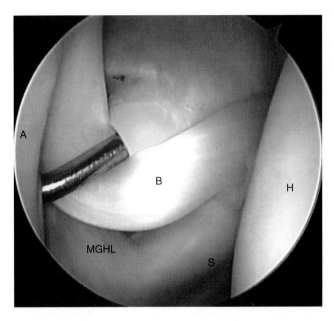

Figure 1-16 Pulling biceps tendon into joint. A, anterior labrum; B, biceps; H, humeral head; MGHL, middle glenohumeral ligament; S, subscapularis.

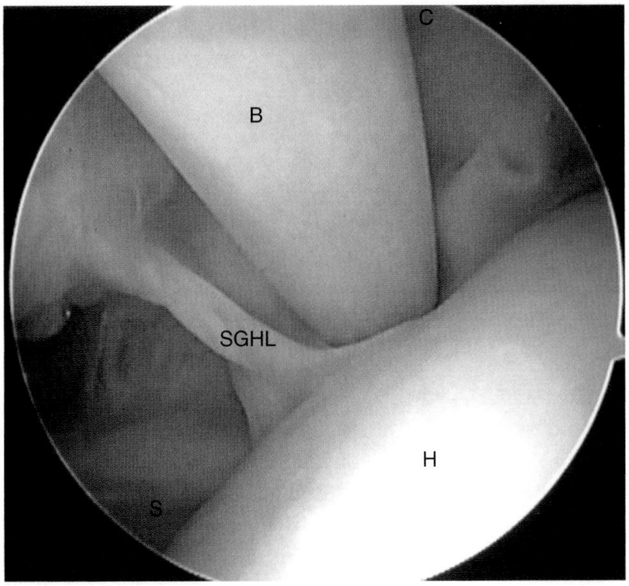

Figure 1-15 Biceps tendon sling (visualized from posterior portal). B, biceps tendon; C, coracohumeral ligament; H, humeral head; S, subscapularis; SGHL, superior glenohumeral ligament.

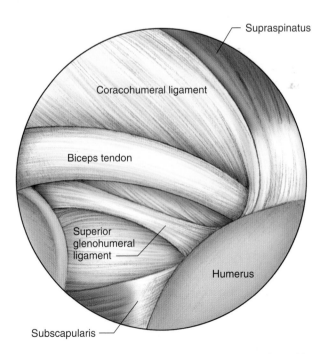

Figure 1-17 Anterior superior structures in relation to biceps tendon and its groove. (From Mazzocca AD, Alberta FG, Cole BJ, Romeo AA. Shoulder: diagnostic arthroscopy. In Miller MD, Cole BJ, eds. Textbook of Arthroscopy. Philadelphia, Elsevier, 2004:80.)

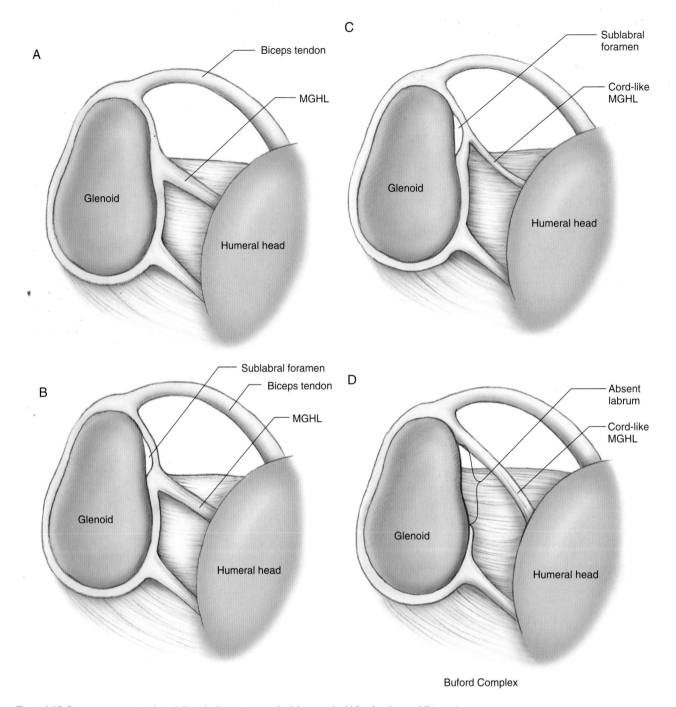

A — Biceps tendon, MGHL, Glenoid, Humeral head

B — Sublabral foramen, Biceps tendon, MGHL, Glenoid, Humeral head

C — Sublabral foramen, Cord-like MGHL, Glenoid, Humeral head

D — Absent labrum, Cord-like MGHL, Glenoid, Humeral head, Buford Complex

Figure 1-18 Four common anatomic variations in the anterosuperior labrum and middle glenohumeral ligament.

3b. Evaluate Anterior Sector

The middle glenohumeral ligament can also be variable in structure. At times, it may seem virtually nonexistent during arthroscopy. Commonly, it ranges from a sheet-like ligament to a robust cord-like structure as seen in a Buford complex (Fig. 1-19). With a Buford complex, the cord-like middle glenohumeral ligament originates high on the glenoid, and the anterior superior labrum is absent. It is important to recognize this as a normal anatomic variant. Erroneous diagnosis of this normal cord-like ligament as a labral tear and repair to the anterosuperior glenoid will result in significant restriction of normal motion.[15]

The subscapularis tendon should be carefully examined for partial-thickness and full-thickness tears. External rotation of the shoulder will allow evaluation of the subscapularis under tension. It is not possible to visualize the entire subscapularis tendon arthroscopically, but most disease tends to occur proximally. Make sure to evaluate the subscapularis recess for loose bodies.

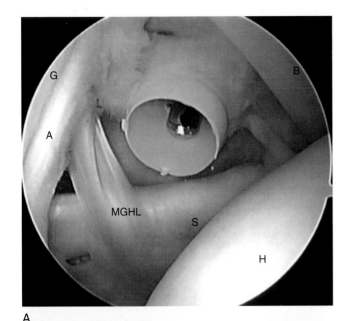

A

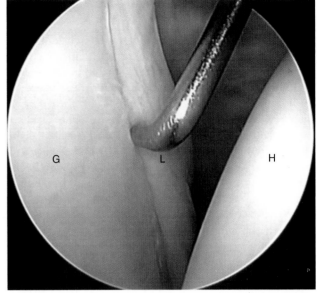

Figure 1-20 Normal anterior labrum. G, glenoid; H, humeral head; L, anterior labrum.

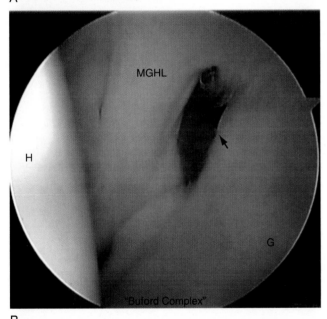

B

Figure 1-19 A, Thin sheet-like middle glenohumeral ligament (right shoulder). **B,** Buford complex: thick cord-like middle glenohumeral ligament (left shoulder) with absent anterosuperior labrum *(arrow)*. A, anterior labrum; B, biceps; G, glenoid; H, humeral head; MGHL, middle glenohumeral ligament; S, subscapularis.

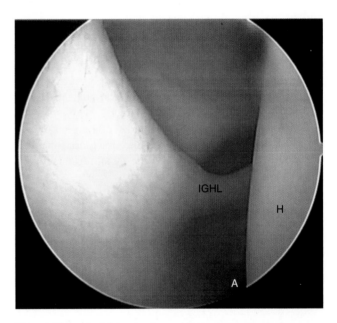

Figure 1-21 Anterior inferior glenohumeral ligament under tension by external rotation. A, axillary pouch; H, humeral head; IGHL, anterior band of inferior glenohumeral ligament.

3c. Evaluate Inferior Sector

The anterior inferior labrum is evaluated with a probe (Fig. 1-20). This area should be inspected for degenerative tearing or scuffing as well as for a true Bankart lesion. In contrast to the anterosuperior labrum, any detachment of the labrum below the equator of the glenoid is considered pathologic. The inferior glenohumeral ligament runs from the glenoid to the anatomic neck of the humerus and can be inspected by externally rotating the shoulder, thereby placing the ligament on tension (Fig. 1-21). The humeral attachment can actually be better visualized by placing the scope in the anterior portal.

By continuing to drive the scope inferior, the anterior axillary pouch is assessed for laxity, loose bodies, and synovitis. In a loose shoulder, one may be able to evaluate the entire axillary pouch at that time. Alternatively, it can be examined after evaluation of the posterior rotator cuff insertion.

3d. Evaluate Rotator Cuff Insertion and Humeral Head

With the arm slightly abducted, forward flexed, and externally rotated and the 30-degree objective pointed laterally, the entire rotator cuff insertion should be inspected, beginning at the anterior supraspinatus just lateral to the bicipital groove (Fig. 1-22). Assess for both partial-thickness and full-thickness tears. If a partial-thickness rotator cuff tear is encountered, a spinal needle can be placed anterolaterally through the subacromial space and into the tear site. This can be marked with a polypropylene (Prolene) suture to evaluate the bursal side of the same region of the tendon.

The rotator cuff insertion can be followed posteriorly with the aid of humeral rotation. The bare area of the humeral head, which often contains remnants of old vascular channels, can be visualized and borders the attachment site of the infraspinatus tendon (Fig. 1-23). Continuing to sweep inferiorly around the posterior rotator cuff insertion will bring the arthroscope into the posterior axillary pouch (Fig. 1-24). Throughout this process, the articular cartilage on the entire humeral head and glenoid should be evaluated (Fig. 1-25).

3e. Evaluate Posterior Sector

In some patients, the posterior labrum can be adequately visualized with the scope in the posterior portal. However, if visualization is inadequate or posterior labral disease is suspected, it is advantageous to place the scope into the anterior portal. This can be accomplished by temporarily placing the arthroscope into the anterior plastic cannula and placing the trocar back into the metal cannula poste-

riorly. The metal cannula can even serve as a probe device to evaluate the posterior labrum and posterior capsule as well as the posterior articular surface (Fig. 1-26). If necessary, a plastic cannula can be placed in the posterior portal to use a probe.

4. Establish Lateral Portal

Once the glenohumeral arthroscopy is complete, the cannula is placed into the subacromial space (see earlier).

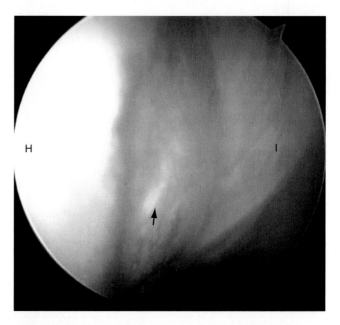

Figure 1-23 Normal bare spot *(arrow)* corresponds to the infraspinatus insertion (I) point. H, humeral head.

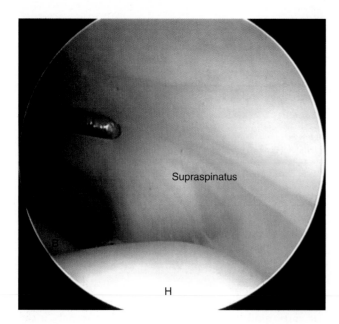

Figure 1-22 Examination of the rotator cuff insertion beginning at the anterior supraspinatus and moving posterior. B, biceps; H, humeral head.

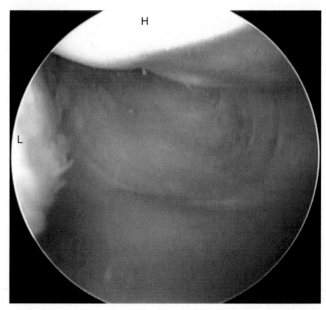

Figure 1-24 Axillary pouch visualized from the posterior portal. H, humeral head; L, labrum.

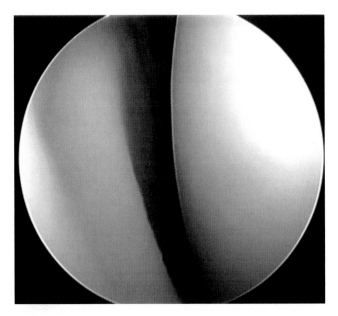

Figure 1-25 Evaluate articular cartilage on the entire glenoid and humeral head.

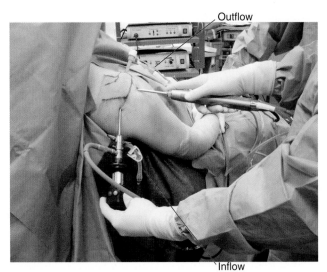

Figure 1-27 Motorized shaver removing bursa through the lateral portal. Inflow is through the scope in the posterior portal. Outflow is through the anterior cannula (green).

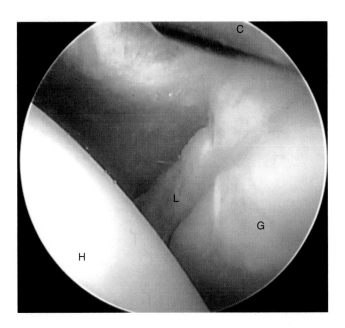

Figure 1-26 Posterior labrum visualized with the scope in the anterior cannula. C, cannula; G, glenoid; H, humeral head; L, labrum.

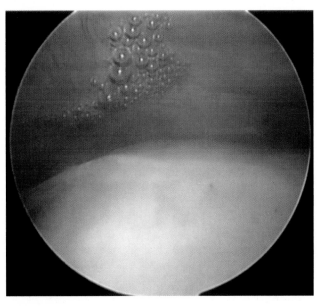

Figure 1-28 Evaluation of the bursal side of the rotator cuff.

If there is a significant amount of subacromial bursal tissue obscuring the view, it may be helpful to reintroduce the trocar into the cannula to sweep and make a potential space. A lateral portal can now be made with the aid of a spinal needle. The portal should be placed distally enough to give adequate access under the acromion but be positioned above the rotator cuff. In the presence of thick bursal tissue, a brightly colored plastic trocar can be helpful to triangulate and begin removal of bursal tissue.

5. Evaluate Subacromial Space

It will likely be necessary to use an oscillating shaver through the lateral portal to remove the subacromial bursa to properly visualize the subacromial structures (Fig. 1-27). A coagulation device often aids in hemostasis. The assistant should apply traction to open the subacromial space. The space is evaluated for bursitis, subacromial adhesions, scuffing of the coracoacromial ligament, acromial morphologic features, and the rotator cuff. The rotator cuff should be completely evaluated by rotating the humeral head (Fig. 1-28). The arthroscope can also be placed into the lateral portal, allowing complete visualization of the posterior rotator cuff.

Complications

- Hemorrhage
- Iatrogenic articular cartilage and rotator cuff injury
- Fluid extravasation
- Neurovascular complications (very rare)
- Infection
- Complications related to anesthesia

References

1. Bishop JY, Sprague M, Gelber J, et al. Interscalene regional anesthesia for shoulder surgery. J Bone Joint Surg Am 2004;86:2135-2142.
2. Blumenthal S, Nadig M, Gerber C, Borgeat A. Severe airway obstruction during arthroscopic shoulder surgery. Anesthesia 2003;99:1455-1456.
3. Davidson PA, Tibone JE. Anterior-inferior (5 o'clock) portal for shoulder arthroscopy. Arthroscopy 1995;11:519-525.
4. Hollinshead WH. Anatomy for Surgeons, vol III, 2nd ed. Philadelphia, Harper & Row, 1969.
5. Klein AH, France JC, Muschler TA, et al. Measurement of brachial plexus strain and arthroscopy of the shoulder. Arthroscopy 1987;3:45-52.
6. Laurencin CT, Detsha, O'Brien SJ, Altchek DW. The superior lateral portal for arthroscopy of the shoulder. Arthroscopy 1994;10:255-258.
7. Lo IK, Lind CC, Burkhart SS. Glenohumeral arthroscopy portals established using an outside-in technique: neurovascular anatomy at risk. Arthroscopy 2004;20:596-602.
8. Mazzocca AD, Cole BJ, Romeo AA. Shoulder: patient positioning, portal placement, and normal arthroscopic anatomy, In Miller MD, Cole BJ, eds. Textbook of Arthroscopy. Philadelphia, Elsevier, 2004:65-77.
9. Mazzocca AD, Alberta FG, Cole BJ, Romeo AA. Shoulder: diagnostic arthroscopy. In Miller MD, Cole BJ, eds. Textbook of Arthroscopy. Philadelphia, Elsevier, 2004:78-85.
10. Morrison DS, Schafer RK, Friedman RL. The relationship between subacromial space pressure, blood pressure and visual clarity during arthroscopic subacromial decompression. Arthroscopy 1995;11:557-560.
11. Pitman MI, Nainzadeh N, Ergas E, et al. The use of somatosensory evoked potentials for detection of neurapraxia during shoulder arthroscopy. Arthroscopy 1988;4:252-255.
12. Rao AG, Kim TK, Chronopoulos E, McFarland EG. Anatomical variants in the anterosuperior aspect of the glenoid labrum: a statistical analysis of seventy-three cases. J Bone Joint Surg Am 2003;85:653-659.
13. Rogerson JS. How to avoid complications in the subacromial space. Presented at the Arthroscopy Association of North America Fall Course; Phoenix, Arizona; December 1, 2005.
14. Urmey WF, Talts KH, Sharrock NE. One hundred percent incidence of hemidiaphragmatic paresis associated with interscalene brachial plexus anesthesia as diagnosed by ultrasonagraphy. Anesth Analg 1991;72:498-503.
15. Williams MM, Snyder SJ, Buford D Jr. The Buford complex—the "cord-like" middle glenohumeral ligament and absent anterosuperior labrum complex: a normal anatomic capsulolabral variant. Arthroscopy 1994;10:241-247.

CHAPTER 2

Knot-Tying and Suture-Passing Techniques

Mary Lloyd Ireland, MD

Adam M. Smith, MD

Indications for less invasive shoulder surgery continue to expand for the treatment of rotator cuff disease, impingement, labral tears, biceps injuries, and glenohumeral instability.[2,3,8,12,13] Techniques are constantly refined for even more difficult procedures, such as capsular release, acromioclavicular instability, and subscapularis tendon repair. Diagnoses that were considered challenging in the past, such as superior biceps–labral complex injuries, are now routinely treated through an all-arthroscopic approach. Shoulder instability can be assessed dynamically under direct visualization to better delineate the bony, labral, or capsular injuries, which can then be treated in the same setting.

Less invasive surgery results in minimal tissue damage, thus allowing earlier return to functional activities, although even with modern techniques a return to prior activity levels cannot be guaranteed. This development has been mostly driven by a combination of factors, including patients' desire for more cosmetic procedures, decreased postoperative pain and morbidity, and outpatient surgery. Innovation by surgeons to accommodate these needs has been enthusiastically backed by the medical device industry.

Initial reports on arthroscopic treatment of shoulder injuries demonstrated inferior results in comparison to open procedures. However, with the development of specialized instruments, improved implants, and new techniques simplifying suture management, more recent studies have suggested at least equivalent outcomes. With rotator cuff, superior labral, and Bankart repair now routine arthroscopic procedures, orthopedic surgeons must have a full understanding of several approaches to tissue fixation and suture management, including a good command of suture passage and arthroscopic knot tying to facilitate minimally invasive techniques.

Anchors

The improvement of suture anchors during the last several years has allowed the continued advancement of all-arthroscopic procedures. Various metal, bioabsorbable, and synthetic anchors are available from several manufacturers. Whereas numerous anchor designs are currently on the market, we believe that the following characteristics are particularly important in choosing an anchor for arthroscopic shoulder surgery.[14] The anchor eyelet should allow the sutures to slide easily and not fray; many designs now incorporate suture eyelets instead of drill holes through the anchor to achieve these goals. Furthermore, we prefer anchors that are preloaded with two multibraided polyester sutures and designed to allow sliding of the second suture even after the first one has been tied. Choosing an anchor that meets these characteristics will allow a more secure and rapid repair with multiple points of suture to anchor fixation.

Anchors have become a mainstay of fixation in shoulder surgery, even with certain open procedures; however, poor bone quality may make the use of anchors difficult and ideally should be noted preoperatively to allow planning for different methods of fixation, such as bone tunnels and augmentation devices. Absorbable or metal anchors can generally be used interchangeably.

Whereas caution should be taken to ensure that all anchors are well seated below the level of any articular surfaces, metal anchors around the shoulder can be problematic.[9] Particularly, care must be taken with the insertion of metal anchors into the glenoid, such as with a superior labral anterior-posterior (SLAP) or Bankart repair, as loosening can cause severe articular cartilage damage.

Sutures

Although there are many suture options, the choice should be based on the type of tissue being repaired and suture characteristics. Monofilament and braided sutures have different indications for use based on their sliding and resorption characteristics (Fig. 2-1).

Modern multibraided polyester sutures have been a key advance in arthroscopic techniques, allowing the repair to be carried out in a more reliable fashion with less risk of suture breakage. FiberWire (Arthrex, Inc., Naples, Fla), Orthocord (DePuy-Mitek, Norwood, Mass), and Ultrabraid (Smith & Nephew, Inc., Memphis, Tenn) are newer types of braided nonabsorbable polyester sutures. These No. 2 size multibraided sutures have demonstrated performance similar to that of the larger diameter No. 5 Ethibond polyester suture.

These sutures are, generally, very strong and resist breaking or fraying with the repeated abrasion of instrument tying through cannulas and stretch minimally. Whereas these sutures do not slide as easily as the conventional Ethibond (Ethicon, Inc., Somerville, NJ) suture, which has a polybutylate coating, their strength characteristics are better suited for point fixation to an anchor.

Monofilament polydioxanone (PDS; Ethicon, Inc., Somerville, NJ) is an absorbable suture that is easily passed through most suture-passing devices.[15] We generally use PDS for capsular plication or rotator interval stitches. PDS loses strength rapidly and maintains only 50% of its initial strength at 4 weeks, which makes it less desirable for rotator cuff or labral repair. PDS suture is also stiffer than braided suture and, in our experience, is more difficult to tie with more frequent suture breakage.

Suture-Passing Techniques

There are many ways to pass suture through tissue. Suture relay and direct suture-grasping techniques using various penetrating devices are effective approaches. The goal of suture passing is the precise placement of sutures to maximize secure tissue fixation and to minimize iatrogenic tissue injury. We advise familiarity with both methods to decrease frustration and operative times, as one technique alone might not always be appropriate for any given pathologic process. Familiarity with the multitude of available suture devices is helpful for efficient arthroscopic repair (Fig. 2-2).

Exposure and visualization are key to any successful surgery. In arthroscopic shoulder surgery, suture management is vastly complicated by inadequate removal of soft tissues. In our experience and observation, the failure to perform an adequate bursectomy before beginning an all-arthroscopic rotator cuff repair is the most common reason for conversion to an open procedure.[1] Care should be taken to resect the bursae laterally, anteriorly, and posteriorly to fully visualize and characterize the tear. This will also facilitate portal placement and maximize visualization and access for repair of the tear.

Suture Relay

Suture relay has been the "workhorse" of arthroscopists from its inception. A cannulated large-bore needle device is passed through the soft tissue in need of repair (Fig. 2-3). A suture lasso such as a nitinol loop is then advanced through the needle and retrieved through a different working portal. The suture end that is to be shuttled through the tissue is retrieved through the same portal.

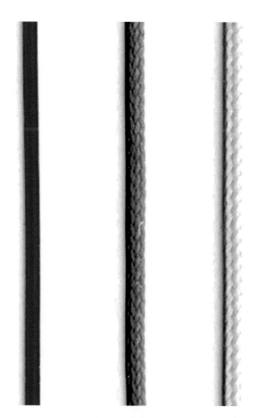

Figure 2-1 Multiple types of sutures are used in the shoulder, including multibraided and monofilament suture. PDS is stiff and loses strength quickly. Ethibond suture slides more easily, and multibraided sutures like FiberWire have the strength of a No. 5 suture. Shown from left to right are PDS, Ethibond, and FiberWire.

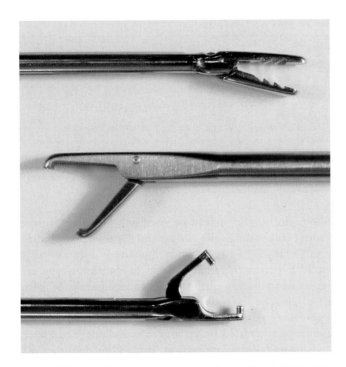

Figure 2-2 Several other devices are necessary for an efficient arthroscopic repair. Suture grasping and retrieving devices are available from several manufacturers. Tissue graspers allow positioning for easier passage of suture. Pictured from top to bottom are serrated grasper, tissue grasper, and ring retriever.

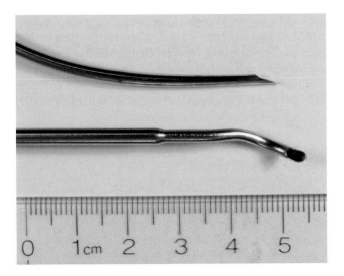

Figure 2-3 Suture lassos are the workhorse of arthroscopic shoulder surgery. Cannulated needles usually come prepackaged and have various bends and angles that assist with suture passage in otherwise difficult locations.

Care should be taken not to entangle the suture that is to be passed with the remaining sutures. This can be avoided by grasping the lasso and the suture in one pass, retrieving them together through the same working portal. We strongly recommend the use of clear plastic cannulas in passing sutures to avoid soft tissue interposition in the suture. Clear cannulas can also be helpful when sutures

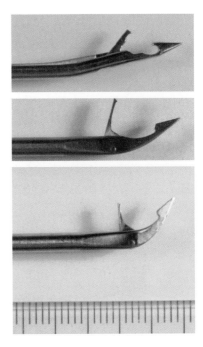

Figure 2-4 Tissue-penetrating devices are extremely valuable and can be used in antegrade or retrograde fashion to pass suture. Various angles are available to facilitate suture passage. Penetrators with a higher angle require a larger bore cannula.

become entangled within the cannula itself. The suture end is then passed through the lasso. Only 10 cm of suture or less should be passed to minimize kinking of the suture or lasso when the lasso is retrieved. The nitinol loop is then retracted through the original portal, retrieving the attached suture limb; this process is repeated until all sutures are retrieved. Suture lasso devices are available from several manufacturers with straight, curved, and corkscrew tips to facilitate suture passage.

Alternatively, devices that pass a monofilament, such as a No. 1 polydioxanone (PDS) or polypropylene (Prolene) suture, can provide a cost-effective alternative to commercially available disposable devices and shuttles. Suture hooks (Linvatec, Largo, Fla) with variable angled tips (i.e., 45-degree right and left) are reusable devices that readily advance a monofilament suture through tissue. The monofilament is then tied around the definitive suture limb by a simple half-hitch and then used to pull the suture through the tissue. When the knot-suture combination reaches the tissue junction, it is helpful to gently tug the monofilament to transfer energy to the level of the knot-suture junction to avoid overloading the monofilament proximally. It is also helpful to shuttle one suture limb at a time from within a cannula to prevent entanglement.

Tissue Penetrators

Tissue-penetrating devices are useful in larger spaces with more robust tissue (Fig. 2-4). These devices have sharp,

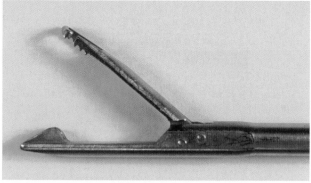

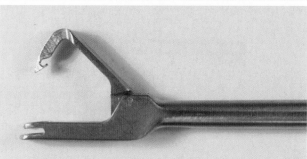

Figure 2-5 One-step suture passers were designed to minimize the number of steps involved in suture passing. In general, a suture is loaded into the end of the device and passed through the tissue. In the ideal situation, the suture is grasped by the same instrument used to pass the suture; however, this can be difficult, and we recommend performing the grasping and retrieving steps through a different portal to avoid pulling the suture out of the tissue. These devices are larger than suture relay or tissue penetrators and can be difficult to use in confined spaces. *Top,* Scorpion (Arthrex, Inc., Naples, Fla). *Bottom,* Caspari suture punch (Arthrotek, Inc., Warsaw, Ind).

pointed ends and are used to grasp or to pass suture directly through tissue. Penetrators can be used in either a retrograde or antegrade fashion to push or to pull suture through tissue and are available with straight and angled tips. Particular care should be taken with these instruments to avoid iatrogenic injury to cartilage or more delicate labral tissue. Obtaining an ideal angle for suture passage can be difficult, and accessory portals should be made if needed to improve instrument orientation.

Antegrade Suture-Passing Devices

More recently, devices have been developed that offer single-step antegrade suture passage and retrieval with the same instrument (Fig. 2-5). The various designs share one common function: to pass suture directly through the tissue and retrieve the limb through the same portal. Convenience, cost-effectiveness, and tissue quality are deciding factors in use of passive penetrators.

Knot-Tying Techniques

A multitude of knots have been described, but there are two basic types of knots: sliding-locking and nonsliding.

Box 2-1 Knot-Tying Terminology

Post	Suture limb around which you make a loop, used to pull knot to tissue
Loop	Suture limb used to make a loop around the post
Half-hitch knot	Single loop around the post
Knot pusher	Mechanical device used to slide a knot or loop down the post limb

Sliding-locking knots can be used only when the suture slides easily through the anchor and the tissue; nonsliding knots may also be used when the suture does not slide easily. Whereas there are benefits to each knot type, we recommend having a thorough understanding of both nonsliding knots and at least one sliding knot.[4-7] The importance of knot security for limiting knot slippage cannot be overstated; only 3 mm of knot slippage or stretch constitutes failed tissue fixation. This section discusses and demonstrates some of the basic knot-tying techniques and principles (Box 2-1).

Nonsliding knots are relatively simple and are composed of simple repeated half-hitches on alternating posts, providing excellent suture fixation.[1]

Sliding knots have a wide range of complexity, depending on whether the knot "locks" to resist slippage. A sliding-locking knot is used whenever possible in our practice. The Samsung Medical Center (SMC) knot[10,11] is one of the most reliable sliding-locking knots, allowing minimal knot slippage (Fig. 2-6); the Weston knot (Fig. 2-7), another reliable knot we routinely use in our practice, allows a secure knot that slides easily.[16]

SUTURE-PASSING PEARLS

- Use of a spinal needle under direct vision allows the surgeon to assess the angle of entry before an accessory portal is made, thus ensuring successful suture passage through tissue.

- An attempt should be made to place the portal in a position that allows a reasonable amount of swelling. For example, placement of the lateral portal too close to the lateral acromion may lead to difficulty in performing adequate acromioplasty and bursectomy.

- Maximize visualization before starting the reparative procedure by performing an extensive bursectomy.

- Obtain adequate hemostasis through use of electrocautery, pump, and blood pressure control. Failure to do so will lead to longer operative times.

- Avoid unloading an anchor by retrieving the lasso and one suture limb simultaneously through the portal. Most problems occur when both suture ends from an anchor are passed through the same portal.

- Tangling of sutures can be a problem when multiple anchors have been placed or when an anchor is loaded with multiple sutures. Keep each suture set "saved" in different cannulas or through the soft tissue.

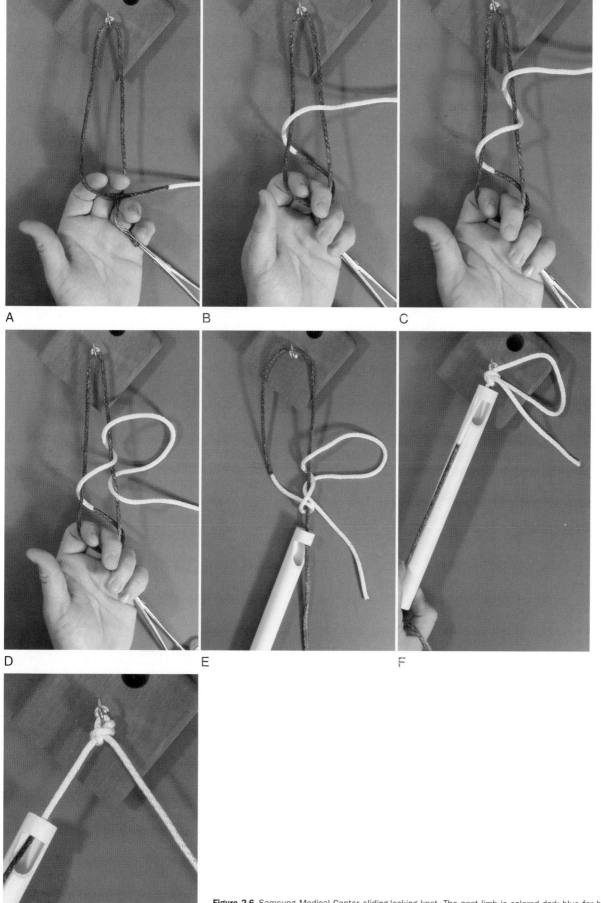

Figure 2-6 Samsung Medical Center sliding-locking knot. The post limb is colored dark blue for better visualization. **A,** The loop strand is passed over the post. **B,** The loop limb is then passed under and over both suture limbs. **C,** The loop limb is then passed under and back over the post limb. **D,** The loop limb is then passed under the post just distal to the first throw. **E,** As tension is pulled on the post, a "locking loop" is formed and should be maintained usually with the index finger. **F,** The post limb is tensioned with a knot pusher, causing the knot to slide distally. Care should be taken to avoid tightening the locking loop until the knot has adequately tensioned the tissue. **G,** While the post limb is tensioned with the knot pusher, the loop strand is then tensioned, tightening the locking loop and effectively securing the knot. This is usually followed with at least two alternating (over and under) half-hitch knots.

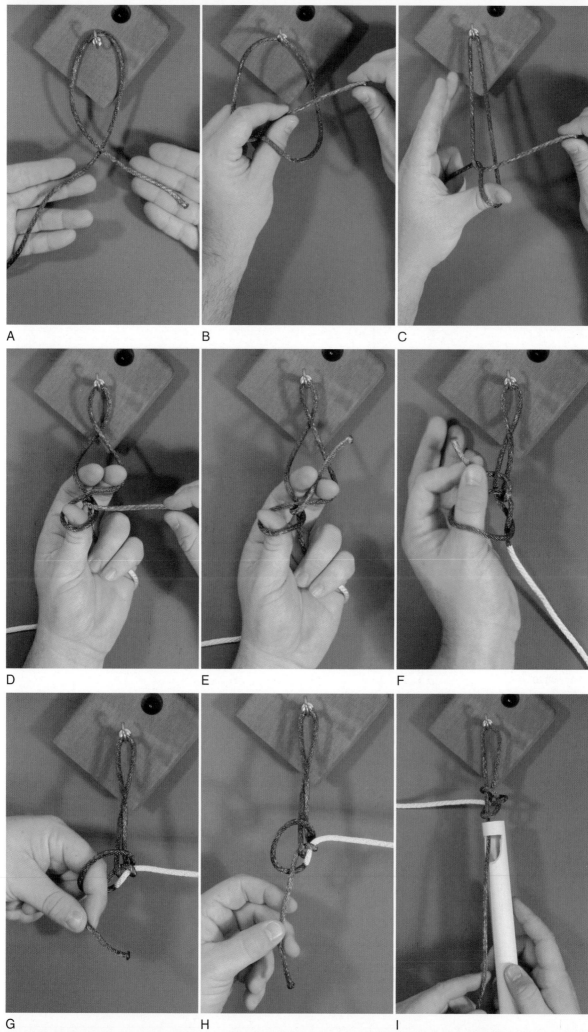

A

B

C

D

E

F

G

H

I

Figure 2-7 Weston knot. **A,** The post limb is placed over the loop limb of suture, making an "open loop." **B,** The index finger of the left hand passes over the open loop, grasping the post limb with index and thumb. The post limb is then passed under and through the open loop, and the end of the suture is grasped with the right hand. **C,** The left thumb is then used to tension the suture loop while the post limb is tensioned by the right hand. **D,** The left index and long fingers are then passed under both limbs of the open loop, over the far strand, and back under the near strand. Tension should be maintained on the post during this maneuver. **E,** The post strand is then passed with the right hand to between the left index and long fingers. **F,** The left index and long fingers are pulled down through the open loop, allowing the post limb to be grasped by the left thumb and index finger. **G,** The post limb is then passed with the left index and thumb through the space occupied by the thumb. **H,** In this figure, the post limb is not yet ready to be tensioned. The knot should be "dressed" so that the post will slide by gently tensioning the post limb only. Tensioning of the loop strand at this stage will lock the knot and thus should be avoided. **I,** The post limb is then tensioned with a knot pusher, sliding the knot to tension the soft tissue. After adequate soft tissue tension has occurred, the loop limb is tensioned, locking the knot. This is typically followed with three alternating half-hitches while alternating the post on at least one throw.

SUTURE-TYING PEARLS

- Be sure to check that the suture slides easily before attempting to tie a sliding knot. If the suture does not slide, a nonsliding knot with reversed half-hitches and throws is necessary to obtain maximum fixation.

- On nonsliding knots, we tie at least six half-hitches, alternating the post and reversing the throws with each knot (underhand and overhand).

- Before the knot is tied, a knot pusher should be passed down each limb to untwist the suture.

- A clear cannula is preferable because it allows visualization of the knot as it slides to the tissue and keeps soft tissue from interfering with the knot.

- Advanced arthroscopists may choose to forego the use of a cannula. If this method is chosen, we recommend that a ring forceps be placed around both suture limbs outside the shoulder and then slid into the shoulder to the cuff or labrum to verify that no soft tissue is intertwined between the sutures.

- Visualize the knot during the tying sequence. An experienced assistant can hold the arthroscope while the knot is being passed to verify adequate soft tissue and knot tensioning.

- Take your time. Allow extra time on all-arthroscopic cases in the beginning. Be patient with yourself to avoid technical difficulties, such as anchor unloading and suture entanglement.

- Practice your knot-tying skills. The time to practice is before the case, when there are no time issues or other stressful situations.

Conclusion

Advances in arthroscopic instruments and techniques have allowed surgeons to perform significantly more complex procedures. Careful planning, preparation, and patience are necessary when the transition is made to arthroscopic techniques. The surgeon must be able to visualize the structures and understand the basic principles of suture passing and knot tying before all-arthroscopic techniques should be considered.

References

1. Altchek DW, Warren RF, Wickiewicz TL, et al. Arthroscopic acromioplasty: technique and results. J Bone Joint Surg Am 1990;72:1198-1207.
2. Burkhart SS. Arthroscopic repair of massive rotator cuff tears: concept of margin convergence. Tech Shoulder Elbow Surg 2000;1:232-239.
3. Burkhart SS, Morgan CD, Kibler WB. The disabled throwing shoulder: spectrum of pathology. Part II: evaluation and treatment of SLAP lesions in throwers. Arthroscopy 2003;19:531-539.
4. Burkhart SS, Wirth MA, Simonich M, et al. Knot security in simple sliding knots and its relationship to rotator cuff repair: how secure must the knot be? Arthroscopy 2000;16:202-207.
5. Burkhart SS, Wirth MA, Simonick M, et al. Loop security as a determinant of tissue fixation security. Arthroscopy 1998;14:773-776.
6. Chan KC, Burkhart SS. How to switch posts without rethreading when tying half-hitches. Arthroscopy 1999;15:444-450.
7. Chan KC, Burkhart SS, Thiagarajan P, et al. Optimization of stacked half-hitch knots for arthroscopic surgery. Arthroscopy 2001;17: 752-759.
8. Geiger DF, Hurley JA, Tovey JA, et al. Results of arthroscopic versus open Bankart suture repair. Clin Orthop 1997;337:111-117.
9. Kaar TK, Schenck RC Jr, Wirth MA, Rockwood CA Jr. Complications of metallic suture anchors in shoulder surgery: a report of 8 cases. Arthroscopy 2001;17:31-37.
10. Kim SH, Ha KI. The SMC knot—a new slipknot with locking mechanism. Arthroscopy 2000;16:563-565.
11. Kim SH, Ha KI, Kim JS. Significance of the internal locking mechanism for loop security enhancement in the arthroscopic knot. Arthroscopy 2001;17:850-855.
12. Lo IK, Burkhart SS. Current concepts in arthroscopic rotator cuff repair. Am J Sports Med 2003;31:308-324.
13. Nam EK, Snyder SJ. The diagnosis and treatment of superior labrum, anterior and posterior (SLAP) lesions. Am J Sports Med 2003;31:798-810.
14. Ritchie PK, McCarty EC. Metal and plastic suture anchors for rotator cuff repair. Oper Tech Sports Med 2004;12:215-220.
15. Trimbos JB, Booster M, Peters AA. Mechanical knot performance of a new generation polydioxanon suture (PDS-2). Acta Obstet Gynecol Scand 1991;70:157-159.
16. Weston PV. A new clinch knot. Obstet Gynecol 1991;78:144-147.

Suture Anchor Fixation for Shoulder Instability

Craig R. Bottoni, MD

Major Brett D. Owens, MD

Recurrent anterior glenohumeral instability is a common sequela of traumatic glenohumeral dislocation or subluxation. The major pathoanatomic features of a traumatic dislocation are the capsulolabral avulsion of the inferior glenohumeral ligament (Bankart-Perthes lesion) and capsular redundancy, which typically worsens with repeated injuries.[1,5,6,17,19] Once recurrent instability affects activities of daily living or precludes return to sporting activities, operative stabilization is typically recommended. However, there is still considerable debate about when to proceed with surgery after the first traumatic dislocation. The orthopedic literature supports early acute arthroscopic stabilization after a traumatic dislocation in a select group of young athletes who are at high risk for repeated shoulder injuries, ostensibly to decrease the risk of recurrence compared with traditional nonoperative management.[2-4,7,8,14] However, patient issues such as player position, time remaining in a season, and time available for rehabilitation may affect the decision of when to undergo surgery.

Before the introduction of arthroscopic techniques in the mid-1980s, shoulder stabilization surgery necessitated a formal deltopectoral approach, through which the subscapularis was either released from its humeral insertion or split longitudinally for access to the glenohumeral joint. The initial technique to reattach the avulsed labrum to bone was through bone tunnels; however, following their introduction in the 1980s, suture anchors quickly became the most commonly used soft tissue repair devices. With the introduction of arthroscopic shoulder techniques, the number as well as the different varieties of fixation devices has exploded.

Arthroscopic shoulder stabilization offers a number of advantages over traditional open repairs. These include smaller incisions, less muscle dissection, less postoperative pain, and better visualization of the entire glenohumeral joint.[10] The first arthroscopic Bankart repairs were performed by transglenoid suture fixation. Sutures were passed across the glenoid and tied over the posterior fascia. As bioabsorbable polymers were developed for use in the shoulder, soft tissue fixation with tacks became popular. The tacks can be inserted arthroscopically over a guide wire to ensure correct placement. Although they are still in use, the tacks have been shown to have limited pullout strength and have for the most part been abandoned for shoulder stabilization. The success of metallic suture anchors in open shoulder surgery led to the development of arthroscopic deployment techniques. Development of longer-lasting polymers and much stronger suture made bioabsorbable anchors the most popular choice for soft tissue repair. The goal of any suture anchor is to repair soft tissue to bone and be able to withstand the forces required for rehabilitation until the normal bone-to-tissue interface is restored. The focus of this chapter is on the technique of arthroscopic anterior shoulder stabilization with use of suture anchors.

Preoperative Considerations

History

It is essential to establish an accurate diagnosis. Important information to elicit includes mechanism of initial injury, frequency and mechanism of dislocation or subluxation episodes, presence of instability during activities of daily living, and prior surgeries.

Recurrent anterior instability typically presents with a limitation of shoulder function due to a subjective feeling that the shoulder is "slipping out of the joint." For anterior instability, shoulder abduction with external rotation most commonly reproduces these symptoms.

Physical Examination

Many shoulder dislocations are reduced by athletic trainers, coaches, or emergency department personnel. The on-field reduction is typically easier and less traumatic than a delayed reduction because of the absence of muscle spasm. Crepitation or pain at the upper arm may be indicative of a proximal humerus fracture. If any question exists, reduction should be delayed until sufficient radiographs are obtained. Plain radiographs will confirm a shoulder dislocation and can assist in identifying any concomitant fractures before a reduction maneuver. Once reduction is obtained, a physical evaluation is repeated to document any neurologic injury or weakness. A radiographic examination is required to confirm reduction and to evaluate the joint for other associated injuries. It is important to determine the presence of an axillary nerve injury, which can be associated with anterior dislocations. It is also imperative to assess the integrity of the rotator cuff, especially in older patients.

Recurrent instability presents with apprehension in the abducted, externally rotated position. Relief of the apprehension with posteriorly directed pressure on the proximal humerus, the relocation sign, is often present. Glenohumeral patholaxity can be assessed and graded in comparison to the contralateral side. This examination should be repeated under anesthesia, when a better comparison to the normal side can be obtained. The examination under anesthesia includes the supine load-shift test with the arm abducted at 70 to 90 degrees to document and to quantify the degree of anterior instability of the glenohumeral joint compared with the contralateral side.

Imaging

- A standard anteroposterior view with the arm in slight internal rotation is used to identify fractures of the greater tuberosity and Hill-Sachs lesions (Fig. 3-1).
- The transscapular Y view can assist with the direction of dislocation before reduction and confirm successful reduction.
- The West Point axillary view can be used to assess glenoid rim fractures (bony Bankart lesion; Fig. 3-2).

Other Modalities

- Computed tomographic scans are occasionally used to assess the extent of bone injuries of the humerus or

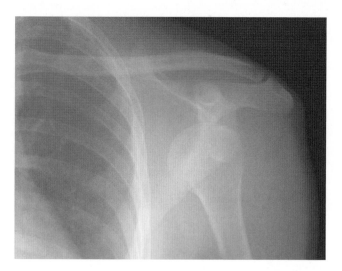

Figure 3-1 An anteroposterior radiograph demonstrating anterior shoulder dislocation.

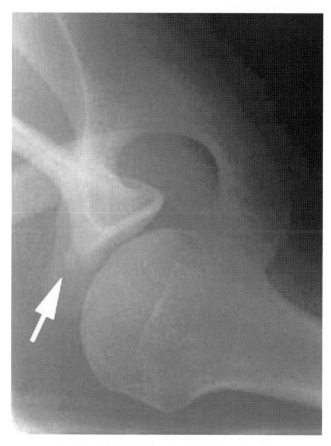

Figure 3-2 A West Point axillary radiograph, best used to evaluate the glenoid. This radiograph reveals an avulsion of the anteroinferior corner of the glenoid (bony Bankart lesion).

glenoid. In addition, they can be used to evaluate the glenoid version.

- Magnetic resonance imaging is the "gold standard" to evaluate intra-articular pathoanatomy. For evaluation of recurrent instability, we prefer magnetic resonance arthrography because the addition of gadolinium improves the visualization of the shoulder pathoanatomy (Fig. 3-3). After an acute dislocation or subluxation, the hemarthrosis serves to distend the joint and obviates the need for contrast agent.

Indications and Contraindications

The primary reason to offer a surgical stabilization procedure is shoulder instability that interferes with activities of daily living or recreational sports. Recurrent dislocation or subluxation episodes can result in additional chondral or osteochondral damage. Contraindications include habitual or voluntary dislocation, a large bony Bankart lesion, and a large engaging Hill-Sachs lesion.

Surgical Technique

Anesthesia and Positioning

Anterior stabilization is typically performed under general anesthesia. An adjunctive regional (interscalene) block may be performed to provide postoperative analgesia. Positioning of the patient is based on the surgeon's preference. Many surgeons believe that the lateral decubitus position allows better visualization and ease of instrumentation with a shoulder distraction system (STaR Sleeve and 3-Point Shoulder Distraction System; Arthrex, Inc., Naples, Fla; Fig. 3-4). However, the beach chair position may allow greater control of the entire arm, especially internal and external rotation. This position also facilitates easier conversion to a traditional open approach.

Surgical Landmarks, Incisions, and Portals

The bone landmarks may be identified with a skin marker to assist in portal position (Fig 3-5). The standard posterior viewing portal is established approximately 2 cm medial and 2 cm inferior to the posterolateral edge of the acromion.

The anterosuperior portal is established by an outside-in technique. An 18-gauge spinal needle is inserted 1 cm anterior to the acromion and 2 cm lateral to the coracoid close to the anterolateral edge of the acromion. The needle should enter the joint high and just medial to the biceps tendon near the root attachment as visualized arthroscopically. A clear 6.5-mm cannula (Stryker Endoscopy, San Jose, Calif) is used for instrumentation.

An anteroinferior portal is established just above the superior edge of the subscapularis and as lateral as possible to obtain the best angle toward the glenoid when suture anchors are inserted. Because of the required instrument passage, a larger 8.25-mm twist-in cannula (Arthrex, Inc., Naples, Fla) is used to establish and to maintain this portal.

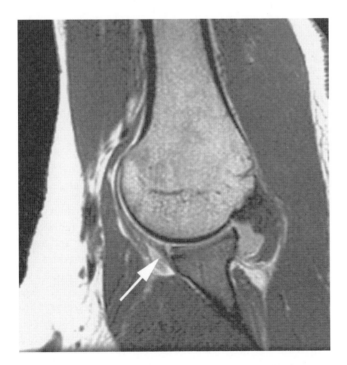

Figure 3-3 Magnetic resonance arthrogram with patient's shoulder in an abducted, externally rotated position to tighten the anterior band of the inferior glenohumeral ligament complex. Note the Bankart lesion (*arrow*).

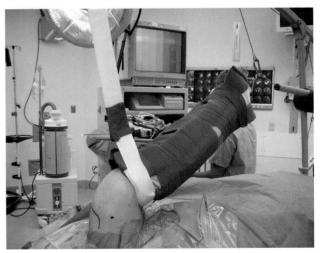

Figure 3-4 Intraoperative photograph of patient in lateral decubitus position. Excellent intra-articular arthroscopic visualization results from the distraction provided by the axillary strap.

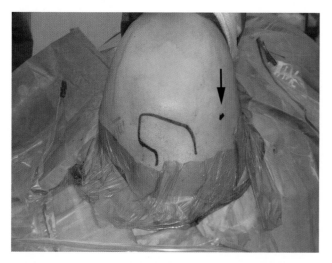

Figure 3-5 Anatomic landmarks identified on skin before arthroscopy. The standard posterior viewing portal is made approximately 2 cm inferior and 2 cm medial to the posterolateral corner of the acromion *(arrow)*.

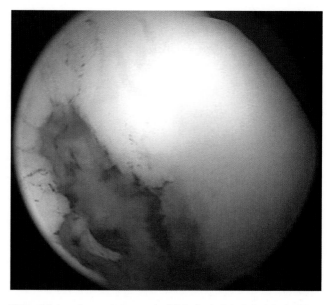

Figure 3-7 An arthroscopic image of a Hill-Sachs lesion of the left shoulder. Note the articular cartilage on both sides of the compression fracture that differentiates it from the normal "bare area" of the posterolateral humeral head.

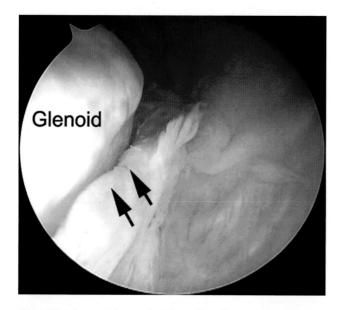

Figure 3-6 Arthroscopic image of a left shoulder with an anterior labral periosteal sleeve avulsion (ALPSA lesion) visualized from the anterosuperior portal.

Box 3-1 Surgical Steps

1. Positioning and portal placement
2. Labral preparation
3. Shuttle suture passage
4. Suture anchor insertion and suture passage
5. Knot tying

then reattached to the articular margin. The anteroinferior glenoid is evaluated for bone and cartilage loss and the posterosuperior humeral head for a bony or cartilaginous Hill-Sachs defect (Fig. 3-7).

Specific Steps (Box 3-1)

For arthroscopic stabilizations to be successfully performed, a reproducible sequence of steps allows the surgeon to properly address the pathoanatomy and avoid the myriad pitfalls that can complicate the procedure.

1. Positioning and Portal Placement

The correct patient positioning and portal placement are critical to allow access to the entire shoulder. For lateral decubitus positioning, the patient is maintained with a deflatable beanbag. It is important to ensure that the patient is well secured to prevent the patient from leaning during the surgery and precluding adequate visualization. The 3-point shoulder system (STaR Sleeve and 3-Point

Arthroscopic Examination

A systematic diagnostic arthroscopy is performed. The superior and posterior labral attachments are inspected. If they are torn, arthroscopic repair is performed as described in Chapters 8 and 22 before anterior pathologic processes are addressed. With anterior instability, the anteroinferior labral attachment is often disrupted (Bankart lesion). Chronic instability often results in a medialized capsulolabral complex (anterior labral periosteal sleeve avulsion [ALPSA lesion]; Fig. 3-6). When it is present, this labral attachment must be sharply reflected from the glenoid and

Shoulder Distraction System) incorporates a strap that wraps under the proximal humerus and allows lateral distraction to improve joint visualization (see Fig. 3-4).

2. Labral Preparation

This step is crucial to prepare the capsulolabral tissue for repair. A sharp arthroscopic elevator (Liberator; ConMed Linvatec, Inc., Largo, Fla) is used to mobilize the capsulolabral tissue from the glenoid attachment (Fig. 3-8). Elevation should be performed until muscle fibers of the subscapularis are visible along the anterior glenoid neck. After mobilization, the capsulolabral tissue will be completely free, thus allowing superior translation for subsequent repair to the articular margin of the glenoid. A mechanical shaver or bur is used to abrade the anterior glenoid and to stimulate a bleeding bed to which the capsulolabral tissue will be reattached (Fig. 3-9). To better visualize the anterior glenoid during preparation, a 70-degree arthroscope may be used from the posterior portal to "look over the edge," or the standard 30-degree arthroscope can be inserted down the anterosuperior portal while instrumenting through the anteroinferior portal.

3. Shuttle Suture Passage

The next step is to pass a temporary suture that will be used subsequently to shuttle one limb of the permanent suture from the anchor through the tissue and labrum, which will secure the capsulolabral tissue back to the glenoid. Several arthroscopic instruments are commercially available to facilitate this step. We prefer to use a 45-degree curved suture shuttle (Spectrum Soft Tissue Repair System; ConMed Linvatec, Inc., Largo, Fla) through which a No. 1 PDS suture (Ethicon, Inc., Somerville, NJ) is passed (Fig. 3-10). It is important to place this shuttle stitch as inferior as possible to allow superior translation and retensioning of the capsulolabral complex onto the articular margin once it is tied. The suture delivery instrument is passed first through the capsule approximately 1 to 2 cm from the labrum. The hook is then passed through the labrum (Fig. 3-10A). The first passage will produce a capsular plication as it forms a pleat in the capsule. The second pass facilitates repair of the labrum back to the glenoid. The primary purpose of the shuttle suture is to serve as a temporary stitch that will then be used to pass one limb of the suture from the suture anchor to be passed through the tissue. Many instruments are available to allow the surgeon to skip this step by passing the instrument through the tissue to retrieve the suture from the previously placed anchor. However, use of a shuttle suture as described allows more precise placement of the sutures through the tissue.

4. Suture Anchor Insertion and Suture Passage

Through the anterosuperior portal, a grasper is used to retrieve the shuttle stitch and pull it out the anterosuperior portal (Fig. 3-10B). At this time, upward retraction of this temporary stitch will allow a determination of how much superior shifting of the capsulolabral tissue is possible and, therefore, where the suture anchor should be correctly placed. Excessive tension on this first stitch will increase the likelihood of a knot's loosening. We prefer the Bio-FASTak suture anchor preloaded with No. 2

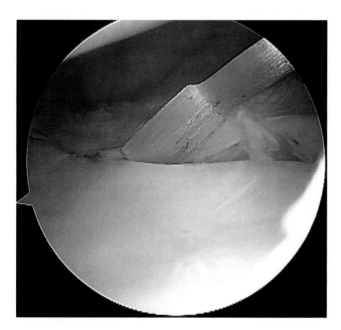

Figure 3-8 An arthroscopic elevator knife is used to mobilize the labrum from the anterior glenoid before repair.

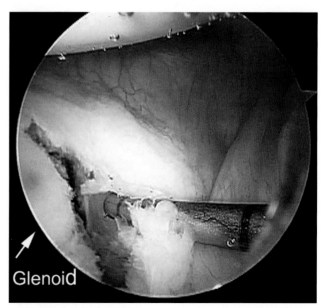

Glenoid

Figure 3-9 Arthroscopic image of a left shoulder visualized from the anterosuperior portal. A mechanical shaver is used to abrade the anterior glenoid in preparation for repair.

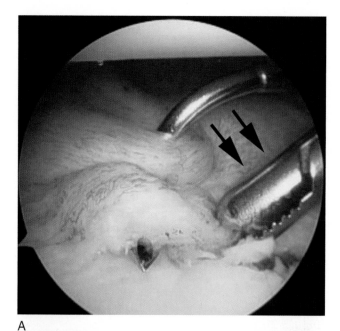

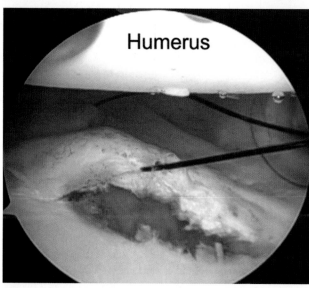

Figure 3-10 A, Through the anteroinferior portal, a curved suture-passing instrument (45-degree Spectrum hook) is passed first through the capsule and then separately through the labrum. A soft tissue grasper *(double arrows)* is used through the anterosuperior portal to maintain tension on the tissue and then to retrieve the PDS suture out the anterosuperior portal once it is passed. **B,** The PDS suture has been passed through the tissue, and one limb exits the anterosuperior portal and the other exits the anteroinferior portal.

FiberWire (Arthrex, Inc., Naples, Fla). The primary advantage of this suture anchor is that the implant can be placed without the use of a drill. The hole is initiated with a sharp trocar and then tapped by hand. The suture anchor is passed through the anteroinferior portal and placed 1 to 2 mm onto the articular margin (Fig. 3-11). After anchor insertion, the suture tails must be separated and cleared of any twists. A knot pusher may be placed on one strand of

the suture and passed down the cannula. While the knot pusher is inserted, the more inferior or anterior limb is identified. This limb is then retrieved through the anterosuperior portal with a ringed grasper (Fig. 3-12). It is imperative to clamp or to hold the opposite limb that is exiting the anteroinferior portal to prevent "unloading" of the suture from the anchor.

At this point, one limb of the PDS shuttle suture and one limb of the permanent suture are exiting each of the anterior cannulas. Outside the anterosuperior portal cannula, the PDS suture is tied to the permanent suture several centimeters from the end (Fig. 3-13). A dilating knot can be made with a simple half-hitch to facilitate passage of the shuttle suture. Once secured, the PDS shuttle suture, along with the attached permanent suture, is pulled through the anteroinferior portal (Fig. 3-14). Arthroscopic visualization of this maneuver is important to ensure that the sutures do not become entangled during passage through the tissue. The PDS suture is now discarded, and both limbs of the permanent suture are exiting the anteroinferior portal, with one limb now through the soft tissue.

5. Knot Tying

The knot pusher is again passed down one limb to ensure that the tails are not twisted around one another. An arthroscopic knot is now tied to secure the capsulolabral tissue back to the glenoid (Fig. 3-15). Many arthroscopic knots have been described; however, the surgeon should become proficient with one sliding-locking knot so it can be tied quickly and reproducibly with little effort. We prefer to use a modified Roeder knot that allows a strong suture buttress. This is backed up with three half-hitches to secure the knot. To reduce the tension on the tissue during tying, an atraumatic tissue grasper can be passed through the anterosuperior portal to translate the tissue while this first knot is tied. The tails of the completed knot are cut with the arthroscopic scissors passed through either the anterosuperior portal or the anteroinferior portal, depending on the optimal angle. This entire process is repeated two or three times to restore the tissue back to the glenoid. The knots should be secure and induce a dimpling effect on the capsulolabral tissue (Fig. 3-16).

Postoperative Considerations

Follow-up

Instability surgery is typically performed on an outpatient basis. A standard sling can be applied postoperatively. We prefer the Cryo/Cuff cooling device (Don Joy, Vista, CA) for additional pain relief. The patients are then seen several days after the procedure for their first dressing change.

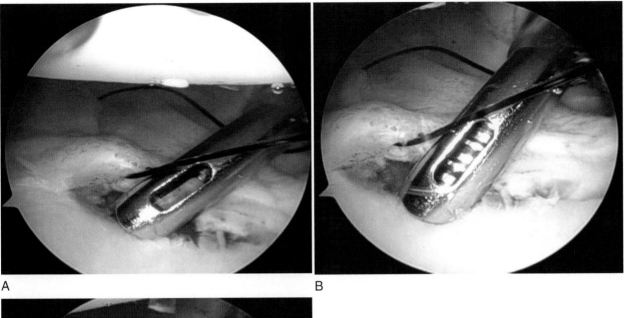

A

B

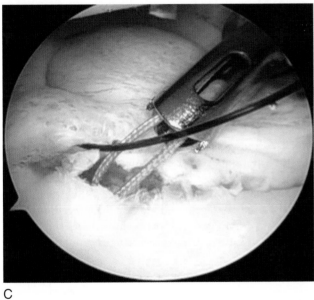

C

Figure 3-11 The bioabsorbable suture anchors (Bio-FASTak; Arthrex, Inc., Naples, Fla) are inserted along the articular margin of the glenoid following shuttle suture passage (purple suture). After the obturator is seated on the edge of the cartilage **(A),** the sharp trocar is used to initiate the hole. The tap is used to deepen the hole **(B),** and then the anchor is inserted **(C).** Note that the suture anchor is placed 1 to 2 mm onto the articular surface.

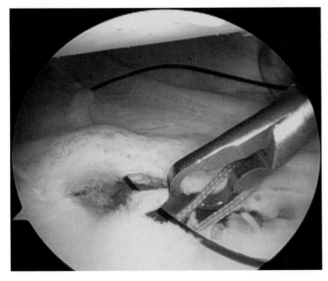

Figure 3-12 A ringed grasper is passed through the anterosuperior portal to pull the inferior limb of the suture through the anterosuperior portal cannula. Now, each cannula has two suture limbs, a purple PDS suture and a permanent limb from the suture anchor.

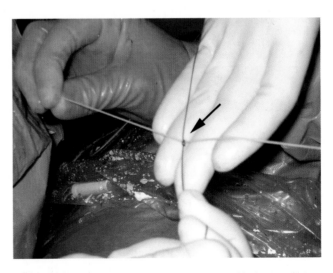

Figure 3-13 The PDS shuttle suture (purple) is tied outside the cannula to the permanent suture with a simple half-hitch *(arrow).* To help facilitate the knot's passage, another half-hitch is tied in the PDS shuttle suture that will serve as a dilation knot.

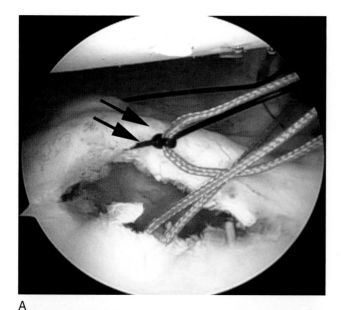

A

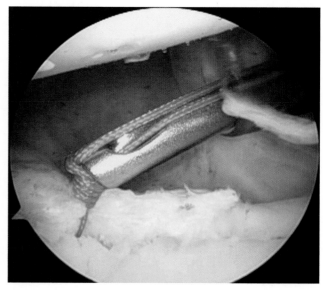

Figure 3-15 An arthroscopic knot is tied outside the cannula and pushed down to abut the tissue. At least three half-hitches are then tied to secure the knot.

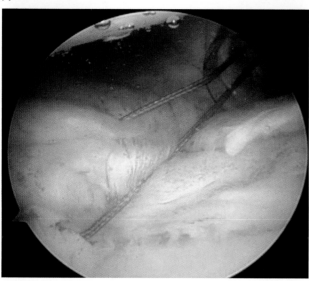

B

Figure 3-14 The PDS shuttle suture is used to pull the one limb of the FiberWire through the tissue (**A,** *arrows*). This step should be done slowly to ensure that the limbs pass freely without entanglement. Once passed, both limbs of the FiberWire will exit the anteroinferior portal, with one limb passing through the capsule and labrum (**B**).

Rehabilitation

The arthroscopic repair, like its open counterpart, requires that the capsulolabral tissue heal back to the glenoid. We have adopted a three-phase rehabilitation program. Each phase lasts approximately 4 weeks but is modified to the patient's individual progress. The first phase consists of immobilization in a standard arm sling with gentle range-of-motion (Codman pendulum) exercises, wrist and elbow motion, and low-resistance isometrics during supervised physical therapy. The sling is worn at all times during this phase except during physical therapy sessions. The second phase consists of progressive resistive exercises and neuromuscular training. We recommend continued sling use during this period. Abduction with external rotation of the shoulder is avoided, but forward elevation with extension is encouraged. The final phase consists of progressive range-of-motion exercises as tolerated, increased resistance, neuromuscular training, and aerobic conditioning. Rubber-band resistance exercises and high-repetition sets are used to regain muscle conditioning. Return to full active duty, contact sports, and activities requiring overhead or heavy lifting is restricted until 4 months postoperatively.

Complications

The complications associated with arthroscopic stabilization include not only problems associated with the actual performance of the steps required to restore the normal anatomy but also problems associated with the equipment required to maintain adequate visualization during the procedure. The camera, arthroscope, and monitor equipment may malfunction, and specialized knowledge by the operating room staff is necessary to troubleshoot problems that inevitably occur. Replacement parts should be readily available to permit continuation of the procedure in the event that some of the equipment becomes damaged.

Complications associated with this procedure include inadequate tissue preparation leading to an inability to properly mobilize the capsulolabral complex. Medialized repairs often result in recurrent instability. Inadequate tensioning of the tissue can lead to suture breakage or

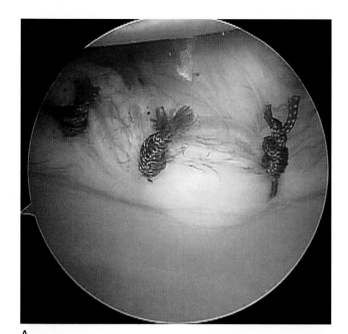

A

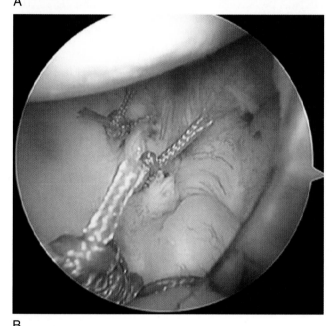

B

Figure 3-16 The completed repair visualized from posterior **(A)** and anterosuperior **(B)** portals.

Table 3-1 Clinical Results of Arthroscopic Bankart Repair with Suture Anchors

Author	Mean Follow-up	Outcome
Warme et al[18] (1999)	25 months	38 shoulders mean Rowe score: 94 3 (8%) recurrence
Kandziora et al[11] (2000)	38 months	55 shoulders mean Rowe score: 85 9 (16%) recurrence
Tauro[16] (2000)	39 months	29 shoulders mean Rowe score: 92 2 (7%) recurrence
Kim et al[13] (2002)	39 months	59 shoulders mean Rowe score: 93 2 (3%) recurrence
Kim et al[12] (2003)	44 months	167 shoulders mean Rowe score: 92 7 (4%) recurrence
Fabbriciani et al[9] (2004)	24 months	30 shoulders mean Rowe score: 91 No recurrence
Mazzocca et al[15] (2005)	37 months	18 shoulders mean ASES score: 90 2 (11%) recurrence
Bottoni et al[7] (2005)	32 months	32 shoulders mean Rowe score: 89 1 (3%) recurrence

ASES, American Shoulder and Elbow Surgeons.

synovitis as they are hydrolyzed. This may be manifested clinically as an increase in shoulder pain at 4 to 6 weeks after surgery and a loss of glenohumeral motion.

Results

Traditionally, compared with open techniques for recurrent instability, results of arthroscopic Bankart repairs have been less favorable. The use of transglenoid fixation, tacks, and nonanatomic repairs resulted in unreasonably high recurrence rates. However, with improved arthroscopic techniques and implants, the results of arthroscopic instability repair have approached and even surpassed those of open techniques (Table 3-1). With comparable rates for recurrent dislocation, arthroscopic stabilization is rapidly becoming the technique of choice, even in the contact and collision athlete. A careful and diligent approach to arthroscopic stabilization can lead to success rates of more than 90%.

recurrent laxity in the tissue, resulting in recurrent instability or failure. Metallic anchors used to secure soft tissue, if left protruding above the articular cartilage, can result in disastrous consequences for the humeral articular surface. Even slight prominence can result in a destruction of the humeral cartilage as the shoulder abrades on the metallic edge. In addition, improperly placed metallic or bioabsorbable anchors can dislodge and become loose bodies that result in destruction of articular cartilage. Some bioabsorbable fixation devices have been associated with a reactive

References

1. Arciero RA, St Pierre P. Acute shoulder dislocation. Indications and techniques for operative management. Clin Sports Med 1995;14:937-953.

2. Arciero RA, Taylor DC. Primary anterior dislocation of the shoulder in young patients. A ten-year prospective study. J Bone Joint Surg Am 1998;80:299-300.

3. Arciero RA, Taylor DC, Snyder RJ, et al. Arthroscopic bioabsorbable tack stabilization of initial anterior shoulder dislocations: a preliminary report. Arthroscopy 1995;11:410-417.

4. Arciero RA, Wheeler JH, Ryan JB, et al. Arthroscopic Bankart repair versus nonoperative treatment for acute, initial anterior shoulder dislocations. Am J Sports Med 1994;22:589-594.

5. Baker CL, Uribe JW, Whitman C. Arthroscopic evaluation of acute initial anterior shoulder dislocations. Am J Sports Med 1990; 18:25-28.

6. Bottoni CR, Arciero RA. Arthroscopic repair of primary anterior dislocations of the shoulder. Tech Shoulder Elbow Surg 2001;2:2-16.

7. Bottoni CR, Smith EL, Berkowitz MJ, et al. Arthroscopic versus open anterior shoulder stabilization: a prospective, randomized clinical trial with preoperative and postoperative magnetic resonance arthrograms. Paper presented at the 31st annual meeting of the American Orthopaedic Society for Sports Medicine; Keystone, Colorado; 2005.

8. DeBerardino TM, Arciero RA, Taylor DC, et al. Prospective evaluation of arthroscopic stabilization of acute, initial anterior shoulder dislocations in young athletes: Two- to five-year follow-up. Am J Sports Med 2001;29:586-592.

9. Fabbriciani C, Milano G, Demontis A, et al. Arthroscopic versus open treatment of Bankart lesion of the shoulder: a prospective randomized study. Arthroscopy 2004;20:456-462.

10. Green MR, Christensen KP. Arthroscopic versus open Bankart procedures: a comparison of early morbidity and complications. Arthroscopy 1993;9:371-374.

11. Kandziora F, Jager A, Bischof F, et al. Arthroscopic labrum refixation for post-traumatic anterior shoulder instability: suture anchor versus transglenoid fixation technique. Arthroscopy 2000;16:359-366.

12. Kim SH, Ha KI, Cho YB, et al. Arthroscopic anterior stabilization of the shoulder: two to six-year follow-up. J Bone Joint Surg Am 2003;85:1511-1518.

13. Kim SH, Ha KI, Kim SH. Bankart repair in traumatic anterior shoulder instability: open versus arthroscopic technique. Arthroscopy 2002;18:755-763.

14. Kirkley A, Werstine R, Ratjek A, et al. Prospective randomized clinical trial comparing the effectiveness of immediate arthroscopic stabilization versus immobilization and rehabilitation in first traumatic anterior dislocations of the shoulder: long-term evaluation. Arthroscopy 2005;21:55-63.

15. Mazzocca AD, Brown FM Jr, Carreira DS, et al. Arthroscopic anterior shoulder stabilization of collision and contact athletes. Am J Sports Med 2005;33:52-60.

16. Tauro JC. Arthroscopic inferior capsular split and advancement for anterior and inferior shoulder instability: technique and results at 2- to 5-year follow-up. Arthroscopy 2000;16:451-456.

17. Taylor DC, Arciero RA. Pathologic changes associated with shoulder dislocations. Arthroscopic and physical examination findings in first-time, traumatic anterior dislocations. Am J Sports Med 1997; 25:306-311.

18. Warme WJ, Arciero RA, Savoie FH 3rd, et al. Nonabsorbable versus absorbable suture anchors for open Bankart repair. A prospective, randomized comparison. Am J Sports Med 1999;27: 742-746.

19. Wheeler JH, Ryan JB, Arciero RA, et al. Arthroscopic versus nonoperative treatment of acute shoulder dislocations in young athletes. Arthroscopy 1989;5:213-217.

CHAPTER 4

Knotless Suture Anchor Fixation for Shoulder Instability

Raymond Thal, MD

Bradley Butkovich, MD, MS

Shoulder instability has been treated by myriad arthroscopic and open techniques. It is well documented that restoration of stability can be reliably obtained by the Bankart repair. Open Bankart procedures are successful; however, there is some morbidity associated with them. In an effort to restore stability to the shoulder while avoiding these morbidities, arthroscopic Bankart repair procedures have been developed. Arthroscopic procedures are not without problems. Some of the poor results of arthroscopic repairs continue to be attributed to labral repair without adequately addressing capsular laxity. Furthermore, early fixation methods (tacks, staples, transglenoid sutures) did not achieve anatomic repairs similar to those of open methods. The use of current suture anchors and arthroscopic knot-tying techniques provides fixation comparable to that of open repair. However, arthroscopic suture anchor repair continues to have pitfalls related to the quality, consistency, and technical challenges associated with arthroscopic knots.

A knotless suture anchor technique that eliminates arthroscopic knot tying has been described and has been found to be successful in addressing shoulder instability. Knotless suture anchors provide a strong, consistent, and low-profile repair with an increased superior capsular shift while eliminating the problems associated with the use of special knot-tying devices, multiple knot designs, and time-consuming techniques of standard suture anchors.

Preoperative Considerations

History

It is essential to obtain a history that is consistent with shoulder instability, including the mechanism of injury, associated injuries, treatment history, chronicity, and disability. Younger patients, increased activity level, and participation in collision sports increase the likelihood of further dislocation and indication for subsequent surgical repair.

Typical History

- Shoulder injury, often an acute traumatic event typically with shoulder in abduction—external rotation and subluxation or frank dislocation of the glenohumeral joint
- Recurrent subluxation or dislocation events despite rehabilitation
- Apprehension or sensation of instability with gesturing or reaching

Physical Examination

- Presence of apprehension sign
- Positive Jobe relocation test result

- Range of motion: usually preserved
- No rotator cuff symptoms or weakness

Imaging

Radiography

- Anteroposterior radiograph
- Scapular Y radiograph
- Axillary radiograph to evaluate the anterior glenoid for a large bony Bankart lesion or glenoid rim fracture

Other Modalities

A history of documented recurrent dislocations precludes the need for other diagnostic studies unless an associated pathologic condition of the shoulder, such as a superior labral anterior-posterior (SLAP) lesion or rotator cuff tear, is suspected.

- Computed tomographic arthrography with reconstruction to assess the bony glenoid, bony Hill-Sachs lesions, and labral pathologic changes
- Magnetic resonance imaging with or without the administration of intra-articular contrast material to assess the glenoid labrum, superior labrum, biceps tendon, and rotator cuff

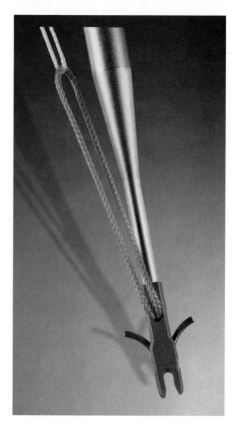

Figure 4-1 Metallic knotless suture anchor design. (From Thal R. Knotless suture anchor fixation for shoulder instability. In Miller MD, Cole BJ, eds. Textbook of Arthroscopy. Philadelphia, Elsevier, 2004.)

Indications and Contraindications

A typical candidate for arthroscopic shoulder stabilization has a history of multiple shoulder subluxations or dislocations, normal strength, and normal range of motion. Associated findings such as rotator cuff tears, SLAP tears, biceps tears, impingement, and acromioclavicular joint arthritis can be addressed at the same time as the index procedure. Capsular redundancy is often addressed with a capsular shift, plication, or resection as indicated.

Significant glenohumeral arthritis, rotator cuff arthropathy, glenoid deficiency, and significant glenoid fracture are contraindications to arthroscopic Bankart repair. A marked glenoid deficiency may require bone grafting. Furthermore, humeral avulsions of the glenohumeral ligament often require open repair.

Knotless Suture Anchor Design

The knotless suture anchor (Fig. 4-1) consists of a titanium body with two nitinol arcs. The arcs have a memory property that creates resistance to anchor pullout after insertion into bone through small drill holes. The knotless suture anchor looks similar to the GII anchor (Mitek Products, Westwood, Mass); however, it differs structur-

ally in several ways. A channel or slot is located at the tip of the knotless suture anchor. A short loop of green No. 1 Ethibond suture (Ethicon, Somerville, NJ), called the anchor loop, is attached to the tail end of the anchor instead of the long strands used in the GII anchor. A second longer loop of white 2-0 Ethibond suture, called the utility loop, is linked to the anchor loop and serves as a passing suture.

The BioKnotless suture anchor (Fig. 4-2), which is an absorbable version of the knotless suture anchor, is also available. The BioKnotless suture anchor looks similar to the Mitek Panalok anchor. The BioKnotless suture anchor has a wedge-shaped, poly-ʟ-lactic acid anchor body with a slot located at the tip. The anchor loop is white No. 1 Panacryl, and the utility loop is green 2-0 Ethibond.

The sides of both anchor designs are flat to create space for the captured suture loop to pass without suture abrasion.

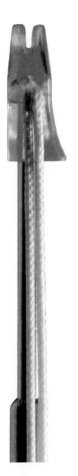

Figure 4-2 BioKnotless suture anchor design. (From Thal R. Knotless suture anchor fixation for shoulder instability. In Miller MD, Cole BJ, eds. Textbook of Arthroscopy. Philadelphia, Elsevier, 2004.)

Surgical Technique

Anesthesia and Positioning

This procedure can be performed under general anesthesia, interscalene block, or a combination of both. The patient can be positioned in either the lateral decubitus position with a 30-degree posterior tilt or the beach chair position. We prefer the lateral decubitus position. The arm is placed in traction in the lateral position and left free in the beach chair position. Additional distraction of the glenohumeral joint can be achieved by manually lifting the proximal humerus laterally. This increases the space between the humeral head and the glenoid, which greatly improves visualization of the anterior glenoid rim, labrum, and anterior inferior glenohumeral ligament (AIGHL).

Surgical Landmarks, Incisions, and Portals

Landmarks

- Acromion
- Posterior soft spot
- Humeral head
- Coracoid

Portals (Fig. 4-3)

- Posterior portal: 3 cm inferior to the posterolateral corner of the acromion at the posterior soft spot. The arthroscope enters the joint in the interval between the infraspinatus and the teres minor muscles.
- Anterior inferior portal: performed under direct visualization with a spinal needle. A cannula should be placed as close as possible to the superior edge of the subscapularis tendon to allow access to the anterior and inferior aspect of the glenoid rim.
- Anterior superior portal: a cannula is placed under direct visualization in the rotator cuff interval, just superior and anterior to the biceps tendon.

Structures at Risk

- Axillary nerve: during mobilization of the anterior inferior labrum
- Musculocutaneous nerve: must stay lateral to coracoid with anterior portal placement

Examination Under Anesthesia and Diagnostic Arthroscopy

Examination under anesthesia should demonstrate instability consistent with physical examination findings and the history. Testing for instability in 90 degrees of abduction with the application of anterior pressure is adequate. Diagnostic arthroscopy should be thorough. Evaluation of the articular surfaces, labrum, biceps tendon, rotator cuff, and glenohumeral ligaments should be completed through both the posterior and anterior portals. Particular attention should be specifically directed toward the anterior labrum and AIGHL.

Specific Steps (Box 4-1)

1. Ligament Preparation and Mobilization

Preparation of the AIGHL is determined by the pathologic findings of the ligament at diagnostic arthroscopy. Visualization is through the posterior portal and instrumentation is through the anterior portals. If visualization

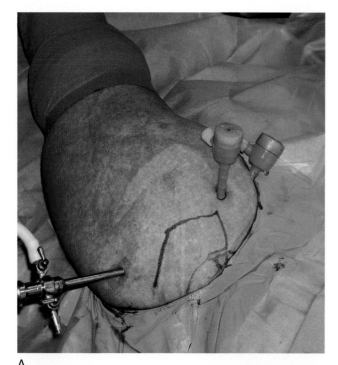

A

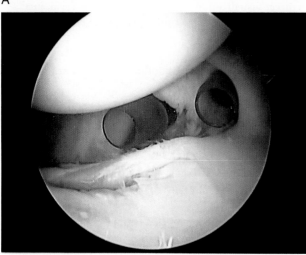

B

Figure 4-3 Arthroscopic portals for knotless fixation. Outside **(A)** and arthroscopic **(B)** views.

Box 4-1 Surgical Steps

1. Ligament preparation and mobilization
2. Glenoid preparation
3. Drill hole placement
4. Suture passage
5. Loop capture and anchor insertion
6. Loop-anchor repair tensioning and completion
7. Closure

is inadequate from the posterior portal, then visualization can be achieved from the anterior superior portal with instrumentation through the anterior inferior portal. The exposed labral edge of the Bankart lesion is débrided with a motorized shaver or bur to promote healing of the ligament to bone after repair.

Commonly, the AIGHL is released and mobilized with care from both the glenoid and the underlying subscapularis with the use of an electrocautery device. If an anterior labroligamentous periosteal sleeve avulsion (ALPSA) lesion is encountered (Fig. 4-4), the periosteum should be incised to release the AIGHL from the anterior glenoid (Fig. 4-5), essentially converting the ALPSA lesion into a Bankart lesion. Once the ligament is mobilized, a grasper is used to pull the ligament superiorly and to the articular margin while capsular tension and mobility are

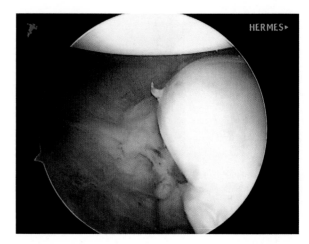

Figure 4-4 ALPSA lesion (anterior view). (From Thal R. Knotless suture anchor fixation for shoulder instability. In Miller MD, Cole BJ, eds. Textbook of Arthroscopy. Philadelphia, Elsevier, 2004.)

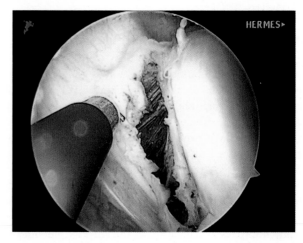

Figure 4-5 ALPSA lesion during mobilization (anterior view). (From Thal R. Knotless suture anchor fixation for shoulder instability. In Miller MD, Cole BJ, eds. Textbook of Arthroscopy. Philadelphia, Elsevier, 2004.)

evaluated. Capsular laxity is also assessed at this time (Fig. 4-6). Complete capsular mobilization allows superior capsular shift that often corrects capsular laxity and stretch. Capsular plication is rarely needed when the capsule is mobilized and adequately shifted superiorly. If concerns about the redundancy of the tissue remain, a small section of the edge of the detached AIGHL can be resected by use of a suction punch to shorten the ligament. The proper amount of ligament to resect is determined by approximating the ligament to the glenoid. Determination of capsular laxity and appropriate tensioning is a critical step and greatly affects the final outcome of the repair.

2. Glenoid Preparation

A motorized bur is used to decorticate the anterior glenoid neck medially 1 to 2 cm through the anterior portals. Abrasion of the articular surface of the anterior glenoid 2 to 4 mm from the edge is also performed to promote appropriate healing of ligament to bone.

3. Drill Hole Placement

The anterior inferior cannula is then replaced by a larger 8-mm cannula to accommodate the drill guide, suture passer, and knotless or BioKnotless suture anchors. Three drill holes are made in the anterior glenoid rim with use of the Mitek drill guide and the Mitek 2.9-mm arthroscopic superdrill (Fig. 4-7). The drilling of the holes is completed in one step because drilling after each anchor is placed is difficult secondary to poor visualization once the shift has been performed. These drill holes are spaced as far apart as possible (1-, 3-, and 5-o'clock positions in the right shoulder) and at the edge of the articular cartilage. It is important to avoid damage to the articular cartilage; as such, the drill bit must be directed medially away from the

articular surface of the glenoid by at least a 15-degree angle. Furthermore, it is critical not to torque the drill in determining hole placement, as this can cause difficulty in placing the anchor; undue tissue tension could distort the inserter rod and lead to an inability to line up the anchor with the drilled hole. The drill holes are marked with a basket forceps, suction punch, or electrocautery to ease hole identification during anchor insertion.

4. Suture Passage

Before implant placement, the utility loop of the knotless suture anchor assembly is passed through the AIGHL at a selected site through the anterior inferior portal (Fig. 4-8). This can be achieved by use of various

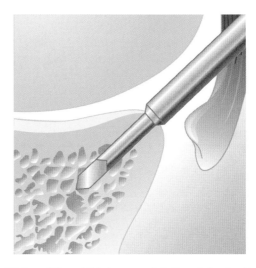

Figure 4-7 Three 2.9-mm drill holes are made in the anterior glenoid rim. (Redrawn from Thal R. Knotless suture anchor fixation for shoulder instability. In Miller MD, Cole BJ, eds. Textbook of Arthroscopy. Philadelphia, Elsevier, 2004.)

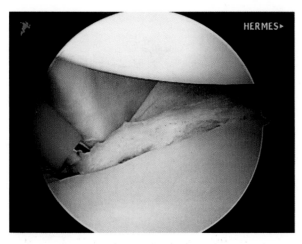

Figure 4-6 A grasper is used to pull the ligament superiorly to the articular margin while capsular tension and mobility are evaluated. The degree of capsular laxity can also be assessed at this time (posterior view). (From Thal R. Knotless suture anchor fixation for shoulder instability. In Miller MD, Cole BJ, eds. Textbook of Arthroscopy. Philadelphia, Elsevier, 2004.)

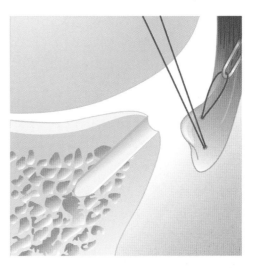

Figure 4-8 The utility loop of the knotless suture anchor assembly is passed through the AIGHL at a selected site. (Redrawn from Thal R. Knotless suture anchor fixation for shoulder instability. In Miller MD, Cole BJ, eds. Textbook of Arthroscopy. Philadelphia, Elsevier, 2004.)

arthroscopic suture-passing instruments and techniques. Our preferred technique for arthroscopic passage of the utility loop is a suture loop shuttle technique (Fig. 4-9). A Shutt suture punch (Linvatec, Largo, Fla) is used in grasping the ligament and pulling it superiorly to the drill hole site while ligament tension is assessed at the most inferior glenoid hole. This allows precision placement of the utility loop through the ligament and simultaneous assessment of proper capsular shift. A 2-0 polypropylene (Prolene) suture loop 48 inches long is then passed through the ligament, by use of the suture punch, and pulled out the

anterosuperior portal. The Prolene suture loop then serves as a suture shuttle and is used to pull the utility loop into the anteroinferior portal, through the AIGHL, and then out the anterosuperior portal. For the inferior two anchors, passing the Prolene suture loop from the intra-articular side of the ligament to the extra-articular side positions the utility loop similarly after shuttling. This helps orient the anchor loop at a better angle and facilitates easy anchor capturing of the anchor loop.

The utility loop is then used to pull the anchor loop through the AIGHL (Fig. 4-10). As the utility loop pulls

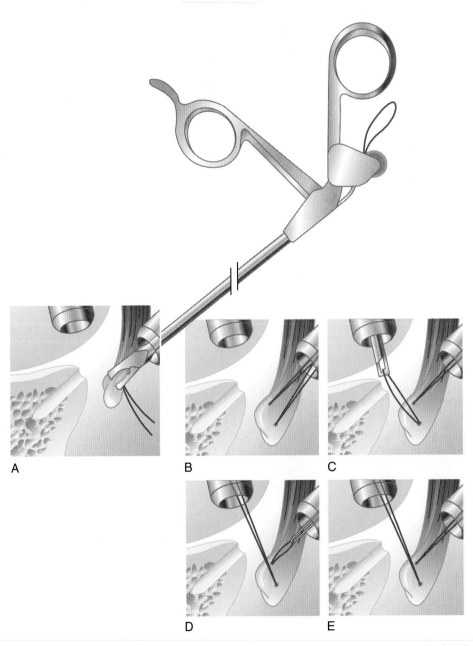

A

B

C

D

E

Figure 4-9 A and **B,** A 48-inch-long, 2-0 Prolene suture loop is passed through the ligament by a suture punch. **C,** The free ends of the Prolene suture loop are pulled out the anterosuperior portal while the loop remains out the anteroinferior portal. **D** and **E,** The Prolene suture loop is used as a suture shuttle to pull the utility loop through the ligament. (Redrawn from Thal R. Knotless suture anchor fixation for shoulder instability. In Miller MD, Cole BJ, eds. Textbook of Arthroscopy. Philadelphia, Elsevier, 2004.)

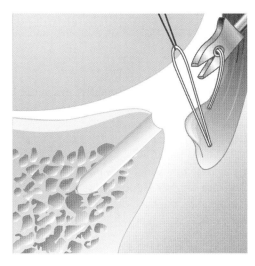

Figure 4-10 The utility loop is used to pull the anchor loop through the AIGHL. (Redrawn from Thal R. Knotless suture anchor fixation for shoulder instability. In Miller MD, Cole BJ, eds. Textbook of Arthroscopy. Philadelphia, Elsevier, 2004.)

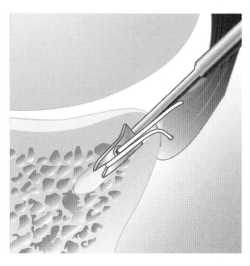

Figure 4-12 The anchor is inserted and tapped into the glenoid drill hole to the desired depth to achieve appropriate tissue tension. (Redrawn from Thal R. Knotless suture anchor fixation for shoulder instability. In Miller MD, Cole BJ, eds. Textbook of Arthroscopy. Philadelphia, Elsevier, 2004.)

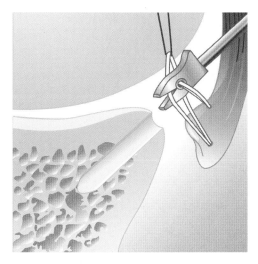

Figure 4-11 One suture strand of the anchor loop is captured or snagged in the channel at the tip of the anchor. (Redrawn from Thal R. Knotless suture anchor fixation for shoulder instability. In Miller MD, Cole BJ, eds. Textbook of Arthroscopy. Philadelphia, Elsevier, 2004.)

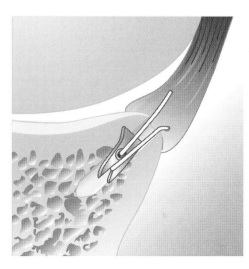

Figure 4-13 The utility loop and inserter rod are removed after a secure, low-profile repair is achieved. (Redrawn from Thal R. Knotless suture anchor fixation for shoulder instability. In Miller MD, Cole BJ, eds. Textbook of Arthroscopy. Philadelphia, Elsevier, 2004.)

the anchor loop through the AIGHL, the attached anchor is brought down the anterior inferior cannula while being controlled with the threaded inserter rod.

5. Loop Capture and Anchor Insertion

After the anchor loop has passed through the AIGHL, one strand of the anchor loop is captured or snagged in the channel at the tip of the anchor (Fig. 4-11). When the metallic knotless anchor is used, the anchor is rotated so the arc positioned inside the anchor loop is facing the utility loop. The anchor is then inserted and tapped into the glenoid drill hole to the desired depth to achieve appropriate tissue tension (Fig. 4-12).

6. Loop-Anchor Repair Tensioning and Completion

Depth of anchor insertion is determined by observing the ligament approximation to the glenoid and by intermittently pulling the utility loop to test the tension of the anchor loop during insertion. The anchor should not bottom out in the drill hole. Overtensioning can cause the anchor loop to tear through the ligament. Once this has been completed, the AIGHL is noted to shift superiorly and securely approximate to the glenoid rim in a low-profile manner (Fig. 4-13). The inserter rod is removed, and suture passage, anchor insertion, and tensioning are repeated for the remaining glenoid drill holes.

7. Closure

Standard closure of the portals is performed.

PEARLS AND PITFALLS

Several Techniques Can Facilitate Capture of the Anchor Loop

- For the inferior two anchors, pass the suture loop from the articular side of the ligament to the extra-articular side. For the superior anchor, pass the suture loop in the opposite direction.
- Use the utility loop through the anterior superior portal to guide and manipulate the anchor loop to the anchor notch and ease loop capture (Fig. 4-14).
- During insertion of the anchor, periodically pull the utility loop to test the tension of the anchor loop.
- Remember, it is critical not to torque the drill in determining hole placement. This can cause difficulty in placing the anchor; undue tissue tension that did not distort the drill could distort the inserter rod and lead to an inability to line up the anchor with the drilled hole.

Placement of the Utility Loop and Anchor Loop in the AIGHL is Critical

- Suture placement should be inferior to the glenoid drill hole so that a superior shift of the ligament is achieved as the anchor is inserted into the drill hole.
- The anchors are inserted in the most inferior hole first, progressing to the most superior hole.

Avoid Breakage of the Anchor Loop

- Several anchor loop configurations can lead to loop breakage with the metallic anchor and should be avoided.
- One arc must be passed through the anchor loop before anchor insertion; otherwise, the anchor loop will be cut on insertion into the bone (Fig. 4-15).
- The anchor loop must pass directly from the base of the anchor into the ligament. If the loop is wrapped around the body of the anchor, the anchor loop will be at risk of being cut by the closing anchor arc as the anchor is inserted into bone (Figs. 4-16 and 4-17).
- The utility loop can be pulled on to hold the anchor loop safely away from the arc during primary anchor insertion. Tension is relaxed once the arcs have entered the bone.

Postoperative Considerations

Follow-up

- 7 to 10 days for initial postoperative evaluation

Rehabilitation

- 0-4 weeks: Use of a sling, with pendulum exercises, range-of-motion exercises of the shoulder and elbow, and isometric exercises of the forearm. External rotation is limited to neutral.

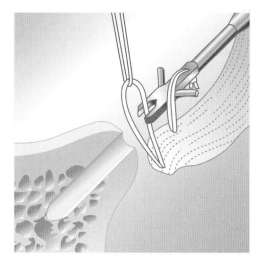

Figure 4-15 One anchor arc has not been passed through the anchor loop and will cut the anchor loop when the anchor is inserted into bone. (Redrawn from Thal R. Knotless suture anchor: arthroscopic Bankart repair without tying knots. Clin Orthop 2001;390:46-47.)

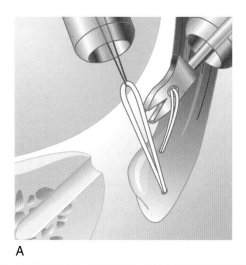
A

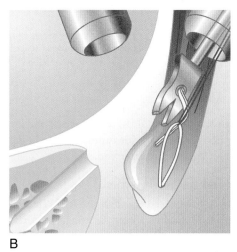
B

Figure 4-14 A, The utility loop is pulled out the anterosuperior portal to orient the anchor loop at a better angle with respect to the anchor and thus facilitate loop capture. **B,** Loop capture is more difficult when the loop is pulled toward the same portal as the anchor. (Redrawn from Thal R. Knotless suture anchor fixation for shoulder instability. In Miller MD, Cole BJ, eds. Textbook of Arthroscopy. Philadelphia, Elsevier, 2004.)

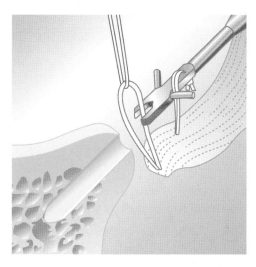

Figure 4-16 The anchor loop is incorrectly wrapped around the anchor. (Redrawn from Thal R. Knotless suture anchor: arthroscopic Bankart repair without tying knots. Clin Orthop 2001;390:46-47.)

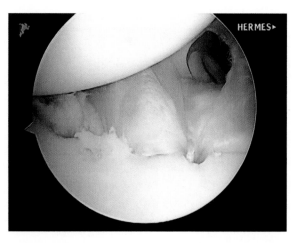

Figure 4-18 Bankart repair with knotless suture anchors. (From Thal R. Knotless suture anchor fixation for shoulder instability. In Miller MD, Cole BJ, eds. Textbook of Arthroscopy. Philadelphia, Elsevier, 2004.)

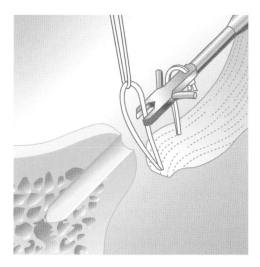

Figure 4-17 The anchor loop is incorrectly wrapped around the anchor. (Redrawn from Thal R. Knotless suture anchor: arthroscopic Bankart repair without tying knots. Clin Orthop 2001;390:46-47.)

- 4 weeks: Progressive active and passive range-of-motion exercises are begun; external rotation is limited to 45 degrees; isometric deltoid and periscapular exercises are begun.
- 6 weeks: Progression to full, active range of motion is allowed.
- 8 weeks: Resistive training with the use of isotonic and isokinetic modalities is performed in a progressive manner with no limitation on the patient.

- Return to contact and overhead sports is not allowed until 5 months postoperatively.

Complications

- Traumatic redislocation
- Incomplete healing of labral repair
- Infection
- Arthrofibrosis
- Anchor loop breakage secondary to improper anchor loop positioning

Results

After arthroscopic Bankart repair with the knotless suture anchor, increased superior capsular shift is attained compared with a standard suture anchor, as the knotless anchor pulls the ligament into the drill hole (Fig. 4-18). The problems associated with tying knots, knot loosening, and complex suture management are eliminated. Suture strength is improved compared with standard suture anchors. Furthermore, satisfactory results are attained with a low recurrence rate, minimal loss of motion, and reliable functional return, even in contact and collision athletes (Table 4-1). The recurrence rate was higher in patients 22 years old or younger.

Table 4-1 Clinical and Biomechanical Results of Knotless Suture Anchor Fixation in Shoulder Instability

Clinical Results		
Author	**Follow-up**	**Outcome**
Thal[2] (2001)	29-month average	21 of 22 (96%) successful
Thal et al[3] (2004)	2-year minimum (range: 2-7 years)	67 of 72 (93%) successful
Garafalo et al[1] (2005)	43 months (range: 36-48 months)	18 of 20 (90%) successful
Biomechanical Results		
Author	**Parameters Tested**	**Results**
Thal[2] (2001)	Suture breakage	Knotless anchor with statistically higher failure load ($P < .0001$)
	Bone pullout of anchor	Increased anchor pullout force in knotless anchor not significant ($P = .195$)
	Average capsular shift	Bankart repair: 4.33 mm Barrel stitch repair: 6.04 mm Plication repair: 6.50 mm* Knotless repair: 6.79 mm*

*Statistically significant.

References

1. Garafalo R, Mocci A, Biagio M, et al. Arthroscopic treatment of anterior shoulder instability using knotless suture anchors. Arthroscopy 2005;21:1283-1289.
2. Thal R. Knotless suture anchor: arthroscopic Bankart repair without tying knots. Clin Orthop 2001;390:42-51.
3. Thal R, Nofzinger M, Bridges M, Kim JJ. Arthroscopic Bankart repair using knotless or BioKnotless suture anchors: 2- to 7-year results. Arthroscopy 2007;23:367-375.

Suggested Readings

Bacilla P, Field LD, Savoie FH. Arthroscopic Bankart repair in a high demand patient population. Arthroscopy 1997;13:51-60.

Bendetto KP, Glotzer W. Arthroscopic Bankart procedure by suture technique: indications, technique, and results. Arthroscopy 1992;8:111-115.

Caspari RB. Arthroscopic reconstruction for anterior shoulder instability. Tech Orthop 1988;3:59-66.

Coughlin L, Rubinovich M, Johansson J, et al. Arthroscopic staple capsulorrhaphy for anterior shoulder instability. Am J Sports Med 1992;20:253-256.

Grana WA, Buckley PD, Yates CK. Arthroscopic Bankart suture repair. Am J Sports Med 1993;21:348-353.

Green MR, Christensen KP. Arthroscopic versus open Bankart procedures: a comparison of early morbidity and complications. Arthroplasty 1993;9:371-374.

Lane JG, Sachs RA, Riehl B. Arthroscopic staple capsulorrhaphy: a long-term follow-up. Arthroscopy 1993;9:190-194.

Loutenheiser TD, Harryman DT II, Yung SW, et al. Optimizing arthroscopic knots. Arthroscopy 1995;11:199-206.

Neviaser TJ. The anterior labroligamentous periosteal sleeve avulsion lesion: a cause of anterior instability of the shoulder. Arthroscopy 1993;9:17-21.

Thal R. A knotless suture anchor: design, function, and biomechanical testing. Am J Sports Med 2001;29:646-649.

Thal R. A knotless suture anchor: technique for use in arthroscopic Bankart repair. Arthroscopy 2001;17:213-218.

Warner JJ, Miller MD, Marks P, Fu FH. Arthroscopic Bankart repair with the Suretac device. Part I: Experimental observations. Arthroscopy 1995;11:2-13.

Warner JJ, Miller MD, Marks P, Fu FH. Arthroscopic Bankart repair with the Suretac device. Part II: Experimental observations. Arthroscopy 1995;11:14-20.

Wolf EM, Wilk RM, Richmond JC. Arthroscopic Bankart repair using suture anchors. Oper Tech Orthop 1991;1:184-191.

CHAPTER 5

Arthroscopic Rotator Interval Capsule Closure

Bradley J. Nelson, MD

Robert A. Arciero, MD

There is growing interest in the role of the rotator interval capsule in shoulder instability. The rotator interval capsule is a triangular area of anterior capsule between the superior border of the subscapularis inferiorly, the anterior margin of the supraspinatus superiorly, the coracoid process medially, and the intertubercular groove laterally (Fig. 5-1). The superior glenohumeral ligament and coracohumeral ligament are structural components of this capsule. Cole et al[6] demonstrated that most of the remaining interval capsule is thin and poorly organized tissue.

Harryman et al[9] demonstrated the importance of the rotator interval capsule in glenohumeral motion and stability. Their study concluded that the role of the interval capsule is to decrease inferior translation in the adducted shoulder and to limit posterior translation in the flexed shoulder. Van der Reis and Wolf[18] demonstrated in a cadaver model that glenohumeral translation and motion could be decreased with arthroscopic rotator interval imbrication.

Imbrication of the rotator interval capsule has become a standard part of open instability procedures since it was first advocated by Neer in 1980.[15] Recent advances in arthroscopic surgery have allowed surgeons to duplicate the open techniques with respect to labral repair and capsular shift. Numerous authors have also described arthroscopic techniques of rotator interval capsular imbrication that are used as part of anterior, posterior, or multidirectional instability procedures.[2,4,5,8,12,14,17] We describe a simple technique of rotator interval capsular imbrication with use of nonabsorbable suture.

Preoperative Considerations

History

A focused history is essential in the diagnosis and management of shoulder instability.

The presence or absence of trauma, the mechanism of injury, and the position of the arm when symptoms occur offer important clues to the direction and extent of the shoulder instability. A history of the arm "dropping out the bottom" is particularly concerning for a lax interval capsule.

Physical Examination

Examination of the cervical spine, areas of tenderness, and range-of-motion and motor strength testing are performed to rule out other sources of shoulder disease. The anterior and posterior apprehension-relocation tests as well as the load and shift test are important in determining the presence and direction of glenohumeral instability. A sulcus sign greater than 2 cm that persists with external rotation of the adducted arm is a crucial indicator of an incompetent rotator interval capsule (Fig. 5-2). The presence of ligamentous laxity may influence the decision to imbricate the rotator interval capsule.

Imaging

Plain radiographs including a true anteroposterior view of the glenohumeral joint and a West Point axillary view are

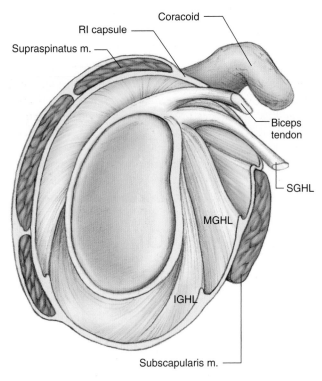

Figure 5-1 Diagram of rotator interval (RI) capsule. IGHL, inferior glenohumeral ligament; MGHL, middle glenohumeral ligament; SGHL, superior glenohumeral ligament.

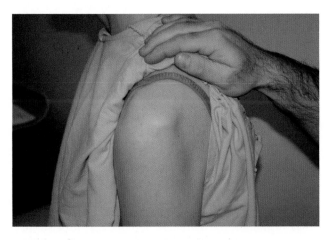

Figure 5-2 Clinical examination demonstrating significant sulcus sign.

obtained for all patients to assess glenoid and humeral head bone loss. Magnetic resonance imaging, with or without the intra-articular administration of gadolinium, is performed to assess for labral disease.

Indications and Contraindications

Rotator interval capsule closure is indicated in conjunction with an arthroscopic stabilization procedure such as a labral repair (anterior, posterior, or superior) or as part of an arthroscopic capsular plication. Patients with a component of inferior instability demonstrated by a significant sulcus sign are proper candidates for an interval capsule imbrication. In addition, most patients with posterior shoulder instability require an interval capsule imbrication as basic science research demonstrates the importance of the interval capsule in resisting posterior translation.

Contraindications include patients who are not candidates for an arthroscopic stabilization. Patients with significant bone loss or true voluntary instability secondary to a psychological disorder are not candidates for rotator interval imbrication. We do not routinely close the rotator interval capsule in patients undergoing stabilization for primary, unidirectional, traumatic instability.

Surgical Planning

Arthroscopic shoulder stabilization and rotator interval capsule closure require a significant amount of specialized equipment. Large disposable cannulas, devices to shuttle suture, suture anchors, and specialized hand-held instruments are required to perform the procedure.

Surgical Technique

Anesthesia and Positioning

Arthroscopic rotator interval capsule closure can be safely performed under general or interscalene regional anesthesia. The patient is positioned in either the lateral decubitus or beach chair position on the basis of the surgeon's preference. A shoulder-specific positioner and arm holder is helpful (Fig. 5-3).

Surgical Landmarks, Incisions, and Portals

Portal location is usually determined by the concomitant procedures performed before the rotator interval capsule closure. Most frequently, a 30-degree arthroscope is used through a standard posterior portal, and dual cannulas are placed anteriorly (Fig. 5-4). One cannula is placed through an anterior superior portal entering the joint just below the biceps tendon. A second cannula is placed through the anterior inferior portal entering the joint just above the subscapularis tendon (Fig. 5-5). These portals allow repair of most anterior labral lesions and anterior capsular plication. Additional accessory portals are often required for superior or posterior labral repairs.

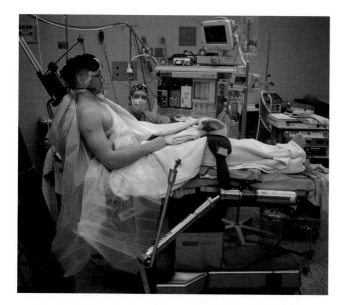

Figure 5-3 The patient in beach chair position with specialized table and arm holder.

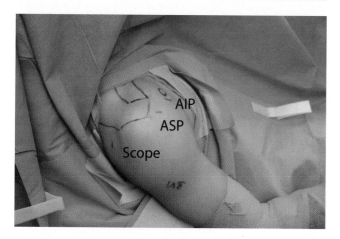

Figure 5-4 Portal sites marked with the patient in the sitting position. AIP, anterior inferior portal; ASP, anterior superior portal.

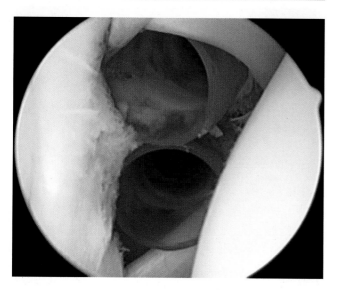

Figure 5-5 Dual anterior cannulas in the right shoulder.

Examination Under Anesthesia and Diagnostic Arthroscopy

An examination under anesthesia is performed to assess range of motion and shoulder stability. The load and shift test is performed to determine anterior and posterior instability. The sulcus test is performed with the arm at neutral rotation and in external rotation to assess inferior instability.

A careful diagnostic arthroscopy is performed to evaluate for evidence of instability, including labral tears, biceps fraying, superior subscapularis fraying, and chondral scuffing. The rotator interval capsule is evaluated arthroscopically, although there is no consensus on what constitutes a lax interval capsule. Fitzpatrick et al[7] suggest that the interval is widened if it is seen extending superior to the biceps tendon.

Specific Steps (Box 5-1)

1. Concomitant Stabilization Procedures

The initial step in arthroscopic stabilization after cannula placement is repair of any associated labral disease. The anterior or posterior capsule is then plicated as indicated. The details of these procedures are discussed elsewhere in this text.

2. Piercing the Middle Glenohumeral Ligament

A No. 2 nonabsorbable suture is loaded into a straight tissue penetrator (Fig. 5-6). The penetrator is placed through the anterior inferior portal cannula (Fig. 5-7) and pierces the middle glenohumeral ligament just above the subscapularis (Fig. 5-8). A suture grasper is placed in the anterior superior portal cannula, and the end of the nonabsorbable suture is transported out the cannula (Fig. 5-9).

3. Piercing the Superior Glenohumeral Ligament

The anterior superior portal cannula is carefully backed out of the glenohumeral joint so it is positioned just outside the capsule. An angled tissue penetrator is placed through this cannula (Fig. 5-10), and the superior glenohumeral ligament is pierced (Fig. 5-11). The limb of the

Box 5-1 Surgical Steps

1. Concomitant stabilization procedures
2. Piercing the middle glenohumeral ligament
3. Piercing the superior glenohumeral ligament
4. Knot tying
5. Closure

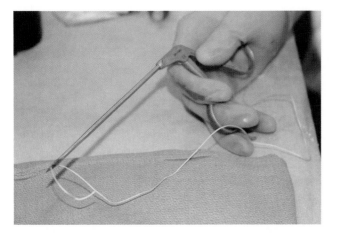

Figure 5-6 No. 2 nonabsorbable suture placed in a tissue penetrator.

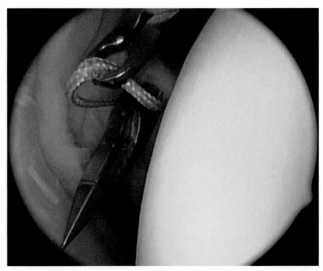

Figure 5-9 Suture grasped from the anterior superior cannula.

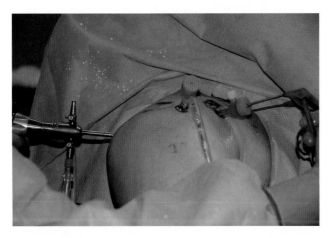

Figure 5-7 Tissue penetrator in the anterior inferior cannula.

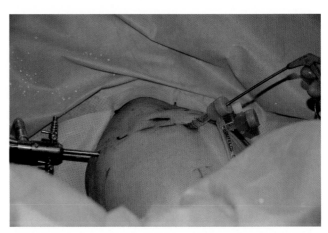

Figure 5-10 Tissue penetrator in the anterior superior cannula.

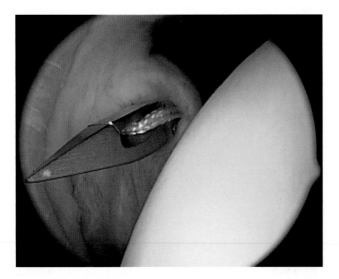

Figure 5-8 Tissue penetrator piercing the middle glenohumeral ligament.

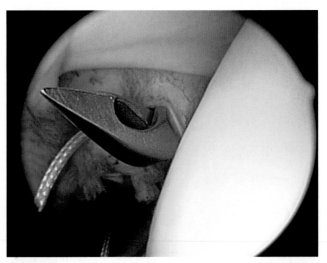

Figure 5-11 Tissue penetrator piercing the superior glenohumeral ligament.

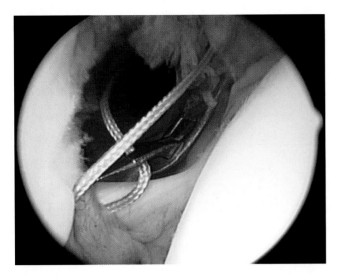

Figure 5-12 Grasping of the suture limb anterior to the middle glenohumeral ligament.

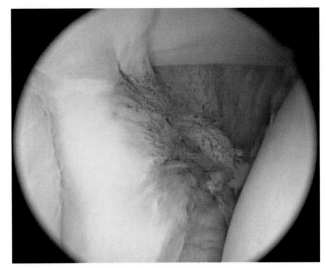

Figure 5-14 Suture tied outside of capsule.

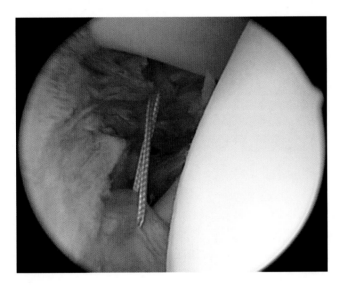

Figure 5-13 Both cannulas repositioned outside of the glenohumeral joint capsule.

suture that is still within the anterior inferior portal cannula is grasped anterior to the middle glenohumeral ligament (Fig. 5-12). This limb of suture is transported out the anterior superior portal.

4. Knot Tying

The anterior inferior portal cannula is removed. Both limbs of the suture are exiting the anterior superior portal cannula, which still traverses the subcutaneous tissue and deltoid muscle but sits just outside the capsule (Fig. 5-13). The shoulder is positioned in 45 degrees of abduction and 45 degrees of external rotation to prevent loss of external rotation, and tension is applied to the sutures (Fig. 5-14). The middle and superior glenohumeral ligaments will be brought together as the rotator interval capsule is imbri-

cated. A sliding-locking arthroscopic knot is tied and advanced until the knot can be felt contacting the capsule. This knot is not visible from within the joint. Two or three half-hitch throws can be placed. An end-cutting suture cutter is slid down the suture and the knot is cut. This is performed with tactile feedback as the knot is extracapsular and not visible. Shoulder range of motion is checked to ensure that there has not been an excessive loss of external rotation.

5. Closure

The portals are closed in a standard fashion. Local anesthetic can be instilled into the joint or a pain pump can be placed, depending on the surgeon's preference. The patient is placed into a shoulder immobilizer in internal rotation and slight abduction if an anterior stabilization procedure was performed. An external rotation sling is used if the posterior labrum was repaired.

Postoperative Considerations

Follow-up

Most patients are sent home the day of surgery. Sutures are removed at 7 to 10 days.

Rehabilitation

The postoperative rehabilitation is determined by the primary stabilization procedure performed. In general, a sling is worn for 4 weeks with the arm in internal rotation after an anterior stabilization or in neutral rotation after a

Table 5-1 Results of Rotator Interval Capsule Closure

Author	Type of Instability	Outcome
Ide et al[11] (2004)	Anterior	50 of 55 (91%) good–excellent
Gartsman et al[8] (1999)	Anterior	49 of 53 (92%) good–excellent
Noojin et al[16] (2000)	Anterior	642 of 662 (97%) good–excellent
Kim et al[13] (2002)	Anterior (revisions)	19 of 23 (83%) good–excellent
Bottoni et al[3] (2005)	Posterior	29 of 31 (94%) good–excellent
Abrams[1] (2003)	Posterior	42 of 49 (88%) good–excellent
Hewitt et al[10] (2003)	Multidirectional	29 of 30 (90%) good–excellent

posterior stabilization procedure. Gentle passive range-of-motion exercises are started on the first day after surgery. Progressive rotator cuff and periscapular muscle strengthening exercises are started at 4 weeks. Full return to sports is allowed at 4 to 6 months, depending on the patient's progress.

Complications

Infection, neurovascular injury, and anesthetic complications are rare serious complications of arthroscopic shoulder stabilization. Recurrent instability and loss of motion are more common complications.

PEARLS AND PITFALLS

- Loss of motion can occur if the interval capsule is closed indiscriminately. Patients should demonstrate a sulcus sign with the arm in external rotation.

- The arm should be positioned in at least 45 degrees of external rotation and 45 degrees of abduction to prevent excessive tightening.

- A sliding knot must be used as the knot is tied on the outside of the capsule.

- An end-cutting suture cutter is required because the suture is cut blindly.

- The superior glenohumeral ligament must be pierced anterior to the biceps tendon or the biceps tendon will be entrapped within the capsular closure.

Results

It is difficult to determine the results of rotator interval capsule closure presented in the literature as the procedure is usually performed secondary to an anterior or posterior labral repair. Results of studies in which rotator interval closure was specifically described are presented in Table 5-1.

References

1. Abrams JS. Arthroscopic repair of posterior instability and reverse humeral glenohumeral ligament avulsion lesions. Orthop Clin North Am 2003;34:475-483.
2. Almazan A, Ruiz M, Cruz F, et al. Simple arthroscopic technique for rotator interval closure. Arthroscopy 2006;22:230.
3. Bottoni CR, Franks BR, Moore JH, et al. Operative stabilization of posterior shoulder instability. Am J Sports Med 2005;33:996-1002.
4. Calvo A, Martinez AA, Domingo J, et al. Rotator interval closure after arthroscopic capsulolabral repair: a technical variation. Arthroscopy 2005;21:765.
5. Cole BJ, Mazzocca AD, Meneghini RM. Indirect arthroscopic rotator interval repair. Arthroscopy 2003;19:E28-31.
6. Cole BJ, Rodeo SA, O'Brien SJ, et al. The anatomy and histology of the rotator interval capsule of the shoulder. Clin Orthop 2001;390:129-137.
7. Fitzpatrick MJ, Powell SE, Tibone JE, et al. The anatomy, pathology, and definitive treatment of rotator interval lesions: current concepts. Arthroscopy 2003;19:70-79.
8. Gartsman GM, Taverna E, Hammerman SM. Arthroscopic rotator interval repair in glenohumeral instability: description of an operative technique. Arthroscopy 1999;15:330-332.
9. Harryman DT, Sidles JA, Harris SL. et al. The role of the rotator interval capsule in passive motion and stability of the shoulder. J Bone Joint Surg Am 1992;74:53-66.
10. Hewitt M, Getelman MH, Snyder SJ. Arthroscopic management of multidirectional instability: pancapsular plication. Orthop Clin North Am 2003;34:549-557.
11. Ide J, Maeda S, Takagi K. Arthroscopic Bankart repair using suture anchors in athletes: patient selection and postoperative sports activity. Am J Sports Med 2004;32:1899-1905.
12. Karas SG. Arthroscopic rotator interval repair and anterior portal closure: an alternative technique. Arthroscopy 2002;18:436-439.
13. Kim SH, Ha KI, Kim YA. Arthroscopic revision Bankart repair: a prospective outcome study. Arthroscopy 2002;18:469-482.
14. Lewicky YM, Lewicky RT. Simplified arthroscopic rotator interval capsule closure: an alternative technique. Arthroscopy 2005;21:1276.

15. Neer CS, Foster CR. Inferior capsular shift for involuntary inferior and multidirectional instability of the shoulder. A preliminary report. J Bone Joint Surg Am 1980;62:897-908.

16. Noojin FK, Savoie FH, Field LD. Arthroscopic Bankart repair using long-term absorbable anchors and sutures. Orthop Today 2000; 4:18-19.

17. Treacy SH, Field LD, Savoie FH. Rotator interval capsule closure: an arthroscopic technique. Arthroscopy 1997;13:103-106.

18. Van der Reis W, Wolf EM. Arthroscopic rotator cuff interval capsular closure. Orthopedics 2001;24:657-661.

CHAPTER 6

Thermal Capsulorrhaphy

Jeffrey R. Dugas, MD
James R. Andrews, MD

Basic Science

With the advent of shoulder arthroscopy in the 1980s came the ability for surgeons to more closely examine the pathologic processes within the shoulder without significantly altering the status of the joint itself. Among the shoulder pathologic processes that became more appreciated with arthroscopy were superior labral tears, posterior capsulolabral injuries, intra-articular biceps disease, and partial rotator cuff tears. In throwing athletes, however, shoulder surgery had yielded only limited success with regard to return to play. Payne et al[13] demonstrated only a 40% return to play in patients treated with rotator cuff débridement who also had increased glenohumeral translation. Similarly, Speer et al[14] demonstrated that return to play was limited in throwers who underwent arthroscopic fixation of anterior labral tears for treatment of anterior instability. It was thought that the inability to control rotational laxity led to the lower rate of return to play.

Capsular and ligamentous tissues are composed predominantly of type I collagen. The application of heat to collagen causes a destruction of the heat-sensitive crosslinks between fibrils, leading the collagen tissue to take on a more gel-like character rather than its normal crystalline-like state. This process, termed denaturation, has been shown to reproducibly occur at approximately 65°C, but the exact effect of heat application depends on exposure time, mechanical stress applied to the tissue during heat application, and method of application.[3] Thermal properties are not uniform in all connective tissues. The response to thermal energy depends on many factors, including species, age, hydration level, fibril orientation, and electrolyte concentration of the surrounding tissues.[4,8] Increased temperatures have been shown to be required to produce denaturation in tissues with increased collagen content and in those under increased tensile loads.[4] The end result of heat application to collagenous tissues is visible shrinkage along the axis of the collagen fibril orientation.[2]

Thermal energy has been used to treat capsular disease of various degrees and causes in the shoulder. As mentioned earlier, thermal energy has been used to decrease rotational laxity in the thrower's shoulder. It has also been used to address shoulder instability and multidirectional instability. Tibone et al[15] demonstrated that both anterior translation and posterior translation were decreased in human cadaveric shoulder specimens after thermal shrinkage of the anterior inferior capsule. In their study, anterior translation decreased more than 40% and posterior translation decreased 35% after application of thermal energy.

Fanton and Khan[6] began using radiofrequency as a modality to decrease capsular volume and capsular laxity in 1996. It was the work of these and other subsequent investigators that led to the increase in popularity of this modality as a means of improving the results of shoulder surgery in the overhead athlete by addressing the rotational laxity. The results of these works are discussed later.

Preoperative Considerations

History

Patients report a history of frank dislocation or, more commonly for this application, experience recurrent subluxation events. Overhead athletes, especially baseball pitchers, often describe a "dead arm" syndrome, with pain and subjective weakness occurring late in the throw.

Physical Examination

A standard shoulder examination is performed, with special focus on assessing stability. Common tests include the apprehension sign, relocation test, sulcus sign, and load and shift test.

Imaging

The diagnostic and imaging work-up includes conventional radiography and cross-sectional imaging modalities such as magnetic resonance imaging and computed tomography. Radiographic studies include standard anteroposterior and axillary lateral views as well as specialized views, such as the Stryker notch view, to rule out bone defects. Magnetic resonance imaging provides visualization of ligamentous and other soft tissue structures, such as the capsulolabral complex and rotator cuff. Computed tomography, especially when it is obtained in conjunction with arthrography, allows assessment of the bony structures to quantify or to rule out a Hill-Sachs defect or bony Bankart lesion.

Indications and Contraindications

Thermal capsulorrhaphy is indicated in mild to moderate cases of instability, especially when patients describe subluxation rather than dislocation events. It can be used as an adjunct to labral repair in patients with a capacious capsule.

Contraindications include bone defects of the glenoid and a compromised capsule.

Technique of Application

Anesthesia and Positioning

This procedure can be performed under general anesthesia, interscalene block, or a combination of both. At our institution, we prefer to perform shoulder arthroscopy in the lateral decubitus position, although thermal capsulorrhaphy can be carried out in the beach chair position as well.

Surgical Landmarks, Incisions, and Portals

Landmarks
- Acromion
- Clavicle
- Coracoid
- Posterior soft spot

Portals
- Posterior portal
- Anterior portal

Structures at Risk
- Axillary nerve during application in the inferior pouch
- Musculocutaneous nerve during placement of the anterior portal

Examination Under Anesthesia and Diagnostic Arthroscopy

After the induction of adequate general or regional anesthesia, examination under anesthesia is carried out on both shoulders to document and to confirm the amount of translation in each direction as well as the end feel of the translation. In addition, with the scapula braced, external rotation and internal rotation are measured with the arm abducted 90 degrees in the plane of the scapula. The patient is then positioned and prepared and draped with the shoulder exposed.

After insufflation of the glenohumeral joint with saline, a standard posterior arthroscopic portal is established and diagnostic arthroscopy is performed. Visualization of the glenoid and humeral articular surfaces is obtained, and the cartilage integrity is noted. Next, the biceps tendon is identified and viewed throughout its entire intra-articular course, including the anchor origin on the visible portion of the labrum. The anterior, posterior, and inferior recesses are viewed from the posterior portal. The undersurface of the rotator cuff is assessed for integrity. Next, a standard anterior portal is established under direct visualization. A blunt trocar is inserted through the cannula, and the rotator cuff, labrum, biceps tendon, and subscapularis tendon are probed to ensure integrity. Specific attention is placed on viewing and assessing the biceps anchor at the superior glenoid rim. In throwing athletes, this area is the most commonly affected as it pertains to the labrum. Careful attention is paid to retract the biceps tendon into the glenohumeral joint to view the most distal portion of the intra-articular tendon as it enters the bicipital groove. The arthroscope is then placed in the anterior portal to view the posterior capsule and posterior labrum and cuff. Any fraying of the articular surface, rotator cuff, or labrum is addressed at this time with use of a standard arthroscopic shaver, and portals are switched as needed to address the pathologic changes. If any labral or rotator cuff detachment is present, these pathologic processes are addressed appropriately before any capsular treatment.

Specific Steps (Box 6-1)

1. Posteroinferior Capsule

Once any other intra-articular pathologic process has been addressed, attention is turned to the joint capsule. If thermal capsulorrhaphy is to be carried out, the arthroscope is first placed in the anterior portal, and a plastic cannula with a flow diaphragm is placed in the posterior portal. The tip of the thermal probe is slightly bent (20 to 30 degrees) several centimeters from the tip to allow easier access to the capsule. The arthroscope is positioned anterior and inferior to the humeral head with the camera directed posteriorly to see the posterior inferior capsule in the region of the posterior band of the inferior glenohumeral ligament. The thermal probe is then directed to the area visualized through the scope, and the capsule is striped from the glenoid to the capsular insertion onto the humerus (Figs. 6-1 and 6-2), leaving intervening normal unshrunk tissue between each stripe. The probe begins at the most inferior position and gradually moves proximally to the posterior portal.

2. Anteroinferior Capsule

The arthroscope is then placed through the posterior portal and the plastic cannula is placed anteriorly. The arthroscope is directed posterior to the humeral head with the camera directed anteriorly to view the anterior band of the inferior glenohumeral ligament. The thermal probe is then inserted through the anterior portal and directed to the area of visualization. By the same technique, the anteroinferior capsule is striped with the probe, and gradual progression is made toward the anterior portal. In general, no thermal energy is used above the middle glenohumeral ligament.

3. Specific Applications

If specific directional laxity is to be addressed with thermal capsular shrinkage, the probe can be used in only the area

Box 6-1 Surgical Steps

1. Posteroinferior capsule
2. Anteroinferior capsule
3. Specific applications
4. Closure and immobilization

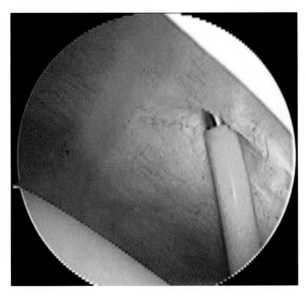

Figure 6-1 Thermal probe contacting the capsular tissue. To the right of the current probe position, a previous pass appears as a more yellow band of shrunken tissue. Untreated tissue should remain between areas of thermal application.

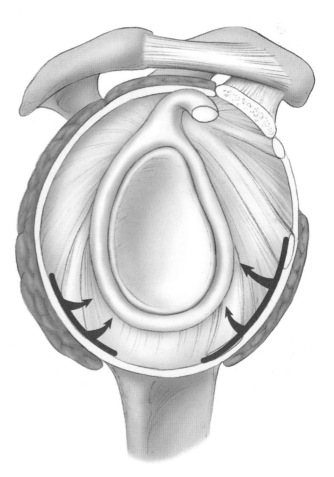

Figure 6-2 Application of thermal energy should focus on the area of the anterior and posterior bands of the inferior glenohumeral ligament as well as the middle glenohumeral ligament. (Redrawn from Fanton GS, Zwahlen BA, Savoie FH III. Radiofrequency technique for shoulder instability. In Miller MD, Cole BJ, eds. Textbook of Arthroscopy. Elsevier, Philadelphia, 2004.)

of interest. For example, in patients in whom anterior instability or anteroinferior capsular redundancy is the main pathologic process, thermal application to only the anterior or anterior inferior capsule may be chosen. Likewise, if the main direction of instability is posterior, thermal shrinkage of the posterior capsule with or without rotator interval closure or shrinkage may be sufficient.

4. Closure and Immobilization

The arthroscopy portals are closed with interrupted or subcuticular stitches. The arm is placed in a shoulder-immobilizing device before transport from the operating room.

Postoperative Considerations

Rehabilitation

Like many shoulder procedures, thermal capsulorrhaphy for the purpose of reducing rotational or directional laxity requires a closely supervised rehabilitation protocol for success to be achieved. Experience with this procedure has taught us that frequent hands-on treatment by a qualified physical therapist is vital to success. In each case, we seek to achieve external rotation in abduction to between 115 and 118 degrees by 12 weeks postoperatively. We do not allow any throwing until 16 weeks postoperatively, with the early rehabilitation focused on range of motion, followed by light strengthening and plyometric drills. By keeping in line with the therapy protocol, difficult situations like overtightening and premature stretching are avoided. Verbal communication of the goals and phases of

the rehabilitation and the obligation of the patient to abide by the therapy protocol is essential.

Complications

Despite the predominance of good results with use of this modality, failure and complications are not uncommon. In our practice, we have decreased the frequency with which we use thermal energy for the treatment of the throwing athlete as we have become more proficient and knowledgeable in capsular plication. Reports of "vanished capsule" or obliterated tissue, chondral damage, and comparatively high recurrence rate have decreased the enthusiasm for this technique.

PEARLS AND PITFALLS

- Slight bending of the probe tip allows easier maneuvering.
- Avoidance of excessive treatment in the axillary pouch will decrease the risk of axillary nerve injury.
- Alternate bands of treated and nontreated tissue optimize the healing response.

Results

Study results with use of thermal energy are summarized in Table 6-1.

Fanton et al[6,12] reported the 2-year results of 42 young, active patients who underwent shoulder arthros-

Table 6-1 Summary of Study Results with Thermal Energy

Author	No. of Subjects	Follow-up	Outcome
Fanton and Khan[6] (2001)	42	28 months	91% returned to preinjury level
Mishra and Fanton[12] (2001)			
Levitz et al[9] (2001)	31	30 months	Thermally treated group: 90% returned to play at same or higher level Traditionally treated group: 67% returned to play at same or higher level
Dugas and Andrews[5] (2002)	170	8.5 months	81% returned to competition
Lyons et al[11] (2001)		24 months	96%
Frostick et al[7] (2000)	28		83%
Levy et al[10] (2001)		40 months 23 months	Laser: 59% better Radiofrequency: 76% better
Anderson et al[1] (2002)	106	6.3 months	14% failure rate

copy with thermal capsulorrhaphy. These patients underwent capsulolabral fixation with tacks or anchors and thermal capsular shrinkage for treatment of recurrent shoulder instability. At an average of 28 months of follow-up, 91% had returned to their preinjury level of sports. These authors also noted similar rate of success with thermal treatment of mild subluxation without the addition of capsulolabral repair.

Levitz et al[9] in 2001 described 31 overhead baseball players who underwent shoulder arthroscopy with thermal capsular shrinkage and compared them with 51 overhead baseball players who underwent shoulder arthroscopy with traditional treatment only, without thermal capsular shrinkage. In this report, at a mean of 30 months postoperatively, the thermal group demonstrated a 90% return to play at the same or higher level, whereas the traditional treatment group had only a 67% return to play at the same or higher level. Early results in this study showed an 80% return to competition at a mean of 7.2 months in the nonthermal group and a 93% return at an average of 8.4 months in the thermal group. In a subsequent review of our patients published in 2002,[5] 138 of the 170 total patients (81%) returned to competition at a mean of 8.5 months. The mean Athletic Shoulder Outcome Rating Scale score was 77 of 90, and the mean stability was rated 9.1 of 10. In the group who had knowledge of their velocity, 76% noted a decreased velocity of 3.4 mph on average.

Reviews on the treatment of multidirectional instability with thermal energy have also been completed. Lyons et al[11] reviewed their experience with arthroscopic laser capsulorrhaphy for the treatment of multidirectional instability. At 2-year follow-up, 96% of the laser-treated group was asymptomatic and had not had any further instability. In another report, Frostick et al[7] showed 83% satisfactory results in 28 patients with use of radiofrequency for the treatment of multidirectional instability.

Levy et al[10] published a combined series of patients in which one group was treated with laser capsulorrhaphy and the other group with radiofrequency capsulorrhaphy. Mean follow-ups were 40 months and 23 months, respectively. In the laser group, early outcome measure averaged a score of 90 of a possible 100 but subsequently declined to an average of 80 at final follow-up. At a mean of 40 months postoperatively, only 59% rated their shoulders much better or better than before surgery. In the radiofrequency group, the mean outcome score throughout the follow-up period averaged 80 of 100, but 76% of patients rated their shoulders much better or better than before surgery.

Anderson et al[1] reported a 14% failure rate in 106 patients at a mean of 6.3 months. In their study, multiple previous dislocations and previous surgery were associated with a higher risk for failure.

References

1. Anderson K, Warren RF, Altchek DW, et al. Risk factors for early failure after thermal capsulorrhaphy. Am J Sports Med 2002;30:103-107.
2. Arnoczky SP, Aksan A. Thermal modification of connective tissues: basic science considerations and clinical implications. J Am Acad Orthop Surg 2000;8:305-313.
3. Chen SS, Wright NT, Humphrey JD. Heat-induced changes in the mechanics of a collagenous tissue: isothermal, isotonic shrinkage. J Biomech Eng 1998;120:382-388.
4. Chvapil M, Jensovsky L. The shrinkage temperature of collagen fibers isolated from the tail tendons of rats of various ages and from different places of the same tendon. Gerontologia 1963;1:18-29.
5. Dugas JR, Andrews JR. Thermal capsular shrinkage in the throwing athlete. Clin Sports Med 2002;21:771-776.
6. Fanton GS, Khan AM. Monopolar radiofrequency energy for arthroscopic treatment of shoulder instability in the athlete. Orthop Clin North Am 2001;32:511-523.
7. Frostick SP, Sinopidis CT, Maskari SA, Richmond JC. Treatment of shoulder instability using electrothermally-assisted capsular shift. Presented at the 67th annual meeting of the American Academy of Orthopaedic Surgeons; Orlando, Fla; March 2000.
8. Le Lous M, Cohen-Solal L, Allain JC, et al. Age related evolution of stable collagen reticulation in human skin. Connect Tissue Res 1985;13:145-155.
9. Levitz CL, Dugas JR, Andrews JR. The use of arthroscopic thermal capsulorrhaphy to treat internal impingement in baseball players. Arthroscopy 2001;17:573-577.
10. Levy O, Wilson M, Williams H, et al. Thermal capsular shrinkage for shoulder instability. J Bone Joint Surg Br 2001;83:640-645.
11. Lyons TR, Griffeth PL, Field LD, Savoie FH. Laser assisted capsulorrhaphy for multidirectional instability of the shoulder. Arthroscopy 2001;17:25-30.
12. Mishra DK, Fanton GS. Two-year outcome of arthroscopic Bankart repair and electrothermal assisted capsulorrhaphy for recurrent traumatic anterior shoulder instability. Arthroscopy 2001;17:844-849.
13. Payne LZ, Altchek DW, Craig EV, Warren RF. Arthroscopic treatment of partial rotator cuff tears in young athletes. Am J Sports Med 1997;25:299-305.
14. Speer K, Warren RF, Pagnani M, et al. Arthroscopic technique for anterior stabilization of the shoulder with a bioabsorbable tack. J Bone Joint Surg Am 1996;78:1801-1807.
15. Tibone JE, Lee TQ, Black AD, et al. Glenohumeral translation after arthroscopic thermal capsuloplasty with a radiofrequency probe. J Shoulder Elbow Surg 2000;9:514-518.

CHAPTER 7

Arthroscopic Management of Rare Intra-articular Lesions of the Shoulder

Felix H. Savoie III, MD

In no other joint is there as much variability in normal anatomy as in the shoulder. Unusual conditions of the shoulder must be differentiated from normal variants. Although most pathologic processes are covered in other chapters, rare lesions such as pigmented villonodular synovitis, osteochondritis dissecans of the glenoid and humerus, traumatic chondral fracture, chondrolysis, synovial osteochondromatosis, ganglion and synovial cysts, blending or bifurcation of the biceps and tearing of the attachment of a Buford complex, reverse humeral avulsion of the glenohumeral ligament with infraspinatus tear, coracoid fracture with extension into the joint, and floating anterior capsule (combined Bankart lesion and humeral avulsion of the glenohumeral ligament) are not commonly encountered within the shoulder.

Each of these entities may require different management. The rarity of these problems complicates diagnosis, preparation, and management. Many are encountered only on entering the joint. It is the goal of this chapter to discuss diagnostic studies and tests that can help preoperatively to identify these conditions correctly and assist with their management.

Preoperative Considerations

History

Most of these patients present with either no trauma or a history of only minor trauma. The exception is the articular fracture, which often has a clear history of a traumatic event, often a dive to the floor during an athletic event, after which pain and limitation of activity occur without physical examination findings. However, in all of these cases, symptoms frequently are not associated with a specific activity. Unlike with rotator cuff disease, the pain and feelings of swelling are not worse at night. Unlike with instability problems, the symptoms are not associated with a particular movement or arm position. Unlike with adhesive capsulitis, there is no consistent loss of motion or pain on inferior glide testing.

Physical Examination

Examination usually reveals palpable swelling within the glenohumeral joint, most easily felt in the area of the rotator interval. There is usually some loss of motion, primarily in internal and external rotation. Crepitation is noted with rotational movements of the glenohumeral joint. In cases in which the Buford complex has been avulsed, results of the anterior superior load and shift examination will be positive.

Imaging

Radiographs are usually normal except in synovial osteochondromatosis, in which multiple loose bodies are noted (Fig. 7-1). Magnetic resonance imaging is helpful in osteochondritis dissecans lesions, cases of synovial cysts (Fig. 7-2), and chondrolysis. Avulsions of a Buford complex, pigmented villonodular synovitis, and articular cartilage

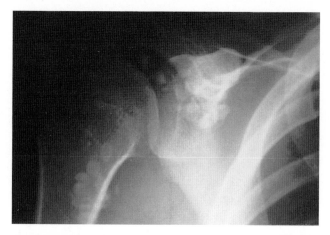

Figure 7-1 Radiologic view of multiple loose bodies in the glenohumeral joint arising from the synovium of the subcoracoid bursa.

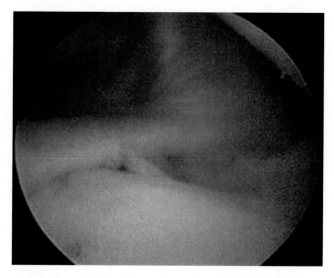

Figure 7-3 A normal Buford complex (cord-like middle glenohumeral ligament) with tearing at the attachment to the glenoid.

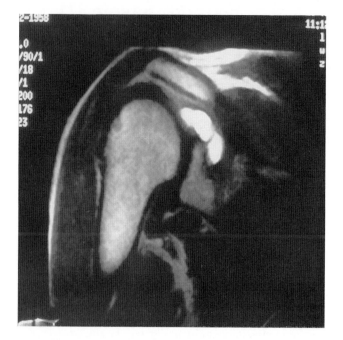

Figure 7-2 Magnetic resonance image of a synovial cyst.

fractures will not show up on most radiographic tests. Glenohumeral avulsions are visualized by arthrography, and the coracoid fracture is best noted on computed tomographic scans.

Indications and Contraindications

Each of these various entities may be managed by arthroscopy. The main contraindications to arthroscopic surgery are in the patient with pigmented villonodular synovitis. Complete excision may require open surgery.

Surgical Technique

Anesthesia and Positioning

Most of these cases require general anesthesia, although experienced regional anesthesiologists may certainly use interscalene block anesthesia. I prefer the lateral decubitus position because of its ability to allow easier access to all areas of the shoulder joint, but the surgeon's preference is usually the rule in these cases.

Diagnostic Arthroscopy

Diagnostic arthroscopy usually reveals the pathologic process. Most of these are readily apparent once the arthroscope is placed within the joint. The avulsion of the Buford complex attachment is the most difficult to differentiate from normal variants. Chondromalacia of the glenoid and fraying of the undersurface of the labrum and outer surface of the glenoid isolated to that area alone and not farther inferior on the glenoid are key findings (Fig. 7-3).

Pigmented villonodular synovitis has the characteristic appearance seen in other joints. However, it is not readily resected as it penetrates through the lining of the joint and expands outward into the surrounding structures (Fig. 7-4). Especially in inferior lesions, the synovial growth may envelope the axillary nerve, requiring its dissection either through open surgery or by arthroscopy.

Synovial cysts (Fig. 7-5) may be related to labral tears or to foreign body reaction. The cyst should be resected and the associated pathologic lesion repaired or removed.

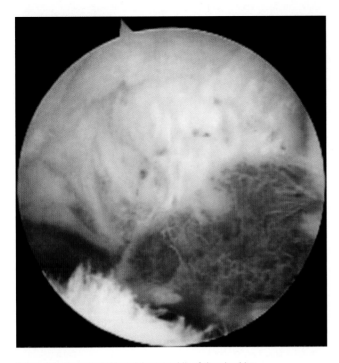

Figure 7-4 Pigmented villonodular synovitis of the shoulder.

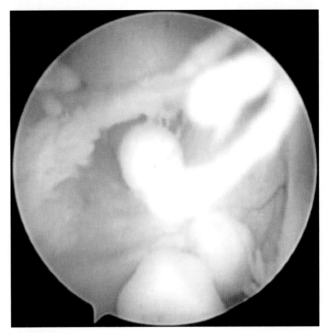

Figure 7-6 Arthroscopic view of the multiple loose bodies of synovial chondromatosis arising from the subcoracoid bursa.

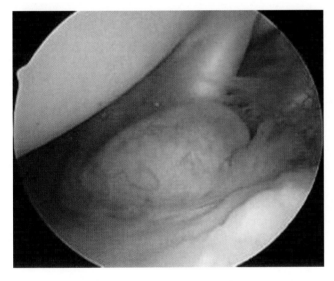

Figure 7-5 Arthroscopic view of a synovial cyst arising from a foreign body near the coracoid.

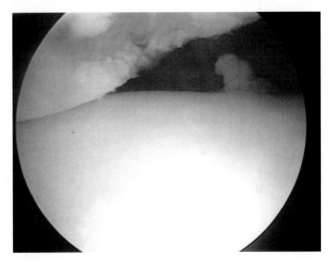

Figure 7-7 Traumatic chondral defect of the humeral head.

In cases of synovial chondromatosis (Fig. 7-6), the multiple loose bodies are readily apparent. It may be useful to place a much larger cannula, such as that used in urologic procedures, to allow the loose bodies to be removed. It is important to find the area of synovium producing the lesions and to excise it. The most common area in which to find this synovium in my experience is the subcoracoid bursa and the bicipital groove.

Traumatic chondral defects and osteochondritis of the humeral head or glenoid result in irritation and swelling within the glenohumeral joint. Finding these loose articular pieces within the shoulder joint and their removal

will help decrease symptoms (Fig. 7-7). The injured bed in the articular surface should also be located and débrided and at least marrow stimulation performed.

The most difficult to manage of these various lesions is chondrolysis of the glenohumeral joint. Although this has been described to follow thermal surgery, the exact cause has yet to be elucidated. Arthroscopy reveals an aggressive destruction of the entire articular surface of the humeral head and glenoid, severe synovitis and capsular damage, and almost an avascular necrosis type of destruction of the humeral head (Fig. 7-8). Biologic glenoid resurfacing with or without humeral head replacement seems to provide the best relief.

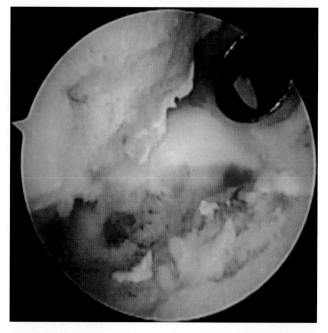

Figure 7-8 Postsurgical avascular necrosis due to thermal chondrolysis.

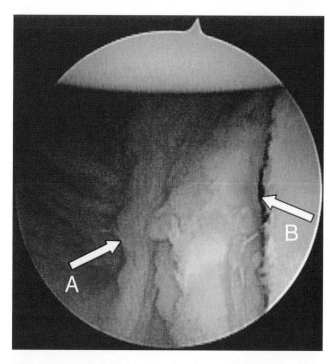

Figure 7-9 Floating anterior capsule; both the Bankart lesion and the humeral avulsion are pictured. A, lateral edge of capsule; B, labrum and medial capsule.

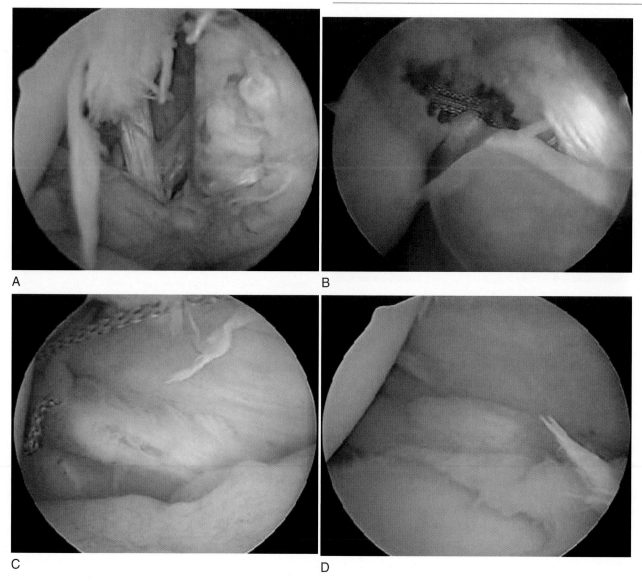

A

B

C

D

Figure 7-10 Reverse humeral avulsion of the glenohumeral ligament. **A,** Arthroscopic view of the capsule and tendon injury. **B,** Anchor placement in preparation for repair. **C,** First set of sutures tied. **D,** Final view of repaired capsule.

Humeral avulsions of the anterior glenohumeral ligaments are covered elsewhere in this text. However, one may occasionally find this lesion in conjunction with a Bankart lesion (Fig. 7-9). In these cases, the Bankart lesion is repaired first, and then the humeral avulsion is repaired. This also represents an excellent indication for open surgery by Matsen's approach to elevate the lateral subscapularis and use the humeral avulsion to access the Bankart lesion. The capsulolabral complex is repaired to the glenoid, and the humeral avulsion is repaired as part of the reattachment of the lateral capsule and subscapularis tendon.

Reverse humeral avulsion of the glenohumeral ligament is even more uncommon. In high-energy trauma, the lateral capsule and the infraspinatus tendon may both be involved, necessitating repair of both the capsule and the tendon with anchors and sutures (Fig. 7-10).

Coracoid fractures are relatively rare lesions in which the fracture may extend into the articular surface of the glenoid. The symptoms are pain, tenderness around the coracoid, and swelling. The fracture is readily visualized on magnetic resonance imaging or computed tomographic scans. Although immobilization often results in union, active individuals may require stabilization. Arthroscopy of the glenohumeral joint may allow monitoring of the articular extension while also allowing reduction and fixation (Fig. 7-11).

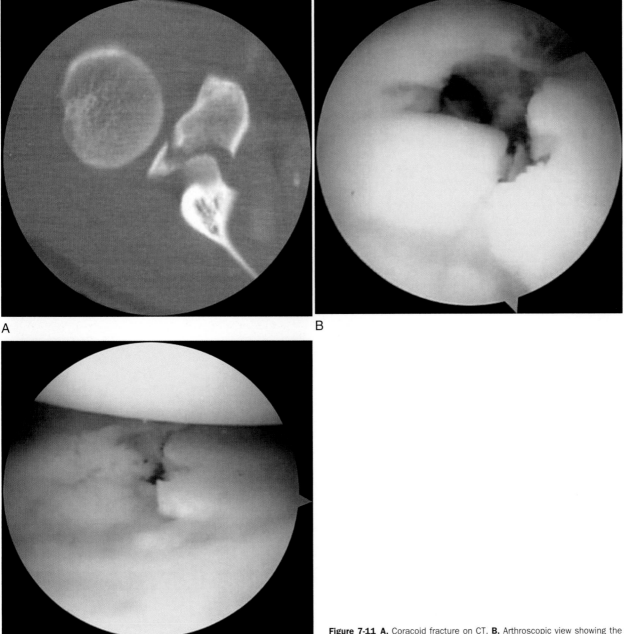

A

B

C

Figure 7-11 A, Coracoid fracture on CT. **B,** Arthroscopic view showing the intra-articular extension. **C,** Arthroscopic view of repaired coracoid.

Summary

There are many more unusual lesions of the shoulder that may or may not require stabilization. Incorporation of all or part of the biceps into the rotator cuff is a normal variant (Fig. 7-12), just like the Buford complex, hypermobile superior labrum, and absent anterior labrum. Before a lesion is repaired, it is incumbent on the surgeon to review the injury, the symptoms, and the physical examination findings to see whether they match the pathologic process that is being viewed. If the mechanism is sufficient to produce the pathologic process being visualized, and the pathologic lesion can produce the symptoms the patient is complaining of, repair is warranted. Elimination of the symptoms after repair may be the only confirmation that the surgeon has performed the correct operation.

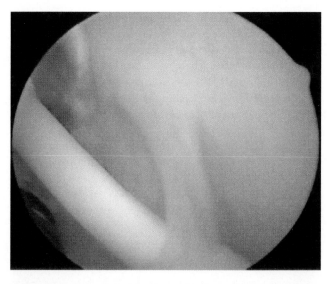

Figure 7-12 Normal variant of the biceps with sling and incorporation into the rotator cuff.

Suggested Readings

Bents RT, Skeete KD. The correlation of the Buford complex and SLAP lesions. J Shoulder Elbow Surg 2005;14:565-569.

Chiffolot X, Ehlinger M, Bonnomet F, Kempf JF. Arthroscopic resection of pigmented villonodular synovitis pseudotumor of the shoulder: a case report with three year follow-up. Rev Chir Orthop Reparatrice Appar Mot 2005;91:470-475.

Debeer P, Brys P. Osteochondritis dissecans of the humeral head: clinical and radiological findings. Acta Orthop Belg 2005;71:484-488.

Hamada J, Tamai K, Doguchi Y, et al. Case report: a rare condition of secondary synovial osteochondromatosis of the shoulder joint in a young female patient. J Shoulder Elbow Surg 2005;14:653-656.

Jerosch J, Aldawoudy AM. Chondrolysis of the glenohumeral joint following arthroscopic capsular release for adhesive capsulitis: a case report. Knee Surg Sports Traumatol Arthrosc 2007;15:292-294. Epub June 24, 2006.

Levine WN, Clark AM Jr, D'Alessandro DF, Yamaguchi K. Chondrolysis following arthroscopic thermal capsulorrhaphy to treat shoulder instability. A report of two cases. J Bone Joint Surg Am 2005;87:616-621.

CHAPTER 8

Arthroscopic Repair of Posterior Shoulder Instability

Steven B. Cohen, MD

James P. Bradley, MD

Posterior instability is relatively uncommon compared with anterior instability of the shoulder. Most authors agree that posterior shoulder instability represents approximately 2% to 10% of shoulder instability cases.[4,8,13] Initial attempts to clarify the distinctions of posterior instability were made in 1962, when McLaughlin recognized that differences exist between "fixed and recurrent subluxations of the shoulder," suggesting that the etiology and treatment of the two are distinctly different.[15] More than 20 years later, in the early 1980s, Hawkins[8] reviewed the difference between true dislocations and subluxations and noted that true recurrent posterior dislocations are rare compared with subluxation episodes. Since that time, additional knowledge has been gained in the differences between unidirectional and multidirectional, traumatic and atraumatic, acute and chronic, and voluntary and involuntary posterior instability. In many respects, each of these may represent a distinct form of posterior instability with its own underlying predispositions, anatomic abnormalities, and treatment algorithms.[16,18] Our collective understanding of posterior shoulder instability continues to evolve.

Pathoanatomy

Recent advances in our understanding of the spectrum of posterior instability have been gained through the study of shoulder injuries in athletes, patients with generalized ligamentous laxity, and patients with post-traumatic injuries. Acute posterior dislocations typically result from a direct blow to the anterior shoulder or indirect forces that couple shoulder flexion, internal rotation, and adduction.[4,8] The most common indirect causes are accidental electric shock and convulsive seizures. Because of incomplete radiographic studies and a failure to recognize the posterior shoulder prominence and mechanical block to external rotation, 60% to 80% of locked posterior dislocations are missed on initial presentation. Additional pathologic processes are frequently associated with posterior instability and include the reverse Hill-Sachs lesion, the reverse bony Bankart lesion, posterior capsular laxity, excessive humeral head retroversion or chondrolabral retroversion, and glenoid hypoplasia.

Preoperative Considerations

History

To diagnose posterior instability, the clinician must perform a thorough history and physical examination as well as maintain a high index of suspicion. A history of a posterior dislocation requiring formal reduction is more obvious; however, patients with recurrent posterior subluxation may present with more subtle findings. The majority of patients with recurrent posterior subluxation complain primarily of pain with specific activities, particularly in the provocative position (90-degree forward flexion, adduction, and internal rotation),[4,8] more so than of instability.

Physical Examination

- Active and passive range of motion
- Palpation for tenderness
- Strength testing
- Evaluation for impingement
- Assessment for generalized ligamentous laxity

Stability Testing

- Load and shift test for anterior and posterior translation (Fig. 8-1)
- Sulcus sign (in both neutral and external rotation) for inferior translation
- Sulcus sign graded as 3+ that remains 2+ in external rotation is pathognomonic for multidirectional instability

Specific Tests

- Jerk test (Fig. 8-2)
- Kim test (Fig. 8-3)
- Circumduction test

Imaging

Plain Radiographs

- Including axillary view
- Evaluate for reverse Hill-Sachs lesions (Fig. 8-4), glenoid pathologic changes (retroversion, fractures, and hypoplasia), bony humeral avulsion of the glenohumeral ligaments

Magnetic Resonance Arthrography

- Evaluate labrum, capsule, biceps tendon, subscapularis integrity (Fig. 8-5)

Computed Tomography

- Evaluate for glenoid version, locked dislocation (Fig. 8-6)

Indications and Contraindications

Many patients with recurrent posterior subluxation can be managed successfully without surgery. Numerous authors have proposed a period of no less than 6 months of physical therapy before surgical treatment is considered. Effec-

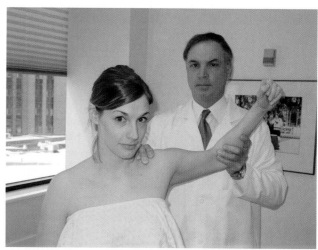

A

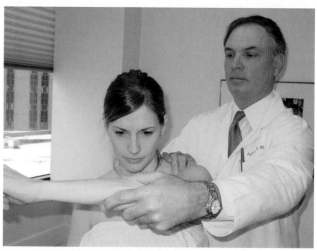

B

Figure 8-2 The jerk test for posterior instability. **A,** The arm is forward flexed and internally rotated. **B,** Posteriorly directed force subluxes the shoulder. Slow abduction of the arm results in a palpable jerk as the joint is reduced. This test has also been described in reverse, by moving the arm from an abducted position forward.

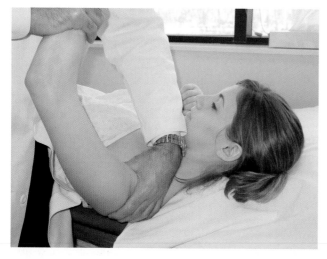

Figure 8-1 The load and shift test is performed by placing the thumb and index or long finger around the humeral head, which is then shifted anteriorly and posteriorly.

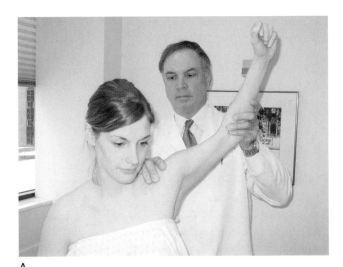

A

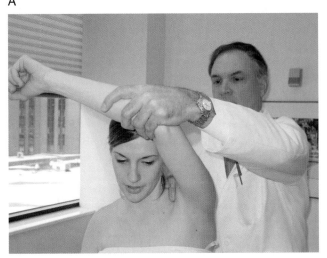

B

Figure 8-3 The Kim test for the detection of posteroinferior labral lesions is performed by applying axial compression to the 90-degree abducted arm **(A)**, which is then elevated and forward flexed in a diagonal direction **(B)**, resulting in pain and a possible clunk.

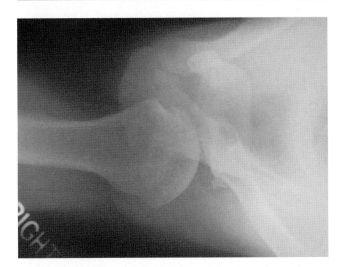

Figure 8-4 A reverse (anterior) Hill-Sachs lesion as demonstrated on an axillary radiograph.

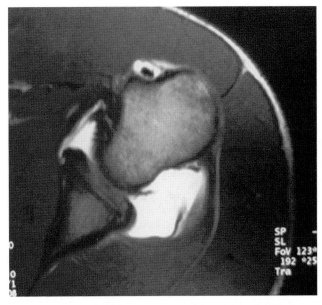

Figure 8-5 Axial magnetic resonance scan through the glenohumeral joint obtained with the intra-articular administration of contrast material demonstrating a capacious posterior capsule.

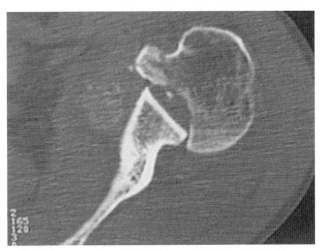

Figure 8-6 Axial computed tomographic scan demonstrating a locked posterior dislocation with large reverse Hill-Sachs lesion and destruction of a significant portion of the articular surface.

tive rehabilitation includes avoidance of aggravating activities, restoration of a full range of motion, and shoulder strengthening. Strengthening of the rotator cuff, posterior deltoid, and periscapular musculature is critical. The premise of such directed physical therapy is to enable the dynamic muscle stabilizers to offset the deficient static capsulolabral restraints. Nearly 70% of patients will improve after an appropriate rehabilitation protocol. The recurrent subluxation, however, is generally not eliminated, but the functional disability is diminished enough that it does not prevent activities. If the disability fails to improve with an extended 6-month period of directed rehabilitation, or in select cases of posterior instability resulting from a macrotraumatic event, surgical intervention should be considered.

Indications

- Patients with continued disabling, isolated, recurrent posterior subluxation after a rehabilitation program
- Recurrent posterior subluxation with a posterior labral tear
- Multidirectional instability with a primary posterior component
- Voluntary positional posterior instability

Relative indications include patients with an antecedent macrotraumatic injury.

Contraindications

- Patients not having completed a reasonable rehabilitation program
- A surgeon's preference for traditional open techniques
- A large engaging reverse Hill-Sachs lesion requiring subscapularis transfer or an osteochondral allograft
- A large reverse bony Bankart lesion
- Patients with voluntary muscle instability
- Underlying psychogenic disorders, and patients unable or unwilling to comply with postoperative limitations

Relative contraindications may include chronic instability resulting in compromised capsulolabral tissue and patients who have undergone previous open surgery.

Because successful results have been achieved after arthroscopic treatment of posterior labral tears in contact athletes, arthroscopic reconstruction is not contraindicated in that population.

Surgical Technique

Anesthesia

The procedure can be performed under interscalene block or general endotracheal anesthesia with an interscalene block for postoperative pain control.

Examination Under Anesthesia

The examination under anesthesia is performed on a firm surface with the scapula relatively fixed and the humeral head free to rotate. A load-and-shift maneuver, as described by Murrell and Warren, is performed with the patient supine.[12] The arm is held in 90 degrees of abduction and neutral rotation while a posterior force is applied in an attempt to translate the humeral head over the posterior

glenoid. A sulcus sign test is performed with the arm adducted and in neutral rotation to assess whether the instability has an inferior component. A 3+ sulcus sign that remains 2+ or greater in external rotation is considered pathognomonic for multidirectional instability. Testing is completed on both the affected and unaffected shoulders, and differences between the two are documented.

Patient Positioning, Landmarks, and Portals

The patient is then placed in the lateral decubitus position with the affected shoulder positioned superior. An inflatable beanbag and kidney rests hold the patient in position. Foam cushions are placed to protect the peroneal nerve at the neck of the fibula on the down leg. An axillary roll is placed. The operating table is placed in a slight reverse-Trendelenburg position. The full upper extremity is prepared to the level of the sternum anteriorly and the medial border of the scapula posteriorly. The operative shoulder is placed in 10 pounds of traction and positioned in 45 degrees of abduction and 20 degrees of forward flexion. The bone landmarks, including the acromion, distal clavicle, and coracoid process, are demarcated with a marking pen.

After preparation and draping, the glenohumeral joint is injected with 50 mL of sterile saline through an 18-gauge spinal needle to inflate the joint. A posterior portal is established 1 cm distal and 1 cm lateral to the standard posterior portal to allow access to the rim of the glenoid for anchor placement (Fig. 8-7). An anterior portal

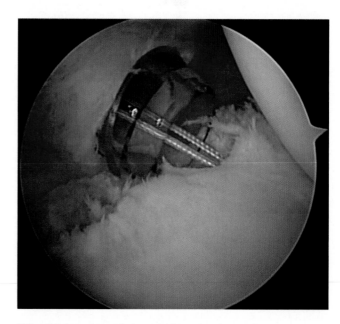

Figure 8-7 Accessory posterior portal for anchor placement.

is then established high in the rotator interval by an inside-to-outside technique with a switching stick. Alternatively, it can also be established by an outside-to-inside technique with the assistance of a spinal needle. Typically, only anterior and posterior portals are required to perform the procedure. An accessory 7-o'clock portal has been described but is not frequently used in our technique.

Diagnostic Arthroscopy

A diagnostic arthroscopy of the glenohumeral joint is then undertaken. The labrum, capsule, biceps tendon, subscapularis, rotator interval, rotator cuff, and articular surfaces are visualized in systematic fashion. This ensures that no associated lesions will be overlooked by poorly directed tunnel vision. Lesions typically seen in posterior instability include a patulous posterior capsule, posterior labral tear, labral fraying and splitting, widening of the rotator interval, and undersurface partial-thickness rotator cuff tears. After the glenohumeral joint is viewed from the posterior portal, the arthroscope is switched to the anterior portal to allow improved visualization of the posterior capsule and labrum. A switching stick can then be used in replacing the posterior cannula with an 8.25-mm distally threaded clear cannula (Arthrex, Inc., Naples, Fla), thus allowing passage of an arthroscopic probe and other instruments through the clear cannula to explore the posterior labrum for evidence of tears.

Specific Steps (Box 8-1)

1. Preparation for Repair

When the posterior labrum is detached, suture anchors are employed in performing the repair. The posterior labrum is visualized from both the posterior and anterior portals to appreciate the full extent of the tear (Fig. 8-8).

- The arthroscope then remains in the anterior portal, and the posterior portal serves as the working portal for the repair.

Box 8-1 Surgical Steps

1. Preparation for repair
2. Placement of suture anchors
3. Labral repair
4. Posterior capsular shift
5. Arthroscopic knot tying
6. Completion of the repair
7. Rotator interval closure

- An arthroscopic rasp or chisel is used to mobilize the torn labrum from the glenoid rim (Fig. 8-9).
- A motorized synovial shaver or meniscal rasp is used to abrade the capsule adjacent to the labral tear and to débride and decorticate the glenoid rim to achieve a bleeding surface.

2. Placement of Suture Anchors

- Suture anchors are then placed at the articular margin of the glenoid rim, rather than down on the glenoid neck, to perform the labral repair (Fig. 8-10).

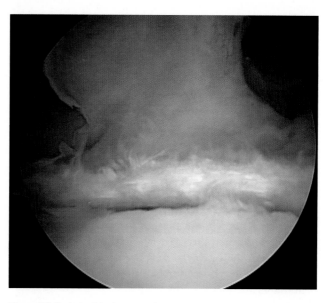

Figure 8-8 Posterior labral tear as viewed through the standard posterior viewing portal; the probe is placed through the accessory posterior portal.

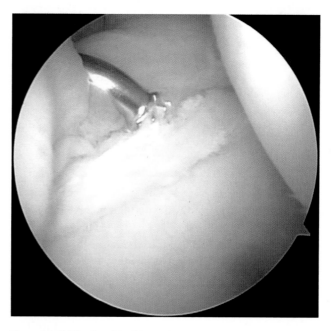

Figure 8-9 Mobilization of the labrum with a rasp.

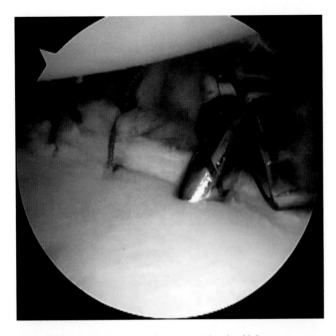

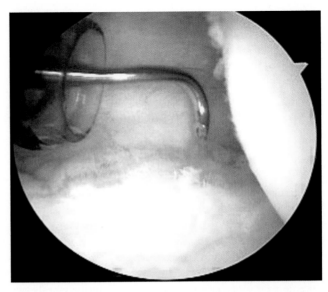

Figure 8-11 A suture-passing device penetrating the labrum.

Figure 8-10 Arthroscopic anchor placement on the glenoid rim.

- A posterior labral tear extending from 6-o'clock to 9-o'clock on a right shoulder is typically repaired with suture anchors at the 6:30, 7:30, and 8:30 positions.

- We prefer the 3.0-mm Bio-Suture Tak suture anchor with No. 2 FiberWire (Arthrex, Inc., Naples, Fla) because of the ease of placing the anchor on the glenoid surface, but a number of other commercially available anchors are also adequate.

- The suture anchor is placed with the sutures oriented perpendicular to the glenoid rim to facilitate passage of the most posterior suture through the torn labrum.

- Avoid inadvertent injury to the articular cartilage.

3. Labral Repair

- After placement of the suture anchors, a 45-degree Spectrum suture hook (Linvatec, Largo, Fla) is loaded with a No. 0 polydioxanone (PDS) suture (Ethicon, Inc., Somerville, NJ). The contralateral side hook is chosen (i.e., a left 45-degree hook for a right shoulder when it is introduced from the posterior portal). Alternatively, there are other commercially available suture passers and suture relays that will also suffice.

- The suture passer is delivered through the torn labrum and advanced superiorly, reentering the joint at the edge of the glenoid articular cartilage (Fig. 8-11).

- Tension must be restored into the posterior band of the inferior glenohumeral ligament to re-establish posterior stability.

- Patients with acute injuries and less evidence of capsular stretching do not require the same degree of capsular advancement as do those with more chronic instability.

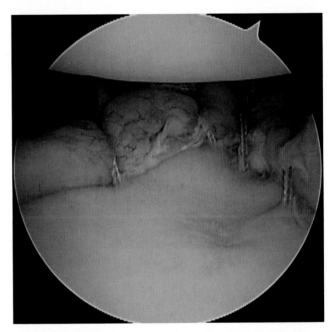

Figure 8-12 Capsular plication (pleat stitch, capsulorrhaphy stitch) can be performed to address capsular redundancy.

- In the setting of a labral tear with some capsular laxity, the suture passer is advanced through the posterior capsule approximately 1 cm lateral to the edge of the labral tear and then underneath the labral tear, to the edge of the articular cartilage, the so-called pleat stitch (Fig. 8-12).

- Placement of as many pleat stitches as necessary in a patulous shoulder capsule can reduce capsular redundancy.

- The PDS suture is then fed into the glenohumeral joint, and the suture passer is withdrawn through the posterior clear cannula.

- An arthroscopic suture grasper is used to withdraw both the most posterior suture in the suture anchor and the end of the PDS suture that has been advanced through the torn labrum. This move detangles the sutures in the cannula.

- The PDS suture is then fashioned into a single loop and tightly tied over the end of the braided suture.

- The most lateral PDS suture, which has not been tied to the braided suture, is then pulled through the clear cannula (Fig. 8-13).

- This advances the most posterior suture in the suture anchor behind the labral tear (Fig. 8-14).

- A labral tear at the 7-o'clock position is advanced to the 7:30 suture anchor, and the 8-o'clock labral tear position is advanced to the 8:30 suture anchor. Additional sutures are then placed in similar fashion to complete the labral repair.

- If the capsule requires further tension, suture capsulorrhaphies can be performed in the intervals between the suture anchors directly to the newly secured labrum.

- Knots are tied after the passage of each suture, which allows continued assessment of the repair and the degree of the capsular shift achieved by each suture

4. Posterior Capsular Shift

- The majority of patients with unidirectional posterior instability and primary posterior multidirectional instability do not have a posterior labral tear and typically display significant capsular laxity at

arthroscopy (Fig. 8-15). An isolated posterior capsulorrhaphy is performed.

- Suture capsulorrhaphies are placed from inferior (6-o'clock) to superior (10-o'clock).

- The 6:30 capsular suture is typically advanced to the 7:30 position, and the reduction in capsular volume is assessed.

- Restoration of adequate tension in the posterior band of the inferior glenohumeral ligament is critical.

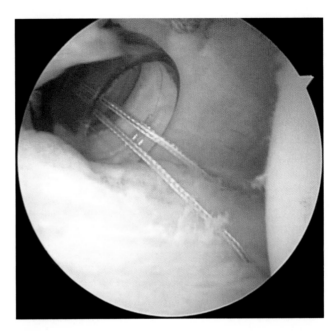

Figure 8-14 Sutures passed through the labrum, before tying.

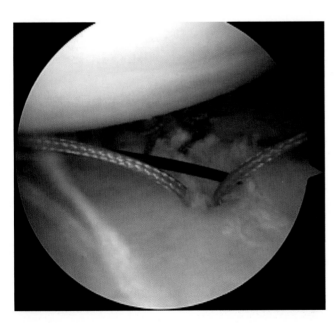

Figure 8-13 Shuttling of the anchor suture through the labrum.

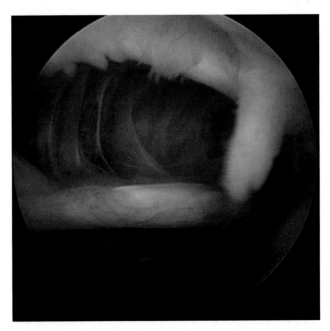

Figure 8-15 Capacious posterior capsule as a sign of posterior instability.

- Additional sutures are then placed at the 7:30, 8:30, and 9:30 positions on the capsule, advancing to the 8:30, 9:30, and 10:30 positions on the glenoid (Fig. 8-16).
- Sutures are tied after each is passed. If the sutures are not tied until the end, one errant suture may necessitate removal of all other sutures to achieve correction.

5. Arthroscopic Knot Tying

- We prefer the sliding-locking Weston knot, but there are a number of arthroscopic knot-tying techniques that work well.
- What is most important is that the surgeon be familiar with the knot used and be skilled in its use.
- The posterior braided suture exiting through the capsule is threaded through a knot pusher, and the end is secured with a hemostat.
- This suture serves as the post, which in effect will advance the capsule and labrum to the glenoid rim when the knot is tightened.
- The knot should be secured posteriorly on the capsule and not on the rim of the glenoid to prevent humeral head abrasion from the knot.
- Each half-hitch must be completely seated before the next half-hitch is thrown.
- Placing tension on the non-post suture and advancing the knot pusher "past point" will lock the Weston knot.
- A total of three alternating half-hitches are placed to secure the Weston knot.

6. Completion of the Repair

- An arthroscopic awl is employed to penetrate the bare area of the humerus, under the infraspinatus tendon, in an effort to achieve some punctate bleeding to augment the healing response.
- The posterior capsular portal incision is then closed by passage of a PDS suture through the crescent Spectrum suture passer and retrieval of the suture with an arthroscopic penetrator.
- Varying the distance of the suture from the portal incision allows titration of the capsulorrhaphy.
- The PDS suture is then tied blindly in the cannula, closing the posterior capsular incision (Fig. 8-17)

7. Rotator Interval Closure

- In the setting of multidirectional instability with a primary posterior component, the rotator interval requires closure (defined by a 2+ or greater sulcus sign that does not improve in external rotation).
- The rotator interval is viewed with the arthroscope in the posterior portal.
- A crescent suture passer is advanced from the anterior portal through the anterior capsule just above the superior border of the subscapularis tendon 1 cm lateral to the glenoid.
- It is then passed through the middle glenohumeral ligament at the inferior border of the rotator interval. This makes up the inferior aspect of the rotator interval closure.
- A No. 0 PDS suture is then fed into the joint and retrieved with a penetrator through the superior glenohumeral ligament.

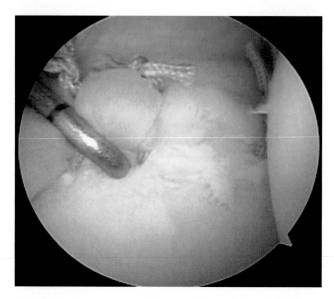

Figure 8-16 Final appearance after capsular advancement.

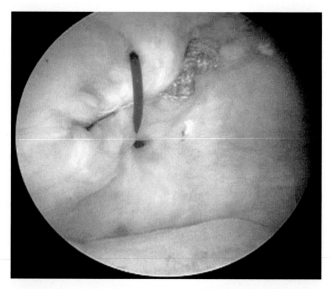

Figure 8-17 Closed posterior portal after cannula removal (as viewed from anteriorly).

The PDS suture is then withdrawn out the anterior cannula, and the knot is tied blindly in the cannula as the closure is visualized through the posterior portal.

Postoperative Considerations

Rehabilitation and Return to Play Recommendations

The rehabilitation program consists of a series of phases. Initially, the posterior capsule must be protected by avoiding extremes of internal rotation.

- Immobilization is maintained in an UltraSling (DonJoy, Carlsbad, Calif) for 6 weeks, abducting the shoulder approximately 30 degrees.
- Immobilization is removed for gentle passive pain-free range-of-motion exercises. We allow 90 degrees forward flexion and external rotation to 0 degrees by 4 weeks after surgery.
- The UltraSling is discontinued 6 weeks after surgery. Active-assisted range-of-motion exercises and gentle passive range-of-motion exercises are progressed, and pain-free gentle internal rotation is instituted.
- At 2 to 3 months after surgery, range of motion and mobilization are progressed to achieve full passive and active motion. Stretching exercises for the anterior and posterior capsule are instituted.
- By 4 months after surgery, the shoulder should be pain free. Concentration on eccentric rotator cuff strengthening is begun.
- At 5 months after surgery, isotonic and isokinetic exercises are advanced.
- At 6 months after surgery, throwing athletes undergo isokinetic testing. When patients are able to achieve at least 80% strength and endurance compared with the uninvolved side, an integrated throwing protocol is instituted.

- Throwers begin an easy-tossing program at a distance of 20 feet without a wind-up. Stretching and the application of heat to increase circulation before throwing sessions are critical.
- By 7 months, light throwing with an easy wind-up to 30 feet is allowed 2 or 3 days per week for 10 minutes per session.
- By 9 months after surgery, long, easy throws from the mid-outfield (150 to 200 feet) are allowed.
- By 10 months, stronger throws from the outfield are allowed, reaching home plate on only one or two bounces.
- At 11 months, pitchers are allowed to throw one-half to three-quarter speed from the mound with emphasis on technique and accuracy.
- By 12 months after surgery, throwers are allowed to throw from their position at three-quarter to full speed. When the throwing athlete is able to perform full-speed throwing for 2 consecutive weeks, return to full competition is permitted.
- Nonthrowing athletes and nonathletes are managed by criteria different from those for the throwing athletes. When patients are able to achieve at least 80% strength and endurance at the 6-month isokinetic testing compared with the uninvolved side, nonthrowing athletes begin a sport-specific program.
- In general, power athletes and contact athletes, such as weightlifters and football players, can return to full competition by 6 to 9 months after surgery. Noncontact athletes such as golfers, basketball players, swimmers, and cheerleaders can generally return to full competition by 6 to 8 months.

Complications

The complications include general risks of surgery, such as infection and hematoma formation, as well as risks particular to arthroscopic posterior shoulder stabilization, such as recurrent instability and stiffness.

PEARLS AND PITFALLS

- There is open debate about whether the lateral decubitus or beach chair position better facilitates shoulder arthroscopy. We prefer the lateral position because we think it allows better access to both the anterior and posterior aspects of the shoulder. Placement of the shoulder in 10 pounds of traction in the position of 45 degrees of abduction and 20 degrees of forward flexion in effect displaces the humeral head anteriorly and inferiorly, bringing the posterior labrum into clear view. We have not been able to achieve such an unimpeded approach to the posteroinferior shoulder capsule in the beach chair position without imparting injury to the articular cartilage of the humeral head in the process.

- We prefer to inject the glenohumeral joint with 40 to 50 mL of sterile saline before placement of the cannula into the glenohumeral joint. It inflates the joint to allow safer insertion of the cannula, limiting risk to the articular cartilage of the humeral head and glenoid.

- After a determination of posterior labral disease or capsular laxity is made, a posterior working portal must be established. Placement of an 8.25-mm distally threaded clear cannula over a switching stick into the posterior portal will allow passage of both the crescent and 45-degree suture hooks. Smaller cannulas will not accommodate the 45-degree suture hook. We also recommend the use of suture anchors for capsulolabral reconstruction instead of suture capsulorrhaphy alone as it results in a more stable repair.

PEARLS AND PITFALLS—cont'd

- Difficulty in the placement of suture anchors can be encountered if the posterior portal is too far superior or medial in the posterior capsule. The conventional posterior portal is near 10-o'clock on the right glenoid, which makes approach to the posteroinferior glenoid difficult for the placement of suture anchors. We therefore place the posterior portal approximately 1 cm inferior and 1 cm lateral to the standard posterior portal in patients with demonstrable posterior instability on examination under anesthesia. When the posterior portal has been made too far superior, an auxiliary posterior portal can then be made inferior and lateral to the existing posterior portal. A spinal needle can be used in positioning the auxiliary portal at 7-o'clock on the glenoid and approximately 1 cm lateral to the glenoid rim on the posterior capsule for approach to the posteroinferior glenoid at a 30- to 45-degree angle in the sagittal plane. Cadaveric studies by Davidson and Rivenburgh[5] have shown the 7-o'clock portal to be a safe distance from the axillary nerve and posterior humeral circumflex artery (39 ± 4 mm) and the suprascapular nerve and artery (29 ± 3 mm). The use of blunt trocars in the placement of the portal further decreases the risk of neurovascular injury.

- We do not routinely close the rotator interval in patients with unidirectional posterior instability. This practice is supported by several other studies in the literature.[13] Harryman et al[7] sectioned the rotator interval and found that in a position of 60 degrees flexion and 60 degrees abduction, a significant increase in posterior translation occurred. However, in posterior instability's provocative position of 60 degrees flexion and 90 degrees internal rotation, no significant increase in posterior translation occurred after sectioning of the rotator interval. Furthermore, although imbrication of the rotator interval significantly decreased posterior translation at a position of 60 degrees flexion and 60 degrees abduction, it did not have a similar effect in the provocative position. A sectioned rotator interval did lead to a significant increase in inferior translation, which was corrected by imbrication of the rotator interval tissue. We do, however, perform rotator interval closure in patients with an inferior component to their instability, as defined by a 2+ or greater sulcus sign that does not improve in external rotation.

Table 8-1 Summary of Studies of Arthroscopic Posterior Shoulder Instability Repair

Author	Follow-up	Outcome
Papendick and Savoie[13] (1995)	10 months	39 of 41 (95%) successful
McIntyre et al[11] (1997)	31 months	15 of 20 (75%) successful
Savoie and Field[15] (1997)	34 months	55 of 61 (90%) successful
Wolf and Eakin[18] (1998)	33 months	12 of 14 (86%) successful
Mair et al[10] (1998)	2-year minimum	9 of 9 (100%) successful
Antoniou et al[1] (2000)	28 months	35 of 41 (85%) successful
Williams et al[17] (2003)	5.1 years	24 of 26 (92%) successful
Kim et al[9] (2003)	39 months	26 of 27 (96%) successful
Fluhme et al[6] (2004)	34 months	15 of 18 (83%) successful
Bottoni et al[2] (2005)	40 months	16 of 18 (88%) successful
Provencher et al[14] (2005)	39 months	26 of 33 (79%) successful
Bradley et al[3] (2006)	27 months	91 of 100 (91%) successful

Results

Results of studies of arthroscopic repair of posterior shoulder instability are presented in Table 8-1.

References

1. Antoniou J, Duckworth DT, Harryman DT II. Capsulolabral augmentation for the management of posteroinferior instability of the shoulder. J Bone Joint Surg Am 2000;82:1220-1230.
2. Bottoni CR, Franks BR, Moore JH, et al. Operative stabilization of posterior shoulder instability. Am J Sports Med 2005;33:996-1002.
3. Bradley JP, Baker CL, Kline AJ, et al. Arthroscopic capsulolabral reconstruction for posterior instability of the shoulder: a prospective study of 100 shoulders. Am J Sports Med 2006;34:1061-1071.
4. Burkhead WZ Jr, Rockwood CA Jr. Treatment of instability of the shoulder with an exercise program. J Bone Joint Surg Am 1992;74:890-896.
5. Davidson PA, Rivenburgh DW. The 7-o'clock posteroinferior portal for shoulder arthroscopy. Am J Sports Med 2002;30:693-696.
6. Fluhme DJ, Bradley JP, Burke CJ, et al. Open versus arthroscopic treatment for posterior glenohumeral instability. Presented at the

American Orthopaedic Society for Sports Medicine annual meeting; Quebec City, Canada; June 24-27, 2004.

7. Harryman DT, Sidles JA, Harris SL, et al. The role of the rotator interval capsule in passive motion and stability of the shoulder. J Bone Joint Surg Am 1992;74:53-66.

8. Hawkins RJ, Koppert G, Johnston G. Recurrent posterior instability (subluxation) of the shoulder. J Bone Joint Surg Am 1984;66:169.

9. Kim SH, Ha KI, Park JH, et al. Arthroscopic posterior labral repair and capsular shift for traumatic unidirectional recurrent posterior subluxation of the shoulder. J Bone Joint Surg Am 2003;85:1479-1487.

10. Mair SD, Zarzour RH, Speer KP. Posterior labral injury in contact athletes. Am J Sports Med 1998;26:753-758.

11. McIntyre LF, Caspari RB, Savoie FH III. The arthroscopic treatment of posterior shoulder instability: two-year results of a multiple suture technique. Arthroscopy 1997;13:426-432.

12. Murrell GA, Warren RF. The surgical treatment of posterior shoulder instability. Clin Sports Med 1995;14(4):903–915.

13. Papendick LW, Savoie FH III. Anatomy-specific repair techniques for posterior shoulder instability. J South Orthop Assoc 1995; 4:169-176.

14. Provencher MT, Bell SJ, Menzel KA, Mologne TS. Arthroscopic treatment of posterior instability: results in 33 patients. Am J Sports Med 2005;33:1463-1471.

15. Savoie FH III, Field LD. Arthroscopic management of posterior shoulder instability. Oper Tech Sports Med 1997;5:226-232.

16. Tibone JE, Bradley JP. The treatment of posterior subluxation in athletes. Clin Orthop 1993;291:124-137.

17. Williams RJ III, Strickland S, Cohen M, et al. Arthroscopic repair for traumatic posterior shoulder instability. Am J Sports Med 2003;31:203-209.

18. Wolf EM, Eakin CL. Arthroscopic capsular plication for posterior shoulder instability. Arthroscopy 1998;14:153-163.

8

Arthroscopic Treatment of Multidirectional Shoulder Instability

Steven B. Cohen, MD

Jon K. Sekiya, MD

Neer and colleagues described the concept of multidirectional instability of the shoulder in detail in 1980. This established the difference between unidirectional instability and global laxity of the capsule inferiorly, posteriorly, and anteriorly. Initial treatments of this condition included open approaches aimed at decreasing capsular laxity by tensioning of the capsule, in particular inferiorly. As the pathoanatomy has become more defined and arthroscopic techniques for shoulder instability have improved, treatment has been more directed at arthroscopic stabilization procedures. Shoulder instability has been found to be a result of several pathologic processes, including capsular laxity, labral detachment, and rotator interval defects. Arthroscopic techniques have evolved from capsular shift by transglenoid sutures, Bankart repair and shift with biodegradable tacks or suture anchors, thermal capsulorrhaphy, rotator interval repair, and capsular plication. For treatment of patients with multidirectional shoulder instability for whom nonoperative attempts have failed, our current method is to perform an arthroscopic capsular shift by reducing capsular volume with capsular plication.

Preoperative Considerations

History

Typically, there is not a history of a traumatic shoulder dislocation, but it may be the inciting event. Most commonly, the instability is due to microtrauma resulting in global capsular laxity. There may be a history of recurrent dislocations or repetitive subluxation events.

Typical History

- Young, active patient
- Pain
- Complaints of shoulder shifting
- Difficulty with overhead activity
- Inability to do sports
- Instability while sleeping
- Trouble with activities of daily living
- Episodes of "dead arm" sensation
- Failed prior attempts at physical therapy

Physical Examination

- Inspection for atrophy
- Glenohumeral active and passive range of motion; scapulothoracic motion (winging)
- Strength testing
- Palpation for tenderness
- Evaluation for ligamentous laxity
- Evaluation for impingement
- Assessment for generalized ligamentous laxity

Stability Testing

- Load and shift test for anterior and posterior translation

- Sulcus sign (in both neutral and external rotation) for inferior translation
- Sulcus sign graded as 3+ that remains 2+ in external rotation is pathognomonic for multidirectional instability

Specific Tests

- Apprehension test
- Relocation test
- O'Brien sign
- Jerk test
- Kim test
- Circumduction test
- Speed test

Imaging

Plain Radiographs

- Anteroposterior view, axillary view, outlet view, Stryker notch view
- Evaluate for Hill-Sachs or reverse Hill-Sachs lesion, glenoid pathologic changes, bony humeral avulsion of the glenohumeral ligaments

Magnetic Resonance Arthrography

- Evaluate for capsular laxity, labral disease, biceps tendon disease, rotator cuff lesions

Computed Tomography

- Evaluate for proximal humeral and glenoid bone defects

Indications and Contraindications

In many patients with atraumatic multidirectional instability, the proper neuromuscular control of dynamic glenohumeral stability has been lost. The goal is to restore shoulder function through training and exercise. Patients with loose shoulders may not necessarily be unstable as evidenced by examination of the contralateral asymptomatic shoulder in patients with symptomatic multidirectional instability. The mainstay of treatment is nonoperative, with attempts to achieve stability by scapular and glenohumeral strengthening exercises. Those patients who have attempted a dedicated program of physical therapy, have functional problems, and remain unstable may then be candidates for surgical treatment.

Patients with a history of multidirectional instability who sustain fractures of the glenoid or humeral head with a dislocation generally require surgical treatment. In addition, significant defects in the humeral head associated with multiple dislocations consistent with Hill-Sachs lesions may require earlier surgical treatment. Glenoid erosion and lip fractures, if significant, can also necessitate surgical intervention if they are associated with recurrent instability.

Contraindications to surgical intervention may include patients with voluntary or habitual instability. In addition, patients who have not attempted a formal physiotherapy program should avoid initial surgical treatment. Furthermore, any patient unable or unwilling to comply with the postoperative rehabilitation regimen should not undergo surgical management.

Surgical Planning

Education of the patient is critical in planning surgical treatment for the individual with an unstable shoulder. The patients should have failed a trial of nonoperative treatment and have persistent instability with functional deficits. The goal of surgical treatment is to reduce capsular volume and to restore glenoid concavity with capsulolabral augmentation. By decreasing capsular volume, range of motion may be decreased as a result. It is important to discuss this possibility with the patient; some more active athletes, such as throwers, gymnasts, and volleyball players, may not tolerate losses of motion to maintain participation in their sport. Additional risks and benefits, including the risk of infection, recurrence of instability, pain, neurovascular injury, persistent functional limitations, and implant complication, should be discussed.

The surgical planning continues with the evaluation under anesthesia and diagnostic arthroscopy. This may alter the plan to include any combination of the following: capsular plication (anterior, posterior, or inferior), rotator interval closure, anterior-posterior labral repair, superior labral anterior-posterior (SLAP) repair, biceps tenodesis or tenotomy, and possible conversion to an open capsular shift.

Surgical Technique

Anesthesia and Positioning

The procedure can be performed under interscalene block or general endotracheal anesthesia with an interscalene block for postoperative pain control.

The patient is then placed in the lateral decubitus position with the affected shoulder positioned superior. An inflatable beanbag and kidney rests hold the patient in position. Pillows are placed to protect the peroneal nerve at the neck of the fibula on the down leg. An axillary roll is placed. The operating table is placed in a slight reverse-

Trendelenburg position. The full upper extremity is prepared to the level of the sternum anteriorly and the medial border of the scapula posteriorly. The operative shoulder is placed in 10 pounds of traction and positioned in 45 degrees of abduction and 20 degrees of forward flexion.

Alternatively, the beach chair position can be used. The head of the bed is raised to approximately 70 degrees with the affected shoulder off the side of the bed with support medial to the scapula. The head should be well supported and all bone prominences padded. The entire arm, shoulder, and trapezial region are prepared into the surgical field. We prefer the lateral decubitus position, which we believe provides an excellent view of the inferior and posterior capsular regions.

Landmarks and Portals

The bone landmarks, including the acromion, distal clavicle, acromioclavicular joint, and coracoid process, are demarcated with a marking pen. After preparation and draping, the glenohumeral joint is injected with 50 mL of sterile saline through an 18-gauge spinal needle to inflate the joint. A posterior portal is established 1 cm distal and 1 cm lateral to the standard posterior portal to allow access to the rim of the posterior glenoid for anchor placement in case a posterior labral or capsular repair is necessary. An anterior portal is then established at the level just superior to the subscapularis tendon lateral to the coracoid to place the most inferior and anterior anchor (5-o'clock portal). An additional anterior superior portal is not typically needed with the technique that we will describe.

Examination Under Anesthesia and Diagnostic Arthroscopy

The examination under anesthesia is performed on a firm surface with the scapula relatively fixed and the humeral head free to rotate. A load-and-shift maneuver, as described by Murrell and Warren, is performed with the patient supine. The arm is held in 90 degrees of abduction and neutral rotation while an anterior or posterior force is applied in an attempt to translate the humeral head over the anterior or posterior glenoid. A sulcus sign test is performed with the arm adducted and in neutral rotation to assess whether the instability has an inferior component. A 3+ sulcus sign that remains 2+ or greater in external rotation is considered pathognomonic for multidirectional instability. Testing is completed on both the affected and unaffected shoulders, and differences between the two are documented.

A diagnostic arthroscopy of the glenohumeral joint is then undertaken. The labrum, capsule, biceps tendon, subscapularis, rotator interval, rotator cuff, and articular surfaces are visualized in systematic fashion. This ensures that no associated lesions will be overlooked by poorly directed tunnel vision. Lesions typically seen in multidirectional instability include a patulous inferior capsule, labral fraying and splitting, widening of the rotator interval, and undersurface partial-thickness rotator cuff tears. After the glenohumeral joint is viewed from the posterior portal, the arthroscope is switched to the anterior portal to allow improved visualization of the posterior capsule and labrum. A switching stick can then be used in replacing the posterior cannula with an 8.25-mm distally threaded clear cannula (Arthrex, Inc., Naples, Fla), thus allowing passage of an arthroscopic probe and other instruments through the clear cannula to explore the posterior labrum for evidence of tears.

Specific Steps (Box 9-1)

1. **Preparation for Repair**

- The arthroscope then remains in the posterior portal, and the anterior portal serves as the working portal for the anterior repair (and vice versa for the posterior repair).

- An arthroscopic rasp or chisel is used to mobilize any torn labrum from the glenoid rim.

- A motorized synovial shaver or meniscal rasp is used to abrade the capsule adjacent to a labral tear and to débride and decorticate the glenoid rim to achieve a bleeding surface for capsular plication (Fig. 9-1).

2. **Multi-Pleated Plication**[15,16]

- A 3.0-mm Bio-Suture Tak anchor loaded with No. 2 FiberWire (Arthrex, Inc., Naples, Fla) is placed in the 5-o'clock position (right shoulder) for the anterior repair and in the 7-o'clock position for the posterior repair, and the sutures are brought out through the working portal (Fig. 9-2).

- A soft tissue penetrator (Spectrum suture hook, Linvatec, Largo, Fla) or crescent suture passer is passed through the labrum directly adjacent to the anchor, and the inferior FiberWire on the anchor is pulled through the labrum (Fig. 9-3).

Box 9-1 Surgical Steps

1. Preparation for repair: mobilization of torn labrum; abrasion of capsule; débridement and decortication of glenoid rim
2. Multi-pleated plication
3. Arthroscopic knot tying
4. Rotator interval closure
5. Posterior portal closure

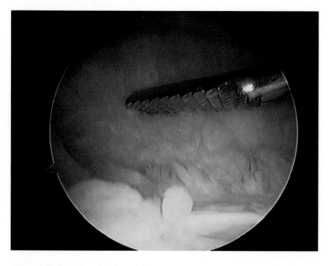

Figure 9-1 Capsular abrasion with a rasp.

- The penetrator is then used to pierce the inferior capsule in the most anterior inferior (5-o'clock anchor) and lateral point or posterior inferior (7-o'clock anchor) and lateral point.
- Once the capsule is pierced through, a No. 1 polydioxanone (PDS) suture (Ethicon, Inc., Somerville, NJ) is shuttled into the joint and the penetrator is removed (Fig. 9-4).
- A suture grasper is then used to grab both the passed PDS suture and the labral suture to pull them out of the working portal.
- The PDS suture is then tied with a simple knot to the FiberWire, and the PDS suture is then used to shuttle the working suture through the inferior tuck of capsule (Fig. 9-5).

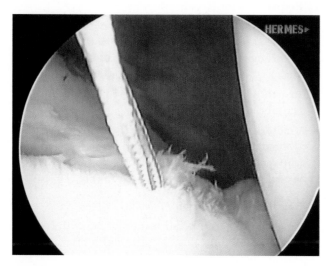

Figure 9-2 Placement of anchor on the rim of the glenoid.

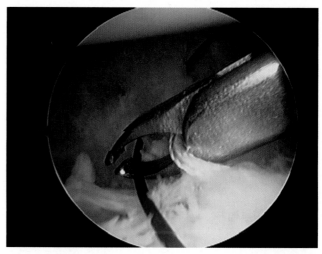

Figure 9-4 Passage of PDS suture into joint.

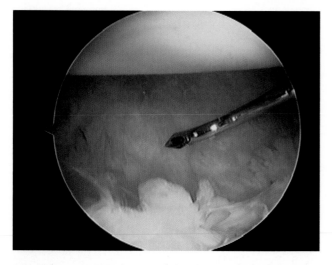

Figure 9-3 Passage of Spectrum suture passer in the capsular tissue and placement of No. 1 PDS suture.

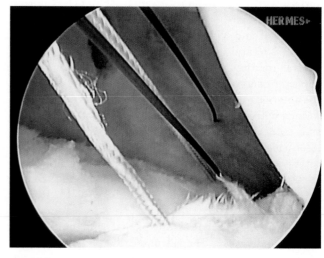

Figure 9-5 Shuttle of FiberWire suture through capsulolabral tissue.

- This simple process is repeated while moving superiorly up the capsule until adequate capsular tension is restored (Fig. 9-6).

- The suture is checked to ensure that it will still slide, then a sliding-locking knot backed with three half-hitches is tied; the remaining suture is then cut (Figs. 9-7 and 9-8).

- This is begun posteriorly and inferiorly (7-o'clock anchor), working posterior with additional anchors as necessary, and then anteriorly and inferiorly (5-o'clock anchor), working up anterior, again using additional anchors as necessary (Fig. 9-9).

- The completed multi-pleated capsular plication reduces volume and improves stability (Fig. 9-10).

3. Arthroscopic Knot Tying

- We prefer the sliding-locking Weston knot, but there are a number of arthroscopic knot-tying techniques that work well.

- What is most important is that the surgeon be familiar with the knot used and be skilled in its use.

- The posterior braided suture exiting through the capsule is threaded through a knot pusher, and the end is secured with a hemostat.

- This suture serves as the post, which in effect will advance the capsule and labrum to the glenoid rim when the knot is tightened.

- The knot should be secured posteriorly on the capsule and not on the rim of the glenoid to prevent humeral head abrasion from the knot.

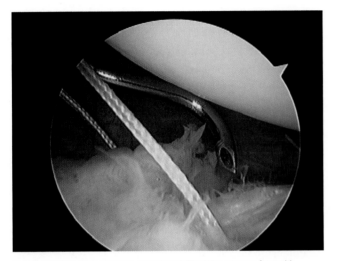

Figure 9-6 Repeated passage of PDS and FiberWire sutures for multi-pleated stitch.

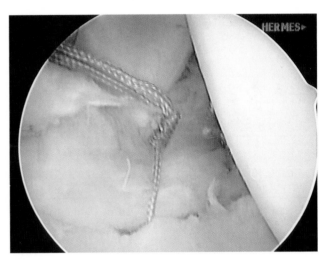

Figure 9-8 Completed tied knot after capsular plication.

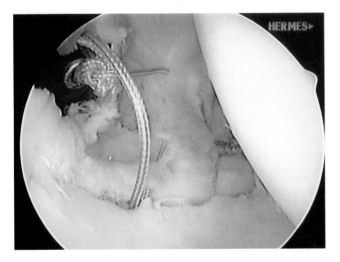

Figure 9-7 Tying of the multi-pleated stitch with an arthroscopic sliding-locking Weston knot.

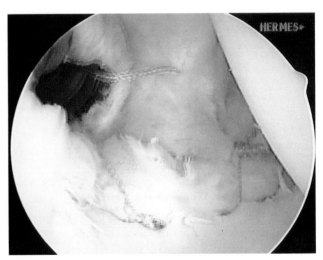

Figure 9-9 Completed plication with multiple anchors.

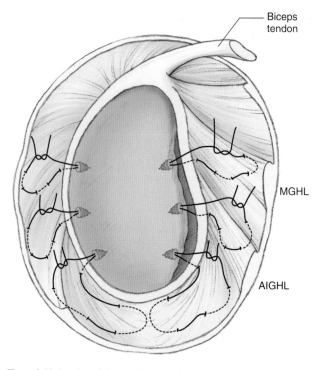

Figure 9-10 Drawing of the anterior multi-pleated plication. AIGHL, anterior inferior glenohumeral ligament; MGHL, middle glenohumeral ligament. (From Sekiya JK. Arthroscopic labral repair and capsular shift of the glenohumeral joint: technical pearls for a multi-pleated plication through a single working portal. Arthroscopy 2005;21:766.)

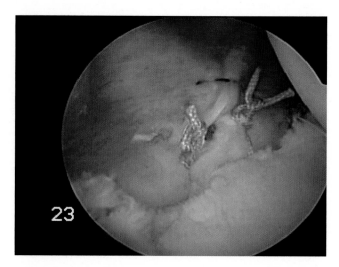

Figure 9-11 Closure of the posterior portal after capsular plication.

- Each half-hitch must be completely seated before the next half-hitch is thrown.
- Placing tension on the non-post suture and advancing the knot pusher "past point" will lock the Weston knot.
- A total of three alternating half-hitches are placed to secure the Weston knot.
- This knot has been found to be biomechanically similar to an open square knot.[4]

4. Rotator Interval Closure

- In this setting of multidirectional instability, the rotator interval may not require closure (defined by a 2+ or greater sulcus sign that does not improve in external rotation) if a multi-pleated repair is performed, plicating both the anterior and posterior bands of the inferior glenohumeral ligament and effectively bringing the entire inferior pouch superiorly.
- If rotator interval closure is required, it is viewed with the arthroscope in the posterior portal.
- A crescent suture passer is advanced from the anterior portal through the anterior capsule–middle glenohumeral ligament just above the superior border of the subscapularis tendon 1 cm lateral to the glenoid.

- It is then passed through the middle glenohumeral ligament at the inferior border of the rotator interval. This makes up the inferior aspect of the rotator interval closure.
- A No. 0 PDS suture is then fed into the joint and retrieved with a penetrator through the superior glenohumeral ligament.
- The PDS suture is then withdrawn out the anterior cannula and switched for a FiberWire suture; the knot is tied blindly in the cannula as the closure is visualized through the posterior portal.

5. Posterior Portal Closure

- A crescent suture passer is advanced from the posterior portal through the posterior capsule just above the superior border of the capsular opening of the posterior portal.
- A No. 0 PDS suture is then fed into the joint and retrieved with a penetrator through the inferior border of the capsular opening in the posterior portal.
- The PDS suture is then withdrawn out the posterior cannula and switched for a FiberWire suture; the knot is tied blindly in the cannula as the closure is visualized through the anterior portal (Fig. 9-11).

Postoperative Care

Follow-up

- The patient is discharged to home on the day of surgery.
- The sutures are removed 6 to 8 days later.

Rehabilitation

- The arm is immobilized in an UltraSling (DonJoy, Carlsbad, Calif) for 6 weeks.
- The arm is maintained in 30 degrees of abduction in neutral rotation.
- The sling is removed for bathing and for gentle pendulum and elbow, wrist, and hand range-of-motion exercises.
- Isometric exercises are started at week 3.
- Passive and active-assisted range of motion is started at week 3.
- Discontinue the sling at week 6.
- Active range of motion is begun at week 6.
- Sport-specific exercises are begun at 4 months.
- Begin overhead sports at 6 months.
- Return to contact sports at 6 to 8 months.

Complications

- Loss of motion
- Recurrence of instability
- Neurovascular injury
- Failure to address missed causes of instability: Large Hill-Sachs lesions that cause instability and

that are not addressed at surgery may lead to recurrence.

Results

Clinical Studies

The details of clinical studies of multidirectional shoulder instability repair are presented in Table 9-1.

PEARLS AND PITFALLS

- History and physical examination are vital.
- Radiographic studies are needed to rule out bony lesion.
- Operative treatment only after trial of rehabilitation.
- Surgical treatment to reduce capsular volume and repair any labral pathology.
- Examination under anesthesia to confirm multidirectional instability.
- Lateral decubitus position allows easier posterior capsular work.
- Bump placed in the axilla can provide a laterally directed force and significantly improve glenohumeral joint visualization, particulary inferiorly (Figure 9-12A-D).
- Technique for surgery = multi-pleated plication
- Underplication or failure to address bony pathology leads to recurrent instability
- Overplication causes loss of motion.

Return to sports at 6 months

Table 9-1 Clinical Studies of Multidirectional Shoulder Instability Repair

Author	Procedure Performed	Follow-up	Outcome
Duncan and Savoie[3] (1993)	Scope inferior capsular shift	1-3 years	100% satisfactory
Pagnani et al[14] (1996)	Scope stabilization by transglenoid sutures	Average: 4.6 years (range: 4-10 years)	74% good–excellent
McIntyre et al[11] (1997)	Scope capsular shift	Average: 34 months	95% good–excellent
Treacy et al[18] (1999)	Scope capsular shift	Average: 5 years	88% satisfactory
Gartsman et al[8] (2000)	Scope labral repair and laser capsulorrhaphy	Average: 33 months (range: 26-63 months)	92% good–excellent
Tauro[17] (2000)	Scope inferior capsular split and advancement	2-5 years	88% satisfactory
Fitzgerald et al[6] (2002)	Scope thermal capsulorrhaphy	Average: 3 years (range: 24-40 months)	76% satisfactory
Favorito et al[5] (2002)	Scope laser-assisted capsular shift	Average: 28 months	81.5% successful
Frostick et al[7] (2003)	Scope laser capsular shrinkage	Average: 26 months (range: 24-33 months)	83% satisfactory
D'Allesandro et al[2] (2004)	Scope thermal capsulorrhaphy	Average: 38 months (range: 2-5 years)	63% satisfactory

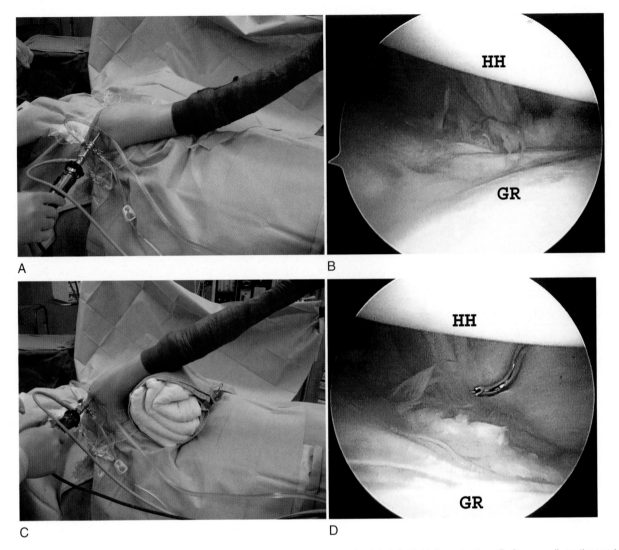

Figure 9-12A-D Placement of an axillary bump significantly improves arthroscopic visualization inferiorly. **A,** No bump in place. **B,** Corresponding arthroscopic view, anterior inferior. **C,** Axillary bump in place. Note the lateral translation of the humeral head. **D,** Significantly improved visualization anterior inferior allowing for precise placement of capsular plication stitches.

Table 9-2 In Vitro Capsular Volume Studies

Author	Type of Capsular Shift	Amount of Volume Reduction
Miller et al[12] (2003)	3 open (medial, lateral, vertical)	Medial: 37% Lateral: 50% Vertical: 40%
Karas et al[9] (2004)	3 arthroscopic (thermal, suture plication, combined)	Scope thermal: 33% Scope plication: 19% Scope combined: 41%
Victoroff et al[19] (2004)	Arthroscopic thermal	Scope thermal: 37%
Luke et al[10] (2004)	Open inferior vs. arthroscopic thermal	Open inferior: 50% Scope thermal: 30%
Cohen et al[1] (2005)	Open lateral vs. arthroscopic plication	Open lateral: 50% Scope plication: 23%
Sekiya et al[15] (2006)	Open inferior vs. arthroscopic multi-pleated plication	Open inferior: 45% Scope multi-pleated: 58%

In Vitro Capsular Volume Studies

During the last several years, multiple studies have investigated the effect of surgical intervention on capsular volume. Comparisons have been made between open capsular shifts with numerous techniques, arthroscopic thermal plication, and arthroscopic suture capsular plications by testing of capsular volume in cadaveric specimens before and after procedures. Table 9-2 summarizes the results and types of shifts performed in these studies.

References

1. Cohen SB, Wiley W, Goradia VK, et al. Anterior capsulorrhaphy: an in vitro comparison of volume reduction—arthroscopic plication versus open capsular shift. Arthroscopy 2005;21:659-664.
2. D'Alessandro DF, Bradley JP, Fleischli JE, Connor PM. Prospective evaluation of thermal capsulorrhaphy for shoulder instability: indications and results, two to five-year follow-up. Am J Sports Med 2004;32:21-33.
3. Duncan R, Savoie FH 3rd. Arthroscopic inferior capsular shift for multidirectional instability of the shoulder: a preliminary report. Arthroscopy 1993;9:24-27.
4. Elkousy HA, Sekiya JK, Stabile KJ, McMahon PJ. A biomechanical comparison of arthroscopic sliding and sliding-locking knots. Arthroscopy 2005;21:204-210.
5. Favorito PJ, Langenderfer MA, Colosimo AJ, et al. Arthroscopic laser-assisted capsular shift in the treatment of patients with multidirectional shoulder instability. Am J Sports Med 2002;30:322-328.
6. Fitzgerald BT, Watson BT, Lapoint JM. The use of thermal capsulorrhaphy in the treatment of multidirectional instability. J Shoulder Elbow Surg 2002;11:108-113.
7. Frostick SP, Sinopidis C, Al Maskari S, et al. Arthroscopic capsular shrinkage of the shoulder for the treatment of patients with multidirectional instability: minimum 2-year follow-up. Arthroscopy 2003;19:227-233.
8. Gartsman GM, Roddey TS, Hammerman SM. Arthroscopic treatment of anterior-inferior glenohumeral instability: two to five-year follow-up. J Bone Joint Surg Am 2000;82:991-1003.
9. Karas SG, Creighton RA, DeMorat GJ. Glenohumeral volume reduction in arthroscopic shoulder reconstruction: a cadaveric analysis of suture plication and thermal capsulorrhaphy. Arthroscopy 2004; 20:179-184.
10. Luke TA, Rovner AD, Karas SG, et al. Volumetric change in the shoulder capsule after open inferior capsular shift versus arthroscopic thermal capsular shrinkage: a cadaveric model. J Shoulder Elbow Surg 2004;13:146-149.
11. McIntyre LF, Caspari RB, Savoie FH 3rd. The arthroscopic treatment of multidirectional shoulder instability: two-year results of a multiple suture technique. Arthroscopy 1997;13:418-425.
12. Miller MD, Larsen KM, Luke T, et al. Anterior capsular shift volume reduction: an in vitro comparison of 3 techniques. J Shoulder Elbow Surg 2003;12:350-354.
13. Murrell GA, Warren RF. The surgical treatment of posterior shoulder instability. Clin Sports Med 1995;14:903.
14. Pagnani MJ, Warren RF, Altchek DW, et al. Arthroscopic shoulder stabilization using transglenoid sutures. A four-year minimum follow-up. Am J Sports Med 1996;24:459-467.
15. Sekiya JK, Willobee JA, Miller MD, et al. Arthroscopic multi-pleated capsular plication compared with open inferior capsular shift for multidirectional instability. Arthroscopy, in press.
16. Sekiya JK. Arthroscopic labral repair and capsular shift of the glenohumeral joint: technical pearls for a multiple pleated plication through a single working portal. Arthroscopy 2005;21:766.
17. Tauro JC. Arthroscopic inferior capsular split and advancement for anterior and inferior shoulder instability: technique and results at 2 to 5-year follow-up. Arthroscopy 2000;16:451-456.
18. Treacy SH, Savoie FH 3rd, Field LD. Arthroscopic treatment of multidirectional instability. J Shoulder Elbow Surg 1999;8: 345-350.
19. Victoroff BN, Deutsch A, Protomastro P, et al. The effect of radiofrequency thermal capsulorrhaphy on glenohumeral translation, rotation, and volume. J Shoulder Elbow Surg 2004;13:138-145.

9

CHAPTER 10

Arthroscopic Treatment of Internal Impingement

Matthew T. Boes, MD

Craig D. Morgan, MD

The term *internal impingement* was initially used by Walch[8] to describe contact of the undersurface of the rotator cuff with the posterior superior labrum in the abducted and externally rotated position. Jobe[5] described progressive internal impingement due to repetitive stretching of anterior capsular structures as the primary cause of shoulder pain in overhead athletes. Our treatment of disability in the throwing shoulder is predicated on the inciting lesion being an acquired contracture of the posteroinferior capsule.[2] The posteroinferior capsular contracture alters the biomechanics of the joint and leads to a progressive pathologic cascade observed in the disabled throwing shoulder.

Due to repetitive overuse, throwers are susceptible to the development of posterior shoulder muscle fatigue and weakness, including the scapular stabilizers and rotator cuff. Posterior muscle weakness leads to failure to counteract the deceleration force of the arm during the follow-through phase of throwing. In the healthy throwing shoulder, a glenohumeral distraction force of up to 1.5 times body weight is generated during the deceleration phase of the throwing motion. This distraction force is counteracted by violent contraction of the posterior shoulder musculature at ball release, which protects the glenohumeral joint from abnormal forces and prevents development of pathologic changes in response to these forces. In the presence of posterior muscle weakness, as seen initially in the disabled thrower, the distraction force becomes focused on the area of the posterior band of the inferior glenohumeral ligament (PIGHL) complex because of the position of the arm in forward flexion and adduction during the follow-through phase of throwing. Fibroblastic thickening and contracture of the PIGHL zone occur as a response to this distraction stress (Fig. 10-1A and B). PIGHL contracture causes a shift of the glenohumeral contact point posteriorly and superiorly in the abducted and externally rotated position[4] (Fig. 10-1C). This shift allows clearance of the greater tuberosity over the posterosuperior glenoid rim, enabling hyperexternal rotation (unlike normal internal impingement). In addition, the posterosuperior shift causes a relaxation of the anterior capsular structures, which manifests as anterior "pseudolaxity" and allows even further hyperexternal rotation around the new glenohumeral rotation point (Fig. 10-1D).

High-level throwing athletes need to achieve extreme external rotation of the humerus in the late cocking phase to maximize the throwing arc in order to generate maximal velocity at ball release. This maneuver creates an abnormal and posteriorly directed force vector on the superior labrum through the long head of the biceps tendon as well as torsion at the biceps anchor. With repetitive stress in the hyperexternally rotated position, the labrum fails and "peels back" from the glenoid rim medially along the posterior superior scapular neck. Failure of rotator cuff fibers in this position can occur through abrasion but, more important, due to twisting and shear failure, which is most pronounced on the articular side of the cuff tendons. Tension failure may ultimately occur in the anterior capsule, causing anterior instability that in our view is a tertiary event and has been erroneously identified as the primary lesion in the disabled thrower.

The collection of symptoms observed in the disabled throwing shoulder has been termed the *dead arm*

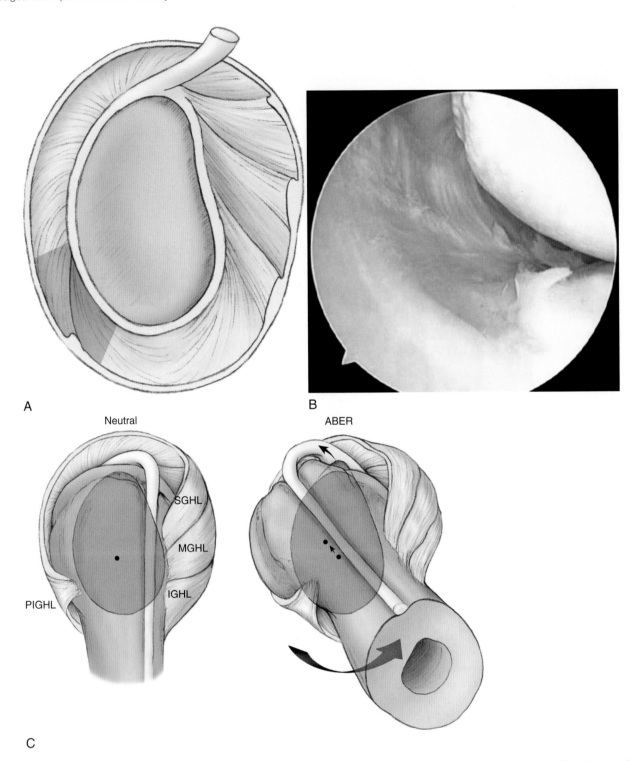

A

B

Neutral

ABER

SGHL

MGHL

IGHL

PIGHL

C

Figure 10-1 A, Diagram showing location of posterior inferior capsular contracture in the area of the PIGHL complex. **B,** Arthroscopic image from the posterior portal with the camera directed inferior to view posterior inferior capsular contracture. **C,** Diagram showing biomechanical effect of posterior inferior capsular contracture. In the abducted–externally rotated (ABER) position, the glenohumeral (GH) contact point is shifted posterosuperior, causing tension on the biceps anchor. IGHL, inferior glenohumeral ligament; MGHL, middle glenohumeral ligament; SGHL, superior glenohumeral ligament.

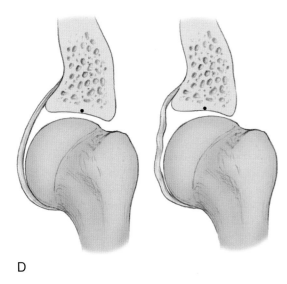

D

Figure 10-1, cont'd D, Diagram showing relative anterior laxity as a result of the posterosuperior shift of the glenohumeral contact point.

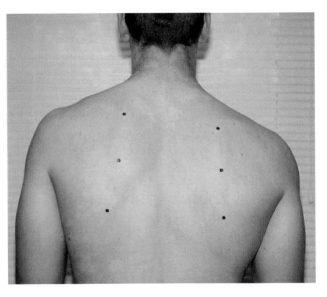

Figure 10-2 Right-hand dominant thrower with significant posterior scapular muscle weakness and resultant scapular asymmetry. Corresponding superior and inferior scapular angles and medial scapular border are marked for comparison.

syndrome. Essentially, the athlete is unable to throw with premorbid velocity and control because of pain and subjective discomfort in the shoulder. Five pathologic components contribute to symptoms in the dead arm syndrome:

1. Posterior muscle weakness, demonstrated by scapular asymmetry
2. PIGHL contracture, the inciting lesion; manifested as a glenohumeral internal rotation deficit (GIRD) in the throwing shoulder versus the nonthrowing shoulder
3. Superior labral anterior-posterior (SLAP) tear, type II, typically the anterior and posterior or posterior subtype (the "thrower's SLAP")[6]
4. Rotator cuff failure, generally partial undersurface and, occasionally, full-thickness tearing in the posterosuperior cuff; and
5. Anterior instability (anterior capsular attenuation or capsulolabral injury), in approximately 10% of cases.

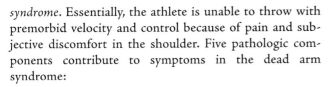

Preoperative Considerations

History

Typical History
- Vague "tightness" in the shoulder
- "Difficulty getting loose"
- Loss of throwing velocity over previous season

- Pain with throwing, particularly in late cocking phase, when the peel-back phenomenon occurs

Symptoms
- Pain, usually posterior superior; described as "deep" in the shoulder
- Mechanical symptoms: painful clicking and popping. These occur after actual injury to the superior labrum or the "SLAP event."

Physical Examination

Inspection
- Both exposed shoulder girdles are inspected from behind.
- Note asymmetry in both shoulder height and scapular position.
- The superior and inferior medial scapular angles are marked as a visual reference.
- Dropped position of the acromion and elevation of the inferomedial angle of the scapula from the chest wall signify scapular protraction and antetilt and are evidence of scapular muscle weakness (Fig. 10-2).

Palpation
- Posterosuperior joint line: superior labral pathology
- Coracoid: protraction of the scapula forces the coracoid into a more lateral position and places

tension on the pectoralis minor tendon, causing tenderness at its insertion.

- Superior scapular angle: scapula infera places tension on the levator scapula muscle insertion, causing similar tenderness.

Range of Motion

- Measurements are made in the supine position with the scapula stabilized by anterior pressure on the shoulder against the examining table. A goniometer is used with carpenter's level bubble chamber attached.
- The arm is abducted 90 degrees to the body, scapular plane; internal rotation and external rotation are measured from a vertical reference point (perpendicular to floor) (Fig. 10-3).
- The throwing shoulder is compared with the nonthrowing shoulder.
- Internal rotation, external rotation, total motion arc, and GIRD of the throwing shoulder versus the nonthrowing shoulder are recorded.

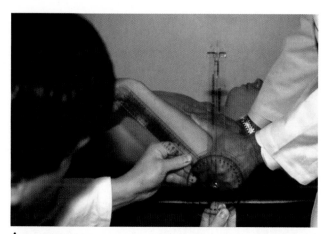

A

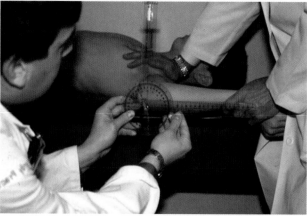

B

Figure 10-3 Measurement of glenohumeral rotation. The scapula is stabilized with posteriorly directed pressure by the examiner against the table to prevent scapulothoracic motion. True glenohumeral internal (**A**) and external (**B**) rotation is recorded from a vertical reference point.

Specificity of clinical tests for type II SLAP tears in these athletes has been determined.[6]

- Modified Jobe relocation test: specific for posterior SLAP lesions (the thrower's SLAP)
- Speed test and O'Brien test: specific for anterior SLAP tears

The Jobe relocation test is performed by placing the arm in maximal abduction and external rotation. Throwers with a posterior SLAP tear will experience pain in this position as a result of the unstable biceps anchor falling into the peel-back position. The discomfort is relieved with a posteriorly directed force to the front of the shoulder, which has been shown under direct arthroscopic visualization to reduce the labrum into the normal position.[1]

Factors Affecting Surgical Planning

- Patients with long-standing GIRD may require a selective posteroinferior quadrant capsulotomy. As outlined later, response to a period of focused internal rotation stretches determines the need for a posterior capsulotomy.
- Extreme hyperexternal rotation (>130 degrees) is associated with attenuation of anterior capsuloligamentous structures. This finding occurs in approximately 10% of all disabled throwers. Patients with this amount of scapular stabilized external rotation require anterior capsular suture plication. We do not perform thermal capsulorrhaphy.

Imaging

Radiographs

- Anteroposterior, scapular lateral, and axillary views to reveal bone abnormalities (e.g., Bennett lesion)

Magnetic Resonance Arthrography

- The intra-articular administration of contrast material allows better resolution of labral pathology and partial-thickness tearing of the rotator cuff.
- Abduction–external rotation views are best for visualization of undersurface rotator cuff tears in throwers.

Indications and Contraindications

Arthroscopic evaluation and treatment are indicated for throwing athletes who present with a history of pain and mechanical symptoms as described earlier with pathologic findings on magnetic resonance arthrography. Once the pathologic cascade has progressed to actual injury to labral and cuff structures, regaining premorbid function is not possible without surgical repair of these structures.

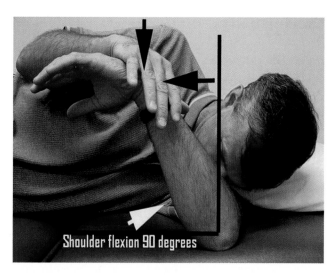

Figure 10-4 Glenohumeral internal rotation or sleeper stretches. The patient lies on the involved side to minimize scapulothoracic motion. The opposite hand provides steady internal rotation pressure.

Table 10-1 Recommended Instruments for Arthroscopic Treatment of Pathologic Processes in the Throwing Shoulder

Instrument	Use
Camera 30-degree lens	

Shoulder arthroscopy set
    (Arthrex)
    Arthroscopic rasp
    Arthroscopic elevator
	Labral detachment

Arthroscopic cannulas
    8 mm
    5 mm
	Anterior working portal
	Anterior accessory portal

Motorized shaver Full-radius blade (Stryker)	Débridement

Motorized burr
    Protective hood; SLAP bur
    (Stryker)
	Preparation of glenoid rim

Arthroscopic bovie
    Long handle, hook tip
    (Linvatec)
	Posterior capsulotomy

BioSuture Tak anchors (Arthrex) No. 1 PDS suture	Labral fixation SLAP fixation Free suture: capsular plication

Lasso suture passer device
    (Arthrex)
    Right-angled
	Suture passage: superior
	    labrum

BirdBeak suture retrievers
    (Arthrex)
    45-degree
    22-degree
	Suture passage
	
	Posterior superior labrum
	Anterior superior labrum

Suture passer set (e.g.,
    Spectrum)
    Straight
    45-degree curved hook
    (left and right)
	Suture passage
	
	Longitudinal rotator cuff tear
	Capsular plication

Patients start internal rotation "sleeper stretches" preoperatively for assessment of the extent of PIGHL contracture (Fig. 10-4). In general, 90% of patients with severe GIRD (>25 degrees) are able to decrease their internal rotation deficit to less than 20 degrees with 10 to 14 days of focused stretching. The remaining 10% are stretch "nonresponders" and are generally older athletes with long-standing GIRD and substantial thickening of the posteroinferior capsule. In these patients, a posteroinferior capsulotomy is indicated to increase internal rotation at the time of surgery.

Contraindications to the procedure are similar to those for other elective arthroscopic shoulder procedures, such as infection and concomitant medical illness.

Surgical Planning

Before the procedure is begun, it is important to have all anticipated instruments and materials needed for the surgery available and on the surgical field so that the procedure can be performed without unnecessary intraoperative delays (Table 10-1). Efficient performance of the procedure will avoid the dreaded scenario of attempting an arthroscopic repair in the distended, "watermelon" shoulder that can severely compromise the quality of the surgery. This cannot be overemphasized. As a general guideline, the type of repair described here should be accomplished in 20 to 40 minutes, depending on the associated pathologic processes. Superior labral tears in throwers may be associated with rotator cuff and anterior capsulolabral pathology. Treatment of these associated pathologic processes must be anticipated at the time of surgery.

Surgical Technique

Anesthesia and Positioning

Patients are administered general anesthesia after placement of an intrascalene nerve block that greatly assists with postoperative pain control.

We perform all arthroscopic repairs in the lateral decubitus position. Positioning is controlled with a beanbag brought to the level of the axilla. The operative extremity is secured in 30 to 40 degrees of abduction by a pulley device with 10 pounds hung to counterweight the arm. The patient is administered antibiotic prophylaxis for skin flora, and the skin is painted with povidone-iodine (Betadine).

Surgical Landmarks, Incisions, and Portals

Repairs in throwing athletes are performed through the following portals:

- Posterior: viewing portal
- Anterior: main working portal; anchor placement in anterior labrum, knot tying
- Posterolateral (portal of Wilmington): anchor placement and suture passage in posterior labrum (Fig. 10-5)
- Anterosuperior: accessory portal; viewing and suture passage in anterior labrum or capsule (depending on associated pathologic changes)

The posterolateral border of the acromion is marked, and a posterior portal is established approximately 2 cm medial and 2 or 3 cm inferior to the corner of the acromion. The blunt camera trocar is directed through the posterior capsule just above the level of the equator of the humeral head. Both the anterior portal and the portal of Wilmington are established by an outside-in technique with an 18-gauge spinal needle.

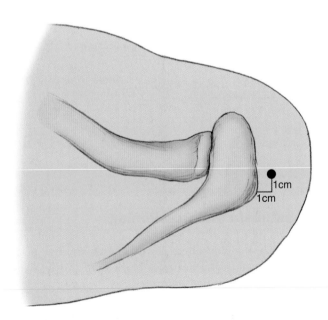

Figure 10-5 Diagram showing location for posterolateral portal or portal of Wilmington. A spinal needle is used for specific localization.

Examination

Diagnostic Arthroscopy and Surgical Tactic

Routine diagnostic arthroscopy is performed to ensure that all portions of the joint are inspected and no pathologic lesion is overlooked. In the disabled throwing shoulder, areas requiring particular attention include

- Superior labrum and biceps anchor
- Rotator cuff insertion
- Anterior labrum and capsuloligamentous structures
- Posterior capsule

Evidence of labral injury must be assessed carefully as findings may be subtle (Box 10-1). An assessment is quickly made of the pathologic areas to be addressed, and a plan is made for the completion of the repair (Box 10-2).

Provocative Tests

Drive-Through Sign

Before other cannulas or instruments are introduced, an assessment is made of laxity in the joint by testing for the drive-through sign. In a normal shoulder, capsular

Box 10-1 Arthroscopic Findings Consistent with Labral Injury or an Unstable Biceps Anchor

Labral Injury
- Frayed labral edge
- Adjacent capsular irritation
- Disruption of the smooth articular contour of the glenoid rim

Unstable Biceps Anchor
- Superior labral sulcus >5 mm
- Displaceable biceps root
- Positive peel-back test result
- Presence of drive-through sign

Box 10-2 Recommended Sequence for Arthroscopic Repairs in Throwing Shoulders with Multiple Pathologic Sites

1. Anterior inferior capsulolabral disruption (if present)
2. Posterior portion SLAP tear
3. Anterior portion SLAP tear
4. Anterior inferior capsular attenuation (if present)
5. PIGHL contracture (if present)
6. Rotator cuff tear (if present)

restraints prevent passage of the arthroscope from posterior to anterior at the midlevel of the humeral head or sweeping of the scope from superior to inferior along the anterior glenoid rim. The drive-through sign may be present in patients with a SLAP tear because of pseudolaxity from the loss of labral continuity around the glenoid rim.[7]

Peel-back Test

The peel-back test is performed by removing the arm from traction and placing it into the abducted and externally rotated position. With a posterior SLAP lesion, the labrum can be observed to fall medially along the glenoid neck during this maneuver (Fig. 10-6). Anterior SLAP lesions will have a negative result of the peel-back test. After assessment of the biceps anchor, the probe is used to assess the undersurface of the rotator cuff and to estimate depth of partial-thickness tears, to determine the stability of the

anterior inferior labrum, and to identify any redundancy in the anterior capsule.[3]

Specific Steps (Box 10-3)

1. Placement of Secondary Portals

An 8-mm cannula is used as a primary anterior working portal. An 18-gauge spinal needle is used to localize the cannula so that it can accommodate all necessary repairs, including anterosuperior anchor placement in the labrum and tying of posterosuperior anchor sutures. The cannula is readied near the skin surface, the spinal needle is used as a guide to the proper insertion angle, the spinal needle is withdrawn, and the cannula is inserted. An accessory 5-mm anterior portal may be placed, depending on the location of associated pathologic lesions requiring treatment.

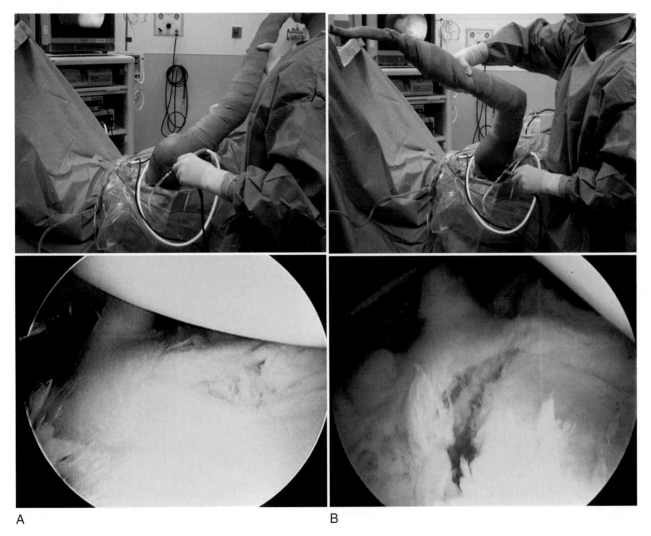

A   B

Figure 10-6 Photographs and corresponding arthroscopic views during dynamic peel-back test. **A,** The superior labrum is reduced in neutral position. **B,** When the shoulder is placed in abduction–external rotation, superior labral instability is revealed, with the labrum falling posteriorly and medially along the scapular neck.

Box 10-3 Surgical Steps

1. Placement of secondary portals
2. Probing of intra-articular structures
3. Intra-articular débridement
4. Preparation of superior labral bone bed
5. Anchor placement, suture passage, and knot tying
6. Dynamic assessment of repair
7. Treatment of associated pathology

2. Probing of Intra-Articular Structures

A probe is introduced in the anterior cannula for more careful assessment of stability of intra-articular structures. Normally, a sublabral sulcus with healthy-appearing articular cartilage can be seen extending up to 5 mm beneath the labrum. An unstable biceps root can easily be displaced with the probe medially along the glenoid neck[3] (Fig. 10-7; see also Box 10-1).

3. Intra-Articular Débridement

A full-radius blade motorized shaver is used to gently débride loose and frayed tissue to prevent snagging of tissue with joint motion or potential loose bodies.

4. Preparation of Superior Labral Bone Bed

An arthroscopic rasp is used to completely separate any remaining attachments in the injury area. A rasp is used because there is less risk of causing intra-substance injury in the labrum than with an elevator. On occasion, some

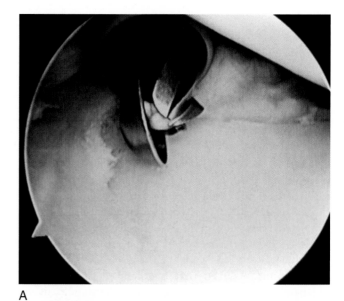

A

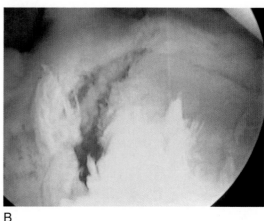

B

Figure 10-8 A and **B,** An arthroscopic burr with protective hood to prevent inadvertent damage to the labrum is used to remove a small amount of cortical bone on the superior glenoid to make a bleeding bone bed for subsequent repair.

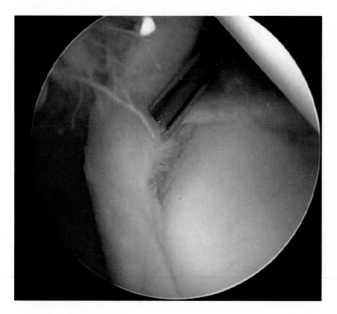

Figure 10-7 Superior labrum and biceps anchor are gently probed to identify evidence of injury or instability.

tenuous attachments from the labrum may be present medially, but the biceps anchor is still unstable. In these cases, we routinely complete the lesion by removing these loose attachments before repair. All loose soft tissue is removed from the repair site carefully with the shaver.

An arthroscopic burr is then used to remove cartilage along the superior glenoid rim to make a bleeding bone bed for labral repair (Fig. 10-8). This step is crucial to allow subsequent healing of the labrum back to the glenoid rim. We prefer a burr with a protective hood that is specifically designed to prevent damage to labral tissue during this step (SLAP burr-Stryker Endoscopy, San Jose, CA). No suction is used while the burr is on to ensure that tissue is not inadvertently sucked into the instrument.

5. Anchor Placement, Suture Passage, and Knot Tying

The portal of Wilmington is used for posterior anchor placement. Only small-diameter instruments are passed through this portal. No cannulas are placed in this portal to prevent damage to the rotator cuff tendons. A spinal needle again is used to localize the portal, which is approximately 1 cm anterior and 1 cm lateral to the posterolateral acromial margin (see Fig. 10-5). The angle of approach for the portal must provide for orientation of the anchor insertion device at 45 degrees to the glenoid rim to ensure solid anchor placement. We prefer to use a biodegradable, tap-in type anchor for superior labral repair (Bio-Suture Tak; Arthrex, Inc., Naples, Fla).

After skin incision, the Spear guide (3.5 mm; Arthrex) is brought into the joint through the portal of Wilmington as described previously for anterior cannula placement. The guide enters medial to the musculotendinous junction of the infraspinatus with minimal damage given its small diameter. The number of anchors to be placed is somewhat subjective but must be sufficient to neutralize peel-back forces.[3] The Spear guide is brought immediately onto the glenoid rim in the area of the previously prepared bone bed. The sharp obturator is removed after proper localization, and a hole is drilled for anchor insertion. The angle of approach of the Spear guide must be meticulously maintained during drilling and subsequent anchor placement to ensure adequate fixation in the bone. We insert anchors until the hilt of the anchor insertion handle abuts the handle of the Spear guide. Gentle twisting in line with the anchor is often needed to remove the insertion handle in dense bone (Fig. 10-9). The Spear guide is removed, and both ends of the suture are brought through the anterior cannula using a looped grasper instrument.

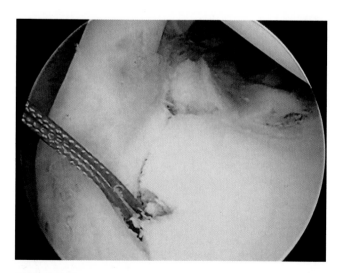

Figure 10-9 After localization with a spinal needle, the Spear guide is introduced into the shoulder through the portal of Wilmington for anchor placement on the posterior superior glenoid rim. The Spear guide is introduced into the joint medial to the rotator cable and in the muscular portion of the cuff. Because of its relatively small diameter (3.5 mm), this causes minimal damage to the rotator cuff.

For passage of a suture limb through the labrum, we use a small-diameter, pointed suture-passing device with a wire loop (Lasso Suture Passer; Arthrex). The passing device is brought through the portal of Wilmington without a cannula (again to minimize cuff damage) and into the joint through the muscle rent made by the Spear guide (Fig. 10-10A and B). The passer is brought through the labrum from superior to inferior, achieving a solid bite of labral tissue, and carefully advanced over the rim to the glenoid face. The wire loop is extended and brought out the anterior cannula (Fig. 10-10C). Next, the suture limb that is closest to the labrum at the anchor site is identified and passed through the wire loop outside the cannula. The wire loop and suture lasso are then carefully removed from the portal of Wilmington, and one of the suture limbs is brought through the labrum and out the portal (Fig. 10-11A). The suture limbs around the anchor are carefully observed as the suture is passed to ensure that no tangling has occurred. Next, the suture that has been passed through the labrum and is now out the portal of Wilmington is brought out the anterior cannula and becomes the post limb of the arthroscopic knot (Fig. 10-11B). Posterior anchors are tied through the anterior portal either medial or lateral to the biceps tendon. Additional suture anchors are placed posterior or anterior to the biceps anchor until it is secure. Posterior anchors are most easily placed through the portal of Wilmington as described before. Anterior anchors may be placed through the anterior cannula. Although we prefer the lasso suture passer for passing sutures, BirdBeak suture retrievers (Arthrex) may alternatively be used, depending on the surgeon's preference. The 45-degree BirdBeak is ideal for passing sutures in the posterior labrum through the anterior superior cannula; the 22-degree BirdBeak works well for the anterior labrum.

6. Dynamic Assessment of Repair

After labral repair, the peel-back and drive-through signs are again assessed to confirm that they are negative and that the pathologic process has been corrected. The peel-back maneuver can be performed for dynamic assessment of whether forces at the biceps anchor have been neutralized (Fig. 10-12). The drive-through sign is performed to assess for additional anterior laxity that may require correction by capsular plication techniques.

7. Treatment of Associated Disease

We generally perform a mini-plication in the anterior capsule when there is a persistent drive-through sign, evidence of anterior capsular tissue attenuation, or more than 130 degrees of external rotation in the 90-degree abducted position. The anterior capsular tissue to be plicated is first abraded with a rasp or "whisker" shaver. Capsular redundancy is then obliterated by suturing a lateral portion of the capsule to the glenoid labrum. The amount of tissue plicated depends on the amount of redundancy observed

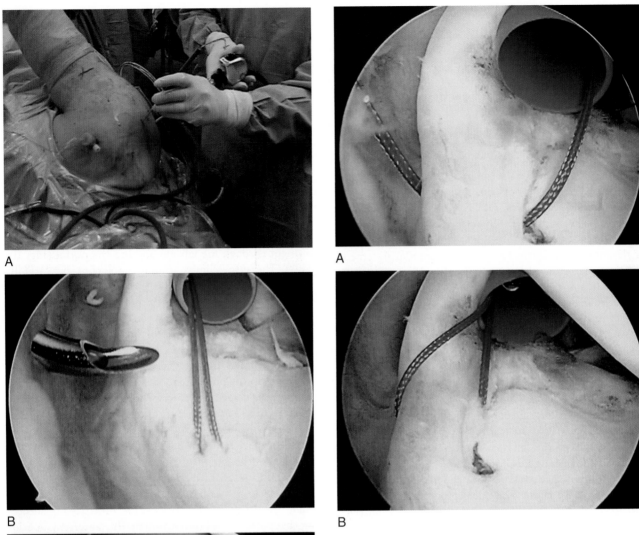

A

B

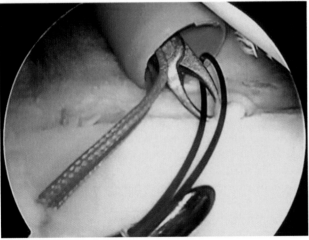

C

Figure 10-10 A and B, The right-angled suture-passing device, which is also small diameter, is brought along the same trajectory and through the same muscle rent made by the Spear guide. **C,** The superior margin to the labrum is pierced with the device, a firm bite of labral tissue is captured, and the pointed device is gently advanced onto the glenoid face. The wire loop is deployed and retrieved from the anterior cannula for passage of the labral post suture.

Figure 10-11 A, The wire loop is carefully retracted to pass a suture limb through the labrum and out the portal of Wilmington. **B,** A looped suture grasper is then used to retrieve this suture limb out the anterior cannula, where it becomes the post limb for the arthroscopic knot. To prevent "snagging" or capturing of the biceps tendon with suture, perform all passage, retrieval, and tying of sutures on one side of the biceps or the other.

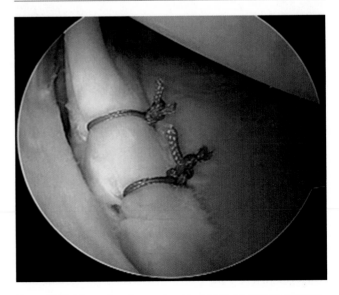

Figure 10-12 After anchor placement and knot tying, the dynamic peel-back maneuver is performed again to confirm stable fixation of the biceps anchor.

on arthroscopic examination (Fig. 10-13). Rarely, a discrete capsulolabral avulsion in the anteroinferior glenoid needs to be repaired as described elsewhere in this text.

A posteroinferior capsulotomy is performed in patients who are selective stretch nonresponders. The response to stretching is assessed preoperatively as outlined earlier. A posterior capsular release is rarely required as part of the treatment of the disabled throwing shoulder. However, for restoration of full motion, the procedure is indicated for patients who display little or no response to stretching. Arthroscopic findings consistent with a patho-logic posteroinferior capsular contracture include inferior recess restriction and a thickened PIGHL complex, which can be up to ½-inch thick in some cases (Fig. 10-14). Biopsy of the capsule in these cases reveals hypocellular and disorganized fibrous scar tissue similar in appearance to end-stage adhesive capsulitis.

Posteroinferior capsular release may be performed by one of two methods:

1. Scope in the anterior portal and instrumentation in the standard posterior portal; or

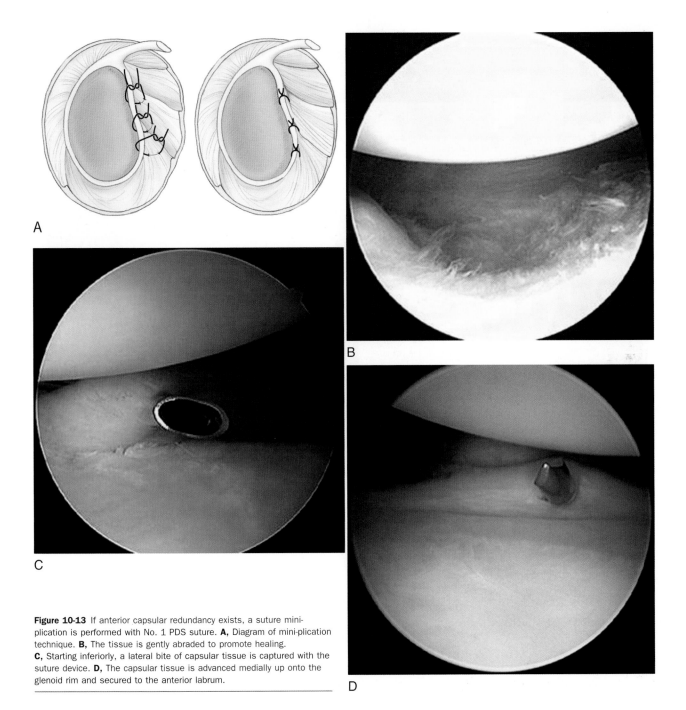

A

B

C

D

Figure 10-13 If anterior capsular redundancy exists, a suture mini-plication is performed with No. 1 PDS suture. **A,** Diagram of mini-plication technique. **B,** The tissue is gently abraded to promote healing. **C,** Starting inferiorly, a lateral bite of capsular tissue is captured with the suture device. **D,** The capsular tissue is advanced medially up onto the glenoid rim and secured to the anterior labrum.

10

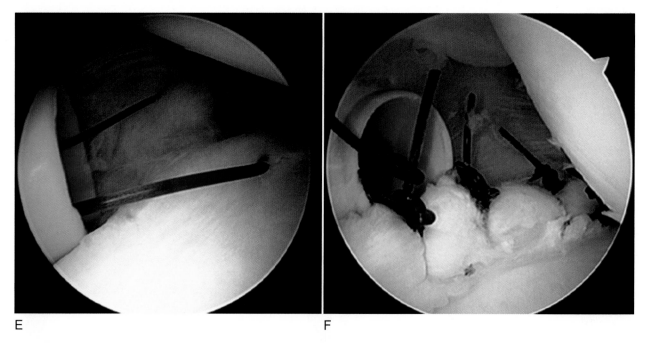

E   F

Figure 10-13, cont'd E, Once the suture is passed, the amount of capsular redundancy is assessed before knot tying, and adjustments are made as needed. **F,** Subsequent sutures are placed advancing superiorly along the anterior labrum until the anterior capsular redundancy is obliterated.

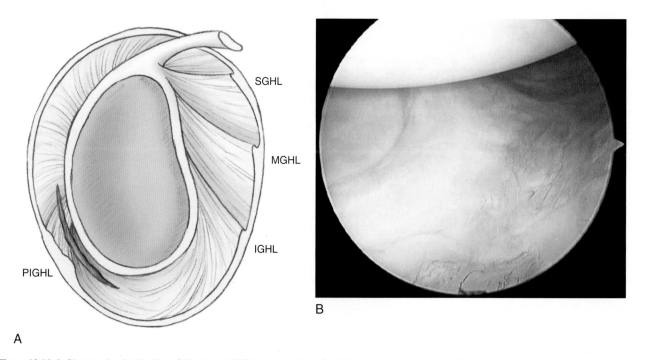

B

A

Figure 10-14 A, Diagram showing location of the posterior inferior capsulotomy. **B,** Arthroscopic photograph from the posterior portal with the camera directed inferiorly shows thickening around the PIGHL and inferior recess restriction.

2. Scope in the standard posterior portal and instrumentation in the posterosuperior portal (portal of Wilmington).

We prefer method 2 as it allows better direct visualization of the capsule during release.

The procedure is performed with electrocautery in a nonparalyzed patient. During the capsulotomy, any twitching of the shoulder musculature will alert the surgeon that the procedure is being performed too close to the axillary nerve, thus placing the nerve at risk for injury. If this occurs, the capsulotomy should be moved to a more superior or medial portion of the capsule or abandoned altogether if no safe zone can be found. A hooked-tip arthroscopic bovie (meniscal bovie; Linvatec, Largo, Fla) with a long shaft is used. The capsulotomy is full thickness and made ¼-inch peripheral to the labrum in the posterior inferior quadrant (6-o'clock to 3- or 9-o'clock). A sweeping technique is used to gently section progressively deeper layers of the capsule under direct visualization (Fig. 10-15). The capsulotomy typically results in a 50- to 60-degree increase in internal rotation immediately (Fig. 10-16).

Postoperative Considerations

Follow-up

All procedures are performed on an outpatient basis. Patients are typically seen 1 day after surgery for dressing change. At 1 week, sutures are removed, and self-directed range of motion is begun under specific guidelines. Patients are seen at regular intervals during the rehabilitation phase to monitor progress with motion and to advance therapy as appropriate.

10

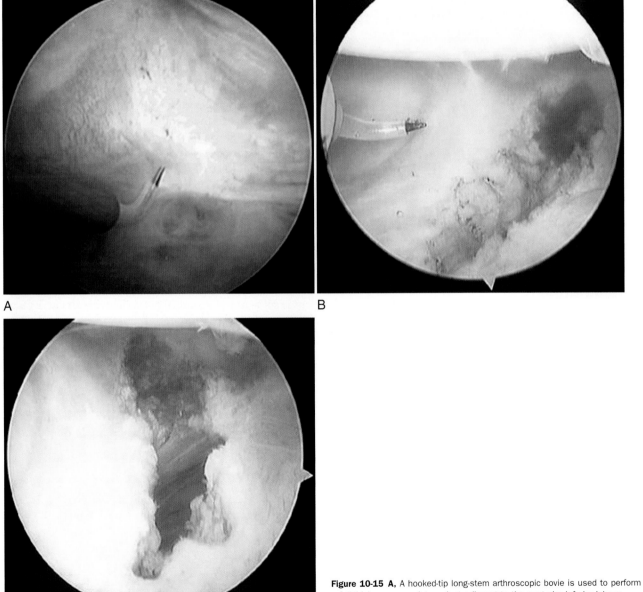

A

B

C

Figure 10-15 A, A hooked-tip long-stem arthroscopic bovie is used to perform a full-thickness capsulotomy just adjacent to the posterior inferior labrum. **B,** Gentle sweeping motions divide the capsule under direct vision. **C,** Completed posterior inferior capsulotomy.

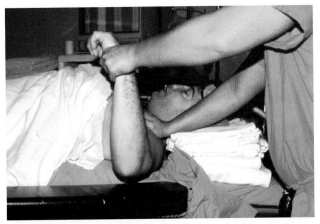

A

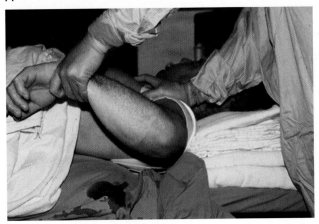

B

Figure 10-16 A, Preoperative internal rotation. **B,** Internal rotation immediately after posterior inferior capsulotomy. A gain of 50 to 60 degrees of internal rotation can be expected immediately intraoperatively.

Rehabilitation

- Immediate: Passive external rotation with arm at the side (not in abduction); flexion and extension of the elbow. Patients undergoing posterior inferior capsulotomy begin internal rotation sleeper stretches on postoperative day 1.
- Weeks 1 to 3: Pendulum exercises. Passive range of motion is begun with a pulley device in forward flexion and abduction to 90 degrees. Shoulder shrugs and scapular retraction exercises are begun in the sling. The sling is worn when the arm is not out for exercises.
- Weeks 3 to 6: The sling is discontinued after 3 weeks. Passive range of motion is advanced to full motion in all planes. Sleeper stretches are started in patients not undergoing capsulotomy.
- Weeks 6 to 16: Stretching and flexibility exercises are continued. Passive external rotation stretching in abduction is begun. Strengthening for rotator cuff, scapular stabilizers, and deltoid is initiated at 6 weeks.

Biceps strengthening is begun at 8 weeks. Continue daily sleeper stretches indefinitely.

- 4 months: Interval throwing program is started on level surface. Stretching and strengthening are continued with emphasis on posterior inferior capsular stretching.
- 6 months: Pitchers start throwing full-speed, depending on progression in interval throwing program. Continue daily sleeper stretches indefinitely.
- 7 months: Pitchers are allowed full-velocity throwing from the mound. Continue daily sleeper stretches indefinitely.

Complications

Complications are similar to those of other procedures involving arthroscopic shoulder reconstruction, including a rare incidence of infection, failed repair, painful adhesion formation, and stiffness. Physicians and therapists working with throwing athletes must be vigilant for the development of postoperative shoulder stiffness through regular follow-up and a directed therapy program. All athletes are instructed to continue daily internal rotation stretches indefinitely to prevent recurrence of the pathologic cascade that will place stress on the repair.

Results

In 182 baseball pitchers (one third professional, one third college, one third high-school) treated during an 8-year period, 92% resumed pitching at the preinjury performance level or better. UCLA scoring averaged 92% excellent results at 1 year and 87% excellent results at 3 years. Pitchers undergoing posteroinferior capsulotomy had an average GIRD reduction of 31 degrees at 6 months and 30 degrees at 2 years and an average increase in fastball velocity of 11 mph at 1 year after the procedure. Results of GIRD reduction for patients treated with SLAP repair with capsular stretching and SLAP repair with capsulotomy are shown with combined UCLA scores in Tables 10-2 to 10-4.

Table 10-2 GIRD reduction SLAP Repair with Posteroinferior Capsular Stretching*

	Preoperative	1 Year	2 Years
GIRD (average degrees)	46	13	15
TMA (throwing shoulder)	120	148	146
TMA (nonthrowing shoulder)	158	160	159

*In 164 baseball pitchers.
GIRD, glenohumeral internal rotation deficit; TMA, total motion arc.

Table 10-3 GIRD Reduction of SLAP Repair with Posterior Inferior Capsulotomy*

	Preoperative	1 Year	2 Years
GIRD (average degrees)	42	12	12
TMA (throwing shoulder)	114	147	147
TMA (nonthrowing shoulder)	158	160	157

*In 18 baseball pitchers.
GIRD, glenohumeral internal rotation deficit; TMA, total motion arc.

Table 10-4 UCLA Scores for Results of SLAP Repair with Capsular Stretching or Capsulotomy*

	1 Year (182)	2 Years (124)	3 Years (86)
Excellent	92%	90%	87%
Good	8%	10%	13%
Fair	0%	0%	0%
Poor	0%	0%	0%

*In 182 baseball pitchers.

10

PEARLS AND PITFALLS

Physical Examination

- The shoulder girdle must be stabilized against the examination table when GIRD measurements are made. Failure to do so will lead to erroneously high values because of scapulothoracic motion.

Positioning and Set-up

- The lateral decubitus position offers a better view of the superior labrum and approach for suture passage because gravity causes superior recess tissue to fall away.
- Repairs are done with use of a pressure device (set at 60 mm Hg) both to widen the field of view and to limit bleeding for better visualization. Significant distention of the soft tissues around the shoulder is possible and must be avoided as it makes manipulation of cannulas and instruments through the tissues difficult and can compromise the procedure.

Steps to Avoid Operating in the Distended Shoulder

- Have an efficient surgical tactic in place.
- Turn the pump off, if necessary, to pause.
- Make sure that cannulas stay in the joint once they are passed through the capsule.
- Have sufficient arthroscopic skill, including suture passage and knot tying.
- Work expeditiously.

Suture Anchors

- For SLAP repair, we now rethread anchors with No. 1 PDS suture, which is resorbable and avoids pain from prominent knots of permanent suture material, as has been our observation with knots in the superior labrum.

Suture Passage

- Tangling of the suture limbs can occur during suture passage and can make sliding of sutures difficult for knot tying. This problem is easily corrected when there is slack in the sutures, so pass the limbs slowly under careful observation to allow corrections.
- When a looped suture-passing device is employed, use one cannula for passing the device and another cannula to retrieve it and thread the suture; otherwise, tangling of sutures will occur. When both sutures are in a cannula that has the best angle of approach for suture passage, use a BirdBeak to penetrate the tissue and retrieve a suture through the same cannula to avoid tangling.
- Have an assistant hold and stabilize the cannulas during suture passage and shuttling or the cannulas will end up out of the joint.

Knot Tying

- Knots must be tied through cannulas (not percutaneously through tissue); otherwise, tissue will become stuck in the knot and prevent sliding and tightening.
- Multiple variations of knot tying are possible. It is important to be proficient with one sliding and one nonsliding knot. We prefer the Duncan loop with a two-hole knot pusher (Arthrex) as it is easily tied, and the two-hole knot pusher allows untwisting of knots during tying.

Peel-Back Test

- A spring-gated carabiner device can be used to link the arm holder with the pulley system so that the arm can be detached during the procedure for this maneuver.

References

1. Burkhart SS. Arthroscopically-observed dynamic pathoanatomy in the Jobe relocation test. Presented at the symposium on SLAP lesions, 18th open meeting of the American Shoulder and Elbow Surgeons; Dallas, Texas; February 16, 2002.
2. Burkhart SS, Morgan CD, Kibler WB. The disabled throwing shoulder: spectrum of pathology. Part I: Pathoanatomy and biomechanics. Arthroscopy 2003;19:404-420.
3. Burkhart SS, Morgan CD, Kibler WB. The disabled throwing shoulder: spectrum of pathology. Part II: Evaluation and treatment of SLAP lesions in throwers. Arthroscopy 2003;19:531-539.
4. Grossman MG, Tibone JE, McGarry MH, et al. A cadaveric model of the throwing shoulder: a possible etiology of superior labrum anterior-to-posterior lesions. J Bone Joint Surg Am 2005;87:824-831.
5. Jobe CM. Posterior superior glenoid impingement: expanded spectrum. Arthroscopy 1995;11:530-537.
6. Morgan CD, Burkhart SS, Palmeri M, et al. Type II SLAP lesions: three subtypes and their relationship to superior instability and rotator cuff tears. Arthroscopy 1998;14:553-565.
7. Panossian VR, Mihata T, Tibone JE, et al. Biomechanical analysis of isolated type II SLAP lesions and repair. J Shoulder Elbow Surg 2005;14:529-534.
8. Walch G, Boileau J, Noel E, et al. Impingement of the deep surface of the supraspinatus tendon on the posterior superior glenoid rim: an arthroscopic study. J Shoulder Elbow Surg 1992;1:238-243.

CHAPTER 11

Open Repair of Anterior Shoulder Instability

Michael J. Pagnani, MD

The shoulder is notable in that it has the greatest range of motion of all the joints in the human body. Bone restraints to motion are minimal. The surrounding soft tissue envelope is the primary stabilizer that maintains the humeral head on the glenoid.

The shoulder capsule is large, loose, and redundant to allow the large range of shoulder motion. There are three main ligaments in the anterior capsule that help prevent subluxation or dislocation. These ligaments are known as the superior glenohumeral ligament, the middle glenohumeral ligament, and the inferior glenohumeral ligament complex (IGHLC). Damage to the IGHLC, which supports the inferior part of the shoulder capsule like a hammock, is related to most cases of anterior instability. The Bankart lesion,[1] involving detachment of the IGHLC insertion on the glenoid, is the most common pathologic lesion associated with traumatic anterior instability (Fig. 11-1). Defects or injuries to the superior and middle glenohumeral ligaments may also contribute to instability.[9]

The primary goals of the surgical treatment of shoulder instability are to restore stability and to provide the patient with nearly full pain-free motion. Older techniques of shoulder stabilization tended to limit shoulder range of motion in exchange for providing stability. We now understand that it is probably more important to preserve motion than it is to stabilize the shoulder. Techniques that limit shoulder motion often lead to osteoarthritis, whereas it is unusual for recurrent dislocation itself to lead directly to osteoarthritis. As a result, any method of open stabilization should be designed to provide full functional use of the shoulder as well as normal stability.

Preoperative Considerations[8]

History

The diagnosis of an anterior dislocation is usually readily apparent. The patient typically gives a history of a specific injury in which the shoulder "popped out." In some cases, dislocation occurs with no history of significant trauma; these patients are frequently noted to have generalized ligamentous laxity and are less likely to demonstrate a Bankart lesion.

The diagnosis of anterior subluxation is often more subtle. The chief complaint may be a sense of movement, pain, or clicking with certain activities. Pain, rather than instability, may be the predominant complaint. In throwers and other overhead athletes, "dead arm" episodes may occur during which the patient experiences a sharp pain followed by loss of control of the extremity.[10]

Physical Examination

Apprehension tests are designed to induce anxiety and protective muscle contraction as the shoulder is brought into a position of instability. The anterior apprehension test is performed with the arm abducted and externally rotated. As the examiner progressively increases the degree of external rotation, the patient develops apprehension that the shoulder will slip out. This test result is uniformly positive in patients with anterior instability.

During the relocation test, the examiner's hand is placed over the anterior shoulder of the supine patient. A

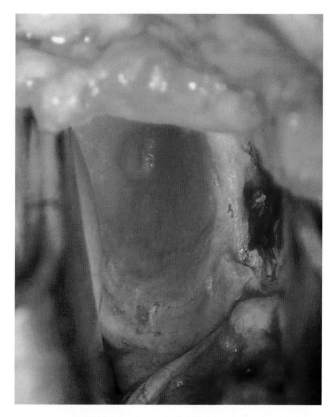

Figure 11-1 The Bankart lesion—detachment of the anteroinferior labrum and the IGHLC insertion from the glenoid.

imaging in determining labral disease is increased with arthrography. Because of the possibility of concomitant rotator cuff injury, magnetic resonance imaging should always be considered in older patients with instability—especially if strength and motion are slow to recover after an episode of dislocation.

Indications and Contraindications

The indications for surgical treatment of recurrent anterior shoulder instability are highly subjective. They include a desire of the patient to avoid recurrent problems with instability (including the necessity of reporting to the emergency department on a frequent basis to have the shoulder reduced), problems with recurrent pain, an inability to perform certain activities because of a fear of further shoulder instability, and the desire to improve athletic performance with improved shoulder stability. Failure of a thorough trial of nonoperative treatment is also an indication for surgical treatment.

There are several relative contraindications to performing a stabilization procedure by an arthroscopic method in patients in whom an operation is deemed advisable. Although there is controversy in this area, reported indications for open stabilization over arthroscopic stabilization include participation in a contact or collision sport, bone defects of the humeral head or glenoid, humeral avulsion of the glenohumeral ligaments, rupture of the subscapularis in association with a traumatic dislocation, failed open or arthroscopic repair, and atraumatic instability.

Contraindications to the open technique include voluntary instability and concomitant psychological issues. Large defects of the humeral head (Hill-Sachs lesions) or glenoid may require supplemental bone grafting to fill the defects.[2] I prefer to use arthroscopic methods of stabilization in throwing athletes. If an open method is used in this group, I recommend the technique of anterior capsulolabral reconstruction described by Jobe,[6] in which the subscapularis tendon is split rather than detached.

posteriorly directed force is applied with the hand to prevent anterior translation of the humeral head. The shoulder is then abducted and externally rotated as it is in the apprehension test. A positive result is obtained when this anterior pressure allows increased external rotation and diminishes associated pain and apprehension. The relocation test seems to be more reliable in overhead athletes, and the result may not be positive in all cases of anterior instability.

The belly press and liftoff tests should also be performed to confirm the integrity of the subscapularis tendon.

Imaging

Routine radiographic examination of the unstable shoulder includes an anteroposterior view (deviated 30 to 45 degrees from the sagittal plane to parallel the glenohumeral joint), a transscapular (Y) view, and an axillary view. In the assessment of more chronic instability, West Point and Stryker notch views are helpful in demonstrating bone lesions of the humeral head and glenoid.

Magnetic resonance imaging is not routinely performed in patients with instability because the findings are usually predictable; however, it may be helpful in preoperative planning. The accuracy of magnetic resonance

Surgical Technique[7]

The basic procedure for the open surgical treatment of recurrent anterior instability is a modification of the Bankart procedure[1] and involves repair of the anterior capsule and labrum to the glenoid. In most cases, the capsular ligaments are stretched as well as detached, and the procedure is also designed to remove any abnormal laxity.

Anesthesia and Positioning

The procedure is performed after placement of an interscalene block. In some cases, the block is supplemented with general anesthesia. The patient is positioned supine with the head of the operating table raised 15 to 30 degrees and the involved upper extremity abducted 45 degrees on an arm board. Folded sheets are placed beneath the elbow and taped to the arm board. The sheets maintain the arm in the coronal plane of the thorax and minimize extension of the shoulder.

The surgeon initially stands in the axilla. Two assistants are used. The first assistant's primary responsibilities are to control arm position and to keep the humeral head reduced during the capsular repair. The first assistant alternates position with the surgeon. When the surgeon is in the axilla, the first assistant stands lateral to the arm. When the surgeon moves to the lateral aspect of the arm, the first assistant shifts to the axilla. The first assistant also holds the humeral head retractor when it is in position. The second assistant stands on the opposite side of the table and holds the medial (glenoid) retractors. The use of a mechanized arm holder can free up the assistants' hands and may facilitate exposure.

Examination Under Anesthesia and Arthroscopic Evaluation

I routinely examine the shoulder under anesthesia to confirm the presence of abnormal anterior translation. Drawer tests are best performed in 90 degrees of abduction and neutral rotation where translation is greatest. Translation is graded 1+ if there is increased translation compared with the opposite shoulder but neither subluxation nor dislocation occurs. If the head can be subluxated over the glenoid rim but then spontaneously reduces, translation is graded 2+. Frank dislocation without spontaneous reduction constitutes 3+ translation.

I also routinely perform an arthroscopic examination of the shoulder in the beach chair position before open stabilization. The arthroscopic examination allows identification and treatment of concomitant injuries to the shoulder, including superior labral and rotator cuff disease that can be difficult to identify through an open approach. In addition, the examination is helpful in planning the specific method of capsular repair.

Specific Steps (Box 11-1)

The skin is incised along the anterior axillary crease (Fig. 11-2) in a longitudinal fashion along Langer's lines. The incision is placed lateral to the coracoid process. The deltopectoral interval is identified (Fig. 11-3), the cephalic vein is retracted laterally, and the interval is developed. The clavipectoral fascia is then incised at the lateral border of the conjoined tendon at its coracoid attachment, and the coracoacromial ligament is divided to facilitate exposure of

Box 11-1 Surgical Steps

1. Incision along the anterior axillary crease
2. Identification of the deltopectoral interval and cephalic vein
3. Takedown of the subscapularis tendon
4. Closure of the rotator interval
5. Horizontal capsulotomy
6. Exposure of Bankart lesion after placement of ring (Fukuda) retractor
7. Débridement of anterior glenoid neck to bleeding bone with a motorized bur
8. Repair of Bankart lesion with inferior capsular flap
9. Lateral T-plasty capsular shift in cases with pronounced capsular laxity
10. Reattachment of subscapularis tendon

11

the superior aspect of the capsule and, particularly, the rotator interval area.

Two self-retaining retractors are then placed in the wound (Fig. 11-4). Placement of these retractors frees the assistants to aid in arm position and shoulder reduction. At this point, the surgeon shifts position from the axilla and stands lateral to the arm. If a mechanized arm holder is used, it is attached to the forearm when the surgeon moves from the axilla.

The bicipital groove and the lesser tuberosity are identified. A vertical tenotomy of the subscapularis tendon is performed with electrocautery approximately 1 cm medial to its insertion on the lesser tuberosity (Fig. 11-5). The medial portion of the tendon is tagged with heavy No. 1 nonabsorbable braided polyester (Ethibond) sutures.

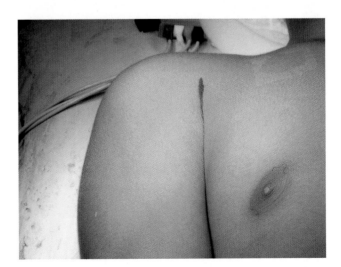

Figure 11-2 Incision along the anterior axillary crease.

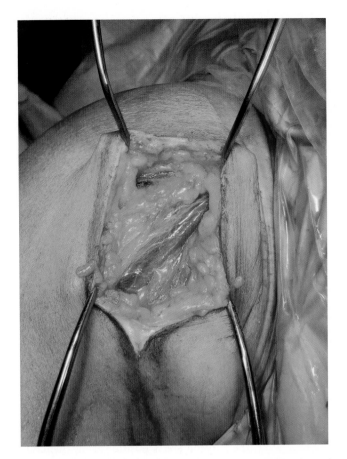

Figure 11-3 Identification of the deltopectoral interval and cephalic vein.

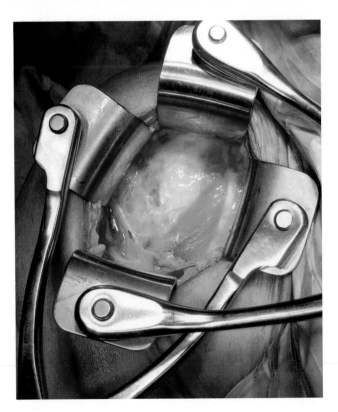

Figure 11-4 Placement of self-retaining retractors.

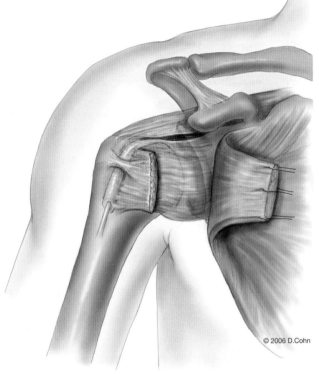

A

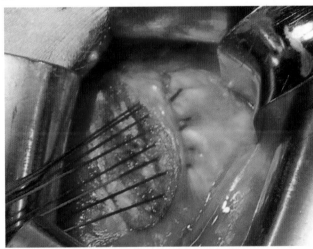

B

Figure 11-5 A and **B,** Takedown of the subscapularis tendon.

The interval between the anterior aspect of the capsule and the subscapularis tendon is then carefully developed with a combination of blunt and sharp dissection.

The laxity and quality of the capsule are then assessed. If there is a lesion in the rotator interval, it is generally closed at this point with No. 1 nonabsorbable braided polyester (Ethibond) sutures (Fig. 11-6). A transverse capsulotomy is then performed (Fig. 11-7), and a ring (Fukuda) retractor is placed intra-articularly. The anterior glenoid neck is explored for evidence of a Bankart lesion. The joint is then irrigated to remove any residual loose bodies.

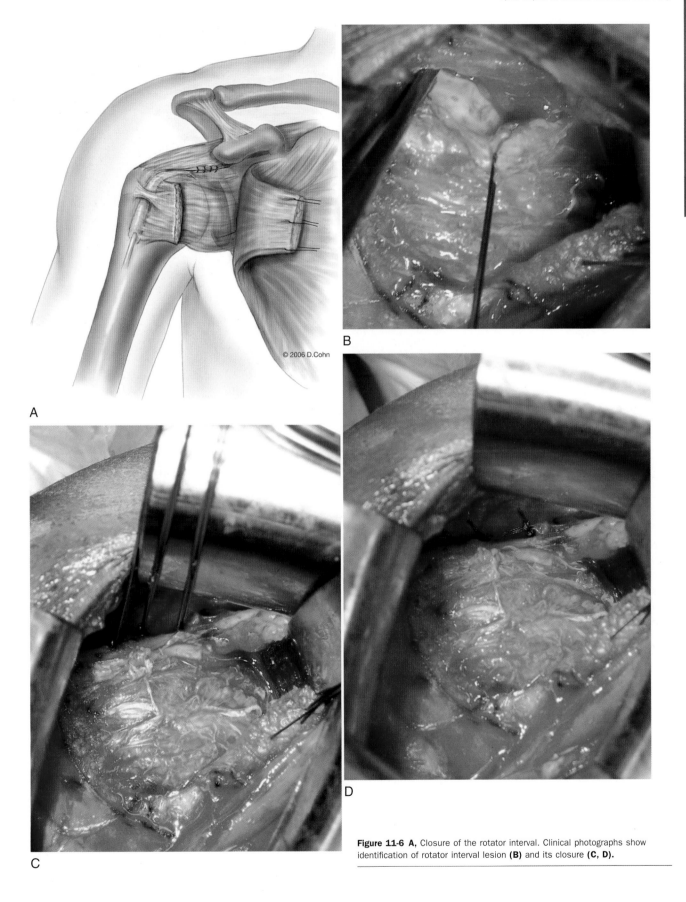

© 2006 D.Cohn

A

B

C

D

Figure 11-6 A, Closure of the rotator interval. Clinical photographs show identification of rotator interval lesion **(B)** and its closure **(C, D).**

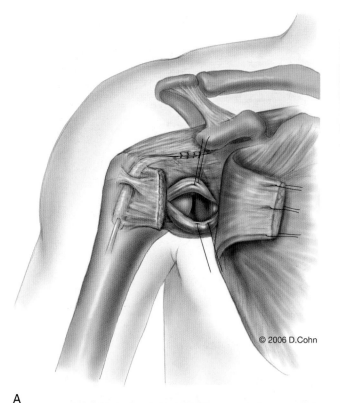

A

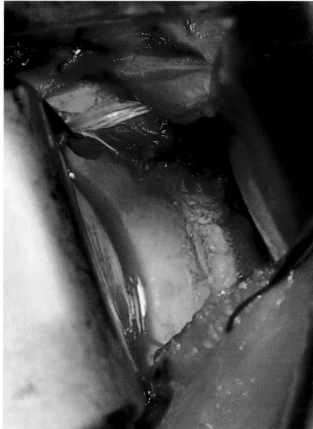

Figure 11-8 Exposure of Bankart lesion after placement of ring (Fukuda) retractor.

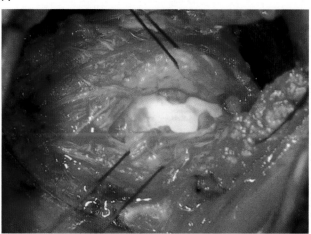

B

Figure 11-7 A and **B,** Horizontal capsulotomy.

If a Bankart lesion is noted, the capsulolabral separation at the anteroinferior glenoid neck is extended medially with use of an elevator or knife to allow placement of a retractor along the glenoid neck (Fig. 11-8). The glenoid neck is then roughened with an osteotome or motorized bur to provide a bleeding surface (Fig. 11-9). Two or three suture anchors are placed in the anteroinferior glenoid neck near but not on the articular margin of the glenoid (Fig. 11-10). The arm is placed in 45 degrees of abduction and 45 degrees of external rotation. The inferior capsular flap is then mobilized slightly medially and

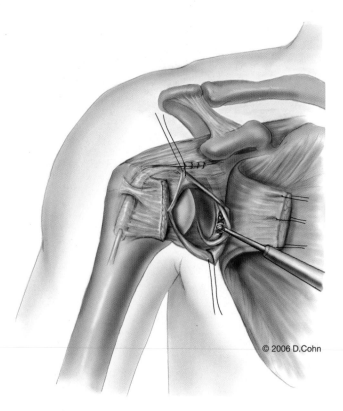

Figure 11-9 Anterior glenoid neck is débrided to bleeding bone with a motorized bur.

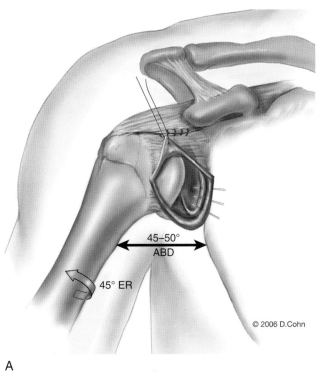

A

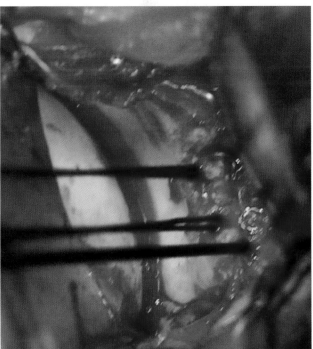

B

Figure 11-10 A and **B,** Placement of suture anchors. ABD, abduction; ER, external rotation.

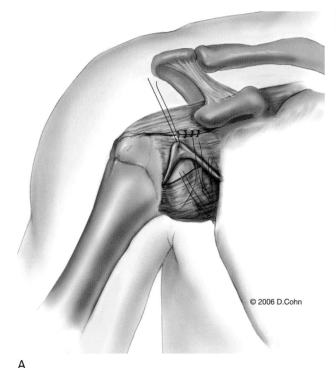

A

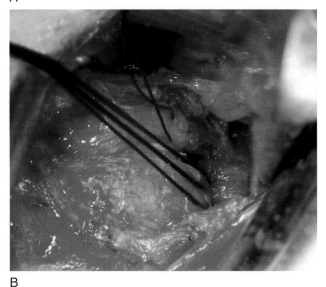

B

Figure 11-11 A and **B,** Inferior capsular flap is used to repair Bankart lesion.

superiorly. The inferior flap is reattached to the anterior aspect of the glenoid to repair the Bankart lesion with use of the suture anchors (Fig. 11-11). The goal is not to reduce external rotation but to obliterate excess capsular volume and to restore the competency of the IGHLC at its glenoid insertion.

After repair of the Bankart lesion (or in the absence of a Bankart lesion), an anterior capsulorrhaphy is performed to eliminate excess capsular laxity. The arm is maintained in 45 degrees of abduction and 45 degrees of external rotation, and the superior and inferior capsular flaps are reapproximated with forceps. The shoulder is held in a reduced position. If the capsular flaps can be overlapped, the capsule is shifted to eliminate excess capsular volume: if there is 5 mm (or less) of overlap, the capsule is imbricated by shifting the superior flap over the inferior flap and passing the sutures a second time through the superior flap (Fig. 11-12); with more than 5 mm of capsular overlap, the capsulotomy is extended in a vertical direction near its lateral insertion on the humeral neck, and a T-plasty capsular shift is performed (Fig. 11-13). The inferior capsular flap is shifted superolaterally, and the superior flap is moved over the inferior flap in an infero-lateral direction. The transverse portion of the capsulotomy is then closed.

After the capsule has been addressed satisfactorily, the subscapularis is reapproximated, but not shortened,

with nonabsorbable suture (Fig. 11-14). The deltopectoral interval is loosely closed with absorbable suture. Routine wound closure is then performed.

Postoperative Considerations

Rehabilitation

The standard rehabilitation protocol is described in Box 11-2. Special situations are noted at the end of Box 11-2.

Complications

Recurrent instability is the greatest concern after any stabilization procedure. Subcutaneous hematoma formation is the most common complication in my experience (1.5% of cases). If a hematoma forms, it may be observed as long as the wound is not draining. When the hematoma causes persistent wound drainage, surgical evacuation is recommended.

Subscapularis rupture has been reported after open anterior stabilization. Although I have no experience with subscapularis rupture in this setting, I recommend meticulous reapproximation of the tendon and restriction of external rotation for 3 months postoperatively as prophylactic measures to prevent its occurrence.

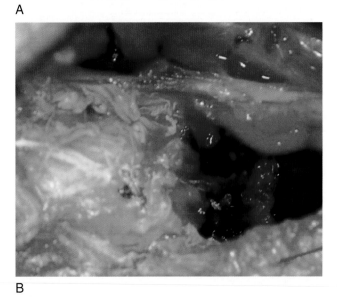

A

B

Figure 11-12 A and **B,** Sutures are passed a second time through the superior capsular flap to double the thickness of the repair and to eliminate excess capsular laxity.

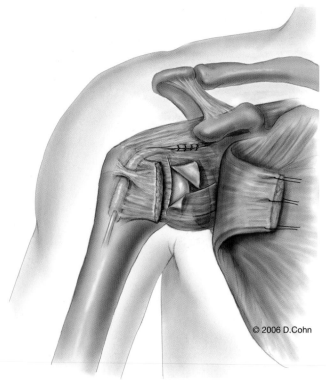

Figure 11-13 Lateral T-plasty capsular shift in cases with pronounced capsular laxity.

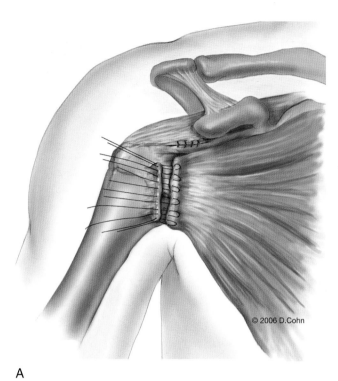

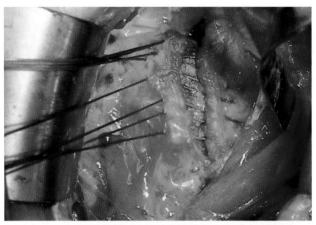

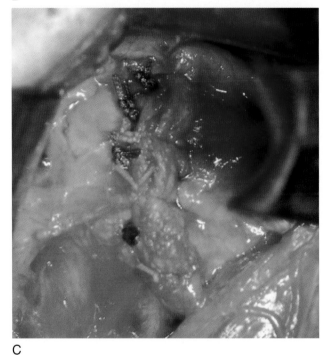

Figure 11-14 A, Reattachment of subscapularis tendon. **B** and **C,** Clinical photographs demonstrate subscapularis reapproximation.

© 2006 D.Cohn

A

B

C

PEARLS AND PITFALLS

- For optimal cosmesis, mark the skin incision in the preoperative holding area by having the patient internally rotate the shoulder. Identify the skin crease extending from the axilla to a point inferior and 1 to 2 cm lateral to the coracoid. Use this crease for your incision.

- Dissect medial to the cephalic vein in developing the deltopectoral interval because branches to the vein enter laterally.

- Use two self-retaining retractors to free your assistants. I prefer the Kolbel self-retaining shoulder retractor with detachable blades (Link America for Waldermar Link, Hamburg, Germany). I use the retractors so that the convex side faces the wound. Blades of an appropriate depth are then attached. The first retractor spreads the wound from medial to lateral. The second retractor is placed so that its base enters from the medial side to spread the wound from inferior to superior. In general, a deeper blade is placed inferiorly than superiorly.

- Avoid overzealous retraction on the conjoined tendon that attaches to the coracoid to prevent injury to the musculocutaneous nerve.

- Make sure that the subscapularis is not tenotomized too far laterally. If you go too far laterally, there will not be a stump to sew back to at closure.

- Externally rotate the shoulder as you take down the inferior aspect of the subscapularis to protect the axillary nerve. Expect to encounter branches of the anterior humeral circumflex artery in this area and be prepared to ligate or coagulate them.

- Pay attention to arm position in tensioning of the capsule. Remind the assistant to keep the arm at the 45-45 position for a standard repair.

- Make sure the assistant has the humeral head reduced in the glenoid when tying your capsular sutures. If the shoulder is not reduced, the capsule will not appose the glenoid neck.

- Be meticulous in closing the subscapularis. Consider use of modified Kessler or Mason-Allen sutures for added strength.

Box 11-2 Standardized Postoperative Rehabilitation Protocol

- Weeks 0-4: Sling immobilization is maintained with the shoulder in internal rotation. Pendulum exercises and elbow range of motion are begun. Shoulder shrugs are started for scapular rotators.

- Weeks 4-8: Passive and active-assisted shoulder range of motion is begun. Limit external rotation to 45 degrees. When 140 degrees of active forward flexion is obtained, begin rotator cuff strengthening (internal and external rotation cuff strengthening with arm at low abduction angles).

- Weeks 8-12: Limit external rotation to 45 degrees. Begin deltoid isometrics with arm at low abduction levels and Bodyblade exercises. If no impingement or rotator cuff symptoms are noted, slowly increase abduction during rotator cuff and deltoid strengthening. Scapular rotator strengthening: press-ups (seated dips), horizontal abduction exercises, open-can exercises.

- Weeks 12-18: Restore terminal external rotation; proprioceptive neuromuscular feedback patterns; plyometric exercises; sport-specific motion with use of pulley, wand, or manual resistance.

- Weeks 18-22: Conventional weight training. Orient for return to sport (progress from field drills to contact drills). Obtain abduction harness, when appropriate, based on the sport and position. Return to full contact when abduction and rotation strength are symmetric on manual muscle testing.

Special Situations

Throwers
- Perform capsular repair at 60 degrees of external rotation.
- Try to get 60 degrees of external rotation by 8 weeks.
- Begin throwing program at 6 months.

Atraumatic instability
- Immobilize for 6 weeks instead of 4 weeks.

Older than 40 years
- Immobilize for 3 weeks instead of 4 weeks.

From Pagnani MJ, Galinat BJ, Warren RF. Glenohumeral instability. In DeLee JC, Drez D, eds. Orthopaedic Sports Medicine. Philadelphia, WB Saunders, 1994:580-622.

Table 11-1 Results of Open Stabilization

Author	N	Recurrence Rate
Cole et al[3] (2000)	24	9%
Gill et al[4] (1997)	60	5%
Hubbell et al[5] (2004)	20	0%
Pagnani and Dome[7] (2002)	58	3%
Uhorchak et al[11] (2000)	66	22%
Wirth et al[12] (1996)	142	3%

Results

The published recurrence rates after open stabilization for anterior instability have generally been low, ranging from 0% to 10% in most series (Table 11-1). However, one report from West Point described a failure rate of 22% in active cadets, indicating that results are not uniformly and predictably good.[11] The outcome of open stabilization in contact athletes appears to be superior to that reported in similar populations with arthroscopic techniques.[5,7] The reported motion loss with current open techniques is also acceptable; in my experience, 84% of patients regained all or nearly all of their motion. No patient lost more than 15 degrees of external rotation compared with the contralateral side. Finally, when the incision is placed in the anterior axillary crease, the cosmetic result is usually satisfactory (Fig. 11-15).

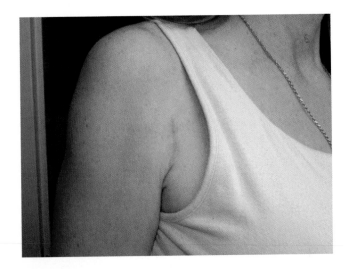

Figure 11-15 Typical cosmetic result.

References

1. Bankart ASB. The pathology and treatment of recurrent dislocation of the shoulder-joint. Br J Surg 1938;26:23-29.
2. Chen AL, Hunt SA, Hawkins RJ, Zuckerman JD. Management of bone loss associated with recurrent anterior glenohumeral instability. Am J Sports Med 2005;33:912-925.
3. Cole BJ, L'Insalata J, Irrgang J, Warner JJP. Comparison of arthroscopic and open anterior shoulder stabilization: a two to six-year follow-up study. J Bone Joint Surg Am 2000;82:1108-1114.
4. Gill TJ, Micheli LJ, Gebhard F, Binder C. Bankart repair for anterior instability of the shoulder. Long-term outcome. J Bone Joint Surg Am 1997;79:850-857.
5. Hubbell JD, Ahmad S, Bezenoff LS, et al. Comparison of shoulder stabilization using arthroscopic transglenoid sutures versus open capsulolabral repairs: a 5-year minimum follow-up. Am J Sports Med 2004;32:650-654.
6. Jobe FW, Giangarra CE, Kvitne RS, Glousman RE. Anterocapsulolabral reconstruction of the shoulder in athletes in overhead sports. Am J Sports Med 1991;19:428-434.
7. Pagnani MJ, Dome DC. Surgical treatment of traumatic anterior shoulder instability in American football players: two- to-six year follow-up in fifty-eight athletes. J Bone Joint Surg Am 2002;84:711-715.
8. Pagnani, MJ, Galinat BJ, Warren RF. Glenohumeral Instability In DeLee JC, Drez D, eds. Orthopaedic Sports Medicine. Philadelphia, WB Saunders, 1994:580-622.
9. Pagnani MJ, Warren RF. Stabilizers of the glenohumeral joint. J Shoulder Elbow Surg 1994;3:173-190
10. Rowe CR, Zarins B. Recurrent transient subluxation of the shoulder. J Bone Joint Surg Am 1981;63:863-872.
11. Uhorchak JM, Arciero RA, Huggard D, Taylor DC. Recurrent shoulder instability after open reconstruction in athletes involved in collision and contact sports. Am J Sports Med 2000;28:794-799.
12. Wirth MA, Blatter G, Rockwood CA Jr. The capsular imbrication procedure for recurrent anterior instability of the shoulder. J Bone Joint Surg Am 1996;78:246-260.

11

CHAPTER 12

Open Repair of Posterior Shoulder Instability

Mark K. Bowen, MD

James P. Sieradzki, MD

Recurrent posterior instability of the glenohumeral joint is less common than anterior instability or multidirectional instability. In most series, isolated posterior instability represents less than 5% of shoulder instability. In some cases in which the posterior instability is primary, there may be a component of inferior laxity. In this chapter, we discuss the clinical syndrome that occurs with recurrent episodes of posterior subluxation. This is distinct from the diagnosis and treatment of acute or fixed (missed) dislocation, which is not discussed in this chapter. The etiology of recurrent subluxation can be direct or indirect macrotrauma, repetitive microtrauma, or atraumatic in association with some generalized ligamentous laxity. The pathologic cause of this condition is unclear and has been attributed to excessive humeral retrotorsion, increased glenoid retroversion, thin and patulous posterior capsule, or decreased tension in the posterior band of the inferior glenohumeral ligament. Increasing evidence suggests that this condition is related to a deficiency of ligamentous-capsular restraints and not to the bony architecture.

Symptoms consist of pain, especially when the shoulder is axially loaded or positioned in forward flexion, adduction, and internal rotation. First-line treatment is physical therapy to develop a stable scapular platform combined with rotator cuff strengthening. Conservative treatment has been most successful in persons with atraumatic causes; surgery is often necessary for traumatic causes. Several open and arthroscopic techniques have been described to treat persistent, symptomatic posterior instability.

Preoperative Considerations

History

A detailed history is mandatory. This includes the injury mechanism, if present; the position of the arm when it is symptomatic; repetitive stresses on the shoulder; the presence of voluntary instability; and previous interventions. In some series, age older than 35 years and previous shoulder surgery, particularly thermal capsulorrhaphy, portended a poorer prognosis with surgical intervention.

Typical History

- The patient is in the second or third decade, with shoulder pain secondary to identifiable trauma or repetitive microtrauma from overhead athletics (particularly tennis, baseball, and swimming).
- Pain or instability is re-created with the arm positioned in an adducted, flexed, and internally rotated position.
- Question the patient about the voluntary ability to "shift" the shoulder in and out of the joint.

Physical Examination

Factors Affecting Surgical Indication

- Preserved range of motion and muscle strength with occasional loss of internal rotation

- Posterior load and shift test grade 2+ to 3+
- Sulcus sign no higher than grade 1
- Anterior translation no higher than grade 1
- Posterior load and shift test reproduces symptoms
- Voluntary "positional" subluxation demonstrated with adduction, flexion, and internal rotation

Imaging

Radiography

- Instability series including anteroposterior with internal rotation, axillary lateral, scapular Y, and Stryker notch views

Other Modalities

- Computed tomographic scan to evaluate glenoid version
- Magnetic resonance arthrography to evaluate posterior capsule and labrum

Indications and Contraindications

This procedure should be considered in a young patient with isolated posterior instability for whom an adequate trial course of physical therapy has failed. The ideal patient has a traumatic cause of the condition and will not have evidence of significant inferior or anterior instability, previous surgery, or degenerative changes. The ability to voluntarily sublux the shoulder by positioning the arm flexed, adducted, and internally rotated and to reduce it with a clunk as the arm is extended does not preclude surgical treatment. However, patients who voluntarily posterior sublux the shoulder with the arm at the side by selective muscle activation should be regarded with caution before proceeding with surgery. Excessive glenoid retroversion is not a contraindication but may affect surgical planning.

Contraindications are few, and most are not absolute. They include multidirectional instability with significant generalized ligamentous laxity and failed previous posterior stabilization. Patients with a psychiatric history, voluntary subluxation, and secondary gain should be avoided.

Surgical Planning

Issues to be considered at the time of surgery include a confirmatory examination under anesthesia and complete arthroscopic examination to evaluate the shoulder for both related and unrelated pathologic processes. The primary direction of instability should be determined on the basis of the patient's history and physical examination findings. The examination under anesthesia should be confirmatory, and rarely should the approach to the instability be changed on the basis of the findings on examination at the time of surgery. The arthroscopic examination will determine whether the posterior labrum will need to be repaired as part of the open stabilization. It may also disclose other anterior or superior labral pathologic processes that might be best treated at that time by arthroscopic repair.

Surgical Technique

Anesthesia and Positioning

This procedure should be performed under a general anesthetic. Regional anesthesia (interscalene block with C4 coverage) may be helpful with postoperative pain management. Positioning for arthroscopy is subject to the surgeon's preference; both the lateral decubitus and beach chair positions are acceptable. Open stabilization can be performed in the beach chair position, but the exposure can be problematic and requires excellent assistance with retraction for adequate visualization, especially in a muscular shoulder. The "floppy" lateral decubitus position with the arm draped free allows easier retraction and manipulation of arm position during the surgical procedure.

Surgical Landmarks and Incisions

Landmarks

- Acromion
- Axillary crease
- Glenohumeral joint
- Posterolateral corner of scapula
- Posterior portal for shoulder arthroscopy centered over the glenohumeral joint

Structures at Risk

- Approach: axillary nerve, posterior humeral circumflex vessels inferior to teres minor
- Capsulotomy: suprascapular nerve, medial to posterior labrum

Examination Under Anesthesia and Diagnostic Arthroscopy

Before positioning of the patient, it is critical to examine both shoulders under anesthesia to assess asymmetry of range of motion and glenohumeral translation. The examination should confirm grade 2 to 3+ posterior translation with limited anterior and inferior translations.

Diagnostic arthroscopy is helpful to evaluate the glenohumeral joint for other intra-articular pathologic changes, including labral tears, rotator cuff injuries, chondral injuries, biceps tendon or anchor tears, and loose bodies.

Specific Steps (Box 12-1)

1. Diagnostic Arthroscopy

Diagnostic arthroscopy evaluates the status of the posterior labrum to determine the need for incorporation of an open labral repair versus capsulorrhaphy only. Other labral pathologic processes (anterior or superior) that are found may be repaired arthroscopically at that time. The rotator cuff, biceps tendon, and articular cartilage may also be evaluated and treated as appropriate.

2. Exposure

A vertically oriented skin incision is planned, centered over the glenohumeral joint (Fig. 12-1). The incision extends from the acromion to the axillary crease and may be shortened with increased experience with the approach. The posterior portal from diagnostic arthroscopy can be incorporated into the middle of the incision. Mentally and visually, the dissection is a direct extension of this portal. The orientation of the deltoid muscle fibers is defined and its fascia split in line with the fibers (Fig. 12-2). The location of the deltoid split is directly over the glenohumeral joint determined by palpation of the joint between the surgeon's thumb posteriorly and long finger anteriorly. Development of the interval in the deltoid exposes the fascia over the infraspinatus and teres minor. The center of the joint is again reassessed by manual palpation. A yellow fat stripe in the infraspinatus muscle is a frequently visible and reliable plane to explore. The overlying fascia is opened horizontally, and a dissection plane is made through infraspinatus muscle (Fig. 12-3). Alternatively, dissection can proceed through the infraspinatus–teres minor interval, but more caution is necessary not to dissect inferior to the teres minor because of the proximity of the axillary nerve.

At this point, it is critical to expose the entire posterior capsule, particularly inferiorly and laterally, where the infraspinatus is most adherent to the capsule. Patient, blunt dissection, deep right-angled retractors, and good assistants are helpful at this stage (Fig. 12-4). Dissection should be limited to 1 cm medial of the glenoid to avoid injury to the suprascapular nerve.

12

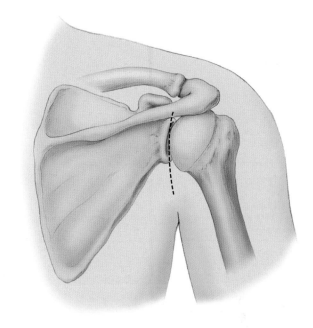

Figure 12-1 Vertical incision over glenohumeral joint.

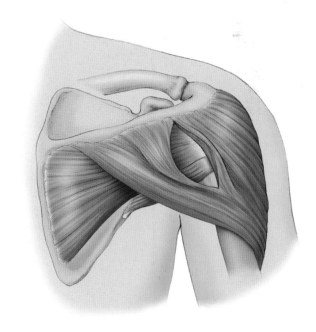

Figure 12-2 Deltoid split in line with fibers.

Box 12-1 Surgical Steps

1. Diagnostic arthroscopy
2. Exposure
3. Capsulotomy
4. Capsulorrhaphy
5. Augmentation (if needed)
6. Closure

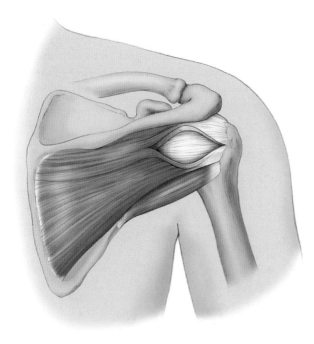

Figure 12-3 Horizontal split through infraspinatus in line with fibers; avoid unnecessary inferior dissection.

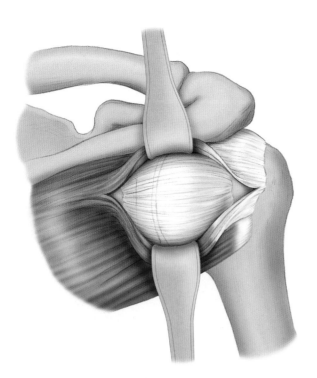

Figure 12-4 Complete exposure of inferior and lateral capsule by blunt dissection and retraction.

3. Capsulotomy

Once the capsule is completely defined, a horizontal incision centered over the middle of the joint is made from the glenoid extending laterally. A vertical incision is made just lateral to the capsular attachment to the glenoid to make a T-shaped pattern and two mobile flaps of capsule (Fig. 12-5). Complete mobilization of the inferior and superior flaps permits successful capsulorrhaphy (Fig. 12-6).

4. Capsulorrhaphy

A humeral head retractor is used to investigate the posterior aspect of the glenohumeral joint. The condition of the

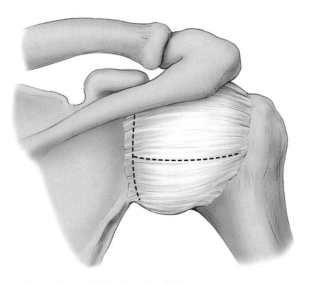

Figure 12-5 T-shaped incision based medially.

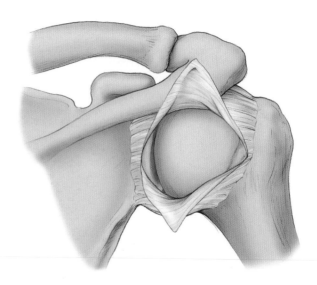

Figure 12-6 Complete mobilization of inferior and superior flaps for proper capsulorrhaphy.

posterior labrum can be difficult to visualize directly and is more accurately confirmed by prior arthroscopy. If the labrum is detached, suture anchors are placed under the labrum, on the posterior glenoid articular margin after débridement and roughening with a rasp or bur (Fig. 12-7). The sutures are placed through the labrum for repair in situ, and these sutures are tied and then used for the medial repair in the capsulorrhaphy. If the labrum is intact, nonabsorbable sutures can be placed through the labrum for repair of the capsule. The medial-based capsular shift is performed with the arm in 20 degrees of abduction and neutral rotation. The inferior flap is first advanced superiorly (Fig. 12-8), and then the superior flap is shifted inferiorly, overlapping the inferior flap (Fig. 12-9). Excessive capsular redundancy is eliminated by imbricating the horizontal capsulotomy during closure or by making a second vertical incision laterally for an H-type repair (Figs. 12-10 and 12-11).

5. Augmentation

In the case of severe capsule deficiency, revision surgery, glenoid hypoplasia, or excessive glenoid retroversion, it may be necessary to augment the repair. Soft tissue augmentation is accomplished by vertically incising the infraspinatus at the level of the glenoid and securing it to the capsule and glenoid with use of the previously placed capsule repair sutures. Rarely, an extracapsular posterior bone block can be added for cases of glenoid deficiency or at revision when repaired capsule tissue is deficient. A

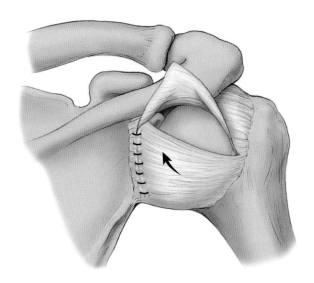

Figure 12-8 Inferior capsular flap is mobilized superiorly first.

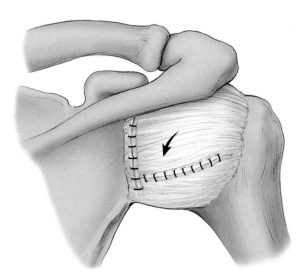

Figure 12-9 Repair is completed with inferior shift of the superior capsular flap.

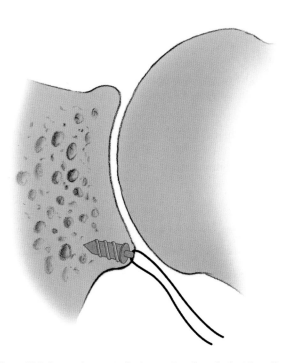

Figure 12-7 Proper placement of suture anchor, if required, at the articular margin.

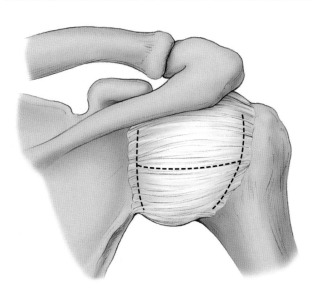

Figure 12-10 H-type incision for excessive capsular laxity.

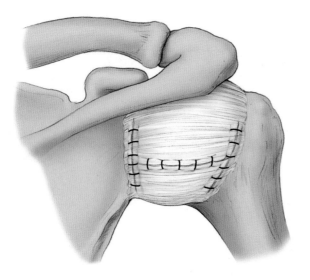

Figure 12-11 Completed H-type repair.

---

tricortical graft 4 × 2.5 cm may be harvested from the scapular spine. The graft and glenoid neck are predrilled before capsular repair to ensure accurate placement. It is placed on the posteroinferior quadrant to increase glenoid depth without impinging on the humeral head. In addition, there are several reports of opening wedge glenoid osteotomy for excessive glenoid retroversion. This is usually reserved for patients with severe instability and glenoid retroversion of more than 10 degrees as determined by computed tomographic scan.

6. Closure

Typically, sutures are not necessary in the infraspinatus split or deltoid fascia. The skin incision is closed in a standard fashion.

SURGICAL PEARLS

- Diagnosis is established by a history suggestive of trauma, arm position, findings of posterior instability on physical examination, and a confirmatory examination under anesthesia.
- Diagnostic arthroscopy evaluates status of the glenoid labrum and any other associated or concomitant pathologic processes.
- The lateral decubitus position and an approach centered over the glenohumeral joint ensure successful exposure of the posterior capsule.
- Consider a muscle-splitting approach through the deltoid and the infraspinatus as deep extension of the posterior arthroscopy portal.
- Expose the capsule completely by developing a plane between muscle and capsule, particularly inferior and lateral.
- Repair the posterior labral tear and shift the capsule sufficiently to remove capsule laxity and restore stability.

Postoperative Considerations

Bracing

- The arm is immediately placed in immobilization in an orthosis that maintains slight abduction, neutral rotation, and neutral flexion-extension. This is maintained for 4 weeks.
- The arm is maintained at neutral rotation for time out of the brace. Passive abduction in neutral rotation, in the plane of the scapula, is allowed.
- Sling protection is continued for weeks 5 and 6.

Rehabilitation

- After week 6, begin active and passive range of motion without stretching internal rotation.
- Goal for range of motion: 90% by 12 weeks.
- Progressive resistance and strengthening exercises for the scapula and rotator cuff are begun and progressed as tolerated.
- Sport-specific and functional exercises are added when sufficient strength is restored.

Complications

- Recurrent instability
- Injury to axillary nerve or posterior humeral circumflex vessels
- Injury to suprascapular nerve and vessels
- Overtightening of glenohumeral joint resulting in decreased range of motion and arthrofibrosis
- Infection
- Intra-articular fracture, nonunion, degenerative arthritis, and osteonecrosis of the glenoid are risks unique to glenoid osteotomy.

Results

Good to excellent results can be achieved in 75% to 90% of patients after most open procedures for isolated posterior instability. Results demonstrate minimal, acceptable decrease in range of motion, dramatic decrease in pain and instability, low rates of recurrence of instability, and ability to return to sport in many cases (Table 12-1).

Table 12-1 Clinical Results of Open Posterior Stabilization Procedures

Author	Follow-up	Procedure	Outcome	Recurrent Instability
Shin et al[8] (2005)	3.9-year mean	Posterior capsular shift 8/17 posterior labral repair through bone tunnels	13/17 (76%) good–excellent	2/17 (11%)
Misamore and Facibene[6] (2000)	45-month mean	Posterior capsular shift 1/14 posterior labral repair with anchor	13/14 (92%) excellent	1/14 (8%)
Fuchs et al[4] (2000)	7.6-year mean	Posterior capsular shift 7/26 posterior labral repair with anchor 3/26 glenoid osteotomy 1/26 posterior bone block	24/26 (92%) good–excellent	6/26 (23%)
Bottoni et al[2] (2005)	40-month mean	Posterior capsular shift	11/12 (91%) good–excellent	0
Rhee et al[7] (2005)	30-month mean	Posterior capsular shift	25/30 (83%) good–excellent	4/30 (13%)
Bigliani et al[1] (1995)	5-year mean	Posterior capsular shift	12/13 (92) good–excellent	NA
Tibone and Ting[9] (1990)	5-year mean	Staple capsulorrhaphy	11/20 (55%) acceptable	6/20 (30%)
Hawkins and Janda[5] (1996)	44-month mean	Posterior capsular shift 1/14 posterior labral repair with suture anchor	13/14 (93%) satisfactory	1/14 (7%)
Bowen et al[3] (1991)	5-year mean	Posterior capsular shift 7/26 with bone block	92% good–excellent	3/26 (12%)
Wolf et al[10] (2005)	7.6-year mean	Variety of posterior capsular plication procedures	32/44 (72%) good–excellent, including 11 patients with multidirectional instability	4/32 (13%)

12

References

1. Bigliani LU, Pollock RG, McIlveen SJ, et al. Shift of the posteroinferior aspect of the capsule for recurrent posterior glenohumeral instability. J Bone Surg Am 1995;77:1101-1120.
2. Bottoni CR, Franks BR, Moore JH, et al. Operative stabilization of posterior shoulder instability. Am J Sports Med 2005;33:996-1003.
3. Bowen MK, Warren FR, O'Brien SJ, Altchek DW. Posterior subluxation of the glenohumeral joint treated by posterior stabilization. Orthop Trans 1991;15:764-765.
4. Fuchs B, Jost B, Gerber C. Posterior-inferior capsular shift for the treatment of recurrent, voluntary posterior subluxation of the shoulder. J Bone Joint Surg Am 2000;82:16-25.
5. Hawkins RJ, Janda DH. Posterior instability of the glenohumeral joint: a technique of repair. Am J Sports Med 1996;24:275-278.
6. Misamore GW, Facibene WA. Posterior capsulorrhaphy for the treatment of traumatic recurrent posterior subluxations of the shoulder in athletes. J Shoulder Elbow Surg 2000;9:403-408.
7. Rhee YG, Lee DH, Lim CT. Posterior capsulolabral reconstruction in posterior shoulder instability. J Shoulder Elbow Surg 2005;9:355-360.
8. Shin RD, Daniel PB, Andrew RS, Zuckerman JD. Posterior capsulorrhaphy for treatment of recurrent posterior glenohumeral instability. Bull Hosp Joint Dis 2005;63:9-12.
9. Tibone J, Ting A. Capsulorrhaphy with a staple for recurrent posterior subluxation of the shoulder. J Bone Joint Surg Am 1990;72:999-1002.
10. Wolf BR, Strickland S, Riley WJ, et al. Open posterior stabilization for recurrent posterior glenohumeral instability. J Shoulder Elbow Surg 2005;14:157-164.

Suggested Reading

Blasier RB, Soslowsky LJ, Malicky DM, Palmer ML. Posterior glenohumeral subluxation: active and passive stabilization in a biomechanical model. J Bone Joint Surg Am 1997;79:433-440.

Fronek J, Warren FR, Bowen M. Posterior subluxation of the glenohumeral joint. J Bone Joint Surg Am 1989;71:205-216.

Hawkins RJ, Koppert G, Johnston G. Recurrent posterior instability (subluxation) of the shoulder. J Bone Joint Surg Am 1984;66:169-174.

Neer CS II, Foster CR. Inferior capsular shift for involuntary inferior and multidirectional instability of the shoulder: a preliminary report. J Bone Joint Surg Am 1980;62:897-908.

Norwood LA, Terry GC. Shoulder posterior subluxation. Am J Sports Med 1984;12:25-30.

Samilson RL. Posterior dislocation of the shoulder in athletes. Clin Orthop 1983;2:369-378.

Santini A, Neviaser R. Long term results of posterior inferior capsular shift. J Shoulder Elbow Surg 1995;4(suppl):S65.

CHAPTER 13

Open Repair of Multidirectional Instability

Pradeep Kodali, MD

Gordon Nuber, MD

Neer and Foster[13] in 1980 described multidirectional instability as the ability to dislocate or to sublux the glenohumeral joint anteriorly, posteriorly, and inferiorly. They also reported that patients were most symptomatic during midrange of motion while performing activities of daily living.

Multidirectional instability is described as global shoulder laxity that can be congenital, acquired, or both, primarily due to combination of a redundant inferior capsular pouch, lax ligaments about the shoulder, and weakened musculotendinous structures.[2,16] Congenital laxity often occurs in multiple joints of the body, such as in Marfan syndrome. Acquired laxity is found in competitive athletes, specifically gymnasts and swimmers. The combination of both is found in individuals who have baseline laxity who become symptomatic after mild to moderate trauma. Diagnosis is largely by clinical examination; however, magnetic resonance imaging can help evaluate the presence and extent of a traumatic component. The mainstay of treatment is nonoperative management focusing on physical therapy that involves strength and neuromuscular coordination of the rotator cuff, deltoid, and scapula.[16] Operative management is reserved for those refractory to conservative measures. The open inferior capsular shift, as originally described by Neer and Foster,[13] has historically been the operative treatment of choice. With advances in arthroscopic techniques, the open procedure is used less frequently.

Preoperative Considerations

History

Most patients present as young adults and can have bilateral symptoms. It is important to ascertain a family history of similar complaints to evaluate for congenital causes. A psychiatric history (i.e., intentional dislocators) may preclude individuals from surgery.[13,16] Pain is invariably the most common presenting complaint. Symptoms are generally provoked by normal daily activities. Also, looseness or the sensation of the shoulder's "slipping out" is a frequent complaint. Rarely, patients may complain of numbness, tingling, and weakness of the affected extremity.

Physical Examination

The mainstay of diagnosis is physical examination. Basic shoulder examination includes inspection for muscle atrophy, palpation for any point tenderness, and active and passive range of motion to evaluate for shoulder biomechanics. As with any complete examination of the shoulder, the physician should evaluate the cervical spine. Signs of global ligamentous laxity, including elbow hyperextension, ability to touch the thumb to the forearm (Fig. 13-1), and patellar subluxation, are frequently observed.

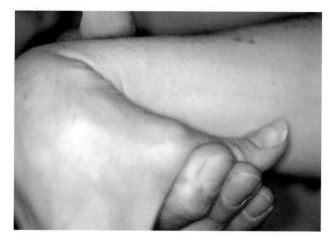

Figure 13-1 Thumb to forearm test demonstrating ligamentous laxity.

A sulcus or apprehension sign is commonly present (Fig. 13-2). We also use the load-shift test to quantify both anterior and posterior laxity (Fig. 13-3).[10] This is done by placing the shoulder off the edge of the table in 90 degrees of abduction and applying an anterior and posterior trans-

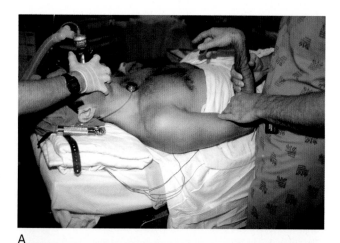

A

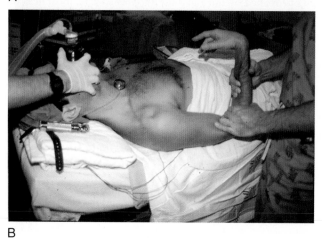

B

Figure 13-2 A, Shoulder before sulcus test. **B,** Sulcus sign with longitudinal pull on the arm.

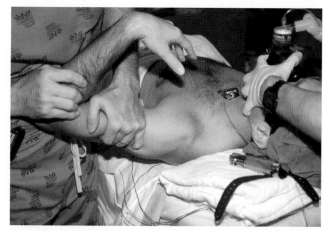

A

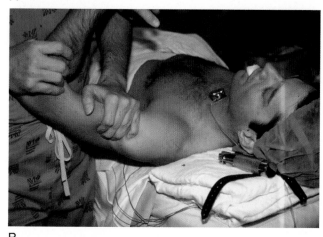

B

Figure 13-3 A, Load-shift test for anterior instability. **B,** Load-shift test for posterior instability.

lational force. It is graded as minimal translation (trace), humeral head translation to the rim (1+), translation over the rim with spontaneous reduction (2+), and dislocation (3+). The contralateral shoulder should be evaluated for laxity as well. Additional maneuvers to demonstrate increased translation include the Fukuda test and the jerk test.[16]

Imaging

Multidirectional instability typically can be diagnosed clinically. However, plain radiographs can be obtained to rule out bone abnormalities, such as a bony Bankart or Hill-Sachs lesion. Computed tomography or magnetic resonance arthrography can be used to evaluate capsular volume.

Indications and Contraindications

Conservative management remains the treatment of choice. Initial management should include a period of immobilization and anti-inflammatory drugs. It is thought that multidirectional instability is due in part to stretching of the static shoulder stabilizers. Therefore, treatment should initially involve strengthening of the shoulder stabilizers, including the rotator cuff muscles and deltoid. Conditioning of the back muscles and the scapular stabilizers is also important for stability.[2] A change in lifestyle to limit pain-provoking activities such as overhead work is recommended. A formal two-phase rehabilitation program including Thera-Band exercises and light weights, focused on strengthening of the rotator cuff and deltoid muscles, has also been described.[4]

The primary indication for operative treatment is a failure of conservative management with persistent pain.[2,6,12,13,16] Conservative management is likely to fail in patients with unilateral involvement, difficulties performing activities of daily living, and higher grades of laxity on initial examination.[12] Contraindications to surgical treatment include noncompliance during a trial of conservative management, voluntary dislocators, and patients with psychiatric abnormalities.[5,13] A poor prognostic indicator, particularly in athletes, is bilateral multidirectional instability requiring bilateral repair.[5]

Historically, surgical options have included thermal capsular shrinkage and glenoid osteotomy.[16] However, the open inferior capsular shift as described by Neer and Foster is the most commonly performed open procedure, with arthroscopic techniques gaining increasing popularity. The inferior capsular shift procedure reduces total capsular volume by releasing the inferior capsule and shifting it superiorly.[6,13]

Surgical Technique

Anesthesia and Positioning

We prefer an interscalene block with sedation, reserving general anesthesia for inadequate block or sedation. Local anesthesia with infiltration of the skin and subcutaneous tissue is also used. The patient can be positioned supine or 20 degrees upright. Although some authors state that all inferior capsular shift procedures can be performed through an anterior approach,[6] others believe the approach should be determined by the primary direction of instability,[5,13,14] as described by the patient or determined by physical examination. If anterior instability is the primary component, we prefer an anterior approach in the supine position with a rolled towel positioned between the thoracic spine and medial border of the scapula.[8] If posterior instability is the primary component, a posterior approach is preferred, keeping in mind that a separate anterior incision may be needed if a Bankart lesion is identified intraoperatively. An examination under anesthesia is performed to confirm surgical decision-making.[10,13,16]

Examination Under Anesthesia

A thorough examination under anesthesia is performed to document motion and direction of instability before surgical stabilization. In addition to a general shoulder examination, an assessment of the degree of capsular redundancy can be accomplished by the sulcus test. This is performed by applying downward traction to the adducted arm (see Fig. 13-2), followed by assessing the degree of downward displacement in varying degrees of external rotation.[10] Persistent inferior displacement with downward traction (sulcus sign) with external rotation may suggest a contribution from the rotator interval. The load-shift test assesses the relative degree of anterior or posterior instability (see Fig. 13-3). Finally, diagnostic arthroscopy can aid in identifying associated Bankart or posterior labral lesions before continuing with the open procedure.

Surgical Landmarks

- Acromion
- Coracoid process
- Axillary fold

Specific Steps

Anterior Approach (Box 13-1)

1. Deltopectoral Approach

The landmark for this approach is the coracoid process. The technique for the inferior capsular shift is similar to that used in the original series by Neer and Foster.[13] Various modifications have been made subsequent to that. The incision is made from the tip of the coracoid process to the axilla along the deltopectoral groove (Fig. 13-4).[9] Develop the deltopectoral interval medial to the cephalic vein, retracting the deltoid laterally and the pectoralis medially (Fig. 13-5). Divide the clavipectoral fascia and retract the coracobrachialis and the short head of the biceps medially. Identify and ligate the anterior humeral circumflex vessels located at the inferior border of the tendinous portion of the subscapularis. Place the arm in

Box 13-1 Surgical Steps: Anterior Approach

1. Deltopectoral approach
2. T-capsulotomy
3. Preparing the reattachment site
4. Capsular shift
5. Subscapularis repair and closure

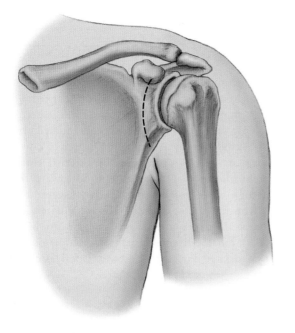

Figure 13-4 Incision for deltopectoral approach.

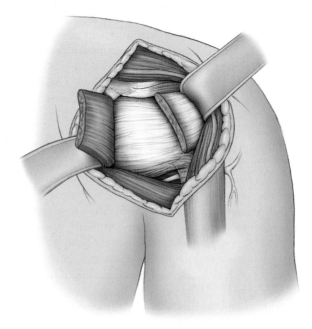

Figure 13-6 Reflect the subscapularis, leaving a stump for reattachment.

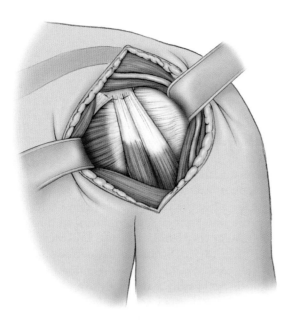

Figure 13-5 The deltopectoral interval is developed now, showing the subscapularis.

external rotation and divide the subscapularis 1 cm medial to its insertion, carefully developing a plane between the subscapularis tendon and capsule. Tag the proximal end and retract medially (Fig. 13-6). In athletes that rely heavily on upper extremity function, consider use of a subscapularis-splitting approach.[3] It has been shown to have a higher rate of return to professional-level activity.

Close the rotator interval between the superior and middle glenohumeral ligaments with absorbable suture if a lesion is present. Identify and protect the axillary nerve as it crosses near the inferior border of the capsule.

2. T-Capsulotomy

Make a T-shaped capsulotomy, starting the horizontal limb medially between the superior and middle glenohumeral ligaments,[10] extending the incision inferolaterally toward the humeral neck (Fig. 13-7). Place the arm in external rotation and release the inferior capsule from the humeral neck, proceeding posteriorly. Tag the inferior flap at its corner. One technique to assess adequate reduction in capsular volume is to place a finger in the inferior capsular pouch and pull the capsular stitch superiorly until the surgeon's finger is extruded. If it does not extrude, then extend the capsular incision around the humeral neck even farther posteriorly.[10,14] Inspect the joint for any loose bodies or labral disease (Fig. 13-8).

3. Preparing the Reattachment Site

With a curet or high-speed bur, decorticate the anterior and inferior sulcus of the humeral neck to obtain a bleeding bed of cancellous bone.

4. Capsular Shift

Suture the capsular flap to the stump of the subscapularis tendon and to the part of the capsule that remains on the humerus. Alternatively, the capsule can be sutured directly into the humerus with the aid of suture anchors. Select the appropriate tension on the flap to eliminate the inferior

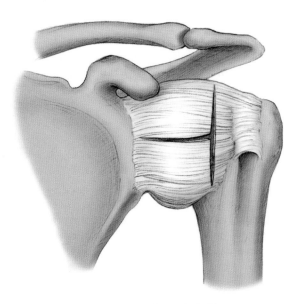

Figure 13-7 The humeral-based T-shaped capsular incision.

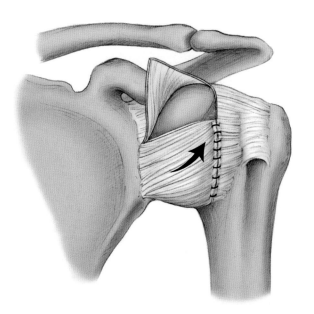

Figure 13-9 The inferior flap is brought up and sutured to the humeral side to decrease the volume of the inferior pouch.

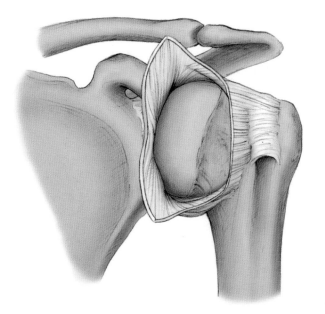

Figure 13-8 The joint is now exposed after the T-shaped capsular incision.

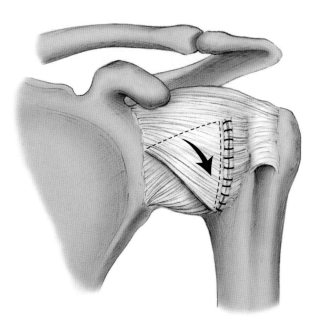

Figure 13-10 After the inferior flap is advanced *(arrow)*, the superior flap is brought down to and sutured to the humeral side.

pouch and reduce the posterior capsular redundancy. Place the arm in 40 degrees of abduction and 40 degrees of external rotation. Advance the inferior flap superiorly such that it is repaired to the bleeding bed of cancellous bone and to the lateral aspect of capsule (Fig. 13-9). Use nonabsorbable sutures in a pants-over-vest fashion.[6] The superior flap is advanced distally and laterally and repaired in a similar fashion to reinforce the anterior capsule (Fig. 13-10). This also allows the middle glenohumeral ligament to reinforce the capsule anteriorly.

5. Subscapularis Repair and Closure

The subscapularis tendon is brought over the capsular shift and then reattached to its usual location with multiple nonabsorbable sutures. Close the deltopectoral interval with absorbable sutures and the skin and subcutaneous tissues in usual fashion.

An alternative to the humeral-based capsular incision is the glenoid-based capsulotomy. Similar concepts apply in regard to capsular advancement (Fig. 13-11).

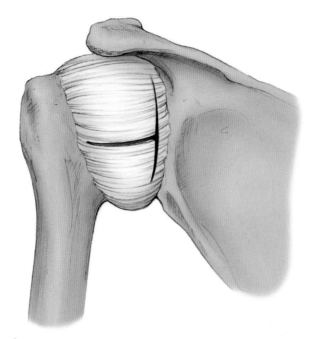

A

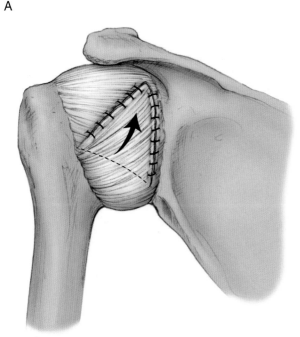

B

Figure 13-11 Glenoid-based capsular shift. (Redrawn from Bowen M, Warren R. Surgical approaches to posterior instability of shoulder. Oper Tech Sports Med 1993;1:301-310.)

However, the flaps are attached to the glenoid margin, commonly with suture anchors.[1,7,11]

Posterior Approach

In our experience, most cases of multidirectional instability can be treated with the anterior approach as patients typically present with anterior instability as the primary component. Cooper and Brems[6] advocate use of the anterior approach for all cases, including those with posterior instability as the primary component. We advocate choosing the approach on the basis of the direction of the primary instability. Refer to Chapter 12 for further details of the posterior approach for instability surgery.

Postoperative Considerations

Rehabilitation

Postoperative care is integral to the healing process. We base our method of immobilization on the primary direction of instability. For anterior instability, patients can typically be discharged in a sling; for posterior instability, we advocate use of a Gunslinger brace. After a 6-week period of immobilization, gradual range-of-motion exercises are initiated according to a strict protocol; the concern is that ambitious patients will do too much too early, resulting in recurrent instability. During weeks 6 through 10, below-the-shoulder exercises are conducted, limiting external rotation to 45 degrees. Beginning in week 10, a stretching program is initiated, focusing on forward elevation and external rotation. At weeks 14 to 16, deltoid and rotator cuff strengthening is added, followed by scapular stabilization exercises at weeks 18 to 20. Contact sports are typically allowed only after complete restoration of strength and condition, usually about 6 months after surgery.

Complications

Reported complications include recurrent instability, persistent symptoms of apprehension, axillary nerve neurapraxia, and infection.

PEARLS AND PITFALLS

- In individuals who are multidirectionally lax, you can cheat the incision toward the axillary crease because the skin is also lax and will stretch superiorly toward the coracoid, thus providing a more cosmetic exposure.

- In peeling the subscapularis off the capsule, use an electrocautery device. The char allows you to see the striations of the tendon better, making the plane between the subscapularis and capsule easier to identify.

- Tag the T-shaped portion of the capsule with a different colored suture to keep it distinct.

- With a bur and Cobb elevator, rough the neck of the glenoid or humerus if suture anchors are used.

- If you are using suture anchors for the glenoid-based capsulotomy, place them at the lip of the glenoid and not medially on the glenoid neck.

Table 13-1 Results of Inferior Capsular Shift

Author	Successful Results/No. of Shoulders	Follow-up	Recurrent Instability
Neer and Foster[13] (1980)	39/40	Variable*	3%
Cooper and Brems[6] (1992)	39/43	2-6 years	9%
Bak et al[3] (2000)	24/26	Median: 54 months	8%
Pollock et al[14] (2000)	46/49	Average: 61 months	4%
Choi and Ogilvie-Harris[5] (2002)	48/53	Average: 42 months	9%
Van Tankeren et al[16] (2002)	14/17	Mean: 39 months	6%[†]

*Less than 12 months (8 shoulders), 12 to 24 months (15 shoulders), and more than 24 months (17 shoulders).
[†]Without any associated injuries.

13

Results

Historical results of the open procedure have been good. However, with increasing success of arthroscopic techniques, the role of the open procedure is diminishing. In Neer and Foster's original series,[13] 39 of 40 shoulders had good results. Cooper and Brems[6] reported that 39 of 48 shoulders functioned well without instability after up to 6 years of follow-up. Four shoulders had recurrent instability, and the patients were subjectively dissatisfied. The authors also stated that if failure occurs, it tends to happen early in the postoperative period. Van Tankeren et al[15] reported excellent results based on objective scores in 14 of 17 shoulders at a mean follow-up of 39 months. Pollock et al[14] described good or excellent results in 46 of 49 shoulders with an average follow-up of more than 5 years (Table 13-1).

References

1. Altchek D, Warren R, Skyhar M, Ortiz G. T-plasty modification of the Bankart procedure for multidirectional instability of the anterior and inferior types. J Bone Joint Surg Am 1991;73:105-112.
2. An Y, Friedman R. Conservative management of shoulder injuries: multidirectional instability of the glenohumeral joint. Orthop Clin North Am 2000;31:275-285.
3. Bak K, Spring B, Henderson I. Inferior capsular shift procedure in athletes with multidirectional instability based on isolated capsular and ligamentous redundancy. Am J Sports Med 2000;28:466-471.
4. Burkhead W, Rockwood C. Treatment of instability of the shoulder with an exercise program. J Bone Joint Surg Am 1992;74:890-896.
5. Choi C, Ogilvie-Harris D. Inferior capsular shift operation for multidirectional instability of the shoulder in players of contact sports. Br J Sports Med 2002;36:290-294.
6. Cooper R, Brems J. The inferior capsular shift procedure for multidirectional instability of the shoulder. J Bone Joint Surg Am 1992;74:1516-1521.
7. Cordasco F, Pollock R, Flatow E, Bigliani L. Management of multidirectional instability. Oper Tech Sports Med 1993;1:293-300.
8. Hoppenfeld S, deBoer P. The shoulder. In Surgical Exposures in Orthopaedics: The Anatomic Approach. Philadelphia, Lippincott-Raven, 1994:2-49.
9. Leslie J, Ryan T. The anterior axillary incision to approach the shoulder joint. J Bone Joint Surg Am 1962;44:1193-1196.
10. Levine W, Prickett W, Prymka M, Yamaguchi K. Repair of athletic shoulder injuries: treatment of the athlete with multidirectional shoulder instability. Orthop Clin North Am 2001;32:475-484.
11. Marquardt B, Potzl W, Witt K, Steinbeck J. A modified capsular shift for atraumatic anterior-inferior shoulder instability. Am J Sports Med 2005;33:1011-1015.
12. Misamore G, Sallay P, Didelot W. A longitudinal study of patients with multidirectional instability of the shoulder with seven- to ten-year follow-up. J Shoulder Elbow Surg 2005;14:466-470.
13. Neer C, Foster C. Inferior capsular shift for involuntary inferior and multidirectional instability of the shoulder. J Bone Joint Surg Am 1980;60:897-908.
14. Pollock R, Owens J, Flatow E, Bigliani L. Operative results of the inferior capsular shift procedure for multidirectional instability of the shoulder. J Bone Joint Surg Am 2000;82:919-928.
15. Schenk T, Brems J. Multidirectional instability of the shoulder: pathophysiology, diagnosis, and management. J Am Acad Orthop Surg 1998;6:65-72.
16. Van Tankeren E, Malefijt M, Van Loon C. Open capsular shift for multidirectional shoulder instability. Arch Orthop Trauma Surg 2002;122:447-450.

CHAPTER 14

Treatment of Bone Defects of Humeral Head and Glenoid

Eric J. Kropf, MD

Jon K. Sekiya, MD

Traumatic anterior glenohumeral dislocation typically results in disruption of the anteroinferior capsulolabral complex (Bankart lesion).[25] To date, anatomic Bankart reconstruction has represented the "gold standard" of treatment and has shown good to excellent results in most series. Although historic treatment protocols have not routinely addressed associated osteoarticular injury, the high prevalence of such lesions is well documented. Compression fractures of the posterior superior humeral head (Hill-Sachs lesion) have been found to occur in 32% to 51% of initial anterior dislocations,[5,17,18,29] and anteroinferior glenoid deficiency has been reported in 22% of primary dislocations.[25] With recurrence rates after soft tissue Bankart reconstruction alone reported as high as 18% to 44% in some series,[2,7,12,13] treatment protocols are evolving. More critical attention is being given to osseous defects of the glenoid and humeral head.

Burkhart and De Beer[4] reviewed 194 cases of arthroscopic Bankart repair, dividing patients into two groups—those with significant bone defects of the glenoid or humeral head and those without such defects. A remarkable difference was seen between the two groups with respect to recurrence rates. Specifically, patients without significant bone defects had a recurrence rate of 4% compared with a 67% failure rate in patients with significant bone defects. Other authors have also demonstrated a strong correlation between the presence of a Hill-Sachs lesion or anterior glenoid erosion and recurrent instability.[4,11,20,25,26]

Historically, the primary goal of treatment has been stable reduction and the prevention of recurrent dislocation. Nonanatomic reconstruction procedures have been employed to constrain the shoulder, including Bristow[16] or Latarjet[1] coracoid transfer, open capsular shift,[24] rotational proximal humeral osteotomy,[32] and transfer of the infraspinatus into the humeral head defect.[8] These procedures yield shoulder stability often at the great expense of motion. Some have been associated with significant long-term complications.[15,33]

The surgical management of shoulder instability is evolving to include anatomic reconstruction of osseous defects of the glenohumeral joint. Success is no longer based on how well the shoulder is "blocked" from dislocation; rather, it is based on restoration of motion and strength with return to a high level of overhead function. Reconstruction of the glenoid has been described with iliac crest autograft or femoral head allograft.[14,19,31] Reconstruction of the humeral head has been performed with large, size- and side-matched allograft,[10,23] a single allograft plug (osteochondral allograft transplantation),[22] and arthroscopic mosaicplasty.[6] Combined reconstructive procedure can be performed in the appropriate setting.

Preoperative Considerations

History

A complete history is obtained. This includes the mechanism of injury; associated injuries; prior treatments, if applicable; and nature of the instability. Specifically, the surgeon should elicit the timing of initial symptoms and the frequency of current symptoms, including pain and instability and their effect on the patient's function. The typical patient initially suffers a high-energy injury secondary to a fall, motor vehicle trauma, or contact sports. Recurrent dislocations or a chronic sense of instability will have followed. Often, the patient will already have undergone multiple instability procedures without success.

Physical Examination

Physical examination proceeds in a systematic fashion. Prior surgical scars should be noted. Active and passive range of motion and rotator cuff strength are tested and compared with the unaffected arm. Instability is assessed in anterior, posterior, and inferior directions and graded on a 3-point scale. Typically, the patient will experience clinically significant apprehension in varying degrees of abduction and external rotation. This factor coupled with significant pain may limit the in-office examination. Therefore, findings should be verified later with a complete examination under anesthesia.

Imaging

Radiography

- Anteroposterior view (internal and external rotation)
- True anteroposterior view of the glenohumeral joint
- Axillary lateral view
- Stryker notch view
- West Point view

Other Modalities

The computed tomographic (CT) scan proves best for assessment of the osseous defect. We have found that plain radiographs will often significantly underestimate the size of the Hill-Sachs or glenoid defect. Multiplanar CT scanning, often with three-dimensional reconstruction, is necessary for the extent of the defect to be truly appreciated. It is essential that CT scans be of high quality and allow accurate preoperative measurements. This allows one to confidently and consistently obtain an appropriately size-matched glenoid or proximal humerus allograft before surgery.

Magnetic resonance imaging with or without the administration of contrast material will aid in assessment of associated soft tissue injury. If possible, the study may prove more valuable if it is performed with the shoulder abducted and externally rotated (ABER view). This may provide clues as to the contribution of the bone defect when the arm is in the position of instability.

Indications and Contraindications

Patients with large osseous defects of the glenoid and humeral head who experience recurrent episodes of instability after anterior capsulolabral reconstruction require a secondary reconstruction procedure. Chronic dislocations and older patients who place less significant demands on the shoulder can probably be treated by more traditional methods (coracoid transfer, capsular shift, subscapularis advancement, or arthroplasty). Throwing athletes and younger patients with significant overhead demands will not tolerate such restricted motion and are ideal candidates for anatomic osteoarticular reconstruction of the glenoid or humeral head as indicated.

Diagnostic arthroscopy provides the most accurate assessment of which lesions will need to be addressed surgically. Significant osseous defects effectively shorten the normal "safe arc" of motion. In a position of athletic function, the humeral head translates anteriorly. With extensive glenoid erosion, the head will "run out" of glenoid and fall off or dislocate.[3,9,11,21,28] Likewise, with large Hill-Sachs lesions, the glenoid will "drop into" the humeral head defect in a similar position when the safe arc of motion is exceeded, causing an abrupt and unsettling sense of instability.[3]

Parameters are being defined to identify those patients who can benefit from osteoarticular reconstruction early at the time of the index procedure. The goal is to avoid foreseeable failure after soft tissue reconstruction and ultimately to spare the patient the repetitive trauma of recurrent instability and the need for revision surgery. Rowe[25] originally described glenoid lesions as significant if they involve 30% of the articular surface. Burkhart and De Beer[4] showed an exceptionally high likelihood of recurrent instability when the anterior-to-posterior glenoid diameter is less below the midglenoid notch than above it ("inverted pear"). Unfortunately, this method of assessment requires information obtained at the time of diagnostic arthroscopy. On the basis of the results of a biomechanical study, Gerber and Nyffeler[11] found that anteroinferior glenoid defects with a total length greater than half the maximum anterior to posterior diameter decreased the resistance to dislocation by 30%. Therefore, they and others have recommended reconstruction for defects of this size.[11,30]

Hill-Sachs lesions that can be seen arthroscopically to engage the anterior glenoid rim in a position of function should be addressed. Conventional guidelines suggest that lesions greater than 25% be addressed, but biomechanical studies have shown that humeral head defects involving as little as 12.5% of the articular surface result in significant biomechanical changes across the glenohumeral joint.[3,9,28]

Contraindications to anatomic reconstruction include arthroscopic or radiographic evidence of advanced degenerative glenohumeral arthritis, avascular necrosis of the humeral head, unaddressed rotator cuff deficiency, and advanced age.

Surgical Planning

By use of CT or magnetic resonance imaging data, the size of the proximal humerus or glenoid allograft is determined. Fresh-frozen or cryopreserved size- and side-matched allograft is obtained from a certified tissue bank. A thorough discussion of potential risks associated with the use of allograft tissue is undertaken with the patient, and informed consent is obtained.

Osteoarticular Allograft Reconstruction of the Glenoid and Humeral Head

For the sake of brevity, we present combined anatomic allograft reconstruction of the glenoid and humeral head in this section. Isolated reconstruction of either defect can be performed in a similar fashion if it is warranted.

Anesthesia and Positioning

After general endotracheal anesthesia is induced, the patient is placed in the beach chair position with the head of the bed raised 30 degrees. A bump is placed under the medial border of the scapula, and the shoulder should be completely free to allow the maximal external rotation and extension that will be needed. An intrascalene block can be used at the discretion of the surgeon and anesthesiologist. The patient is prepared in the usual sterile fashion with the arm draped free.

Surgical Landmarks, Incisions, and Portals

Landmarks

- Anterior, lateral, and posterior borders of the acromion
- Coracoid process
- Distal clavicle
- Acromioclavicular joint
- Deltopectoral groove

Portals and Approaches

- Posterior portal
- Anterior portal
- Deltopectoral approach to glenohumeral joint

Examination Under Anesthesia and Diagnostic Arthroscopy

Examination under anesthesia is performed, and findings are compared with the contralateral limb with specific attention to degree and position of instability. Instability should be graded anteriorly, posteriorly, and inferiorly and compared with the unaffected side.

Diagnostic arthroscopy is extremely useful in this setting. Soft tissue and chondral injury can be assessed, and the size and position of the glenoid or humeral head defect can be thoroughly inspected. In the most common clinical scenario, the surgeon may have underestimated the size of the defect. As a result, appropriate consent will not have been signed and allograft tissue will not be available. Therefore, it is not uncommon for diagnostic arthroscopy to be performed alone before the definitive procedure.

Specific Steps

1. Exposure

A 6- to 10-cm skin incision is made in line with the deltopectoral groove from the tip of the coracoid directed distally. Subcutaneous tissue is dissected sharply with meticulous hemostasis down to the level of the deltopectoral fascia. The deltopectoral interval is identified and developed, retracting the pectoralis major medially and the deltoid laterally. The cephalic vein can be taken medially or laterally, depending on the situation. If it is traumatized, the vein should be tied off before proceeding with deep dissection. The lateral border of the conjoint tendon is identified and retracted medially. The subscapularis tendon is then tagged with stay sutures and incised perpendicular to its fibers approximately 5 mm from its insertion point on the lesser tuberosity, ensuring that adequate tissue is left for later repair. When the subscapularis tendon is incised, it is important to externally rotate the humerus to minimize the risk of iatrogenic injury to the axillary nerve. A lateral humeral-based capsulotomy incision is made, again leaving a small cuff of tissue for later repair (Fig. 14-1).

2. Preparation of the Recipient Humeral Head Site

The humerus is maximally externally rotated and extended, exposing the Hill-Sachs lesion. Once it is exposed, a microsagittal saw or high-speed bur is used to reshape the defect and to make a bed of bleeding subchondral bone. Ultimately, a wedge-shaped defect needs to be made that can be press fitted with the allograft wedge. The final dimensions of the finished defect are measured with respect to length, width, and height and recorded.

3. Allograft Preparation

The corresponding anatomic quadrant of the humeral head is identified and marked to best conform to the

14

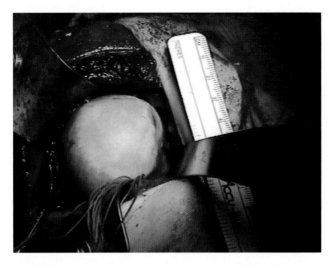

Figure 14-1 A deltopectoral approach is taken to the glenohumeral joint. The subscapularis has been detached from the lesser tuberosity and a laterally based capsulotomy performed. The humerus is maximally extended and externally rotated. The Hill-Sachs defect is well exposed in the working field.

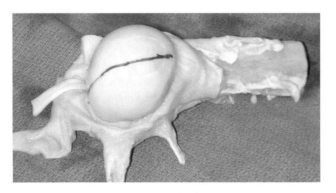

Figure 14-2 The allograft humeral head and associated soft tissue structures are shown. The recipient site has been prepared, and the allograft is marked in the corresponding quadrant of the humeral head.

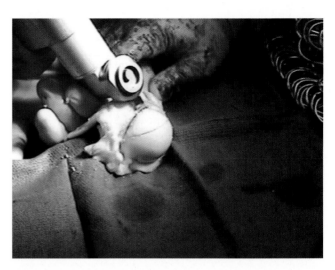

Figure 14-3 With an oscillating saw, a size- and side-matched allograft is made. The allograft should be roughly 2 mm larger in all dimensions compared with the recipient defect. The final allograft can be trimmed to fit as necessary.

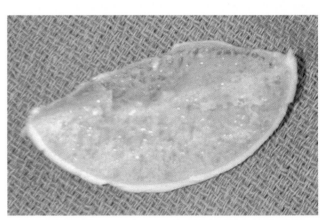

Figure 14-4 The final size- and side-matched allograft is depicted here. Final adjustments to height, width, and length have been made with a microsagittal saw.

dimensions of the recipient defect (Fig. 14-2). A wedge is then cut from the allograft humeral head approximately 2 to 3 mm larger in all dimensions than the measured recipient defect (Fig. 14-3). It is best to err on the side of making too large an allograft plug as little can be done if the piece is too small. The allograft is then provisionally tried in the Hill-Sachs defect. Final adjustments in length, height, or width of the graft are made with a high-speed bur or microsagittal saw (Fig. 14-4). This is done in one dimension at a time with careful attention to detail, realizing that adjustments in one plane will affect the final size of the graft in all dimensions.

4. Allograft Fixation

Once the surgeon is satisfied with the final size and configuration, the allograft is seated in the recipient defect and provisionally held with two 0.045 Kirschner wires (Fig. 14-5). The wires are then sequentially replaced with

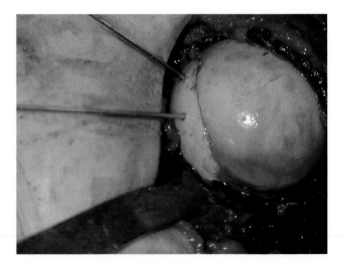

Figure 14-5 The allograft is seated in the prepared humeral head defect. Provisional fixation is achieved with two 0.045 Kirschner wires.

headless, variable pitch compression screws. Either way, it is absolutely essential that the screw heads be countersunk below the surface of the adjacent articular cartilage (Fig. 14-6).

5. Preparation of the Glenoid Rim

The humeral head is retracted posteriorly with a humeral retractor (Fukuda), and the glenoid rim is exposed. A curved osteotome is used to subperiosteally strip the soft tissues medially off of the anteroinferior glenoid rim. The full extent of the anteroinferior glenoid rim defect can then be appreciated; a direct measurement is taken and correlated with the preoperative CT scan estimate of the defect. The glenoid defect is then prepared with a high-speed bur to make a surface of fresh bleeding bone.

6. Allograft Preparation

The appropriately size- and side-matched allograft glenoid or scapula with intact soft tissue attachments is obtained (Fig. 14-7). The in vivo measurement of the defect is compared with preoperative CT estimates of the glenoid rim defect. In the same anteroinferior position on the allograft glenoid, a piece is cut at least 2 or 3 mm larger than desired (Fig. 14-8). The glenoid is tried in the desired position and trimmed with a high-speed bur as necessary (Fig. 14-9). It is technically easier to perform subsequent capsulolabral repair if suture is provisionally passed through the allograft before implantation. We prefer to do so with two No. 0 Ethibond sutures (Fig. 14-10).

7. Allograft Fixation

The prepared allograft is then placed in the appropriate anatomic position. When the surgeon is satisfied, it is held provisionally with two 0.045 Kirschner wires, which are

sequentially exchanged for two AO 4.0 partially threaded cortical screws (Fig. 14-11).

8. Capsular Shift

The glenohumeral joint is reduced, and capsular redundancy is addressed as necessary by capsular shift. The previously passed Ethibond sutures in the glenoid allograft are passed through the intact capsule in a horizontal mattress fashion and tied on the outside of the capsule. This anchors the glenohumeral capsule to the newly secured glenoid allograft. The humeral-based shift is then completed in a standard fashion, with the arm placed in 30 degrees of abduction and external rotation. Often mere placement of the allograft will greatly reduce the size of

14

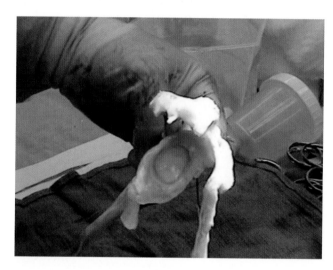

Figure 14-7 Side- and size-matched scapular allograft with intact soft tissue attachments is pictured here.

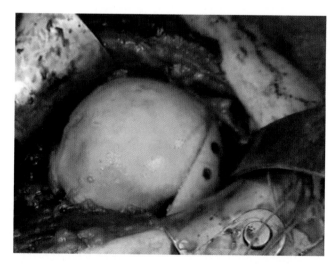

Figure 14-6 K-wires are sequentially exchanged for headless, variable pitch compression screws. Excellent purchase and compression are achieved, and the screws are sunk below the level of articular cartilage.

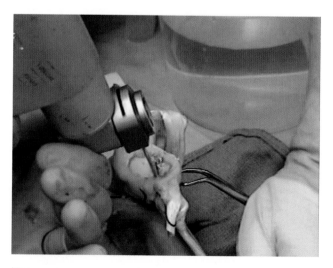

Figure 14-8 After measurements have been made, the allograft is cut from the anteroinferior aspect of the glenoid roughly 2 or 3 mm larger than needed to fill the defect.

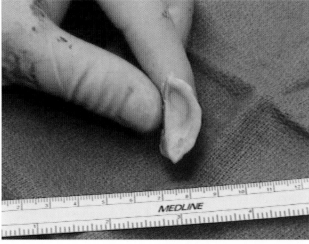

A

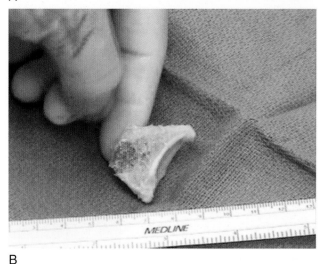

B

Figure 14-9 A and **B,** The allograft is trimmed with a high-speed bur to best fit the recipient bed.

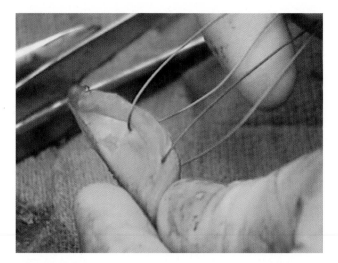

Figure 14-10 Two No. 0 Ethibond sutures are passed through the allograft before implantation in anticipation of their later use during capsular shift.

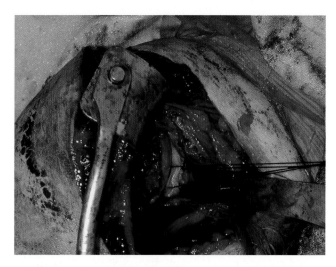

Figure 14-11 Allograft glenoid depicted fixed to native glenoid rim in anterior inferior position.

the infraglenoid recess as the void has now been filled by graft.

9. Closure

The wound is then copiously irrigated with antibiotic solution. The shoulder is taken through a complete range of motion to ensure smooth articulation between the native humeral head, allograft, and glenoid. The joint capsule is closed with absorbable suture, and the subscapularis is repaired anatomically back to a cuff of tissue with a nonabsorbable suture. The conjoint tendon and deltopectoral interval are allowed to fall back into their native position. A 2-0 absorbable subcutaneous stitch and running 4-0 absorbable subcuticular suture are used to approximate the skin.

Postoperative Considerations

Immobilization, Follow-up, and Rehabilitation

The patient is placed immediately into a shoulder immobilizer. At the first postoperative visit, 6 to 8 days later, the wound is inspected and the patient is allowed to begin pendulum exercises only. At 1 month, active and passive range of motion is initiated under the guidance of an experienced physical therapist. Strengthening begins at 4 to 6 months. The patient is generally not cleared for return to sport or strenuous overhead activity until at least 7 to 12 months after the date of surgery.

Radiographs

Radiographs are taken at 2, 6, 12, and 24 weeks postoperatively to ensure maintained position of the allograft. If it is clinically warranted, a CT scan can be performed to ensure incorporation of the allograft (Fig. 14-12).

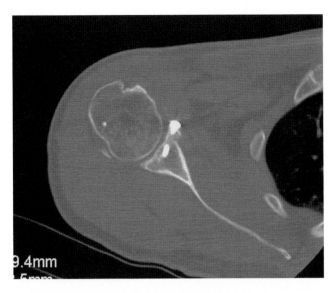

Figure 14-12 Single axial CT scan image of the shoulder 6 weeks after allograft reconstruction of anterior glenoid rim and Hill-Sachs defect of the humeral head. The image shows maintained joint space and smooth transition from native to allograft glenoid rim.

Box 14-1 Surgical Steps

1. Exposure
2. Preparation of the recipient bed
3. Preparation of the allograft plug
4. Allograft transplantation

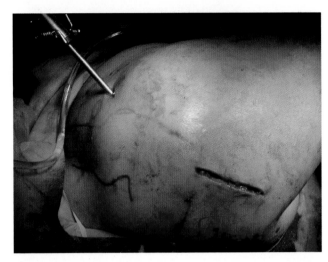

Figure 14-13 After diagnostic arthroscopy, a 6-cm incision is made from the posterolateral corner of the acromion directed distally in line with the deltoid fibers.

Osteoarticular Allograft Reconstruction of Humeral Head Defects

The method of anatomic allograft reconstruction of the humeral head described in the preceding section requires an extensive deltopectoral approach and maximal external rotation of the humerus to present the Hill-Sachs lesion into the working field. If allograft reconstruction of the glenoid rim is planned concomitantly, such an approach is logical. However, a second population of patients exists—those with only a soft tissue Bankart lesion and an associated Hill-Sachs lesion. These patients will often be treated by open or arthroscopic Bankart repair yet remain symptomatic secondary to engagement of a large humeral head defect.[4] If the anterior soft tissue reconstruction is intact or if it is desired to perform an arthroscopic anterior capsulolabral repair, we believe that the humeral head defect can best be addressed through a limited posterior approach to the humeral head and osteochondral allograft transplantation.[22]

Anesthesia and Positioning

After general anesthesia is induced, an examination of the affected extremity is performed and findings are compared with the contralateral side. The patient is placed in the lateral decubitus position with the arm held in 10 pounds of traction. Diagnostic arthroscopy is performed and pathologic change is noted, confirming the size and location of the humeral head defect. If the glenoid does not show significant erosion, we choose to address the labral injury and capsular laxity arthroscopically. An anterior working portal is established by needle localization; arthroscopic labral repair and capsular shift by multi-pleated plication technique are then performed through a single working portal.[19]

Specific Steps (Box 14-1)

1. Exposure

A skin incision is made from the posterolateral corner of the acromion directed distally in line with the deltoid fibers for approximately 6 cm (Fig. 14-13). Superficial dissection is carried down to the deltoid fascia and split in line with its fibers to the level of the upper border of the teres minor. The infraspinatus is split at the level of its tendinous raphe and retracted superiorly and inferiorly to expose the posterior joint capsule. Careful attention is given to protect the axillary nerve inferiorly. A vertical capsulotomy incision is made. The Hill-Sachs lesion can be easily visualized in its superior posterior position without the need to excessively rotate the humerus (Fig. 14-14).

2. Preparation of the Recipient Bed

Once the humeral head is exposed, osteoarticular allograft transplantation is performed by use of the allograft

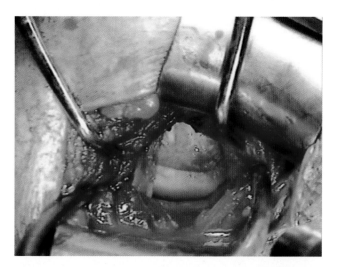

Figure 14-14 A posterior approach to the humeral head is carried down. After a vertical capsulotomy incision, the Hill-Sachs defect is seen in its posterosuperior position without the need to excessively rotate the humerus.

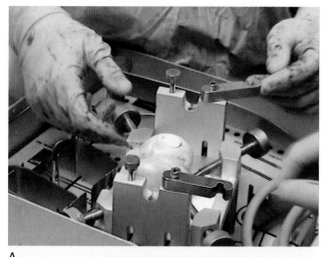

A

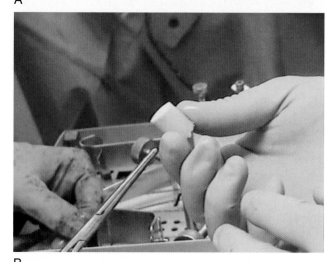

B

Figure 14-16 **A,** The allograft humeral head is placed in the OATS allograft workstation and drilled full-length in the corresponding position. **B,** The graft is then trimmed with a microsagittal saw to mirror the measured dimensions of the recipient socket.

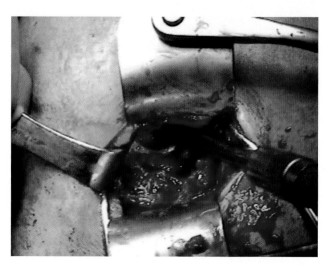

Figure 14-15 The humeral head defect is reamed down to the level of bleeding subchondral bone. The defect is measured in four quadrants, and measurements are recorded.

Osteoarticular Transplantation System (OATS; Arthrex, Naples, Fla). A cannulated sizing guide is placed to size the lesion in a posterior inferior location, which will prevent "engagement" with the glenoid when it is filled with a single large allograft plug. The plug functionally serves as a block to engagement, so it is not necessary to completely fill the defect. While the sizer is held in the desired position, a drill tip guide pin is fired through the center, and orientation is marked. A calibrated cutting blade is passed over the guide wire, and the recipient site defect is reamed until a bleeding bed of subchondral bone is encountered (Fig. 14-15). The recipient socket has been made and should be measured in four quadrants.

3. Preparation of the Allograft Plug

The allograft humeral head is secured in the allograft OATS workstation. The same sizer previously used to measure the Hill-Sachs lesion is placed over the corresponding location on the allograft and circumferentially marked, noting orientation. When the surgeon is satisfied with positioning, the donor harvesting drill is drilled through the entire length of the graft. It is important to drill the entire length of the allograft humeral head as it is relatively simple to trim the graft, but little can be done if the graft is too short. The harvested allograft is then measured and trimmed with an oscillating saw to mirror the depth of the defect (Fig. 14-16).

4. Allograft Transplantation

The allograft plug is then press fitted in the prepared socket and gently tapped into position until all edges are flush with the surrounding native cartilage rim (Fig. 14-17). No fixation is required. The posterior capsule is closed with absorbable suture, and subcutaneous tissue and skin are closed in a routine fashion.

Postoperative Considerations

Immobilization, Follow-up, and Rehabilitation

The shoulder is placed in a sling, and the sling is worn at all times including sleep. Pendulum exercises begin at 1 week. Passive and active-assisted range of motion begins at 1 to 2 months, avoiding stress on the posterior capsule (no adduction or internal rotation). The sling is discontinued at 2 months. Range of motion is gradually liberalized, and if the patient has full motion at 4 to 5 months, shoulder and periscapular strengthening is initiated. A functional training or throwing program begins at 6 to 7 months. Return to sport or full work duty is allowed when full functional pain-free range of motion and reasonable strength are achieved.

Complications

To date, long-term follow-up is not available for these treatment protocols, making prediction of potential complications difficult. Theoretical complications are those of allograft or autograft procedures, including nonunion, failed incorporation of the graft, and hardware failure. Long-term prospective data are needed to determine the rate of progression to degenerative arthritis.

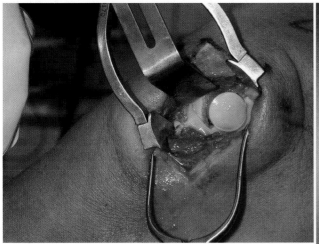

A

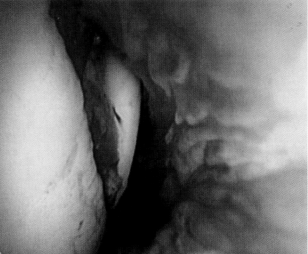

B

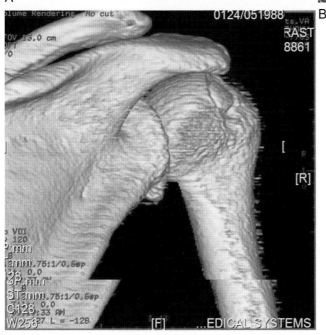

C

Figure 14-17 The allograft plug is tapped gently into position until it is flush with the native surrounding cartilage rim. **A,** Cadaveric model of allograft plug seated in final position. **B,** Arthroscopic image of allograft in place. **C,** Three-dimensional CT reconstruction of allograft plug at 3-month follow-up visit in an active 19-year-old man.

PEARLS AND PITFALLS

- The CT scan, although it is not normally a component of an instability work-up, is essential if a significant bone defect is suspected. Radiography and magnetic resonance imaging will routinely underestimate the size of these lesions.

- Functional diagnostic arthroscopy must be performed to appreciate the potential contribution of osteoarticular defects to recurrent instability. For example, the arm must be placed in a position of function (usually abduction–external rotation) to determine whether a Hill-Sachs lesion truly "engages" in a functional position.

In Humeral Head Reconstruction

- In preparing the allograft, err on the side of oversizing the graft by 1 or 2 mm compared with the measured, prepared defect. Trim the graft accordingly with an oscillating saw. Alterations in one plane will affect the final dimensions of the graft in all planes.

- Use variable pitch compression screws for final fixation. Be sure that the screw heads are countersunk below the articular surface. Take the shoulder through a range of motion to be sure.

- To gain exposure to the posterolateral humeral head if the anterior approach is being used, a generous inferior (taken all the way up posteriorly) capsular release off the humeral side is needed to externally rotate the humeral head sufficiently for exposure. We also recommend releasing (then repairing at the completion of the procedure) the upper 1 to 2 cm of the pectoralis major tendon on the humerus.

In Glenoid Reconstruction

- Use a curved osteotome or elevator to strip the medial soft tissues back a few millimeters off the glenoid rim. If this is not done, the full extent of anterior inferior glenoid bone loss may be underappreciated.

- Before positioning the allograft in the native recipient bed, pass two No. 0 Ethibond sutures through the graft. These will be used for later reattachment of the native capsule. It is significantly easier to do this before fixing the graft in place.

- Be cautious of overly aggressive capsular shift once the glenoid allograft is in place. The allograft will restore size to the glenoid and fill the previous void. Once the native capsule is attached to the allograft, redundancy is partially addressed, and the humeral-based shift need not be as aggressive as may have been anticipated.

Table 14-1 Clinical Results of Glenoid Reconstruction

Author	Procedure	Follow-up	Outcome
Warner et al[31] (2006)	Iliac crest autograft	33-month mean	No recurrence (N = 11) 7-degree loss of flexion 14-degree loss of external rotation
Hutchinson et al[19] (1995)	Iliac crest autograft (N = 6) Femoral head allograft (N = 9)	32-month mean	No recurrence Average motion loss: 16 to 26 degrees of external rotation
Haaker et al[14] (1993)	Iliac crest autograft	6 to 42 months	No recurrence (N = 24) 10-degree loss of external rotation
Scheibel et al[27] (2004)	Anatomic screw fixation of large bony Bankart lesion	30-month mean	No recurrence (N = 10) 12-degree loss of external rotation

Results

Published reports of osteoarticular allograft reconstruction of osseous defects of the glenohumeral joint are limited. Most are case reports or small case series. The best follow-up data range from 2 to 5 years. Still, early biomechanical and clinical results are promising. To date, recurrent instability that follows these reconstruction procedures has not been reported. Satisfaction rates of patients and functional assessment scores are greatly improved and loss of motion is minimal compared with more historic procedures. Logic suggests that with greater stability, the progression of degenerative arthritis will be slowed, but more data and time are required to validate this claim. We believe that anatomic reconstruction of the humeral head and glenoid represents a viable alternative to Bristow and Latarjet procedures in the young, high-demand patient with a significant osseous lesion (Tables 14-1 and 14-2).

Table 14-2 Clinical Results of Reconstruction of Humeral Head Defects

Author	Procedure	Follow-up	Outcome
Gerber[10] (1997)	Chronic locked anterior dislocation; large anatomic graft	4 patients	No recurrence Forward flexion of 145 degrees
Miniaci and Gish[23] (2004)	Large anatomic allograft	Average of 50 months	No recurrence (N = 18) 2 of 18 required later hardware removal
Chapovsky and Kelly[6] (2005)	Arthroscopic mosaicplasty	Case report (1 year)	No recurrence Return to sport (basketball)
Kropf and Sekiya[22] (2006)	Humeral head osteochondral allograft transplantation	Case report (1 year)	No recurrence Return to active military duty

14

References

1. Allain J, Goutallier D, Glorion C. Long-term results of the Latarjet procedure for the treatment of anterior instability of the shoulder. J Bone Joint Surg Am 1998;80:841-852.
2. Bacilla P, Field LD, Savoie FH. Arthroscopic Bankart repair in a high demand athletic population. Arthroscopy 1997;13:51-60.
3. Burkhart SS, Danaceau SM. Articular arc length mismatch as a cause of failed Bankart repair. Arthroscopy 2000;16:740-744.
4. Burkhart SS, De Beer JF. Traumatic glenohumeral bone defects and their relationship to failure of arthroscopic Bankart repairs: significance of the inverted-pear glenoid and the humeral engaging Hill-Sachs lesion. Arthroscopy 2000;16:677-694.
5. Calandra JJ, Baker CL, Uribe J. The incidence of Hill-Sachs lesions in initial anterior shoulder dislocations. Arthroscopy 1989;5:254-257.
6. Chapovsky F, Kelly JD. Osteochondral allograft transplantation for treatment of glenohumeral instability. Arthroscopy 2005;21:1007.
7. Cole BJ, L'Insalata J, Irrgang J, Warner JJP. Comparison of arthroscopic and open anterior shoulder stabilization: a two to six-year follow-up study. J Bone Joint Surg Am 2000;82:1108-1114.
8. Connolly JF. Humeral head defects associated with shoulder dislocations—their diagnostic and surgical significance. AAOS Instr Course Lect 1972;21:42-54.
9. Flatow EL, Warner JJP. Instability of the shoulder: complex problems and failed repairs. J Bone Joint Surg Am 1998;80:122-140.
10. Gerber C. Chronic locked anterior and posterior dislocations. In Warner JJP, Ianotti JP, Flatow EL, eds. Complex Revision Problems in Shoulder Surgery, 2nd ed. Philadelphia, Lippincott, 2005:89-103.
11. Gerber C, Nyffeler RW. Classification of glenohumeral joint instability. Clin Orthop 2002;400:65-76.
12. Grana WA, Buckley PD, Yates CK. Arthroscopic Bankart suture repair. Am J Sports Med 1993;21:348-353.
13. Green MR, Christensen KP. Arthroscopic Bankart procedure: two to five year followup with clinical correlation to severity of glenoid labral lesion. Am J Sports Med 1995;23:276-281.
14. Haaker RG, Eickhoff U, Klammer HL. Intraarticular autogenous bone grafting in recurrent shoulder dislocations. Mil Med 1993;158:164-169.
15. Hawkins RJ, Angelo RL. Glenohumeral osteoarthritis: a late complication of the Putti-Platt repair. J Bone Joint Surg Am 1990;72:1193-1197.
16. Helfet AJ. Coracoid transplantation for recurring dislocation of the shoulder. J Bone Joint Surg Br 1958;40:198-202.
17. Hill HA, Sachs MD. The groove defect of the humeral head. A frequently unrecognized complication of dislocations of the shoulder joint. Radiology 1940;35:690-700.
18. Hovelius L. Anterior dislocation of the shoulder in teenagers and young adults. J Bone Joint Surg Am 1987;69:393-399.
19. Hutchinson JW, Neumann L, Wallace WA. Bone buttress operation for recurrent anterior shoulder dislocation in epilepsy. J Bone Joint Surg Br 1995;77:928-932.
20. Itoi E, Lee SB, Amrami KK, et al. Quantitative assessment of classic anteroinferior bony Bankart lesions by radiography and computed tomography. Am J Sports Med 2003;31:112-118.
21. Itoi E, Lee SB, Berglund LJ, et al. The effect of a glenoid defect on anteroinferior stability of the shoulder after Bankart repair: a cadaveric study. J Bone Joint Surg Am 2000;82:35-46.
22. Kropf EJ, Sekiya JK. Osteoarticular allograft transplantation for large humeral head defects in glenohumeral instability. Arthroscopy 2007;23(3):322.e1–5.
23. Miniaci A, Gish MW. Management of anterior glenohumeral instability associated with large Hill-Sachs defects. Tech Shoulder Elbow Surg 2004;5:170-175.
24. Neer CS, Foster CR. Inferior capsular shift for involuntary inferior and multidirectional instability of the shoulder. A preliminary report. J Bone Joint Surg Am 1980;62:897-908.
25. Rowe CR, Patel D, Southmayd WW. The Bankart procedure; a long-term end-result study. J Bone Joint Surg Am 1978;60:1-16.
26. Rowe CR, Zarins B, Ciullo JV. Recurrent anterior dislocation of the shoulder after surgical repair. J Bone Joint Surg Am 1984;66:159-168.
27. Scheibel M, Magosch P, Lichtenberg S, Habermeyer P. Open reconstruction of anterior glenoid rim fractures. Knee Surg Sports Traumatol Arthrosc 2004;12:568-573.
28. Sekiya JK, Wickwire AC, Stehle, JH, Debski RE. Biomechanical analysis of Hill-Sachs lesions in a joint compression model: injury and repair using articular allograft transplantation. Arthroscopy Association of North America, unpublished data, 2006.
29. Simonet WT, Cofield RH. Prognosis in anterior shoulder dislocation. Am J Sports Med 1984;12:19-24.
30. Tjoumakaris FP, Knopf EJ, Sekia JK: Osteoarticular allograft reconstruction of a large glenoid and humeral head defect in recurrent shoulder instability. Tech Shoulder Elbow Surg 2007;8(2):98–104.
31. Warner JP, Gill TJ, O'Holleran JD, et al. Anatomical glenoid reconstruction for recurrent anterior glenohumeral instability with glenoid deficiency using an autogenous tricortical iliac crest bone graft. Am J Sports Med 2006;34:205-212.
32. Weber BG, Simpson LA, Hardegger F. Rotational humeral osteotomy for recurrent anterior dislocation of the shoulder associated with a large Hill-Sachs lesion. J Bone Joint Surg Am 1984;66:1443-1446.
33. Young CD, Rockwood CA Jr. Complications of a failed Bristow procedure and their management. J Bone Joint Surg Am 1991;73:969-981.

CHAPTER 15

Coracoid Transfer: The Modified Latarjet Procedure for the Treatment of Recurrent Anterior Inferior Glenohumeral Instability in Patients with Bone Deficiency

David P. Huberty, MD

Stephen S. Burkhart, MD

Traumatic anterior inferior glenohumeral instability is a frequent problem in an active youthful population. Fortunately, primary surgical stabilization of the patient with recurrent traumatic dislocations, whether arthroscopic or open, has been predictably gratifying for both the patient and the surgeon. The best results have been obtained with accurate identification and treatment of the pathologic lesions without alteration of normal anatomy. In most cases, this involves repair of the avulsed anterior inferior labrum and inferior glenohumeral ligament to the glenoid rim. This "essential lesion" or Bankart lesion is present in as many as 97% of traumatic dislocations.[18] Successful correction of recurrent instability has been reported in more than 90% of patients by surgeons using both arthroscopic and open techniques to repair the Bankart lesion. However, the most frequently reported complication after both arthroscopic and open surgery for traumatic anterior instability is recurrent instability.[12,16] Undoubtedly a significant number of treatment failures are related to a failure to recognize and to treat the full extent of the pathologic process.

In the senior author's experience, arthroscopic treatment of patients with recurrent traumatic anterior insta-

bility has been successful in all patients except those with significant bone deficiency. Problematic bone deficiency may occur on either the glenoid or humeral side of the shoulder joint. We believe that loss of more than 25% of the inferior glenoid diameter (inverted pear) or an engaging Hill-Sachs lesion (a Hill-Sachs lesion that engages the anterior glenoid rim in the position of overhead athletic function, that is, 90 degrees of abduction and 90 degrees of external rotation) constitutes problematic bone deficiency (Figs. 15-1 to 15-3). In a series of 194 patients, Burkhart and De Beer reported a 4% recurrence rate for arthroscopic suture anchor Bankart repair in patients without significant bone deficiency. However, 67% of the 21 patients with significant bone deficiency (by the preceding criteria) had recurrent instability after an arthroscopic Bankart repair.[3] This clinical dilemma, the young active patient with recurrent traumatic anterior instability and a significant bone deficiency, presents the orthopedist with a difficult therapeutic challenge. We have found a modified Latarjet reconstruction to be the most effective form of treatment. The original Latarjet procedure, developed and reported in 1954, transfers a large segment of the coracoid (2.5 to 3 cm in length) as bone

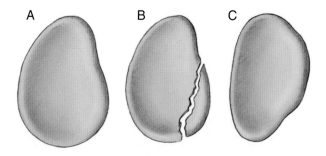

Figure 15-1 A, The normal shape of the glenoid is that of a pear, larger diameter inferior than superior. **B,** A bony Bankart lesion can cause an inverted-pear configuration. **C,** A compression (impression) Bankart lesion from numerous dislocations can also cause an inverted-pear configuration. (Redrawn with modification from Burkhart SS, De Beer JF. Traumatic glenohumeral bone defects and their relationship to failure of arthroscopic Bankart repairs: significance of the inverted-pear glenoid and the humeral engaging Hill-Sachs lesion. Arthroscopy 2000;16:677-694.)

graft to the anterior inferior glenoid rim.[11] We have incorporated several modifications to the original Latarjet procedure that we believe will improve the long-term results.

The modified Latarjet coracoid transfer is a technically demanding operation that can provide a safe and reliable solution with lasting positive results in a challenging population of patients. We recommend this treatment for young active patients with recurrent anterior inferior shoulder instability associated with the inverted-pear configuration of glenoid bone deficiency or an engaging Hill-Sachs lesion. Graft placement and orientation are critical to both the short-term and long-term success of this operation.

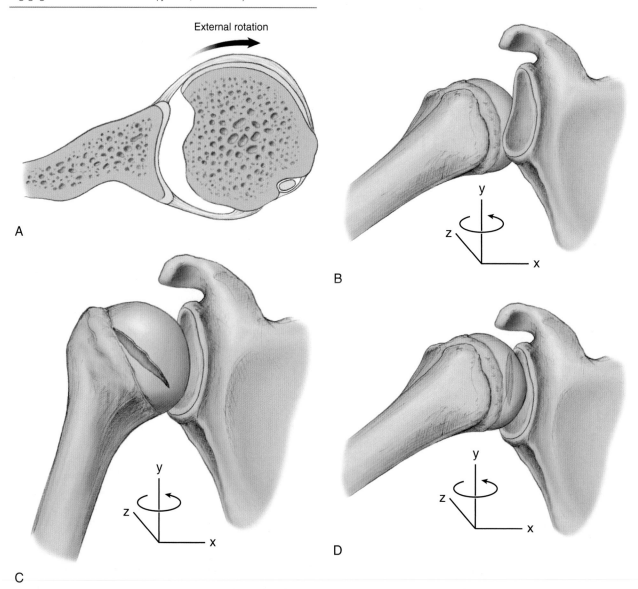

Figure 15-2 Engaging Hill-Sachs lesion. **A,** In a functional position of abduction and external rotation, the long axis of the Hill-Sachs lesion is parallel to the glenoid and engages its anterior cortex. **B,** Creation of lesion in a left shoulder with arm in abduction and external rotation. **C,** Orientation of Hill-Sachs lesion. **D,** Engagement of Hill-Sachs lesion in functional position of abduction and external rotation.

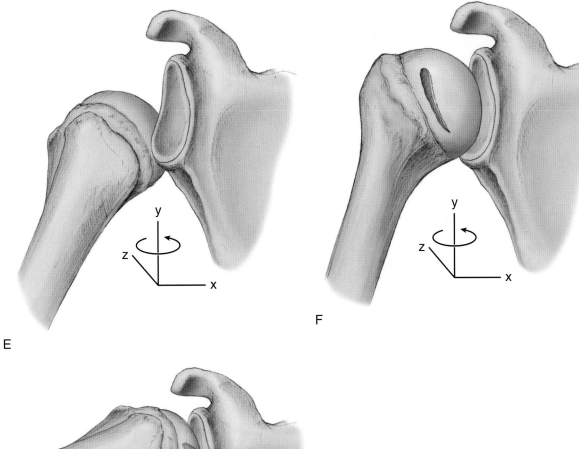

E

F

G

Figure 15-2, cont'd E, The Hill-Sachs lesion is nonengaging with the arm at the side and in some extension; it will engage only with the arm at the side with external rotation and extension, which is not a functional position. **F,** Orientation of a nonengaging Hill-Sachs lesion. **G,** In a functional position of abduction and external rotation, the Hill-Sachs lesion is diagonal to the anterior margin of the glenoid and does not engage. (Redrawn with modification from Burkhart SS, De Beer JF. Traumatic glenohumeral bone defects and their relationship to failure of arthroscopic Bankart repairs: significance of the inverted-pear glenoid and the humeral engaging Hill-Sachs lesion. Arthroscopy 2000;16:677-694.)

Rationale for Efficacy

The efficacy of this procedure can be explained by the combination of four main effects. First, the large bone graft replaces glenoid bone loss and augments the concavity of the glenoid articular arc. This effect diminishes the shoulder's propensity for dislocation during off-axis loads (Fig. 15-4). Second, in the case of the engaging Hill-Sachs lesion, the extended articular arc provided by the coracoid graft prevents engagement of the humeral bone defect. The

shoulder is not able to externally rotate to the degree necessary for engagement over the front of the graft (Fig. 15-5). Third, the transferred conjoined tendon acts as a tether, restricting external rotation to some extent, and the posterior capsule restricts anterior translation of the humeral head over the augmented glenoid concavity. Finally, the transferred conjoined tendon forms a sling across the anterior inferior capsule when the shoulder is abducted and externally rotated, serving as an additional constraint to anterior inferior translation.

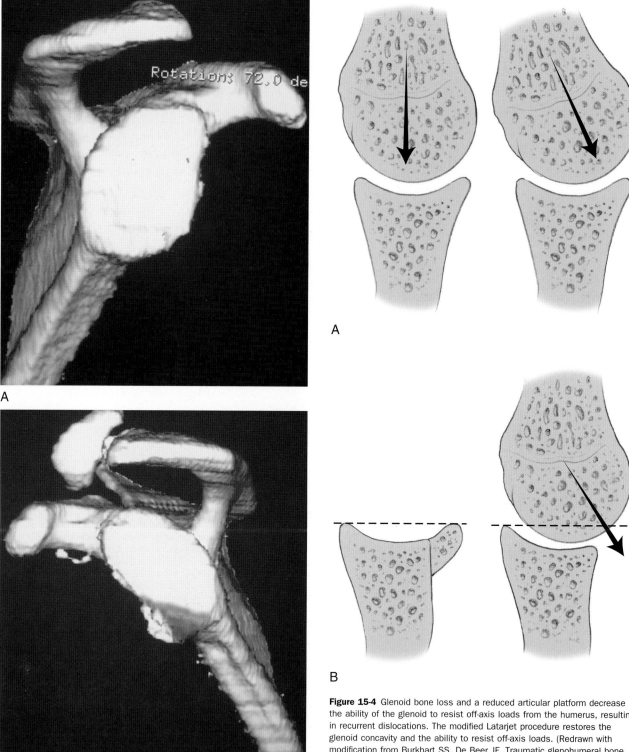

A

B

Figure 15-3 Three-dimensional computed tomographic scans of bilateral shoulders. **A,** The normal right glenoid demonstrates the normal pear shape when it is viewed en face. **B,** The abnormal left glenoid appears in the shape of an inverted pear because of a bony Bankart lesion.

A

B

Figure 15-4 Glenoid bone loss and a reduced articular platform decrease the ability of the glenoid to resist off-axis loads from the humerus, resulting in recurrent dislocations. The modified Latarjet procedure restores the glenoid concavity and the ability to resist off-axis loads. (Redrawn with modification from Burkhart SS, De Beer JF. Traumatic glenohumeral bone defects and their relationship to failure of arthroscopic Bankart repairs: significance of the inverted-pear glenoid and the humeral engaging Hill-Sachs lesion. Arthroscopy 2000;16:677-694.)

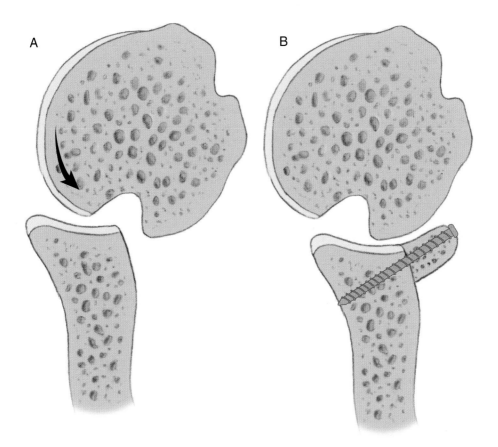

Figure 15-5 The modified Latarjet procedure will lengthen the glenoid articular arc to prevent engagement of an engaging Hill-Sachs lesion. **A,** Engagement of Hill-Sachs lesion. **B,** Prevention of engagement by lengthening of the glenoid articular arc. (Redrawn with modification from Burkhart SS, De Beer JF. Traumatic glenohumeral bone defects and their relationship to failure of arthroscopic Bankart repairs: significance of the inverted-pear glenoid and the humeral engaging Hill-Sachs lesion. Arthroscopy 2000;16:677-694.)

Preoperative Considerations

History

A thorough history is essential and should elicit the mechanism of injury and prior treatments received. Previous operative reports should be obtained and reviewed; they often yield valuable information about areas of bone deficiency, tissue quality, and fixation devices used. The physical examination determines the position and direction of instability as well as identifies or eliminates factors that contribute to instability.

Essential Components of the History
- Age
- Mechanism of dislocations
- Number of dislocations
- Position of shoulder during dislocation
- Reduction efforts (self- or physician-reduced)
- Dominant arm
- Sport and work requirements
- Prior treatments
- Patient's goals

Physical Examination
- Muscle tone or wasting
- Range of motion, active and passive
- Strength assessment (rule out concomitant rotator cuff tear)
- Position of apprehension
- Relocation relief
- Direction of instability (load and shift test)
- Generalized ligamentous laxity
- Neurovascular examination

Imaging

Preoperative radiographs give valuable information about various areas of bone deficiency. However, quantification of bone loss based on plain radiographs is difficult. Three-dimensional computed tomographic scans of bilateral shoulders have been extremely valuable in allowing accurate quantification of glenoid and humeral bone loss (see Fig. 15-3). The magnetic resonance imaging scan is also essential to allow accurate identification of the spectrum of pathologic lesions responsible for instability (Bankart, SLAP, humeral avulsion of the glenohumeral ligament, capsular redundancy, and bone defects).

Radiography

- True anteroposterior view of shoulder: evaluation of glenohumeral joint space
- Anteroposterior view, internal and external rotation: Hill-Sachs lesions, tuberosity fractures
- Stryker notch view: Hill-Sachs lesion
- Axillary lateral view: concentric reduction, anterior glenoid bone loss
- West Point view: anterior inferior glenoid fracture or bone loss

Indications and Contraindications

Indications

Surgery is indicated for active patients with recurrent anterior inferior instability and bone deficiency defined by at least one of the following:

- Inverted-pear glenoid, determined arthroscopically (more than 25% loss of inferior diameter of glenoid)
- Engaging Hill-Sachs lesion, determined arthroscopically (posterior superior humeral head defect that engages the anterior rim of the glenoid in a functional position of 90 degrees of abduction and 90 degrees of external rotation)

Contraindications

- Active infection in or around the shoulder joint
- Intentional and voluntary dislocations (relative contraindication)

Surgical Technique

Anesthesia and Positioning

The procedure is usually performed under a combination of general anesthesia with endotracheal intubation or laryngeal mask ventilation and regional anesthesia through an interscalene nerve block. The patient is positioned in the beach chair or lateral decubitus position for the arthroscopic part of the procedure. The coracoid transfer is best performed in the beach chair position.

Surgical Landmarks, Incisions, and Portals

Similar to standard arthroscopy, the anatomic landmarks should be drawn out. Diagnostic arthroscopy uses the standard anterior and posterior portals; the coracoid transfer is performed through a standard deltopectoral approach.

Examination Under Anesthesia and Diagnostic Arthroscopy

Accurate identification of the full extent of the pathologic process is the first major goal. Examination under anesthesia should confirm the degree and position of laxity. We believe it is essential to begin with diagnostic arthroscopy so that any bone deficiency can be identified and quantified and concomitant pathologic lesions (SLAP lesions) may be treated arthroscopically before the open coracoid transfer.

The posterior, anterior, and anterior superior portals are generally used for diagnostic arthroscopy. Glenoid bone deficiency is evaluated by viewing from the anterior superior portal while using a calibrated probe through the posterior portal. The shape of the glenoid is assessed, and the probe is used to quantify the amount and location of bone loss (Fig. 15-6). The normal inferior glenoid has an average anterior-posterior diameter of 23 mm, and the bare spot normally lies in the center of this measurement.[5] This information gives the surgeon a simple method of quantifying the percentage of glenoid bone deficiency (Box 15-1). Our data have shown that 25% or greater glenoid bone loss is significant, and in this scenario, the glenoid assumes the shape of an inverted pear.

To assess the humerus for a significant bone defect, previously defined as an engaging Hill-Sachs lesion, we sequentially view from the posterior portal and then the anterosuperior portal with the arm removed from traction. The arm is placed in the position of apprehension, usually 90 degrees of abduction and 90 degrees of external rotation, and we observe whether the humeral head defect slides onto or engages the anterior rim of the glenoid (see Fig. 15-2). If the humeral head defect is oriented such that it is oblique to and does not engage the anterior glenoid rim in the 90-90 position, it is a nonengaging and less significant lesion.

If a significant bone deficiency is identified on either the glenoid or humerus, we proceed with the modified

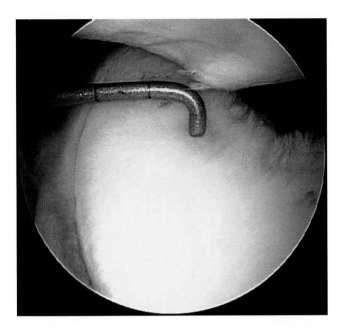

Figure 15-6 Arthroscopic view of a left shoulder through an anterosuperior portal demonstrating an inverted-pear glenoid. Note how the inferior aspect of the glenoid appears narrower than the superior aspect of the glenoid.

Latarjet procedure, after first treating other concomitant pathologic lesions (such as a SLAP lesion) arthroscopically. However, if the bone defect does not meet these criteria for significance, we treat identified intra-articular disease including the Bankart lesion arthroscopically.

The Modified Latarjet Procedure

Specific Steps (Box 15-2)

1. Superficial Exposure

A standard deltopectoral approach is used to begin the modified Latarjet procedure. The cephalic vein is carefully dissected and generally retracted laterally, preserving the major branches to the deltoid. The clavipectoral fascia is divided and the coracoid is exposed to its base where the coracoclavicular ligaments insert. The coracoacromial ligament is released from the lateral tip of the coracoid, and the pectoralis minor tendon is sharply dissected free from the medial surface of the coracoid (Fig. 15-7). It is this

Box 15-1 Estimation of Glenoid Bone Deficiency

1. Measure inferior diameter of glenoid/23 mm
2. Measure distance from bare spot to anterior glenoid rim *(A)* and from bare spot to posterior glenoid rim *(B)*. $$\text{Percentage of bone loss} = \frac{2B - (A+B)}{2B} \times 100$$

Box 15-2 Surgical Steps

1. Superficial exposure
2. Coracoid osteotomy
3. Graft mobilization and preparation
4. Second-level exposure
5. Recipient site preparation
6. Graft placement, orientation, and fixation
7. Closure

medial surface of the coracoid that will later be approximated to the anterior glenoid neck.

2. Coracoid Osteotomy

Next, a 70-degree angled sagittal saw blade is used to osteotomize the coracoid at its base, just distal to the insertion of the coracoclavicular ligaments (Fig. 15-8). In general, 2.5 to 3 cm of coracoid graft is obtained. We think that use of an angled saw simplifies the osteotomy by allowing an easier angle of approach and makes scapular or glenoid fracture much less likely. Neurovascular structures are protected with Chandler elevators placed medially and inferiorly.

3. Graft Mobilization and Preparation

It is crucial that the conjoined tendon be left attached to the coracoid graft. This preserves some blood supply to the

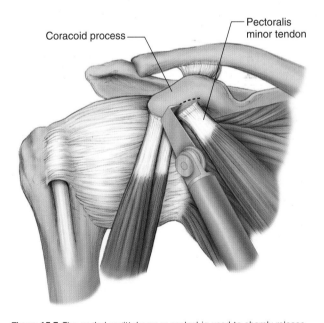

Figure 15-7 The angled sagittal saw or scalpel is used to sharply release the pectoralis minor tendon from the coracoid neck. (Redrawn with modification from Burkhart SS, De Beer JF. Traumatic glenohumeral bone defects and their relationship to failure of arthroscopic Bankart repairs: significance of the inverted-pear glenoid and the humeral engaging Hill-Sachs lesion. Arthroscopy 2000;16:677-694.)

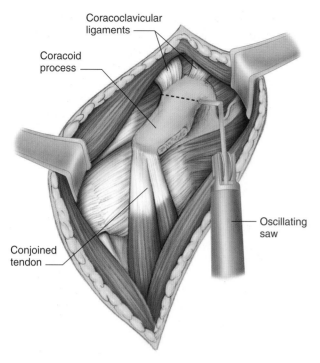

Figure 15-8 The coracoid osteotomy is made proximal to the neck of the coracoid. An angled saw blade simplifies the osteotomy by more easily achieving the proper angle of approach. (Redrawn with modification from Burkhart SS, De Beer JF. Traumatic glenohumeral bone defects and their relationship to failure of arthroscopic Bankart repairs: significance of the inverted-pear glenoid and the humeral engaging Hill-Sachs lesion. Arthroscopy 2000;16:677-694.)

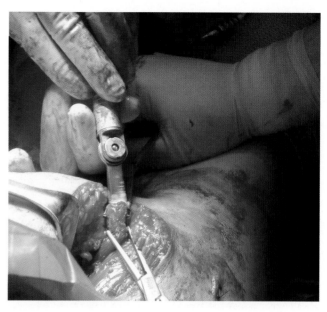

Figure 15-9 The coracoid graft is held with two Kocher clamps while the sagittal saw is used to shave off a thin layer of cortical bone from the medial coracoid surface (pectoralis minor insertion site). This produces a bleeding cancellous surface to optimize later graft consolidation.

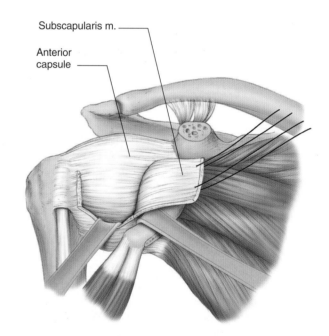

Figure 15-10 The superior half of the subscapularis tendon is detached, and a plane between the inferior half of the tendon and the capsule is developed. (Redrawn with modification from Burkhart SS, De Beer JF. Traumatic glenohumeral bone defects and their relationship to failure of arthroscopic Bankart repairs: significance of the inverted-pear glenoid and the humeral engaging Hill-Sachs lesion. Arthroscopy 2000;16:677-694.)

graft (a vascularized graft) and, we believe, speeds consolidation. The transferred coracoid graft will continue to serve as a stable attachment for the short head of the biceps and coracobrachialis muscles. The conjoined tendon and graft must be mobilized for transfer to the anterior glenoid neck. Great care must be maintained during this step so as not to cause stretch injury to the musculocutaneous nerve, which enters the coracobrachialis muscle a variable distance (approximately 5 cm) distal to the coracoid attachment.[7] Next, the medial coracoid surface (pectoralis minor insertion site) is prepared to a bleeding cancellous surface by shaving off the thin cortical layer with the sagittal saw (Fig. 15-9). The graft is tucked in the medial tissue for later use.

4. Second-Level Exposure

An excellent exposure of the anterior shoulder is obtained once the coracoid has been osteotomized. The superior half of the subscapularis tendon is detached distally from just medial to the biceps tendon while preserving the underlying capsule (Fig. 15-10). Tagging sutures (No. 2 FiberWire; Arthrex, Inc., Naples, Fla) are placed in the superior half of the subscapularis with a grasping stitch and are used to assist with dissection between tendon and capsule as well as for later repair. This portion of the subscapularis tendon is reflected medially, and the lower half

of the tendon is preserved intact throughout. (Although it is conceptually tempting to perform this operation through a simple split in the subscapularis, the exposure gained by reflecting the superior half of subscapularis is much more reproducible for glenoid preparation, graft orientation, and fixation.) Next, the plane between the remaining lower subscapularis and capsule is developed, and a vertical capsular incision is made 1 cm medial to the glenoid rim. The capsule and underlying labrum are reflected laterally by sharp subperiosteal dissection (Fig. 15-11). Maximal length of the capsular flap is necessary for later repair.

5. Recipient Site Preparation

The anterior glenoid neck and rim are prepared as the recipient bone bed for grafting by use of curets and high-speed bur (a light dusting). The goal here is to establish a bleeding bone surface devoid of fibrous tissue while removing as little bone structure as possible. Three suture anchors (3.0 mm Bio-Suture Tak; Arthrex, Naples, Fla) are placed at the native glenoid rim at the 3-, 4-, and 5-o'clock positions (right shoulder) and are used later for capsular repair (Fig. 15-12).

6. Graft Placement, Orientation, and Fixation

The coracoid seems perfectly formed for placement as an anterior glenoid bone graft. The curved contour of the coracoid bone (original inferior surface) seems to perfectly match the radius of curvature of the anterior inferior glenoid. The prepared medial surface of the coracoid graft is placed against the recipient anterior inferior glenoid neck with the long axis of the graft oriented superior to inferior (Fig. 15-13). Minor graft rotation and trimming are performed as necessary for best fit. Proper positioning

of the coracoid graft relative to the glenoid rim is critically important for success in preventing recurrent dislocation and for the avoidance of late degenerative arthritis (Fig. 15-14). The graft is placed not as a bone block but rather so that it functions as an extension of the glenoid articular arc. The graft is temporarily fixed in place with guide pins for the 4.0-mm cannulated screws. If the graft is sufficiently large, we prefer to use the 4.5-mm cannulated screw set as the guide pin is considerably more robust. When the surgeon is satisfied with orientation and fit, the graft is permanently secured with two cannulated screws, achieving purchase in the far glenoid cortex. Screw lengths have been remarkably consistent at 36 and 34 mm, although intraoperative radiographs are always obtained to confirm graft position and fixation (Fig. 15-15). At this point, before capsular closure, we generally irrigate the joint copiously and take the shoulder through range of motion to assess stability. Once the coracoid graft has been secured, we have found that dislocation is virtually impossible even in the most provocative position. Finally, the previously reflected capsule is repaired by means of the suture anchors to the native glenoid rim. This places a synovium-lined tissue layer between the coracoid graft and humeral head, preventing the humeral articular surface from abrading against the coracoid graft.

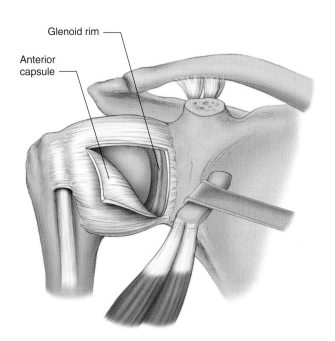

Figure 15-11 Capsulotomy is performed by dissecting 1 cm medial to the glenoid rim to preserve as much capsular length as possible for later reattachment. (Redrawn with modification from Burkhart SS, De Beer JF. Traumatic glenohumeral bone defects and their relationship to failure of arthroscopic Bankart repairs: significance of the inverted-pear glenoid and the humeral engaging Hill-Sachs lesion. Arthroscopy 2000;16:677-694.)

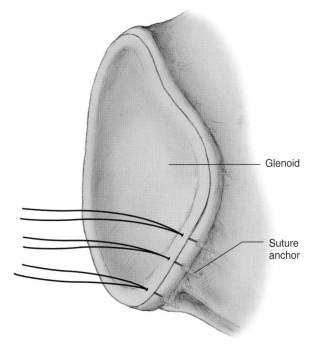

Figure 15-12 Suture anchors are placed along the glenoid rim for later reattachment of the capsulolabral tissue. The later capsulolabral repair ensures that the coracoid bone graft remains extra-articular. (Redrawn with modification from Burkhart SS, De Beer JF. Traumatic glenohumeral bone defects and their relationship to failure of arthroscopic Bankart repairs: significance of the inverted-pear glenoid and the humeral engaging Hill-Sachs lesion. Arthroscopy 2000;16:677-694.)

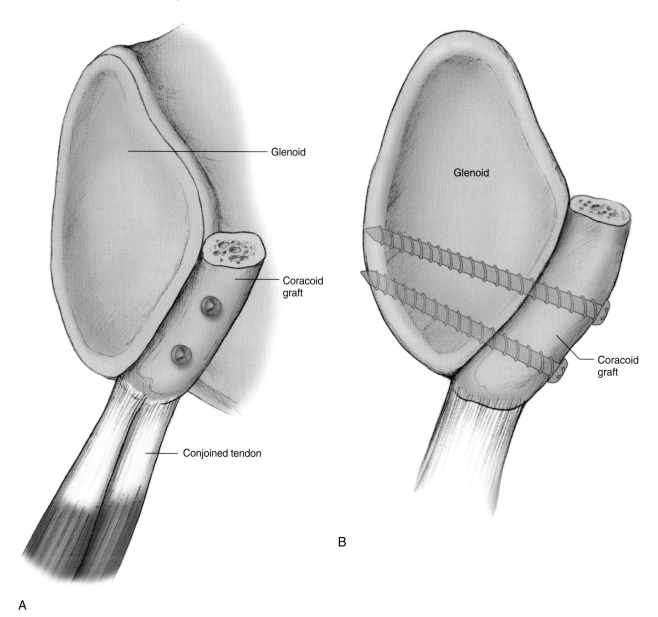

Glenoid

Coracoid graft

Conjoined tendon

A

Glenoid

Coracoid graft

B

Figure 15-13 The coracoid graft is fixed to the glenoid with two bicortical screws. **A,** The raw bone surface where the pectoralis minor was removed will usually provide the best fit against the glenoid, and the graft can be further contoured with a power bur to fit the curve of the anterior inferior glenoid. **B,** After graft fixation, the glenoid again resembles the shape of a pear. (Redrawn with modification from Burkhart SS, De Beer JF. Traumatic glenohumeral bone defects and their relationship to failure of arthroscopic Bankart repairs: significance of the inverted-pear glenoid and the humeral engaging Hill-Sachs lesion. Arthroscopy 2000;16:677-694.)

7. Closure

The superior half of the subscapularis tendon is repaired to its insertion by means of the previously placed Fiber-Wire tagging sutures. The conjoined tendon, remaining attached to the coracoid graft, now passes through the remaining horizontal split in the subscapularis tendon (Fig. 15-16). Finally, the wound is thoroughly irrigated, and standard closure of the subcutaneous and subcuticular layers is performed. The patient is placed in a sling with a small pillow. A consistent postoperative rehabilitation protocol is followed.

Postoperative Considerations

Rehabilitation

- A padded sling is worn for the first 4 weeks. It is removed three times daily for passive external rotation to neutral.
- The immobilizer is discontinued at 4 weeks, and passive overhead motion is encouraged.
- Gentle external rotation stretching is initiated at 6 weeks.

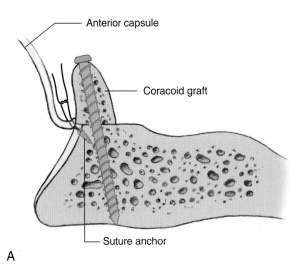

Anterior capsule

Coracoid graft

Suture anchor

A

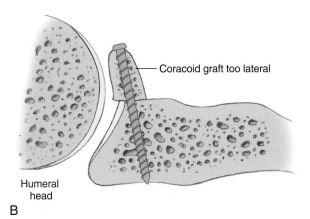

Coracoid graft too lateral

Humeral head

B

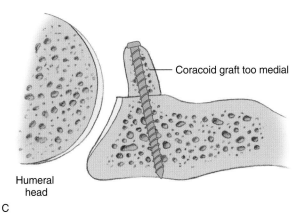

Coracoid graft too medial

Humeral head

C

Figure 15-14 A, The graft is placed so that it becomes an extra-articular platform that acts as an extension of the articular arc of the glenoid. **B,** If the graft is incorrectly placed too lateral, it will act as a bone block and predispose to early degenerative arthritis. **C,** If the graft is incorrectly placed too medial along the glenoid neck, this may predispose to recurrent subluxation. (Redrawn with modification from Burkhart SS, De Beer JF. Traumatic glenohumeral bone defects and their relationship to failure of arthroscopic Bankart repairs: significance of the inverted-pear glenoid and the humeral engaging Hill-Sachs lesion. Arthroscopy 2000;16:677-694.)

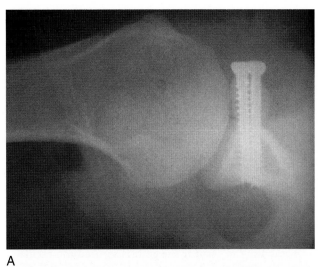

A

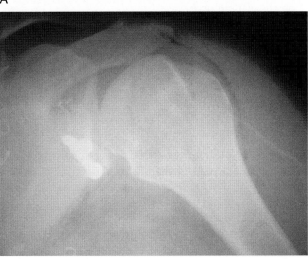

B

Figure 15-15 Intraoperative axillary lateral **(A)** and anteroposterior **(B)** radiographs demonstrate ideal graft placement and fixation.

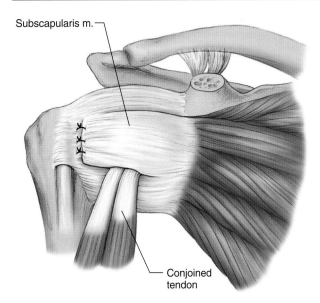

Subscapularis m.

Conjoined tendon

Figure 15-16 The subscapularis is repaired with No. 2 FiberWire suture along the superior margin; the conjoined tendon passes through the split in the subscapularis tendon. (Redrawn with modification from Burkhart SS, De Beer JF. Traumatic glenohumeral bone defects and their relationship to failure of arthroscopic Bankart repairs: significance of the inverted-pear glenoid and the humeral engaging Hill-Sachs lesion. Arthroscopy 2000;16:677-694.)

15

- The surgically repaired shoulder should have 50% of the normal shoulder's external rotation at 3 months.
- Strengthening exercises are delayed until there is radiographic evidence of early graft consolidation (usually 3 to 4 months).
- Heavy labor and sporting activity are generally allowed at 6 months.

Complications

The majority of the reported complications are related to the coracoid graft harvest and the position of graft fixation along the glenoid.

- Instability can recur if the graft is secured too medial on the glenoid neck.
- Scapula fracture has been reported during graft harvest with the osteotome.
- Late graft fracture and recurrent dislocation have occurred after traumatic athletic injury.
- Fibrous union or nonunion of the graft may result.
- Postoperative infection has occurred in 0% to 5% of patients.
- Significant glenohumeral arthritis developed in 20% of patients at 14 years of follow-up.

PEARLS AND PITFALLS

- Take the time to carefully expose the base of the coracoid so that a coracoid graft of maximal length can be obtained. A maximal length (usually 2.5 to 3 cm) will allow graft fixation with two screws. This is optimal with regard to compressive and rotational stability of the graft. Coracoid graft fracture can occur in trying to obtain dual screw fixation in a shorter length.
- Use of a 70-degree angled sagittal saw blade (as opposed to a curved osteotome) has significantly simplified the coracoid osteotomy. The cut can be made with more precision, and scapular fracture is much less likely to occur.
- If coracoid graft diameter is sufficient, we recommend use of the 4.5-mm cannulated screws. The guide wire is more robust and less likely to be sheared off in overdrilling through the dense cortical bone of the coracoid.

Results

To date, there have been only four reports of the Latarjet procedure in the English language literature (Table 15-1),[1,3,4,19] although there are many reports of the Bristow procedure (often called the Latarjet-Bristow procedure), which is a significantly different procedure that transfers only the coracoid tip to the glenoid neck. Regarding the Latarjet procedure, Burkhart et al[3] reported the results of 104 patients an average of 39 months after reconstruction. Six complications were reported, including one hematoma that required evacuation, one fibrous union with loose screws, and four recurrent dislocations and one recurrent subluxation (4.9% recurrence rate). All recurrent dislocations were related to violent trauma in the early postoperative period and occurred with graft dislodgement. Patients achieved an average of 179.6 degrees of forward elevation (2.4 degrees improved from preoperative range) and an average of 48.1 degrees of external rotation with the arm at the side (7.3 degrees less than preoperative range). The authors concluded that this is a safe and effective procedure for a challenging clinical problem.

Allain et al[1] retrospectively reviewed 56 patients an average of 14.3 years after the Latarjet procedure for recurrent anterior instability. The primary purpose of this research was to determine the prevalence of glenohumeral arthritis and factors related to its development. At the latest follow-up, there were no cases of postoperative dislocation despite presence of the apprehension sign in six patients. Eleven patients (20%) were thought to demonstrate significant glenohumeral arthritis. The authors concluded that the development of glenohumeral arthritis is most closely related to a preoperative tear of the rotator cuff and too lateral placement of the coracoid graft.

Table 15-1 Results of Studies of the Latarjet Procedure

Author	Follow-up	Outcome	Conclusion
Allain et al[1] (1998)	14.3 years mean (range: 10-23)	88% good and excellent results by grading system of Rowe 1 of 58: persistent instability	Precise graft placement is critical to avoid recurrent instability and late glenohumeral arthritis.
Burkhart and De Beer[4] (2000)	39 months (range: 12-88)	5 of 104: recurrent instability 4 of 5 failures related to violent trauma with graft dislodgement	Modified Latarjet procedure is a safe and reliable treatment of patients with recurrent instability and bone deficiency.

References

1. Allain J, Goutallier D, Glorion C. Long-term results of the Latarjet procedure for the treatment of anterior instability of the shoulder. J Bone Joint Surg Am 1998;80:841-852.

2. Bigliani LU, Newton PM, Steinmann SP, et al. Glenoid rim lesions associated with recurrent anterior dislocation of the shoulder. Am J Sports Med 1998;26:41-45.

3. Burkhart S, De Beer J, Barth J, et al. Results of modified Latarjet reconstruction in patients with anteroinferior instability and significant bone loss. Arthroscopy; in press.

4. Burkhart SS, De Beer JF. Traumatic glenohumeral bone defects and their relationship to failure of arthroscopic Bankart repairs: significance of the inverted-pear glenoid and the humeral engaging Hill-Sachs lesion. Arthroscopy 2000;16:677-694.

5. Burkhart SS, De Beer JF, Tehrany AM, Parten PM. Quantifying glenoid bone loss arthroscopically in shoulder instability. Arthroscopy 2002;18:488-491.

6. Churchill RS, Moskal MJ, Lippett SB, Matsen FA III. Extracapsular anatomically contoured anterior glenoid bone grafting for complex glenohumeral instability. Tech Shoulder Elbow Surg 2001;2:210-218.

7. Eglseder WA Jr, Goldman M. Anatomic variations of the musculocutaneous nerve in the arm. Am J Orthop 1997;26:777-780.

8. Helfet AJ. Coracoid transplantation for recurring dislocation of the shoulder. J Bone Joint Surg Br 1958;40:198-202.

9. Itoi E, Lee SB, Berglund LJ, et al. The effect of a glenoid defect on anteroinferior stability of the shoulder after Bankart repair: a cadaveric study. J Bone Joint Surg Am 2000;82:35-46.

10. Kim SH, Ha KI, Kim YM. Arthroscopic revision Bankart repair: a prospective outcome study. Arthroscopy 2002;18:469-482.

11. Latarjet M. Apropos du traitement des luxations récidivantes de l'epaule. Lyon Chir 1954;49:994-1003.

12. Lazarus M, Harryman D. Complications of open anterior stabilization of the shoulder. J Am Acad Orthop Surg 2000;8:1222-1132.

13. Lo IK, Parten PM, Burkhart SS. The inverted pear glenoid: an indicator of significant glenoid bone loss. Arthroscopy 2004;20;169-174.

14. Maynou C, Cassagnaud X, Mestdagh H. Function of subscapularis after surgical treatment for recurrent instability of the shoulder using a bone-block procedure. J Bone Joint Surg Br 2005;87:1096-1101.

15. Mazzocca AD, Brown FM, Carreira DS, et al. Arthroscopic anterior shoulder stabilization of collision and contact athletes. Am J Sports Med 2005;33:52-60.

16. Stein DA, Jazrawi L, Bartolozzi AR. Arthroscopic stabilization of anterior shoulder instability: a review of the literature. Arthroscopy 2002;18:912-924.

17. Tauber M, Resch H, Forstner R, et al. Reasons for failure after surgical repair of anterior shoulder instability. J Shoulder Elbow Surg 2004;3:279-285.

18. Thomas S, Matsen FA III. An approach to the repair of avulsion of the glenohumeral ligaments in the management of traumatic anterior glenohumeral instability. J Bone Joint Surg Am 1989;71:506-513.

19. Walch G, Boileau P. Latarjet-Bristow procedure for recurrent anterior instability. Tech Shoulder Elbow Surg 2000;1:256-261.

15

Arthroscopic Rotator Cuff Repair: Single-Row Technique

Andreas H. Gomoll, MD
Brian J. Cole, MD, MBA

Arthroscopic treatment of rotator cuff tears has become a routine procedure following a general trend toward less invasive surgery. Proponents of this technique emphasize the decreased risk of complications, such as infection, stiffness, and deltoid avulsions; critics mention the lack of long-term studies, the controversy about the strength of fixation, and the technical challenge of all-arthroscopic repair of large tears for nonspecialists. The goal of arthroscopic rotator cuff repair is to relieve pain and to improve shoulder function while addressing all concomitant intra-articular disease in a minimally invasive manner. Many technical aspects of arthroscopic rotator cuff surgery are evolving as our understanding of failure mechanisms and patient outcomes grows. Many issues remain controversial, such as the need for routine acromioplasty, management of incomplete tears, optimal suture management, and anchor configuration (single row versus double row). The successful arthroscopic treatment of rotator cuff tears depends on recognition of tear patterns, appropriate use of releases, secure fixation with restoration of the footprint under minimal tension, and proper rehabilitation. This and the following chapter provide an overview of the indications, surgical technique, rehabilitation, and results of arthroscopic rotator cuff repair. To provide a balanced perspective, we present the standard single-row technique here; Chapter 17 discusses double-row and suture bridge techniques, which we currently use in all but small and uncomplicated tears.

Preoperative Considerations

History

- The pain is commonly insidious in onset, extending over the lateral arm and shoulder, often radiating toward the deltoid insertion.

- The pain is often dull at rest.

- Overhead and reaching activities exacerbate the pain, which then frequently takes on a sharp character.

- The pain frequently increases at night and may awaken the individual from sleep.

- Patients frequently describe difficulties in combing their hair, holding a hair dryer, and reaching their back pocket.

- Weakness with the inability to abduct and elevate the arm is seen in more advanced cases.

- Acute onset of weakness, especially in association with trauma, may indicate an acute or acute-on-chronic tear. The acute tear, especially in young patients without preexisting shoulder problems, should be addressed more expediently, with early magnetic resonance imaging and surgical fixation.

Physical Examination

Factors Affecting Surgical Indication

- The patient's age, functional status, expectations or demands, and comorbidities
- Pain and shoulder dysfunction resistant to conservative management
- Acute traumatic weakness in a younger patient should be treated expediently; older patients can undergo a trial of conservative management.

Factors Affecting Surgical Planning

- Associated pathologic processes: assess biceps tendon, capsulolabral complex, acromioclavicular joint, acromion, and subscapularis tendon
- Chronicity of the tear: tissue quality and muscle atrophy
- Morphologic features and size of the tear

Imaging

Radiography

- True anteroposterior view of the shoulder assesses for degenerative changes, calcific tendinitis, and humeral head elevation in massive rotator cuff tears.
- Axillary view demonstrates joint space narrowing and the rare but occasionally symptomatic os acromiale.
- Outlet view demonstrates acromial morphologic features.

Ultrasonography

- Noninvasive, readily available and inexpensive, but operator dependent
- Sensitivities of 58% to 100% and specificities of 78% to 100% for full-thickness tears; less accurate for partial-thickness tears with sensitivities from 25% to 94%

Magnetic Resonance Imaging and Magnetic Resonance Arthrography (Fig. 16-1)

- Sensitivities close to 100% for full-thickness tears
- Allows evaluation of soft tissue envelope, especially for tear retraction and muscle degeneration, which influence surgical decision-making
- Magnetic resonance arthrography improves sensitivity, especially for the detection of partial tears, to more than 90%

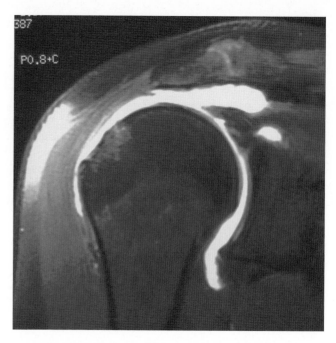

Figure 16-1 Magnetic resonance image depicting large rotator cuff tear with retraction of the tendon edge almost to the level of the glenoid.

Tear Classification

Partial Tears

Partial tears generally involve less than 50% of the tendon thickness and do not lead to retraction of the muscle. On the basis of location within the tendon, partial tears are classified as intrasubstance, bursal sided, or articular sided (undersurface); the last constitutes approximately 90% of partial tears. Weakness is uncommon in partial-thickness tears but can arise from pain, which is often greater than in complete tears.

Full-thickness Tears

In contrast, full-thickness tears represent complete discontinuity of rotator cuff fibers, resulting in communication between the articular and bursal spaces. The extent of the lesion on imaging studies is described in both anteroposterior and mediolateral directions; 1 cm is generally considered small, 1 to 3 cm medium, 3 to 5 cm large, and more than 5 cm massive. Tears that involve two or more tendons are automatically classified as massive and occasionally require more complex reconstruction. Larger tears with chronic tendon retraction lead to fatty degeneration of the associated muscle that may be irreversible, making results of direct repair less predictable.

Rotator cuff tears can be further classified on the basis of tear configuration. Crescentic, L-shaped, and U-shaped tears have been described, all of which require slight modifications in repair technique (see later).

Indications and Contraindications

The primary indication for surgical treatment is persistent pain unresponsive to nonoperative measures or, more rarely, acute weakness due to a traumatic tear in a younger individual; poor function and diminished strength are relative indications with less reliable outcomes. The ideal surgical candidate is a compliant patient with few comorbidities and adequate tendon quality who can follow a rigorous postoperative rehabilitation program. All patients should recognize that the results are dependent on many factors, including size and retraction of the tear, tissue quality, muscle degeneration and atrophy, and overall health of the patient.

Contraindications include active or recent infection, medical comorbidities that preclude surgery, and advanced glenohumeral arthritis. Relative contraindications may include significant muscle degeneration and fixed superior migration of the humeral head.

Surgical Technique

Anesthesia and Positioning

Arthroscopic rotator cuff repair is usually performed under general anesthesia with endotracheal intubation or laryngeal mask ventilation, regional anesthesia through an interscalene nerve block, or a combination thereof. The decision is made in collaboration with the patient and anesthesiologist. Regional anesthesia has been found especially helpful for pain management in outpatient procedures because its effects commonly continue for several hours. Preemptive analgesia with anti-inflammatory drugs given before the operation is increasingly being used and is usually continued for several days postoperatively. This treatment will have to be re-evaluated in light of emerging reports of potential detrimental effects of anti-inflammatory drugs on early tendon healing.

On the basis of the surgeon's preference, the patient is placed in either the beach chair or lateral decubitus position. Whereas each position has unique advantages and limitations, both are acceptable choices for arthroscopic rotator cuff repair.

Surgical Landmarks, Incisions, and Portals

Landmarks
- Clavicle
- Acromion
- Acromioclavicular joint
- Coracoid process
- Scapular spine

Portals and Approaches
- Anterior portal
- Posterior portal
- Standard lateral portal
- Posterolateral portal

A portal that we have recently described and find particularly useful is the posteromedial portal, which is placed approximately 3 cm medial to the standard posterior portal. This portal allows in-line passage of a suture-retrieving instrument (i.e., penetrating suture grasper).

When it is necessary to achieve ideal anchor orientation, the surgeon can make accessory portals that deviate from the standard portals. These portals should be kept as small as possible to minimize trauma to the deltoid muscle and be used only for percutaneous anchor placement without the use of a cannula.

Structures at Risk
- Deltoid muscle and axillary nerve with lateral portals
- Musculocutaneous nerve with anterior portals
- Suprascapular nerve with Neviaser portal

Examination Under Anesthesia and Diagnostic Arthroscopy

Before preparation and draping, the shoulder joint is put through a range of motion to assess for stiffness, which, if significant, requires additional capsular releases.

A brief diagnostic glenohumeral arthroscopy is performed through standard anterior and posterior portals to evaluate potentially associated pathologic processes, such as biceps tendinitis, chondral damage, and labral disease. After the rotator cuff tear is visualized, it is often helpful to mark the exact location by percutaneous passage of a suture through the tear, especially in small and partial tears, which can be difficult to localize from the subacromial space.

Specific Steps (Box 16-1)

After routine glenohumeral arthroscopy to evaluate for and address any associated pathologic process, the arthroscope is placed into the subacromial space through either a standard posterior portal or a separate posterolateral portal.

1. Acromioplasty and Bursectomy
Currently, many surgeons routinely perform an acromioplasty before rotator cuff repair, which can improve

Box 16-1 Surgical Steps

1. Acromioplasty and bursectomy

2. Releases

3. Tear patterns and margin convergence

4. Footprint preparation and anchor placement

5. Suture management

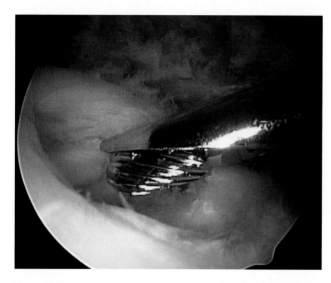

Figure 16-2 A bur or shaver is used to prepare the footprint by removal of any soft tissue and roughening of the cortex.

visualization and may reduce potential external compression of the cuff from an anterolateral spur. A complete release of the coracoacromial ligament should be avoided, especially in large and massive rotator cuff tears, because it provides a restraint to superior escape of the humeral head in the rotator cuff–deficient shoulder. An adequate acromioplasty, however, can easily be performed even without complete release of the coracoacromial ligament. A bursectomy and limited acromioplasty are performed with an arthroscopic bur and radiofrequency ablation device through the lateral portal with visualization from posteriorly, or vice versa; this is described in more detail in Chapter 23. Next, the footprint on the greater tuberosity is prepared to obtain an optimal environment for healing (Fig. 16-2). This can be performed with the shaver or a bur; however, extensive decortication has largely been abandoned because it does not appear to improve healing and can compromise secure anchor fixation.

2. Releases

Adhesions frequently form between retracted rotator cuff tears and surrounding tissues. It is necessary to release these adhesions before attempting to reduce and repair the cuff to the footprint. To assess cuff mobility, the surgeon can apply traction to the tendon edge with either a grasper or traction suture through the lateral portal. A thorough release should be performed if the tendon edge cannot be reduced to the footprint in a tension-free manner. We prefer to visualize through the posterior portal while using a Bankart elevator or electrothermal device through the lateral and anterior portals to release any adhesions. Most commonly, it is necessary to release both upper and lower aspects of the rotator cuff; adhesions form superiorly with the acromion and inferiorly with the capsulolabral complex, glenoid, and glenoid neck. In long-standing tears, where the cuff is adherent to the glenoid neck, release of the capsule adjacent to the superior and posterior labrum is particularly useful. However, the suprascapular nerve and vessels are at risk during this dissection, which should not extend farther than 1 cm medial to the glenoid rim. Anterior releases along the rotator interval can separate adhesions between the supraspinatus and the coracoid and subscapularis. Rarely, posterior release between the supraspinatus and infraspinatus is required.

3. Tear Patterns and Margin Convergence

Several tear configurations have been described. Crescentic tears are more commonly found acutely or subacutely and usually are easily mobilized and repaired directly to bone with suture anchors (Fig. 16-3). U-shaped tears are generally larger and may require side-to-side repair (i.e., margin convergence) to reduce tear size and decrease tension on the leading edge, thus allowing a more stable repair to the tuberosity (Fig. 16-4). L-shaped tears are best addressed with a side-to-side repair of the longitudinal limb before the horizontal limb is secured to bone with suture anchors (Fig. 16-5).

Side-to-side repairs are performed in a medial to lateral progression with free sutures that can be passed through the tendon substance by a variety of instruments and techniques (Fig. 16-6). Our preference is to use a straight penetrating suture grasper when working in the posterior two thirds of the cuff as well as during repair of the more medial extent of the side-to-side component of a tear. Laterally and anteriorly, a shuttle-type suture-passing device is more effective. Sutures should generally be tied directly after passing and before anchor placement to reduce the risk of suture entanglement (Fig. 16-7).

4. Footprint Preparation and Anchor Placement

In general, suture anchors are placed in the medial aspect of the footprint for a single-row technique; they should be placed in a systematic fashion to help with suture management, often from posterior to anterior. After placement, the corresponding sutures are stored in unused cannulas to avoid entanglement. Anchor placement can be performed either through the standard portals or through additional percutaneous stab incisions as needed to obtain the optimal anchor orientation of 45 degrees, tilted laterally (dead man's angle).

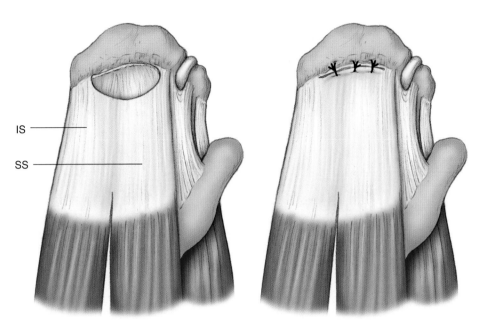

Figure 16-3 Crescentic tears are directly repaired to the rotator cuff insertion (footprint) with suture anchors. Releases are performed as necessary to ensure a tension-free repair. IS, infraspinatus tendon; SS, supraspinatus tendon. (Redrawn from Lo IK, Burkhart SS. Arthroscopic repair of crescent-shaped, U-shaped, and L-shaped rotator cuff tears. In Miller MD, Cole BJ, eds. Textbook of Arthroscopy. Philadelphia, Elsevier, 2004:217-240.)

For the repair of large crescentic tears or U-shaped tears after margin convergence (Fig. 16-8A and B), we place our initial anchor medial (in the frontal plane) and central (in the sagittal plane), approximately 5 mm off the articular margin. We consecutively retrieve all four suture limbs with a penetrating suture grasper, thus forming two independent horizontal mattress sutures, which further converge the two leaves of the tear (Fig. 16-8C). Next, we place at least two additional anchors, one more posterior and lateral to the first, and the final anchor is typically placed just behind the bicipital groove. A combination of horizontal mattress and simple stitches can be used, constructing a modified Mason-Allen equivalent (Fig. 16-8D and E).

5. Suture Management

The senior author prefers a low-profile penetrating suture grasper for the posterior cuff in combination with a 45-degree ipsilateral (i.e., right curve for right shoulder) curved suture shuttle device for the more anterior aspect of the tear. Alternatively, various devices are available that can be passed with a loaded suture through the anterolateral or lateral portal (while viewing from posteriorly) and antegrade directly through the lateral tendon edge. Whether a shuttle or a suture-passing device is used, only one suture limb should be kept within a cannula at any given time to avoid entanglement.

Most tears of the supraspinatus and infraspinatus tendons retract in a posteromedial rather than purely medial direction. Therefore, sutures should be placed more posteriorly into the tendon relative to the anchor to prop-erly restore the tendon edge to its original, more anterior insertion site.

Arthroscopic knot tying is a crucial technical aspect of a successful repair. Although many different sliding and nonsliding techniques have been described, the senior author prefers simple half-hitches on alternating posts. This reliable and simple method does not require sliding of the suture through the tissue, which has been associated with suture cutout. Irrespective of the technique used, care must be taken to ensure that the knot tightly reduces the tendon to the anchor and bony bed of the footprint to allow healing.

Postoperative Considerations

Rehabilitation

Postoperative rehabilitation is of crucial importance in achieving a good outcome. Postoperatively, patients are placed in a sling with a supportive abduction pillow, which is worn at all times except for showering and therapy. The rehabilitation program is divided into three phases on the basis of the progression of tendon healing.

Phase 1 (weeks 0-4): Exercises are restricted to passive range of motion only. Restrictions are based on intraoperative assessment of construct stability, commonly limiting passive external rotation to 40 degrees and forward flexion to 90 degrees. Therapeutic exercises during this phase include pendulum exercises; elbow, wrist, and hand

Text continued on p. 166.

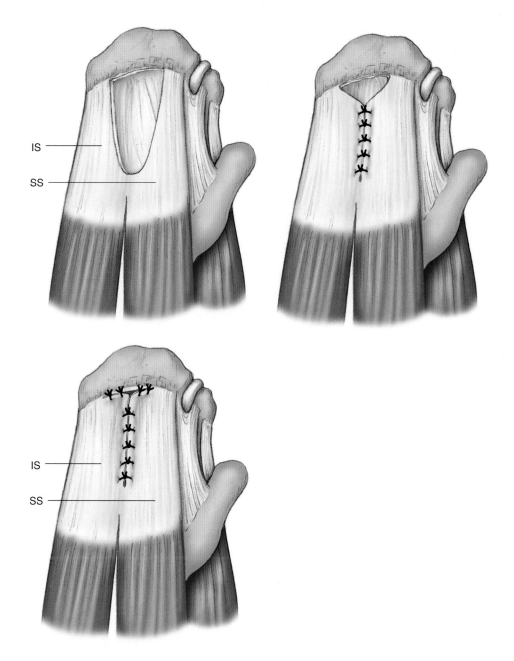

Figure 16-4 A U-shaped tear is repaired by side-to-side margin convergence sutures. The residual defect is then secured to the footprint with suture anchors. IS, infraspinatus tendon; SS, supraspinatus tendon. (Redrawn from Lo IK, Burkhart SS. Arthroscopic repair of crescent-shaped, U-shaped, and L-shaped rotator cuff tears. In Miller MD, Cole BJ, eds. Textbook of Arthroscopy. Philadelphia, Elsevier, 2004:217-240.)

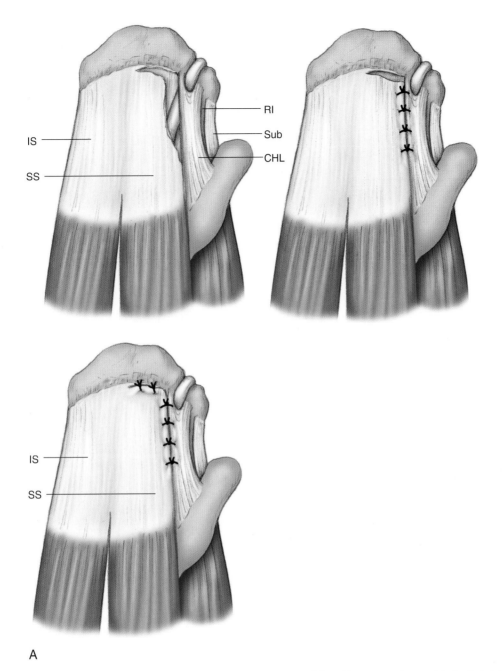

A

Figure 16-5 A, Acute L-shaped tears are repaired with margin convergence of the long limb, followed by suture anchor repair to the footprint. IS, infraspinatus tendon; SS, supraspinatus tendon; Sub, subscapularis tendon; RI, rotator interval; CHL, coracohumeral ligament.

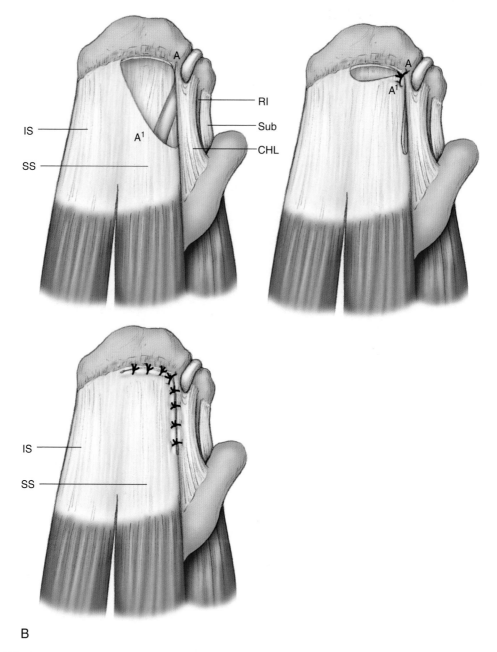

B

Figure 16-5, cont'd B, Chronic L-shaped tear that has assumed a U-shaped configuration. The posterior leaf is usually more mobile. The corner (A¹) should be reduced to its original position (A) before side-to-side repair. Finally, the free edge is repaired to bone with suture anchors. CHL, coracohumeral ligament; IS, infraspinatus tendon; RI, rotator interval; SS, supraspinatus tendon; Sub, subscapularis tendon. (Redrawn with modification from Lo IK, Burkhart SS. Arthroscopic repair of crescent-shaped, U-shaped, and L-shaped rotator cuff tears. In Miller MD, Cole BJ, eds. Textbook of Arthroscopy. Philadelphia, Elsevier, 2004:217-240.)

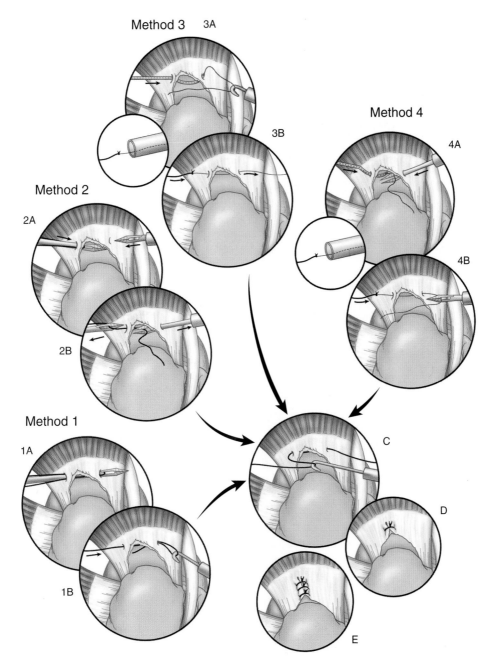

Figure 16-6 Side-to-side repair techniques for margin convergence. Method 1, A suture penetrator delivers the suture through both anterior and posterior leaves. Method 2, Handoff technique: a suture penetrator delivers the suture through the posterior leaf, then penetrates the anterior leaf to retrieve the suture. Method 3, Suture shuttle technique: a monofilament suture is delivered through both leaves with a shuttle device. The monofilament suture is then used to shuttle a nonresorbable braided suture through the tear. Method 4, Modified handoff technique using a suture shuttle device in the posterior leaf and a suture penetrator anteriorly.

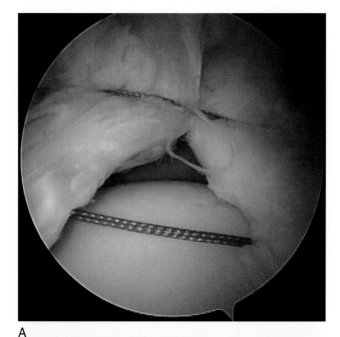

A

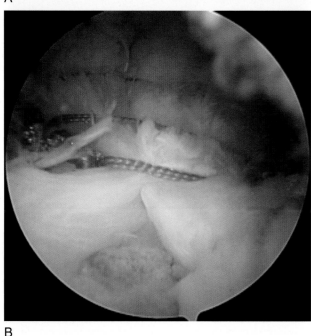

B

Figure 16-7 Margin convergence, view from the lateral portal. The humeral head is visible through the residual defect. **A,** A medial margin convergence suture was tied before the more lateral suture was passed. **B,** Both sutures have been tied, significantly reducing the tear size.

range of motion; grip strengthening; and isometric scapular stabilization.

Phase 2 (weeks 4-8): The sling is discontinued, and range of motion is progressed to 140 degrees of forward flexion, 40 degrees of external rotation, abduction to 60 to 80 degrees, and posterior capsular stretching to maintain or to improve internal rotation. Therapeutic exercises are advanced to gentle active-assisted exercises in the supine position with progression to active exercises with resis-

tance at 6 weeks. Deltoid and biceps strengthening is initiated, with the arm kept close to the side to minimize lever arm forces on the rotator cuff.

Phase 3 (approximately weeks 8-12) is characterized by progression to full motion, as tolerated. Scapular strengthening is continued, and internal and external rotation isometric exercises are added to the program. During the final phase of rehabilitation, sport-specific activities are initiated, flexibility is maintained, and strengthening exercises are continued. Formal physical therapy is usually discontinued after approximately 4 months, with return to unrestricted athletic activities at 6 months.

Complications

Complications are relatively rare, with reported infection rates of less than 1%. Significant fluid extravasation with subcutaneous edema has been implicated in airway obstruction. More common are hypotensive episodes in up to 20% of patients undergoing shoulder arthroscopy with interscalene block in the sitting position. These potentially serious episodes are reportedly caused by activation of the Bezold-Jarisch reflex and can be addressed by preemptive beta-blockade.

The incidence of minor complications related to edema from fluid extravasation is unknown and is typically inconsequential. However, there have been reports of subcutaneous emphysema causing serious pulmonary complications during shoulder arthroscopy, which emphasizes the need for continued monitoring of the patient's shoulder and neck for excessive swelling or crepitation.

PEARLS AND PITFALLS

- The biceps tendon, capsulolabral complex, acromioclavicular joint, acromion, and subscapularis tendon are structures that may require additional interventions that could considerably prolong and complicate an all-arthroscopic procedure; as such, they should be assessed preoperatively.

- Preoperative recognition of the tissue quality and morphologic features of a tear is crucial to successful rotator cuff repair, but it is also of importance to better manage patients' expectations.

- Sparing the most anterior attachment of the coracoacromial ligament and the deltoid fascia during subacromial decompression helps minimize fluid extravasation during subacromial arthroscopy.

- Extensive removal of bursal tissue both laterally and posteriorly allows easier suture retrieval and anchor placement.

- Do not hesitate to place anchors through additional percutaneous stab incisions if needed to obtain good orientation.

- Only one suture should be kept in a working cannula during knot tying; the knot pusher can be slid along the suture limbs to ensure free passage down to the anchor before knot tying.

- Visualize the anchor during suture passing to reduce the risk of unloading.

- Rotation of the arm aids in achieving correct anchor location and alignment.

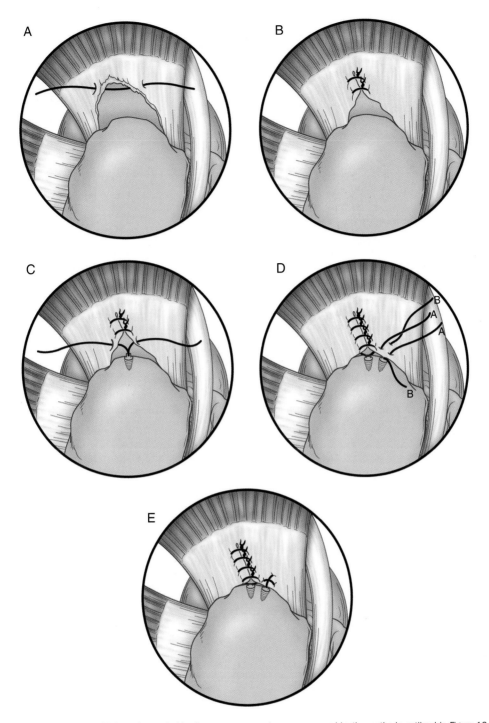

Figure 16-8 Repair of a large crescentic or U-shaped tear. **A,** Margin convergence sutures are passed by the methods outlined in Figure 16-6. **B,** The sutures are tied individually after passing. **C,** A double-loaded anchor is placed (only one suture is depicted), and one limb from each suture is retrieved through the anterior and posterior leaves. These sutures are tied, effectively forming additional, but anchored, margin convergence sutures. **D,** Additional anchors are placed anterior and posterior to the first anchor. Both limbs of one suture (A) are passed through the tendon, but only one limb of the other suture (B) is passed. **E,** Suture limbs A are tied as a horizontal mattress suture, then suture limbs B are tied over the top as a simple stitch, forming a modified Mason-Allen equivalent. The procedure is repeated for the remaining anchor to secure the other leaf of the tear.

Table 16-1 Clinical Outcomes after Arthroscopic Rotator Cuff Repair

Author	Follow-up	Patients	Outcome
Youm et al[6] (2005)	3 years	42	95% good–excellent results
Wilson et al[5] (2002)	5 years	100	88% good–excellent results
Murray et al[4] (2002)	3.3 years	48	95% good–excellent results
Burkhart et al[1] (2001)	3.5 years	59	95% good–excellent results
Gartsman et al[3] (1998)	2.5 years	73	84% good–excellent results

Results

Clinical outcomes after arthroscopic rotator cuff repair have been comparable to those of open reconstruction, despite the fact that radiologic investigations have demonstrated a comparatively higher rate of recurrent tears on magnetic resonance imaging follow-up (Table 16-1). Between 77% and 98% of patients are satisfied with their outcome after rotator cuff repair, with excellent pain relief and functional improvement in more than 80%. Benefits of arthroscopic repair versus open or mini-open techniques include smaller incisions with less soft tissue dissection, avoidance of deltoid detachment, improved visualization of the entire glenohumeral joint for evaluation and treatment of concomitant pathologic processes, and decreased postoperative pain. However, arthroscopic repair has been associated with a significant rate of recurrent tears.[2] Our results have demonstrated a recurrent tear rate of up to 47% at 2 years on magnetic resonance imaging examination. Nonetheless, clinical results do not seem to suffer in these patients. We have found significantly improved functional and pain scores, as well as improved strength, even in the setting of a recurrent tear; patients rated the postsurgical shoulder at 85% of the normal, contralateral side.

References

1. Burkhart SS, Danaceau SM, Pearce CE. Arthroscopic rotator cuff repair: analysis of results by tear size and repair technique—margin convergence versus direct tendon-to-bone repair. Arthroscopy 2001;17:905-912.
2. Galatz LM, Ball CM, Teefey SA, et al. The outcome and repair integrity of completely arthroscopically repaired large and massive rotator cuff tears. J Bone Joint Surg Am 2004;86:219-224.
3. Gartsman GM, Khan M, Hammerman SM. Arthroscopic repair of full-thickness tears of the rotator cuff. J Bone Joint Surg Am 1998;80:832-840.
4. Murray TF Jr, Lajtai G, Mileski RM, Snyder SJ. Arthroscopic repair of medium to large full-thickness rotator cuff tears: outcome at 2- to 6-year follow-up. J Shoulder Elbow Surg 2002;11:19-24.
5. Wilson F, Hinov V, Adams G. Arthroscopic repair of full-thickness tears of the rotator cuff: 2- to 14-year follow-up. Arthroscopy 2002;18:136-144.
6. Youm T, Murray DH, Kubiak EN, et al. Arthroscopic versus mini-open rotator cuff repair: a comparison of clinical outcomes and patient satisfaction. J Shoulder Elbow Surg 2005;14:455-459.

Suggested Readings

Burkhart SS, Athanasiou KA, Wirth MA. Margin convergence: a method of reducing strain in massive rotator cuff tears. Arthroscopy 1996;12:335-338.
Gartsman GM, O'Connor DP. Arthroscopic rotator cuff repair with and without arthroscopic subacromial decompression: a prospective, randomized study of one-year outcomes. J Shoulder Elbow Surg 2004;13:424-426.
Lo IK, Burkhart SS. Double-row arthroscopic rotator cuff repair: re-establishing the footprint of the rotator cuff. Arthroscopy 2003;19:1035-1042.
Loutzenheiser TD, Harryman DT 2nd, Yung SW, et al. Optimizing arthroscopic knots. Arthroscopy 1995;11:199-206.

CHAPTER 17

Arthroscopic Rotator Cuff Repair: Double-Row Techniques

Christopher S. Ahmad, MD

Neal S. ElAttrache, MD

The persistent tear rate after open and arthroscopic rotator cuff repair is concerning[3-7] and has stimulated development of improved rotator cuff repair techniques. Arthroscopic repair techniques currently emphasize proper recognition of tear pattern, adequate mobilization of retracted tendons, restoration of the native insertional footprint, and adequate repair strength. The techniques for arthroscopic rotator cuff repair have evolved from single-row suture anchors to double rows of suture anchors in the greater tuberosity. Studies have also shown that transosseous tunnel repair techniques provide improved footprint coverage,[2] pressurized contact area at the footprint,[11] and reduced motion at the footprint tendon-bone interface.[1] It is believed that improved contact characteristics will help maximize healing potential between repaired tendons and the greater tuberosity. The most recent techniques developed in double-row rotator cuff repair now replicate transosseous tunnel techniques and create tissue compression against the tuberosity to enhance healing.[10] These new techniques have been referred to as suture bridge techniques.

Preoperative Considerations

History

- Anterolateral shoulder pain exacerbated with overhead activity
- Patients may report specific trauma
- Night pain when sleeping on the affected side
- Weakness with overhead activity

Physical Examination

- Spinati atrophy
- Subacromial crepitation
- Decreased active range of motion
- Tenderness over greater tuberosity
- Weakness to forward elevation indicates supraspinatus tear.
- Weakness to external rotation indicates infraspinatus tear.
- Presence of impingement signs
- Liftoff test performed with the hand behind the back and then lifted off the back indicates subscapularis tear.
- Belly press is performed for patients who have limited internal rotation. The hand is used to press into the patient's abdomen, and the elbow is brought forward past the body midline. Inability to pass the midline indicates subscapularis tear.

Imaging

- Plain radiographs may indicate proximal humerus migration and sclerosis on the greater tuberosity or undersurface of the acromion for massive chronic tears.

- Magnetic resonance imaging is the standard imaging study. It delineates which tendons are involved, degree of retraction, muscle atrophy, and fatty infiltration of the muscle bellies.

Indications and Contraindications

- Several factors affecting surgical indications include age and health of the patient, activity level, size and chronicity of the tear, degree of pain and disability, and the patient's expectations.
- Young age, high activity, and relative acuteness of the tendon tear are features supporting early operative treatment.
- Older age, low demands, mild symptoms, and relative chronicity of the tendon tear are features supporting nonoperative treatment.

Surgical Technique

Anesthesia and Positioning

The surgeon's, anesthesiologist's, and patient's preferences determine the type of anesthesia administered. The procedure may be performed under regional anesthesia, general anesthesia, or a combination. The patient may be positioned in either the beach chair or the lateral decubitus position. The beach chair position is more familiar to many surgeons and is often easier to convert to an open procedure. The lateral decubitus position provides traction on the arm, which enhances visualization in the subacromial space.

Surgical Landmarks and Portals

Landmarks
- Clavicle
- Acromion
- Scapular spine
- Acromioclavicular joint
- Coracoid process

Portals
- Posterior portal
- Posterolateral portal
- Lateral portal
- Anterior portal
- Neviaser portal

Examination Under Anesthesia and Diagnostic Arthroscopy

Examination under anesthesia confirms passive range of motion. Diagnostic arthroscopy is performed in a stepwise fashion to evaluate the following:

- Anterior, posterior, and superior labrum
- Proximal biceps tendon
- Rotator cuff, including subscapularis
- Cartilage surfaces of the humeral head and glenoid

Specific Steps (Box 17-1)

1. Tear Pattern Recognition

A standard posterior portal is established, and glenohumeral diagnostic arthroscopy is performed with appropriate intra-articular procedures carried out. The camera is then introduced into the subacromial space, and a lateral working portal is made 2 cm lateral to the midanterior acromion. A bursectomy is performed, and the tear pattern is identified (crescent-shaped, L-shaped, U-shaped, combined). An acromioplasty is performed as necessary.

2. Tear Mobilization

The lateral mobility of the tear is assessed by grasping the tear edge and pulling laterally. Crescent-shaped tears mobilize easily to the lateral aspect of the greater tuberosity footprint with minimal tension and do not require releases or mobilization techniques (Figs. 17-1 to 17-3). With the camera in the lateral portal, anterior and posterior tear mobility is assessed by pulling the anterior rotator cuff tear limb posterior and the posterior rotator cuff tear limb anterior. For U-shaped tears, the anterior and posterior tear limbs both have mobility. L-shaped tears have asymmetric limb mobility; typically, the posterior limb is more mobile than the anterior limb.

Box 17-1 Surgical Steps

1. Tear pattern recognition
2. Tear mobilization
3. Greater tuberosity preparation
4. Margin convergence if necessary
5. Medial-row suture anchor placement
6. Medial suture passing
7. Lateral-row suture anchor placement
8. Lateral suture passing
9. Knot tying

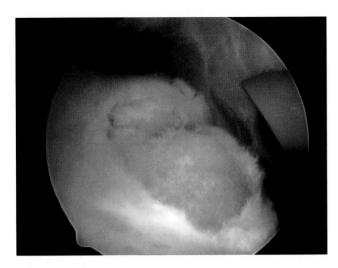

Figure 17-1 Crescent-shaped tear with greater tuberosity débrided.

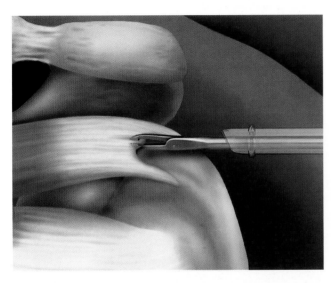

Figure 17-2 Soft tissue grasper from lateral portal to assess lateral mobility.

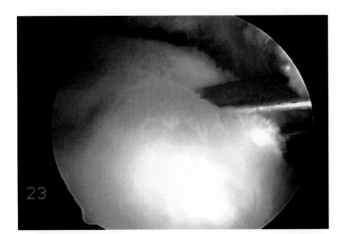

Figure 17-3 Crescent-shaped tear with soft tissue grasper demonstrating full mobility to lateral footprint.

Many chronic tears are immobile, and mobilization techniques are performed as necessary, including anterior interval slide, posterior interval slide, and capsular releases. A double-row repair requires adequate lateral mobilization of the tendon so that it may cover the entire footprint in the lateral direction (see Fig. 17-3).

3. Greater Tuberosity Preparation

The greater tuberosity footprint is débrided with removal of soft tissue, and the cortical bone is abraded to stimulate healing. Decortication is avoided because it may compromise suture anchor fixation strength (see Fig. 17-1).

4. Margin Convergence

U- and L-shaped tears often have poor lateral mobility, and margin convergence sutures are necessary (Figs. 17-4 and 17-5). While viewing from the lateral portal, free No. 2 sutures are passed through the anterior limb of rotator cuff and then the posterior limb to form a simple suture configuration (Fig. 17-6). The suture-passing sequence is repeated for the necessary number of sutures to convert the U- or L-shaped component to a crescent-shaped tear. Two to four sutures are typically placed. Knot tying for these sutures is delayed until after the medial row of suture anchors is placed to avoid restricting exposure to the medial tuberosity. Tying of the margin convergence sutures converts the U-shaped tear to a crescent-shaped tear, and the techniques for crescent-shaped tear repair are then carried out (Fig. 17-7).

17

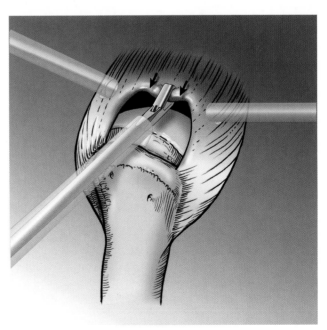

Figure 17-4 Illustration demonstrating U-shaped tear with poor lateral mobility at apex of tear.

5. Medial-Row Suture Anchor Placement

The repair sequence involves placement of a medial row of suture anchors followed by suture passing through the tendon in a mattress fashion. The medial-row anchors are positioned as medial as possible adjacent to the articular

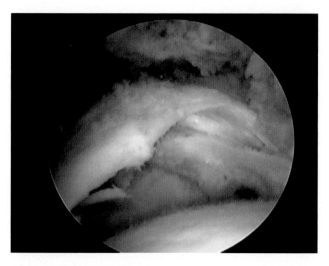

Figure 17-5 U-shaped tear visualized from lateral portal.

surface of the humeral head (Fig. 17-8). For a typical crescent-shaped supraspinatus tear, two anchors are placed, one in the anterior third and one in the posterior third of the footprint (Fig. 17-9). For larger tears, more anchors are placed as necessary. Suture anchors that are double loaded with two sutures are preferred.

6. Medial Suture Passing

If margin convergence sutures are placed, they are tied before medial anchor suture passing. Medial suture anchor passing is then performed, creating medial mattress suture configurations, ideally 10 to 12 mm medial to the lateral edge of the rotator cuff tear. This requires suture-passing instrumentation that will facilitate medial placement of the suture (Fig. 17-10). This maximizes the tendon available for contact with the footprint. The sutures are passed with the surgeon's preferred suture-passing device. The second suture from the anchor, if it is double loaded, may also be placed as a second mattress suture.

7. Lateral-Row Suture Anchor Placement

Next, the lateral row of suture anchors is placed. On the basis of the size of the footprint repair site, one or two lateral suture anchors are placed. The anchors are placed

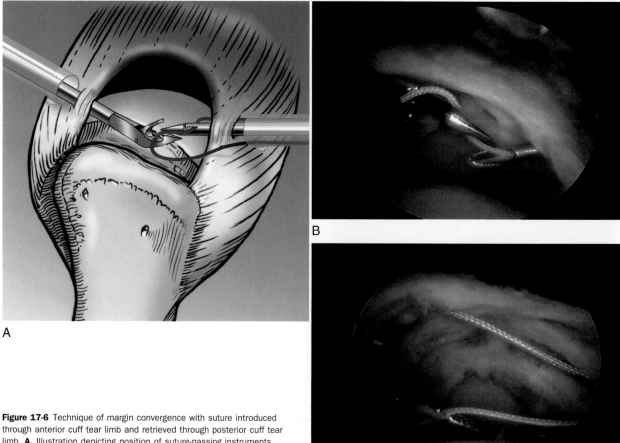

A

B

C

Figure 17-6 Technique of margin convergence with suture introduced through anterior cuff tear limb and retrieved through posterior cuff tear limb. **A,** Illustration depicting position of suture-passing instruments. **B,** First suture placed with visualization from lateral portal. **C,** Second suture placed with visualization from lateral portal.

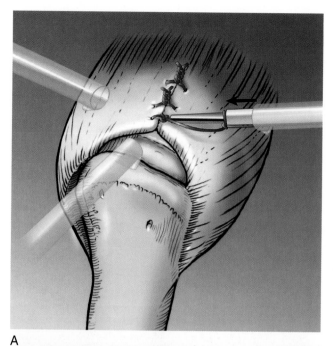

A

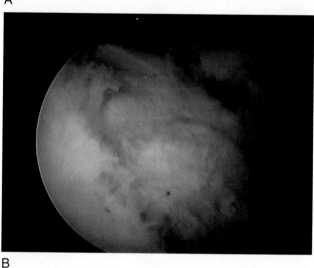

B

Figure 17-7 A, After margin convergence sutures are tied, a crescent-shaped tear is obtained. **B,** After margin convergence sutures are tied, a crescent-shaped tear is obtained as visualized from posterior portal.

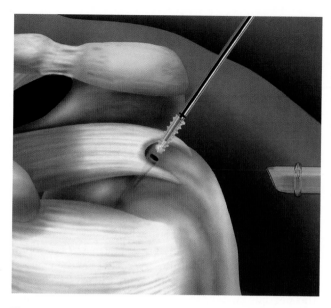

Figure 17-8 Medial-row anchor placement adjacent to articular surface.

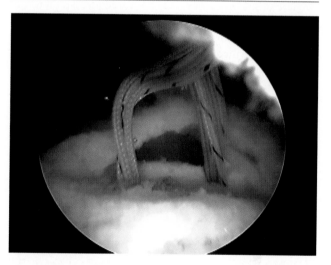

Figure 17-9 Medial-row anchors in place adjacent to articular surface.

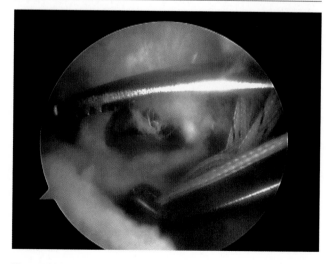

Figure 17-10 Suture passing that allows medial placement of the sutures through the tendon.

lateral to the lateral edge of the footprint to fully maximize the tendon-to-footprint contact.

8. Lateral Suture Passing

For non–suture bridge double-row repair, the lateral sutures are placed in a simple fashion with the surgeon's preferred suture-passing devices. Typically, 5 to 8 mm of tissue is captured in the simple sutures.

9. Knot Tying

Knot tying is typically performed in the following sequence: lateral sutures working from posterior to anterior; medial sutures working from posterior to anterior. Figure 17-11 demonstrates a completed double-row repair.

Alternative Techniques: Suture Bridge Methods

Suture Shuttle Through Lateral Anchor

Techniques have been developed to make suture bridges that are equivalent to transosseous tunnel compression stitches. Several variations exist to form a suture bridge, and early methods made use of existing implants and instruments. The medial suture anchors are placed as previously described for a double-row technique. One suture from each anchor is placed in a horizontal mattress fashion. The second suture limbs from each anchor are then passed together just medial to the horizontal mattress sutures. This not only makes a suture bridge but also approximates a modified Mason-Allen suture construct. Either one or two lateral suture anchors may be placed just lateral to the edge of the greater tuberosity (Fig. 17-12). After all sutures are passed, the horizontal mattress sutures are tied. One limb from the medial compression suture and one suture from the lateral anchor are retrieved outside the lateral cannula. The suture from the medial anchor is then sewn through the lateral suture with a free needle (Fig. 17-13). The lateral suture, acting as a shuttle with the medial suture attached to it, is pulled through the eyelet. A second suture may be shuttled through each anchor to make a cruciate-type suture bridge, if desired, to enhance the repair (Fig. 17-14). After the sutures are shuttled, knot tying is performed (Fig. 17-15).

PushLock

A new implant has been developed to facilitate placement of compression sutures and to reduce knot tying. For the PushLock (Arthrex, Naples, Fla) device, medial suture anchor placement and suture passing are performed as previously described for the double-row repair technique. A hole is then punched at the intended site for the lateral implant, just lateral to the lateral edge of the tuberosity. The medial sutures to be used for compression (one suture from the anterior medial anchor and one suture from the posterior medial anchor) are then passed through the eyelet of the implant outside the cannula (Fig. 17-16). Manual tension is applied to the suture bridge sutures as they are delivered into the tunnel to achieve the desired compression (Fig. 17-17). The implant is advanced over the inserter and captures the eyelet, which fixes the sutures in place and eliminates the need for knot tying. The sutures are then cut. Cruciate suture configurations can be made with a second PushLock anchor to further enhance the

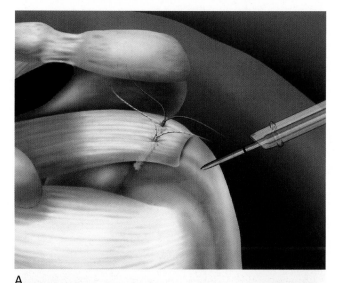

A

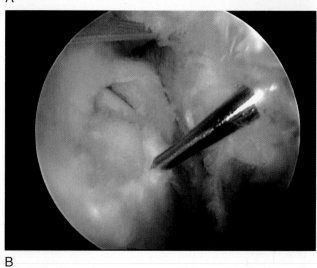

B

Figure 17-12 A, Punch placed at lateral margin of greater tuberosity. **B,** Punch for lateral anchor just lateral to edge of tuberosity as visualized from posterior portal.

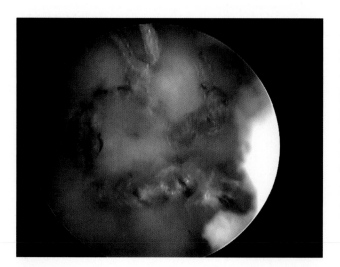

Figure 17-11 Completed double-row rotator cuff repair visualized from lateral portal.

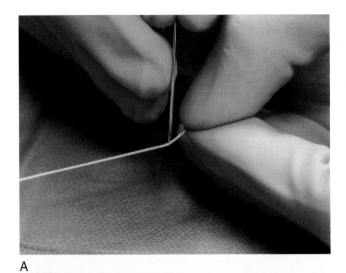

A

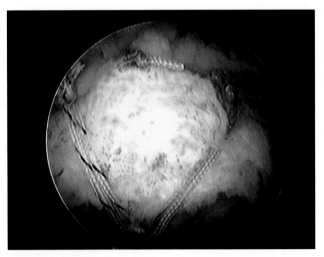

Figure 17-15 Completed rotator cuff repair with two suture bridges from two medial-row anchors passed through single lateral suture anchor.

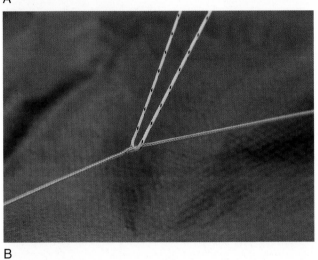

B

Figure 17-13 Medial suture is sewn through lateral suture to facilitate shuttling through lateral suture anchor. **A,** Needle penetrating suture. **B,** Medial suture passed through lateral suture.

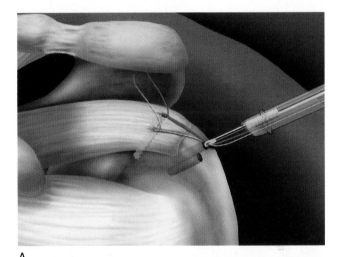

A

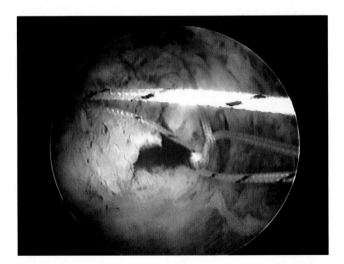

Figure 17-14 Medial sutures are shuttled through lateral suture anchor eyelet.

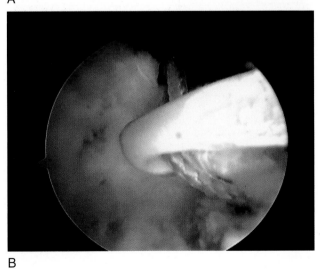

B

Figure 17-16 A, Eyelet of implant controls medial sutures and is delivered into lateral tunnel. **B,** Eyelet controlling medial sutures.

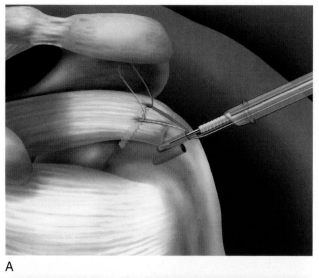

A

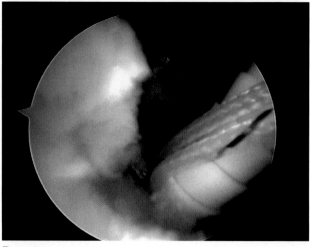

B

Figure 17-17 A, Sutures are tensioned into tunnel and implant is driven down shaft of inserter. **B,** Implant is driven down shaft of inserter into tunnel.

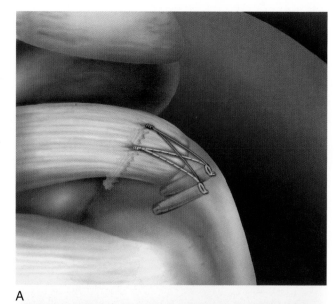

A

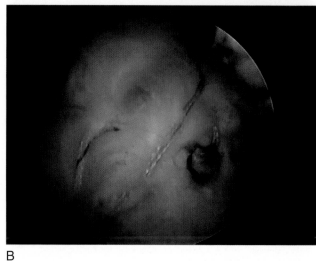

B

Figure 17-18 A, Completed repair with four suture bridges; lateral knot tying is avoided. **B,** Clinical visualization of completed repair from lateral portal.

repair (Fig. 17-18). Figure 17-19 demonstrates a case example of a crescent-shaped tear repaired with a four–suture bridge technique.

Postoperative Considerations

Patients are placed in a sling with a small abduction pillow. The sling is worn continuously for 6 weeks except for bathing. During the first 6 weeks, active elbow, wrist, and hand exercises are performed. From 6 to 12 weeks, passive and active-assisted range of motion is initiated. After 12

weeks, active motion and gentle strengthening are initiated. More aggressive strengthening is initiated at 4 months.

Complications

- Failure of tendon to heal
- Stiffness
- Missed pathologic changes: acromioclavicular joint arthritis, biceps tendinitis
- Infection

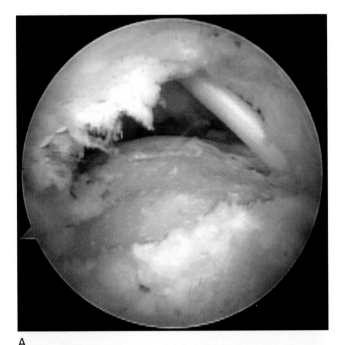

A

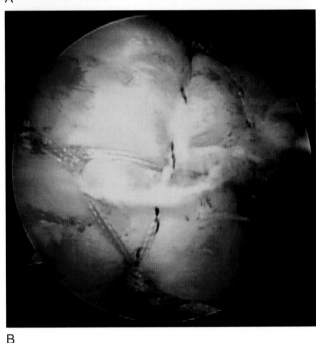

B

Figure 17-19 Case example of cruciate suture bridge technique with four suture bridges. **A,** Crescent-shaped tear. **B,** Completed repair.

PEARLS AND PITFALLS

- The rotator cuff tear pattern must be recognized for an appropriate strategy to be designed for mobilization and repair of the tear.
- Margin convergence should be performed for U-shaped tears to avoid tension overload of the central sutures.
- The medial-row suture anchors must be placed as medial as possible, which is adjacent to the articular cartilage, to maximize and reproduce contact at the repair site and to avoid overcrowding of the greater tuberosity with implants.
- The lateral-row suture anchors must be placed as lateral as possible to avoid overcrowding of the tuberosity with implants and to maximize repair site contact.
- Suture bridge repair constructs create optimal footprint restoration and rotator cuff to tuberosity contact mechanics.

Results

To date, no clinical studies specifically report the outcome of double-row suture anchor repair techniques or suture bridge repair techniques for management of rotator cuff tears. Several laboratory studies indicate improved strength of fixation to cyclic loading for double-row rotator cuff repairs compared with single-row rotator cuff repairs.[8,9] Other studies have demonstrated that traditional transosseous repair techniques have superior restoration of footprint coverage,[2] pressurized footprint contact area,[11] and decreased motion at the footprint tendon-bone interface.[1] In the laboratory, we have compared suture bridge rotator cuff repairs with double-row rotator cuff repairs that are currently employed clinically.[10] For strength of fixation, the four–suture bridge technique had significantly higher ultimate load to failure with no difference in gap formation to cyclic loading. Furthermore, the suture bridge rotator cuff repair provided more pressurized contact area and mean pressure over the repaired rotator cuff tendon insertion compared with a double-row technique.

References

1. Ahmad CS, Stewart AM, Izquierdo R, Bigliani LU. Tendon-bone interface motion in transosseous suture and suture anchor rotator cuff repair techniques. Am J Sports Med 2005;33:1667-1671.

2. Apreleva M, Ozbaydar M, Fitzgibbons PG, Warner JJ. Rotator cuff tears: the effect of the reconstruction method on three-dimensional repair site area. Arthroscopy 2002;18:519-526.

3. Bishop J, Lo I, Klepps S, et al. Cuff integrity following arthroscopic versus open rotator cuff repair: a prospective study. Proceedings, American Academy of Orthopaedic Surgeons 71st annual meeting; San Francisco, Calif; 2004.

4. Galatz LM, Ball CM, Teefey SA, et al. The outcome and repair integrity of completely arthroscopically repaired large and massive rotator cuff tears. J Bone Joint Surg Am 2004;86:219-224.

5. Gazielly DF, Gleyze P, Montagnon C. Functional and anatomical results after rotator cuff repair. Clin Orthop 1994;304:43-53.

6. Harryman DT, Mack LA, Wang KY, et al. Repairs of the rotator cuff. Correlations of functional results with integrity of the cuff. J Bone Joint Surg Am 1991;73:982-989.

7. Jost B, Pfirrmann CWA, Gerber C. Clinical outcome after structural failure of rotator cuff repairs. J Bone Joint Surg Am 2000;82:304-314.

8. Kim DH, ElAttrache NS, Tibone JE, et al. Biomechanical comparison of a single-row versus double-row suture anchor technique for rotator cuff repair. Am J Sports Med 2006;34:407-414.

9. Ma CB, Comerford L, Wilson J, Puttlitz CM. Biomechanical evaluation of arthroscopic rotator cuff repairs: double-row compared with single-row fixation. J Bone Joint Surg Am 2006;88:403-410.

10. Park M, ElAttrache N, Tibone J, et al. Footprint contact biomechanics for a new arthroscopic transosseous-equivalent rotator cuff repair technique compared to a double-row technique arthroscopic rotator cuff repair. American Shoulder and Elbow Surgeons Specialty Day meeting; Chicago, Ill; 2006.

11. Park MC, Cadet ER, Levine WN, et al. Tendon-to-bone pressure distributions at a repaired rotator cuff footprint using transosseous suture and suture anchor fixation techniques. Am J Sports Med 2005;33:1154-1159.

CHAPTER 18

Arthroscopic Subscapularis Repair

Ammar Anbari, MD

Anthony A. Romeo, MD

An all-arthroscopic repair of the subscapularis tendon has seen significant interest in the past 10 years. As we refine our knowledge and arthroscopic techniques in repairing other rotator cuff tears, we are now more capable of addressing subscapularis tears in an all-arthroscopic fashion as well. The main advantages of an all-arthroscopic repair of the subscapularis tendon are smaller incisions, less postoperative pain, and the ability to better visualize and address coexisting pathologic processes, including labral tears and posterior superior rotator cuff tears. This chapter addresses the preoperative considerations and the techniques involved in performing an arthroscopic subscapularis repair.

Preoperative Considerations

History

In most cases, isolated high-grade subscapularis tears are a result of trauma. Most patients describe an event with excessive external rotation of the shoulder or with resistance to forceful external rotation. Some patients hear a "pop" and others feel the shoulder "slipping out of place." In older individuals, tears may be associated with shoulder dislocations. Presenting complaints include anterior shoulder pain and difficulty reaching behind the back or tucking in a shirttail. These complaints can be relatively nonspecific, and it is important to consider the multiple causes of anterior shoulder pain, including acromioclavicular joint arthrosis or dislocation, biceps tendon tears or inflammation, anterior capsulolabral damage, and fractures of the lesser tuberosity.

Physical Examination

As with all shoulder conditions, physical examination begins with a thorough examination of the shoulder including observation, range of motion, and strength testing. The two most common physical examination findings associated with subscapularis tears are increased external rotation compared with the opposite side and weakness of internal rotation. External rotation is evaluated with the arm at the side and compared with the opposite extremity.

Because other muscles, such as the pectoralis major, are strong internal rotators of the shoulder, special tests can isolate the subscapularis for assessment of internal rotation strength. The belly press test is performed by asking the patient to press the ipsilateral hand on the abdomen, maintaining the elbow anterior to the body. If the patient is not able to keep the elbow anterior to the trunk or if the wrist is flexed in attempting to press into the abdomen, the belly press test result is considered positive and the subscapularis is not functioning. The liftoff test requires the patient to be able to place the ipsilateral hand behind the back. The patient is asked to lift the hand off the back; if the patient is unable to do so, the test result is considered positive. A modification to this test, also known as the subscapularis lag test, involves placing the patient's ipsilateral hand in maximum internal rotation off the back. The examiner asks the patient to keep the hand off the back as the hand is released. If the patient is not able to maintain the hand away from the body and the hand falls onto the back, the lag test result is considered positive.

Imaging

A standard shoulder imaging series including an axillary view is obtained to assess for alternative pathologic changes, such as fractures and glenohumeral arthritis. Magnetic resonance imaging is the "gold standard" imaging modality for diagnosing subscapularis tendon tears. Magnetic resonance arthrography improves the sensitivity of diagnosis of questionable tears. The magnetic resonance image provides information about the quality of the muscle belly, the amount of fatty infiltration, and any displacement of the long head of the biceps tendon (Fig. 18-1). The tendon should be assessed on both axial and sagittal images with verification of its insertion on the lesser tuberosity.

Indications and Contraindications

The most common indication for subscapularis repair is pain nonresponsive to conservative management. In younger individuals, consideration for repair in the absence of pain should be given to restore normal shoulder mechanics. Important secondary indications are restoration of shoulder function and, in selected cases, treatment of recurrent shoulder instability.

Relative contraindications to surgery include lack of pain, severe atrophy, retraction or significant fatty degeneration on magnetic resonance imaging, and rotator cuff tear arthropathy. Absolute contraindications are severe medical illness precluding anesthesia and ongoing active infection. The decision to perform an open or arthroscopic procedure should be based on the surgeon's individual comfort level with the chosen technique. Open repair and arthroscopic repair are simply different techniques, and the ultimate surgical goals are the same regardless of which technique is chosen.

Surgical Technique

Anesthesia and Positioning

Most patients are placed under general anesthesia. We prefer to supplement every case with an interscalene block. This reduces the amount of anesthetic required during the case and improves pain control in the postoperative period. If the patient's medical condition does not allow general anesthesia, regional anesthesia can be performed alone with sedation. Maintenance of a mean arterial pressure of 70 to 90 mm Hg or a systolic pressure near 100 mm Hg allows maximal visualization and minimizes bleeding. We have also used epinephrine in the arthroscopic solution to help control bleeding and to maximize visualization.

We prefer the beach chair position for arthroscopic repairs of the subscapularis (Fig. 18-2). It is a familiar position and allows the surgeon to attend to other pathologic lesions at the same time. The upper extremity can be easily moved and rotated to better visualize the subscapularis and its insertion. Furthermore, the beach chair position allows the surgeon to convert to an open procedure if necessary.

The patient is aligned on the edge of the table so that the affected shoulder and scapula are exposed. We place two folded towels on the medial edge of the scapula to

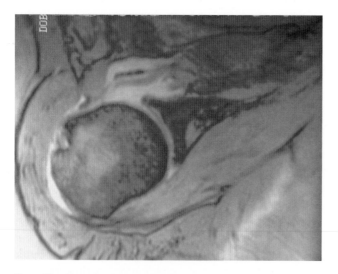

Figure 18-1 Magnetic resonance image of a torn subscapularis.

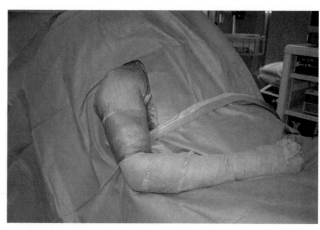

Figure 18-2 Positioning of the patient.

retract it farther laterally. The back of the table is elevated completely to position the acromion parallel to the floor. The head is secured to the operating table with tape, or an optional head rest may be used if the table allows it. Care should be taken to prevent excessive flexion or extension in the neck.

Surgical Landmarks, Incisions, and Portals

We begin every case by outlining the bony landmarks on the skin. The posterior and anterior corners of the acromion as well as the soft spot between the posterior clavicle and anterior scapular spine are marked first. A line is drawn between the two corners of the acromion. The anterior and posterior edges of the clavicle are marked next along with the scapular spine. The acromioclavicular joint is palpated and marked. Finally, a circle is drawn over the prominence of the coracoid.

The posterior portal is the first portal to be established. With use of a three-finger shuck, the index finger of the same hand as the shoulder being operated on is placed in the soft spot between the clavicle and scapular spine. The middle finger is placed on the coracoid, and the thumb feels the interval between the infraspinatus and teres minor. This helps the surgeon find the best location for the posterior portal.

The anterior portal is generally placed just lateral to the coracoid and below the coracoacromial ligament. Although this portal can easily be established in outside-in technique by use of a spinal needle, we prefer to establish it through an inside-out technique. This involves driving the arthroscope anteriorly beneath the biceps tendon and gently pushing against the anterior capsule. The arthroscope is removed, and a Wissinger rod is pushed through the scope cannula to make a puncture hole in the rotator interval. The skin is tented anteriorly, and a No. 11 knife blade is used to make the skin incision. The rod is pushed through the skin incision, and a 6-mm clear cannula equipped with an outflow attachment is placed over the rod into the joint. The Wissinger rod is withdrawn, and the arthroscope is reintroduced.

An accessory anterolateral portal is made in all subscapularis repairs. This portal is located in the rotator interval anterior and medial to the anterolateral corner of the acromion. This places it about 1 to 2 cm superior and 2 cm lateral to the standard anterior portal. A spinal needle is used to localize this portal, with an intra-articular entrance site just posterior to the native biceps tendon (Fig. 18-3). After the portal is made, it is enlarged to allow the placement of a threaded 6-mm clear cannula. It is important not to place the two anterior portals too close to each other. This portal is established after sufficient anterior débridement is performed and the lesser tuberos-

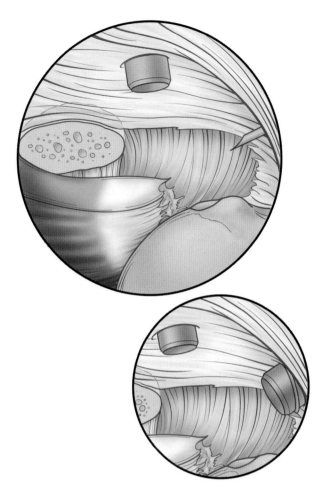

Figure 18-3 Accessory anterolateral portal. (Redrawn from Fox JA, Noerdlinger MA, Sasso LM, Romeo AA. Arthroscopic subscapularis repair. In Miller MD, Cole BJ, eds. Textbook of Arthroscopy. Philadelphia, Elsevier, 2004.)

ity is exposed. In most cases, the biceps tendon is released for later tenodesis as discussed later.

Examination Under Anesthesia and Diagnostic Arthroscopy

A thorough examination of both shoulders under anesthesia is performed on every patient after induction of anesthesia but before positioning. Range of motion, signs of instability, and arthritis are documented. Any previous surgical scars are marked and reused if possible.

We always start our procedures by performing a diagnostic glenohumeral arthroscopy. Any intra-articular pathologic process is addressed. If a coexisting superior cuff tear is present, we prefer to complete our subacromial work and superior cuff repair first before proceeding with subscapularis repair. This helps limit swelling of the shoulder and provides an easier working environment in the subacromial space.

A dynamic examination of the subscapularis insertion is performed by advancing the arthroscope to the anterior aspect of the glenohumeral joint. The lens is pointed to look laterally and the shoulder is internally rotated. If significant retraction has occurred, it is possible to see the conjoined tendons and note the medial displacement of the long head of the biceps. A probe or a grasper can be used to examine the extent of the tear (Fig. 18-4).

Specific Steps (Box 18-1)

1. Biceps Tendon

In many cases of significant subscapularis tear, the biceps tendon anchor within the bicipital groove has been disrupted, and the tendon itself is subluxed medially. We have not attempted to resuspend the biceps within the intertubercular groove. Rather, in almost all cases, our preference is to release the biceps tendon intra-articularly at the superior labrum and to perform an open subpectoral biceps tenodesis once the subscapularis repair has been completed. This approach is helpful for two reasons. First, it allows increased visualization and working area within the anterior shoulder as the biceps is now absent. Second, it eliminates any possibility of recurrent biceps subluxation or persistent pain from stenosis of the tendon or from a biceps tendon abnormality within the groove.

2. Coracoidplasty

This step is somewhat analogous to performing a subacromial decompression. By removal of bone from the postero-lateral tip of the coracoid, two goals are met. First, there is extra space for the technical aspect of the subscapularis repair to be performed. Second, it provides the repaired subscapularis more space, with no mechanical impingement from the coracoid.

We start with débridement of the capsular tissue of the rotator interval at the superior edge of the subscapularis to expose the coracoid (Fig. 18-5), by use of a combination of a mechanical shaver and a radiofrequency device, working through the anterior portal. This area can be quite vascular, and prompt attention to any bleeding is required to maintain visualization. By keeping the shaver on the lateral edge of the coracoid, no neurovascular structures will be violated. Once the coracoid is reached, an electro-

Box 18-1 Surgical Steps

1. Biceps tendon
2. Coracoidplasty
3. Mobilization of subscapularis
4. Preparation of the tendon edge and lesser tuberosity
5. Anchor placement
6. Suture management and passage
7. Additional anchor placement
8. Knot tying

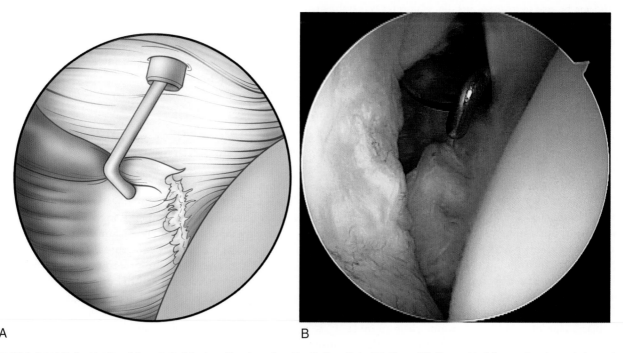

A   B

Figure 18-4 A and **B,** Examination of the extent of the tear. (**A** redrawn from Fox JA, Noerdlinger MA, Sasso LM, Romeo AA. Arthroscopic subscapularis repair. In Miller MD, Cole BJ, eds. Textbook of Arthroscopy. Philadelphia, Elsevier, 2004.)

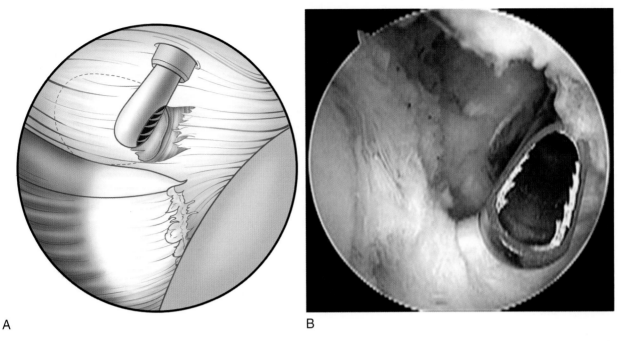

A   B

Figure 18-5 A and **B,** Exposure of the coracoid by débridement of the capsular tissue of the rotator interval. (**A** redrawn from Fox JA, Noerdlinger MA, Sasso LM, Romeo AA. Arthroscopic subscapularis repair. In Miller MD, Cole BJ, eds. Textbook of Arthroscopy. Philadelphia, Elsevier, 2004.)

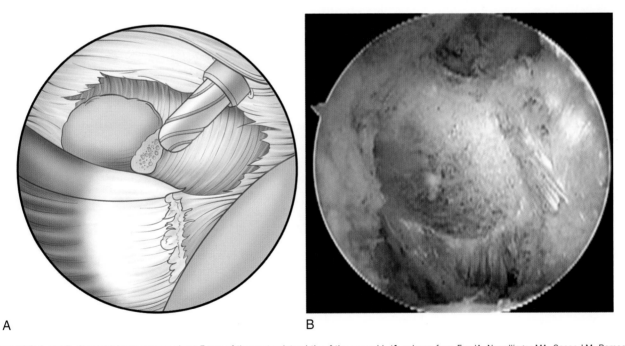

A   B

Figure 18-6 A and **B,** Coracoidplasty: remove about 5 mm of the posterolateral tip of the coracoid. (**A** redrawn from Fox JA, Noerdlinger MA, Sasso LM, Romeo AA. Arthroscopic subscapularis repair. In Miller MD, Cole BJ, eds. Textbook of Arthroscopy. Philadelphia, Elsevier, 2004.)

thermal device is used to further remove the soft tissue attachment on the tip of the coracoid and expose the undersurface. A 4.0-mm bur is then used to remove about 5 mm of the posterolateral tip of the coracoid, again working through the anterior portal (Fig. 18-6).

3. Mobilization of Subscapularis

By use of a grasper or a probe placed through the anterior portal, the mobility of the torn subscapularis is assessed. If the tendon can be reduced to the lesser tuberosity relatively tension free, one can proceed directly to the repair.

If, on the other hand, the tendon is not mobile, soft tissue dissection must be performed, most commonly by use of a radiofrequency device. This involves first releasing the soft tissue fibrous attachments between the coracoid and subscapularis. A release of the coracohumeral ligament and the anterior capsule is also helpful. Finally, the middle glenohumeral ligament, which crosses at a 45-degree angle to the tendon, should be released by a shaver or an electrothermal device.

4. Preparation of the Tendon Edge and Lesser Tuberosity

A 5.0-mm shaver is inserted through the anterior portal and used to freshen up and remove the frayed edges of the torn subscapularis. Next, the shoulder is internally rotated and slightly abducted to visualize the lesser tuberosity. A 4.0-mm bur is placed through the anterolateral portal and used to prepare the bony bed for placement of suture anchors (Fig. 18-7). In most cases, the tendon insertion is slightly medialized, and a small amount of the articular surface is included in the resection.

5. Anchor Placement

The suture anchors are placed through the anterior portal (Fig. 18-8). This portal allows optimal anchor placement at a 45-degree angle to the bone (dead man's angle). We prefer to use double-loaded anchors because they provide better stability for the repair. We place the anchors initially at the inferior edge of the subscapularis footprint before proceeding superiorly, which allows us good visualization throughout the repair process. We separate the anchors by 5 to 8 mm. In general, partial repairs can be accomplished with one or two anchors; a maximum of three anchors is required for complete ruptures.

6. Suture Management and Passage

To aid in suture management, a switching stick is placed through the anterior cannula, and the cannula is removed. The sutures are then pulled out of the cannula, and a hemostat is placed on them. The cannula is placed back over the switching stick into the joint (Fig. 18-9). This leaves the anterior cannula empty to facilitate the use of shuttling devices. To perform the repair, we use a 30-degree suture lasso (Arthrex, Naples, FL), a curved Spectrum device (Linvatec, Utica, NY), or a penetrator (Arthrex, Naples, Fla).

The suture limb that will be placed in the subscapularis is pulled from the anterior portal out through the anterolateral portal by a crochet hook (Fig. 18-10). The suture lasso or the Spectrum device is placed through the anterior portal and used to penetrate the tendon. The suture should be passed at an angle from lateral to medial through the entire thickness of the tendon.

Once the passage device has penetrated through the tendon, its nitinol loop or polydioxanone (PDS) suture is advanced (Fig. 18-11) and retrieved with the crochet hook through the anterolateral portal.

The anchor suture is then fixed to the passing wire or suture and shuttled through the tendon and back out the anterior portal (Fig. 18-12). Care must be taken not to unload the anchor.

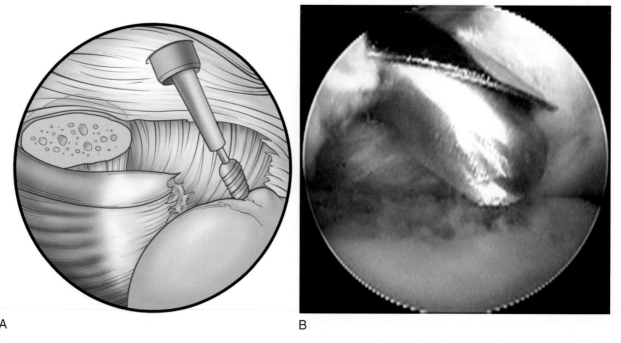

A   B

Figure 18-7 A and **B,** Preparation of the lesser tuberosity. (**A** redrawn from Fox JA, Noerdlinger MA, Sasso LM, Romeo AA. Arthroscopic subscapularis repair. In Miller MD, Cole BJ, eds. Textbook of Arthroscopy. Philadelphia, Elsevier, 2004.)

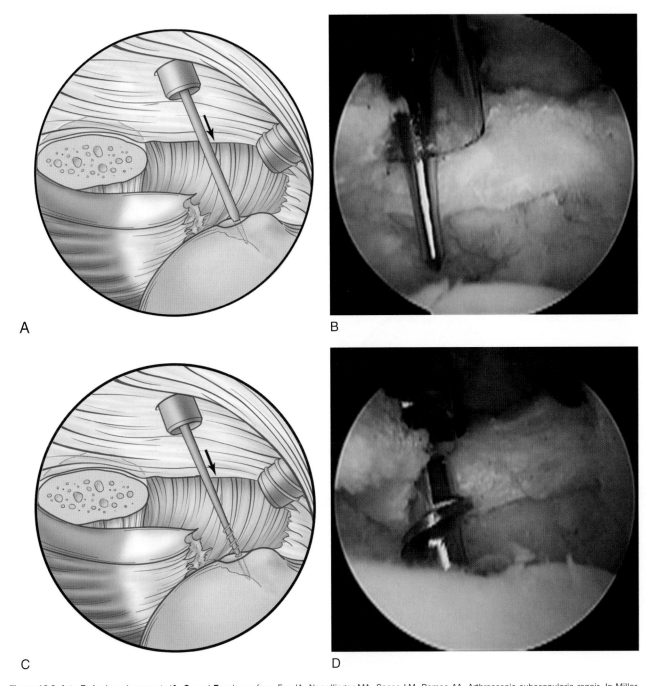

A

B

C

D

Figure 18-8 A to **F,** Anchor placement. (**A, C,** and **E** redrawn from Fox JA, Noerdlinger MA, Sasso LM, Romeo AA. Arthroscopic subscapularis repair. In Miller MD, Cole BJ, eds. Textbook of Arthroscopy. Philadelphia, Elsevier, 2004.)

The same process is repeated for the other suture limb, resulting in a mattress configuration in the subscapularis tendon (Fig. 18-13). Once both limbs have been retrieved, they are placed outside of the anterior cannula by the switching stick technique (Fig. 18-14). A hemostat is again placed to secure the two limbs, and the process is repeated for the next anchor. At the end of this process, two mattress sutures should be passed through the subscapularis tendon. It is important to place the sutures at least 5 mm apart to achieve optimal fixation.

7. Additional Anchor Placement

It is up to the surgeon's preference to tie sutures immediately or after placement of all remaining anchors. We prefer to tie the sutures last because in our hands, this allows better visualization and thus improved placement of the remaining anchors and sutures.

The same process is repeated to place the sutures through the upper edge of the tendon. Only one limb of the second suture on the last anchor is placed through the tendon (Fig. 18-15). This will be the first suture to be tied and will allow restoration of the height of the tendon.

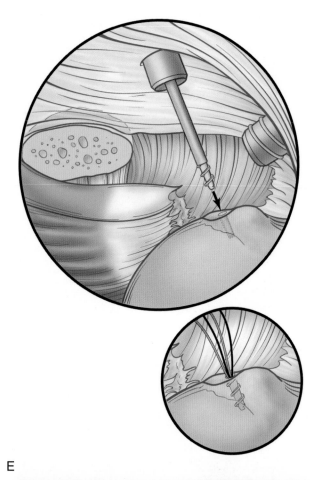

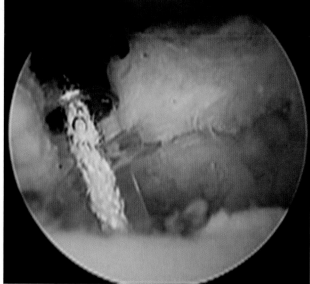

E

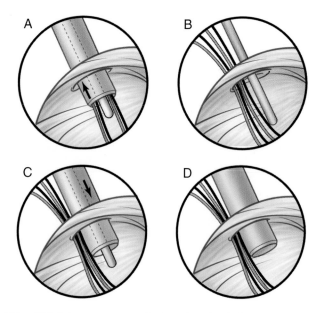

Figure 18-9 Suture management. (Redrawn from Fox JA, Noerdlinger MA, Sasso LM, Romeo AA. Arthroscopic subscapularis repair. In Miller MD, Cole BJ, eds. Textbook of Arthroscopy. Philadelphia, Elsevier, 2004.)

8. Knot Tying

The anterolateral portal is used for arthroscopic knot tying as it allows the surgeon to pass-point the knots and provides a better angle of approach to the tendon. We start by tying the most superior suture to set the position of the remaining sutures.

A crochet hook is used to retrieve the two limbs of the most superior suture out of the anterolateral portal. The arm is internally rotated and forward flexed to better visualize the knots. Multiple alternating half-hitches with alternating posts are placed, and the suture ends are cut (Fig. 18-16). The process is repeated for the second suture on the proximal anchor, followed by the inferior anchor. Ideally, the sutures are tied to place the knot on the tendon side of the repair, not the tuberosity (Fig. 18-17).

The arm is gently rotated to inspect the security of the repair and the tied knots. If necessary, gentle débridement can be performed with a shaver. Motion is assessed to determine limits for the postoperative rehabilitation program. Wounds are closed in a standard fashion, and the arm is placed into an abduction pillow sling.

Postoperative Considerations

Rehabilitation

The postoperative rehabilitation program is individualized on the basis of the quality and security of the repair and

F

Figure 18-8, cont'd

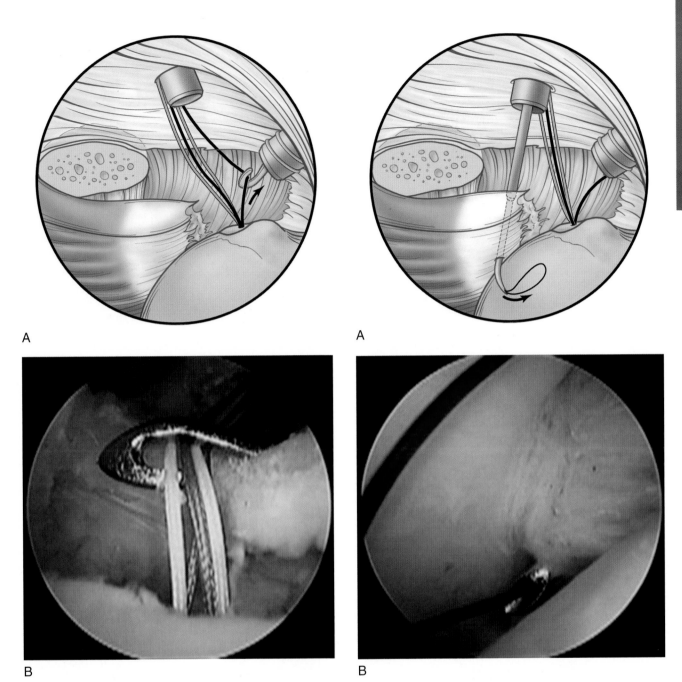

A

A

B

B

Figure 18-10 A and **B,** One suture is pulled from the anterior portal out through the anterolateral portal. (**A** redrawn from Fox JA, Noerdlinger MA, Sasso LM, Romeo AA. Arthroscopic subscapularis repair. In Miller MD, Cole BJ, eds. Textbook of Arthroscopy. Philadelphia, Elsevier, 2004.)

Figure 18-11 A and **B,** Passing a suture through the subscapularis. (**A** redrawn from Fox JA, Noerdlinger MA, Sasso LM, Romeo AA. Arthroscopic subscapularis repair. In Miller MD, Cole BJ, eds. Textbook of Arthroscopy. Philadelphia, Elsevier, 2004.)

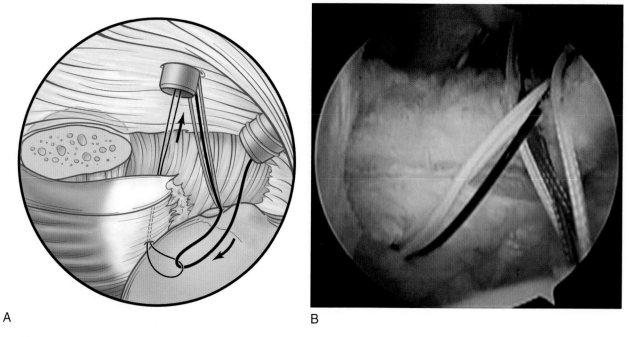

A

B

Figure 18-12 A and **B,** Suture shuttling. (**A** redrawn from Fox JA, Noerdlinger MA, Sasso LM, Romeo AA. Arthroscopic subscapularis repair. In Miller MD, Cole BJ, eds. Textbook of Arthroscopy. Philadelphia, Elsevier, 2004.)

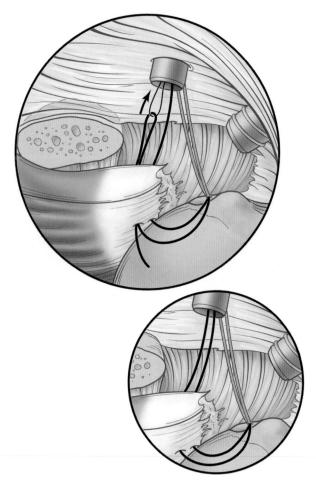

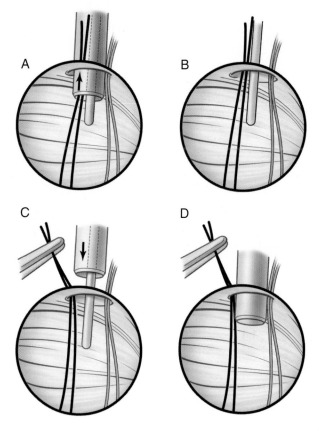

Figure 18-14 Suture management. (Redrawn from Fox JA, Noerdlinger MA, Sasso LM, Romeo AA. Arthroscopic subscapularis repair. In Miller MD, Cole BJ, eds. Textbook of Arthroscopy. Philadelphia, Elsevier, 2004.)

Figure 18-13 Mattress suture. (Redrawn from Fox JA, Noerdlinger MA, Sasso LM, Romeo AA. Arthroscopic subscapularis repair. In Miller MD, Cole BJ, eds. Textbook of Arthroscopy. Philadelphia, Elsevier, 2004.)

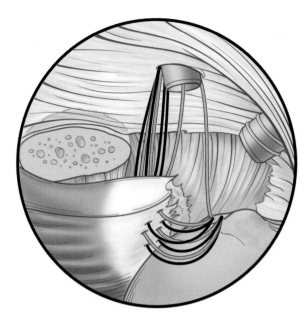

Figure 18-15 Only one limb of the second suture on the last anchor is placed through the tendon. (Redrawn from Fox JA, Noerdlinger MA, Sasso LM, Romeo AA. Arthroscopic subscapularis repair. In Miller MD, Cole BJ, eds. Textbook of Arthroscopy. Philadelphia, Elsevier, 2004.)

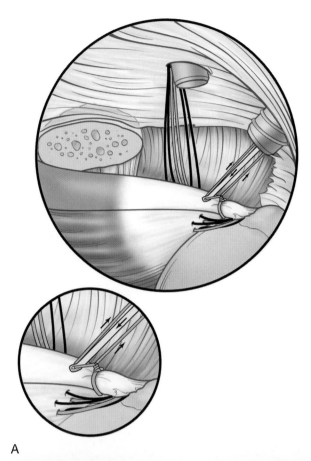

A

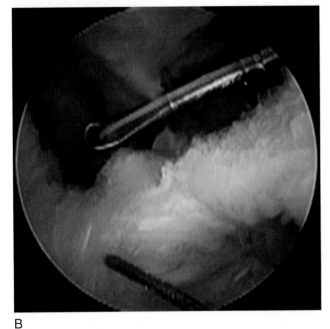

B

Figure 18-16 A and B, Suture tying. (A redrawn from Fox JA, Noerdlinger MA, Sasso LM, Romeo AA. Arthroscopic subscapularis repair. In Miller MD, Cole BJ, eds. Textbook of Arthroscopy. Philadelphia, Elsevier, 2004.)

the biologic quality of the torn tendon. However, our general rehabilitation protocol is described here.

Initially, for the first 2 weeks, we allow forward elevation to 90 degrees and internal rotation to the abdomen. We limit external rotation to 40 degrees to prevent stretching of the repair. From 2 to 6 weeks, we allow the patient to increase external rotation as tolerated; however, we do not permit stretching or manipulation by a physical therapist. Forward elevation is increased to 140 degrees.

At 6 weeks, the sling is discontinued, and we begin active range of motion with progression to full motion as tolerated. We do not start strengthening until 12 weeks after surgery.

Sports-related rehabilitation is initiated at 5 months postoperatively. We allow return to collision sports at 9 months. Patients should expect maximal improvement to occur by about 12 months postoperatively.

Complications

Complications are those seen with arthroscopic shoulder surgery and rotator cuff repair. These include infection, nerve damage, stiffness, repair failure, and complications from fluid extravasation.

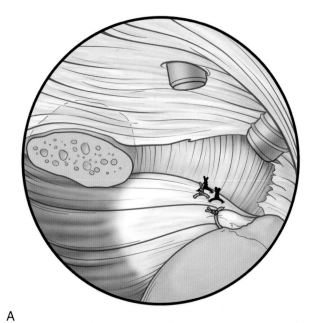

A

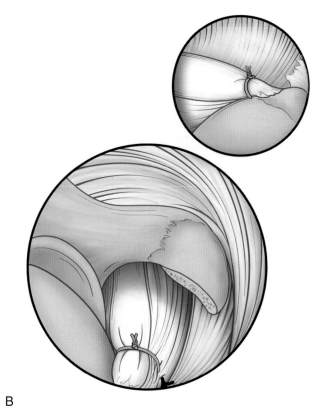

B

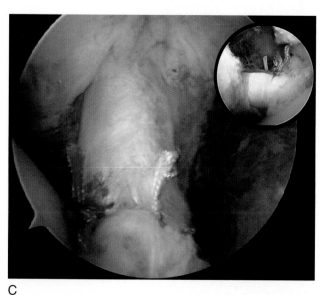

C

Figure 18-17 A to **C,** Final results. (**A** and **B** redrawn from Fox JA, Noerdlinger MA, Sasso LM, Romeo AA. Arthroscopic subscapularis repair. In Miller MD, Cole BJ, eds. Textbook of Arthroscopy. Philadelphia, Elsevier, 2004.)

PEARLS AND PITFALLS

- An interscalene block reduces the amount of anesthetic required during the case and improves pain control in the postoperative period.
- The anterior portal is generally placed just lateral to the coracoid and below the coracoacromial ligament.
- The accessory anterolateral portal is located in the rotator interval anterior and medial to the anterolateral corner of the acromion.
- It is important not to place the two anterior portals too close to each other.

- Consider releasing the long head of the biceps and performing a subpectoral tenodesis.
- A coracoidplasty provides extra space for the technical aspect of the repair and allows the repaired subscapularis more space with no mechanical impingement from the coracoid.
- We place the anchors initially in the inferior edge of the subscapularis footprint, then proceed superiorly, which allows us good visualization throughout the repair process.
- Suture management is crucial in all rotator cuff repairs.
- Suture tying starts with the most proximal suture to set the position for the remaining sutures.

Table 18-1 Clinical Results of Arthroscopic Subscapularis Repairs

Author	Follow-up	Outcome
Romeo (2005)	27 months	Forward elevation improved from 138 to 161 degrees External rotation improved from 70 to 86 degrees ASES score improved from 46 to 82 Simple Shoulder Test score improved from 7 to 10/12 79% good to excellent results
Bennett[1] (2003)	Minimum of 2 years	Constant score improved from 43 to 74 ASES score improved from 16 to 74 VAS for pain dropped from 9 to 2/10 Function improved from 25% to 82%
Burkhart and Tehrany[2] (2002)	10.7 months	Forward elevation improved from 96 to 146 degrees UCLA score improved from 10.7 to 30.5 92% good to excellent results

ASES, American Shoulder and Elbow Surgeons; VAS, visual analogue scale.

Results

Arthroscopic subscapularis repair is a relatively new procedure; therefore, very little information is available in the literature regarding its results. Open repair of the subscapularis has been reported with acceptable results.

The senior author (A. A. R.) has reviewed the results of 14 patients with subscapularis tendon tears treated arthroscopically (Table 18-1). The average follow-up was 27 months. Three patients had an associated supraspinatus tear. One patient fell 2 weeks after surgery and required a revision arthroscopy. No neurovascular complications were noted. Forward elevation improved from 138 to 161 degrees, external rotation from 70 to 86 degrees. The American Shoulder and Elbow Surgeons (ASES) score improved from 46 to 82. The Simple Shoulder Test score improved from 7 to 10 on a 12-point scale. The unadjusted Constant score was 75 of 100 for the surgical side and 79 for the unaffected side, suggesting a functional result similar to that of the unaffected shoulder. On the Rowe function subscale, 79% of patients rated their results good to excellent.

Bennett[1] reviewed the results of eight patients with isolated subscapularis tears treated arthroscopically. The patients were observed for a minimum of 2 years. The Constant score improved from 43 to 74. The ASES score improved from 16 to 74. The visual analogue scale for pain dropped from 9/10 to 2/10. The percentage of function improved from 25% to 82%.

Burkhart and Tehrany[2] reported the results of 25 patients with subscapularis tears treated arthroscopically; 8 patients had isolated complete tears, 6 patients had other rotator cuff disease, and 11 patients had partial tears with other rotator cuff tears. The average follow-up was 10.7 months. Forward elevation improved from 96 to 146 degrees. The UCLA scores improved from 10.7 to 30.5; 92% of patients reported good to excellent results. UCLA scores were similar between isolated and combined tears and between complete and partial tears.

These studies suggest excellent early results and restoration of the force couples, leading to stable, painless glenohumeral joint motion. Although arthroscopic subscapularis repair is a technically demanding technique, we believe that a secure repair can be accomplished arthroscopically and that outcomes after all-arthroscopic repair are similar to those of traditional open techniques.

References

1. Bennett WF. Arthroscopic repair of isolated subscapularis tears: a prospective cohort with 2- to 4- year follow-up. Arthroscopy 2003;19:131-143.

2. Burkhart SS, Tehrany AM. Arthroscopic subscapularis tendon repair: technique and preliminary results. Arthroscopy 2002;18:454-463.

Suggested Readings

Edwards TB, Walch G, Sirveaux F, et al. Repair of tears of the subscapularis. J Bone Joint Surg Am 2005;87:725-730.

Fox JA, Noerdlinger MA, Romeo AA. Arthroscopic subscapularis repair. Tech Shoulder Elbow Surg 2003;4:154-168.

Gerber C, Krushell RJ. Isolated rupture of the tendon of the subscapularis muscle. Clinical features in 16 cases. J Bone Joint Surg Br 1991;73:389-394.

Gerber C, Hersche O, Farron A. Isolated rupture of the subscapularis tendon. J Bone Joint Surg Am 1996;78:1015-1023.

Lo IK, Burkhart SS. Subscapularis tears: arthroscopic repair of the forgotten rotator cuff tendon. Tech Shoulder Elbow Surg 2002;3:282-291.

Lyons RP, Green A. Subscapularis tendon tears. J Am Acad Orthop Surg 2005;13:353-363.

Nerot C. Rotator cuff ruptures with predominant involvement of the subscapularis tendon. Chirurgie 1993-94;291:103-106.

Richards DP, Burkhart SS, Lo IK. Subscapularis tears: arthroscopic repair techniques. Orthop Clin North Am 2003;34:485-498.

Tennent TD, Beach WR, Meyers JF. A review of the special test associated with shoulder examination. Part I: The rotator cuff tests. Am J Sports Med 2003;31:154-160.

CHAPTER 19

Mini-Open Rotator Cuff Repair

Vonda J. Wright, MD
Edward V. Craig, MD

The goals of rotator cuff surgery are to reduce pain and to improve shoulder function. To maximize benefit and to minimize surgical morbidity, surgical techniques for rotator cuff repair have shifted from full open techniques, with detachment of the anterior deltoid, to less invasive methods in which more surgery is performed through smaller incisions. Currently, most surgeons approach the rotator cuff through an arthroscopically assisted mini-open technique or a completely arthroscopic procedure. Whichever approach is selected, the fundamental operative aims of satisfactory decompression and secure tendon repair to bone are identical.

Preoperative Considerations

History

Whether the cause of a patient's shoulder pain is intrinsic tendon degeneration or extrinsic pressure (anatomy of the acromial arch), patients with impingement and rotator cuff irritation generally present with pain during overhead use of the arm. This motion compresses the supraspinatus tendon between the curvatures of the humeral head and acromial arch. This pain is aggravated by use at initial presentation but may progress until patients feel discomfort even at rest. Pain at rest and at night may usually be more indicative of a full-thickness cuff tear. The pain is generally localized to the lateral deltoid and radiates down from the acromion to the deltoid insertion. In addition to pain, patients may experience mechanical symptoms such

as popping or clicking as the humeral head rotates against a thickened bursa or coracoacromial ligament.

Physical Examination

On objective physical evaluation, clinicians may observe atrophy of the supraspinatus and infraspinatus, long head of the biceps rupture, or acromioclavicular joint ganglion. Patients may have decreased active range of motion as a result of cuff weakness. The weakness is especially pronounced with external rotation of the arm near the body and with resisted forward flexion. With larger tears, the rotator cuff no longer stabilizes the humeral head, and the deltoid will pull the humeral head up in the form of a shrug. Whereas passive range of motion is usually preserved in full-thickness tears, long-standing immobilization may lead to secondary stiffness.

Imaging

Typically, patients with a presentation consistent with impingement or rotator cuff tear are evaluated initially with plain radiographs. A complete series includes anteroposterior, lateral outlet (a lateral view of the scapula taken with a 10-degree caudal tilt of the beam), and axillary views.[2] Cystic changes of the supraspinatus insertion and a subacromial traction spur may be apparent. When large rotator cuff tears exist and the humeral head is no longer depressed by the cuff, the acromiohumeral interval may be narrowed. Radiographic changes in the acromioclavicular joint may be seen, and there is an association between cuff disease and persistent unfused os acromiale.

Both magnetic resonance imaging and ultrasonography have been useful in diagnosis of cuff tears. Findings may include changes to the acromioclavicular joint, acromion, or humeral head. On magnetic resonance imaging, the key finding of rotator cuff disease is increased signal in both T1- and T2-weighted images. It is possible to identify not only full-thickness lesions but also partial tears, tendon delamination, muscle atrophy or fat infiltration, tendon retraction, and muscle scarring.

Indications

The indications for performing rotator cuff repair are generally well established. Dunn et al[4] queried members of the American Academy of Orthopaedic Surgeons as to their indications for rotator cuff repair and preferred technique. They found that surgeons who performed a high volume of shoulder surgeries were more likely to recommend cuff repair over conservative treatment and were more positive about the outcomes of surgical intervention versus closed treatment. Of the respondents, 46.2% preferred the mini-open repair versus 14.5% and 36.6% for all-arthroscopic and open repair, respectively. When the decision to fix the rotator cuff has been made, the approach—open, mini-open, or all-arthroscopic—depends on the surgeon's preference and ability to achieve secure tendon repair.

Whereas all-arthroscopic techniques are increasing as technical methods of fixation improve, there are a number of clinical scenarios in which the open repair may have advantages over the more technically difficult arthroscopic method. These include retracted cuffs, larger tears, and tears involving the subscapularis and biceps dislocation as well as revision cuff surgery. In cases in which a mini-open repair is chosen, an expeditious arthroscopic acromioplasty is usually essential as fluid infiltration can make a mini-open repair difficult.

The advantages of the mini-open technique over a traditional open procedure include anterior deltoid preservation, improved joint visualization, decreased pain, and more rapid return to work or sports. In addition, this approach allows more extensive cuff mobilization and more secure fixation with transosseous sutures compared with the all-arthroscopic technique.[3]

Surgical Technique

Positioning and Anesthesia

In most instances, anesthesia is achieved by an interscalene block. Additional local anesthesia is used to cover the area overlying the posterior glenohumeral portal that is not anesthetized by the block. After regional anesthesia, the patient is positioned for surgery.

At our institution, shoulder arthroscopy is accomplished with the patient in a beach chair position. The patient is secured by a beanbag device or an operating room table with a head stabilizer. All bone prominences are protected, as is the peroneal nerve distally. This position allows access to the shoulder from a point medial to the scapula. The arm is prepared and draped free in the normal sterile fashion.

The mini-open rotator cuff repair is a hybrid of arthroscopic evaluation and débridement of the glenohumeral joint, subacromial space, bursa, and rotator cuff followed by a small open approach to relocation of the cuff tendon back down to bone.

Surgical Landmarks and Incisions

Mini-open rotator cuff repair is initiated after an expeditious subacromial decompression (described elsewhere). Although the lateral portal may be simply extended, an anterior superior skin incision following Langer's lines is more aesthetic and avoids the "dimpling" frequently seen with a lateral portal extension. This incision may extend from lateral to the coracoid process past the anterolateral corner of the acromion. The length of the incision is approximately 3 to 4 cm (Fig. 19-1). Before incision, the skin is infiltrated with a 1:500,000 concentration of epinephrine to minimize bleeding.

Specific Steps (Box 19-1)

The soft tissue is dissected off the deltoid fascia to develop small full-thickness flaps. The previous portal site is easily visualized, and the deltoid is split in line with its fibers to the level of the anterior acromion (Fig. 19-2). The distal extent of the deltoid split is limited by placement of a stay suture (No. 1 Tevdek) to avoid damage to the axillary nerve.

Self-retaining retractors are placed deep under the anterior and posterior edges of the deltoid split to reveal the underlying bursal tissue. Subdeltoid scarring may prevent retractor insertion, requiring blunt dissection before retractor placement. Although much of the subacromial bursa will have previously been excised arthroscopically, any remaining bursa is dissected off the rotator cuff tendon sharply for optimal visualization. At this point, it is easy to palpate the acromion and to evaluate the adequacy of the acromioplasty. The acromion can be modified at this point if necessary.

The cuff tear may be readily apparent in the wound at this point. If it is not or the tendon is retracted, rotation of the arm will bring it into view. The supraspinatus insertion, the most frequent site of tendon disease, is readily

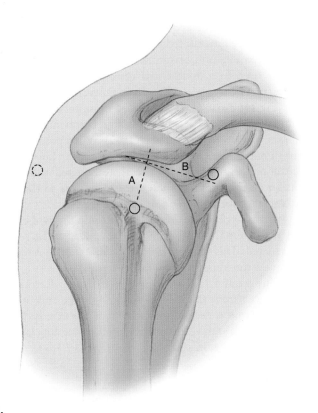

A

Box 19-1 Surgical Steps

1.	Subacromial decompression
2.	Anterior superior incision
3.	Development of skin flaps
4.	Splitting of deltoid
5.	Dissection of subdeltoid scarring
6.	Removal of subacromial bursa
7.	Exposure of cuff tear
8.	Freshening of tendon edge
9.	Reattachment of cuff tendons
10.	Evaluation of repair
11.	Wound irrigation
12.	Closure

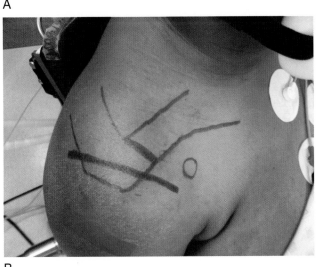

B

Figure 19-1 A and **B,** The skin incision extends from just lateral to the coracoid process and passes over the lateral acromion parallel to Langer's lines. (**A** redrawn from Craig E. Mini-open and open techniques for full-thickness rotator cuff repairs. In Craig E, ed. The Shoulder. Master Techniques in Orthopaedic Surgery. Philadelphia, Lippincott Williams & Wilkins, 2004:309-340.)

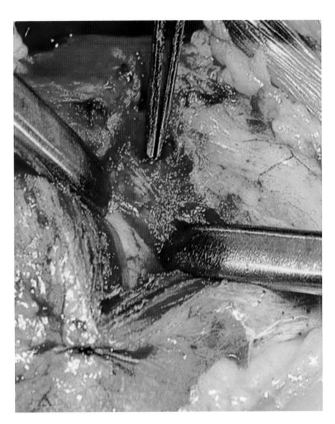

Figure 19-2 The deltoid is split from the acromioclavicular joint laterally for a total length of 5 cm. The distal extent of the split is marked with a stay suture. (From Craig E. Mini-open and open techniques for full-thickness rotator cuff repairs. In Craig E, ed. The Shoulder. Master Techniques in Orthopaedic Surgery. Philadelphia, Lippincott Williams & Wilkins, 2004:309-340.)

seen by this method. At this point, it is possible to precisely identify the rotator cuff anatomy, the shape of the tendon tear, and the involved tendons and their positions relative to the glenoid. The supraspinatus tendon is sometimes retracted by the pull of the coracohumeral ligament and superior capsule. If necessary, the tendon can be mobilized by the release of the extra-articular and intra-articular adhesions or by the release of the coracohumeral ligament and rotator interval.

A nonabsorbable stay suture, such as No. 2 Ethibond, is passed through the tendon edge to facilitate traction during this process. This avoids crushing of the tendon with clamps (Fig. 19-3).

Once the tendon is mobilized, the frayed edge of the tendon may be freshened. Care should be taken to avoid excessive tendon removal. A shaver or rasp is used to remove any remaining soft tissue from the rotator cuff footprint. Establishment of a bleeding bed may not be essential, however, as Fealy et al[5] reported that the lowest cuff vascularity is at the anchor site or cancellous trough. The key blood supply for healing appears to be in the peritendinous region.

The rotator cuff tendons are then reattached to their original bone insertions by drill holes through bone, by use of suture anchors, or by a combination of both. Suture anchors are placed at appropriate intervals in the tuberosity, and the tendon is tied securely to the original footprint. When bone tunnels are used, holes are drilled with a 1/8-inch drill bit through the lateral side of the greater tuberosity. Matching holes are made in the footprint with the tunnels communicating. Sutures are passed through the tunnels and in a Mason-Allen or figure-of-eight pattern

through the tendon edge (Fig. 19-4). Sutures are placed approximately 1 cm apart. A typical supraspinatus tear requires three interrupted sutures.

A combination of suture anchors and bone tunnels may be used in a double-row configuration to secure a larger surface area of tendon back down to bone. In this case, the suture anchors are placed more medially at the anatomic neck, with the bone tunnels providing lateral fixation of the tendon edge (Fig. 19-5). When possible, the arm should be kept at the patient's side during knot tying. Repair of the tendon with the arm abducted will place tension on the fixation when the arm returns to the side and increase the likelihood of failure.

At this point, the arm is brought into forward elevation and external rotation, and the adequacy of the repair is evaluated. This also provides assurance of safe range of motion in the initial postoperative period.

The wound is then copiously irrigated. Retractors are removed from the deltoid edges, as is the stay stitch, and the deltoid edges are approximated. The skin is closed in two layers, a sterile dressing is placed, and a sling is used to protect the repair.

Postoperative Considerations

Rehabilitation

Early passive range of motion is initiated postoperatively with protection of the cuff repair on day 1. Supine passive forward flexion and supine external rotation begin on day 1 with the assistance of a therapist. The patient is taught to perform circular Codman exercises while bending over to 90 degrees at the waist. All exercises in the immediate postoperative period must be done passively. At 6 weeks postoperatively, active exercises and light activity are permitted. Resistive exercises for the deltoid and rotator cuff are allowed after 3 months.

Complications

Several complications can accompany the mini-open rotator cuff repair.[3] Terminal branches of the axillary nerve may be injured if the deltoid split extends more than 4 to 5 cm distal to its origin. This danger can be minimized by placement of a stay suture at the distal extent of the split to prohibit progression.

Care must be taken to firmly secure the rotator cuff tendon down to bone. Insecure repair of rotator cuff tendon may lead to repeated rupture or tissue gapping, inadequate healing, continued pain, and weakness. Finally, an excessively long arthroscopic portion of the procedure will lead to the distention of the soft tissues and skin, subcutaneous tissue, and deltoid. This obscures the bone landmarks and makes subdeltoid dissection difficult.

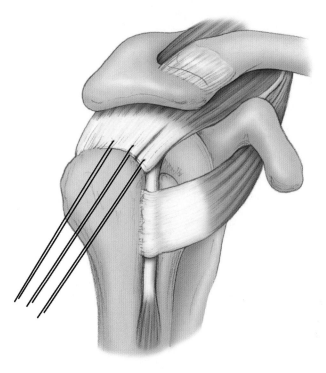

Figure 19-3 The supraspinatus tendon is mobilized, and nonabsorbable stay sutures, such as No. 2 Ethibond, are passed through the tendon edge to facilitate traction during this process. This avoids crushing of the tendon with clamps. (Redrawn from Craig E. Mini-open and open techniques for full-thickness rotator cuff repairs. In Craig E, ed. The Shoulder. Master Techniques in Orthopaedic Surgery. Philadelphia, Lippincott Williams & Wilkins, 2004:309-340.)

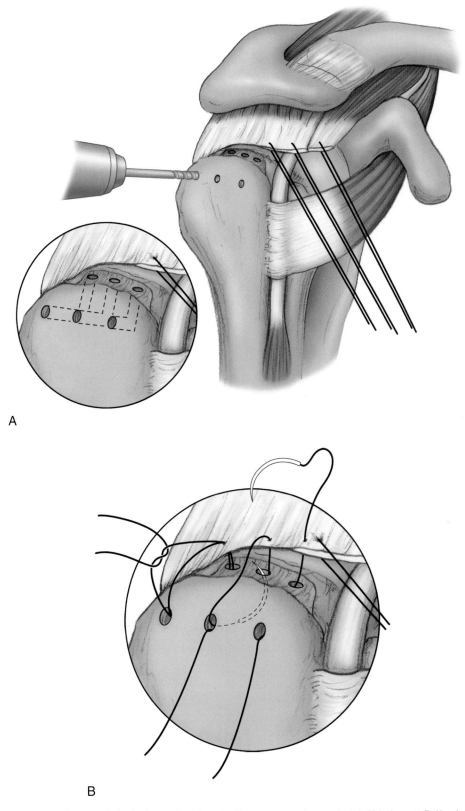

A

B

Figure 19-4 A, A ⅛-inch drill is used to make holes in the greater tuberosity. These are spaced approximately ½ inch apart. **B,** Nonabsorbable sutures are then passed through the cuff tendon in a figure-of-eight fashion. (Redrawn from Craig E. Mini-open and open techniques for full-thickness rotator cuff repairs. In Craig E, ed. The Shoulder. Master Techniques in Orthopaedic Surgery. Philadelphia, Lippincott Williams & Wilkins, 2004:309-340.)

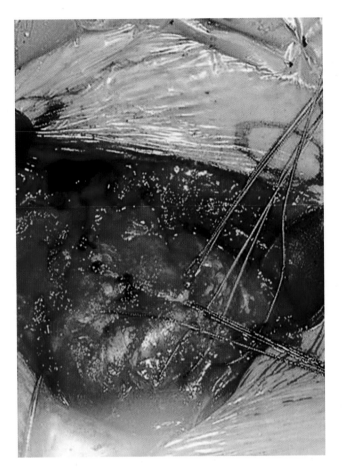

Figure 19-5 The tendon is secured down to bone by the stay sutures to take tension off the repair during knot tying. Any loose or insecure sutures should be passed again. (From Craig E. Mini-open and open techniques for full-thickness rotator cuff repairs. In Craig E, ed. The Shoulder. Master Techniques in Orthopaedic Surgery. Philadelphia, Lippincott Williams & Wilkins, 2004:309-340.)

Table 19-1 Results

Author	Follow-up	Outcomes
Baysal et al[1] (2005)	>1 year	AACR: 96% satisfied or very satisfied; 78% returned to unmodified work by 1 year
Sauerbrey et al[9] (2005)	3 years	No difference between AACR and MOR
Warner et al[11] (2005)	27 months	No difference between AACR and MOR
Kim et al[7] (2003)	Mean: 39 months	No difference between AACR and MOR
Fealy et al[6] (2002)	Minimum of 2 years	AACR: 75 patients; no detectable difference by tear size
Shinners et al[10] (2002)	3 years	AACR: 93% good or excellent

AACR, all-arthroscopic cuff repair; MOR, mini-open cuff repair.

Results

Most investigators report success of more than 80% for mini-open rotator cuff repair in terms of pain control and return of function (Table 19-1). In 2005, Baysal et al[1] documented functional outcomes and quality of life in 84 patients undergoing a mini-open cuff repair. Of their group, 96% of the patients were satisfied or very satisfied with surgical outcome, and 78% returned to unmodified work by 1 year postoperatively. Interestingly, neither the patient's age nor the size of the cuff tear affected outcomes, and most improvement was seen by the 6-month postoperative visit with continued improvement until 1 year. Shinners et al[10] described 67 patients undergoing mini-open cuff repair; 93% received good or excellent outcomes ratings, with all patients experiencing decreased pain and improved function postoperatively. Again, tear size and age of the patient did not affect outcome. A double-row mini-open technique was found effective for the treatment of cuff tears of all sizes by the Hospital for Special Surgery group.[6] Seventy-five consecutive patients underwent arthroscopically assisted mini-open cuff repair and were observed for a minimum of 24 months. There was no detectable difference in outcomes between patients with small, moderate, or large cuff tears.

More studies have compared rotator cuff repair by the mini-open approach and an all-arthroscopic approach. Warner[11] retrospectively summarized his initial experience with mini-open cuff repair versus all-arthroscopic cuff repair. He found no difference in outcomes between the two groups in terms of clinical outcomes, satisfaction of patients, or recovery time and suggested that the approach is based on the preference of the surgeon or patient. Another retrospective comparison looked at 54 patients undergoing cuff repair with an average of 36 months of follow-up. By use of the American Shoulder and Elbow Surgeons (ASES) score, improvements in pain, satisfaction, and functional outcomes were not significantly different between mini-open cuff repair and all-arthroscopic cuff repair groups.[9] Kim et al[7] reported their retrospective case series of 76 patients treated for full-thickness cuff tears by all-arthroscopic techniques or mini-open salvage of unsuccessful arthroscopic repairs. The mean follow-up was 39 months. All patients in both groups had improved ASES scores, with no significant difference in scores, pain, or return to activity between the groups. This study found outcomes to be dependent on tear size and not treatment technique.

The current literature examining the outcomes of rotator cuff surgery is composed of level III and IV studies, and these do not conclusively answer the question of whether all-arthroscopic or mini-open repairs provide better outcomes for patients with small or moderate-sized rotator cuff tears. A large national multicenter study is being undertaken in Canada to answer this question in a prospective manner.[8]

References

1. Baysal D, Balyk R, Otto D, et al. Functional outcome and health-related quality of life after surgical repair of full-thickness rotator cuff tear using a mini-open technique. Am J Sports Med 2005;33:1346-1355.
2. Craig E. Impingement and rotator cuff tear: treatment by anterior acromioplasty and repair. In Craig E, ed. Clinical Orthopaedics. Philadelphia, Lippincott Williams & Wilkins, 1999:213-221.
3. Craig E. Mini-open and open techniques for full-thickness rotator cuff repairs. In Craig E, ed. The Shoulder. Master Techniques in Orthopaedic Surgery. Philadelphia, Lippincott Williams & Wilkins, 2004:309-340.
4. Dunn W, Schackman B, Walsh C, et al. Variation in orthopedic surgeons' perceptions about the indications for rotator cuff surgery. J Bone Joint Surg Am 2005;87:1978-1984.
5. Fealy S, Adler R, Drakos M, et al. Patterns of vascular and anatomical response after rotator cuff repair. Am J Sports Med 2006;34:120-127.
6. Fealy S, Kingham TP, Altchek DW. Mini-open rotator cuff repair using a two-row fixation technique: outcomes analysis in patients with small, moderate, and large rotator cuff tears. Arthroscopy 2002;18:665-670.
7. Kim SH, Ha KI, Park JH, et al. Arthroscopic versus mini-open salvage repair of the rotator cuff tear: outcome analysis at 2 to 6 years' follow-up. Arthroscopy 2003;19:746-754.
8. MacDermid J, Holtby R, Razmjou H. All-arthroscopic versus mini-open repair for small or moderate-sized rotator cuff tears: a protocol for a randomized trial [NCT00128076]. BMC Musculoskelet Disord 2006;7:25.
9. Sauerbrey A, Getz C, Piancastelli M, et al. Arthroscopic versus mini-open rotator cuff repair: a comparison of clinical outcome. Arthroscopy 2005;21:1415-1420.
10. Shinners T, Noordsij P, Orwin J. Arthroscopically assisted mini-open rotator cuff repair. Arthroscopy 2002;18:21-26.
11. Warner J, Tetreault P, Lehtinen J, Zurakowski D. Arthroscopic versus mini-open rotator cuff repair: a cohort comparison study. Arthroscopy 2005;21:328-332.
12. Youm T, Murray D, Kubiak E, et al. Arthroscopic versus mini-open rotator cuff repair: a comparison of clinical outcomes and patient satisfaction. J Shoulder Elbow Surg 2005;14:455-459.

CHAPTER 20

Open Rotator Cuff Repair

John W. Sperling, MD, MBA

Multiple facets need to be incorporated to arrive at a successful rotator cuff repair. The process starts with a thorough understanding of the patient's symptoms, motivation, and ability to comply with postoperative restrictions. Careful examination together with appropriate imaging studies allows proper surgical planning.

Preoperative Considerations

History

Evaluation of the patient with a rotator cuff tear begins with a thorough history. It is critically important to understand the severity of the symptoms and the patient's ability to comply with postoperative restrictions. The surgeon also needs to elucidate the primary complaint, whether it is pain, weakness, or loss of motion, to better determine and guide the patient's expectations.

The history ascertains the patient's dominant extremity as well as occupation. The duration of pain and dysfunction is determined and whether it started with a specific traumatic event. To understand the severity of pain and the degree to which it interferes with the quality of life, patients are asked to rate the pain on a scale of 1 to 10 at rest, with activities, and at night. The patient is also asked about specific alleviating and aggravating factors. Last, patients are asked to localize the pain—whether it occurs over the anterolateral aspect of the shoulder or radiates in a more radicular pattern down the entire arm, possibly consistent with a neurologic component of pain.

If possible, the results of prior studies are obtained, and prior treatment attempts and their results are reviewed. With a history of prior shoulder surgery, operative notes and images can help further delineate the pathologic process.

A focused review of systems is performed to rule out the possibility of other pathologic processes that frequently cause or mimic shoulder pain, such as inflammatory arthritis, cervical radiculopathy, and even thoracic neoplasias. A list of medications and associated medical problems should be recorded.

Physical Examination

Physical examination includes inspection and palpation of the entire shoulder, followed by specialized functional tests. Inspection assesses soft tissue swelling, deformity, or atrophy. Palpation comprises an examination of the cervical spine, acromioclavicular joint, and bicipital groove. The neurovascular examination of the extremities includes assessment of strength, sensation, and reflexes.

Subsequently, active and passive shoulder motion is recorded for forward flexion, abduction, internal rotation, and external rotation. Strength is graded on a scale of 1 to 5 for internal rotation, external rotation, flexion, extension, and abduction. Impingement tests have been found to be fairly nonspecific but can help elucidate a diagnosis of subacromial impingement; weakness is suggestive of a tear of the rotator cuff. More specialized tests include the liftoff and belly press tests for subscapularis function, as well as external rotation strength, and the lag sign for infraspinatus function; these allow more sensitive assessment of muscle strength.

Imaging

Radiography

Three radiographic views are routinely obtained: 40-degree posterior oblique views with internal and external rotation and an axillary view. One may observe superior subluxation of the humeral head and a decrease in the acromial-humeral distance with significant rotator cuff deficiency. One caveat is that with posterior subluxation, there can be the false appearance of superior humeral head subluxation. There may be sclerosis or rounding of the greater tuberosity with rotator cuff disease as well. The axillary view allows assessment of glenohumeral cartilage loss and subluxation. In addition, one may choose to obtain a Neer outlet view to evaluate acromial morphologic features.

Advanced Imaging Studies

Multiple options are available to further investigate the integrity of the rotator cuff, including arthrography, computed tomographic arthrography, magnetic resonance imaging, and ultrasonography. The decision of which test to perform is based on the individual surgeon's preference. Magnetic resonance imaging provides important additional information about tear size and configuration, degree of retraction, and muscle atrophy or degeneration.

Indications and Contraindications

After the information obtained from the history, physical examination, and imaging studies is integrated, one determines the diagnosis and can present treatment options to the patient. It is critical to understand the patient's goals and expectations for surgery. Clearly, the primary indication for rotator cuff surgery is pain relief; recovery of strength and function is less predictable. Contraindications include active or recent infection, significant medical comorbidities, and an inability to follow the postoperative restrictions and rehabilitation.

A detailed conversation with the patient then occurs concerning treatment options. The risk, benefits, and alternatives to surgical repair are discussed in detail. The decision to employ specific techniques, such as open versus arthroscopic repair, is based on the individual surgeon's preference and familiarity with each technique. I individualize this decision for each patient on the basis of the age of the patient, the physical demands on the shoulder, the size and configuration of the tear, and a primary or revision setting. My practice consists primarily of performing arthroscopic rotator cuff repair. However, the technique of open repair may be particularly useful in the revision setting when multiple anchors are already present within the humeral head. In addition, open repair may be considered in the young, active heavy laborer with a large rotator cuff tear.

Surgical Technique

Anesthesia and Positioning

A combination of regional anesthesia and light sedation or general anesthesia is commonly used for rotator cuff repair, which increasingly is being performed on an outpatient basis. The patient is carefully padded and placed in the beach chair position. The waist should be in approximately 45 degrees of flexion and the knees in 30 degrees of flexion. The table may be slightly rolled away from the surgical shoulder.

Surgical Landmarks

In nearly all patients, regardless of size, one can palpate the posterior scapular spine. The lateral border of the acromion, the anterior border of the acromion, and the anterior portion of the clavicle and coracoid are then marked with a sterile marker (Fig. 20-1). If one is performing an arthroscopy before the open repair, one may wish to mark out the standard anterior incision and attempt to place the incision for the anterior portal in line with this future incision.

Specific Steps (Box 20-1)

There is significant variability in the skin incision used for open rotator cuff repair, including oblique incisions, horizontal incisions, and vertical incisions. The choice of which incision to use is based on the individual surgeon's preference.

1. Incision

An incision is made over the anterior superior aspect of the shoulder parallel with the lateral border of the acro-

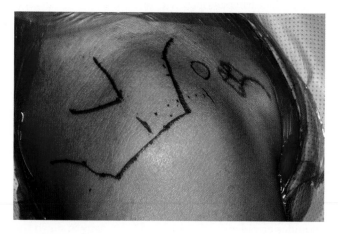

Figure 20-1 The landmarks on the shoulder are identified and marked. A 4- to 5-cm incision is made parallel to the lateral border of the acromion.

Box 20-1 Surgical Steps

| 1. Incision |
| 2. Deltoid split |
| 3. Rotator cuff repair |
| 4. Deltoid repair |

mion in line with Langer's lines. The length of the skin incision is typically 4 to 5 cm. The skin is incised as well as the fat. The skin flaps are carefully developed and mobilized.

2. Deltoid Split

The deltoid muscle insertion into the acromion is clearly identified. There is significant variability among surgeons in regard to the technique with which they take down the deltoid (Fig. 20-2). In this example, the deltoid is taken down off the anterior aspect of the acromion with full-thickness sleeves (Fig. 20-3). One must take great care to ensure that this includes both the deep and superficial fascia of the deltoid. The surgeon then has the option

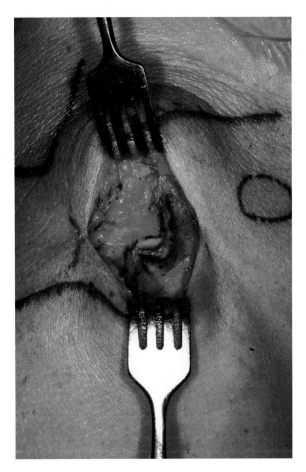

Figure 20-3 Full-thickness flaps of the deltoid including the superficial and deep layers of fascia are taken down.

either of splitting the deltoid in line with the fibers starting from the acromioclavicular joint anteriorly for approximately 3 cm or of extending the deltoid detachment posteriorly over the lateral border of the acromion. The extent of the deltoid detachment over the lateral acromion border can be modified on the basis of the size of the rotator cuff tear. One must be careful to avoid splitting the deltoid laterally in line with its fibers more than 4 or 5 cm from the acromial border to protect the axillary nerve. However, in most cases, no more than a 2-cm split in line with the fibers of the deltoid is necessary. One can mark the area where the proximal deltoid split is made with a retention stitch (Fig. 20-4). An additional stitch is usually placed distally in the deltoid split to prevent propagation (Fig. 20-5).

3. Rotator Cuff Repair

On the basis of the surgeon's preference, an acromioplasty may then be performed (Fig. 20-6). The torn rotator cuff edges are identified, and retention stitches are placed (Fig. 20-7). Systematic releases are then performed to mobilize the tendon. Specifically, one releases overlying bursal adhesions from the torn rotator cuff. Frequently, there is

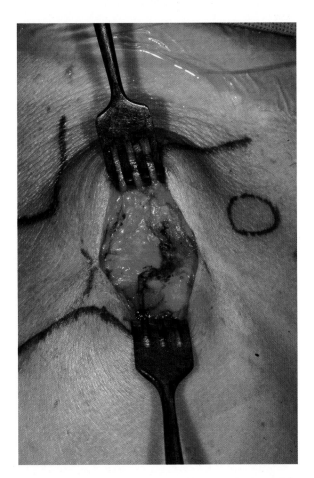

Figure 20-2 The area of deltoid to be taken off the acromion is carefully outlined.

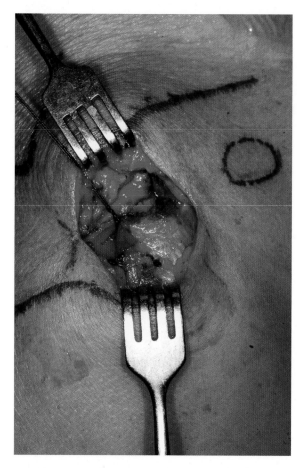

Figure 20-4 A marking stitch is placed in the corner of the deltoid to ensure proper alignment of the deltoid at the time of repair.

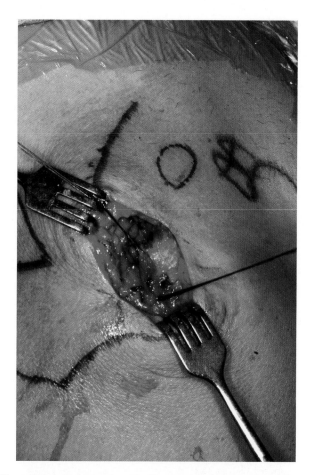

Figure 20-5 A stitch is placed in the distal deltoid split to prevent propagation.

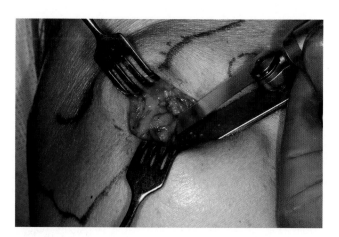

Figure 20-6 An acromioplasty may be performed on the basis of the surgeon's preference.

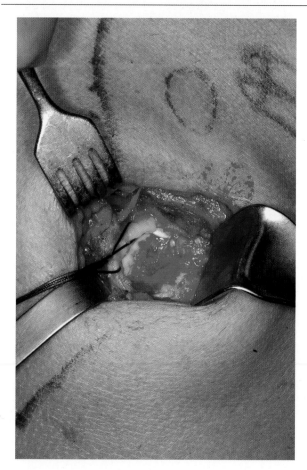

Figure 20-7 Retention stitches are placed in the rotator cuff tear.

scarring of the coracohumeral ligament to the rotator cuff that must be released. One may also perform intra-articular releases between the labrum and rotator cuff. Care must be taken not to injure the suprascapular nerve in performing medial releases.

The tendon edges are freshened. The rotator cuff repair can then be performed on the basis of the tear configuration (Fig. 20-8). It is my preference in performing a tendon to bone repair to use modified Mason-Allen stitches placed through bone tunnels.

4. Deltoid Repair

For closure, a meticulous repair of the deltoid is required. At the end of the procedure, the deltoid is repaired back in a tendon to tendon as well as a tendon to bone manner (Figs. 20- 9 to 20-11). Drill holes are placed through the acromion with tendon to bone stitches. In addition, the split within the deltoid itself is repaired with multiple side-to-side stitches. Complications in this approach may be related to deltoid dehiscence postoperatively.

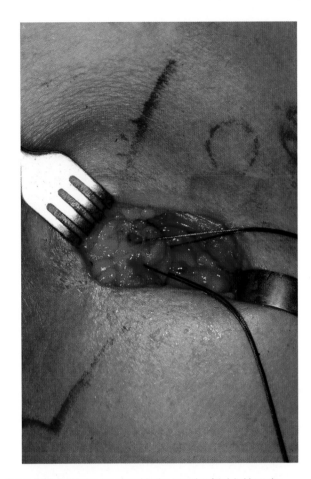

Figure 20-9 Drill holes are placed in the acromion for deltoid repair.

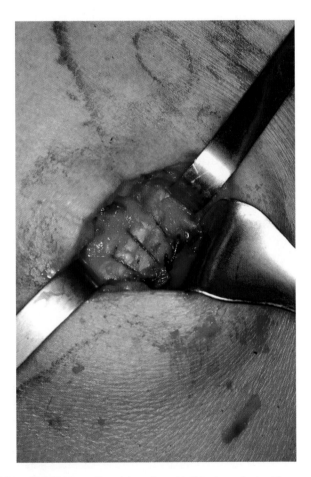

Figure 20-8 Rotator cuff repair is performed in this circumstance with tendon to bone stitches.

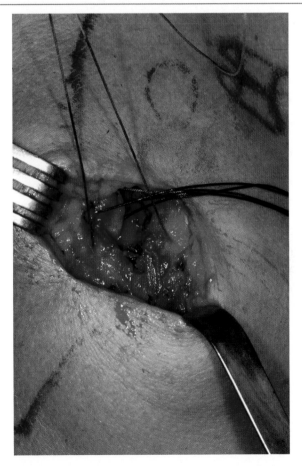

Figure 20-10 The corner of the deltoid is sutured back to its anatomic location.

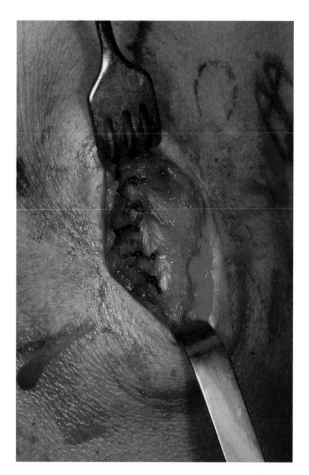

Figure 20-11 Final deltoid repair.

Postoperative Considerations

Rehabilitation

The patient is placed in a shoulder immobilizer. Passive range-of-motion exercises are started with parameters determined at the time of surgery. Pulley and wand exercises are incorporated into the rehabilitation program from week 3 to week 6 on the basis of the individual patient. The patient then progresses to gentle isometric strengthening exercises.

Results

Results of selected series of open rotator cuff repairs are listed in Table 20-1.

A study by Hawkins et al[3] of 100 rotator cuff repairs at a mean follow-up of 4.2 years revealed that 86% had no or slight pain. All patients had an acromioplasty in addition to the rotator cuff repair. The average abduction improved from 81 to 125 degrees postoperatively. Of 100 patients, 94 considered themselves improved with the surgery. Ellman et al[2] reported the results of open rotator cuff repair in 50 patients with a mean follow-up of 3.5 years. The results were satisfactory in 84% and unsatisfactory in 16%.

Neer et al[4] reviewed the results of 245 shoulders that underwent rotator cuff repair. Acromioplasty was also performed in 243 of 245 shoulders. Excellent or satisfactory results were obtained in 91% of the shoulders. Cofield et al[1] reviewed the results of 105 shoulders with a chronic rotator cuff tear that underwent open surgical repair and acromioplasty and were observed for an average of 13.4 years. There was satisfactory pain relief in 96 of 105 shoulders. The most frequent complication was apparent failure of rotator cuff healing. Five patients underwent repeated repair. Tear size was found to be the most important determinant of outcome with regard to active motion, strength, rating of the result, satisfaction of the patient, and need for reoperation.

Table 20-1 Results of Open Rotator Cuff Repair

Author	No. of Patients	Follow-up (Mean)	Age of Patient (Mean)	Outcome
Cofield et al[1] (2001)	105	13.4 years	58 years	80% satisfactory–excellent results
Hawkins et al[3] (1985)	100	4.2 years	51 years	94% subjective improvement
Ellman et al[2] (1986)	50	3.5 years	60 years	84% satisfactory results
Neer et al[4] (1988)	233	NA	59 years	91% satisfactory–excellent results

References

1. Cofield RH, Parvizi J, Hoffmeyer PJ, et al. Surgical repair of chronic rotator cuff tears: a prospective long-term study. J Bone Joint Surg Am 2001;83:71-77.
2. Ellman H, Hanker G, Bayer M. Repair of the rotator cuff: end-result study of factors influencing reconstruction. J Bone Joint Surg Am 1986;68:1136-1144.
3. Hawkins RJ, Misamore GW, Hobeika PE. Surgery for full thickness rotator cuff tears. J Bone Joint Surg Am 1985;67:1349-1355.
4. Neer CS, Flatow EL, Lech O. Tears of the rotator cuff—long term results of anterior acromioplasty and repair. Orthop Trans 1988;12:735.

CHAPTER 21

Tendon Transfers for Rotator Cuff Insufficiency

Brett S. Sanders, MD

Scott D. Pennington, MD

Thomas F. Holovacs, MD

Jon J. P. Warner, MD

Direct primary repair achieves reliable pain relief and functional improvement in the majority of rotator cuff tears.[13,22,49] However, less commonly, very large musculotendinous defects, static superior subluxation of the humeral head, chronicity, and poor bone or tendon tissue quality may preclude successful primary repair.[3,4,16,20,22] In such cases, alternative reconstructive surgical techniques should be considered. Historically, the management of irreparable massive rotator cuff tears had encompassed a wide range of surgical procedures, including open or arthroscopic débridement, muscle or tendon transposition (upper subscapularis, teres minor, teres major, latissimus dorsi, pectoralis major, trapezius, deltoid, biceps, and triceps), tendon allografts, synthetic graft material, xenograft, and arthroplasty.[1,2,5,8,12,36-38]

Although débridement may allow pain relief in the low-demand patient,[42,43] function is not reliably restored.[6,22] Bridging of tendinous gaps with allografts and xenografts has not gained widespread acceptance because of variable functional results and inability to re-establish the length-tension relationship of the rotator cuff.[11] If the coracoacromial arch is intact, hemiarthroplasty may offer some relief in the setting of rotator cuff arthropathy,[26,30] but this treatment rarely addresses functional limitations.[25] Recently, reverse total shoulder arthroplasty has offered a promising solution for pain relief and concomitant functional improvement in older patients with irreparable tears; however, long-term data on the longevity of these prostheses are not available in the United States. Furthermore, a reverse prosthesis alone will not restore an external rotation deficit, which can be a persistent source of disability. For younger, high-demand patients, local or regional muscle and tendon transfers are viable treatment options that provide a vascularized, functional replacement of the affected musculotendinous unit when other repair methods are likely to fail.

When a musculotendinous unit has become torn and retracted from its insertion, the constituent muscle fibers undergo atrophy secondary to disuse. Concomitantly, fatty infiltration of the muscle interstitium results from macroarchitectural changes in the muscle fiber pennation angle.[32] Once these changes have occurred, the muscle may not generate the strength and excursion necessary for normal function, even after successful primary repair.[13,18,16,22,32] Even if excursion is sufficient to allow primary repair, fatty infiltration appears to be an irreversible event that may permanently compromise mechanical integrity of the musculotendinous unit.

Several donor muscles about the shoulder girdle have been shown to possess a suitable vector of pull, with adequate strength and amplitude to act as a surrogate rotator cuff tendon.[7,9,19,24,27,28,31,44,51] Empirically derived functional tendon transfers, of proven efficacy in foot and hand surgery, have been used to restore shoulder function after obstetric palsy in children.[10,27] The analogous situation in the adult can result from brachial plexopathy and iatrogenic, inherited, or degenerative injury to the neuromusculotendinous unit of the rotator cuff. Advancement or transposition of local and regional muscles has been described to treat commonly occurring massive degenerative rotator cuff tears.[8,16,37] The two patterns of massive, irreparable rotator cuff tears are posterior superior and anterior superior configurations. Posterior superior rotator cuff tears are the most common type and involve the supraspinatus and infraspinatus (and occasionally the teres minor) tendons. Anterior superior rotator cuff tears involve the supraspinatus and the subscapularis. In this chapter, we review two reliable regional tendon transfers for treatment of the most commonly occurring deficits in the rotator cuff: the irreparable, massive posterior superior rotator cuff tear and the irreparable subscapularis tear (Table 21-1).

Latissimus Dorsi Transfer for Posterior Superior Rotator Cuff Tears

Preoperative Considerations

The latissimus dorsi transfer is primarily indicated for patients with unacceptable pain and functional deficits caused by a chronic, irreparable, massive tear of the posterosuperior rotator cuff. Because there is no strict preoperative definition of an irreparable tear, the clinician must use a constellation of findings on the history, physical examination, and radiographic work-up to ascertain the feasibility of primary rotator cuff repair. Size of the tear, chronicity, and tendon and bone quality are preoperative

Table 21-1 Local and Regional Tendon Transfer Options for Muscle Deficits About the Shoulder

Deficit	Transfer Option
Infraspinatus (posteroinferior cuff)	Latissimus ± teres major Teres alone
Supraspinatus	Subscapularis Teres minor Anterior deltoid
Subscapularis (anterosuperior cuff)	Pectoralis major (split, clavicular head or sternal head) Teres major
Serratus anterior	Pectoralis major (split, sternal head)
Trapezius	Rhomboid, levator advancement (Eden-Lange)

risk factors that may mitigate the success of primary cuff repair.

History

- Insidious onset of shoulder pain and loss of function during months to years
- Fatigue or pain with use of the arm in abduction
- External rotation weakness
- Prior failed surgery on the rotator cuff

Physical Examination

- Atrophy of the spinati may be noted, indicating a chronic, massive tear.
- Active forward flexion and external rotation are limited compared with the contralateral side. Motor testing of the supraspinatus and infraspinatus demonstrates weakness.
- Passive motion should be well maintained in the tendon transfer candidate.
- External rotation lag (a difference in passive and active external rotation arc) is indicative of a massive posterior cuff tear. An external rotation lag sign that persists in abduction, termed the *signe du clarion* (hornblower sign), indicates extension of the tear into the teres minor[23] (Fig. 21-1).
- Subscapularis function is intact (Gerber liftoff test).
- It may be advantageous to perform an impingement test with a lidocaine injection into the subacromial space to test rotator cuff strength if the examination is limited by pain.

Imaging

- True anteroposterior, scapular Y, and axillary lateral views of the shoulder
- Plain films may demonstrate static superior subluxation of the humeral head. An acromiohumeral distance of less than 7 mm (normal, 10.5 mm) suggests an irreparable tear of the infraspinatus (Fig. 21-2A).
- Magnetic resonance imaging is performed to characterize the status of the rotator cuff tendons and to evaluate muscle atrophy and fatty infiltration.
- A massive tear, defined as a tear encompassing two or more tendons, with grade 3 or 4 fatty infiltration of the rotator cuff musculature on magnetic resonance imaging or computed tomography, portends a poor prognosis for a successful primary repair and as such is an indication for tendon transfer (Fig. 21-2B).[20]

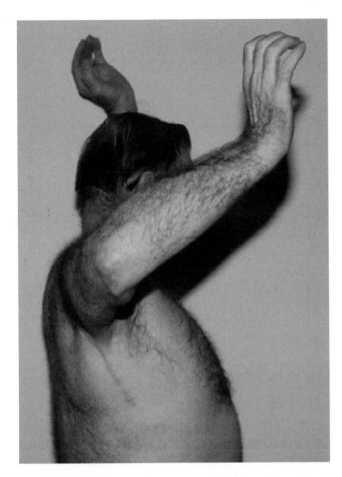

Figure 21-1 The hornblower sign is pathognomonic of a massive posterior cuff tear.

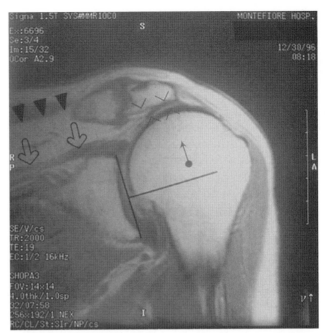

A

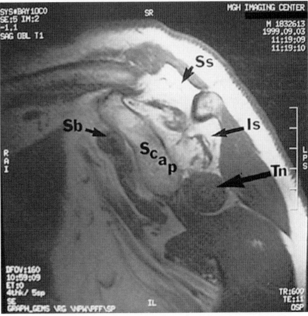

B

Figure 21-2 A, Magnetic resonance image demonstrates superior subluxation of the humeral head, indicating massive rotator cuff tear. **B,** Grade 4 fatty infiltration of two rotator cuff tendons. IS, infraspinatus tendon; Sb, subscapularis tendon; scap, scapula; SS, supraspinatus tendon; Tn, teres minor. (**B** from Warner JJP. Management of massive irreparable rotator cuff tears: the role of tendon transfer. Instr Course Lect 2001;50:63-71.)

Contraindications

Not all patients with massive, irreparable rotator cuff tears require surgery. Some patients with massive cuff tears experience minimal pain and maintain good overall shoulder function. Reconstructive efforts in such patients are unnecessary.

Patients with massive, irreparable rotator cuff tears often demonstrate pseudoparalysis, or the inability to initiate abduction. This finding is a contraindication to latissimus dorsi tendon transfer. Isolated loss of forward elevation alone is not reliably restored by this technique. In addition, patients with anterosuperior rotator cuff tears involving the subscapularis, such that the liftoff test result is positive, are not good candidates for latissimus transfer.

Prior failed attempts at primary rotator cuff repair are not necessarily contraindications to a latissimus transfer, but more limited gains in satisfaction and function should be expected.[48] Other relative contraindications include deltoid dysfunction, shoulder stiffness, severe rotator cuff tear arthropathy, and infection.

Surgical Technique

Anesthesia and Positioning

The patient is assessed by the anesthesiologist preoperatively for the use of an interscalene block and catheter. However, because the interscalene block does not extend to the axilla, general anesthesia is necessary. We have had experience in positioning one of two ways—beach chair or lateral decubitus.

If the beach chair position is selected, the patient is placed onto a custom beach chair device with retractable kidney rests, providing maximal exposure (T-Max Shoulder Positioner; Tenet Medical Engineering, Calgary, Canada). The beach chair position is relatively contraindicated in obese patients because of difficulty with surgical field exposure in the axilla. After induction, the patient is placed as far laterally on the table as possible to facilitate positioning of the surgeon during exposure. A first-generation cephalosporin is administered for prophylaxis. The operative limb and hemi-torso are prepared and draped in the usual sterile fashion and then secured by means of a sterile pneumatic arm holder (Spider Limb Positioner; Tenet Medical Engineering, Calgary, Canada). In this position, the surgeon may easily approach the superior shoulder and the axilla without the need of an assistant to hold the extremity (Fig. 21-3).

Alternatively, the lateral decubitus position may be used. After induction, the patient is placed into the lateral decubitus position on the far lateral side of a standard operating table. A full-length beanbag supports the patient's body, with an axillary roll in place on the contralateral side. The Tenet arm holder is positioned at the midportion of the bed on the ventral side of the patient. Preparation and draping proceed in the standard fashion, with care taken to provide adequate exposure superiorly and posteriorly (Fig. 21-4).

Surgical Landmarks and Incisions

Landmarks

- Anterosuperior exposure: acromion, acromioclavicular joint, clavicle, and coracoid process. The incision is placed in relation to these landmarks parallel to Langer's lines over the lateral third of the acromion, beginning at the posterior edge of the acromion and extending anteriorly 1 cm lateral to the coracoid process.
- Posteroinferior exposure: anterior border of the latissimus, triceps muscle belly, posterior deltoid. The posteroinferior incision of the latissimus dorsi is drawn parallel to the anterior border of the latissimus approximately 6 to 8 cm distal to the axillary fold. Proximally, the incision is curved superiorly parallel to the posterior axillary line to allow access to the posterior aspect of the deltoid (Fig. 21-5).

Structures at Risk

- Latissimus transfer: axillary nerve, radial nerve, brachial artery, thoracodorsal neurovascular pedicle

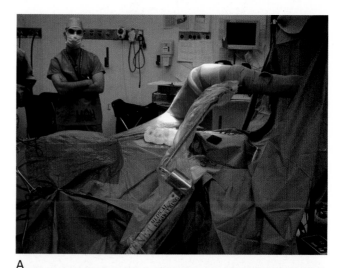

A

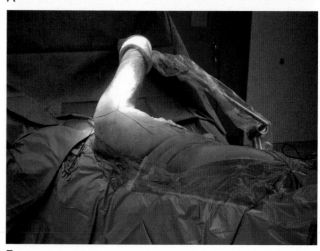

B

Figure 21-4 Lateral decubitus position.

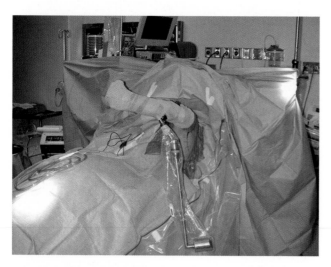

Figure 21-3 Beach chair position.

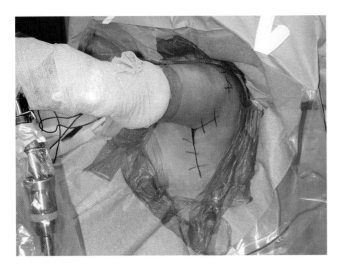

Figure 21-5 Posterior incision for latissimus dissection.

Box 21-1 Surgical Steps of Latissimus Transfer

1. Superior exposure, cuff assessment, and mobilization

2. Greater tuberosity preparation (with anchor placement)

3. Posteroinferior exposure and mobilization of the latissimus tendon

4. Tendon transfer

5. Tendon fixation

6. Closure

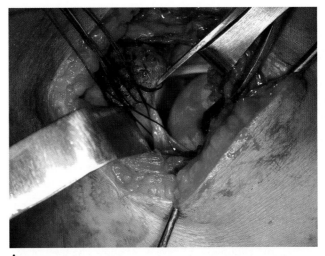

A

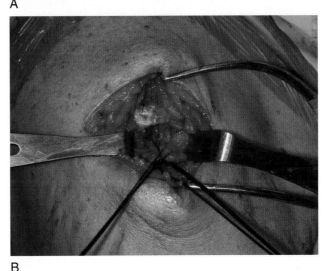

B

Figure 21-6 Mobilization (**A**) and assessment (**B**) of cuff excursion.

Specific Steps (Box 21-1)

1. Superior Exposure, Cuff Assessment, and Mobilization

We approach the rotator cuff first during the procedure to allow assessment of cuff tissue and placement of anchors before harvesting of the latissimus. A No. 10 scalpel is used to incise skin and subcutaneous tissue to the level of the deltoid fascia. Sharp dissection with the scalpel is used to develop skin flaps at this level adequate to allow visualization of the lateral acromion and interval between the anterior and middle deltoid. Electrocautery is used to secure hemostasis, and self-retaining retractors are placed.

Next, the electrocautery is used to split the deltoid in line with its fibers for a distance of 4 to 5 cm between the anterior and middle heads of the deltoid. The anterior deltoid may be reflected subperiosteally off the acromion by means of the electrocautery to provide visualization of the rotator cuff, if necessary. The interval between the anterior deltoid and coracoacromial arch is identified, and the coracoacromial ligament attachment to the acromion

is preserved. The subacromial bursa is excised. Placement of Army-Navy retractors or a self-retaining subacromial spreader may be useful for exposure of the rotator cuff. The torn edges of the rotator cuff are then tagged with No. 3 Ethibond, and a systematic release of the rotator cuff is performed. A No. 15 scalpel is employed to release the coracohumeral ligament, extra-articular subacromial adhesions, and the superior capsule of the glenohumeral joint just deep to the rotator cuff. Care is taken not to release more than 1.8 cm medial to the glenoid to avoid iatrogenic injury to the suprascapular nerve. If the biceps tendon is present, it is released from the supraglenoid tubercle and tenodesed in the biceps groove. Once releases have been performed, the compliance and excursion of the cuff are assessed for the possibility of primary repair (Fig. 21-6).

2. Greater Tuberosity Preparation (with Anchor Placement)

If primary repair is deemed to be not feasible, the rotator cuff tendon edges are freshened with a scalpel and the greater tuberosity is prepared with a rongeur on its antero-lateral surface. The footprint must be placed laterally enough to allow creation of an external rotation moment for the transferred tendon. Suture anchors are then placed to allow multiple fixation points and to re-establish the rotator cuff footprint, depending on the tear pattern. A moistened saline gauze is then packed into the wound, and attention is turned to the posteroinferior exposure (Fig. 21-7).

3. Posteroinferior Exposure and Mobilization of the Latissimus Tendon

With the arm holder in a position of abduction and maximal internal rotation, attention is turned to the posteroinferior incision. The skin is incised with a No. 10 scalpel, and skin flaps are developed above the level of the superficial fascia (Fig. 21-8A). By sharp dissection, the anterior border of the latissimus is defined. Posteriorly, the teres major, long head of the triceps, and posterior deltoid are identified. Careful dissection anteriorly will identify the neurovascular pedicle of the latissimus approximately 10 cm from the musculotendinous junction. If the muscle portion of the teres major is distinct from the latissimus posteriorly, this interval may be developed distally to further isolate the latissimus. However, the bellies of these two muscles are often confluent. In this case, dissection is carried superiorly just off the anterior border of the latissimus to its insertion, which is identified by the long, flat tendon insertion on the anterior humerus. Exposure is facilitated by maximal internal rotation and abduction of the brachium. Once the insertion has been identified, the tendon is released under direct vision with a No. 15 scalpel, with care taken to avoid the radial and axillary nerves, which are close. The rest of the muscle belly may then be liberated of any adhesions to the chest wall in a retrograde fashion (Fig. 21-8B).

4. Tendon Transfer

After the latissimus has been identified and mobilized, a running locking stitch of No. 3 Ethibond is placed in the tendon, and final releases are performed distally (Fig. 21-9A). Adequate excursion of the tendon may be tested by the ability to elevate the tendon superior to the level of the acromion (Fig. 21-10A). If this maneuver cannot be performed, further dissection of the thoracodorsal neuro-vascular pedicle may be performed as necessary, remembering that the average length of the pedicle is 8.4 cm. Alternatively, consideration may be given to augmentation of the graft with autogenous tissue (i.e., hamstring tendons) or soft tissue allografts to gain more length (Fig. 21-9B).

Once it has been determined that the tendon has enough length and excursion to reach the insertion site on the greater tuberosity, a subdeltoid tunnel is developed by a curved clamp inserted proximal to distal from the antero-superior exposure to the posteroinferior exposure. The

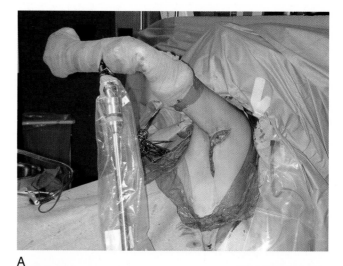

A

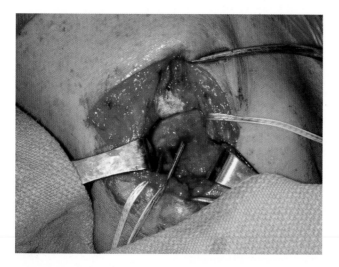

Figure 21-7 Preparation of the greater tuberosity for tendon insertion. Note lateral placement of anchors on tuberosity.

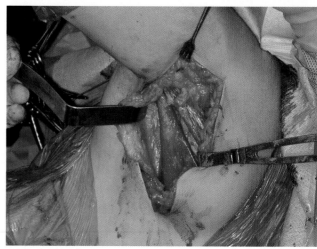

B

Figure 21-8 A, Posteroinferior incision. **B,** Mobilization of latissimus tendon.

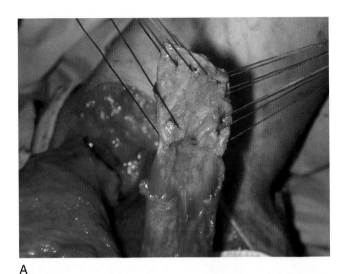

A

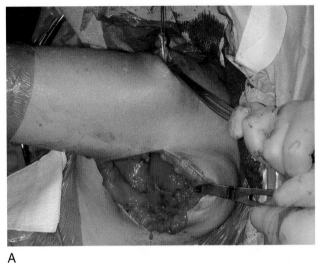

A

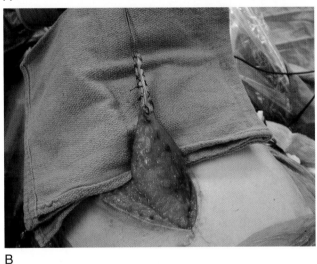

B

Figure 21-9 A, Preparation of latissimus tendon. **B,** Latissimus with the addition of fascia lata graft to reinforce tendon and attain length.

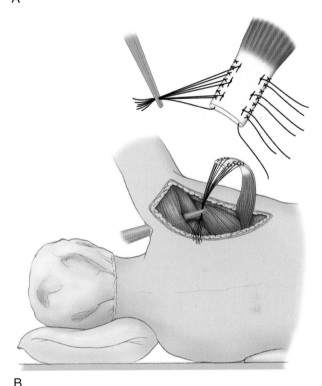

B

Figure 21-10 A, Testing adequate mobilization and excursion of the tendon transfer. **B,** Passage of tendon. (**B** redrawn from Warner JJP. Management of massive irreparable rotator cuff tears: the role of tendon transfer. Instr Course Lect 2001;50:63-71.)

plane between the deltoid and teres minor is bluntly dissected, and the previously placed tagging sutures are drawn proximally through the soft tissue tunnel in an anterograde fashion. The axillary nerve is lateral to the passage of the tendon. Adequate excursion within the tunnel is confirmed by placing the tendon on the intended insertion site (Fig. 21-10B).

5. Tendon Fixation

Tendon fixation is performed to the insertion site with the arm in 45 degrees of abduction and 30 degrees of external rotation by means of horizontal mattress sutures from the suture anchors. Frequently, slight external rotation may be needed to secure the tendon without too much tension. If the mobilized remnant of the rotator cuff will reach the insertion site, it may be incorporated into the fixation of the latissimus tendon or secured with No. 5 FiberWire sutures in a Mason-Allen configuration through bone tunnels to the greater tuberosity (Fig. 21-11).

6. Closure

The deltoid is then repaired to the acromion through bone tunnels with No. 5 FiberWire (Fig. 21-12). All wounds are closed with 2-0 Vicryl sutures, followed by 3-0 Monocryl. Drains may be left in the wounds if it is deemed necessary. Before the patient is extubated, the SOBER brace (Laboratoire SOBER, Crolles, France) is fashioned to the patient in a position of 45 degrees of abduction and 45 degrees of external rotation (Fig. 21-13).

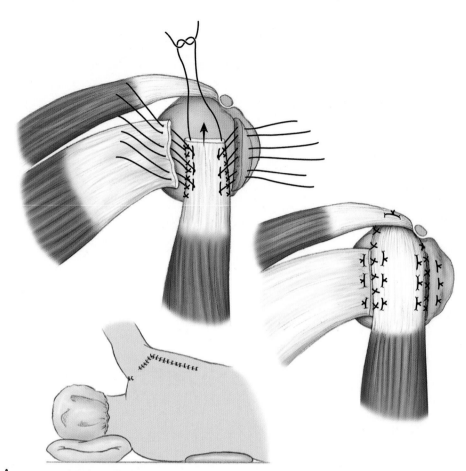

Figure 21-11 Tendon fixation. **A**, Schematic. **B**, At time of surgery. (**A** [redrawn] and **B** from Higgins LD, Warner JJP. Massive tears of the posterosuperior rotator cuff. In Warner JJP, Iannotti JP, Flatow EL, eds. Complex and Revision Problems in Shoulder Surgery, 2nd ed. Philadelphia, Lippincott Williams & Wilkins, 2005:129-160.)

A

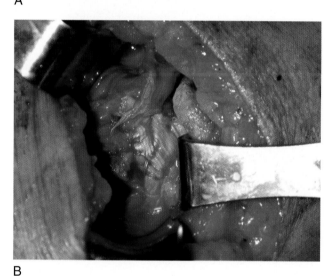

B

Postoperative Considerations

Rehabilitation

The postoperative protocol is designed to protect tendon healing to bone while maintaining adequate excursion of the tendon through the submuscular tunnel and prevent-ing glenohumeral stiffness and postsurgical adhesions. The patient is instructed to wear the SOBER brace continuously in abduction and external rotation for 6 weeks. During this time, passive abduction with external rotation above the plane of the brace (greater than 45 degrees) is instituted with physical therapy. Internal rotation and adduction are not permitted. At 6 weeks, the brace is removed, and gentle activities of daily living are allowed

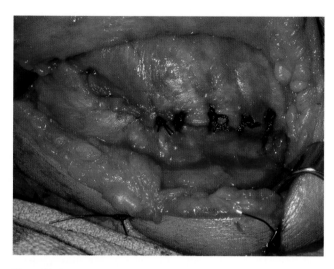

Figure 21-12 Deltoid repair.

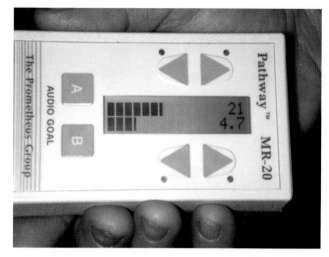

Figure 21-14 A biofeedback device is used to retrain the latissimus in its transferred location. (Pathway Biofeedback Device; Prometheus Group, Dover, NH.)

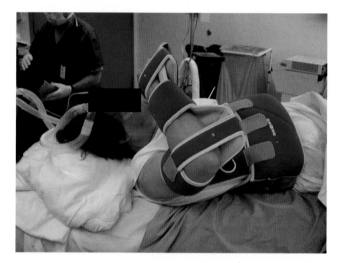

Figure 21-13 Application of SOBER brace in 45 degrees of abduction and external rotation before extubation. (From Higgins LD, Warner JJP. Massive tears of the posterosuperior rotator cuff. In Warner JJP, Iannotti JP, Flatow EL, eds. Complex and Revision Problems in Shoulder Surgery, 2nd ed. Philadelphia, Lippincott Williams & Wilkins, 2005:129-160.)

with gentle mobilization of the extremity in physical therapy.

At the 3-month mark, active strengthening of the rotator cuff and tendon transfer is allowed. The normal vector of the latissimus is one of adduction, internal rotation, and extension. However, in its new position, the transfer must act out of phase as an external rotator. Therefore, muscle re-education is performed with the aid of a biofeedback device (Fig. 21-14). An electrode is placed on the latissimus, which senses contraction and provides auditory and visual feedback to the patient. With the shoulder positioned in the midrange of abduction, the patient is instructed to adduct the arm, causing contraction of the latissimus. The therapist then assists the arm into forward flexion and external rotation during this

maneuver, making a J shape in space. With time, the patient learns how to contract the latissimus to execute abduction and external rotation. Full retraining of the muscle may take up to 12 months.

Complications

Complications of latissimus dorsi transfer include infection, scar tenderness (contraction of the axillary scar if it crosses perpendicular to the axilla), and pseudoparesis of the shoulder. As with any rotator cuff surgery, deltoid injury and axillary nerve injury may occur as well. Late failure of the transfer has been variably reported, but if this is an intraoperative concern, the tendon may be augmented with autogenous fascia lata.[48]

Results

Results of the latissimus dorsi transfer have been reported by Gerber,[15] Aoki et al,[2] Miniaci and MacLeod,[35] Warner and Parsons,[49] and Habermeyer et al.[21] Good to excellent subjective results have been demonstrated in 13 of 16 patients[15] and 8 of 12 patients.[2] In Gerber's series, pain relief at rest was satisfactory in 94% of patients, and pain with exertion was 75% at 65 months postoperatively. Functionally, average improvement has ranged from 36 to 53 degrees in flexion and 14 degrees in external rotation. Habermeyer found an increased Constant score from 46 to 76 at 32 months postoperatively with a single-incision technique.

More recent midterm results (53 months) by Gerber[17] have shown that patients maintained improvements in pain and function (subjective shoulder value increase from 28% to 66%; age- and gender-matched Constant score increase from 55 to 73).

Results in the setting of a failed prior attempt at rotator cuff repair have been less predictable. Warner and Parsons found that only 8 of 16 patients had adequate pain relief in the setting of a revision surgery, with an average gain in flexion of 44 degrees. In contrast, a satisfactory outcome was obtained in five of six patients who had the transfer as a primary procedure. Negative prognostic factors in the setting of a revision included prior deltoid injury, stiffness, and poor tendon quality of the remaining rotator cuff.

Irreparable rotator cuff tears continue to be a challenging problem for the reconstructive shoulder surgeon. For the appropriately chosen patient, latissimus dorsi transfer has been shown to provide reliable pain relief and improved function. Further study is necessary to delineate the future role of tendon transfers in the setting of prior arthroplasty or revision surgery, especially when patients have continued weakness of the external rotators (Table 21-2).

Pectoralis Major Transfer for Subscapularis Insufficiency

Preoperative Considerations

The pectoralis major transfer is primarily indicated for patients with unacceptable pain and functional deficits caused by a chronic, irreparable tear of the subscapularis. Pectoralis major transfer to the lesser tuberosity has proved to be a useful salvage procedure for subscapularis insufficiency when its primary repair is precluded by subscapularis muscle atrophy, fatty infiltration, or poor tendon quality. Multiple techniques have been described for this transfer, including transfer of one or both heads of the

Table 21-2 Results of the Latissimus Dorsi Transfer

Author	No. of Patients	Follow-up	Outcomes
Aoki et al[2] (1996)	12	35 months	66% good–excellent UCLA score Forward flexion improved 36 degrees
Miniaci and MacLeod[35] (1999)	17 revision	51 months	82% satisfactory UCLA score Forward flexion improved 59 degrees External rotation improved 12 degrees
Warner and Parsons[49] (2001)	16 revision	29 months	Postoperative score of 70% Forward flexion improved 60 degrees External rotation improved 37 degrees
	6 primary	25 months	Postoperative score of 55% Forward flexion improved 43 degrees External rotation improved 29 degrees
Gerber et al[19] (1988)	4	14 months	75% good–excellent results Forward flexion improved 88 degrees Abduction improved 75 degrees External rotation improved 23 degrees
Gerber[15] (1992)	16	33 months	Postoperative normal age-adjusted Constant score of 73 Adequate pain relief in 94% of patients Forward flexion improved 52 degrees External rotation improved 13 degrees
Gerber et al[17] (2006)	69	53 months	Subjective shoulder value improved from 28% to 66% Age- and gender-matched Constant score improved from 55 to 73 Pain improved from 6 to 12 (of a possible 15 points) Forward flexion improved 19 degrees External rotation improved 7 degrees
Habermeyer et al[21] (2006)	14	32 months	Constant score improved from 46 to 74 Forward flexion improved 51 degrees External rotation improved 14 degrees

tendon superficial or deep to the conjoined tendon to insert on the lesser tuberosity.[12,41,50] Our preferred method, transfer of the sternal head of the pectoralis superficial to the conjoined tendon, is described here.[46]

History

- Insidious onset of shoulder pain and loss of function
- Remote traumatic injury (external rotation)
- Prior surgical injury to the subscapularis

Physical Examination

- Positive liftoff test result, positive belly press test result
- Internal rotation weakness
- Increased passive external rotation compared with the contralateral side

Imaging

Routine studies are as described for the latissimus dorsi transfer. Pertinent positive findings are the following:
- Static anterior subluxation on an axillary plain film or complete anterosuperior escape of the humeral head on a true anteroposterior view may indicate subscapularis insufficiency.
- Greater than grade 2 fatty infiltration of subscapularis on computed tomography or magnetic resonance imaging

Contraindications

Primary subscapularis tendon repair is preferable, if possible. If the subscapularis insufficiency is a component of a massive irreparable anterosuperior rotator cuff tear, the patient may be best served by a reverse shoulder prosthesis if he or she meets the criteria for that salvage procedure. Combined latissimus and pectoralis major tendon transfers have not yielded satisfactory results in our experience.[1] Concurrent infection, stiffness, and medical comorbidities may preclude pectoralis major transfer.

Surgical Technique

Anesthesia and Positioning

Anesthesia and beach chair positioning are as described for the latissimus dorsi transfer.

Examination Under Anesthesia

Before draping, the passive external rotation of the unaffected contralateral arm is assessed.

Surgical Landmarks and Incisions

- Deltopectoral approach: the lateral aspect of the coracoid and the deltoid insertion serve as the boundaries of the deltopectoral incision.

Structures at Risk

- The axillary nerve courses over the belly of the subscapularis and is at risk throughout the mobilization of the subscapularis.
- The medial pectoral nerve is at risk during dissection and mobilization of the sternal head of the pectoralis if dissection is carried too medially. Injury to this nerve results in denervation of the transferred muscle.
- Axillary artery

Specific Steps (Box 21-2)

1. Deltopectoral Approach

With the arm in slight forward flexion, abduction, and neutral rotation, a standard deltopectoral approach, extending from the lateral aspect of the coracoid toward the insertion of the deltoid, is employed for initial exposure. Taking the cephalic vein laterally, the interval between the pectoralis major and deltoid is exposed and maintained with self-retaining retractors. The clavipectoral fascia is incised, and the conjoined tendon is retracted medially. Externally rotate the arm to expose the lesser tuberosity.

2. Evaluation and Mobilization of the Subscapularis Tendon

The subscapularis tendon deficiency may initially be difficult to appreciate as the lesser tuberosity is often enveloped in scar tissue. After this scar is excised and the bone of the lesser tuberosity is exposed, identification of the torn edge of the subscapularis tendon is attempted. The remnant tendon is tagged with 3-0 braided suture and mobilized from under the conjoined tendon with a combination of blunt and sharp dissection. Care is taken to

Box 21-2 Surgical Steps of Pectoralis Transfer

1. Deltopectoral approach
2. Evaluation and mobilization of the subscapularis tendon
3. Harvest of sternal head of the pectoralis major tendon
4. Transfer under the clavicular head
5. Fixation to the humeral head

protect the axillary nerve on the anterior inferior aspect of the subscapularis during dissection. If the subscapularis tendon is of poor quality or irreparable, proceed with the pectoralis major transfer.

3. Harvest of Sternal Head of the Pectoralis Major Tendon

The interval between the sternal and clavicular heads of the pectoralis major tendon is best delineated at its humeral insertion. Placement of the muscle under tension by abducting and externally rotating the shoulder facilitates the differentiation of the sternal and clavicular portions of the pectoralis major. Often, a stripe of fatty tissue may be present in the plane between the two muscles (Fig. 21-15A). A Cobb elevator, No. 15 scalpel blade, or Metzenbaum scissors are used to isolate the tendon of the sternal head as it inserts inferior and deep to the clavicular head (Fig. 21-15B and C). The tendon is then detached

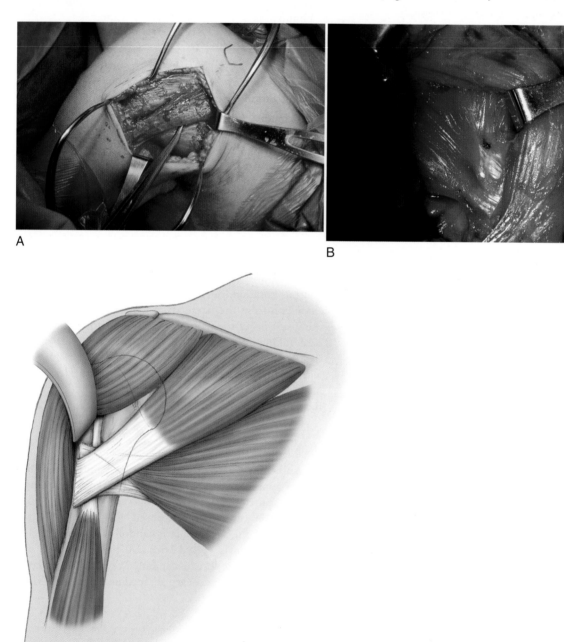

A

B

C

Figure 21-15 A, Identification of sternal and clavicular heads of pectoralis major. **B,** Sternal head of pectoralis major. **C,** Schematic of relationship of clavicular and pectoral head insertions.

sharply off the bone. After No. 2 braided nonabsorbable traction sutures are placed into the tendon in a Mason-Allen fashion, blunt dissection between the muscle bellies of the sternal and clavicular heads proceeds medially. The medial and lateral pectoral nerves are safe as long as one stays lateral to the pectoralis minor and less than 8.5 cm from the humeral insertion of the pectoralis major.

4. Transfer under the Clavicular Head

After the sternal head is sufficiently mobilized, a Kelly clamp is passed from superior to inferior, deep to the clavicular head of the pectoralis major and lateral to the conjoined tendon. The traction sutures are grasped with this clamp to transfer the sternal head under the clavicular head (Fig. 21-16).

5. Fixation to the Humeral Head

The arm is then placed into the patient's physiologic amount of passive external rotation, as determined by the nonoperative arm during the examination under anesthesia. The transferred sternal head of the pectoralis major is then fixed to the lesser tuberosity by anchors or transosseous sutures.

Postoperative Considerations

Rehabilitation

- A sling is worn for 6 weeks with only passive range of motion to protect the transfer and to limit scarring.

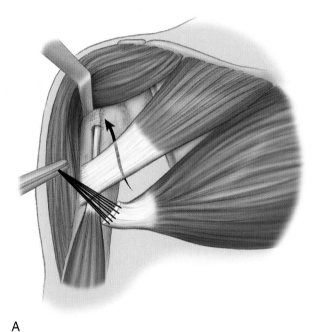

A

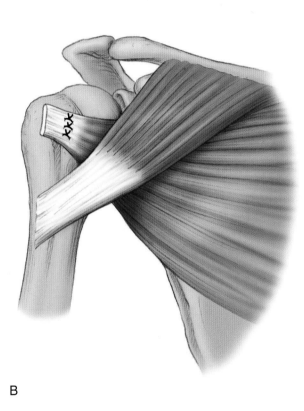

B

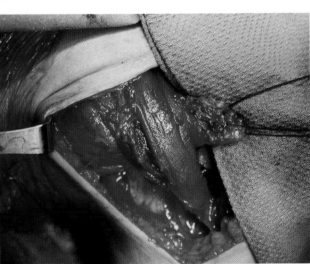

C

Figure 21-16 Transfer of tendon under clavicular head. (**A** and **B** redrawn from Warner JJP. Management of massive irreparable rotator cuff tears: the role of tendon transfer. Instr Course Lect 2001;50:63-71.)

Table 21-3 Results of the Pectoralis Major Transfer

Author	No. of Patients	Follow-up	Outcomes
Warner (2004)	11	38 months	ASES score improved from 42 to 61 81% of patients satisfied
Aldridge et al[1] (2004)	11	31 months	Constant score improved from 21 to 36 63% of patients satisfied
Gerber et al[14] (2004)	30	32 months	Constant score improved from 47 to 70 82% good–excellent results
Galatz et al[12] (2003)	14	18 months	79% of patients satisfied
Noerdlinger et al[39] (2002)	15	64 months	Improved Rowe scores Improved Constant scores Return to preinjury activities
Resch et al[42] (2000)	12	28 months	Constant score improved from 27 to 67 75% good–excellent results

ASES, American Shoulder and Elbow Surgeons.

- Begin active-assisted range of motion after 6 weeks.
- Start active range of motion at 2 months.
- Strengthening may begin after 3 months.
- Return to sport or work after 6 months.

Complications

- Recurrent instability
- Avulsion of transferred pectoralis tendon
- Infection
- Deep venous thrombosis
- Coracohumeral impingement

PEARLS AND PITFALLS

Latissimus

- Position latissimus tendon laterally over tuberosity to achieve a greater external rotation moment about the glenohumeral joint.
- Add a fascia lata graft if there is concern about the quality or length of the tendon.
- Consider placing the obese patient in the lateral decubitus position instead of the beach chair position to optimize exposure.
- Supervise postoperative rehabilitation to avoid late rupture.

Pectoralis

- Do not dissect too medially to avoid nerve injury to the sternal head of the pectoralis. Partial subscapularis repair is helpful to improve results.

Results

After split pectoralis major tendon transfer, good to excellent results are achieved in nearly 80% of patients. Although patients usually have improvement in function and a decrease in pain, many will not have a negative liftoff test result postoperatively. Better results are obtained if the subscapularis tendon can be partially or completely repaired concomitantly with the pectoralis major transfer (Table 21-3).

References

1. Aldridge JM, Atkinson TS, Mallon WJ. Combined pectoralis major and latissimus dorsi tendon transfer for massive rotator cuff deficiency. J Shoulder Elbow Surg 2004;13:621-629.
2. Aoki M, Okamura K, Fukushima S, et al. Transfer of latissimus dorsi for irreparable rotator cuff tears. J Bone Joint Surg Br 1996;78:761-766.
3. Apoil A, Augereau B. Reparation par lambeau de deltoid des grandes pertes de substance de la coiffe des rotateurs de l'epaule. Chirurgie 1985;11:287-290.
4. Arntz CT, Matsen FA III, Jackins S. Surgical management of complex irreparable rotator cuff deficiency. J Arthroplasty 1991;6:363-370.
5. Beauchamp M, Beaton DE, Barnhill TA, et al. Functional outcome after L'Episcopo procedure. J Shoulder Elbow Surg 1998;7:90-96.
6. Burkhart SS. Arthroscopic débridement and decompression for selected rotator cuff tears: clinical results, pathomechanics, and patient selection based on biomechanical parameters. Orthop Clin North Am 1993;24:111-123.

7. Cleeman E, Hazrati Y, Auerbach JD, et al. Latissimus dorsi tendon transfer for massive rotator cuff tears: a cadaveric study. J Shoulder Elbow Surg 2003;12:539-543.

8. Cofield RH. Subscapularis muscle transposition for repair of chronic shoulder cuff tears. Surg Gynecol Obstet 1982;154:667-672.

9. Comtet JJ, Herzberg G, Naasan IA. Biomechanical basis of transfers for shoulder paralysis [review]. Hand Clin 1989;5:1-14.

10. Covey DC, Riordan DC, Milstead ME, et al. Modification of the L'Episcopo procedure for brachial plexus birth palsies. J Bone Joint Surg Br 1992;74:897-901.

11. DeFranco MJ, Derwin K, Iannotti JP. New therapies in tendon reconstruction. J Am Acad Orthop Surg 2004;12:298-304.

12. Galatz LM, Connor PM, Calfee RP, et al. Pectoralis major transfer for anterior-superior subluxation in massive rotator cuff insufficiency. J Shoulder Elbow Surg 2003;12:1-5.

13. Gazielly DF, Gleyze P, Montagnon C. Functional and anatomical results after rotator cuff repair. Clin Orthop 1994;304:43-53.

14. Gerber A, Clavert P, Millett PJ, et al. Split pectoralis major and teres major tendon transfers for reconstruction of irreparable tears of the subscapularis. Tech Shoulder Elbow Surg 2004;5:5-12.

15. Gerber C. Latissimus dorsi transfer for the treatment of irreparable tears of the rotator cuff. Clin Orthop 1992;275:152-160.

16. Gerber C, Hersche O. Tendon transfers for the treatment of irreparable rotator cuff defects. Orthop Clin North Am 1997;28:195-203.

17. Gerber C, Maquieira G, Espinosa N. Latissimus dorsi transfer for the treatment of irreparable rotator cuff tears. J Bone Joint Surg Am 2006;88:113-120.

18. Gerber C, Meyer DC, Schneeberger AG, et al. Effect of tendon release and delayed repair on the structure of the muscles of the rotator cuff: an experimental study in sheep. J Bone Joint Surg Am 2004;86:1973-1982.

19. Gerber C, Vihn TS, Hertel R, et al. Latissimus dorsi transfer for treatment of massive tears of the rotator cuff: a preliminary report. Clin Orthop 1988;232:51-61.

20. Goutallier D, Postel JM, Bernageau J, et al. Fatty muscle degeneration in cuff ruptures: pre- and postoperative evaluation by CT scan. Clin Orthop 1994;304:78-83.

21. Habermeyer P, Magosch P, Rudolph T, et al. Transfer of the tendon of latissimus dorsi for the treatment of massive tears of the rotator cuff: a new single incision technique. J Bone Joint Surg Br 2006;88:208-212.

22. Harryman DT, Mack LA, Wang KY. Repairs of the rotator cuff: correlation of functional results with integrity of the cuff. J Bone Joint Surg Am 1991;73:982-989.

23. Hertel R, Ballmer FT, Lombert SM, et al. Lag signs in the diagnosis of rotator cuff rupture. J Shoulder Elbow Surg 1996;5:307-313.

24. Herzberg G, Urien JP, Dimnet J. Potential excursion and relative tension of muscles in the shoulder girdle: relevance to tendon transfers. J Shoulder Elbow Surg 1999;8:430-437.

25. Hettrich CM, Weldon E 3rd, Boorman RS, et al. Optimizing the glenoid contribution to the stability of a humeral hemiarthroplasty without a prosthetic glenoid. J Bone Joint Surg Am 2004;86:2022-2029.

26. Hockman DE, Lucas GL, Roth CA. Role of the coracoacromial ligament as restraint after shoulder hemiarthroplasty. Clin Orthop 2004;419:80-82.

27. Hoffer MM, Wickenden R, Roper B. Brachial plexus birth injuries: results of tendon transfer of the rotator cuff. J Bone Joint Surg Am 1978;60:691-695.

28. Jonsson B, Olofsson BM, Steffner LC. Function of the teres major, latissimus dorsi, and pectoralis major muscles: a preliminary study. Acta Morphol Neerl Scand 1971;9:275.

29. Jost B, Puskas GJ, Lustenberger A, et al. Outcome of pectoralis major transfer for the treatment of irreparable subscapularis tears. J Bone Joint Surg Am 2003;85:1944-1951.

30. Laudicina L, D'Ambrosia R. Management of irreparable rotator cuff tears and glenohumeral arthritis. Orthopedics 2005;28:382-358.

31. L'Episcopo JB. Tendon transplantation in obstetrical paralysis. Am J Surg 1934;25:122-125.

32. Meyer DC, Hoppeler H, von Rechenberg B, Gerber C. A pathomechanical concept explains muscle loss and fatty muscular changes following surgical tendon release. J Orthop Res 2004;22:1004-1007.

33. Meyer DC, Pirkl C, Pfirrmann WA, et al. Asymmetric atrophy of the supraspinatus muscle following tendon tear. J Orthop Res 2005;23:254-258.

34. Miller BS, Joseph TA, Noonan TJ, et al. Rupture of the subscapularis tendon after shoulder arthroplasty: diagnosis, treatment, and outcome. J Shoulder Elbow Surg 2005;14:492-496.

35. Miniaci A, MacLeod M. Transfer of the latissimus dorsi muscle after failed repair of a massive tear of the rotator cuff. J Bone Joint Surg Am 1999;81:1120-1127.

36. Neer CS, Flatow EL, Lech O. Tears of the rotator cuff: long term results of anterior acromioplasty and repair. Orthop Trans 1988;12:735.

37. Neviaser JS, Neviaser RJ, Neviaser TJ. The repair of chronic massive ruptures of the rotator cuff of the shoulder by use of a freeze-dried rotator cuff. J Bone Joint Surg Am 1978;60:681-684.

38. Neviaser RJ, Neviaser TJ. Transfer of the subscapularis and teres minor for massive defects of the rotator cuff. In Bayley IL, Kessel L, eds. Shoulder Surgery. Berlin, Springer, 1982:60-63

39. Noerdlinger MA, Cole BJ, Stewart M, Post M. Results of pectoralis major transfer with fascia lata autograft augmentation for scapula winging. J Shoulder Elbow Surg 2002;11:345-350.

40. Ozaki J, Fujimoto S, Masuhara K. Reconstruction of chronic massive rotator cuff tears with synthetic materials. Clin Orthop 1986;202:173-183.

41. Phipps GJ, Hoffer MM. Latissimus dorsi and teres major transfer to rotator cuff for Erb's palsy. J Shoulder Elbow Surg 1995;4:124-129.

42. Resch H, Povacz P, Ritter E, et al. Transfer of the pectoralis major muscle for the treatment of irreparable rupture of the subscapularis tendon. J Bone Joint Surg Am 2000;82:372-382.

43. Rockwood CA, Burkhead WZ. Management of patients with massive rotator cuff débridement. Orthop Trans 1988;12:12:190.

44. Rockwood CA Jr, Williams GR Jr, Burkhead WZ Jr. Débridement of degenerative, irreparable lesions of the rotator cuff. J Bone Joint Surg Am 1995;77:857-866.

45. Schoierer O, Herzberg G, Berthonnaud E, et al. Anatomical basis of latissimus dorsi and teres major transfers in rotator cuff tear surgery with particular reference to the neurovascular pedicles. Surg Radiol Anat 2001;23:75-80.

46. Shiino K. Über die Bewegungen im Schultergelenk und die Arbeitsleistung der Schultermuskeln. Arch Anat Physiol Anat 1913;Suppl:1-89.

47. Warner JJP. Management of massive irreparable rotator cuff tears: the role of tendon transfer. AAOS Instr Course Lect 2001;50:63-71.

48. Warner JJP, Gerber C. Treatment of massive rotator cuff tears: posterior-superior and antero-superior. In Iannotti JP, ed. The Rotator Cuff: Current Concepts and Complex Problems. Rosemont, Ill, American Academy of Orthopaedic Surgeons, 1998:59-94.

49. Warner JJP, Parsons M. Latissimus dorsi transfer: a comparative analysis of primary and salvage reconstruction of massive, irreparable rotator cuff tears. J Shoulder Elbow Surg 2001;10:514-521.

50. Watson M. Major ruptures of the rotator cuff: the results of surgical repair in 89 patients. J Bone Joint Surg Br 1985;67:618.

51. Wirth MA, Rockwood CA Jr. Operative treatment of irreparable rupture of the subscapularis. J Bone Joint Surg Am 1997;79:722-731.

52. Zachary RB. Transplantation of teres major and latissimus dorsi for loss of external rotation at shoulder. Lancet 1947;2:757.

Arthroscopic Repair of SLAP Lesions by the Single-Anchor Double-Suture Technique

Max Tyorkin, MD
Stephen J. Snyder, MD

SLAP (superior labrum anterior and posterior) tears were largely underappreciated before the advent of shoulder arthroscopy and modern magnetic resonance imaging techniques. In 1985, Andrews et al[1] described superior glenoid labral lesions related to the long head of the biceps in 73 throwing athletes. In 1990, Snyder et al[14] proposed the name SLAP lesion to describe a more complex injury involving the superior labrum extending from anterior to posterior in relation to the biceps tendon anchor.

Mechanisms causing SLAP lesions range from tensile failure at the biceps root to compression loading with the shoulder in the flexed and abducted position.[1] More recently, Burkhart and Morgan[3] have described a peel-back mechanism of the superior labrum with progressive enlargement in overhead athletes.

Snyder's original classification consists of four subgroups (types I to IV) based on the condition of the superior labrum and the attachment of the biceps anchor to the superior labrum and superior glenoid tubercle.[14] Combined and complex lesions have frequently been observed. Maffet et al[7] expanded the original classification of SLAP lesions, introducing what they have labeled types V to VII.

Preoperative Considerations

History

A thorough history is essential in elucidating an injury to the superior labrum. Typically, the patients are teenage male athletes who complain of shoulder pain exacerbated by overhead activity. This is often associated with popping, snapping, catching, or locking, similar to mechanical symptoms associated with a meniscal tear.[7,14] SLAP lesions must be differentiated from other pathologic processes of the shoulder, such as instability, impingement, rotator cuff tear, and acromioclavicular joint disease.

Physical Examination

Both the comprehensive physical examination and the history are essential in raising the index of suspicion for a possible SLAP lesion. A complete examination is important but not accurate in predicting with certainty the existence of a SLAP lesion, although there are several tests that may prove useful. The biceps tension (Speed) test was the most accurate in our study.[5,12,16] The Speed test result is positive when pain is elicited with resisted forward elevation of the fully supinated arm with the elbow extended and the arm flexed to 90 degrees. The compression-rotation sign described by Andrews et al[1] is demonstrated with the patient supine, the shoulder elevated to 90 degrees, and the elbow flexed to 90 degrees. An axial load is then applied to the humerus to compress the glenohumeral joint while the arm is rotated. A positive test result is pain as well as mechanical symptoms elicited during this test. The O'Brien sign, or the active compression test, is elicited by first placing the arm in 90 degrees of forward flexion and 10 to 20 degrees of adduction. The arm is then fully internally rotated into the thumb-down position. The patient is then asked to resist downward pressure to the arm that is applied by the examiner. Pain is produced when an unstable superior labrum is present. The test is then repeated but with the arm in full supination; the pain should be decreased in this position compared with the initial position for the test result to be considered positive.[10]

Imaging

As with most shoulder disease, standard radiographic evaluation includes four views of the shoulder (anteroposterior, axillary, outlet, and acromioclavicular joint views). Although plain radiographs are not specific for labral disease, they are important to rule out other coexisting pathologic processes of the shoulder.

Magnetic resonance imaging has been popular in evaluating labral lesions. Nonenhanced magnetic resonance imaging has proved to be unreliable in determining the presence of SLAP tears unless a superior paralabral cyst is present. It is, however, useful to evaluate for concomitant pathologic changes, such as rotator cuff tears, acromioclavicular joint disease, and biceps disease. Standard magnetic resonance imaging is also valuable in detecting a paralabral cyst encroaching on the spinoglenoid notch, a finding that is often associated with superior and posterior labral tears. The use of gadolinium contrast medium for magnetic resonance arthrography offers improved visualization of intra-articular structures and is known to improve the ability to detect SLAP tears accurately; however, reported results continue to be somewhat unpredicable.[2,17]

Indications and Contraindications

Because physical findings and magnetic resonance imaging scans are often equivocal, a high index of suspicion for a SLAP lesion should exist, especially when a patient is symptomatic after an appropriate amount of conservative treatment and an associated mechanism of injury (i.e., abrupt traction or a throwing athlete). If the patient fits the diagnostic criteria and is not able to function at his or her desired level, consideration should be given to diagnostic arthroscopy.

Indications

- Mechanical symptoms and magnetic resonance imaging diagnosis of superior labral disease
- Suspected labral disease in the face of known coexisting shoulder abnormalities
- Refractory intra-articular symptoms with inconclusive diagnostic studies

Relative Contraindications

- Arthritis or shoulder stiffness
- Patients with anatomic variants such as Buford complex or a sublabral foramen must be identified.
- Repair in the population of older patients should be undertaken with caution because their symptoms are usually due to other causes.

Surgical Technique

Anesthesia and Positioning

Once general endotracheal anesthesia is achieved, the patient is placed in lateral decubitus position supported with a beanbag. The arthroscopic video equipment tower is on the anterior side of the table in clear view of the surgeon. Once the patient is prepared and draped, the arm is suspended in a traction device. A sterile suspensory arm-holding traction sleeve is applied and connected to the overhead device by a sterile S hook. Approximately 10 pounds of weight is applied to hold the arm in a position of approximately 70 degrees of abduction and 10 degrees of forward flexion.

Surgical Landmarks, Incisions, and Portals

The bone landmarks of the acromion, clavicle, and acromioclavicular joint are outlined with a marking pen. A bursal orientation line is drawn; this begins at the posterior aspect of the acromioclavicular joint and extends laterally across the acromion onto the deltoid.

The posterior portal is established first. It is usually located 2 cm inferior and 1 cm medial to the posterolateral corner of the acromion. A small stab incision is made through the skin and subcutaneous tissues with a No. 11 scalpel blade. A blunt obturator in an arthroscopic sheath is used to enter the glenohumeral joint.

Next, the anterior superior portal is established by an outside-in technique. This portal is placed just superior to the biceps tendon in the rotator interval with use of a spinal needle to confirm proper location. This is the *most crucial portal* because it must be located to allow insertion of the suture anchor into the superior glenoid on the posterior aspect of the biceps anchor.

The third portal is the anterior midglenoid portal. This portal is made by the outside-in method as well. A spinal needle enters the skin approximately 2 cm inferior to the anterior superior portal and penetrates the capsule through the rotator interval at the superior edge of the subscapularis tendon. It is important to maximize the distance between the anterior superior and midglenoid portals to facilitate instrumentation.

Examination Under Anesthesia and Diagnostic Arthroscopy

Examination under anesthesia is performed to evaluate the mobility and stability of the joint. This is followed by a complete diagnostic arthroscopy from both anterior and posterior portals. The superior labrum is best visualized from the posterior portal and palpated with a probe from the anterior superior portal. When a SLAP lesion is present, the labrum may be frayed, torn, or detached or a combination. As categorized by Snyder et al,[14] there are four basic types. A type I SLAP lesion has a frayed superior labrum, but the biceps anchor attachment to the superior glenoid is intact. Type II lesions have a separation of the superior labrum and biceps anchor from the superior glenoid with or without fraying of the superior labrum. Type III lesions appear similar to a bucket-handle tear of the meniscus; the superior labrum is torn, but it may or may not be displaced with an otherwise normal biceps anchor. Type IV is similar to type III with a bucket-handle labral tear, but the tear extends into the biceps tendon.

Specific Steps

Type I and type III SLAP lesions in which the biceps anchor is otherwise stable are treated by débridement alone. We use a 4.0-mm full-radius shaver and débride the labrum to a smooth edge. The shaver is used from both anterior and posterior portals on viewing from the opposite side. After shaving, a probe is used to evaluate the remaining labrum and the biceps anchor.

Type II lesions are repaired by a single-anchor double-suture technique as outlined in Box 22-1.

Type IV lesions are treated similarly to type II lesions unless the biceps tendon split is severe. When more than about 30% of the tendon is included with the displaced labral tear, one must consider repairing the tendon, releasing it, and repairing the labrum as with a type II SLAP lesion or performing a biceps tenodesis. In most cases, we prefer to excise the labral fragment along with the attached portion of torn biceps. If the remaining tendon appears healthy and the anchor is stable, then it is left alone. If the tendon appears degenerative, it will be released and tenodesed, especially in the young active patient.

Single-Anchor Double-Suture SLAP Repair

1. Establish Portals

With the arthroscope in the standard posterior portal, we establish the anterior superior portal with an outside-in technique. A spinal needle determines the ideal location. Insert the needle approximately 2 cm from the anterolateral corner of the acromion so that it enters the joint in the superior edge of the rotator interval behind the biceps tendon (Fig. 22-1). Ensure that the needle can readily reach the superior neck of the glenoid on passing posterior to the biceps. After an incision is made with a No. 11 blade in Langer's lines, insert a clear, smooth, plastic 6-mm operating cannula along the chosen path.

Next, establish an anterior midglenoid portal with the same outside-in technique as outlined before, entering through the rotator interval just above the subscapularis tendon.

2. Prepare the Labrum and Glenoid

Débride any remaining soft tissue off the superior glenoid below the detached labrum–biceps anchor. Trim any fraying of the labrum (Fig. 22-2). The posterior portion of the lesion and glenoid are best trimmed with the shaver in the posterior portal and the arthroscope anteriorly. The superior glenoid rim and neck are only slightly decorticated, with care taken not to remove excessive bone. The bone here is often relatively soft, and use of a bur is seldom necessary.

Box 22-1 Surgical Steps

1. Establish portals
2. Prepare the labrum and glenoid
3. Insert anchor
4. Pass and manage sutures
5. Tie the sutures to fix the labrum
6. Close portals

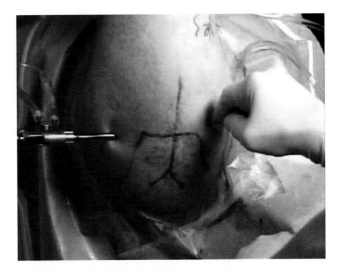

Figure 22-1 Establishment of the anterior superior portal with an outside-in technique. A spinal needle is used to determine the ideal location. The needle is inserted approximately 2 cm from the anterolateral corner of the acromion so that it enters the joint in the superior edge of the rotator interval behind the biceps tendon.

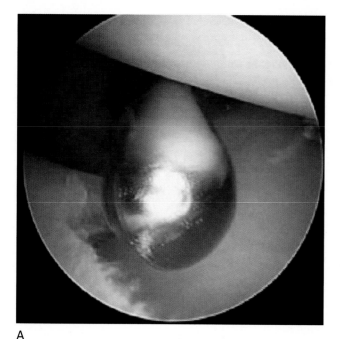

A

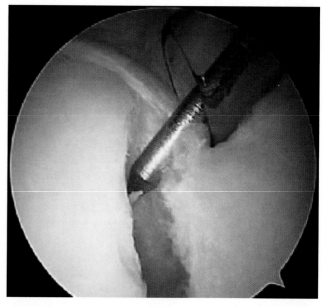

Figure 22-3 Making the pilot hole for an anchor. A 2-mm punch is inserted into the anterior superior portal and posterior to the biceps to make a pilot hole for the double-suture 4-mm anchor.

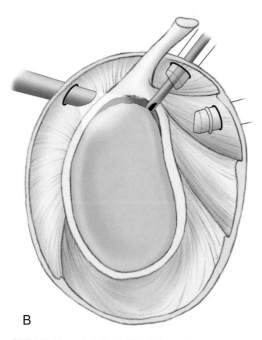

B

Figure 22-2 Débridement of the SLAP lesion.

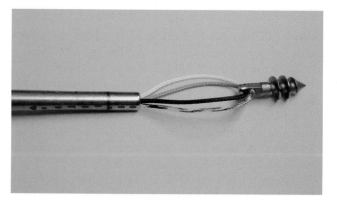

Figure 22-4 The 4-mm anchor. By convention, the green suture is at the upper end of the eyelet and the white suture is at the lower portion of the eyelet closer to the screw threads. To facilitate suture management, half of each suture limb is colored purple with a surgical marking pen.

3. Anchor Placement

Insert a 2-mm Revo punch into the anterior superior portal and posterior to the biceps to make a pilot hole for the double-suture 4-mm Big Eye Revo anchor (Linvatec, Largo, Fla). The punch must penetrate the superior glenoid exactly at the center of the biceps anchor just below the edge of the cartilage angled 45 degrees relative to the glenoid surface. Extreme caution must be exercised to ensure that the punch is completely within the bone and does not skive off posteriorly or medially above the glenoid (Fig. 22-3).

We use a titanium 4-mm × 12-mm threaded anchor. The vertically oriented eyelet is first loaded with two strands of nonabsorbable No. 2 suture in a specific manner. One suture is white and the other is dark green. By convention, the green suture is at the upper end of the eyelet and the white suture is at the lower portion of the eyelet closer to the screw threads. To facilitate suture management, we color half of each suture limb purple with a surgical marking pen. The anchor is then loaded on the inserter such that the purple suture ends exit on the same side of the eyelet (Fig. 22-4). The anchor is then inserted into the pilot hole until the horizontal seating line is below bone and the purple limbs of the suture are toward the biceps tendon. Seating the anchor so that the opening of the eyelet is toward the biceps allows easier sliding of suture. The screwdriver is removed, and sutures are tested for security by gentle traction (Fig. 22-5).

4. Suture Management

With a crochet hook, retrieve the two unmarked suture limbs through the anterior midglenoid portal (Fig. 22-6). Place the suture outside the cannula by use of a switching rod. Next retrieve the two purple-dyed suture limbs through the anterior midglenoid cannula (Fig. 22-7).

5. Labrum Fixation

Insert a Spectrum (Linvatec) medium-sized crescent hook loaded with a Shuttle Relay suture passer (Linvatec) through the anterior superior cannula (Fig. 22-8). Puncture the superior labrum on the posterior edge of the center of the biceps attachment. Pass the needle through the root of the biceps and under the labrum directly in line with the anchor. The Shuttle Relay is advanced into the joint and retrieved with a grasper through the anterior midglenoid cannula. The two purple suture limbs inside the cannula are loaded into the Shuttle eyelet and shuttled through the superior labrum and the anterior superior cannula (Fig. 22-9).

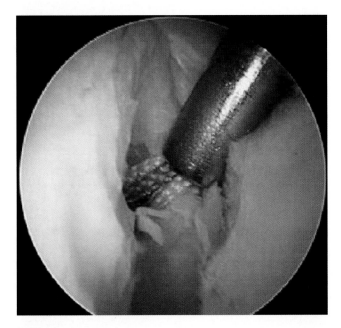

Figure 22-5 Anchor in place.

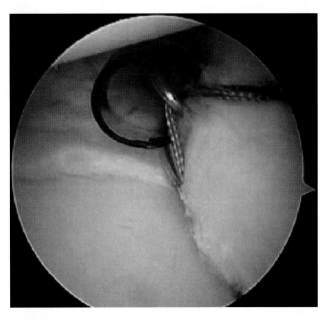

Figure 22-7 Retrieval of the two purple sutures.

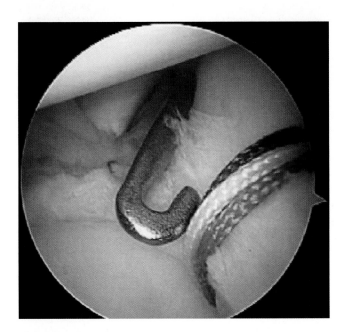

Figure 22-6 Retrieval of the two non-purple sutures.

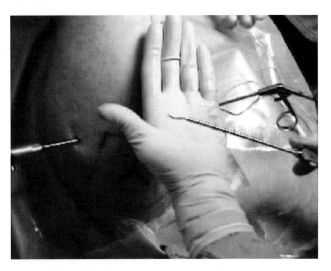

Figure 22-8 A medium-sized crescent hook loaded with a suture passer is passed through the anterior superior cannula.

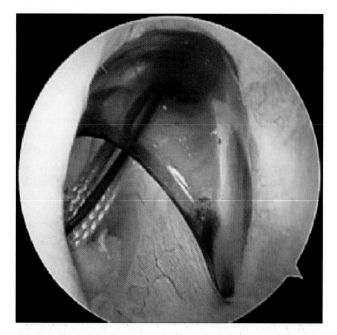

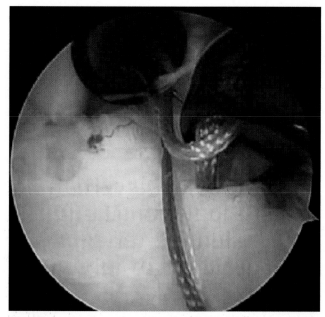

Figure 22-9 Suture shuttle with two purple sutures. The shuttle is advanced into the joint and retrieved with a grasper through the anterior midglenoid cannula. The two purple suture limbs inside the cannula are loaded into the eyelet and shuttled through the superior labrum and the anterior superior cannula.

Figure 22-10 The purple-white suture is transferred from the anterior superior portal into the midglenoid cannula with a crochet hook anterior to the biceps tendon.

Next, the purple-white suture is transferred from the anterior superior portal into the midglenoid cannula with a crochet hook anterior to biceps tendon (Fig. 22-10). This will avoid tangling of the purple-white suture when the green sutures are tied. Then retrieve the purple-green suture into the anterior superior portal posterior to the biceps tendon with a crochet hook (Fig. 22-11). Pull the purple-green suture (the one through the labral tissue) to make it the shorter limb and use it as the initial post strand. Tie the green suture with a sliding-locking knot and three alternating half-hitches (Fig. 22-12).

Retrieve both limbs of the white suture anterior to the biceps into the anterior superior cannula with a crochet hook (Fig. 22-13). Pull the purple-white strand to make it the shorter limb and tie it with a sliding knot. Evaluate the repair by pulling on the biceps tendon with a probe, checking for tension and stability (Fig. 22-14).

6. Closure

The portals are closed with a single 3-0 subcutaneous stitch supplemented with a Steri-Strip. A sterile dressing is applied.

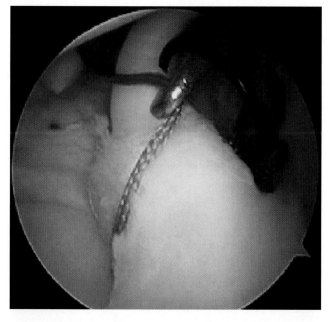

Figure 22-11 The purple-green suture is retrieved into the anterior superior portal posterior to the biceps tendon with a crochet hook.

Postoperative Considerations

Rehabilitation

The shoulder is protected in a 15-degree UltraSling (DJ Orthopedics, Carlsbad, Calif). The patient should begin elbow, wrist, and hand exercises immediately, with gentle pendulum exercises after 1 week. The shoulder should be protected from excess stress on the biceps tendon for 12 weeks. Progressive resistance exercises are allowed at 6 weeks. Vigorous throwing or strenuous lifting is allowed after 3 months if there are no limitations on motion and the patient is asymptomatic.

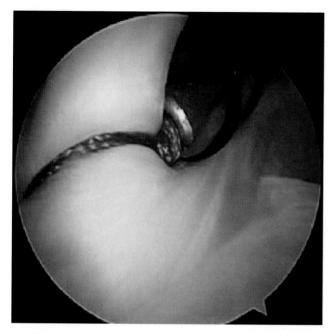

Figure 22-12 The purple-green suture (the one through the labral tissue) is pulled to make it the shorter limb, and it is used as the initial post strand. The green suture is tied with a sliding-locking knot and three alternating half-hitches.

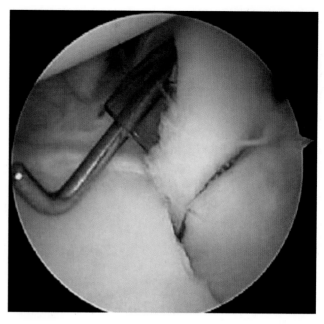

Figure 22-14 Evaluate the repair by pulling on the biceps tendon with a probe, checking for tension and stability.

Complications

- Missed coexisting shoulder disease
- Failure to insert anchor properly
- Failure to recognize anatomic variants (e.g., Buford complex, sublabral hole)
- Stiffness with loss of external rotation

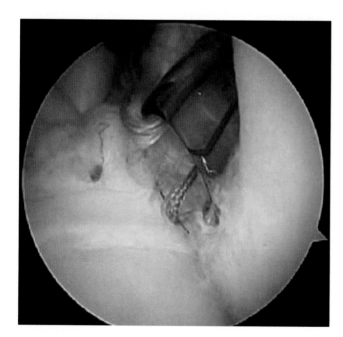

Figure 22-13 Both limbs of the white suture are retrieved anterior to the biceps into the anterior superior cannula with a crochet hook. The purple-white strand is pulled to make it the shorter limb and tied with a sliding knot.

PEARLS AND PITFALLS

- Be sure to identify normal versus pathologic anatomy (e.g., sublabral foramen, meniscoid-type attachment, Buford complex as normal variants).
- Repair of lesions in the older population (older than 40 years) should be undertaken only for true symptomatic lesions.
- Establish anterior portals with appropriate distance between them to prevent cannula crowding.
- Make sure to place anchor in appropriate position at the center of biceps attachment off the glenoid articular surface.
- Make sure to stage your suture passing, especially with an anchor that is double loaded, to avoid suture tangling.
- All related pathologic processes must be addressed.

Results

Good to excellent results are achieved in nearly 80% of cases, and patients exhibit a measurable decrease in pain and increase in return to preinjury activity level (Table 22-1). However, the outcome depends on concurrent pathologic changes and the treatment rendered.

Table 22-1 Clinical Results of SLAP Lesion Repair

Author	Follow-up	Outcome
Yoneda et al[18] (1991)	24 months minimum	80% good–excellent
Field and Savoie[5] (1993)	21 months mean (range: 12-42 months)	20 of 20 (100%) good–excellent (Rowe)
Resch et al[12] (1993)	18 months mean (range: 6-30 months)	12 of 14 (86%) successful
Pagnani et al[11] (1995)	1 year minimum	19 of 22 (86%) satisfied
Morgan et al[8] (1998)	12 months mean	84% excellent
Stetson et al[16] (1998)	3.8 years mean (range: 14 months-8 years)	82% good–excellent (Rowe)
Samani et al[13] (2001)	35 months mean (range: 24-51 months)	88% successful
O'Brien et al[9] (2002)	3.7 years mean (range: 2-7.4 years)	23 of 31 (74%) good–excellent
Kim et al[6] (2002)	33 months mean (range: 24-49 months)	94% satisfactory (UCLA)
Cohen et al[4] (2006)	44 months mean (range: 25-97 months)	71% good–excellent

References

1. Andrews JR, Carson WG Jr, McLeod WD. Glenoid labrum tears related to the long head of the biceps. Am J Sports Med 1985; 13:337-341.
2. Bencardino JT, Beltran J, Rosenberg ZS, et al. Superior labrum anterior-posterior lesions: diagnosis with MR arthrography of the shoulder. Radiology 2000;214:267-271.
3. Burkhart SS, Morgan CD. The peel-back mechanism: its role in producing and extending posterior type II SLAP lesions and its effect on SLAP repair rehabilitation. Arthroscopy 1998;14:637-640.
4. Cohen DB, Coleman S, Drakos MC, et al. Outcomes of isolated type II SLAP lesions treated with arthroscopic fixation using a bioabsorbable tack. Arthroscopy 2006;22:136-142.
5. Field LD, Savoie FH III. Arthroscopic suture repair of superior labral detachment lesions of the shoulder. Am J Sports Med 1993;21: 783-790.
6. Kim SH, Ha KI, Kim SH, et al. Results of arthroscopic treatment of superior labral lesions. J Bone Joint Surg Am 2002;84:981-985.
7. Maffet MW, Gartsman GM, Moseley B. Superior labrum–biceps tendon complex lesions of the shoulder. Am J Sports Med 1995;23:93-98.
8. Morgan CD, Burkhart SS, Palmeri M, et al. Type II SLAP lesions: three subtypes and their relationship to superior instability and rotator cuff tears. Arthroscopy 1998;14:553-565.
9. O'Brien SJ, Allen AA, Coleman SH, et al. The trans–rotator cuff approach to SLAP lesions: technical aspects for repair and a clinical follow-up of 31 patients at a minimum of 2 years. Arthroscopy 2002;18:372-377.
10. O'Brien SJ, Pagnani MJ, Fealy S, et al. The active compression test: a new and effective test for diagnosing labral tears and acromioclavicular joint abnormality. Am J Sports Med 1998;26:610-613.
11. Pagnani MJ, Speer KP, Altchek DW, et al. Arthroscopic fixation of superior labral lesions using a biodegradable implant: a preliminary report. Arthroscopy 1995;11:194-198.
12. Resch H, Golser K, Thoeni H, et al. Arthroscopic repair of superior glenoid labral detachment (the SLAP lesion). J Shoulder Elbow Surg 1993;2:147-155.
13. Samani JE, Marston SB, Buss DD. Arthroscopic stabilization of type II SLAP lesions using an absorbable tack. Arthroscopy 2001;17: 19-24.
14. Snyder SJ, Karzel RP, Del Pizzo W, et al. SLAP lesions of the shoulder. Arthroscopy 1990;6:274-279.
15. Snyder SJ. Shoulder Arthroscopy, 2nd ed. Philadelphia, Lippincott Williams & Wilkins, 2003:147-165.
16. Stetson WB, Snyder SJ, Karzel RP, et al. Long-term clinical follow-up of isolated SLAP lesions of the shoulder. Presented at the 65th annual meeting of the American Academy of Orthopaedic Surgeons; March 1998.
17. Waldt S, Burkart A, Lange P, et al. Diagnostic performance of MR arthrography in the assessment of superior labral anteroposterior lesions of the shoulder. AJR Am J Roentgenol 2004;182:1271-1278.
18. Yoneda M, Hirooka A, Saito S, et al. Arthroscopic stapling for detached superior glenoid labrum. J Bone Joint Surg Br 1991;73: 746-750.

CHAPTER 23

Arthroscopic Subacromial Decompression and Distal Clavicle Excision

Mark Rodosky, MD

Joanne Labriola, MD

The supraspinatus tendon traverses a bony canal or outlet, the size of which is strongly affected by the morphologic features of the undersurface of the anterior acromion and the acromioclavicular joint. During supraspinatus tendon excursion within this outlet, the acromion may apply compressive forces to the tendon. The subacromial bursa serves to mitigate these forces, but repetitive application of these forces or a single macrotraumatic force may traumatize the subacromial bursa and supraspinatus tendon, leading to painful inflammatory changes. This painful process, termed impingement, is hypothesized to compromise the health of the tendon, leading to tearing of the rotator cuff. Therefore, the impingement syndrome includes a spectrum of pathologic changes from subacromial bursitis to full-thickness tears of the rotator cuff (Box 23-1). A subacromial decompression may be performed to relieve the forces placed on the rotator cuff tendons or to protect tendon repairs.

Surgical techniques for subacromial decompression have evolved from open to mini-open to all-arthroscopic techniques. Advantages of arthroscopic techniques include decreased trauma to the deltoid, decreased surgical pain, and improved cosmesis.

Shoulder pain due to degenerative changes in the acromioclavicular joint is a common problem. In addition, osteophytes from a hypertrophic degenerative acromioclavicular joint can result in impingement of the underlying rotator cuff. Both problems can be relieved through distal clavicle excision. Distal clavicle excision can be performed

at the same time as an arthroscopic subacromial decompression through an indirect approach, or it can be performed alone through direct techniques. In patients with isolated acromioclavicular arthritis, the direct approach is preferred to prevent unnecessary instrumentation of the noninvolved subacromial space.

Preoperative Considerations

History

Preoperative evaluation begins with a thorough history. This includes the position in which symptoms occur, athletic activities, antecedent trauma or injury, and previous treatments.

Patients with subacromial bursitis or rotator cuff tendinitis have a common pattern of pain and activities that elicit symptoms. Patients often complain of lateral shoulder pain, pain with overhead activities, pain with abduction and internal rotation maneuvers (e.g., turning the steering wheel), and night pain. The pain is typically improved with nonsteroidal anti-inflammatory agents and steroid injections and may resolve after a course of physical therapy and activity restriction.

Patients with acromioclavicular degenerative joint disease typically have more anterior superior pain that worsens on crossing of the arm in front of the body or on

Box 23-1 Stages of Subacromial Impingement Syndrome

Stage I	Edema and hemorrhage of the subacromial bursa and rotator cuff
Stage IIa	Fibrosis and inflammation of the rotator cuff
Stage IIb	Partial-thickness tears of the rotator cuff
Stage III	Full-thickness tears of the rotator cuff tendons

reaching behind the back. Patients may describe a previous injury to the acromioclavicular joint or fall on the tip of the shoulder. Similarly, the pain is typically improved with nonsteroidal anti-inflammatory agents and steroid injections and may resolve after a course of physical therapy and activity restriction.

Physical Examination

Typical Findings

Impingement Syndrome

- Painful arc of motion (70 to 120 degrees)
- Tenderness at greater tuberosity
- Pain with passive abduction and internal rotation (Neer sign, Hawkins sign)
- Relief of pain with subacromial lidocaine (Xylocaine) injection (Neer test)

Acromioclavicular Degenerative Joint Disease

- Painful arc of motion (120 to 180 degrees)
- Prominent acromioclavicular joint
- Tenderness at acromioclavicular joint
- Pain with cross-body adduction or maximal internal rotation

Factors Affecting Surgical Indications and Planning

- Decreased range of motion (adhesive capsulitis)
- Tenderness of the acromion, motion of distal unfused acromion (os acromiale)
- Tenderness at the glenohumeral joint (degenerative changes of glenohumeral joint)
- Tenderness of long head of biceps tendon, O'Brien sign (biceps tendinitis, SLAP tear)
- Apprehension, ligamentous laxity (glenohumeral instability)
- Increased motion of distal clavicle (acromioclavicular joint instability)
- Atrophy, weakness in abduction and external rotation, liftoff test (rotator cuff tear)
- Abnormal neurologic evaluation, Hoffman sign (cervical radiculopathy)

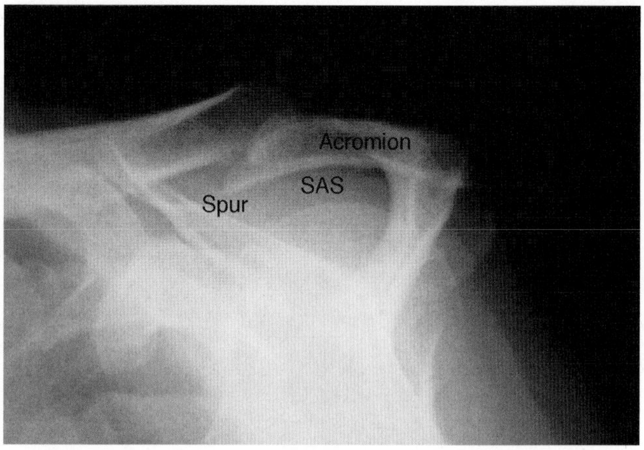

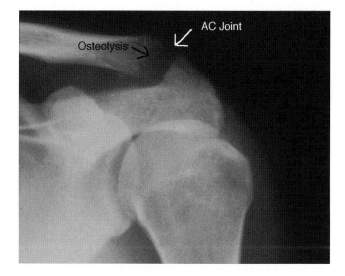

Figure 23-1 Outlet view radiograph shows encroachment of subacromial space (SAS) with an anterior undersurface acromial spur.

Figure 23-2 Anteroposterior radiograph (Zanca view) showing osteolysis of the acromioclavicular (AC) joint.

Imaging

Radiography

A radiographic series of the shoulder typically includes an anteroposterior radiograph of the glenohumeral joint (30 degrees from anteroposterior of shoulder) to look for glenohumeral arthritis; an outlet view for evaluation of acromial morphologic features (Fig. 23-1); an axillary lateral view, which is the best view to rule out an os acromiale (unfused acromion); and a Zanca view, which is the best view for evaluation of degenerative changes or osteolysis of the acromioclavicular joint (Fig. 23-2).

Other Modalities

Magnetic resonance imaging may be performed to assess the condition of the rotator cuff and associated pathologic

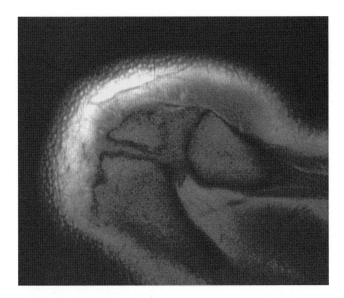

Figure 23-3 Magnetic resonance image shows widening at site of an unstable os acromiale.

changes. It can be helpful in evaluation of an os acromiale by showing the presence of fluid and widening at the site, indicating instability of the os acromiale (Fig. 23-3).

Indications and Contraindications

Surgery is indicated in patients for whom 3 to 6 months of nonoperative management has failed; this includes anti-inflammatory medications (nonsteroidal anti-inflammatory drugs and steroid injections), physical therapy (must include strengthening of the rotator cuff in nonimpingement positions), and activity modification. At the time of surgery, the patient should have full passive range of motion of the shoulder, or a manipulation under anesthesia should be considered before the arthroscopic procedure. In younger patients, ligamentous laxity and glenohumeral instability may be the primary pathologic processes, and these conditions should be addressed before a subacromial decompression is performed. If a symptomatic os acromiale is identified, it should be repaired or excised at the time of surgery. If the os is excised as part of the subacromial decompression, the distal clavicle should be preserved to maintain sufficient deltoid attachment.

If the patient has an irreparable rotator cuff tear or cuff arthropathy, disruption of the coracoacromial ligament is contraindicated. If the patient has instability of the acromioclavicular joint secondary to a grade III or higher injury, distal clavicle excision without a concomitant stabilizing procedure is contraindicated.

Surgical Planning

Concomitant Procedures

Associated pathologic processes, such as os acromiale, rotator cuff tear, labral tear, biceps disease, and loose bodies, should be addressed.

Indirect Versus Direct Distal Clavicle Excision

The approach to the distal clavicle should be determined preoperatively. If subacromial pathologic changes and acromioclavicular degenerative joint disease coexist, an indirect approach to the distal clavicle through the subacromial space is preferable. If the acromioclavicular joint disease is isolated, the distal clavicle may be approached directly.

Surgical Technique

Anesthesia and Positioning

These procedures can be performed under general anesthesia, regional anesthesia, or a combination. Hypotensive anesthesia is recommended to minimize bleeding and to maximize visualization. The patient may be positioned in either the lateral decubitus or beach chair position. The senior author prefers the patient to be seated in an upright beach chair position with the acromion parallel to the floor (Fig. 23-4).

Surgical Landmarks, Incisions, and Portals

Landmarks

- Clavicle
- Acromion
- Scapular spine
- Coracoid

Portals and Approaches

Subacromial Decompression and Indirect Acromioclavicular Resection

- Anterior working portal
- Posterior scope portal
- Lateral working portal

Direct Acromioclavicular Resection

- Anterior portal
- Posterior portal

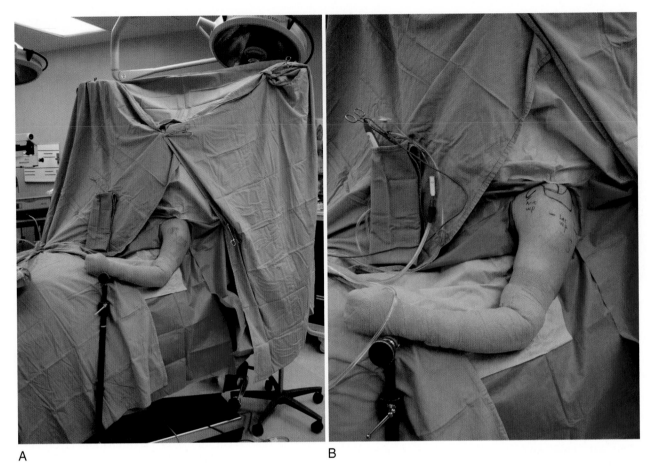

A   B

Figure 23-4 A and **B,** Patient is placed in an upright beach chair position.

Structures at Risk

Subacromial Decompression and Indirect Acromioclavicular Resection

- Anterior portal: brachial plexus, axillary artery
- Posterior portal: axillary nerve, posterior circumflex humeral artery
- Lateral portal: axillary nerve

Direct Acromioclavicular Resection

- Anterior portal: brachial plexus, axillary artery

Examination Under Anesthesia and Diagnostic Arthroscopy

Examination under anesthesia evaluates range of motion and ligamentous laxity. Diagnostic arthroscopy investigates possible associated intra-articular or subacromial pathologic changes, such as os acromiale, rotator cuff tear, labral tear, biceps disease, and loose bodies.

Box 23-2 Surgical Steps in Subacromial Decompression

1. Set-up and equipment

2. Glenohumeral arthroscopy

3. Acromial exposure

4. Acromioplasty

Specific Steps

Subacromial Decompression (Box 23-2)

1. Set-up and Equipment

The senior author prefers a beach chair position (see Fig. 23-4) and the use of an interscalene nerve block for anesthesia. The block is performed in the holding area, and the patient is brought into the operating room and transferred awake onto the already set up beach chair. The patient is secured in the upright position, and after protective goggles and extremity padding are placed, the patient is sedated.

Medications are used to maintain a hypotensive state whenever it is safe for the patient. An arthroscopic fluid pump is extremely helpful in maintaining an adequate arthroscopic fluid pressure to optimize visualization in the hypervascular subacromial space. The patient's neck should be observed by the anesthesia staff for evidence of fluid extravasation, which can lead to collapse of the softer portions of the airway and respiratory compromise. This is rarely a problem, even at very high levels of pressure, when the procedure is less than 60 minutes. In the beach chair position, gravity helps widen the subacromial space for improved viewing.

2. Glenohumeral Arthroscopy

Glenohumeral arthroscopy is an important part of the subacromial decompression procedure. Because most rotator cuff tears begin on the articular side, the surgeon will miss the pathologic process unless the undersurface of the rotator cuff is evaluated from within the glenohumeral joint. The arthroscope is introduced through the posterior portal. The skin incision is made parallel to the lateral edge of the acromion and approximately 2 to 3 cm inferior to the posterolateral corner of the acromion. This position correlates with the softest area of the posterior shoulder, or soft spot (Fig. 23-5). This posterior portal position allows the surgeon to use the same posterior portal for easier visualization of the subacromial space, where most of the work is to be done. The skin and deltoid are simply translated medially to line up with the glenohumeral joint line. Before placement of the scope, it is advantageous to mark the site of the anterior portal, which is immediately lateral to the tip of the coracoid (see Fig. 23-5). This site will almost always be colinear with the

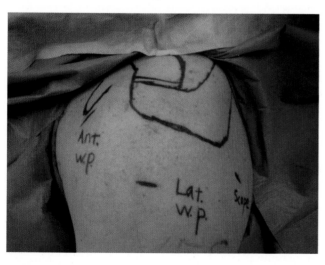

Figure 23-5 Close-up view of the patient showing the three standard protocols for the procedure: anterior working portal (Ant. w.p.), lateral working portal (Lat. w.p.), and posterior arthroscope portal (Scope). The anterior portal is immediately lateral to the tip of the coracoid process. The lateral working portal is immediately posterior and inferior to the anterior edge of the acromion.

glenohumeral joint line and serves as an aiming point when the arthroscope is introduced into the glenohumeral joint through the posterior portal. When an arthroscopic acromioclavicular resection is performed as an additional procedure, the surgeon should verify that the portal is parallel to the acromioclavicular joint. This is almost always true when the portal is placed immediately lateral to the coracoid tip.

The anterior portal is always lateral to the coracoid and conjoined tendon. However, it may be positioned superior or inferior, depending on the suspected pathologic process. For instance, in the presence of a full-thickness supraspinatus tendon tear, the portal can be placed between the subscapularis and superior glenohumeral ligament to prevent an additional defect immediately adjacent to the tear. In the presence of a superior labral tear, the anterior portal can be placed more lateral and above the superior glenohumeral ligament to facilitate concomitant repair of the superior labrum. Once inside the glenohumeral joint, the surgeon should systematically evaluate the cartilage, labrum, ligaments, capsule, rotator cuff, and biceps (Fig. 23-6).

3. Acromial Exposure

After completion of the glenohumeral arthroscopy, the joint fluid is evacuated with suction, and the arthroscope and anterior cannula are removed. The arthroscope is placed through the posterior portal into the subacromial space with an attempt to keep it immediately below the acromion to keep as much bursa as possible below the site of entry. It is helpful to use the trocar of the arthroscope to bluntly break up subacromial adhesions, moving it in a sweeping motion beneath the acromion. The anterolateral corner of the acromion is visualized before establishment of the lateral working portal. This portal is established with the help of a spinal needle to verify that the portal is parallel and slightly below the undersurface of the anterior third of the acromion, while at the same time allowing the front edge of the working instruments to be in line with the front edge of the acromion (Fig. 23-7). The anterior position of the portal places it closer to the area of work (i.e., the front third of the acromion), where the acromioplasty will be performed, and adjacent to the leading edge of the supraspinatus tendon, where most rotator cuff tears are found. It is better to err slightly lower than to be too high. A low portal can be corrected by abducting the arm, whereas a high portal makes it impossible to access the medial acromion and limits visualization of the acromioclavicular joint. The surgeon needs to make sure that the portal is no more than 3 to 4 cm from the edge of the acromion to avoid damage to the axillary nerve.

A small stab wound through skin only is used to establish the lateral portal; a semiaggressive shaver with teeth on the inner blade is used to perform a bursectomy and to expose the undersurface of the acromion (Fig. 23-8). It is best to start in the safer anterolateral aspect of the

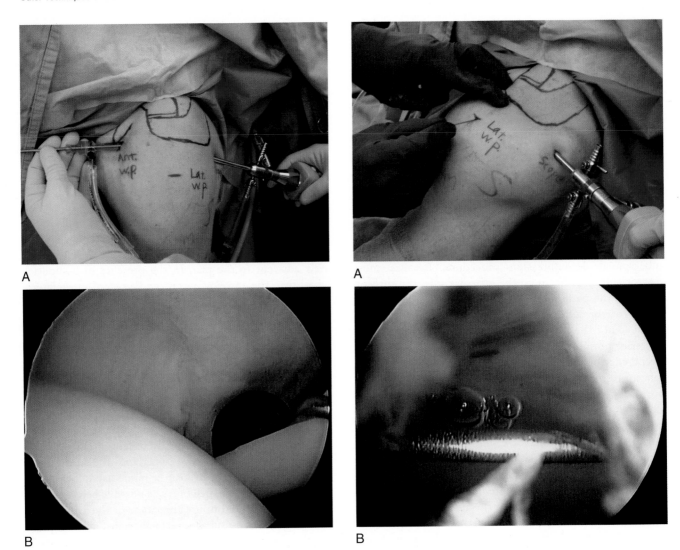

A

B

Figure 23-6 A, Outside view during glenohumeral arthroscopy with the arthroscope in the posterior portal and the cannula in the anterior working portal. **B,** Inside view showing evaluation of the rotator cuff immediately posterior to the biceps tendon (seen to the left of the biceps tendon).

A

B

Figure 23-7 A, Outside view demonstrating localization of the lateral working portal with an 18-gauge spinal needle. The arthroscope is in the posterior portal, beneath the acromion. **B,** Inside view showing the needle coming inside the subacromial space, beneath the acromion from the lateral direction.

subacromial space, beneath the anterior third of the acromion, and to expose it first to properly identify the position of the working instruments. This will allow the surgeon to avoid doing damage to the undersurface of the deltoid. The débridement proceeds in a posterior and medial direction, until the spine of the scapula is identified. This will allow exposure of the front two thirds of the scapula, making it easier to flatten the acromion without leaving a hidden ridge at the margin of resection. The acromioclavicular joint capsule is not violated unless a combined distal clavicle excision or removal of prominent osteophytes is planned.

In cases in which the rotator cuff is deficient or not repairable, the coracoacromial ligament is preserved. In most other cases, the ligament is released from the front edge of the acromion with the use of an electrocautery device. This is best performed by first incising the ligament at the anterolateral corner of the acromion in a line parallel with the deltoid fibers to safely establish the depth of the muscle fibers without risk of severing the deltoid fibers perpendicular to their length. Once the depth of the muscle is known, the surgeon can safely begin to release the deltoid around the front edge of the acromion. The acromion is now exposed and ready for the acromioplasty (Fig. 23-9).

4. Acromioplasty

The acromioplasty is easily and efficiently performed with an oval bur placed through the lateral working portal, avoiding the extra step of switching portals (Fig. 23-10A). The surgeon starts at the front edge of the anterolateral aspect of the acromion, burring down and flattening the

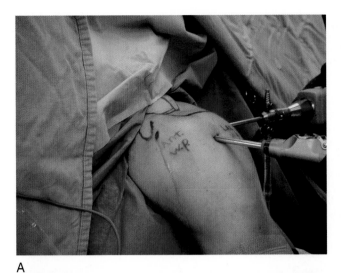

A

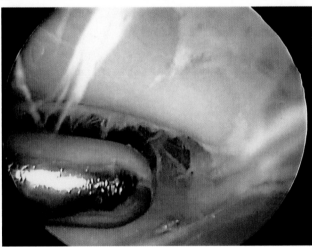

B

Figure 23-8 A, Outside view during subacromial arthroscopy with the motorized shaver entering the subacromial space through the lateral working portal and the arthroscope in the posterior portal. **B,** Inside view with the motorized shaver exposing the spine of the scapula.

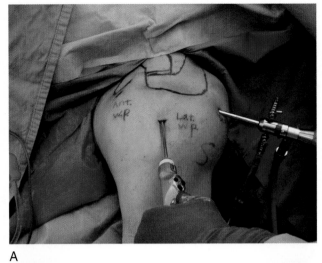

A

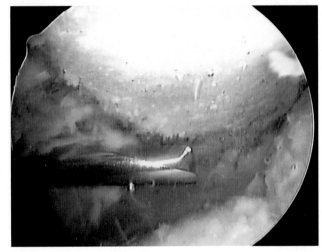

B

Figure 23-9 A, Outside view depicting the arthroscope in the posterior portal and the motorized cylindrical bur entering the subacromial space through the lateral working portal. **B,** The inside view demonstrating that the bur is parallel to the undersurface of the anterior third of the acromion and immediately posterior to its anterior edge.

lateral half of the anterior third of the acromion until it is linear with the middle third of the acromion, which has been fully exposed (Fig. 23-10B). This is performed in most patients with the entire width of the bur. The lateral half is then used as a template for the medial half. The medial half is resected in the same way with another sweep of the oval bur until the entire front third of the acromion is flattened to the level of the middle third of the acromion (Fig. 23-10C). At completion, all bone particles are evacuated with suction, and the bursal surface of the rotator cuff is fully inspected. Postoperative radiographs will reveal removal of the acromial spur and conversion to a type I acromion (Fig. 23-11).

Alternatively, a "cutting block" technique can be used, in which the anterolateral spur of the acromion is burred down from the lateral working portal first. Subsequently,

the arthroscope is placed into the lateral portal and the bur into the posterior portal. The acromioplasty now proceeds from posterior to anterior, with use of the just prepared posterior part of the acromion as a template for resection of the next, more anterior, part.

At completion, all bone particles are evacuated with suction, and the bursal surface of the rotator cuff is fully inspected.

Distal Clavicle Excision, Indirect Approach
(Box 23-3)

1. Subacromial Approach

After completion of the subacromial decompression, the acromioclavicular joint is exposed. While the arthroscope is still in the posterior portal, an anterior working portal is established. In most people, the routine anterior

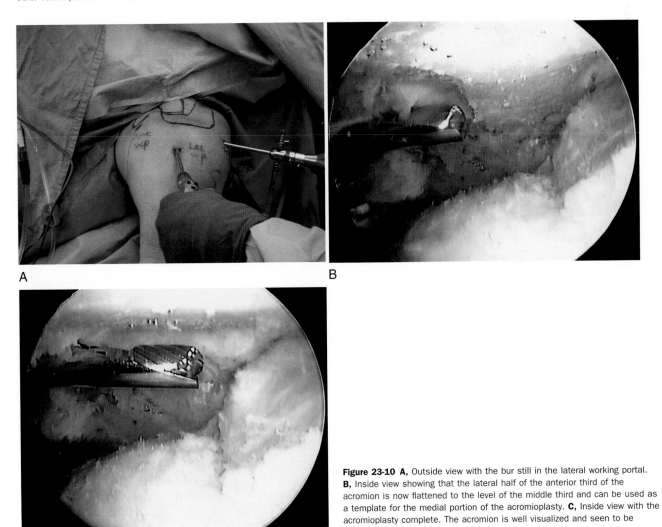

Figure 23-10 A, Outside view with the bur still in the lateral working portal. **B,** Inside view showing that the lateral half of the anterior third of the acromion is now flattened to the level of the middle third and can be used as a template for the medial portion of the acromioplasty. **C,** Inside view with the acromioplasty complete. The acromion is well visualized and seen to be entirely flat with no hidden ridges.

Figure 23-11 A, Outlet view radiograph in a patient with a preoperative spur. **B,** Outlet view radiograph in same patient after the spur has been removed during the subacromial decompression with acromioplasty.

glenohumeral portal placed immediately adjacent to the coracoid process will line up directly with the acromioclavicular joint. It is important to verify this preoperatively. The portal is established by placing a blunt medium trocar through the anterior portal and immediately beneath the acromioclavicular joint. With the trocar in position, the arthroscope is quickly switched from the posterior portal to the lateral working portal to provide a direct end-on view of the acromioclavicular joint and distal clavicle.

2. Exposure of the Distal Clavicle

The trocar is removed, and an aggressive shaver is placed through the anterior portal to resect the inferior and

Box 23-3 Surgical Steps in Distal Clavicle Excision, Indirect Approach

1. Subacromial approach

2. Exposure of the distal clavicle

3. Resection of the distal clavicle

intra-articular fibrocartilaginous disk anterior capsule of the acromioclavicular joint (Fig. 23-12A). The arthritic distal clavicular cartilage is exposed and scraped away with the shaver. Next, an electrocautery device is used to elevate the capsule from the edge of the clavicle. The superior posterior capsule is elevated with a hook-type electrocautery device, preserving it, as it is important for stability of the acromioclavicular joint. Exposure of the superior aspect of the distal clavicle is important to ensure that the entire width of the distal clavicle is resected without leaving any small parcels of bone that can hypertrophy and lead to residual pain in the acromioclavicular joint.

3. Resection of the Distal Clavicle

After exposure of the distal clavicle, a high-speed oval bur is brought in through the anterior portal and used to resect 1 cm of the distal clavicle to a smooth flat surface. Before resection, it is important to identify the orientation of the acromioclavicular joint on radiographs. This helps the surgeon identify the morphologic features of the joint, including its orientation and osteophytes. The usual

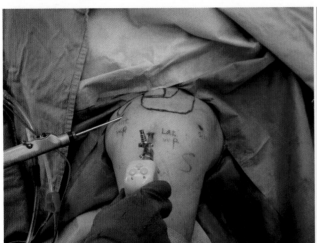

A

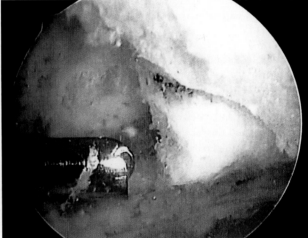

B

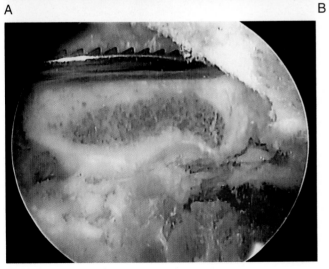

C

Figure 23-12 A, Outside view during indirect acromioclavicular excision with the arthroscope in the lateral working portal and the motorized instrument in the anterior working portal. **B,** Inside view demonstrating the position of the motorized bur at the distal clavicle. The front half of the distal clavicle has been resected. **C,** Inside view depicting the rasp verifying the width and angle of the resection.

Box 23-4 Surgical Steps in Distal Clavicle Excision, Direct Approach

| 1. Portals |
| 2. Exposure |
| 3. Distal clavicle resection |

orientation is a sloping surface from superolateral to inferomedial. Removal of a few millimeters of bone from the acromial facet of the acromioclavicular joint will facilitate visualization and subsequent resection.

The front half of the clavicle should be resected first (Fig. 23-12B). The initial resection allows the surgeon to measure the depth of resection against the intact posterior half and use it as a template for its resection. Studies have shown that between 5 and 10 mm of distal clavicle resection is necessary to successfully eliminate pain. No more than 1 cm of the distal clavicle should be removed to maintain the integrity of the superior and posterior capsule, which provides anteroposterior stability of the acromioclavicular joint, as well as that of the coracoclavicular ligaments, which provide stability against superior migration of the distal clavicle. Resection level and orientation can be verified with the use of a flat rasp with known dimensions (Fig. 23-12C).

Distal Clavicle Excision, Direct Approach (Box 23-4)

1. Portals

In the direct approach, the arthroscope and instruments are placed directly into the acromioclavicular joint through anterosuperior and posterosuperior portals (Fig. 23-13A). Because the acromioclavicular joint is variably inclined and may be extremely narrow, it is important to determine the precise joint location and inclination with a 22-gauge needle (Fig. 23-13B). The needle is placed in the center of the joint, and it is insufflated with arthroscopy fluid. Next, the positions of the anterior and posterior portals are verified with two additional 22-gauge needles, by verifying free outflow of fluid through the needles. The portals are aligned with the joint line, approximately 1 to 2 cm from the anterior and posterior joint edges. Instruments should enter the joint at an angle of approximately 30 degrees from the horizontal (Fig. 23-13C).

Once the position and angle of the acromioclavicular joint are confirmed with the needles, a No. 11 blade scalpel is used to incise the skin portals and to puncture the joint capsule. The blade is guided into the joint by sliding against the needle. The anterior aspect of the acromioclavicular joint is wider than the posterior aspect, and therefore the anterior portal is established first. A standard arthroscope is placed through a trocar with sheath into the wider anterior joint edge. The posterior portal is established under direct vision by placing a 3- to 4-mm shaver directly into the joint. Cannulas are not used as they are too restrictive and space is limited.

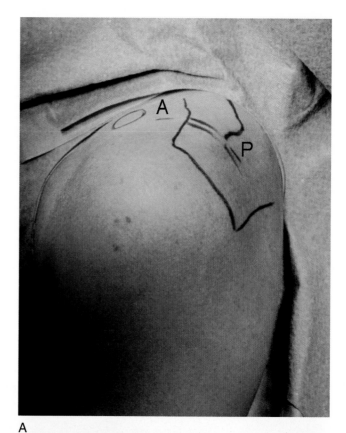

A

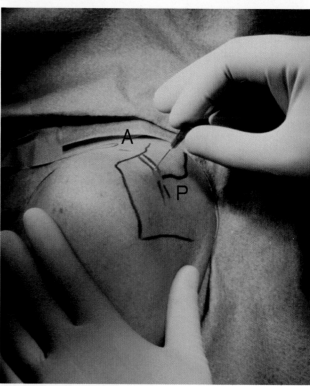

B

Figure 23-13 A, Direct acromioclavicular resection portal sites for a left shoulder, which include the anterior (A) and posterior (P) portals. **B,** A 22-gauge spinal needle is used to localize the precise position of the acromioclavicular joint.

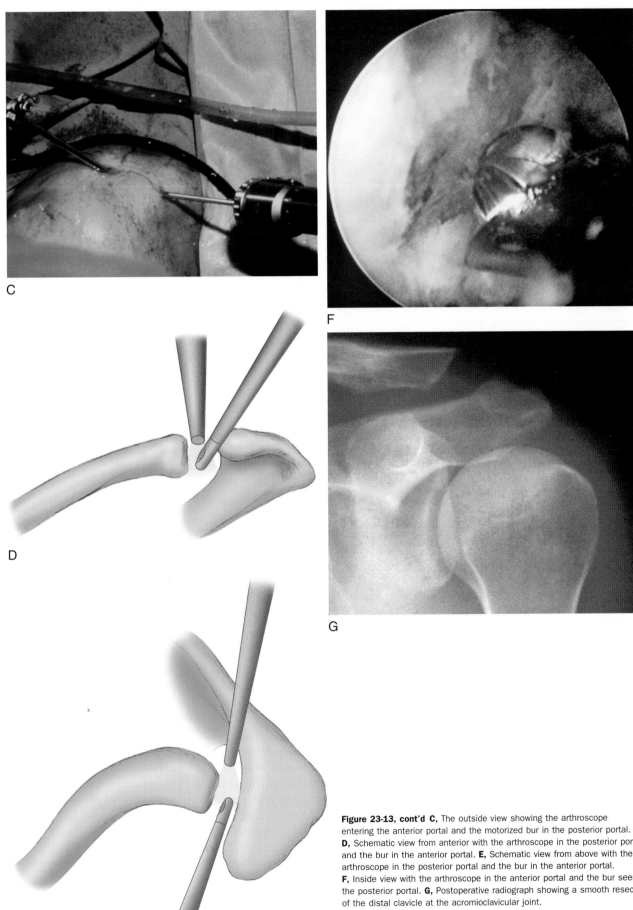

C

D

E

F

G

Figure 23-13, cont'd C, The outside view showing the arthroscope entering the anterior portal and the motorized bur in the posterior portal. **D,** Schematic view from anterior with the arthroscope in the posterior portal and the bur in the anterior portal. **E,** Schematic view from above with the arthroscope in the posterior portal and the bur in the anterior portal. **F,** Inside view with the arthroscope in the anterior portal and the bur seen in the posterior portal. **G,** Postoperative radiograph showing a smooth resection of the distal clavicle at the acromioclavicular joint.

2. Exposure

Under direct vision with the shaver in the posterior portal, intervening disk and synovial tissue are resected to expose the arthritic cartilage surfaces (Fig. 23-13D and E). The cartilage is scraped away with the shaver. A hook-tipped electrocautery device is used to elevate the joint capsule from the edge of the distal clavicle in a circumferential fashion. The capsule should be released and not excised, as it is important to the postoperative stability of the joint.

3. Resection of the Distal Clavicle

A 5- to 6-mm oval bur is placed through the posterior portal and the resection begins (Fig. 23-13F). The posterior one half to two thirds of the joint is resected first; 5 to 10 mm is removed from the posterior aspect. This allows precise measurement of resection by use of the known dimensions of the bur as a guide. The instruments are switched, with the arthroscope being placed into the posterior aspect of the joint. Before resecting the front portion of the distal clavicle, the surgeon verifies that the joint capsule has been sufficiently released from the front portion of the joint. Once satisfied, the surgeon places the bur through the anterior portal and removes the front portion of the clavicle. The posterior resection is used as a template, and the clavicle is resected to a smooth flat surface. Bone debris is removed by suction, and the distal clavicle is inspected to make certain that there are no retained particles of bone adherent to the joint capsule. Postoperative radiographs demonstrate smooth resection of the distal clavicle at the acromioclavicular joint (Fig. 23-13G).

Postoperative Considerations

Follow-up

Patients are seen after 7 to 10 days for suture removal and wound inspection.

Rehabilitation

Patients wear a sling and compressive cold device for comfort during the first 48 hours. Pendulum exercises are started immediately, and a formal rehabilitation program begins within the first 24 to 48 hours. This program includes passive and active range-of-motion exercises in all planes of motion. Strengthening exercises are initiated within the first few weeks after surgery, when the patients have regained close to full range of motion and their comfort level will tolerate the stress. Return to most activities is expected within 6 weeks, and full return to strenuous activities is expected by 3 to 6 months.

Complications

- Incomplete resection of acromion or distal clavicle
- Regrowth of acromion or distal clavicle
- Infection
- Adhesive capsulitis
- Neurovascular injury

PEARLS AND PITFALLS

Subacromial Decompression

- Correct portal placement is the most important aspect of arthroscopic subacromial decompression; in heavier patients, it is a common mistake to make the portals too high. The surgeon can avoid improper placement by paying strict attention to bone landmarks and using a spinal needle to localize the lateral working portal under direct vision.
- The use of an arthroscopic pump is helpful. It allows the surgeon to change the pressure to adjust for variability in the patient's blood pressure.

Acromioclavicular Resection

- Make certain that the anterior working portal is parallel to the acromioclavicular joint. This will make the resection easier to perform.
- Avoid leaving small parcels of bone behind in the joint capsule by making certain that the capsule is fully released from the edge of the clavicle and by resecting the clavicle from the top edge first; as the surgeon moves inferiorly, the bur resects from lateral to medial. Bone left attached to the capsule will grow to become larger and may leave the patient with residual pain.

Results

After arthroscopic acromioplasty and subacromial decompression, good to excellent results are achieved in nearly 80% of patients, demonstrated by decreased pain with activities and improved function. However, less than 70% of throwing athletes return to their sport postoperatively (Table 23-1). In patients with both subacromial impingement syndrome and painful acromioclavicular degenerative joint disease, concomitant subacromial decompression and distal clavicle excision produce good to excellent results in nearly 90% of patients. However, patients who have an extended duration of symptoms before surgery or damage to the rotator cuff tendons have poorer outcomes (Table 23-2). For isolated acromioclavicular joint disease without acromioclavicular hypermobility, direct distal clavicle excision through a superior approach yields good to excellent results in more than 90% of patients (Table 23-3).

Table 23-1 Clinical Results after Subacromial Decompression

Author	Follow-up	No. of Patients	Outcome
Ellman[5] (1987)	17 months (12-36 months)	49	88% good–excellent
Esch et al[6] (1988)	19 months (12-36 months)	71	77% good–excellent
Gartsman[8] (1990)	29 months (24-48 months)	126	87% no rotator cuff tear 83% partial-thickness rotator cuff tear
Roye et al[14] (1995)	41 months (2-7 years)	88	89% nonthrowing athletes 68% throwing athletes
Stephens et al[15] (1998)	8 years 5 months (6-10 years)	82	81% good–excellent 67% throwing athletes

Table 23-2 Clinical Results after Subacromial Decompression and Distal Clavicle Excision

Author	Follow-up	No. of Patients	Outcome
Kay et al[9] (2003)	6 years (3.9-9 years)	20	100% good–excellent 25% re-formed distal clavicle
Lozman et al[11] (1995)	32 months (minimum 2 years)	18	89% good–excellent
Levine et al[10] (1998)	32.5 months (24-70 months)	24	88% good–excellent
Martin et al[12] (2001)	4 years 10 months (3-8 years)	31	100% good–excellent

Table 23-3 Clinical Results after Direct Distal Clavicle Excision

Author	Follow-up	No. of Patients	Outcome
Auge and Fischer[1] (1998)	18.7 months (12-25 months)	10	100% good–excellent 100% osteolysis
Flatow et al[7] (1995)	31 months (24-49 months)	41	93% osteoarthritis or osteolysis 58% acromioclavicular hypermobility

References

1. Auge W, Fischer R. Arthroscopic distal clavicle resection for isolated atraumatic osteolysis in weight lifters. Am J Sports Med 1998;26:189-192.
2. Bigliani L, Levine W. Subacromial impingement syndrome. J Bone Joint Surg Am 1997;79:1854-1868.
3. Blazar P, Iannotti J, Williams G. Anteroposterior instability of the distal clavicle after distal clavicle resection. Clin Orthop 1998;348:114-120.
4. Debski R, Fenwick J, Vangura A, et al. Effect of arthroscopic procedures on the acromioclavicular joint. Clin Orthop 2003;406:89-96.
5. Ellman H. Arthroscopic subacromial decompression: analysis of one- to three-year results. Arthroscopy 1987;3:173-181.
6. Esch J, Ozerkis L, Helgager J, et al. Arthroscopic subacromial decompression: results according to the degree of rotator cuff tear. Arthroscopy 1988;4:241-249.
7. Flatow E, Duralde X, Nicholson G, et al. Arthroscopic resection of the distal clavicle with a superior approach. J Shoulder Elbow Surg 1995;4:41-50.
8. Gartsman G. Arthroscopic acromioplasty for lesions of the rotator cuff. J Bone Joint Surg Am 1990;72:169-180.
9. Kay S, Dragoo J, Lee R. Long-term results of arthroscopic resection of the distal clavicle with concomitant subacromial decompression. Arthroscopy 2003;19:805-809.
10. Levine W, Barron O, Yamaguchi K, et al. Arthroscopic distal clavicle resection from a bursal approach. Arthroscopy 1998;14:52-61.
11. Lozman P, Hechtman K, Uribe J. Combined arthroscopic management of impingement syndrome and acromioclavicular arthritis. J South Orthop Assoc 1995;4:177-181.
12. Martin S, Baumgarten T, Andrews J. Arthroscopic resection of the distal aspect of the clavicle with concomitant subacromial decompression. J Bone Joint Surg Am 2001;83:328-335.
13. McFarland E, Selhi H, Keyurapan E. Clinical evaluation of impingement: what to do and what works. J Bone Joint Surg Am 2006;88:432-441.
14. Roye R, Grana W, Yates C. Arthroscopic subacromial decompression: two to seven-year follow-up. Arthroscopy 1995;11:301-306.
15. Stephens S, Warren R, Payne L, et al. Arthroscopic acromioplasty: a 6- to 10-year follow-up. Arthroscopy 1998;14:382-388.

23

CHAPTER 24

Arthroscopic Management of Glenohumeral Arthritis

C. Benjamin Ma, MD

Shoulder arthroscopy has allowed clinicians to better diagnose and treat abnormalities of the glenohumeral joint. Arthroscopic stabilization and rotator cuff repairs are commonly performed shoulder procedures.[1,6,13] The use of arthroscopy has expanded to the treatment of osteoarthritis of various causes.[2,10,11] Most patients can tolerate advanced arthritis of the shoulder because it is not a weight-bearing joint. Arthroscopic débridement of the shoulder can be beneficial for removal of loose cartilage fragments, osteophytes, and loose bodies and for synovectomy. Despite the mixed results of arthroscopic débridement of knee arthritis, reports of arthroscopic débridement for shoulder arthritis have been favorable.[3,7,12,14] Whereas shoulder arthroplasty is considered the "gold standard" for the treatment of shoulder osteoarthritis, arthroscopic débridement can be an alternative, especially for young and active patients, to delay the need for prosthetic replacement.

Preoperative Considerations

History

Most patients with shoulder osteoarthritis present with typical shoulder pain that is worse at night. Pain is related to activity. Shoulder osteoarthritis rarely presents with rest pain, with the exception of night pain. The patients also complain of restricted movement of the involved shoulder. A common complaint is difficulty reaching to the back and above the head. Severe forms of osteoarthritis of

the shoulder will also have painful crepitation. Patients may also complain of a locking and clicking sensation if loose bodies are present.

It is extremely important to determine what the perceived limitations are for the patient. If the patient's main complaint is stiffness, arthroscopic débridement alone may not suffice, and arthroscopic cheilectomy or capsulotomy may be needed to improve postoperative motion. If the patient also shows symptoms of subacromial bursitis, subacromial decompression should be performed to address disease in the subacromial space.

Physical Examination

Physical examination usually demonstrates limited range of motion. Most patients who have a large inferior humeral spur will have limited forward flexion. Patients with a flattened humeral head will have limited external and internal rotation. Strength of the rotator cuff tendons is usually preserved; however, strength testing can be limited secondary to pain. Patients can also exhibit bursitis-type symptoms. As with all shoulder complaints, a full cervical examination should be performed to rule out referred pain from degenerative disease of the cervical spine.

Imaging

Plain radiographs demonstrate narrowing of the glenohumeral joint space. Orthogonal views can demonstrate the location of the humeral osteophytes. Standard radiographs include anteroposterior (Fig. 24-1A), axillary lateral (Fig. 24-1C), and scapula Y views of the glenohumeral joint and an anteroposterior view of the acromioclavicular joint. For patients presenting with predominantly arthritic symptoms, weight-bearing views of the glenohumeral joint

should be performed to better diagnose the amount of joint space narrowing (Fig. 24-1B). For the weight-bearing view, an anteroposterior glenohumeral joint radiograph is taken with the patient holding a 1-pound weight in the hand with the shoulder abducted at around 30 to 45

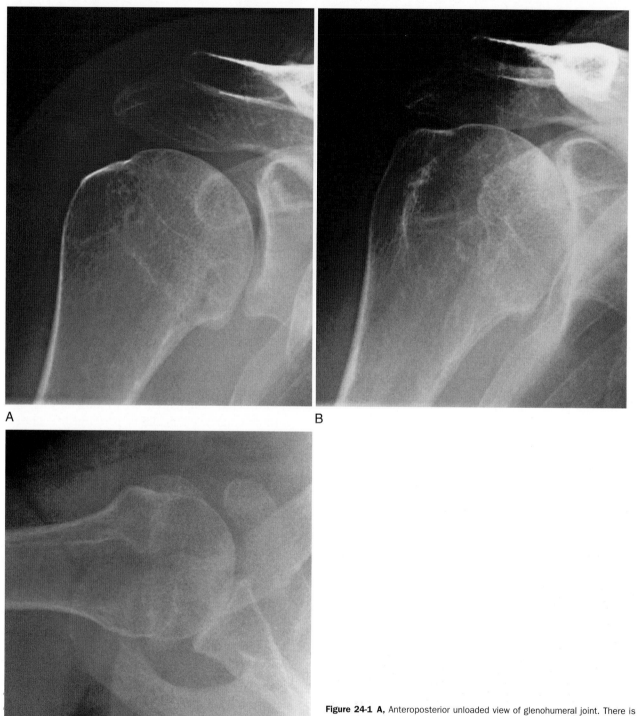

A

B

C

Figure 24-1 A, Anteroposterior unloaded view of glenohumeral joint. There is space between the glenoid and the humerus. **B,** Anteroposterior weight-bearing view of glenohumeral joint. For the same patient holding a 1-pound weight, there is complete obliteration of the joint space demonstrating bone-on-bone arthritis. **C,** Axillary lateral view of the glenohumeral joint demonstrating joint space narrowing.

degrees. This is analogous to the weight-bearing view of the lower extremities to demonstrate true joint space under load. This is extremely helpful for patients with inflammatory arthritis, where there can be absence of large osteophytes.

Magnetic resonance imaging can be obtained but is usually not required; it is, however, useful to investigate early arthritis to demonstrate the presence of cartilage wear. It can also show labral and rotator cuff disease. These lesions can be addressed concomitantly during surgery. Magnetic resonance imaging can also demonstrate the significance of posterior wear of the glenoid. The axial images from this three-dimensional analysis can help quantify the amount of glenoid deficiency.

Preoperative radiographic studies can be extremely helpful to define the size and position of osteophytes; a three-dimensional study like magnetic resonance imaging or computed tomography is best to achieve this. Another important evaluation is the shape of the glenoid. A bilobed glenoid, representing significant posterior wear, may require glenoidplasty or indicate less favorable outcome (Fig. 24-2).

Preoperative injections can be helpful to predict the patient's response to surgery. Selective injection to the glenohumeral and subacromial space can be performed to determine the relative contribution of each compartment to the patient's symptoms.

Indications and Contraindications

Understanding the etiology of shoulder osteoarthritis is extremely important. Patients with concentric glenoid wear may benefit from débridement and synovectomy, whereas patients with large osteophytes may benefit from cheilectomy and capsulotomy. The patient's complaints are

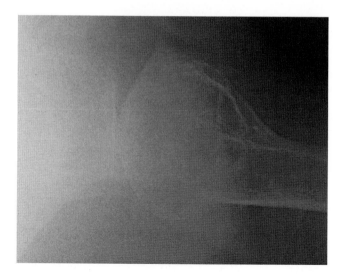

Figure 24-2 Bilobed glenoid. These patients can benefit from glenoidplasty to restore the concavity of the glenohumeral joint.

the most important guide as to which structural abnormalities need to be addressed surgically. Especially severe posterior wear of the shoulder with a bilobed glenoid may not benefit from surgical débridement and glenoidplasty. Patients who have anterior superior migration with acetabulization of the glenoid may also not benefit significantly from arthroscopic surgeries. In my practice, I have found that selective injection to the glenohumeral and subacromial space can help predict the response of the patients to arthroscopic treatment.

Surgical Techniques

Anesthesia and Positioning

Most of the patients receive an interscalene block with general anesthesia. The interscalene block minimizes the use of narcotics intraoperatively and will decrease the incidence of postoperative nausea and complications. The block is also helpful for postoperative pain control so that the patients can transition smoothly to oral pain medication.

Arthroscopic débridement of the shoulder can be performed in either the beach chair or lateral position. In this chapter, the set-up for a beach chair position is outlined.

For the beach chair position, I use a regular operating room table with a full-length beanbag (Fig. 24-3). I prefer this set-up as it can accommodate patients with various body habitus and weights. A beach chair position add-on device to the operating table can make set-up easy and quick; however, patients who are large or small may not fit as well as with a beanbag.

The patient is first positioned with the bed in a reflex position with the foot of the table flexed. The back of the table is then raised up to the beach chair position. The reflex position will prevent the patient's slipping toward the end of the bed. The beanbag is then folded in to expose the operative shoulder. The operative shoulder is exposed up to the medial border of the scapula. The beanbag is then wrapped around the head and the lower torso while it is being inflated. This set-up allows excellent control of the body and the head during the operation. After the beanbag is inflated, the patient and the beanbag are then shifted over to the edge of the table to expose the operative shoulder. Because the full-length beanbag is cradling the patient, this is a stable set-up and will expose the operative shoulder nicely (see Fig. 24-3). An arm-holding device facilitates positioning and traction of the shoulder.

Surgical Landmarks, Incisions, and Portals

For arthroscopic débridement of the shoulder, standard shoulder arthroscopy portals can be used. A posterior

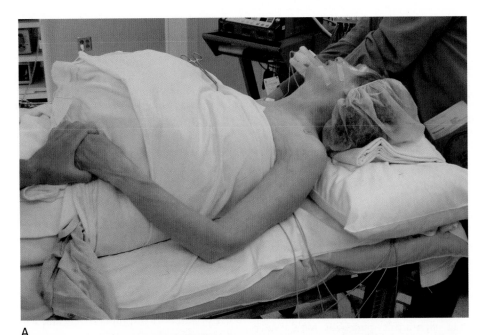

A

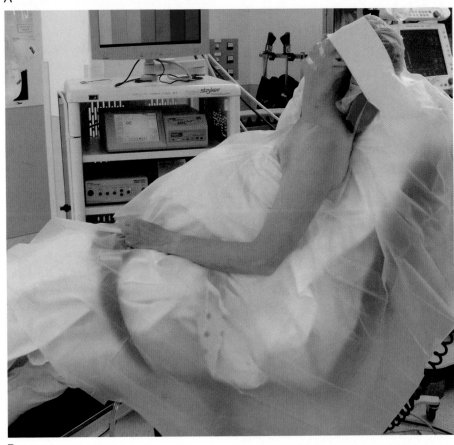

B

Figure 24-3 A, The beach chair set-up is shown with a full-length beanbag as a positioning aid. **B,** The operating table is first reflexed, followed by lowering of the foot of the table. The back is then raised up to the beach chair position. The reflex position prevents the patient from sliding toward the end of the bed.

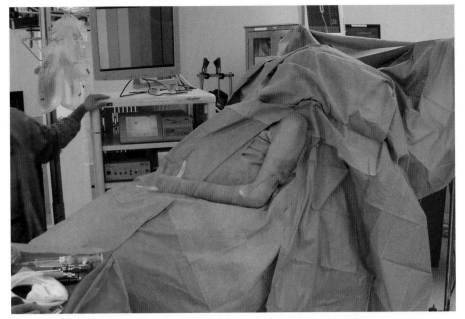

C

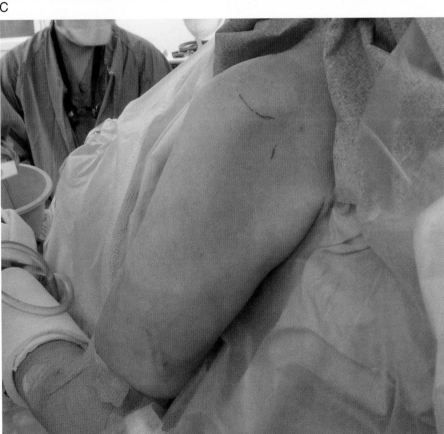

D

Figure 24-3, cont'd C, The patient and the beanbag are then slid over toward the edge of the table to allow excellent exposure of the operative shoulder. The shoulder is then prepared and draped accordingly. An arm holder will be used for traction and positioning. **D,** Posterior view of the shoulder. The shoulder is draped up to the medial border of the scapula. This versatile position and draping can accommodate easy transition to open anterior and posterior approaches to the shoulder.

arthroscopy portal is used for diagnostic arthroscopy. The landmark for the portal is the posterior soft spot of the shoulder. An anterior portal is used as the working portal. The landmark of the anterior portal is just lateral to the tip of the coracoid process. An accessory posterior portal can be used for access to the inferior part of the shoulder for removal of loose bodies and inferior osteophytes. The landmark for the accessory posterior portal is 2 cm below and in line with the standard posterior portal.[4,5] The accessory portal should be established by spinal needle localization under direct visualization (Fig. 24-4).

Diagnostic Arthroscopy

Diagnostic arthroscopy is performed to reveal any labral or rotator cuff tears, which can be addressed concomitantly. A torn labrum or frayed rotator cuff can be débrided with a mechanical shaver or repaired if appropriate.

Specific Steps (Box 24-1)

1. Débridement, Synovectomy, and Removal of Osteophytes

A thermal coagulation device is used to remove any inflamed synovium. Biceps tendon tears affecting more than 50% of the tendon width should be treated with a biceps tenotomy or tenodesis, depending on the activity level of the patient. This portion of the operation should

be discussed with the patient preoperatively regarding the incidence of biceps deformity after tenotomy. After débridement of the soft tissues, excessive osteophytes can be removed with a narrow osteotome or mechanical bur. The accessory posterior portal can be helpful for access to the inferior portion of the shoulder (Fig. 24-5). Previous cadaveric studies have shown that the accessory portal provides safe access to the inferior capsule; the average distance between the portal and the axillary nerve is approximately 3 cm. When cheilectomy of the inferior osteophyte is performed, a mechanical bur can be used. The lateral attachment of the inferior capsule represents the inferior part of the anatomic neck of the humerus. An inferior osteophyte will be medial but inferior to the reflection of the capsule (Fig. 24-5B). I usually use the attachment of the inferior capsule to define where the normal anatomic neck is; cheilectomy can be performed safely medial to it. Frequent intraoperative radiographic or fluoroscopic evaluation is extremely helpful to determine the extent of the excision (Fig. 24-6). Large loose bodies can also be removed through the accessory posterior portal (Fig. 24-7).

Box 24-1 Surgical Steps

1. Débridement, synovectomy, and removal of osteophytes

2. Capsular release

3. Subacromial decompression

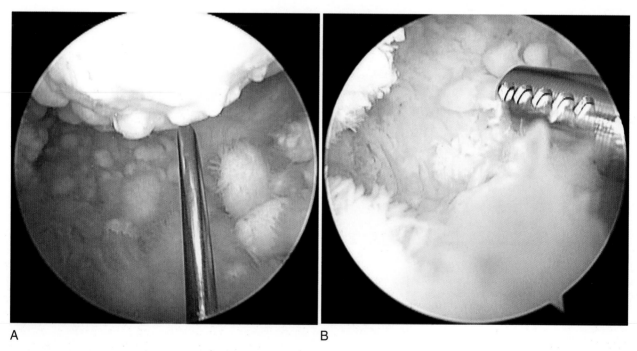

A   B

Figure 24-4 An accessory posterior portal is useful for access to the inferior aspect of the shoulder. The landmark of the portal is 2 cm directly inferior to the standard posterior portal. **A,** The accessory posterior portal is localized by a spinal needle. **B,** A shaver is introduced through the accessory posterior portal.

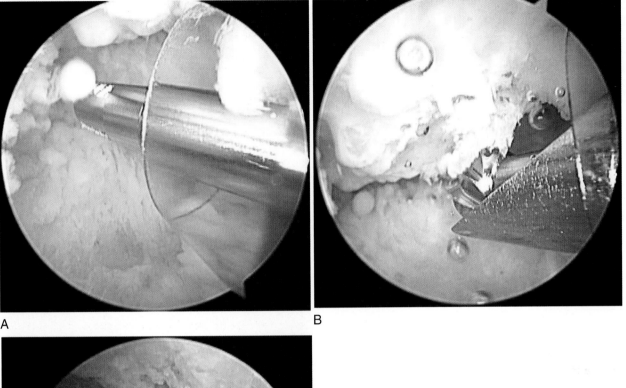

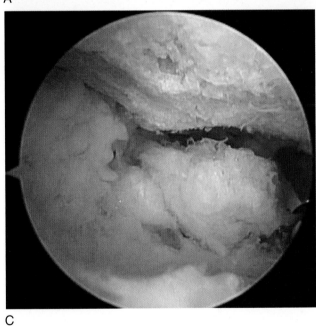

Figure 24-5 Dissection along the axillary pouch. **A,** A shaver is introduced into the axillary pouch through the accessory posterior portal. Synovectomy is performed. **B,** A bur is introduced to remove the inferior spur. **C,** Inferior bone spur can be osteotomized and removed from the axillary pouch.

Microfracture can be performed on contained lesions on the humerus and glenoid; however, the outcome of this procedure in the shoulder has not been well documented. Glenoidplasty can also be performed to reshape the concavity of the shoulder. This is a more extensive procedure, and in my experience, I have not found significant benefit.

2. Capsular Release

For stiff shoulders, capsulotomy can also be performed arthroscopically to increase range of motion. Following standard procedure for capsular release as outlined elsewhere in greater detail, this is usually performed with a thermal coagulation device at a low temperature setting. The anterior capsule is cut close to the glenoid from the rotator interval superiorly to the 5-o'clock position inferiorly.[8,15] The axillary nerve is closest to the capsule in this location, and it is usually safer first to elevate the capsule off the inferior musculature and then carefully to cut it under direct visualization. This can also be performed with the thermal coagulation device under the capsule, cutting toward the joint to protect the axillary nerve that is

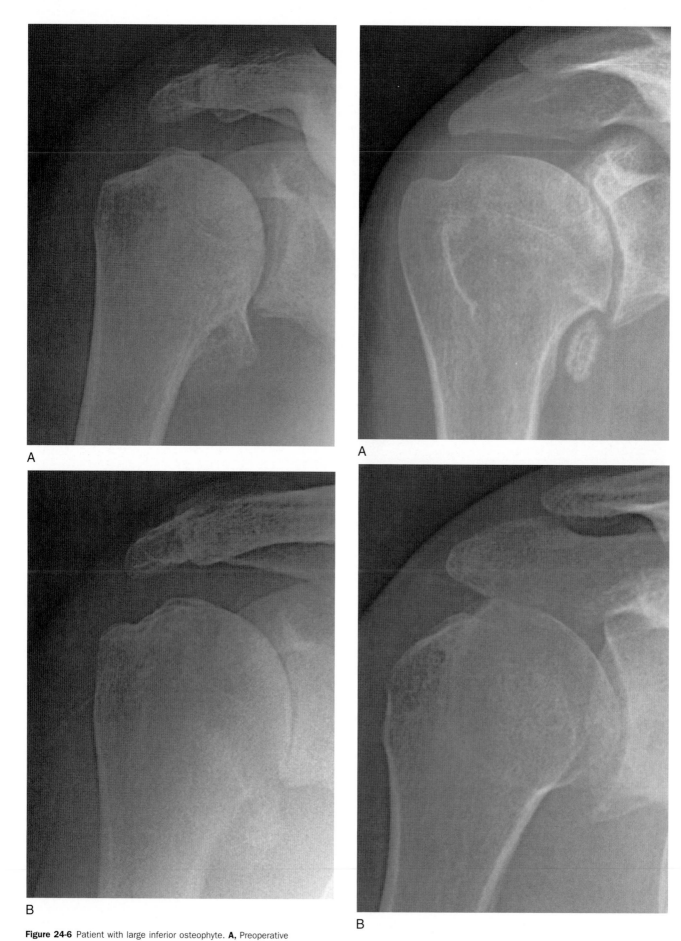

A

B

Figure 24-6 Patient with large inferior osteophyte. **A,** Preoperative anteroposterior glenohumeral joint radiograph demonstrating large protruding inferior spur. **B,** Postoperative anteroposterior glenohumeral joint radiograph demonstrating excision of inferior spur.

A

B

Figure 24-7 A, Preoperative anteroposterior glenohumeral joint radiograph demonstrating osteoarthritis and large intra-articular loose body. **B,** Postoperative anteroposterior glenohumeral joint radiograph demonstrating removal of loose body and excision of inferior humeral spur.

Table 24-1 Outcomes of Arthroscopic Débridement for Shoulder Osteoarthritis

Author	No. of Patients	Follow-up	Treatment	Outcome
Ellman et al[7] (1992)	18	6 months-3 years	Arthroscopic subacromial decompression	Subjective improvement
Weinstein et al[14] (2000)	25	30 months	Lavage, débridement, bursectomy	80% good–excellent
Kelly et al[9] (2000)	14	34 months	Glenoidplasty	80% good–excellent
Cameron et al[3] (2002)	61	45 patients with minimum of 2 years	Débridement with and without capsular release	87% would have surgery again 88% improvement in pain
Safran et al[12] (2002)	17	Prospective 4-year study, minimum of 1 year	Débridement plus bursectomy	85% good to excellent at 6 months 70% at 2-4 years

24

inferior to the capsule. The arthroscope is then switched to the anterior portal to complete the posterior capsulotomy through the posterior portal.

3. Subacromial Decompression

After intra-articular examination and dissection, I proceed to the subacromial space. If a significant amount of bursitis is present, a subacromial bursectomy is performed. Acromioplasty is not needed unless the patient has a large acromial spur and had signs of impingement symptoms preoperatively.

Rehabilitation

The patients are allowed full range of motion after débridement. They are encouraged to work on end range of motion early, especially after capsulotomy and removal of osteophytes. Strengthening of the rotator cuff tendons usually begins 3 to 4 weeks after surgery.

Complications

The risk of arthroscopic débridement is similar to the risk of any shoulder arthroscopic surgery. With the excision of osteophytes and glenoidplasty, there is a higher risk of bleeding and potential injury to the axillary nerve in dissecting inferiorly. Regional anesthesia is helpful in this

setting as the patient should not be paralyzed and the axillary nerve can react if any dissecting equipment is close.[15]

PEARLS AND PITFALLS

- Use a spinal needle to localize the accessory posterior portal.
- Use a twist-in or lip cannula over the posterior port to allow easy access through the portal and to avoid backing out.
- The bur can be used at the axillary pouch, but do not have the suction on to avoid injury to the inferior capsule and axillary nerve.
- An anterior inferior portal can be used, but the risk of axillary nerve injury is much higher than with the posterior accessory portal.
- Intraoperative fluoroscopic imaging is helpful to determine the extent of resection.
- The axillary nerve is closest to the glenoid rim (1 cm away) at the 5-o'clock position.
- Turn down the power of the coagulation device in performing capsulectomy of the inferior capsule.

Results

There has been a paucity of long-term results on arthroscopic débridement of the shoulder; most of the reports are case series without any comparison or control group. There are also a variety of recommendations regarding the need for glenoidplasty and subacromial decompressions. The results are summarized in Table 24-1.

References

1. Bishop J, Klepps S, Lo IK, et al. Cuff integrity after arthroscopic versus open rotator cuff repair: a prospective study. J Shoulder Elbow Surg 2006;15:290-299.
2. Bishop JY, Flatow EL. Management of glenohumeral arthritis: a role for arthroscopy? Orthop Clin North Am 2003;34:559-566.
3. Cameron BD, Galatz LM, Ramsey ML, et al. Non-prosthetic management of grade IV osteochondral lesions of the glenohumeral joint. J Shoulder Elbow Surg 2002;11:25-32.
4. Davidson PA, Rivenburgh DW. The 7-o'clock posteroinferior portal for shoulder arthroscopy. Am J Sports Med 2002;30:693-696.

5. Difelice GS, Williams RJ 3rd, Cohen MS, Warren RF. The accessory posterior portal for shoulder arthroscopy: description of technique and cadaveric study. Arthroscopy 2001;17:888-891.

6. Edwards TB, Walch G, Nove-Josserand L, et al. Arthroscopic débridement in the treatment of patients with isolated tears of the subscapularis. Arthroscopy 2006;22:941-946.

7. Ellman H, Harris E, Kay SP. Early degenerative joint disease simulating impingement syndrome: arthroscopic findings. Arthroscopy 1992;8:482-487.

8. Esmail AN, Getz CL, Schwartz DM, et al. Axillary nerve monitoring during arthroscopic shoulder stabilization. Arthroscopy 2005;21:665-671.

9. Kelly EW, Steinmann SP, O'Driscoll SW. Arthroscopic glenoidplasty for advanced glenohumeral osteoarthritis. Presented at the 67th annual meeting of the American Academy of Orthopaedic Surgeons; Orlando, Fla; 2000.

10. McCarty LP 3rd, Cole BJ. Nonarthroplasty treatment of glenohumeral cartilage lesions. Arthroscopy 2005;21:1131-1142.

11. Parsons IM 4th, Weldon EJ 3rd, Titelman RM, Smith KL. Glenohumeral arthritis and its management. Phys Med Rehabil Clin N Am 2004;15:447-474.

12. Safran MR, Wolde-Tsadik G, Crawford D. Prospective outcome study of arthroscopic débridement of grade IV glenohumeral arthritis. Presented at the annual meeting of the American Academy of Orthopaedic Surgeons; Dallas, Texas; 2002.

13. Verma NN, Dunn W, Adler RS, et al. All-arthroscopic versus mini-open rotator cuff repair: a retrospective review with minimum 2-year follow-up. Arthroscopy 2006;22:587-594.

14. Weinstein DM, Bucchieri JS, Pollock RG, et al. Arthroscopic débridement of the shoulder for osteoarthritis. Arthroscopy 2000;16:471-476.

15. Wong KL, Williams GR. Complications of thermal capsulorrhaphy of the shoulder. J Bone Joint Surg Am 2001;83(suppl 2 pt 2):151-155.

CHAPTER 25

Arthroscopic Management of Shoulder Stiffness

Gregory P. Nicholson, MD

The diagnosis of shoulder stiffness, also termed frozen shoulder or adhesive capsulitis, is one of exclusion. It is a clinical syndrome characterized by painful restricted passive and active range of motion. It is associated with night pain and pain with activities.[1,5-7,11] This clinical entity has been difficult to classify and follows an unpredictable clinical course.[1,2,6,15] The pathophysiologic mechanism of the disease can include idiopathic, post-traumatic, and postsurgical etiologic factors and diabetes; it can even occur as a consequence of prolonged impingement syndrome.[7,10,11,16-18] It appears that susceptible shoulders respond to an insult in a common pathway of expression; this is glenohumeral synovitis. If this process continues unabated, the capsule will become thickened and disorganized in its collagen structure and actually become contracted.[3,13] The time course of the process and recovery is unpredictable. The true etiology, diagnostic criteria, pathophysiology, treatment methods, and natural history of this condition are under debate and investigation.[1,2,7,10-12,14,15,19] There are patients who do not respond to time, proper therapy, injections, or anti-inflammatory medications and are profoundly affected by the shoulder stiffness. These patients can be offered an arthroscopic capsular release.

Preoperative Considerations

History

The majority of patients with adhesive capsulitis of idiopathic etiology are women between the ages of 35 and 60 years. A history should be taken for other contributing factors, especially endocrine abnormalities such as diabetes and hypothyroidism. A history of trauma or surgery is important to note. A neurologic history is important to note for possible involvement of cervical disease. The type of prior surgical procedure on or around the shoulder is important, and a previous operative note can be helpful.

Physical Examination

Adhesive capsulitis, or frozen shoulder, is a limitation of motion without an obvious clinical reason for the loss of motion, such as arthritis or previous fracture of the shoulder. Thus, a comprehensive examination of the shoulder and cervical spine needs to be performed. The examiner should evaluate passive motion and active motion in forward elevation in the plane of the scapula, external rotation at the side, and internal rotation. In a stiff shoulder, internal rotation behind the back can be painful. It is helpful to evaluate internal rotation with the arm abducted in the scapular plane approximately 40 degrees and then let the forearm drop toward the floor. Thus, rotation can be evaluated and measured, and the early movement of the scapula is easily seen in those patients with posterior capsular involvement. The affected side should always be compared with the nonaffected side, and the shoulder girdle should be inspected for atrophy. Evaluation for acromioclavicular joint pain, impingement-type pain, and cervical radicular symptoms must be done. In this systematic fashion, the examiner can determine the motion planes that are involved and evaluate any contributing factors to the loss of motion and pain patterns.

It can be helpful to perform differential injections around the shoulder to determine pathologic locations and contributions. A subacromial injection of anesthetic can remove subacromial pain generators and allow the examiner to evaluate the shoulder with that area temporarily "eliminated." An injection in the glenohumeral joint itself can eliminate glenohumeral pain, thus allowing the examiner to evaluate shoulder motion again with pain eliminated. If the motion is remarkably improved, it may not be a true shoulder stiffness problem. Most times, however, the injections help the pain aspect, but the range of motion is not improved, confirming a diagnosis of stiffness.

Imaging

Plain radiographs evaluate conditions such as arthritis of the glenohumeral joint, calcific tendinitis, and subacromial impingement. A true anteroposterior view of the glenohumeral joint, an axillary view, and an outlet view should be performed.

Magnetic resonance imaging can evaluate for rotator cuff disease; but in a true adhesive capsulitis picture, magnetic resonance imaging will exclude other pathologic processes. Bone scan, computed tomographic scan, and electromyography are rarely necessary for the evaluation of frozen shoulder. Arthrography with limited joint volume was at one time thought to be a "gold standard" type of test,[6] but it is not necessary for the diagnosis of shoulder stiffness if a proper history and physical examination are performed.

Conservative Treatment

Conservative treatment should always be attempted. As mentioned previously, injections can relieve pain and facilitate therapy. The pathophysiologic process is that of glenohumeral inflammation. Corticosteroid injections into the glenohumeral joint can decrease the inflammatory response, relieve pain, and allow better motion. An oral steroid medication can also be administered. Gentle range of motion and stretching are instituted. Nonsteroidal antiinflammatory medication can be prescribed after or in conjunction with steroids. If the pain is relieved, most patients can accept the limitations of motion.[2,15] This allows more time to restore motion and function. A patient not responding to or becoming worse with a therapy program designed specifically for shoulder stiffness can be a candidate for arthroscopic capsular release.

Indications and Contraindications

Indications for Surgical Intervention

There are those patients who do not respond to conservative management. A recalcitrant frozen shoulder is one that has had symptoms for more than 4 months and has not responded to a surgeon-designed therapy program directed toward the diagnosis of shoulder stiffness. This program should be given at least 6 weeks to show progress. If patients still have sleep disturbance, pain, and limitation of motion that affects their occupation, recreation, and sleep, it is time to consider an arthroscopic capsular release.[7-9] The etiology of the stiffness was not found to have a significant effect on the outcome of arthroscopic capsular release; thus, it is equally effective across causes.[7]

Contraindications for an Arthroscopic Capsular Release

If the patient has motion loss and a shoulder prosthesis in place, an open approach may be preferred. If there is motion loss and a history of an open instability repair that used a subscapularis shortening procedure, an open approach may be preferred.

Surgical Technique

Anesthesia and Positioning

By definition, there is restricted range of motion of the shoulder; thus, there is small joint volume, and small movements can help intra-articular exposure. For this reason, the preference is for the beach chair position with the arm free. The lateral position with the arm in traction will restrict the ability to rotate the shoulder during the procedure, and traction will not open up the contracted joint. A combined anesthetic technique, such as a light general anesthetic with a scalene regional block for intraoperative and postoperative pain relief, is preferred. If the patient is going to be admitted for therapy, an indwelling scalene catheter can be used for prolonged pain control. The surgeon should choose the best option on the basis of the patient and the experience of the anesthesia and surgical team.

The patient is placed in the beach chair position with a small towel roll under the medial border of the scapula. The landmarks of the scapular spine, acromion, and coracoid are marked after standard preparation and draping. An assessment of motion is made under anesthesia (Fig. 25-1). No manipulation is performed at this time because it would cause bleeding within the glenohumeral joint and make for a more difficult procedure.

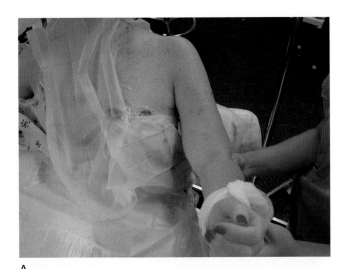

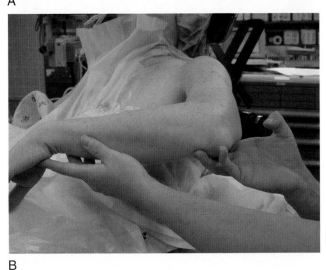

Figure 25-1 Preoperative assessment of range of motion in a left shoulder in the beach chair position under anesthesia. **A,** External rotation is markedly limited at the side to only approximately 10 degrees. **B,** Internal rotation with the arm in 40 degrees of abduction in the scapular plane reveals that the forearm falls only to parallel to the floor. This represents approximately 20 degrees of internal rotation motion.

Box 25-1 Surgical Steps

1. Limited synovectomy
2. Rotator interval and anterosuperior release
3. Inferior release
4. Portal change and posterior superior release
5. Gentle manipulation

25

devices have been used to perform the capsular release, including monopolar devices, basket cutters, and shavers.[4,7-12,14,17] A combination of release tools can be used, depending on the surgeon's preference.

Specific Steps (Box 25-1)

1. Limited Synovectomy

After motion assessment, the glenohumeral joint is insufflated with saline with an 18-gauge spinal needle from the posterior portal. The posterior portal is placed approximately 2 cm medial and inferior to the posterolateral corner of the acromion. A stab wound is made at this spot, and the blunt obturator for the arthroscopic sheath is introduced into the joint. The joint is contracted and the capsule is thickened. The tip of the scope sheath is aimed at the superior aspect of the glenoid toward the long head of biceps origin. This will allow the arthroscopic sheath to enter a more open area of the joint and avoid articular cartilage damage.

The arthroscope is connected, and visualization of the arthroscopic triangle is achieved. The arthroscopic triangle formed by the long head of the biceps tendon, the glenoid, and the top of the subscapularis tendon is typically contracted and involved with a red, gelatinous synovitis (Fig. 25-2). The spinal needle is inserted anteriorly just lateral to the tip of the coracoid and into the arthroscopic triangle. A stab wound is made anteriorly, and a smooth cannula is placed into the joint through the arthroscopic triangle. Fluid flow will allow visualization. The shaver is brought in to débride the accessible synovitis. This gelatinous synovium is easily débrided without significant bleeding. At this point, the smooth cannula is removed and the ArthroWand is brought in anteriorly down the track created by the cannula. There is no need to attempt to bring the device through the cannula because it will restrict mobility.

2. Rotator Interval and Anterosuperior Release

The arthroscopic capsular release must begin superiorly and proceed inferiorly, thus "unzipping" the shoulder. The cautery device begins the release just below the biceps tendon in the rotator interval (Fig. 25-3). The "base" of the

Equipment and Instruments

The surgeon's knowledge of the chosen pump is underrated but important. Proper fluid management during the case facilitates a clear field and prevents unnecessary swelling. It is helpful to use a 1 : 300,000 dilution of epinephrine in the fluid, which helps decrease bleeding. My preference for the release instrument is the ArthroWand bipolar cautery device (ArthroCare, Sunnyvale, Calif). The 3.5-mm, 90-degree (non–turbo vac) model allows a 3.5-mm swath of tissue to be cut without bleeding. It is a stiff instrument that allows the surgeon to cut and to manipulate the tissue by both pushing away and pulling back toward the portal. The right angle at the tip allows the surgeon to cut into tissue and around corners. Other

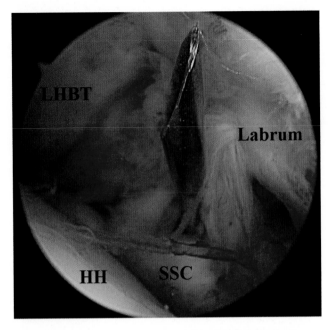

Figure 25-2 The initial arthroscopic view of the contracted arthroscopic triangle in a left shoulder. A spinal needle is in the middle of the interval. Note the gelatinous synovitis over the biceps and anterior capsule. HH, humeral head; LHBT, long head of biceps tendon; SSC, subscapularis tendon.

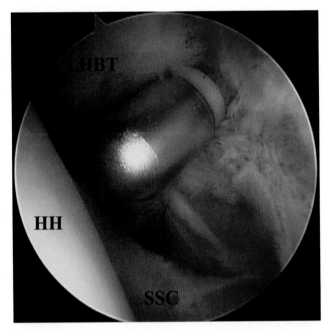

Figure 25-3 The ArthroWand device begins the release at the biceps root. The tip is turned into the tissue. The release will be carried down the glenoid rim in an extralabral fashion. HH, humeral head; LHBT, long head of biceps tendon; SSC, subscapularis tendon.

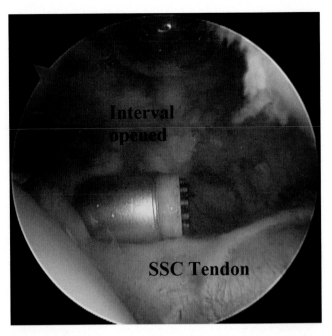

Figure 25-4 The left shoulder, viewing from the posterior portal after release of the rotator interval. The subscapularis (SSC) tendon is clearly visible, and the triangle size is larger. The interval release allows improved external rotation and the ability to continue the release inferiorly.

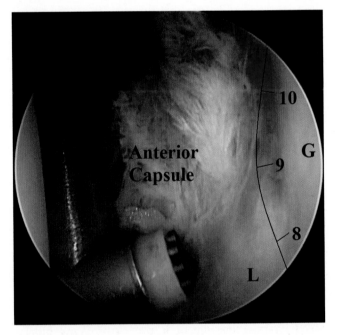

Figure 25-5 In this left shoulder, the arthroscope is moved inferiorly and the ArthroWand begins to release the anterior capsule. The tip of the cautery device is turned into the tissue. G, glenoid; L, labrum. An advantage of the ArthroWand is its stiffness, allowing the surgeon to cut the tissue by either pulling back toward or pushing away from the portal entry site.

triangle is released and then carried across the top of the subscapularis tendon (Fig. 25-4). This provides mobility to proceed inferiorly. An extralabral capsular release is performed (Fig. 25-5). The thickened capsule is cut or released by the cautery device. Mobility and visualization in the inferior aspect of the joint improve as the release continues from superior to inferior down the anterior capsule (Fig. 25-6).

3. Inferior Release

As the ArthroWand cautery device gets down inferiorly (from the 5- to 7-o'clock position), the device is turned facing superiorly to cut the capsule (Fig. 25-7) while preventing injury to the axillary nerve. The device is also kept along the rim of the glenoid; drifting away from the glenoid rim can endanger the axillary nerve.

4. Posterior Superior Release

Once the 5- or 6-o'clock position is reached, the arthroscope is switched to the anterior portal and the cautery device to the posterior portal. The capsular release is now repeated from superior to inferior and extralabral, but along the posterior capsule (Fig. 25-8). The region above the biceps origin, the posterosuperior recess, should be addressed and released if it is found to be contracted. This capsular area can restrict the excursion of the supraspinatus tendon unit.

After the capsule has been circumferentially released, the subacromial space is evaluated. In patients with previous surgery or impingement, the subacromial space can be involved, in which case[7-9,11,18] any adhesions should be débrided and an acromioplasty performed. If the patient has developed acromioclavicular joint pain during the stiffness process, it should be addressed at this time.

5. Gentle Manipulation

Finally, the shoulder is put through a gentle manipulation. A sequence of forward elevation in the plane of the scapula, external rotation at the side, abduction, and internal rotation is performed holding the proximal humerus, thus lowering the moment arm and decreasing the risk of a

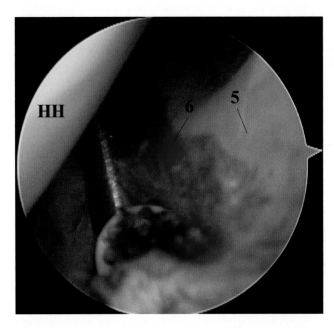

Figure 25-7 The cautery has stayed along the glenoid (G) and released the capsule down around and beyond the 6-o'clock position. HH, humeral head.

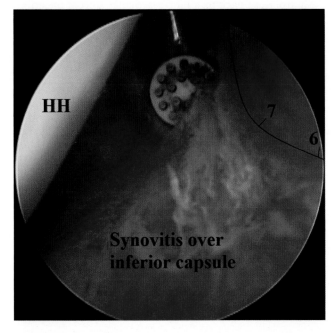

Figure 25-6 As the release reaches the 7-o'clock position (5-o'clock in a right shoulder), the cautery tip is turned up, facing away from the axillary nerve. The bipolar device can still cut the capsule or debulk it in this method. Note the extensive red synovitis on the inferior capsule. HH, humeral head.

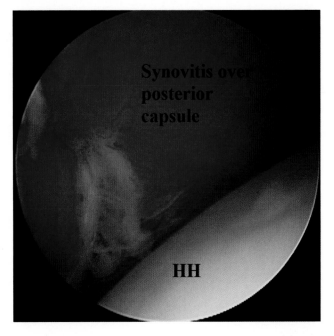

Figure 25-8 The arthroscope is now in the anterior portal looking posteriorly in this left shoulder. The posterior capsule is thickened and covered with the typical synovitis material seen in adhesive capsulitis. The posterior capsule will be released in a fashion similar to the anterior capsule. HH, humeral head.

humerus fracture. A few soft releases may be felt, representing the last few contractures being lysed. This is not a true manipulation. The capsular release provides for a controlled, bloodless, atraumatic manipulation with this range of motion at the end of the procedure (Fig. 25-9).

Postoperative Considerations

The majority of patients are admitted for a 24-hour stay to allow physical therapy while the scalene regional block is in effect. This provides an opportunity for pain-free motion exercises. It also shows the patients that motion has been restored and can be achieved without pain. This is a big psychological step for many patients who have battled pain, poor motion, and dysfunction for a prolonged time. If the surgeon elects in-hospital treatment in this fashion, it is recommended to try to schedule the case early in the morning, so that the therapist can see the patient while the block is still in effect. Analgesics and nonsteroidal anti-inflammatory medications are routinely prescribed to control pain and inflammation. I have used a derotation sling and wedge (Apex sling; EBI Inc., Parsippany, NJ) to place the shoulder in a neutral position and avoid the internally rotated position typically seen with a traditional sling.

Outpatient therapy emphasizing motion for forward elevation, external rotation, and internal rotation is performed 3 days a week for 3 weeks, then 2 days a week for 3 weeks more. Patients are to perform daily range-of-motion exercises at home for 20 to 30 minutes, three times a day. Isometric strength and resistive strength exercises are not prescribed until motion is pain free, flexible, and consistent, approximately after 6 to 8 weeks. The time to final pain-free range of motion is approximately 6 to 10 weeks.[7,14,17,19] The need for home continuous passive motion therapy is rare, but it should be considered in those patients who may be at higher risk for slow progress, such as diabetic patients with profound motion loss (external rotation at side less than 0 degrees) and those for whom a previous stiffness procedure (manipulation or release procedure) has failed.

Pitfalls and Complications

The goal is a balanced capsular release. This cannot be accomplished with manipulation alone. One of the pitfalls is to not accomplish the balanced release and to leave one of the areas not addressed. Thus, the surgeon should always assess and address the anterior, inferior, and posterior capsular regions. The interval should always be released and the subacromial space evaluated. Even with good technique, I have found that approximately 20% of patients will develop a transient decrease in motion 3 to 5 weeks after the procedure. The shoulder motion becomes less flexible and can actually become "rubbery" and painful. This is an inflammatory flare-up and has been described by other authors.[7,19] It should be recognized and the patient reassured and treated with patience, anti-inflammatory medication, and, if it is not contraindicated, either a Medrol dose pack or an intra-articular steroid injection. It will resolve in 3 to 6 weeks.

Other potential complications include injury to the axillary nerve, fracture of the humerus, damage to the joint surface, and recurrent stiffness. There is also the risk of complications from the scalene block. In my experience, the complication rate has been low, and no patient has developed recurrent stiffness after arthroscopic capsular release.

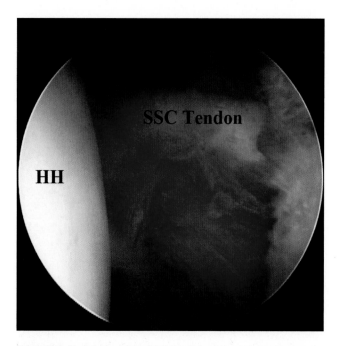

Figure 25-9 The left shoulder looking anteriorly after complete release and placement of the shoulder through a full range of motion. The subscapularis muscle belly is now seen with the shoulder in external rotation. The contracted capsule is no longer seen. HH, humeral head; SSC, subscapularis.

PEARLS

- This type of arthroscopy is technically challenging because of the contracted joint space. The surgeon must be patient.
- Knowledge of the pros and cons of the chosen pump system is critical to visualization and success.
- The use of the ArthroWand bipolar cautery device allows a bloodless capsular release. It also ablates a 3.5-mm section of capsule. The right angle allows the device to cut through the thickened capsule completely.
- The goal is a balanced release of the capsule, and thus a circumferential extralabral release is recommended.
- Stiff shoulder can be initiated by or maintained by the capsule, the interval, or the subacromial space.
- The capsular release technique as described allows the surgeon to address all areas of potential pathologic change.

Results

Arthroscopic capsular release has shown the ability to consistently restore range of motion, to improve shoulder function, and to relieve pain for a variety of shoulder stiffness causes (Table 25-1 and Fig. 25-10).[4,7,10-12,14,16-19] It has the potential to shorten the natural history of this still not fully understood clinical entity. Reports on outcomes have shown a time to achieve final pain-free range of motion between 6 and 10 weeks. The time in formal therapy has averaged 2.5 months. The recurrence of stiffness has not been seen. The average improvement in range of motion has been 73 degrees for forward elevation, 44 degrees in external rotation, and 8 spinal segments in internal rotation. The etiology of the stiffness did not have an effect on motion, pain, or satisfaction of the patient. Diabetic frozen shoulder did show a trend toward a longer time to achieve final range of motion but had significant improvement in motion, pain, and function.[7]

Table 25-1 Results of Arthroscopic Capsular Release

Author	Follow-up	Results
Watson et al[19] (2000)	12 months	8 of 73 patients had recurrence of pain or stiffness Final motion averaged 90% of contralateral side
Harryman et al[4] (1997)	Average of 33 months (12-56 months)	3 of 30 patients had recurrence of shoulder stiffness Final motion averaged 93% of contralateral side
Warner et al[17] (1996)	Average of 39 months (24-64 months)	23 patients with average improvement of 48 points in the Constant score Motion returned to within 7 degrees of contralateral side
Segmuller et al[14] (1995)	13.5 months	76% of 24 patients (26 shoulders) returned to near-normal motion 88% of patients very satisfied with procedure

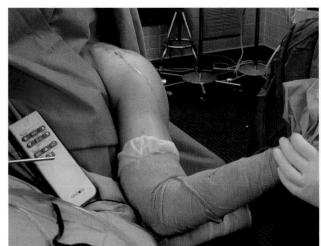

A

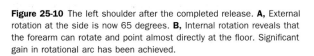

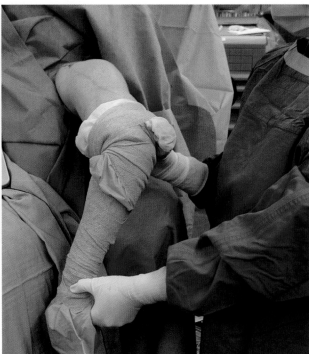

B

Figure 25-10 The left shoulder after the completed release. **A,** External rotation at the side is now 65 degrees. **B,** Internal rotation reveals that the forearm can rotate and point almost directly at the floor. Significant gain in rotational arc has been achieved.

References

1. Grey RG. The natural history of "idiopathic" frozen shoulder. J Bone Joint Surg Am 1978;60:564.

2. Griggs SM, Ahn A, Green A. Idiopathic "adhesive capsulitis": a prospective functional outcome study of non-operative treatment. J Bone Joint Surg Am 2000;82:1398-1407.

3. Hannafin JA, DiCarlo EF, Wickiewicz TL. Adhesive capsulitis: capsular fibroplasia of the glenohumeral joint. J Shoulder Elbow Surg 1994;3:S5.

4. Harryman DT, Matsen FA, Sidles JA. Arthroscopic management of refractory shoulder stiffness. Arthroscopy 1997;13:133-147.

5. Murnaghan JP. Frozen shoulder. In Rockwood CA, Matsen FA, eds. The Shoulder, vol 2. Philadelphia, WB Saunders, 1993:837-861.

6. Neviaser RJ, Neviaser TJ. Frozen shoulder: diagnosis and management. Clin Orthop 1987;223:59-64.

7. Nicholson GP. Arthroscopic capsular release for stiff shoulders. Effect of etiology on outcomes. Arthroscopy 2003;19:40-49.

8. Nicholson GP. Adhesive capsulitis. Manipulation or arthroscopic capsular division. In Barber FA, Fischer SP, eds. Surgical Techniques for the Shoulder and Elbow. New York, Thieme, 2003:127-130.

9. Nicholson GP, Ticker JB. Arthroscopic capsular release. In Imhoff AB, Ticker JB, Fu F, eds. Atlas of Shoulder Arthroscopy. London, Martin Dunitz, 2003:343-351.

10. Ogilivie-Harris DJ, Myerthall S. The diabetic frozen shoulder: arthroscopic release. Arthroscopy 1997;13:1-18.

11. Ozaki J, Nakagawa Y, Sukurai G, Tomai S. Recalcitrant chronic adhesive capsulitis of the shoulder. J Bone Joint Surg Am 1989;71: 1511-1515.

12. Pearsall AW, Osbahr DC, Speer KP. An arthroscopic technique for treating patients with frozen shoulder. Arthroscopy 1999;15: 2-11.

13. Rodeo SA, Hannafin JA, Tom J, et al. Immunolocalization of cytokines in adhesive capsulitis of the shoulder. J Orthop Res 1997;15:427-436.

14. Segmuller HE, Taylor DE, Hogan CS, et al. Arthroscopic treatment of adhesive capsulitis. J Shoulder Elbow Surg 1995;4:403-408.

15. Shaffer B, Tibone JE, Kerlan RK. Frozen shoulder: a long term follow-up. J Bone Joint Surg Am 1992;74:738-746.

16. Ticker JB, Beim GM, Warner JJP. Recognition and treatment of refractory posterior capsular contracture of the shoulder. Arthroscopy 2000;16:27-34.

17. Warner JJP, Allen A, Marks P, Wong P. Arthroscopic release of chronic refractory capsular contracture of the shoulder. J Bone Joint Surg Am 1996;78:1808-1816.

18. Warner JJP, Allen A, Marks PH, Wong P. Arthroscopic release of postoperative capsular contracture of the shoulder. J Bone Joint Surg Am 1997;79:1151-1158.

19. Watson L, Dalziel R, Story I. Frozen shoulder: a 12-month clinical outcome trial. J Shoulder Elbow Surg 2000;9:16-22.

CHAPTER 26

Arthroscopic and Open Management of Scapulothoracic Disorders

Kevin M. Doulens, MD

John E. Kuhn, MD

Knowledge about the interplay of structures and biomechanics surrounding the scapula and its role in shoulder motion is evolving steadily. The result is that our understanding of shoulder disease is also increasing. It is becoming clear that processes affecting the scapula in turn greatly influence the function of the shoulder.[8] Conditions of the scapulothoracic articulation can be broadly divided into four main disease processes: bursitis, crepitus, dyskinesis, and winging. Each of these is a unique entity, but they are often seen in combination.

Scapulothoracic bursitis presents as posterior shoulder pain with range of motion. The patient can often localize the pain under the scapula. There are two major bursae that are consistently identified, the infraserratus bursa between the serratus and the chest wall and the supraserratus bursa between the subscapularis and the serratus (Fig. 26-1). In addition, four minor adventitial bursae have been described.[9] Clinically significant bursitis tends to affect two areas most commonly—the superior medial angle and the inferior angle. The bursae at these locations are minor adventitious bursae that may become apparent only when they are inflamed. Through a process that is similar to subacromial bursitis, repetitive motion of the scapula over the rib cage causes inflammation and edema in the bursae. As with other types of bursitis, this process can be initially treated with rehabilitation and judicious corticosteroid injections. This is often sufficient to quiet the process and relieve the patient's symptoms. On occasion, the bursitis is refractory to medical management, and surgical intervention in the form of a bursectomy is required.

Scapular crepitus is a process whereby palpable and often audible noises are generated under the scapula. Of significance in this process is that not all crepitus is painful or pathologic, and the volume of the noise does not correlate with the severity of the pain. Crepitus ranges from mild, painless subscapular crunching to painless but loud snapping and from minimal discomfort to disabling pain. In most patients, symptomatic scapulothoracic crepitus is associated with bursitis.

Winging of the scapula is a finding that may result from many causes. In athletes, winging is typically seen as an isolated palsy of the serratus due to a long thoracic nerve neurapraxic injury. Winging may also be seen with profound scapular bursitis or may manifest as part of scapular dyskinesis. Scapular dyskinesis is defined as abnormal motion of the scapula characterized by medial border or inferior angle prominence, early excessive scapular elevation and shrugging, or rapid downward rotation during lowering of the arm.[8] A static abnormality of scapular position, called the SICK scapula, probably represents a more severe state of this condition.[2] Whereas dyskinesis is likely to be the most common finding in the athlete with shoulder pain, it is best treated with appropriate rehabilitation and will not be explored in detail in this chapter. Winging due to bursitis typically resolves with treatment of bursitis. Winging due to long thoracic nerve injury resolves spontaneously in most athletes; when it persists, surgical intervention can be considered.

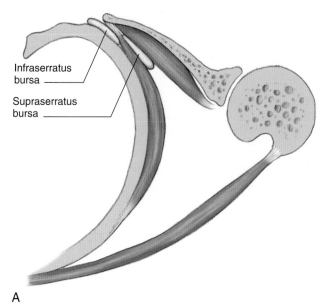

A

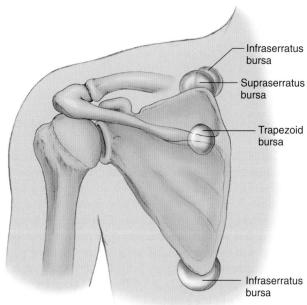

B

Figure 26-1 Bursae about the scapula. A number of bursae have been described about the scapula, including the two major bursae (infraserratus and supraserratus) and the four minor or adventitial bursae. (Redrawn from Kuhn JE, Hawkins RJ. Evaluation and treatment of scapular disorders. In Warner JJP, Iannotti JP, Gerber C, eds. Complex and Revision Problems in Shoulder Surgery. Philadelphia, Lippincott-Raven, 1997:357-375.)

Preoperative Considerations

History

Many scapulothoracic conditions in athletes are related to other pathologic processes in the shoulder, and as such, the history should include a thorough orthopedic review of systems. A typical history of the patient with a scapulothoracic disorder includes the following:

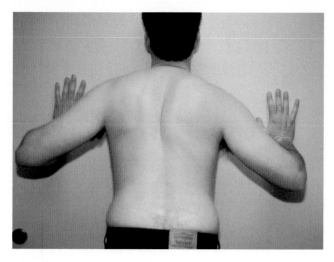

Figure 26-2 Winging of the scapula. Winging can be accentuated by pushing off from a wall or by resisting forward elevation.

- Pain with activity greater than pain at rest
- Painful crepitus
- Increased pain on carrying or lifting objects away from the body
- Pain at the superior angle of the scapula
- Pain near other scapulothoracic muscles

Physical Examination

The physical examination for scapulothoracic disorders requires the physician to stand behind the patient, who is disrobed or wearing a sports bra. The scapular position at rest should be noted. A scapula that is depressed, anteriorly tilted, and internally rotated suggests a SICK scapula and typically has tenderness at the pectoralis minor insertion on the coracoid.[2] Patients are asked to elevate and then lower the arms while the physician looks for dyskinesis. Crepitus can be heard, and the location of crepitus (superomedial angle or inferior angle) frequently can be determined by careful palpation. Provocative testing to elicit winging can be performed by having the patient push off from the wall or elevate the arms against resistance (Fig. 26-2).

Imaging

Radiography

Radiographs are helpful to find subscapular bone prominences (Fig. 26-3) and include the following views:

- True anteroposterior view
- Axillary view
- Scapular Y view (Fig. 26-3A).

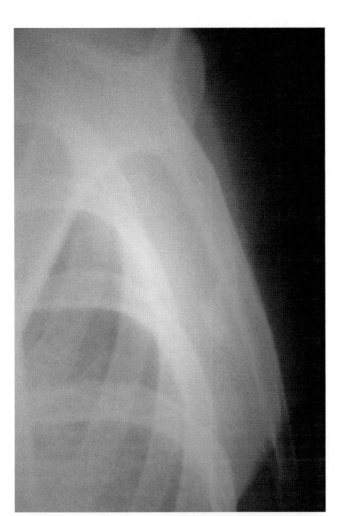

A

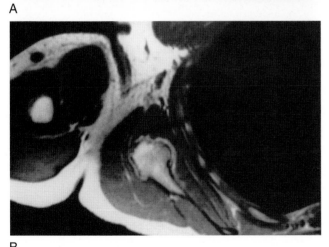

B

Figure 26-3 Subscapular bone prominences associated with scapulothoracic disorders. The osteochondroma **(A)** is the most common tumor of the scapula. The corresponding magnetic resonance image demonstrates reactive bursal tissue with high signal around the osteochondroma **(B)**.

Other Modalities

Magnetic resonance imaging and computed tomographic scans are usually not necessary but can be helpful in identifying soft tissue and bone lesions (Fig. 26-3B).

Electromyography

If winging of the scapula is thought to be of neurologic origin, electromyography will assist in the diagnosis. Serial studies every 3 to 4 months can document recovery of an injured long thoracic nerve.

Indications and Contraindications

Most scapulothoracic problems in athletes are not treated surgically. Rehabilitation focused on pectoralis minor stretching, serratus and lower trapezius strengthening, posterior capsule stretching, and core strengthening will treat the SICK scapula and scapular dyskinesis.[2] Patients with scapular bursitis and milder forms of crepitus will often respond to similar rehabilitation and the judicious use of corticosteroid injections. By mixing steroid and local anesthetic, injections can be therapeutic and diagnostic, perhaps giving an indication of potential postsurgical results. Athletes with long thoracic nerve injury can be monitored for many months with serial electromyography as the nerve typically recovers spontaneously, occasionally taking up to 2 years. Bracing may help with symptom relief while the nerve recovers. In patients for whom nonoperative approaches fail, surgery may be considered for these conditions.

There are no absolute contraindications to surgery of the scapula; however, physicians must be cautious of the patient with less than obvious pathologic changes, the patient with questionable responses to therapy and injection, and the patient who may have a voluntary component to the complaint. Scapulothoracic crepitus often exists without symptoms. In addition, some patients who have secondary gain develop voluntary scapular winging. Patients with secondary gain, unrecognized scapular dyskinesis, and voluntary winging will have predictably poor postsurgical outcomes.

Surgical Technique: Bursectomy and Partial Scapulectomy

Anesthesia and Positioning

Positioning of the patient is similar for both bursectomy and partial scapulectomy. The prone position is used, often with a bolster under the lateral chest to cause the rib cage to rise and the shoulder to fall forward, thereby making the scapula more prominent. The surgical preparation should extend from C5 to L1 and include the entire back and the arm of the involved side.

Specific Steps

Bursectomy (Box 26-1)

Scapulothoracic bursectomy can be performed in an open or an endoscopic fashion. The open procedure has a distinct advantage in that it allows direct visualization of adventitial bursae whose position and plane of dissection might be anatomically variable.

In the open procedure for a superior medial bursectomy, the incision is placed medial to the superior vertebral border of the scapula. The trapezius is split in line with its fibers, and the levator scapulae and rhomboids are exposed. The levator and rhomboids are then incised off of the medial border of the scapula in a subperiosteal fashion. A plane is then developed between the serratus anterior under the scapula and the chest wall. The thickened bursa can be dissected from this space. The levator, rhomboids, and trapezius are then reapproximated to the scapula, and the skin is closed. Postoperatively, the patient uses a sling for comfort and begins passive physical therapy immediately. Once the periscapular muscles have healed adequately at approximately 3 to 4 weeks, active motion is initiated. Strengthening can begin at 12 weeks. For symptomatic inferior angle bursae, the incision can be made along the inferior medial border just distal to the angle. The trapezius and then the latissimus dorsi are split in line with their fibers, allowing direct access to the inferior angle and the bursa. After the bursa is excised, the muscles are reapproximated and skin is closed. Postoperative care and rehabilitation are the same.

The endoscopic approach to scapulothoracic bursitis involves the use of two or three portals to access the subscapular space.[11] The patient may be positioned in either the prone or lateral position. All portals must be kept at least 2 cm medial to the medial border of the scapula to prevent injury to the dorsal scapular nerve (Fig. 26-4). The first portal is inserted medial to the scapula and midway between the scapular spine and the inferior angle. Insufflation of the infraspinatus bursa with injection will help identify the plane of surgery. The blunt obturator and endoscope can then be inserted into the bursa. The second portal can be either superior or inferior, depending on the location of the pathologic process. The superior portal is made, once again at least 2 cm medial to the medial border of the scapula at the level of the scapular spine. This will allow access to the superior medial angle. If required, a third portal can be made at the inferior angle of the scapula in a similar fashion to access the inferior portion.[15] In all these portals, landmarks are few, and hemostasis is critical to allow adequate visualization. Once the bursectomy is performed, the portals are closed and the patient is placed into a sling. Activity is performed as tolerated.

Partial Scapulectomy (Box 26-2)

Painful scapulothoracic crepitus and its most dramatic presentation, the snapping scapula, are both treated with a partial scapulectomy when conservative measures fail. The pathologic lesion is generally at the superior medial angle, and so excision of this corner of the scapula is often

Box 26-1 Bursectomy, Open or Arthroscopic

- Skin incision medial to scapula.
- Levator and rhomboids dissected subperiosteally off medial scapula (open only).
- Plane between subscapularis and chest wall developed and bursae resected.
- Muscles reapproximated to scapula and skin closed.

Box 26-2 Surgical Steps: Scapulectomy

Partial scapulectomy

- The skin is incised.
- The trapezius is split and dissected from the spine of the scapula.
- The superomedial angle is dissected free.
- The superomedial angle is resected with a saw.
- The medial border of the supraspinatus is repaired to the rhomboid-serratus-subscapularis flap, and the inferior border and trapezius are repaired to bone.

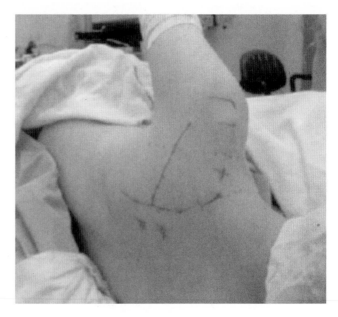

Figure 26-4 Endoscopic portals for scapulothoracic bursectomy. (From Pavlik A, Ang K, Coghlan J, Bell S. Arthroscopic treatment of painful snapping of the scapula by using a new superior portal. Arthroscopy 2003;19:608-612.)

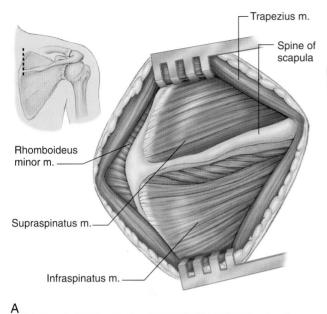

Trapezius m.

Spine of scapula

Rhomboideus minor m.

Supraspinatus m.

Infraspinatus m.

A

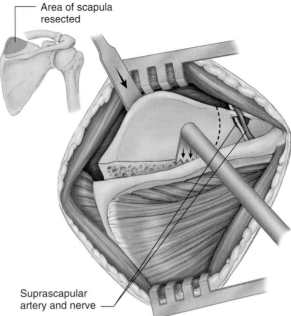

Area of scapula resected

Suprascapular artery and nerve

B

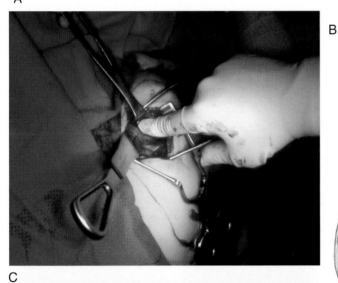

C

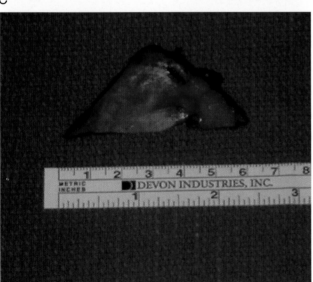

DEVON INDUSTRIES, INC.

D

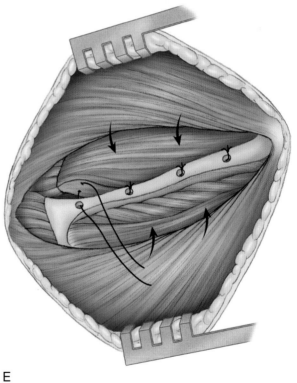

E

26

Figure 26-5 Partial scapulectomy. **A,** The skin incision is made in Langer's lines, and the trapezius is dissected from the spine of the scapula. **B,** The superomedial angle is resected after it has been dissected in a subperiosteal fashion in the plane between supraspinatus and the rest of the scapular muscles. **C,** An acromial retractor is placed between the subscapularis and the scapula, and the superomedial angle is cut with a saw. **D,** The resected superomedial angle is triangular with a base of about 5 cm. **E,** The medial border of the supraspinatus is repaired to the rhomboid-serratus-subscapularis flap, and the inferior border and trapezius are repaired to bone. (**A, B,** and **E** redrawn from Kuhn JE, Hawkins RJ. Evaluation and treatment of scapular disorders. In Warner JJP, Iannotti JP, Gerber C, eds. Complex and Revision Problems in Shoulder Surgery. Philadelphia, Lippincott-Raven 1997:357-375.)

successful at relieving symptoms. As in the bursitis procedures, the patient is placed prone.

The incision is placed along the medial border of the scapula from the level of the scapular spine inferiorly to the superomedial angle (Fig. 26-5). The skin is elevated in a subcutaneous plane, exposing the spine of the scapula laterally. The trapezius is split in line with its fibers and elevated from the spine of the scapula, and the plane between the undersurface of the trapezius and the supraspinatus is developed. Starting along the spine, the supraspinatus is then dissected free from medial to lateral in a subperiosteal fashion until the edge of the scapular notch can be palpated. It is important to not extend farther lateral as damage to the suprascapular nerve and artery can occur. Starting once again along the medial border, the levator and rhomboids are elevated off subperiosteally. With the superior medial border exposed, the dissection is carried subperiosteally around the border and under the scapula to peel the serratus and subscapularis off the bone. This is most easily done with a Cobb elevator. Once both sides of the scapula have been exposed, the superior corner can be resected. This cut is made with an oscillating saw and runs from the base of the scapular spine to approximately 4 or 5 cm lateral along the superior edge of the scapula. Once again, care must be taken to not disturb the contents of the scapular notch. With the superior medial angle resected, the plane between the supraspinatus and the combined muscle flap are sutured together with No. 2 permanent suture. The trapezius is secured to the spine of the scapula. Skin is closed, and the patient is placed into a sling.

Passive range of motion can begin immediately. Active exercises start at 6 weeks, and strengthening begins at 12 weeks.

Scapular Winging

Operative treatment of scapular winging for patients whose therapy fails and who remain symptomatic is an attempt to restore stability in the face of a known deficiency. Because restoration of normal anatomy is not possible, these surgeries will have varying degrees of success and probably will not be able to return athletes to high levels of function.

Transfer of the sternal head of the pectoralis major muscle is the most popular therapy for permanent serratus anterior palsy (Fig. 26-6). For this procedure, the patient is placed in the lateral decubitus position. Either one or two incisions can be used. For a single incision, it is made across the axilla from the border of the pectoralis major anteriorly to the inferior angle of the scapula. The sternocostal head lies under the clavicular head at the insertion into the humerus. The sternocostal head is released and redirected back toward the inferior tip of the scapula. Because this muscle alone is generally not long enough to reach without excessive tensioning, an autologous fascia lata or hamstring tendon graft from the ipsilateral leg is harvested. The fascia lata graft is tubularized and sewn into the end of the pectoralis major tendon. The distal tip of the scapula is then cleared of soft tissues, and a small hole is made in the tip. The fascia lata graft is then passed through the hole and sutured back onto itself. Enough tension is applied so that the end of the pectoralis tendon is in contact with the scapula.

The patient is placed into a sling, and postoperative passive range of motion is begun immediately. Active motion is begun at 6 weeks, and strengthening begins at 12 weeks.

Postoperative Considerations

Rehabilitation

The patient is kept in immobilization for up to 6 weeks after muscle transfer or fascial sling reconstructions. Passive therapy is begun immediately to avoid stiffness, and active motion is allowed at week 6. After these procedures, strengthening rehabilitation is begun around 12 weeks.

Complications

Any surgery that involves dissection under the scapula has the potential for chest wall complications, most notably pneumothorax. Postoperative radiographs will help identify any involvement of the lungs. Incisions and portals made midline to the medial border of the scapula can lead to dorsal scapular nerve injury. Splitting of the trapezius does not interfere with its innervation. If the superomedial angle of the scapula is resected too far laterally, the suprascapular nerve and artery are at risk.

PEARLS AND PITFALLS

Partial Scapulectomy

- A superior-inferior incision gives better access and is in Langer's lines, leaving a nicer scar.
- When the muscles from the superior angle are dissected, a towel clip in the spine can draw the scapula out of the wound to improve visualization.
- A broad blunt retractor placed between the scapula and subscapularis muscle will protect the muscle when the saw is used to remove the bone.
- Before cutting the bone, palpate to be certain that you are not near the scapular notch.

Pectoralis Transfer for Scapular Winging

- Work near the humerus carefully to dissect the sternal head from the clavicular head of the pectoralis. The sternal head is more superior and lies behind the clavicular head.
- In making the hole in the scapula for the tendon, make certain that the hole is placed only in the thin membrane-like bone and does not violate the thicker peripheral bone.
- The scapula must be positioned so the edge of the native pectoralis tendon meets the scapula bone. This allows better healing and may prevent stretching of the graft that is used primarily for augmentation.

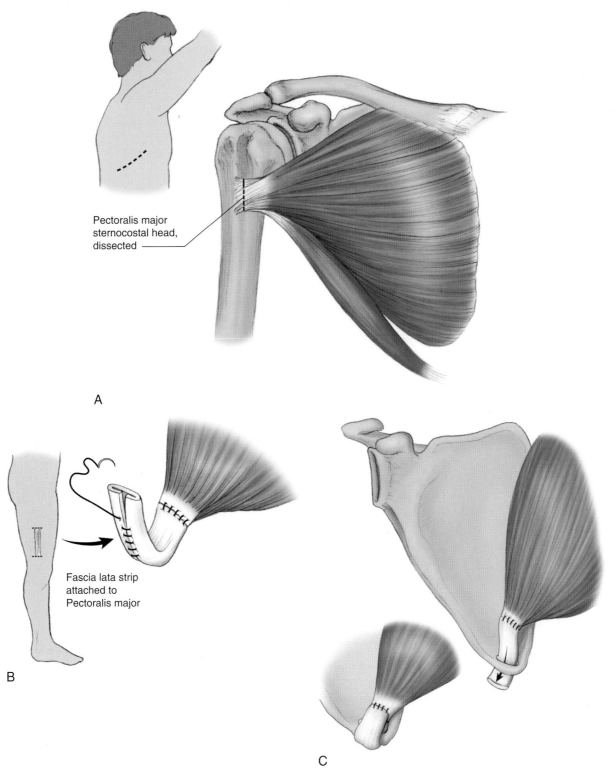

Pectoralis major sternocostal head, dissected

A

B

Fascia lata strip attached to Pectoralis major

C

Figure 26-6 Pectoralis major transfer for serratus anterior palsy. (Redrawn from Kuhn JE, Plancher KD, Hawkins RJ. Scapular winging. J Am Acad Orthop Surg 1995;3:319-325.)

Table 26-1 Results of Scapulothoracic Bursectomy*

Author	N and Technique	Outcome
Ciullo and Jones[3] (1993)	13 arthroscopic bursectomy	100% return to preinjury activity
McCluskey and Bigliani[12] (1991)	9 open bursectomy	89% good–excellent
Nicholson and Duckworth[13] (2002)	17 open bursectomy	100% relief of pain
Sisto and Jobe[17] (1986)	4 open bursectomy	4/4 return to professional pitching

*All are level 4 case series.

Table 26-2 Results of Partial Scapulectomy for Scapulothoracic Crepitus*

Author	N and Technique	Outcome
Arntz and Matsen[1] (1990)	12 patients, 14 shoulders	86% complete relief
Harper et al[6] (1999)	7 arthroscopic resections	6 successful, 1 failure
Lehtinen et al[11] (2004)	6 open, 6 combined open and scope, 2 scope, 2 bursectomy	13/16 (81%) satisfied
Pavlik et al[15] (2003)	10 arthroscopic resections	4 excellent, 5 good, 1 fair
Richards and McKee[16] (1989)	3 open resections	100% success in pain relief

*All reports are level 4 case series.

Table 26-3 Results of Pectoralis Major Transfers for Serratus Anterior Palsy*

Author	N	Outcome
Connor et al[4] (1997)	11 pectoralis transfers	10/11 satisfactory
Gozna and Harris[5] (1979)	3 pectoralis transfers	3/3 successful
Iceton and Harris[7] (1987)	15 pectoralis transfers	9 satisfactory, 2 fair, 4 failures
Noerdlinger et al[14] (2002)	15 pectoralis transfers	2 excellent, 5 good, 4 fair, 4 poor
Steinmann and Wood[17] (2003)	9 pectoralis transfers	4 excellent, 2 good, 3 poor

*All reports are level 4 case series.

Results

The results of these different procedures vary (Tables 26-1 to 26-3). Bursectomy and partial scapulectomy are surgeries with high success rates and satisfaction of patients. Muscle transfers and sling procedures have lower and less predictable results but may still be beneficial to the patient in terms of pain relief and improved function.

References

1. Arntz CT, Matsen FA III. Partial scapulectomy for disabling scapulothoracic snapping. Orthop Trans 1990;14:252-253.
2. Burkhart SS, Morgan CD, Kibler WB. The disabled throwing shoulder: spectrum of pathology. Part III: the SICK scapula, scapular dyskinesis, the kinetic chain, and rehabilitation. Arthroscopy 2003;19:641-661.
3. Ciullo JV, Jones E. Subscapular bursitis: conservative and endoscopic treatment of "snapping scapula" or "washboard syndrome." Orthop Trans 1992-1993;16:740.
4. Connor PM, Yamaguchi K, Manifold SG, et al. Split pectoralis major transfer for serratus anterior palsy. Clin Orthop 1997;341:134-142.
5. Gozna ER, Harris WR. Traumatic winging of the scapula. J Bone Joint Surg Am 1979;61:1230-1233.
6. Harper GD, McIlroy S, Bayley JI, Calvert PT. Arthroscopic partial resection of the scapula for snapping scapula: a new technique. J Shoulder Elbow Surg 1999;8:53-57.
7. Iceton J, Harris WR. Treatment of winged scapula by pectoralis major transfer. J Bone Joint Surg Br 1987;69:108-110.

8. Kibler WB, McMullen. Scapular dyskinesis and its relation to shoulder pain. J Am Acad Orthop Surg 2003;11:142-151.

9. Kuhn JE, Plancher KD, Hawkins RJ. Symptomatic scapulothoracic crepitus and bursitis. J Am Acad Orthop Surg 1998;6:267-273.

10. Kuhn JE, Plancher KD, Hawkins RJ. Scapular winging. J Am Acad Orthop Surg 1995;3:319-325.

11. Lehtinen JT, Macy JC, Cassinelli E, Warner JJP. The painful scapulothoracic articulation. Clin Orthop 2004;423:99-105.

12. McCluskey GM III, Bigliani LU. Surgical management of refractory scapulothoracic bursitis. Orthop Trans 1991;15:801.

13. Nicholson GP, Duckworth MA. Scapulothoracic bursectomy for snapping scapula syndrome. J Shoulder Elbow Surg 2002;11:80-85.

14. Noerdlinger MA, Cole BJ, Stewart M, Post M. Results of pectoralis major transfer with fascia lata autograft augmentation for scapula winging. J Shoulder Elbow Surg 2002;11:345-350.

15. Pavlik A, Ang K, Coghlan J, Bell S. Arthroscopic treatment of painful snapping of the scapula by using a new superior portal. Arthroscopy 2003;19:608-612.

16. Richards RR, McKee MD. Treatment of painful scapulothoracic crepitus by resection of the superomedial angle of the scapula: a report of three cases. Clin Orthop 1989;247:111-116.

17. Sisto DJ, Jobe FW. The operative treatment of scapulothoracic bursitis in professional pitchers. Am J Sports Med 1986;14:192-194.

18. Steinmann SP, Wood MB. Pectoralis major transfer for serratus anterior paralysis. J Shoulder Elbow Surg 2003;12:555-560.

26

CHAPTER 27

Proximal Biceps Tenodesis

Albert Tom, MD

Augustus D. Mazzocca, MD

Biceps tendinopathy rarely occurs in isolation. Rather, it is usually associated with a spectrum of concomitant shoulder disorders, including subacromial impingement, rotator cuff tears, biceps instability, and SLAP tears. A diligent work-up is essential for correct identification and treatment of these associated pathologic entities.

The role of the long head of the biceps tendon has been heavily debated in the literature. Electromyography literature and biomechanical cadaver studies provide evidence of a role as a secondary humeral head depressor[7,18]; this function appears more pronounced in the unstable shoulder.[1] Others, however, argue that the long head of the biceps tendon is a vestigial structure.

Although there is no clear consensus on the surgical treatment of symptomatic, refractory, isolated biceps tendinopathy, it is generally agreed that débridement is indicated for partial tears affecting 30% to 50% of the tendon substance.[1,3,19] Advocates of tenotomy base their approach on the benign natural history and good functional outcomes of traumatic biceps ruptures. However, complications such as cosmetic ("Popeye") deformity due to distal retraction of the muscle belly, supination weakness, and muscle spasm have led to the development of numerous tenodesis techniques.[5] Recent series have reported a 70% incidence of Popeye deformity and 38% incidence of elbow flexion fatigue with tenotomy alone.[13]

Arthroscopic biceps tenodesis techniques are plentiful in the literature (Table 27-1). Described techniques include proximal fixation with interference screws, suture anchors, and suturing to the conjoined tendon, rotator cuff, and even transverse humeral ligament. Interference screw tenodesis demonstrated failure loads before tendon migration that were three times higher than after tenotomy alone in a cadaver model.[21] Failure of proximal stabi-

lization has been attributed to the retention of diseased, inflamed, pain-generating tendon and synovium within the fixed confines of the intertubercular groove.[15] Securing the biceps tendon distal to the intertubercular groove with a subpectoral tenodesis approach removes the diseased tendon entirely and restores the proper biceps length-tension relationship to ensure optimal bicipital function. Biceps tenodesis is therefore recommended over biceps tenotomy for three reasons:

1. maintenance of the length-tension relationship of the biceps muscle by establishment of a new origin of biceps attachment at the appropriate length to prevent muscle atrophy;

2. maintenance of elbow flexion and supination strength for maximum elbow function; and

3. better cosmetic appearance.

Multiple biomechanical cadaver and animal studies have shown increased load to failure with biotenodesis techniques over suture anchor, keyhole, and tunnel techniques.[14] Our preferred surgical technique for the treatment of isolated biceps tendinopathy is an open subpectoral tenodesis with a biotenodesis screw,[10,11,17] which is discussed in this chapter.

Preoperative Considerations

History

A typical history includes the following:

- Anterior shoulder pain radiating to biceps muscle
- Pain that awakens the patient from sleep

Table 27-1 Studies of Arthroscopic Tenodesis Techniques

Author		Study	Results
Richards and Burkhart[16] (2005)	Biomechanical cadaver study Load to failure	7-mm biotenodesis screw vs. 2 Mitek GII anchors	7-mm biointerference screw: 233.5 ± 55.5 N 2 Mitek G2 anchors: 135.5 ± 37.8 N
Wolf et al[21] (2005)	Biomechanical cadaver study Load to failure	Tenodesis vs. tenotomy	Tenotomy: 110.7 N Tenodesis: 310.8 N
Ozalay et al[14] (2005)	Biomechanical cadaver study Load to failure	Tunnel vs. interference screw vs. suture anchor vs. keyhole	Tunnel: 229 ± 44.1 N Interference screw: 243.3 ± 72.4 N Suture anchor: 129.0 ± 16.6 N Keyhole: 101.4 ± 27.9 N
Jayamoorthy et al[5] (2004)	Biomechanical sheep study Load to failure	Keyhole vs. biointerference screw vs. metal interference screw	Keyhole: 303 N 8-mm biointerference screw: 234 N Metal interference screw: 201 N
Mazzocca et al[9] (2005)	Biomechanical cadaver study Load to failure and cyclic gap formation	Subpectoral bone tunnel (SBT) vs. arthroscopic suture anchor (SA) vs. subpectoral interference screw (SIS) vs. arthroscopic interference screw (AIS)	Cyclic gap formation: SBT: 9.39 ± 2.82 mm AIS: 5.26 ± 2.60 mm SIS: 1.53 ± 0.60 mm SA: 3.87 ± 2.11 mm No differences in load to failure
Osbahr et al[13] (2002)	Retrospective review	Tenodesis vs. tenotomy	No difference in cosmesis, pain, or spasm
Gill et al[4] (2001)	Case series	30 biceps tenotomy, 19 months of follow-up	90% return to sports 96.7% return to work 13.3% complication rate (Popeye sign)
Boileau et al[2] (2002)	Case series	Biceps tenodesis with interference screw fixation (8 or 9 mm)	90% strength of normal side No elbow motion loss 2 initial failures (7-mm screw)
Nord et al[12] (2005)	Case series	Tenodesis with anchor through subclavian port	11 patients, 2-year follow-up: 90% good–excellent results
Kelly et al[6] (2005)	Case series	Tenotomy	68% good, very good, or excellent result 70% Popeye sign 38% fatigue with resisted elbow flexion

- Pain with forward shoulder elevation and forearm supination. Anteromedial pain is indicative of acromioclavicular joint disease.
- Association with other shoulder disease, typically rotator cuff tear

Physical Examination

- Pain in intertubercular groove that moves laterally with external rotation

- No pain with cross-arm adduction or acromioclavicular joint palpation
- Positive result of O'Brien, Speed, and Yergason tests
- Positive result of subpectoral biceps tenderness test[5]: pain with palpation of the biceps tendon under the inferior border of the pectoralis major tendon. With the arm in neutral rotation, resisted internal rotation tensions the pectoralis major tendon. The biceps tendon can be palpated just distal to the inferior border of the pectoralis major, pressing laterally. Specificity of the subpectoral biceps tenderness test

can be improved if a glenohumeral lidocaine injection provides symptomatic relief.

Imaging

- Anteroposterior, scapular oblique, and axillary views
- Magnetic resonance arthrography, if indicated
- Ultrasonography, if available

Indications and Contraindications

The decision to treat biceps disease surgically is predicated on a clinical presentation of bicipital groove pain, provocative test results, response to injection, and failed nonoperative management. Findings on arthroscopic examination may include biceps tendinosis occurring with or without concurrent rotator cuff disease, biceps tendinosis in association with superior labral anterior-posterior (SLAP) lesions, and tendinosis secondary to instability of the biceps tendon. Instability of the biceps tendon can occur with disruption of the lateral aspect of the superior glenohumeral ligament and coracohumeral ligament, as observed in association with anterior supraspinatus tendon tears, or with disruption of the medial aspect of the coracohumeral ligament, often seen with a subscapularis tear. Instability of the biceps tendon is generally treated with a biceps tenodesis because reconstruction of the coracohumeral ligament attachment on the humerus has generally not been satisfactory.

Absolute contraindications to biceps tenodesis include any medical condition that precludes the safe administration of anesthesia or renders the patient unstable for operative intervention.

Surgical Technique

Anesthesia and Positioning

The senior author prefers beach chair positioning with interscalene block plus general anesthesia; the regional block alone is insufficient to anesthetize the axillary incision adequately. A complete examination under anesthesia is performed on both upper extremities to examine for concurrent pathologic processes of the shoulder or elbow.

Surgical Landmarks, Incisions, and Portals

Landmarks

- Coracoid
- Acromion
- Clavicle
- Pectoralis major tendon

Portals and Approaches

- Posterior portal
- Anterior portal
- Axillary fold incision at inferior border of pectoralis major tendon

Structures at Risk

- Axillary fold incision at inferior border of pectoralis major tendon: cephalic vein, musculocutaneous nerve (overzealous retraction), pectoralis major insertion (retraction)

Examination Under Anesthesia and Diagnostic Arthroscopy

Examination under anesthesia is performed to ensure full range of motion and glenohumeral stability.

Diagnostic arthroscopy evaluates the intra-articular biceps tendon, rotator cuff, glenoid labrum, glenohumeral ligaments, and chondral surface.

Specific Steps (Box 27-1)

1. Arthroscopic Preparation

Glenohumeral arthroscopy is begun with a standard posterior viewing portal (Fig. 27-1). A dry inspection of the intra-articular biceps tendon is performed initially because the pump pressure will result in vascular compression, causing the tenosynovitis to be "washed out." Injection or tendon fraying is indicative of bicipital disease. It is unknown how much biceps fraying can be accepted without the need for intervention, but some authors have proposed up to 30% to 50%. Additional inspection of the more distal tendon portions is accomplished by pulling the biceps tendon into the glenohumeral joint with a probe.

Box 27-1 Surgical Steps

1. Arthroscopic preparation
2. Biceps tenotomy
3. Exposure
4. Tendon preparation
5. Tunnel preparation
6. Tenodesis
7. Closure

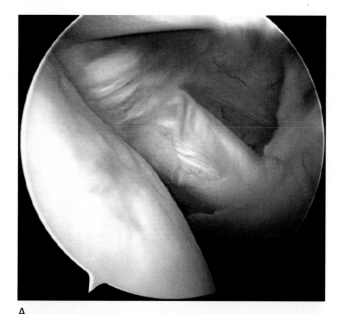

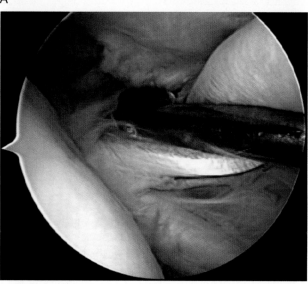

Figure 27-1 Glenohumeral arthroscopy. **A,** Dry inspection. **B,** Inspection of the more distal tendon portions is accomplished by pulling the biceps tendon into the glenohumeral joint with a probe.

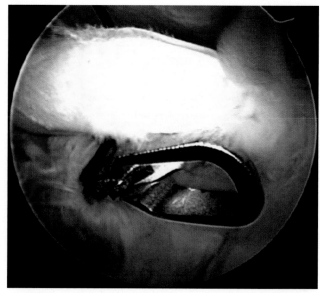

Figure 27-2 A basket forceps inserted through the anterior cannulated portal to transect the biceps tendon at the superior labral junction.

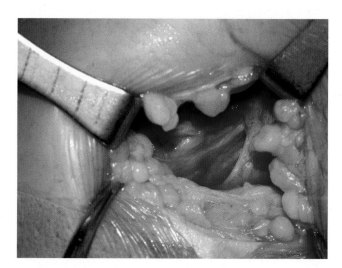

Figure 27-3 Exposure of the pectoralis major muscle.

2. Biceps Tenotomy

A basket forceps is inserted through the anterior cannulated portal to transect the biceps tendon at the superior labral junction (Fig. 27-2). Care is taken to avoid inadvertent damage to the superior glenoid labrum.

3. Exposure

With the arm slightly abducted and externally rotated, the inferior border of the pectoralis major tendon is palpated. A 3- to 4-cm incision is performed in line with the axillary fold, with one quarter of the incision above and three quarters of the incision below the inferior border of the pectoralis major tendon. A No. 15 blade scalpel is used to incise the subcuticular tissues. After hemostasis has been achieved with the electrocautery, Gelpi or Weitlaner self-retaining retractors are inserted to improve exposure. The overlying fatty tissue is cleared until the fascia overlying the pectoralis major, coracobrachialis, and biceps is identified (Fig. 27-3). Once the inferior border of the pectoralis major has been identified, the fascia overlying the coracobrachialis and biceps is incised in line with the incision. If these anatomic landmarks are not easily identified, the dissection is probably too lateral, especially if the cephalic vein is seen in the deltopectoral groove, in which case the dissection is also too proximal.

Blunt dissection with Mayo scissors and finger dissection sweep posterior to the pectoralis major tendon. The biceps tendon can be palpated in the intertubercular groove behind the pectoralis major tendon. A pointed curved Hohman retractor is placed on the lateral humeral cortex to retract the pectoralis tendon insertion superior and lateral. A blunt Chandler retractor is positioned on the medial cortex to retract the coracobrachialis and short head of the biceps. Vigorous medial retraction should be avoided to prevent injury to the musculocutaneous nerve. The long head of the biceps musculotendinous junction should be visualized. A right-angled clamp is then used to bluntly open the biceps sheath and deliver the tendon into the wound (Fig. 27-4).

4. Tendon Preparation

A No. 2 FiberWire (Arthrex, Inc., Naples, Fla) is used to sew a modified Krakow stitch starting 2.5 cm proximal to the musculotendinous junction (Fig. 27-5). The remaining

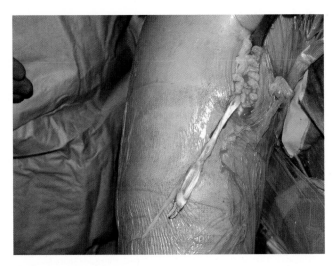

Figure 27-4 Delivery of the diseased biceps.

tendon is removed sharply with a No. 15 blade scalpel. The two ends of FiberWire exiting the biceps tendon are tied together with a square knot.

5. Tunnel Preparation

The periosteum 1 cm proximal to the pectoralis major tendon is reflected sharply off the humerus, forming a rectangle measuring approximately 2 × 1 cm (Fig. 27-6). A 2.4-mm threaded guide pin is drilled up to but not penetrating the far cortex. The starting point is just proximal to the inferior edge of the pectoralis major tendon and situated in the intertubercular groove, centered in the medial to lateral direction on the humerus (Fig. 27-7A). Subsequently, an 8-mm reamer is used to overream the guide pin without violating the posterior cortex. The reamer is then carefully backed out by hand to avoid tunnel widening on exiting (Fig. 27-7B). A headlight may be used to assist with illumination. An Arthrex 8- × 12-mm biotenodesis screw is loaded on the tip of the cannulated tenodesis screwdriver. A nitinol loop retrieves a strand of FiberWire through the cannulated screwdriver. The retrieved FiberWire tensions the biceps tendon to the screwdriver tip, and a needle driver secures the FiberWire tightly against the handle of the screwdriver.

6. Tenodesis

The biceps tendon is pushed into the humeral tunnel and secured in place by the advancing biotenodesis screw until the screw head is countersunk. The tunnel may be tapped before screw insertion if dense cortical bone is encountered. After screw insertion, the biceps tendon should be draped over and covering the tenodesis screw. A right-angled clamp can be used to elevate the biceps tendon to ensure complete seating of the screw.

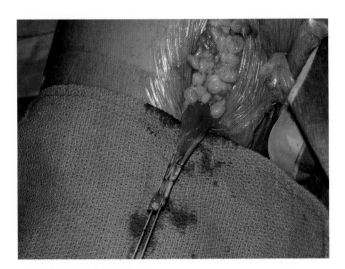

Figure 27-5 A modified Krakow stitch is sewn 2.5 cm proximal to the musculotendinous junction.

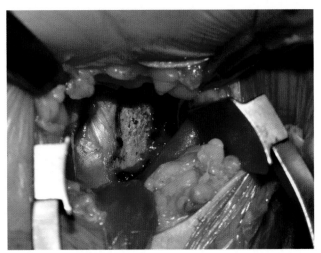

Figure 27-6 Elevation of the periosteum.

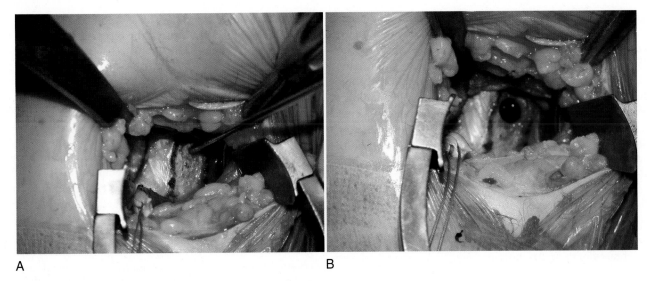

A   B

Figure 27-7 A, A threaded guide pin is drilled up to but not penetrating the posterior cortex. An 8-mm reamer is used to overream the guide pin, avoiding violation of the posterior cortex. **B,** The reamer is carefully backed out by hand to avoid tunnel widening on exiting.

7. Closure

After copious irrigation, 3-0 Monocryl buried sutures close the deep subcutaneous tissue. Steri-Strips are applied to the skin. The wound is injected with 5 mL of 0.25% bupivacaine (Marcaine).

Postoperative Considerations

Follow-up

Sutures are removed on the seventh postoperative day. The three-view radiographic examination is repeated to assess tunnel placement.

Rehabilitation

Postoperative management is dictated by concomitant procedures.

Isolated Biceps Tenodesis

- Progression from passive to active-assisted to full range of motion
- Strengthen at 12 weeks
- Full activity at 4 to 6 months
- If the intraoperative construct is resilient: return to work in 2 weeks
- Early full range of motion
- Functional rehabilitation

Rotator Cuff Repair

- Passive range of motion first 6 weeks, then progression from active-assisted to active range of motion
- Immediate elbow range of motion and grip strengthening

Acromioplasty

- Passive range of motion with rapid progression to active-assisted and active range of motion
- Immediate elbow range of motion and grip strengthening
- Follow isolated biceps tenodesis protocol

Complications

- Infection
- Spitting of subcutaneous sutures due to the very thin skin
- Construct failure
- Persistent pain
- Musculocutaneous or axillary nerve injury
- Humerus fracture
- Potential reaction to biodegradable screw
- Hematoma or seroma
- Functional tenotomy

PEARLS AND PITFALLS

- Make the incision more inferior, if desired, for dissection closer to the axilla. The fat stripe marks the inferior pectoralis border. The biceps tendon is under the pectoralis tendon.

- Place a curved Hohman retractor inferior to the pectoralis tendon and around the lateral cortex to retract the pectoralis superolaterally.

- Inadvertent placement of the Hohman retractor in the intertubercular groove may sweep the biceps medially and out of view. Remove and reposition the retractor if the biceps tendon is not visible.

- Place retractors before locating the tendon.

- Be careful not to plunge medially with the Chandler retractor—the brachial artery is at risk.

- Feel the intertubercular groove and the medial and lateral cortex to ensure centered guide pin placement.

- Ream 8-mm hole through near cortex only.

- For thick cortical bone, a tap is available for near cortex.

- Begin the modified Krakow stitch and transect the biceps tendon 2.5 cm from the musculotendinous junction. (Measurement from

unpublished anatomic studies; the natural biceps contour dips down under the pectoralis. The biceps muscle peak is three or four fingerbreadths from the inferior edge of the pectoralis.)

- It is better to err too short rather than too long. It is difficult to overtighten the construct.

- Tie the ends of the modified Krakow stitch together before loading the tenodesis driver.

- The 8- × 12-mm biotenodesis screw is built for cortical fixation. The small taper makes it difficult to start.

- Ream to far cortex but do not ream on the way out, which widens the tunnel. Unchuck reamer at far cortex and reverse reamer out by hand.

- During screw insertion, the biceps tendon rotates around the screw. This is to be expected. The tendon drapes the screw when it is seated.

- The pectoralis major covers the biceps when the Hohman retractor is removed.

- Coagulate superficial bleeding vessels.

27

Results

Our experience includes 20 patients with more than 2 years of follow-up. The preoperative to postoperative scores averaged the following increases: Rowe score, 57 to 91; American Shoulder and Elbow Surgeons score, 42 to 86; Simple Shoulder Test score, 5 of 12 to 10 of 12; Constant-Murley score, 45 of 75 to 67 of 75.

References

1. Barber FA, Byrd JW, Wolf EM, Burkhart SS. How would you treat the partially torn biceps tendon? Arthroscopy 2001;17:636-639.
2. Boileau P, Krishnan SG, Coste JS, Walch G. Arthroscopic biceps tenodesis: a new technique using bioabsorbable interference screw. Arthroscopy 2002;18:1002-1012.
3. Eakin CL, Faber KJ, Hawkins RJ, Hovis WD. Biceps tendon disorders in athletes. J Am Acad Orthop Surg 1999;7:300-310.
4. Gill TJ, McIrvin E, Mair S, Hawkins RJ. Results of biceps tenotomy for treatment of pathology of the long head of the biceps brachii. J Shoulder Elbow Surg 2001;10:247-249.
5. Jayamoorthy T, Field JR, Costi JR, et al. Biceps tenodesis: a biomechanical study of fixation methods. J Shoulder Elbow Surg 2004;3:160-164.
6. Kelly AM, Drakos MC, Fealy S, et al. Arthroscopic release of the long head of the biceps tendon. Am J Sports Med 2005;33:208-213.
7. Kilicoglu O, Koyuncu O, Demirhan M, et al. Time-dependent changes in failure loads of 3 biceps tenodesis techniques. Am J Sports Med 2005;33:1536-1544.
8. Kim SH, Ha KI, Kim HS, Kim SW. Electromyographic activity of the biceps branchii muscle in shoulders with anterior instability. Arthroscopy 2001;17:864-868.
9. Mazzocca AD, Bicos J, Santangelo S, et al. The biomechanical evaluation of four fixation techniques for proximal biceps tenodesis. Arthroscopy 2005;21:1296-1306.
10. Mazzocca AD, Rios CG, Romeo AA, Arciero RA. Subpectoral biceps tenodesis with interference screw fixation. Arthroscopy 2005;21:896.
11. Mazzocca AD, Romeo AA. Arthroscopic biceps tenodesis in the beach chair position. Oper Tech Sports Med 2003;11:6-14.
12. Nord KD, Smith GB, Mauck BM. Arthroscopic biceps tenodesis using suture anchors through the subclavian port. Arthroscopy 2005;21:248-252.
13. Osbahr DC, Diamond AB, Speer KP. The cosmetic appearance of the biceps muscle after long-head tenotomy versus tenodesis. Arthroscopy 2002;18:483-487.
14. Ozalay M, Akpinar S, Karaeminogullari O, et al. Mechanical strength of four biceps tenodesis techniques. Arthroscopy 2005;21:992-998.
15. Pfahler M, Branner S, Refior HJ. The role of the bicipital groove in tendopathy of the long biceps tendon. J Shoulder Elbow Surg 1999;8:419-414.
16. Richards DP, Burkhart SS. A biomechanical analysis of two biceps tenodesis fixation techniques. Arthroscopy 2005;21:861-866.
17. Romeo A, Mazzocca AD, Tauro JC. Arthroscopic biceps tenodesis. Arthroscopy 2004;20:206-213.
18. Sakurai G, Ozaki J, Tomita Y, et al. Electromyographic analysis of shoulder joint function of biceps brachii muscle during isometric contraction. Clin Orthop 1998;354:123-131.
19. Sethi N, Wright R, Yamaguchi K. Disorders of the long head of the biceps tendon. J Shoulder Elbow Surg 1999;8:644-654.
20. Verma NN, Drakos M, O'Brien SJ. Arthroscopic transfer of the long head biceps to the conjoint tendon. Arthroscopy 2005;21:764.
21. Wolf RS, Zheng N, Weichel D. Long head biceps tenotomy versus tenodesis: a cadaveric biomechanical analysis. Arthroscopy 2005;21:182-185.

CHAPTER 28

Anatomic Acromioclavicular Joint Reconstruction

Albert Tom, MD

Augustus D. Mazzocca, MS, MD

Acromioclavicular joint separation represents one of the most common shoulder injuries in general orthopedic practice. The most common mechanism of this injury is a fall with a direct force to the lateral aspect of the shoulder and with the arm in an abducted position. Depending on the magnitude of injury to the acromioclavicular joint capsule and ligaments as well as to the coracoclavicular ligaments, these injuries can be classified by increasing severity as type I through type VI. Typically, the first- and second-degree sprains of the acromioclavicular joint, otherwise known as type I and type II injuries, are treated conservatively; most return to preinjury status. Whereas the treatment of type III dislocations remains controversial, high-grade injuries—typically types IV, V, and VI—with greater than 100% displacement in either a posterior or inferior direction are typically treated surgically.

The literature is replete with surgical techniques to address complete acromioclavicular dislocations, including primary repair of the coracoclavicular ligaments, augmentation with autogenous tissue (coracoacromial ligament), augmentation with absorbable and nonabsorbable suture as well as with prosthetic material, and coracoclavicular stabilization with metallic screws. The Weaver-Dunn technique with transfer of the coracoacromial ligament has been the most popular procedure in the acute and chronic injury. Several more recent reports have described good results with modifications of the Weaver-Dunn technique. However, studies observed compromised results in patients who had residual subluxation or dislocation after surgery.

From a biomechanical perspective, the importance of the coracoclavicular ligaments and acromioclavicular ligaments in controlling superior and horizontal translation of the distal clavicle has been elucidated. In fact, failure to surgically reproduce the conoid, trapezoid, and acromioclavicular ligament function with current techniques may explain the observed incidence of recurrent instability and pain.

I advocate use of a separate, more robust graft source, rather than the coracoacromial ligament, to improve surgical results. The use of a free autogenous or allograft tendon has been further supported in our biomechanics laboratory.

Preoperative Considerations

The pain associated with acromioclavicular joint injury may be difficult to localize because of the complex sensory innervation of the joint. An acute injury as described before is an important indicator in the diagnosis. Conversely, the lack of a discrete injury with acromioclavicular joint pain and joint separation is more consistent with a degenerative condition. Given an acute injury, it is important to obtain the level of perceived pain, its location, and any history of previous shoulder injuries. During examination, the patient should be upright so that the weight of the arm helps exaggerate any deformities.

History

- Acute traumatic event
- Distal clavicular fracture (not always obvious)
- Age of the patient—physeal fracture
- Prior surgical procedures (distal clavicle resection)
- Current physical limitations and disability
- Reconstruction for instability, not pain
- Failure of at least 3 months of conservative treatments
- Pain with forward elevation
- Posterior headache (nuchae)

Physical Examination

Acromioclavicular joint examination

- Inspection (Fig. 28-1)
- Tenderness to palpation
- Anterior-posterior translation or mobility
- Superior-inferior translation or mobility
- Reduction of the distal clavicle with shoulder shrug differentiates type III from type V (distal clavicle buttonhole through deltotrapezial fascia)

Range of motion

- Arm positioning limitation
- Inability to lift arm
- Pain with forward elevation and wing out

Strength testing

Differential Diagnosis

Other causes of pain must be ruled out:

- Cervical spine disease: trapezial spasm
- Thoracic outlet syndrome
- Scapular dyskinesis
- Hyperlaxity
- Coracoid fracture

Factors Affecting Surgical Planning

- Prior surgeries, incisions

Imaging

- Zanca view: 10- to 15-degree cephalad tilt (Fig. 28-2)
- Axillary, outlet, and anteroposterior views of the shoulder in the scapular plane
- Cross-arm adduction view: anteroposterior shoulder—measure clavicle override

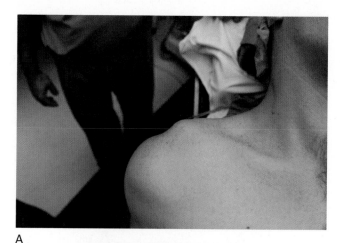

A

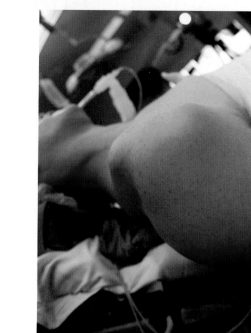

B

Figure 28-1 A, Anteroposterior view, type V. **B,** Lateral view, type V.

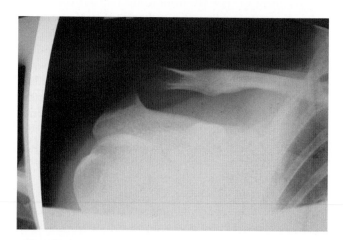

Figure 28-2 Preoperative radiograph, type V.

- Magnetic resonance imaging: labral injury masquerading as acromioclavicular joint pain
- Computed tomographic scan: nondisplaced lateral clavicle or acromion fracture

Indications

- Advocate reconstruction even for symptomatic type III injuries in laborers, throwers, and overhead athletes
- Instability after distal clavicle excision
- No absolute indications

Contraindications

Reconstruction is contraindicated in painless, functional grade III separation and with regional pain syndrome, unclear diagnosis, adhesive capsulitis, and other shoulder problems.

Surgical Planning

- Semitendinosus allograft or autograft
- Reasonable expectations of the patient and compliance with postoperative regimen
- Postoperative sling immobilization for 6 weeks

Surgical Technique

Anesthesia and Positioning

The patient is placed in the beach chair position after induction of general anesthesia. Be sure the head is mobile for possible repositioning. A small towel bump is placed on the medial scapular edge to elevate the coracoid anterior. Drape wide to expose the sternoclavicular joint and posterior clavicle. The arm is draped free.

Surgical Landmarks and Portals

Landmarks
- Clavicle
- Acromion
- Coracoid process

Portals
- Scope first
- Standard posterior arthroscopy port
- Anterior rotator interval port

Examination Under Anesthesia

- Evaluate anterior-posterior translation as well as superior-inferior translation of the distal clavicle.
- Evaluate glenohumeral range of motion and stability.

Specific Steps (Box 28-1)

1. Exposure

A No. 10 blade scalpel is used to make a 6-cm longitudinal incision, centered over or slightly medial to the coracoid. Medial and lateral skin flaps are elevated with a needle-tipped bovie. Gelpi retractors assist with exposure. A transverse incision is made along the midaxis of the clavicle extending into the acromioclavicular joint. Full-thickness flaps of the superior acromioclavicular joint capsule are elevated superiorly and inferiorly with a needle-tipped bovie. The anterior and posterior portion of the distal clavicle is completely exposed (Fig. 28-3). If acromioclavicular joint arthrosis is present, 5 mm of distal

Box 28-1 Surgical Steps

1. Exposure
2. Passing under the coracoid
3. Clavicular tunnels
4. Graft preparation
5. Graft passage
6. Biotenodesis fixation
7. Acromioclavicular joint capsular ligament repair
8. Closure

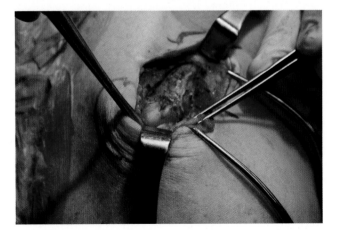

Figure 28-3 Initial exposure.

clavicle is resected. Many surgeons perform a distal clavicle resection (Fig. 28-4). However, there is tremendous variability in the acromioclavicular joint, and there seems to be tremendous stability from an intact acromioclavicular joint. For that reason, I believe that it may be advantageous to preserve the distal clavicle and have done so in select patients.

The medial and lateral coracoid base is exposed with a Cobb elevator. A headlight may be useful for this portion of the procedure. Care is taken to avoid excessive medial dissection to prevent musculocutaneous nerve injury.

2. Passing under the Coracoid

A specially designed cannulated passing device (Arthrex, Inc., Naples, Fla) is passed medial to lateral around the coracoid. A FiberWire or FiberStick (Arthrex, Inc., Naples, Fla) is then shuttled through the cannulated handle and retrieved laterally at the tip. This passing stitch is later used for graft passage around the coracoid (Fig. 28-5).

An alternative means of coracoid graft fixation is biotenodesis screw fixation of the looped end of the semitendinosus graft in a coracoid base bone tunnel. This is best achieved by positioning the 7-mm offset ACL guide on the medial coracoid base and reaming an 8- or 9-mm bone tunnel.

3. Clavicular tunnels

The conoid ligament tunnel is established with a guide pin drilled 4.5 cm medial from the intact lateral distal clavicle edge. This is positioned along the posterior superior cortex and is marked before distal clavicle resection. The pin is directed at 30 degrees anterior, aiming toward the coracoid. A second guide pin from the Arthrex biotenodesis set is drilled central on the clavicle's anteroposterior dimension and 1.5 cm lateral to the medial pin. This tunnel will be used to reconstruct the trapezoid ligament and is again directed 30 degrees anterior toward the coracoid (Figs. 28-6 and 28-7). A 5.5-mm reamer is used to ream both tunnels (Fig. 28-8). The reamer is removed by hand twisting after penetration of the far cortex to avoid tunnel widening.

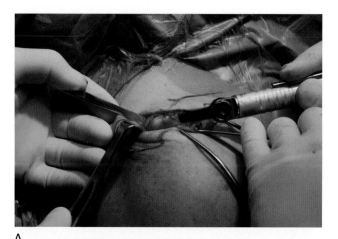

A

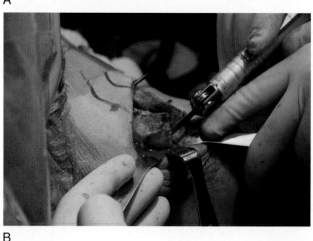

B

Figure 28-4 A, Resection of the distal clavicle. **B,** Beveling of the posterior edge of the distal clavicle.

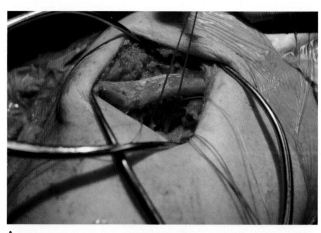

A

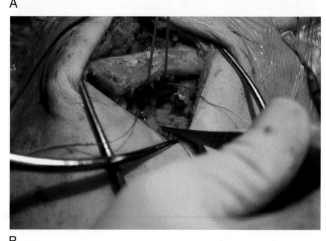

B

Figure 28-5 A, FiberWire around the coracoid. **B,** Close-up view.

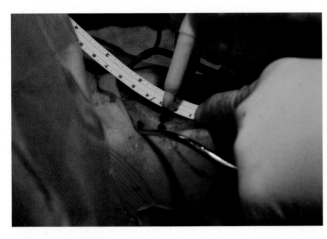

Figure 28-6 Marking the clavicular tunnels.

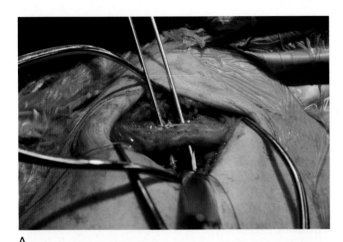

A

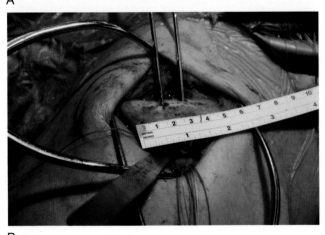

B

Figure 28-7 A, Guide pins in the tunnels. **B,** Measuring the guide pins.

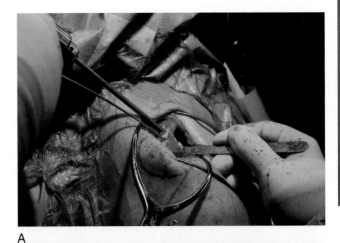

A

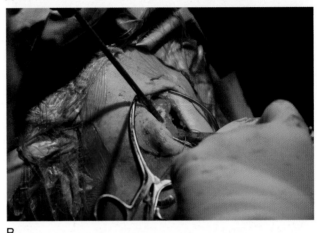

B

Figure 28-8 A, Reaming the coracoid tunnel. **B,** Reaming the trapezoid tunnel.

5. Graft Passage

The initially passed FiberWire or FiberStick is used to shuttle the prepared semitendinosus graft along with an additional No. 2 FiberWire around the coracoid process. The accessory FiberWire will provide secondary fixation. The free ends of the semitendinosus graft along with the free No. 2 FiberWire are shuttled into the respective clavicular bone tunnels by use of a suture-passing device (Fig. 28-10).

6. Biotenodesis Fixation

A 5.5 × 8-mm PEEK (polyetheretherketone) tenodesis screw is then loaded onto the biotenodesis screwdriver (Arthrex, Inc., Naples, Fla). The nitinol loop retriever is used to pass the FiberWire through the cannulated screwdriver system. With countertension on the opposite graft end, the PEEK screw is inserted flush to the cortical surface. The clavicle is then overreduced with downward pressure from a Cobb elevator. A superiorly directed force on the humerus will also assist in reducing the clavicle. If the distal clavicle is preserved, I avoid overreducing the acromioclavicular joint.

4. Graft Preparation

An allograft semitendinosus graft is contoured to fit through a 5.5-mm tunnel. No. 2 FiberWire is used to place baseball stitches at each end of the graft (Fig. 28-9).

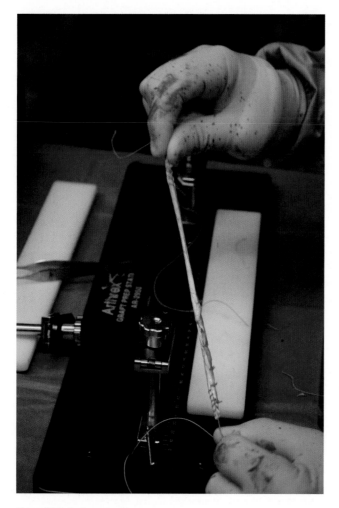

Figure 28-9 Graft preparation.

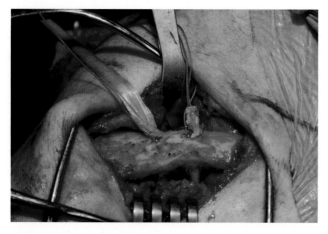

Figure 28-10 Passage of the graft.

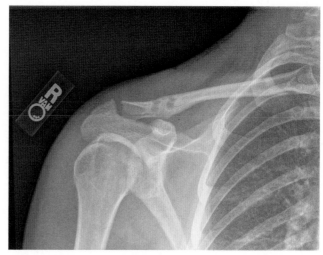

Figure 28-11 Postoperative radiograph.

A second PEEK tenodesis screw is inserted into the second clavicular tunnel through the FiberWire suture. The graft is tensioned as the screw is inserted. The order of tunnel fixation does not matter. The FiberWire is tensioned and tied with surgeon knots. The graft ends are then sutured to one another, and the excess graft is excised.

7. Superior Acromioclavicular Joint Capsular Ligament Repair

No. 2 FiberWire stitches are used to imbricate the superior acromioclavicular joint capsular ligaments in a pants-over-vest configuration. This will offer additional anteroposterior stability to the reconstruction. The deltotrapezial fascia is also repaired in this step if full-thickness flaps of fascia and acromioclavicular joint capsular ligament were elevated in a single layer.

8. Closure

After copious wound irrigation, the subcutaneous tissues are closed with 2-0 Vicryl sutures. A 3-0 Monocryl is used to perform a subcutaneous skin closure. The wound is injected with bupivacaine (Marcaine).

Postoperative Considerations

Follow-up

- Sutures are removed at 1 week.
- Patients are seen at 1, 2, 3, and 6 months and then annually.

- Postoperative radiographs include bilateral Zanca views to measure coracoid-clavicular distance (Fig. 28-11).

Rehabilitation

- A platform brace (Lehrman) is worn for 6 weeks.
- Immediate pendulum exercises are begun, with limitation of passive external rotation to 30 degrees and passive forward flexion to 90 degrees.
- Active range of motion is started at 8 weeks.
- Strengthening is started at 12 to 16 weeks.
- Sports-specific activities and return to full athletics are allowed at 16 to 24 weeks.
- Return to heavy labor is allowed at 6 months.

Complications

- Infection
- Sterile abscess from FiberWire or PEEK screw reaction
- Potential clavicle fracture from stress riser effect on bone tunnels. Unpublished three- and four-point load data revealed diminished stress riser effect when clavicular tunnels are filled with tenodesis screws.
- Construct failure
- Potential musculocutaneous nerve injury
- Persistent pain

PEARLS

- Include the sternoclavicular joint in the operative field to allow wide exposure.
- Place a small towel bump under the medial scapular edge.
- Bullet the semitendinosus ends to allow easy graft passage.
- Make sure the head of the patient can be repositioned to the side, allowing room for conoid tunnel drilling.
- Instead of repositioning the head, the clavicle can be displaced anteriorly with a towel clip to allow access for conoid tunnel drilling.
- The skin incision is over the coracoid process, more medial than usual (not over the acromioclavicular joint).
- The medial skin incision allows direct visualization of the coracoclavicular ligament and coracoid.
- Tag the deltoid and trapezial fascia for good repair.
- Pass sutures under the coracoid either medial to lateral or lateral to medial.
- If sutures are passed lateral to medial, make sure the medial coracoid base is exposed and position a Darrach retractor on the medial base to "catch" the passing device.
- Do not power-spin the reamer out to avoid tunnel widening.
- Overreduce the acromioclavicular joint if the distal clavicle is resected, abutting the clavicle to the coracoid process.
- Do not overreduce the clavicle if the distal clavicle is preserved.
- The 5.5 × 8-mm PEEK screws are inserted into a 5.5-mm bone tunnel (line to line).
- Drill up by 0.5 mm if the graft is too big for screw fixation.
- Insert the screw anterior to the graft to adequately re-create the posteriorly positioned coracoclavicular ligaments.
- A postoperative platform brace (Lehrman) is prescribed for 6 weeks.

Results

Results of studies of acromioclavicular joint reconstruction are shown in Table 28-1.

Table 28-1 Results of Studies of Acromioclavicular Joint Reconstruction

Author	Study	Native Coracoclavicular Ligament	Anatomic Coracoclavicular Ligament Reconstruction	Coracoacromial Transfer
Lee et al[6] (2003)	Cadaver	650 N (load to failure)	700 N (load to failure) Semitendinosus	150 N (load to failure)
Costic et al[1] (2004)	Cadaver	60.8 ± 5.2 N/mm (stiffness) 560 ± 206 N (load to failure)	23.4 ± 5.2 N/mm (stiffness) 406 ± 60 N (load to failure) Semitendinosus	
Grutter and Petersen[3] (2005)	Cadaver	815 N	774 N Flexor carpi radialis	483 N
Mazzocca et al[7] (2006)	Cadaver		396.4 ± 136.42 N	354.3 ± 100.26 N

References

1. Costic RS, Labriola JE, Rodosky ME, Debski RE. Biomechanical rationale for development of anatomical reconstruction of coracoclavicular ligaments after complete acromioclavicular joint dislocations. Am J Sports Med 2004;32:1929-1936.

2. Debski RE, Parson IM, Woo S, Fu FH. Effect of capsular injury on acromioclavicular joint mechanics. J Bone Joint Surg Am 2001;83:1344-1351.

3. Grutter PW, Petersen SA. Anatomical acromioclavicular ligament reconstruction. Am J Sports Med 2005;31:1-6.

4. Jari R, Costic RS, Rodosky MW, Debski RE. Biomechanical function of surgical procedures for acromioclavicular joint dislocations. J Arthroscopy 2004;20:237-245.

5. Jones HP, Lemos MJ, Schepsis AA. Salvage of failed acromioclavicular joint reconstruction using autogenous semitendinosus tendon from the knee. Am J Sports Med 2001;29:234-237.

6. Lee SJ, Nicholas SJ, Akizuki KH, et al. Reconstruction of the coracoclavicular ligaments with tendon grafts. Am J Sports Med 2003;31:648-654.

7. Mazzocca AD, Santangelo SA, Johnson ST, et al. A biomechanical evaluation of an anatomical coracoclavicular ligament reconstruction. Am J Sports Med 2006;34:236-246.

CHAPTER 29

Management of Pectoralis Major Muscle Injuries

LCDR Christopher I. Ellingson, MD

Jon K. Sekiya, MD

First described in 1822 by Patissier, pectoralis major ruptures are an uncommon injury. During the past 30 years, small case series have increased awareness of this injury, and meta-analyses of these studies have shown that operative repair results in significantly better outcomes than nonoperative treatment.[1,2] The pectoralis major consists of two muscle heads that converge and insert lateral to the bicipital groove as two distinct laminae.[8,16] The inferior sternocostal head fibers rotate and insert posterior and superior to the clavicular fibers, placing them at a mechanical disadvantage at the extremes of humeral extension.[16] Ruptures can be classified as complete or incomplete and may occur as avulsions from the humerus or rupture of the tendon, musculotendinous junction, or muscle belly.[1,7,8,10]

Techniques for repair include sutures through drill holes in the humerus, barbed staples, and suture anchors.[1,2,6,8,11,14,16] The senior author prefers the use of a bone trough with tunnels to reapproximate the laminae to their native insertions.

Preoperative Considerations

History

Given the relative rarity of pectoralis major ruptures, knowledge of their mechanism and physical findings is essential to ensure timely and accurate diagnosis of this injury. In a series by Hanna et al,[7] 50% of unrepaired ruptures were initially misdiagnosed or diagnosed late. Peak incidence of this injury occurs in male athletes between 20 and 40 years old.[1,2,8] Indirect injury mechanisms are most common, although rupture has been reported with direct blows and trauma.[2,8,16] Bench press is the most common activity associated with pectoralis major ruptures. Eccentric contraction with the arm abducted and externally rotated places the inferior fibers of the sternocostal head at a mechanical disadvantage and results in their failure first.[16]

Patients report a tearing or searing pain often associated with a "pop" when the injury occurs. This is usually accompanied by the acute onset of swelling, ecchymosis, and painful motion of the affected arm. Patients may not seek treatment immediately but will usually present with continued weakness, pain with movement of the arm, and deformity with muscle contraction.

Physical Examination

Ecchymosis is usually present over the anterior chest, axilla, or proximal arm of the injured patient. The anterior chest and axilla are examined for asymmetry with the contralateral side. Loss of chest wall contour can be accentuated by abducting the arm 90 degrees or having the patient adduct against resistance (Fig. 29-1). A cord of remaining fascia may still be present on the lateral chest wall and may be mistaken for an intact pectoralis major tendon. This cord represents the intact fascia of the pectoralis major and its continuation with the fascia of the brachium and medial antebrachial septum. Direct palpation of the axilla

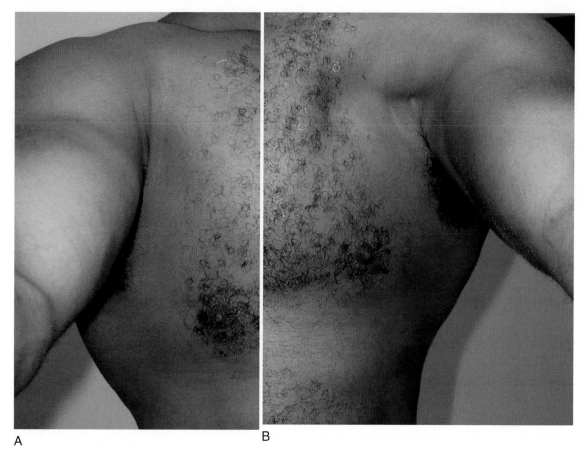

Figure 29-1 Physical examination of a patient with a pectoralis major muscle rupture with the arm forward elevated and under resisted adduction. **A,** Uninjured side. **B,** Chronic pectoralis major muscle injury.

will often reveal a defect, particularly in the inferior lateral aspect of the chest wall just at the medial border of the axilla. However, this can be masked by the intact fascia, hematoma or edema, or intact clavicular head of the pectoralis major. Serial examinations may be necessary during a short period, but the diagnosis of a pectoralis major rupture is usually made clinically.

Imaging

Plain radiographs of the injured shoulder are obtained to evaluate for associated fractures or possible bone avulsions; however, no gross abnormalities are usually appreciated.[15] Other studies described Cybex testing, ultrasonography, and computed tomographic evaluation, but magnetic resonance imaging is the optimal imaging technique for delineation of pectoralis major injuries.[4,5,9,11-13] T2-weighted axial images are most helpful in evaluating acute injuries, and magnetic resonance imaging may help distinguish between complete, partial, and intramuscular ruptures.[12] In cases with equivocal physical examination findings, magnetic resonance imaging may prevent a delay in diagnosis.[11]

Indications and Contraindications

Nonoperative treatment may be pursued for intrasubstance muscle tears of the pectoralis major or in elderly patients.[3] Complete tears of the pectoralis major, including isolated tears of the sternocostal head, should be treated surgically in young, healthy patients. Residual deformity and weakness will remain in such tears treated nonoperatively.[8,10,14]

Surgical Technique

Anesthesia and Positioning

General anesthesia is preferred to allow complete muscle relaxation and mobilization of the torn pectoralis major tendon. The patient is placed in the modified beach chair position with the head and body elevated approximately 30 to 45 degrees. A sandbag or small roll of sheets may be placed under the patient's scapula to allow more motion of the shoulder during repair. The arm and shoulder are prepared and draped free to allow intraoperative manipulation and positioning.

Surgical Landmarks

Standard landmarks for a deltopectoral approach are used. The proximal extent of the incision may be placed slightly medially for better mobilization of the often retracted pectoralis tendon and muscle. The distal portion of the incision may be placed slightly laterally on the arm to allow easier access to the humeral insertion during repair.

Examination Under Anesthesia

An evaluation under anesthesia of the affected shoulder is performed with attention directed to the anterior chest wall and axilla. Comparison to the contralateral side is made, and deformity or defects are noted.

Specific Steps (Box 29-1)

1. Exposure

A standard longitudinal incision is made for a deltopectoral approach. Once the incision is made through the skin, hemostasis is obtained, and subcutaneous dissection is performed to identify and free the pectoralis major from the subcutaneous tissues. The interval between the pectoralis and deltoid is identified, and the cephalic vein is mobilized and protected as this interval is developed. The retracted end of the torn pectoralis is often identified medially in the wound where it has retracted. In the case of an isolated rupture of the sternocostal head, this is identified inferior to the intact clavicular head of the pectoralis major (Fig. 29-2).

2. Tendon-Muscle Mobilization

The end of the torn tendon may be grasped and a temporary suture placed to allow traction of the muscle during mobilization. A combination of sharp and blunt dissection is used to free the muscle and tendon from both the chest wall and subcutaneous tissues. The difficult dissection encountered in chronic tears is facilitated by anesthesia, providing complete muscle relaxation during dissection.

Box 29-1 Surgical Steps

1. Exposure
2. Tendon-muscle mobilization
3. Tendon reattachment
4. Closure

Once the tendon is mobilized, a double laminar repair is performed with a No. 2 or No. 5 braided nonabsorbable suture. A Krackow stitch is used to place two or three sutures in the lamina of the sternocostal and clavicular heads, with up to six sutures total (Fig. 29-3). In the case of an intrasubstance muscle tear, a three-layered, modified Kessler technique is used to reapproximate the posterior fascia, middle muscle, and anterior fascia.

3. Tendon Reattachment

Once the tendon has been mobilized and sutures have been placed, the insertion site is identified and prepared for reattachment. The insertion of the pectoralis major tendon is located just lateral to the bicipital groove. A retractor holds the deltoid and cephalic vein out of the field. The biceps tendon is identified on the anterior humerus, and a longitudinal incision in the periosteum is

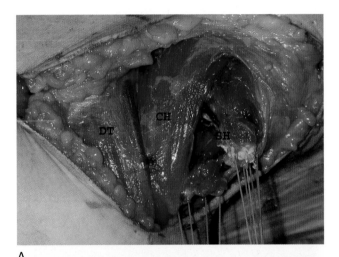

A

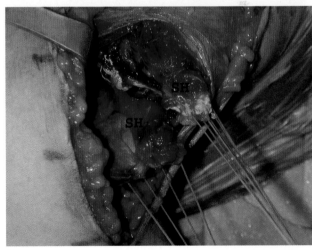

B

Figure 29-2 Intraoperative photograph of an intact clavicular head (CH) and torn sternal head (SH). **A,** Note the unretracted deltoid (DT) and cephalic vein. **B,** Same case with the deltoid and intact clavicular head retracted. The sternal head is tagged for repair in two layers.

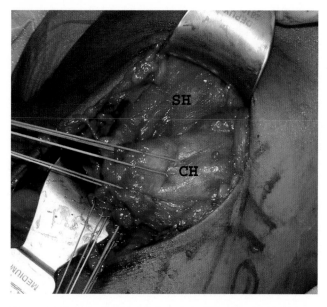

Figure 29-3 Rupture of both the clavicular head (CH) and sternal head (SH) of the pectoralis major. The orientation of the muscle is reproduced with the sternal head placed deep to the clavicular head.

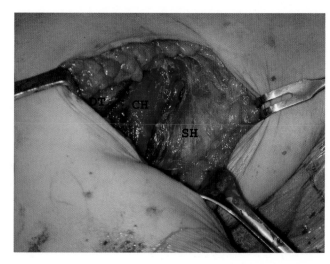

Figure 29-5 Isolated repair of the sternal head of the pectoralis major (SH). Note that this attachment is deep to the intact attachment of the clavicular head (CH). DT, deltoid.

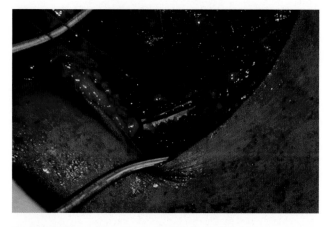

Figure 29-4 A groove is made by a bur lateral to the biceps in the anatomic attachment of the pectoralis major tendon. The sutures are then passed through bur holes and tensioned before being tied.

made directly lateral to this. In the case of an isolated sternocostal head rupture, the intact lamina of the clavicular head will need to be retracted cephalad and lateral to allow placement of the sternocostal head just medially. A trough is made with a bur lateral to the biceps groove for insertion of the tendon, with care taken not to breach the cortex fully. A bur or drill is then used to make three holes in the cortex approximately 10 mm apart in a longitudinal manner along this trough. Matching holes are made approximately 5 mm more lateral to the first holes to allow tying of the sutures over a bone bridge (Fig. 29-4). Internal and external rotation of the humerus will aid in exposure and access for placement of these holes.

A needle or suture passer is then used to place each paired suture strand through separate holes, and these sutures are tied over the bone bridges with the arm placed in neutral adduction and rotation. The repair is visually inspected and palpated while the arm is gently internally and externally rotated to ensure coordinated movement of the pectoralis muscle and tight reapproximation to its insertion site (Fig. 29-5).

4. Closure

A standard closure is performed with reapproximation of the subcutaneous tissue followed by skin closure of the surgeon's choice. We prefer a subcuticular closure with absorbable suture for optimal cosmesis.

Postoperative Considerations

The patient is placed in a sling on the operative side, and physical therapy is initiated on postoperative day 1 for pendulum exercises. Only passive motion consisting of passive forward elevation of the adducted arm to 130 degrees is allowed for the first 6 weeks. The patient is instructed to avoid any active forward elevation or abduction during these 6 weeks. After 6 weeks, passive range of motion is advanced, and a periscapular strengthening regimen is begun to include isometric exercises. The patient is monitored and at 3 months should have full motion of the affected shoulder. The strengthening regimen is then advanced, and at 6 months the patient may resume light-weight press exercises and pushups. Full activity is allowed approximately between 9 and 12 months. Single-rep maximum bench pressing is discouraged indefinitely.

Complications

Proper tensioning of the repair is necessary to avoid stiffness or residual weakness of the pectoralis major. Neutral positioning of the arm helps reduce the risk of inappropriate tensioning. The risk of complications increases in chronic injuries as a result of increased difficulty with surgical exposure secondary to increased retraction and scarring of the ruptured tendon.[2]

Results

Because of the relative rarity of pectoralis major tears, outcome studies are limited to small case series and meta-analyses. Overall surgical outcomes are better than nonsurgical treatment in both acute and chronic tears (Fig. 29-6 and Table 29-1).[1,2,7,14,16]

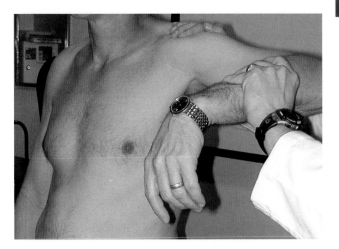

Figure 29-6 A patient more than 1 year after surgical repair of pectoralis major muscle injury. The patient is back to full active duty in the U.S. Navy, which requires biannual pushup tests to maintain physical readiness.

PEARLS AND PITFALLS

- Look for deformity with the arm forward flexed and adducted against resistance.
- Palpable cord often represents fascia that may hinder diagnosis—do not mistake for an intact pectoralis major tendon.
- The patient is placed in a beach chair position with a scapular bump.
- Look for isolated sternocostal head tears inferior to the intact clavicular head.
- Insert lateral to the biceps tendon.
- The neutral arm position allows proper tensioning.
- Anticipate difficult exposure or mobilization in chronic cases.

Table 29-1 Outcomes of Pectoralis Major Muscle Rupture

Author	Study	Results

Aarimaa et al[1] (2004)	33 repairs
	Meta-analysis of 73 cases
		33 repairs: 13 excellent, 17 good, 3 fair
		Meta-analysis of 73 cases
		    32 acute repairs (<3 weeks): 18 excellent, 12 good
		    19 delayed (>3 weeks): 8 excellent, 11 good
		    22 nonoperative: 1 excellent, 16 good, 5 fair

Hanna et al[7] (2001)	22 ruptures	10 repaired: peak torque 99% of uninjured side 12 nonoperative: peak torque 56% of uninjured side
Bak et al[2] (2000)	Meta-analysis of 72 cases	Surgical repair: 88% excellent-good (statistically better if repaired within 8 weeks of injury) Nonoperative: 27% excellent-good
Schepsis et al[14] (2000)	17 ruptures	6 acute repairs (<2 weeks from injury): 96% subjective, 102% isokinetic strength 7 chronic repairs (>2 weeks from injury): 93% subjective, 94% strength 4 nonoperative: 51% subjective, 71% strength
Wolfe et al[16] (1992)	8 ruptures	4 repaired: peak torque 105.8% compared with normal side 4 nonoperative: peak torque deficit 29.9% compared with normal side

References

1. Aarimaa V, Rantanen J, Heikkila J, et al. Rupture of the pectoralis major muscle. Am J Sports Med 2004;32:1256-1262.

2. Bak K, Cameron EA, Henderson IJP. Rupture of the pectoralis major: a meta-analysis of 122 cases. Knee Surg Sports Traumatol Arthrosc 2000;8:113-119.

3. Beloosesky Y, Hendel D, Weis A, et al. Rupture of the pectoralis major muscle in nursing home residents. Am J Med 2001;111:233-235.

4. Carrino JA, Chandnanni VP, Mitchell DB, et al. Pectoralis major muscle and tendon tears: diagnosis and grading using magnetic resonance imaging. Skeletal Radiol 2000;29:305-313.

5. Connell DA, Potter HG, Sherman MF, Wickiewicz TL. Injuries of the pectoralis major muscle: evaluation with MR imaging. Radiology 1999;210:785-791.

6. Egan TM, Hall H. Avulsion of the pectoralis major tendon in a weight lifter: repair using a barbed staple. Can J Surg 1987; 30:434-435.

7. Hanna CM, Glenny AB, Stanley SN, Caughey MA. Pectoralis major tears: comparison of surgical and conservative treatment. Br J Sports Med 2001;35:202-206.

8. Kretzler HH, Richardson AB. Rupture of the pectoralis major muscle. Am J Sports Med 1989;17:453-458.

9. Liu J, Wu JJ, Chang CY. Avulsion of the pectoralis major tendon. Am J Sports Med 1992;20:366-368.

10. McEntire JE, Hess WE, Coleman SS. Rupture of the pectoralis major muscle: a report of eleven injuries and review of fifty-six. J Bone Joint Surg Am 1972;54:1040-1045.

11. Miller MD, Johnson DL, Fu FH, et al. Rupture of the pectoralis major muscle in a collegiate football player: use of magnetic resonance imaging in early diagnosis. Am J Sports Med 1993;21:475-477.

12. Ohashi K, El-Khoury GY, Albright JP, Tearse DS. MRI of complete rupture of the pectoralis major muscle. Skeletal Radiol 1996; 25:625-628.

13. Pavlik A, Csepai D, Berkes I. Surgical treatment of pectoralis major rupture in athletes. Knee Surg Sports Traumatol Arthrosc 1998; 6:129-133.

14. Schepsis AA, Grafe MW, Jones HP, Lemos MJ. Rupture of the pectoralis major muscle: outcome after repair of acute and chronic injuries. Am J Sports Med 2000;28:9-15.

15. Simonian PT, Morris ME. Pectoralis tendon avulsion in the skeletally immature. Am J Orthop 1996;25:563-564.

16. Wolfe SW, Wickiewicz TL, Cavanaugh JT. Ruptures of the pectoralis major muscle: an anatomic and clinical analysis. Am J Sports Med 1992;20:587-593.

CHAPTER 30

Nonarthroplasty Options for Glenohumeral Arthritis: Meniscal Allograft Resurfacing

L. Pearce McCarty III, MD
Brian J. Cole, MD, MBA

Glenohumeral arthritis in young patients poses a particularly difficult treatment challenge. Nevertheless, independent of the patient's age, nonoperative treatment is often initially effective. Accordingly, nonsteroidal anti-inflammatory medications, intra-articular injections of cortisone or commercially available hyaluronate solutions,* appropriate activity modification, and physical therapy represent first-line therapy for patients with symptomatic glenohumeral degenerative joint disease.

Given the inherent problems with prosthetic glenoid resurfacing in this population (i.e., concerns about early glenoid loosening) and the difficulties with revision surgery posed by limited glenoid bone stock, prosthetic glenoid resurfacing is problematic in young, active patients. Arthroscopic débridement with capsular release often represents initial surgical therapy for this demanding population but can fail to provide long-term satisfactory results.[4,15] Furthermore, traditional hemiarthroplasty and humeral head resurfacing offer reasonable treatment options for select young individuals with unipolar disease, such as osteonecrosis of the humeral head, but may not result in significant pain relief or functional improvement for those with bipolar processes.

In this challenging population, a growing number of techniques have evolved to address bipolar glenohumeral disease with biologic resurfacing of the glenoid. Several biologic interpositional options have been proposed with limited success, including use of the anterior capsule, Achilles tendon allograft, meniscal allograft, and, more recently, various soft tissue rotator cuff augmentation devices.[1,3,5,10,16] This chapter presents one such technique in which glenoid resurfacing is accomplished by an allograft meniscus combined with conventional humeral prosthetic replacement. The technique of glenoid resurfacing with a meniscal allograft tissue is well described.[5,16] The premise behind the use of a human meniscus is that it provides a conforming biomechanical construct of fibrocartilaginous tissue with peripheral "liftoff," theoretically decreasing contact forces across an otherwise arthritic glenohumeral joint.[5]

Preoperative Considerations

History

Patients often present with a history of previous surgical intervention. It is therefore essential to obtain all pertinent operative reports and intraoperative records detailing types of implants used. A typical history might include the following[12]:

---

*Note that use of commercially available hyaluronate solutions in the glenohumeral joint is not an indication approved by the Food and Drug Administration.

- Labral repair by use of a headed, bioabsorbable tack
- Labral repair by use of multiple bioabsorbable, knotless anchors[6]
- Labral repair by use of multiple metallic suture anchors
- Use of "thermal capsulorrhaphy" technique[11]
- Use of postoperative intra-articular continuous pain catheters with local anesthetic agents
- Postoperative course after labral repair in which the patient does well during the initial 6 to 9 months, then develops increasing shoulder pain, particularly at rest and at night with associated loss of glenohumeral motion
- Open, nonanatomic stabilization, such as a Magnuson-Stack or Putti-Platt procedure
- Traumatic anterior or posterior instability with subsequent pain after adequate rehabilitation or operative stabilization
- History of proximal humerus fracture with or without open reduction and internal fixation

Physical Examination

Typical findings include the following:

- Loss of both active and passive range of motion, typically most pronounced in external rotation
- Glenohumeral crepitation with range of motion
- Weakness with testing of the rotator cuff secondary to pain inhibition

Particular attention should be paid to the status of the axillary nerve after previous surgical intervention or traumatic instability.

Imaging

Radiography

- True anterior-posterior view in plane of scapula (Grashey view) to assess glenohumeral joint and to permit preoperative templating for humeral head replacement
- Axillary lateral view to assess glenohumeral joint and to permit preoperative templating in the case that prosthetic humeral head replacement is planned
- West Point axillary view to identify bone loss along the anterior inferior glenoid rim (i.e., a "bony Bankart" lesion)
- Stryker notch view to evaluate volume of bone loss with Hill-Sachs lesions

Other Modalities

Magnetic resonance imaging without contrast enhancement is performed to assess for the following:

- Presence of joint effusion
- Presence of loose bodies
- Synovitis
- Capsular thickening
- Status of glenohumeral cartilage (Fig. 30-1)
- Status of the rotator cuff
- Evidence of inflammatory reaction to bioabsorbable implants
- Glenoid version and evidence of posterior wear pattern

Computed tomography with multiplanar and three-dimensional reconstructions is performed to assess for the following:

- Prominent metallic hardware
- Volume of humeral head osteochondral loss in cases of Hill-Sachs or reverse Hill-Sachs lesions
- Volume of glenoid bone loss in cases of bony Bankart lesions
- Glenoid version and evidence of posterior wear pattern

Indications and Contraindications

The ideal candidate for biologic resurfacing is relatively young (younger than 50 years) and active and has well-preserved deltoid and rotator cuff musculature. Indications include the following:

- Symptomatic, bipolar glenohumeral degenerative joint disease
- Relatively concentric joint space loss without significant glenoid version or structural abnormalities
- Failure of nonoperative treatment options as well as less aggressive operative modalities (e.g., arthroscopic débridement)

Relative contraindications include the following:

- Infection
- Significant glenoid version abnormalities or structural loss of glenoid anatomy (i.e., biconcave glenoid)
- Significant neural injury or neuromuscular disorder
- Uncorrected instability
- Voluntary dislocators
- Patients unable or unwilling to comply with postoperative rehabilitation and restrictions
- Shoulder pain that is not limited to the glenohumeral joint

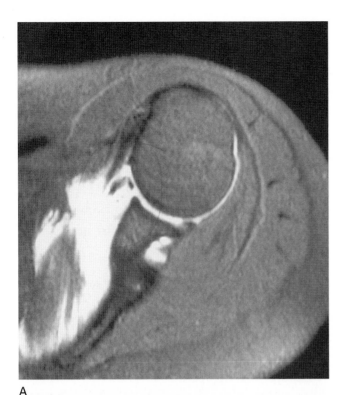

A

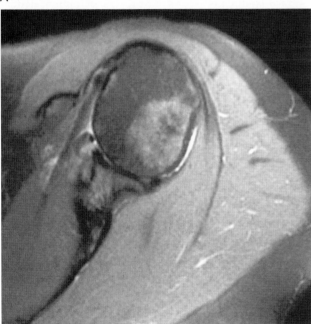

B

Figure 30-1 A, Preoperative axial magnetic resonance image of a 37-year-old patient before a labral repair performed at an outside institution. A bioabsorbable, headed poly-L-lactic acid labral tack was used for the repair. **B,** Postoperative axial magnetic resonance image of same patient at 9 months. Severe degeneration of both humeral and glenoid articular cartilage is demonstrated.

Arthroscopic débridement permits evaluation of the humeral and glenoid joint surfaces, removal of chondral loose bodies, and synovectomy when indicated. Selective capsular release, in the authors' opinion, should always precede more significant operative treatment (Fig. 30-2).

At times, particularly in the setting of the shoulder that has had multiple operations, it can be difficult to determine whether the glenohumeral joint is the sole or primary pain generator on the basis of history, physical examination findings, and imaging studies. In these cases, a fluoroscopically guided glenohumeral injection of local anesthetic is potentially diagnostic of the cause of the patient's pain. If significant pain relief is not received from the injection, the patient may not respond well to a resurfacing procedure. Furthermore, it is particularly important in a young population that the patient accept the limited-goals nature of the proposed procedure, that is, the intent is to provide reasonable pain relief and functional range of motion, not to restore normal shoulder function. The patient should understand that such a procedure may represent a temporary or "bridging" solution to the problem and that revision to conventional total shoulder arthroplasty may be indicated in the future. Most important, although the procedure may improve the patient's symptoms, albeit to a lesser degree compared with glenohumeral replacement, it does not prevent or compromise this later revision to conventional total shoulder arthroplasty.

30

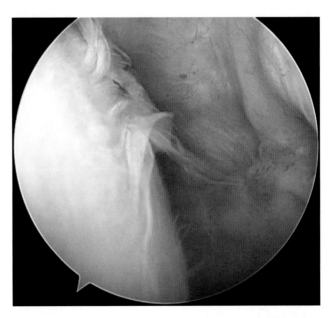

Figure 30-2 Intraoperative image of the patient depicted in Figure 30-1 at the time of diagnostic arthroscopy and débridement, demonstrating grade III-IV changes across the humeral head as well as glenohumeral synovitis.

Surgical Planning

Allograft Sizing, Processing, and Preservation

The smallest available lateral meniscal allograft should be requested for glenoid resurfacing. The anterior and posterior horns of the lateral meniscus are situated relatively close to one another, giving it a smaller radius of curvature and making it a better geometric match for the glenoid than the medial meniscus. Fresh-frozen allografts that have tested free of viral and bacterial contamination are preferred. Theoretically, a contralateral lateral meniscus can be chosen and positioned such that the indentation for the popliteus tendon is superior near the biceps insertion. However, specific differences in surgical technique have not been well elucidated, and thus the surgeon's preferences often prevail in determining exact graft position relative to the glenoid anatomy. Recipients should be educated about the small but finite risk of disease transmission with implantation of any allograft tissue. This risk is strongly mitigated through diligent donor screening policies and polymerase chain reaction testing for viral contaminants.

Surgical Technique

Anesthesia and Positioning

General anesthesia with endotracheal airway is preferred. Depending on the experience of the anesthesiology staff, regional anesthesia in the form of an interscalene block can serve as a useful adjunct, both for minimizing the need for intraoperative inhaled anesthetics and for reducing the need for postoperative, narcotic pain medication.

The patient is placed in a well-padded, modified beach chair position. The medial border of the scapula on the operative side is roughly aligned with the edge of the operating table; a small, rolled towel can be useful to protract the scapula further, facilitating intraoperative access to the face of the glenoid. The patient is positioned such that full glenohumeral extension and some degree of glenohumeral adduction is possible. An articulated arm-holding device, such as the McConnell arm holder (McConnell Orthopedic Manufacturing Company, Greenville, Texas), can be a useful adjunct.

Surgical Landmarks, Incisions, and Portals

Landmarks

- Coracoid process
- Acromion
- Deltoid insertion
- Axillary crease

Portals and Approaches

- Deltopectoral approach

Structures at Risk

- Cephalic vein
- Musculocutaneous nerve
- Axillary nerve

Examination Under Anesthesia and Diagnostic Arthroscopy

Passive range of motion and stability are evaluated carefully and documented.

Specific Steps (Box 30-1)

1. Deltopectoral Approach

Surface landmarks—coracoid process, acromion, deltoid insertion—are marked on the skin. An 8- to 10-cm incision is made from a point immediately lateral to the lateral tip of the coracoid process in the direction of the deltoid insertion. The fat stripe indicating the interval between the medial border of the anterior deltoid and the superior border of the pectoralis major is located. The cephalic vein is identified, preserved, and taken laterally with the deltoid. Medial mobilization of the cephalic vein may be preferred to avoid inadvertent laceration as many of the surgical steps are performed medially with prolonged posterior displacement of the proximal humerus. The blades of a self-retaining retractor, such as a Kolbel retractor, are placed beneath the deltoid and pectoralis major. A Hohman retractor is placed superior to the coracoacromial ligament. The tip of the coracoid process is visualized, and the "red stripe" that marks the lateral border of the conjoined tendon is identified. By use of blunt dissection, a plane is developed deep to the conjoined tendon. The musculocutaneous nerve is palpated at its entry into the deep surface

Box 30-1 Surgical Steps

1. Deltopectoral approach
2. Lesser tuberosity osteotomy
3. Humeral preparation
4. Inferior capsular release
5. Glenoid preparation and meniscal allograft implantation
6. Humeral implant, lesser tuberosity repair, and closure

of the conjoined tendon. If the entry point is distal, then one of the blades of the self-retaining retractor may be safely placed deep to the conjoined tendon. Otherwise, gentle, intermittent manual retraction is used to avoid traction injury to the nerve.

2. Lesser Tuberosity Osteotomy

The arm is forward flexed and internally rotated. The long head of the biceps tendon is transected in its groove and sutured to the superior aspect of the pectoralis major insertion. The remnant of the long head of the biceps tendon is used as a guide to open the rotator interval and is then transected at its junction with the superior labrum. A 1-inch flat osteotome is then used to osteotomize the lesser tuberosity. A 5-mm-thick wafer of bone is taken, permitting reflection of the subscapularis (Fig. 30-3). Traction sutures are placed around the tuberosity fragment to assist with release. The axillary nerve is identified by palpation. If there is any doubt about its location, gentle dissection can be used along the inferior border of the subscapularis to visualize the nerve directly. A "360-degree release" of the subscapularis tendon is then performed, with release of the coracohumeral ligament superiorly, release of the anterior capsular reflection posteriorly, and release of subdeltoid and subcoracoid adhesions. The final element of the release—the inferior glenohumeral capsule—is addressed after humeral preparation.

3. Humeral Preparation

The humerus is maintained in a position of adduction and neutral flexion or extension as the capsular attachment to the humerus is released and the humerus is progressively externally rotated. Osteophytes are removed from the humerus, permitting identification of the anatomic neck. A freehand cut is made to match the native version and inclination of the proximal humerus, and a third-generation system that permits precise recapitulation of the native anatomy is used. As an alternative to the traditional stemmed component, a humeral head resurfacing implant can be used, permitting even greater preservation of proximal humeral bone stock but making access to the glenoid more challenging in some cases.

4. Inferior Capsular Release

Release of the inferior capsule completes the 360-degree release of the subscapularis and permits the posterior translation of the proximal humerus that is necessary for broad access to the glenoid. The traction sutures placed through the lesser tuberosity are pulled in a superior direction to put the inferior border of the subscapularis under tension. A plane is developed between the lower muscle border of the subscapularis and the anterior inferior capsule. This maneuver permits clear visualization along both the superior and inferior surfaces of the inferior glenohumeral capsule, allowing it to be released in a safe, controlled manner, with minimal risk to the axillary nerve.

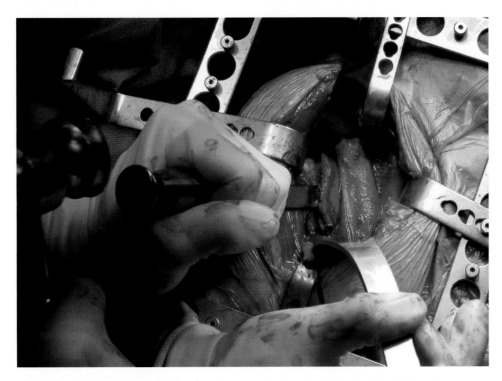

Figure 30-3 The lesser tuberosity osteotomy is initiated at the bicipital groove and continued medially with a broad, flat osteotome.

For additional safety, the release is performed at the capsulolabral junction, and a finger is maintained superior and posterior to the nerve. The inferior capsule typically is released until the triceps origin can be visualized.

5. Glenoid Preparation and Meniscal Allograft Implantation

A Fukuda or similar type of retractor is then placed behind the posterior rim of the glenoid, and the humerus is placed in a position of slight external rotation, relaxing the posterior capsule and facilitating glenoid exposure. An anterior glenoid retractor is placed into the subscapularis recess, and a Hohman retractor is placed along the superior edge of the glenoid. The labrum is débrided. The glenoid face is reamed lightly. A microfracture awl is used to make multiple perforations across the glenoid, spaced 5 mm apart. The lateral meniscal allograft is removed from its bony attachment, and the ends of the meniscus are sutured over one another with a heavy, nonabsorbable suture (Fig. 30-4). The degree of overlap is judged to allow the size of the prepared meniscus to approximate the size of the recipient glenoid. A Bankart awl or small drill bit is used to prepare the glenoid for transosseous sutures. A total of eight heavy, nonabsorbable sutures are used, starting at 12-o'clock and progressing in 90-minute intervals (Fig. 30-5). The meniscal allograft is marked similarly (Fig. 30-6). Posterior sutures can be difficult to place in transos-

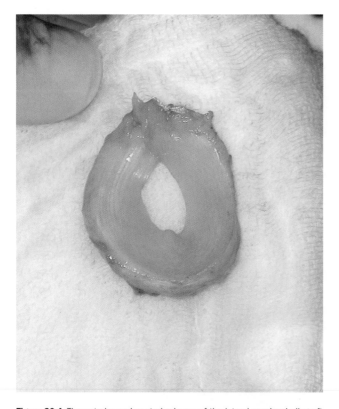

Figure 30-4 The anterior and posterior horns of the lateral meniscal allograft are overlapped and sutured together to approximate the surface area and shape of the glenoid recipient site.

seous fashion, and suture anchors can be used instead, placed in percutaneous fashion as one would do during an arthroscopic posterior labral repair (Fig. 30-7). By use of a small trocar-tipped or cutting needle, these sutures are now passed through the meniscal allograft, which is then advanced down the sutures and onto the face of the glenoid (Fig. 30-8). Sutures are tied in balanced fashion (12-o'clock, then 6-o'clock, and so on).

6. Humeral Implant, Lesser Tuberosity Repair, and Closure

The humeral head protector is removed and replaced with the humeral trial. The subscapularis is reduced to its insertion, and soft tissue balance is assessed. The trial is then removed, and a series of four holes are drilled through the bicipital groove along the lateral edge of the lesser tuberosity footprint. A series of three holes are drilled medial to the footprint. Four No. 5 nonabsorbable sutures are then placed through the holes in horizontal fashion. The superior-most of these sutures will pass through a lateral drill hole and then around the neck of the implant rather than through a matching medial drill hole. The humeral implant is then inserted. A small amount of cement can be used along the proximal aspect of the implant, but given the future possibility of conversion to total shoulder arthroplasty, the humeral stem is not cemented in its entirety. The previously placed No. 5 sutures are then passed around the lesser tuberosity wafer and tied down securely (Fig. 30-9). The humerus is internally and externally rotated to assess the security of the tuberosity repair. There should be no observable motion at the repair site. If desired, the rotator interval can be closed with the humerus in maximal external rotation. Motion, stability, and soft tissue balance are assessed once again. A drain is not used routinely. The deltopectoral interval is closed loosely with 2-0 Ethibond (Ethicon, Inc., Somerville, NJ) nonabsorbable sutures. Colored sutures can serve as a useful landmark in the event of future revision to total shoulder arthroplasty.

Postoperative Considerations

Follow-up

- At 7 to 10 days for wound check and radiographs (true anteroposterior view in plane of scapula and outlet view)

Rehabilitation

0-6 weeks

- Pendulum exercises are begun.
- Lesser tuberosity osteotomy precautions: No active internal rotation, backward extension, or passive external rotation beyond the safe limit determined intraoperatively is allowed.

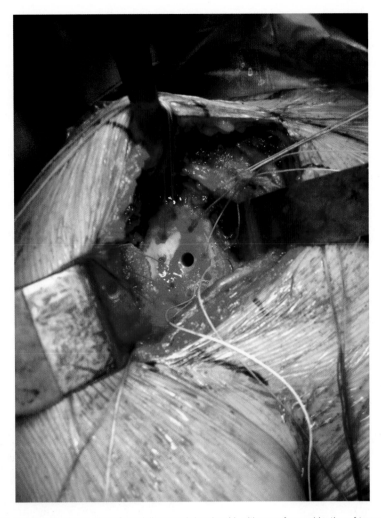

Figure 30-5 Heavy, nonabsorbable sutures are placed circumferentially around the glenoid, with use of a combination of transosseous sutures and suture anchors.

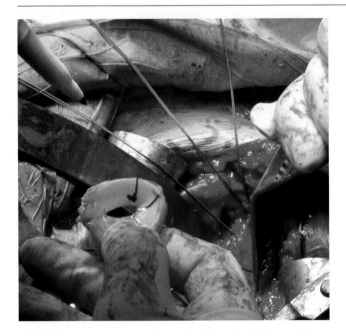

Figure 30-6 The meniscal allograft is marked circumferentially to match placement of the glenoid sutures.

- A simple sling is worn for weeks 0 to 4.
- Active use of the elbow, wrist, and hand is encouraged.
- Active-assisted range of motion is permitted up to 120 degrees of forward flexion, 75 degrees of abduction.

7-12 weeks

- Active-assisted range of motion is progressed to active range of motion for internal rotation and backward extension as tolerated.
- Active-assisted range of motion is progressed to active range of motion in forward flexion, abduction, and external rotation as tolerated.
- Begin gentle deltoid and rotator cuff isometrics, with the exception of internal rotation.
- Start periscapular strengthening exercises.

13 weeks and beyond

- Progress strengthening, including resisted internal rotation.
- Perform gentle end-range stretching.

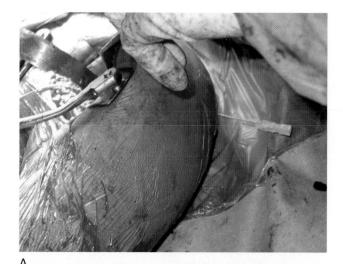

A

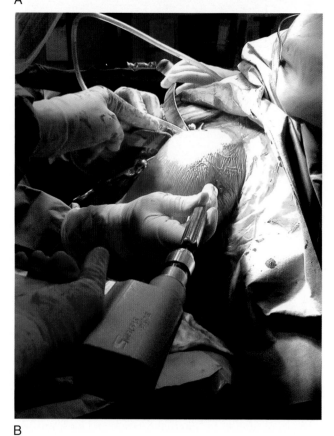

B

Figure 30-7 A, Spinal needle localization determines the appropriate direction and angle for placement of suture anchors along the posterior glenoid rim. **B,** Suture anchors are placed along the glenoid rim by use of a cannulated guide through a posterior stab incision.

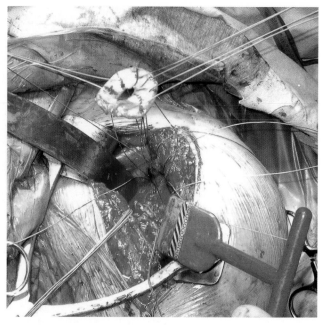

Figure 30-8 Sutures are placed through the meniscal allograft at marked positions, and the allograft is pushed down the sutures onto the face of the glenoid.

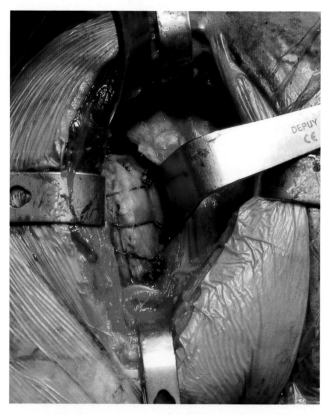

Figure 30-9 The lesser tuberosity osteotomy is repaired with heavy, nonabsorbable suture through transosseous tunnels.

Table 30-1 Clinical Results of Biologic Glenohumeral Resurfacing

Author	Procedure	Follow-up	Outcome
Burkhead and Hutton[3] (1995)	Humeral hemiarthroplasty Biologic resurfacing of glenoid with either fascia lata autograft or anterior capsule	34 months	Range of motion in forward flexion improved from 81 to 137 degrees Neer's full exercise rating system: 8 excellent, 2 satisfactory results
Krishnan et al[10] (2004)	Humeral hemiarthroplasty Biologic resurfacing of glenoid and acromion with Achilles tendon allograft	3 years	ASES score improved from 25 to 75 Range of motion in forward flexion improved from 35 to 95 degrees
Argo et al[1] (2005)	Arthroscopic interposition grafting with porcine xenograft	13 months	VAS for pain dropped from 8 to 2 Range of motion in forward flexion improved from 90 to 150 degrees Range of motion in abduction improved from 70 to 120 degrees

ASES, American Shoulder and Elbow Surgeons; VAS, visual analogue scale.

30

PEARLS AND PITFALLS

- At times, particularly in the setting of the shoulder that has had multiple operations, it can be difficult to determine whether the glenohumeral joint is the sole or primary pain generator on the basis of the history and physical examination findings alone. In these cases, a fluoroscopically guided glenohumeral injection of local anesthetic can serve as a valuable diagnostic aid. Those patients who obtain minimal symptomatic relief from such an injection may not respond well to a resurfacing procedure.

- When releasing the inferior capsule, rotate the inferior border of the Fukuda retractor laterally to increase the tension placed on the capsule, making it easier to visualize and to isolate. This can also facilitate tension on the posterior capsule if release is required to facilitate internal rotation.

- When placing suture anchors along the posterior glenoid rim, first use percutaneous spinal needle localization from a posterior approach to establish direction and angle, then make a small stab incision and advance one of several commercially available cannulated guides with a sharp obturator through the incision onto the glenoid. After anchor placement, collect sutures out through the anterior deltopectoral approach. The same stab incision can be used to place two or three anchors.

- A lesser tuberosity osteotomy probably does a better job of preserving anatomy and function than does a transtendinous approach through the subscapularis. Given the likelihood of future procedures in this young population, this approach may facilitate preservation of function in the shoulder with multiple operations.

- Failure to comply with postoperative activity restrictions, particularly for the first 6 weeks, not only endangers the lesser tuberosity repair but may also impair healing of the meniscal allograft to the face of the glenoid.

- Significant popping or clicking or the sensation of a "clunk" during the early postoperative period is likely to signify failure of fixation at the meniscus-glenoid interface.

Complications

Complications are similar to those of total shoulder arthroplasty:

- Injury to the axillary nerve
- Injury to the musculocutaneous nerve
- Failure of the lesser tuberosity repair
- Infection
- Incomplete relief of pain
- Failure of the meniscus-glenoid interface

Results

Published and presented results of biologic resurfacing procedures are limited, and those available reflect only short- and intermediate-term outcomes (Table 30-1).

References

1. Argo D, Savoie FH, Field LD. Arthroscopic treatment of glenohumeral arthritis with interpositional grafting. Presented at Arthroscopy Association of North America, 24th annual meeting; Vancouver, BC, Canada; 2005.

2. Athwal G, Shridharani S, O'Driscoll SW. Osteolysis and arthropathy of the shoulder after use of bioabsorbable knotless suture anchors. J Bone Joint Surg Am 2006;88:1840-1845.

3. Burkhead WZ Jr, Hutton KS. Biologic resurfacing of the glenoid with hemiarthroplasty of the shoulder. J Shoulder Elbow Surg 1995;4:263-270.

4. Cameron BD, Galatz LM, Ramsey ML, et al. Non-prosthetic management of grade IV osteochondral lesions of the glenohumeral joint. J Shoulder Elbow Surg 2002;11:25-32.

5. Creighton RA, Cole BJ, Nicholson GP, et al. Effect of lateral meniscal allograft on shoulder articular contact areas and pressures. J Shoulder Elbow Surg; Epub Nov 8, 2006.

6. Freehill MQ, Harms DJ, Huber SM, et al. Poly-L-lactic acid tack synovitis after arthroscopic stabilization of the shoulder. Am J Sports Med 2003;31:643-647.

7. Gerber C, Lambert SM. Allograft reconstruction of segmental defects of the humeral head for the treatment of chronic locked posterior dislocation of the shoulder. J Bone Joint Surg Am 1996;78:376-382.

8. Hamada S, Hamada M, Nishiue S, Doi T. Osteochondritis dissecans of the humeral head. Arthroscopy 1992;8:132-137.

9. Johnson DL, Warner JJ. Osteochondritis dissecans of the humeral head: treatment with a matched osteochondral allograft. J Shoulder Elbow Surg 1997;6:160-163.

10. Krishnan SG, Burkhead WZ Jr, Nowinski RJ. Humeral hemiarthroplasty with biologic resurfacing of the glenoid and acromion for rotator cuff tear arthropathy. Tech Shoulder Elbow Surg 2004;5:51-59.

11. Levine WN, Clark AM Jr, D'Alessandro DF, Yamaguchi K. Chondrolysis following arthroscopic thermal capsulorrhaphy to treat shoulder instability. A report of two cases. J Bone Joint Surg Am 2005;87:616-621.

12. Petty DH, Jazrawi LM, Estrada LS, Andrews JR. Glenohumeral chondrolysis after shoulder arthroscopy: case reports and review of the literature. Am J Sports Med 2004;32:509-515.

13. Scheibel M, Bartl C, Magosch P, et al. Osteochondral autologous transplantation for the treatment of full-thickness articular cartilage defects of the shoulder. J Bone Joint Surg Br 2004;86:991-997.

14. Siebold R, Lichtenberg S, Habermeyer P. Combination of microfracture and periostal-flap for the treatment of focal full thickness articular cartilage lesions of the shoulder: a prospective study. Knee Surg Sports Traumatol Arthrosc 2003;11:183-189.

15. Weinstein DM, Bucchieri JS, Pollock RG, et al. Arthroscopic débridement of the shoulder for osteoarthritis. Arthroscopy 2000;16:471-476.

16. Yamaguchi K, Ball C, Galatz L. Meniscal allograft interposition arthroplasty of the arthritic shoulder: early results and a review of the technique. Presented at the 18th open meeting of the American Shoulder and Elbow Surgeons; Dallas, Texas; 2002.

PART 2

The Elbow

CHAPTER **31**

Patient Positioning and Portal Placement

Frederick M. Azar, MD
Bradley D. Dresher, MD

As advances in technology and technique allow better visualization and navigation of the elbow joint, indications for elbow arthroscopy are expanding. Descriptions of new portals, instrumentation, and techniques are frequent in the literature and continue to increase the use of the arthroscope for diagnosis and treatment of a number of elbow injuries and disorders. A thorough understanding of portal placement and normal arthroscopic anatomy is essential for use of the arthroscope in the elbow joint to be mastered and for complications to be avoided.

Preoperative Considerations

History

A comprehensive history discerns whether a single traumatic event or repetitive traumatic episodes occurred before the onset of symptoms. The circumstances under which symptoms occur and whether they are related to activities of daily living, occupational activities, or athletic activities are noted.

Typical History

- Loss of velocity and control in a throwing athlete
- Repetitive episodes versus traumatic event
- Acute versus chronic pain
- Mechanical symptoms: popping, locking, catching
- Instability
- Neurovascular symptoms

Physical Examination

All three elbow compartments (medial, lateral, posterior) are carefully examined. Elbow stability, range of motion, and neurovascular status are evaluated.

Medial Compartment

- Check for valgus instability. With the elbow flexed to 30 degrees to relax the anterior capsule and to free the olecranon from its bony articulation in the olecranon fossa, apply valgus stress with the arm in full supination. Discomfort along the medial aspect of the elbow may indicate ulnar collateral ligament injury.
- Palpate the proximal flexor-pronator mass and medial epicondyle.
- Test resisted wrist flexion and forearm pronation; pain with these maneuvers may indicate medial epicondylitis or flexor-pronator tendon disease.
- Palpate the ulnar nerve in the cubital tunnel; flex and extend the elbow as the nerve is palpated to detect nerve subluxation.
- Assess the Tinel sign over the ulnar nerve.

Posterior Compartment

- Palpate the triceps muscle insertion and the posterolateral and posteromedial joint to check for bone spurs or impingement.
- "Clunk" test for posterior olecranon impingement: Grasp the patient's upper arm to stabilize the arm as the elbow is brought into full extension. Pain with this

maneuver may indicate compression of the olecranon into the fossa (valgus extension overload).

Lateral Compartment

- Palpate the lateral epicondyle and extensor origin to identify lateral epicondylitis or tendon disease.
- Pain with resisted wrist dorsiflexion and forearm supination is indicative of lateral epicondylitis.
- Palpate the radiocapitellar joint while the forearm is pronated and supinated to check for crepitus or catching, which may indicate chondromalacia.
- Inspect the "soft spot" to check for synovitis or effusion.

Stability

- The O'Driscoll posterolateral instability test can be performed to evaluate posterolateral rotatory instability. However, because of the patient's apprehension, the test result is usually negative. This test is best done under general anesthesia.

Range of Motion

- Flexion, extension, pronation, and supination are determined and compared with the opposite extremity.

Imaging

Radiography

Review carefully for fractures, subluxation, dislocation, degenerative changes, osteophytes, and loose bodies.

- Anteroposterior view with elbow in full extension
- Lateral view with elbow flexed 90 degrees
- Axial view (best for identifying posteromedial osteophytes)
- Gravity stress test view (detects valgus laxity)

Magnetic Resonance Imaging

- Evaluation of osteochondral lesions in radiocapitellar joint
- Detection of early vascular changes
- Assessment of extent of lesion and displacement of fragments
- Evaluation of soft tissue structures
- Detection of partial-thickness undersurface tears or full-thickness tears of the ulnar collateral ligament (magnetic resonance arthrography with saline contrast or gadolinium)
- Detection of loose bodies

Indications and Contraindications

Common indications include removal of loose bodies, resection of symptomatic plicae, capsular release in patients with contracture, removal of osteophytes, synovectomy in patients with inflammatory arthritis, treatment of osteochondritis dissecans, débridement for lateral epicondylitis, and treatment of some elbow fractures (Steinmann et al). The primary contraindication to elbow arthroscopy is any severe distortion of normal bone or soft tissue anatomy that jeopardizes safe entry of the arthroscope into the joint. Local soft tissue infection in the area of portal sites also is a contraindication.

Surgical Technique

Anesthesia and Positioning

We prefer to use a general anesthetic because it is reliable, provides muscle relaxation, allows positioning without discomfort to the patient, and permits the use of a tourniquet when it is needed. Local and intravenous blocks have the disadvantage of making neurovascular evaluation unreliable postoperatively.

Supine Position (Fig. 31-1; authors' preference)

The patient is placed supine on the operating table with the scapula at the edge of the table and the shoulder abducted 90 degrees. The operative extremity is placed in a prefabricated wrist gauntlet, stockinette, or finger traps. Enough traction is applied to suspend the elbow away from the table at 90 degrees of flexion (10 pounds is the standard amount). A well-padded tourniquet is placed high on the operative arm to allow proper portal placement and instrument manipulation. Use of a traction setup allows access for medial and lateral approaches and eliminates the need for an assistant to hold the extremity. Flexing the elbow 90 degrees relaxes the neurovascular

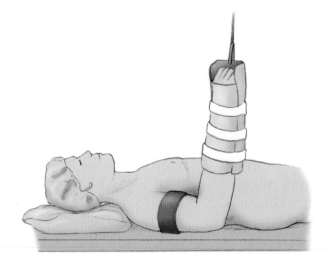

Figure 31-1 Supine position for elbow arthroscopy. (Redrawn from Baker CL Jr, Jones GL. Current concepts. Arthroscopy of the elbow. Am J Sports Med 1999;27:251-264.)

structures, making portal placement safer, and the forearm can be supinated and pronated during the procedure.

If a suspension device is not available, two arm boards can be used to support the operative extremity. This requires an assistant to hold the arm at 90 degrees of elbow flexion at all times. This set-up is more stable but does require more operative personnel.

Prone Position (Fig. 31-2)

After intubation, the patient is placed prone, with care taken to place chest bolsters to assist in torso and airway care. The patient is then positioned near the edge of the table; with a rolled towel or arm holder, the operative extremity is positioned with the shoulder abducted 90 degrees, the elbow flexed 90 degrees, and the hand pointed toward the floor. Before the extremity is prepared, a well-padded tourniquet is placed high on the arm, and the elbow is moved through a full range of motion to ensure that complete flexion and extension can be obtained and the shoulder is not hyperextended. Baker noted several advantages of the prone position. First, because of the weight of the arm over a bolster, no traction is needed because gravity assists in joint distraction. Second, the arm is stable during the procedure, unlike in the supine position, in which the arm may tend to swing during portal placement and instrument introduction. Third, the neurovascular structures are protected by being farther away from the capsule as a result of gravity and fluid distention of the joint. Next, if it is needed, conversion to an open procedure can be done through a medial or lateral exposure. Finally, the elbow can be fully extended during the procedure if necessary.

Lateral Decubitus Position (Fig. 31-3)

This position is similar to the prone position but allows access to the posterior compartment and also provides easy maintenance of anesthesia during the procedure. Again, a tourniquet is applied high on the arm, and the arm is positioned with a bump or bolster attached to the bed.

Surgical Landmarks, Incisions, and Portals

General Principles of Portal Placement

- Mark all portal sites before surgery, when the elbow is not distended or edematous.
- Mark all surface landmarks with a pen (lateral epicondyle, medial epicondyle, radial head, capitellum, and olecranon).
- Palpate the ulnar nerve and mark its location; check that it does not subluxate from the cubital tunnel.
- Identify the location and course of any visible superficial cutaneous nerves and mark them; when necessary, use a retractor to expose and protect these nerves.
- Distend the joint by an 18-gauge needle through the direct lateral portal site (soft spot) with 20 to 40 mL of lactated Ringer solution.
- Initiate an anterolateral portal (authors' preference) or anteromedial portal after placing a second 18-gauge needle in the anticipated portal site.
- A blunt or conical trocar and cannula are used to trap the capsule over the radial head for anterolateral portal placement.
- The 18-gauge needle is left in the soft spot to be used as an outflow.
- Once the initial portal is made, all subsequent portals should be made under direct vision with use of an 18-gauge needle.

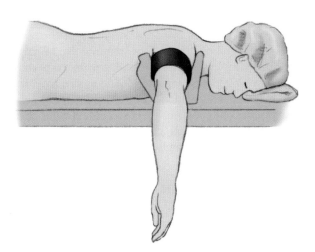

Figure 31-2 Prone position for elbow arthroscopy. (Redrawn from Baker CL Jr, Jones GL. Current concepts. Arthroscopy of the elbow. Am J Sports Med 1999;27:251-264.)

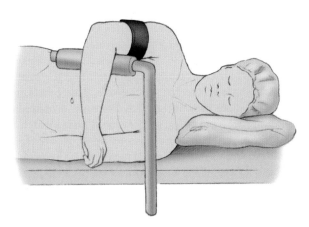

Figure 31-3 Lateral decubitus position for elbow arthroscopy. (Redrawn from Baker CL Jr, Jones GL. Current concepts. Arthroscopy of the elbow. Am J Sports Med 1999;27:251-264.)

- When making portals, avoid "stab" incisions. Instead, lay the tip of the blade against the skin and pull the skin across the blade; this allows subcutaneous tissue and sensory nerves to fall away to a safe distance and reduces the risk of nerve injury. Spread the subcutaneous tissues with a mosquito hemostat to prevent damage to the superficial cutaneous nerves.

- A switching stick is a helpful alternative to establishing the anteromedial from the anterolateral portal or the anterolateral from the anteromedial portal by driving the arthroscope directly to the second portal site from inside and then cutting down on the switching stick from outside and placing a cannula over the exposed tip.

- Pump pressures should be maintained at 35 to 45 mm Hg to prevent fluid extravasation and possible compartment syndrome. The use of nonvented cannulas decreases fluid extravasation into the soft tissues.

After general anesthesia has been administered, bone anatomy and landmarks are palpated and marked (Fig. 31-4). The radial head, found by supination and pronation of the forearm, is outlined, as are the medial and lateral epicondyles and the olecranon. The course of the ulnar nerve through the cubital tunnel also should be outlined.

Specific Portal Placement

Lateral Portals (Fig. 31-5)

The direct lateral portal lies in the center of a triangle formed by the lateral epicondyle, radial head, and olecranon. This soft spot is easily palpated before distention. This approach passes through the anconeus muscle; it is used for initial joint distention and for lateral portal viewing. Watch for the posterior antebrachial cutaneous nerve, which passes within 7 mm.

The anterolateral portal lies 2 to 3 cm distal and 1 to 2 cm anterior to the lateral humeral epicondyle, within the sulcus between radial head and capitellum anteriorly. These measurements may vary, depending on the size of the patient, and portal placement depends on locating the radiocapitellar articulation. The anterolateral portal passes through the extensor carpi radialis brevis and the supinator muscle before reaching the capsule. This portal provides an excellent view of the medial capsule, medial plica, coronoid process, trochlea, and coronoid fossa. Watch for the posterior antebrachial cutaneous nerve, an average of 2 mm from the sheath; the radial nerve, which is usually 7 to 11 mm anteromedial to the portal but may be as close as 2 or 3 mm; and the posterior interosseous nerve, 1 to 13 mm from the portal, depending on the degree of forearm pronation.

The middle anterolateral portal, located 1 cm directly anterior to the lateral epicondyle, provides access to the radiocapitellar joint and lateral compartment and is a good working portal for instrumentation. It also functions as a good viewing portal for the anterior ulnohumeral joint.

The proximal anterolateral portal is made 1 to 2 cm proximal and 1 cm anterior to the lateral epicondyle. Stothers et al described this portal as being safer than the middle anterolateral portal, which was safer than the standard distal anterolateral portal.

Medial Portals (Fig. 31-6)

The anteromedial portal is placed 2 cm anterior and 2 cm distal to the medial epicondyle. It is usually placed under direct visualization with the use of an 18-gauge needle. The anteromedial portal passes between the radial aspect of the flexor digitorum sublimis and the tendinous portion of the pronator teres before entering the joint capsule. It allows examination of the radiocapitellar and humeroulnar joints, the coronoid fossa, the capitellum, and the superior capsule. Watch for the medial antebrachial cutaneous nerve, which is an average of 6 mm from the portal but may be as close as 1 mm; the median nerve, which is 19 mm anterolateral to the portal with the joint distended and 12 mm without distention; and the ulnar nerve, located an average of 21 mm from the portal. The portal lies 17 mm posteromedial to the brachial artery.

The proximal medial (superomedial) portal is placed 1 cm anterior and 1 to 2 cm proximal to the medial epicondyle and passes through a tendinous portion of the flexor-pronator group. This portal provides excellent viewing of the anterior compartment of the elbow, particularly the radiocapitellar joint. Watch for the median nerve, which is 22.3 mm from the portal.

Posterior Portals (Fig. 31-7)

The posterolateral portal is placed 2 to 3 cm proximal to the olecranon tip and just lateral to the lateral border of the triceps muscle. This portal allows examination of the olecranon tip, olecranon fossa, and posterior trochlea.

The straight posterior portal is located over the center of the triceps tendon, 2 cm medial to the posterolateral portal and 3 cm proximal to the tip of the olecranon. This portal is helpful for removal of impinging olecranon osteophytes and loose bodies from the posterior elbow joint. Watch for the posterior and medial antebrachial cutaneous nerves, which lie on the lateral and medial aspects of the upper arm 23 to 25 mm medial to the straight posterior portal, and the ulnar nerve, located within 25 mm of the straight posterior portal.

Normal Arthroscopic Anatomy

Anterior Compartment

Through the anterolateral portal (Fig. 31-8), the coronoid and its articulation with the trochlea can be viewed. Flexion and extension of the elbow bring the anterior trochlea into view. The brachialis tendon insertion can be evaluated on

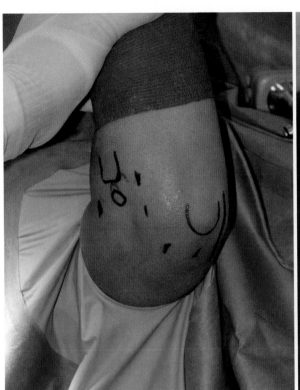

A

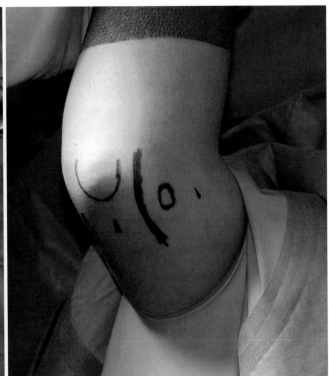

B

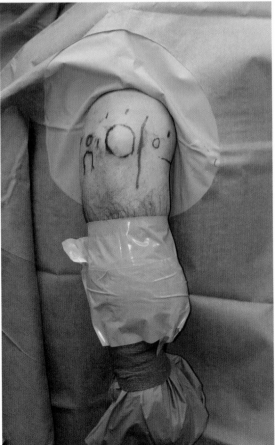

C

Figure 31-4 Bone anatomy and landmarks outlined before distention of the joint: radial head, medial and lateral epicondyles, olecranon, and course of the ulnar nerve.

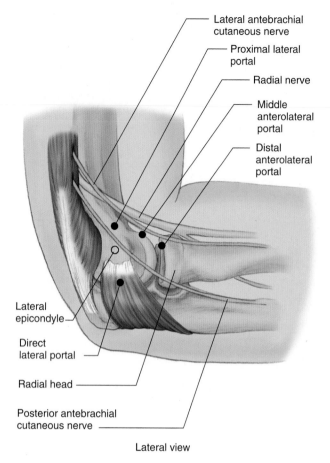

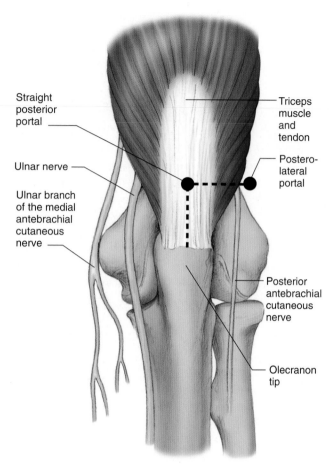

Figure 31-5 Lateral portals. (Redrawn from Baker CL Jr, Jones GL. Current concepts. Arthroscopy of the elbow. Am J Sports Med 1999;27:251-264.)

Posterior view

Figure 31-7 Posterior portals. (Redrawn from Baker CL Jr, Jones GL. Current concepts. Arthroscopy of the elbow. Am J Sports Med 1999;27:251-264.)

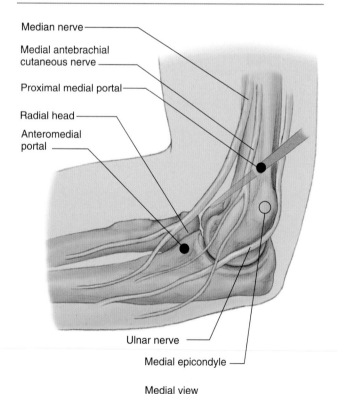

Medial view

Figure 31-6 Medial portals. (Redrawn from Baker CL Jr, Jones GL. Current concepts. Arthroscopy of the elbow. Am J Sports Med 1999;27:251-264.)

the coronoid process. The coronoid fossa can be seen proximal in the compartment. With the arthroscope directed medially, the medial portion of the capsule can be examined, including the anterior third of the anterior bundle of the ulnar collateral ligament. With proper orientation of the scope, the proximal ulna and medial gutter can be viewed. The sublime tubercle, with the intersection of the anteromedial capsule and the proximal medial ulna, can be evaluated.

Through the anteromedial portal (Fig. 31-9), established under direct vision by initial placement of an 18-gauge needle, the radial head and the radiocapitellar articulation can be identified. Supination and pronation of the forearm allow viewing of 75% of the surface of the radial head. The annular ligament can be noted crossing the radial neck, and the radial fossa can be evaluated with proximal viewing of the scope. The attachment of the capsule to the humerus can be seen superiorly. The scope can then be advanced to examine the lateral gutter, the undersurface of the capsule, and the origin of the extensor muscles to the lateral epicondyle. The articulations of the radius, ulna, and distal humerus can be viewed by placing

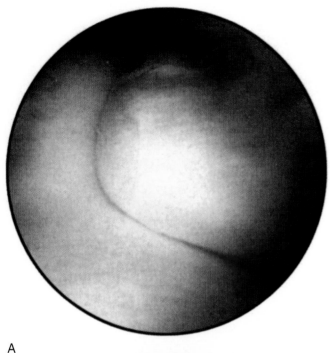

A

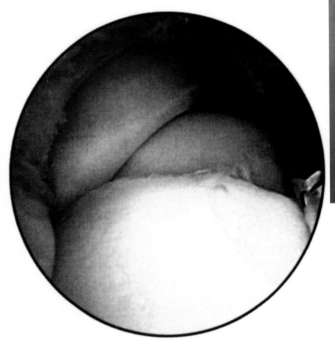

Figure 31-9 Anteromedial portal, anterior aspect of elbow. The coronoid and trochlea are in the foreground and the radiocapitellar joint is in the background, with the shaver just proximal to the radiocapitellar joint. The annular ligament is clearly seen. (From Phillips BB. Arthroscopy of upper extremity. In Canale ST, ed. Campbell's Operative Orthopaedics, 10th ed. St. Louis, Mosby, 2003.)

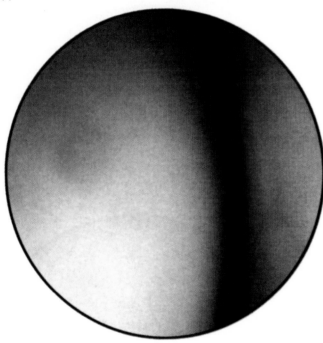

B

Figure 31-8 Anterolateral portal. **A,** Medial side of elbow; the coronoid process is on the right and the trochlea is on the left. **B,** Radiocapitellar joint with varus stress applied to expose the undersurface of the radial head. (From Phillips BB. Arthroscopy of upper extremity. In Canale ST, ed. Campbell's Operative Orthopaedics, 10th ed. St. Louis, Mosby, 2003.)

the scope between the trochlear and capitellar ridges up to the medial border of the radial head.

Lateral Compartment

Through the direct lateral portal (Fig. 31-10), the articulation of the olecranon, radial head, and capitellum can be seen. Again, supination and pronation of the forearm allow viewing of 75% of the radial head articular surface. The capitellum can be seen and most of the smooth convex surface can be examined through this portal. The olecranon fossa can also be evaluated at this position. The scope can then be positioned posterior into the groove formed by the olecranon and trochlea. The entire olecranon can be seen from this vantage. The apophyseal scar can be viewed at the midpoint as a bare area of roughened articular cartilage. The undersurface of the trochlea should be visible when the scope is turned anteriorly. The posterolateral corner and capsule are viewed by looking posteriorly from the olecranon-trochlear groove. The posterior compartment can then be viewed for establishment of the posterior portals. If the 4-mm arthroscope is too large for this portal, a 2.7-mm arthroscope can be used.

Posterior Compartment

The olecranon tip will be the first landmark seen through the posterolateral portal (Fig. 31-11). The triceps tendon insertion will be seen at the olecranon tip, where osteophyte formation may be noted posteromedially in patients with posterior impingement due to valgus extension overload. The olecranon fossa and posterior trochlear surface also can be seen from this position. Normally 50% to 60% of the ulnar collateral ligament can be seen when the scope is pushed medially and the posteromedial corner of the

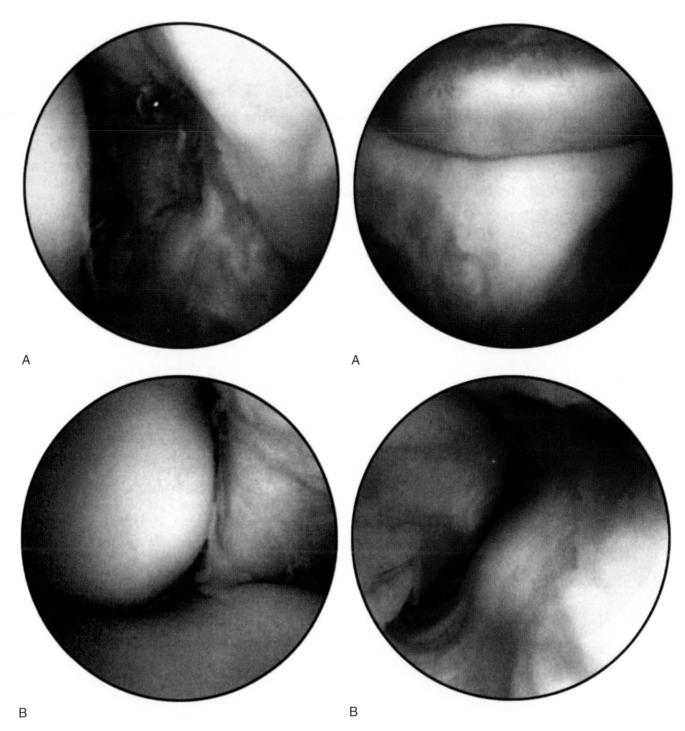

A

A

B

B

Figure 31-10 Direct lateral portal. **A,** Bare area of olecranon is right inside with trochlea on left. **B,** With the elbow flexed 90 degrees (patient supine), the articular surface of three bones can be seen. Radial head is superior left, ulna is superior right, and capitellum is inferior. (From Phillips BB. Arthroscopy of upper extremity. In Canale ST, ed. Campbell's Operative Orthopaedics, 10th ed. St. Louis, Mosby, 2003.)

Figure 31-11 Posterolateral portal. **A,** Posterior compartment; tip of olecranon is superior, trochlea is inferior, and olecranon fossa is in foreground. **B,** Medial gutter with posterior aspect of ulnar collateral ligament on the right and distal humerus on the left. (From Phillips BB. Arthroscopy of upper extremity. In Canale ST, ed. Campbell's Operative Orthopaedics, 10th ed. St. Louis, Mosby, 2003.)

elbow is seen. The ulnar nerve is superficial to this area of the elbow and must be identified and protected.

Postoperative Considerations

Complications

- Neurovascular: superficial or deep
- Infection
- Articular cartilage damage
- Fluid extravasation and compartment syndrome
- Synovial-cutaneous fistula

- Arthrofibrosis
- Complex regional pain syndrome

The most common complication related to portal placement is nerve damage, which occurs in about 3% of procedures. Most of these injuries are to cutaneous nerves and are transient, although there have been isolated reports of major neurovascular injuries. These include irreparable damage to the ulnar nerve; transection of the ulnar, radial, and posterior interosseous nerves; and compression neuropathy of the radial nerve.

Drainage from a portal site occurs in approximately 2.5% of patients, but deep infection is less frequent (~1%).

31

Suggested Reading

Andrews JR, Baumgarten TE. Arthroscopic anatomy of the elbow. Orthop Clin North Am 1995;26:671-677.

Baker CL, Brooks AA. Arthroscopy of the elbow. Clin Sports Med 1996;15:261-281.

Baker CL, Jones GL. Arthroscopy of the elbow. Am J Sports Med 1999;27:251-264.

Baker CL Jr. Normal arthroscopic anatomy of the elbow: prone technique. In McGinty JB, Burkhart SS, Jackson RW, et al, eds. Operative Arthroscopy, 3rd ed. Philadelphia, Lippincott Williams & Wilkins, 2003.

Baker CL Jr, Shalvoy RM. The prone position for elbow arthroscopy. Clin Sports Med 1991;10:623-628.

Field LD, Altchek DW, Warren RF, et al. Arthroscopic anatomy of the lateral elbow: a comparison of three portals. Arthroscopy 1994; 10:602-607.

Haapaniemi T, Berggren M, Adolfsson L. Case report. Complete transection of the medial and radial nerves during arthroscopic release of post-traumatic elbow contracture. Arthroscopy 1999;15:784-787.

Kelly EW, Morrey BF, O'Driscoll SW. Complications of elbow arthroscopy. J Bone Joint Surg Am 2001;83:25-34.

Kim SJ, Jeong JH. Technical note. Transarticular approach for elbow arthroscopy. Arthroscopy 2003;19:E27.

Kim SJ, Jeong JH. Transarticular approach for elbow arthroscopy. Arthroscopy 2003;19:E37.

Meyers JF, Carson WG Jr. Elbow arthroscopy: supine technique. In McGinty JB, Burkhart SS, Jackson RW, et al, eds. Operative Arthroscopy, 3rd ed. Philadelphia, Lippincott Williams & Wilkins, 2003.

Micheli LJ, Luke AC, Mintzer CM, Waters PM. Elbow arthroscopy in the pediatric and adolescent population. Arthroscopy 2001;17:694-699.

Miller CD, Jobe CM, Wright MH. Neuroanatomy in elbow arthroscopy. J Shoulder Elbow Surg 1995;4:168-174.

Morrey BF. Complications of elbow arthroscopy. Instr Course Lect 2000;49:255-258.

Papilion JD, Neff RS, Shall LM. Compression neuropathy of the radial nerve as a complication of elbow arthroscopy: a case report and review of the literature. Arthroscopy 1988;4:284-286.

Phillips BB, Strasburger S. Arthroscopic treatment of arthrofibrosis of the elbow joint. 1998;Arthroscopy 14:38-44.

Reddy AS, Kvitne RS, Yocum LA, et al. Arthroscopy of the elbow: a long-term clinical review. Arthroscopy 2000;16:588-594.

Savoie FH III, Field LD. Arthrofibrosis and complications in arthroscopy of the elbow. Clin Sports Med 2001;20:123-129.

Selby RM, O'Brien SJ, Kelly AM, Drakos M. The joint jack: report of a new technique essential for elbow arthroscopy. Arthroscopy 2002; 18:440-445.

Soffer SR. Diagnostic arthroscopy of the elbow. In Andrews JR, Timmerman LA. Diagnostic and Operative Arthroscopy, Philadelphia, WB Saunders, 1997.

Steinmann SP, King GJW, Savoie FH III. Arthroscopic treatment of the arthritic elbow. J Bone Joint Surg Am 2005;87:2114-2121.

Stothers K, Day B, Regan WR. Arthroscopy of the elbow: anatomy, portal sites, and a description of the proximal lateral portal. Arthroscopy 1995;11:449-457.

Takahashi T, Iai H, Hirose D, et al. Distraction in the lateral position in elbow arthroscopy. Arthroscopy 2000;16:221-225.

Thomas MA, Fast A, Shapiro D. Radial nerve damage as a complication of elbow arthroscopy. Clin Orthop 1987;215:130-131.

Arthroscopic Management of Osteochondritis Dissecans of the Elbow

Jason W. Levine, MD

Larry D. Field, MD

Felix H. Savoie III, MD

Osteochondritis dissecans, a localized condition involving the articular surface, results in the separation of a segment of articular cartilage and subchondral bone. The most common site of osteochondritis dissecans of the elbow is the capitellum. Lesions have been reported in the trochlea and radial head as well as in the olecranon and olecranon fossa.[17]

Osteochondritis dissecans generally occurs in athletes aged 11 to 21 years who report a history of overuse.[4,24] The osteonecrotic lesion involves only a segment of capitellum, primarily at a central or anterolateral position.[13,27] Appropriate treatment of this disorder remains controversial. Often treated with benign neglect, this condition is a potentially sport-ending injury for an athlete, with long-term sequelae of degenerative arthritis.[1,27] The surgical option that we present and have studied is fragment excision with débridement of the necrotic lesion.

Preoperative Considerations

History

Osteochondritis dissecans is primarily a disorder of the young athlete and rarely occurs in adults. The typical patient is between the ages of 11 and 21 years; the majority fall between 12 and 14 years.[4,21,24] Male athletes are more affected, but this disorder is prevalent among female gymnasts. The dominant arm is almost always involved, and bilateral involvement has been reported in some 5% to 20%.[25] A history of overuse is often described with common sport activities such as baseball, gymnastics, weightlifting, racket sports, and cheerleading.[22]

Physical Examination

Pain, the most common complaint, is usually insidious and progressive in nature. Pain is often localized over the lateral aspect of the elbow, but it may also be poorly defined.[25] The pain is associated with activities and relieved by rest. Clinically, tenderness can be palpated laterally over the radiocapitellar joint.

Range of motion is limited, particularly extension. It is not uncommon to see flexion contractures of 5 to 23 degrees.[3,4,15,23,31] Loss of flexion is less likely; supination and pronation are rarely altered. Clicking, catching, grinding, or locking suggests fragment instability or loose bodies. Crepitus and swelling may be present as well.[4,22,24,25] Provocative tests, such as the active radiocapitellar compression test, may help make the diagnosis.[2] As the patient actively pronates and supinates the forearm with the elbow in full extension, the dynamic muscle forces compress the radiocapitellar joint and reproduce the symptoms.

Imaging

Radiographs are the initial diagnostic test of choice. Standard anteroposterior and lateral views of the elbow usually show the classic findings of radiolucency and rarefaction of the capitellum with flattening or irregularity of the articular surface. A rim of sclerotic bone often surrounds the radiolucent crater, which is typically in the central or anterolateral aspect of the capitellum (Fig. 32-1). Loose bodies may be present if the necrotic segment becomes detached.

Additional studies may be needed to further evaluate osteochondritis dissecans. Computed tomography is useful in determining the extent of the osseous lesion as well as the presence and location of loose bodies. Computed tomographic arthrography more accurately defines the integrity of the articular surface.[10]

Magnetic resonance imaging has become the standard modality for further evaluation.[4,28] Not only can magnetic resonance imaging assess the articular surface, but it can also define both size and extent of the lesion (Fig. 32-2). Early, stable lesions show changes on T1-weighted images, but T2-weighted images remain normal. On the other hand, advanced lesions show changes on both T1- and T2-weighted images.[4,8] Loose in situ lesions have a cyst under the lesion. Magnetic resonance arthrography can improve the diagnosis with leakage of dye beneath the disrupted cartilage.[8,28]

Progress and healing can be followed by plain radiographs. If the fragment remains stable, the central sclerotic fragment gradually becomes less distinct and the surrounding area of radiolucency slowly ossifies. A nonhealing lesion in a patient who remains symptomatic despite conservative treatment should prompt the clinician to evaluate further.[4,27]

Indications and Contraindications

Treatment of osteochondritis dissecans is a highly debated topic. Options vary from nonoperative measures to fragment excision to fixation of the fragment. Management decisions are based primarily on the integrity of the articular cartilage and status of the involved segment, whether it is stable, unstable but attached, or detached and loose.

Stable lesions with intact cartilage and in situ subchondral fragments are managed conservatively.[4,25,28] Sports and other aggravating activities are stopped until symptoms subside, approximately for 3 to 6 weeks. We recommend protecting the elbow in a hinged elbow brace without restriction. The athlete can usually return to

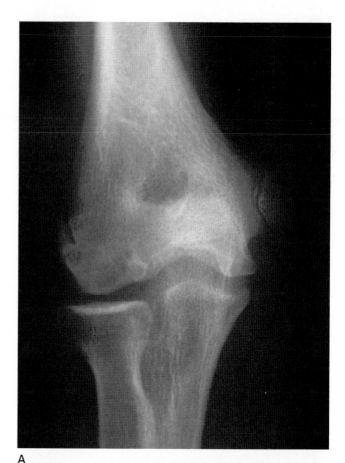

A

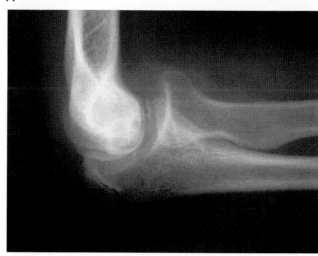

B

Figure 32-1 Anteroposterior **(A)** and lateral **(B)** radiographs demonstrating radiolucency and rarefaction typical of osteochondritis dissecans of the elbow.

sports unrestricted 3 to 6 months after treatment is begun.[22] Patients with intact lesions detected early and treated conservatively have the best prognosis. However, it is prudent for the clinician to inform the family of possible long-term sequelae.[1,11,25-28,31]

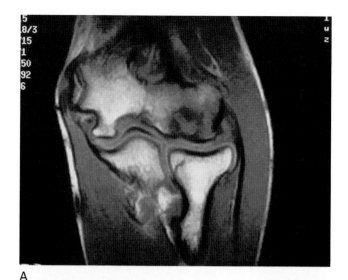

A

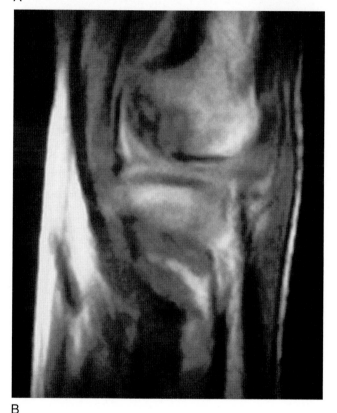

B

Figure 32-2 Coronal **(A)** and sagittal **(B)** magnetic resonance images of the same lesion shown in Figure 32-1. Increased signal of the T2 image indicates disruption of the articular surface.

Box 32-1 Surgical Steps

1. Establishment of arthroscopy portals
2. Drilling
3. Débridement or abrasion
4. Fragment removal or abrasion
5. Fixation

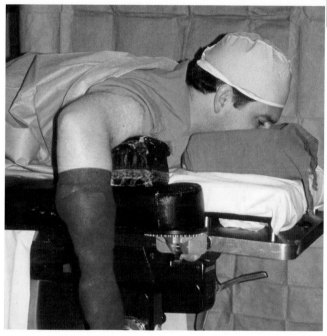

Figure 32-3 Prone position for arthroscopic treatment of the elbow.

ment. One method is to excise the unstable fragment with or without subchondral drilling or abrasion chondroplasty.[†] The other method is to attempt fixation of the segment with or without bone graft.[9,12,14,19,20,29]

Surgical Technique

Specific Steps (Box 32-1)

Excision and Drilling

We use general anesthesia and the prone position for arthroscopic evaluation of the elbow. The patient is placed prone on the operating table over chest rolls to ensure adequate ventilation. The shoulder is abducted to 90 degrees, and the arm is supported by an arm positioner or an arm board (Fig. 32-3). The arm board is placed parallel to the operating table, centered at the shoulder. A sandbag,

Surgical indications are persistent or worsening symptoms despite prolonged conservative care, loose bodies, and evidence of instability including violation of intact cartilage or detachment.[4,7,18,25] The only universally accepted regimen is the removal of loose bodies.[*] Otherwise, debate continues over two types of surgical manage-

*References 1-4, 7, 16-18, 23, 25, 26, 28, 30, 31.

†References 1, 3, 4, 6, 7, 11, 15, 16, 18, 22, 25-27, 30.

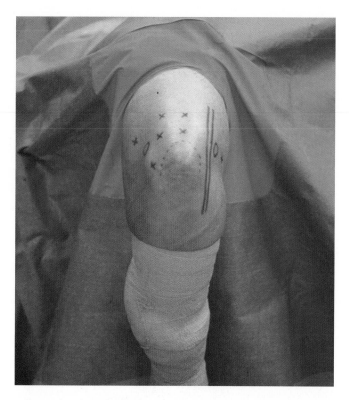

Figure 32-4 Common arthroscopic elbow portals.

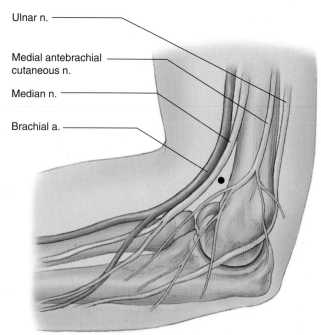

Ulnar n.

Medial antebrachial cutaneous n.

Median n.

Brachial a.

Figure 32-5 Illustration demonstrating anatomic positioning of the proximal anteromedial portal.

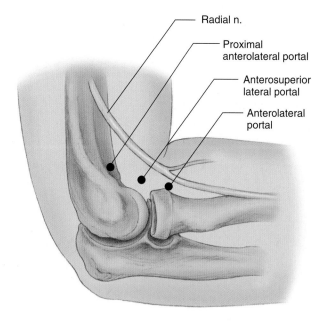

Radial n.

Proximal anterolateral portal

Anterosuperior lateral portal

Anterolateral portal

Figure 32-6 Illustration demonstrating anatomic positioning of common lateral arthroscopic portals.

foam support, or rolled blankets placed under the upper arm elevate the shoulder and allow the elbow to rest in 90 degrees of flexion.

Surface landmarks are marked on the skin before portals are established. Important landmarks to outline are the radial head, olecranon, lateral epicondyle, medial epicondyle, and ulnar nerve (Fig. 32-4). Before the portals are made, the joint must be distended with 20 to 30 mL of sterile saline. This can be done by placing an 18-gauge spinal needle in either the olecranon fossa or the soft spot bounded by the lateral epicondyle, olecranon, and radial head. Neurovascular structures are displaced away from the joint with distention of the joint, which gives an additional margin of safety.[5,15]

The arthroscope is introduced through the proximal anteromedial portal. This portal is 2 cm proximal to the medial epicondyle and just anterior to the medial intermuscular septum (Fig. 32-5). The medial intermuscular septum is identified by palpation, and the portal is made anterior to the septum so that the ulnar nerve is not injured. The blunt trocar is introduced into the portal, anterior to the septum, and aimed toward the radial head while contact is maintained with the anterior surface of the humerus. This allows the brachialis muscle to remain anterior and protect the median nerve and brachial artery. The trocar enters the elbow through the tendinous origin of the flexor-pronator group and medial capsule.[17]

Once entrance into the joint is confirmed, the anterior aspect of the capitellum is evaluated. Loose bodies are removed through a proximal anterolateral portal. The proximal anterolateral portal is positioned 2 cm proximal and 1 to 2 cm anterior to the lateral epicondyle (Fig. 32-6). This portal may be used as the initial portal in elbow arthroscopy. The blunt trocar is aimed toward the center of the joint while contact is maintained with the anterior humerus and pierces the brachioradialis muscle, brachialis muscle, and lateral joint capsule before entering the anterior compartment. The coronoid fossa is a common place for loose bodies to be localized (Fig. 32-7). Although the osteochondritic lesion may be noted on the anterior aspect of the capitellum (Fig. 32-8), it is most commonly noted on the posterior aspect and can be barely visualized with the scope in the anterior portal. One should always perform a varus and valgus stress test while the scope is in the anterior portal to document any concomitant instability of the elbow. Once a complete diagnostic arthroscopy of the anterior compartment of the elbow and removal of any associated loose bodies have been completed, the inflow is left in the proximal anteromedial portal and the scope is transferred to a straight posterior portal. The straight posterior or trans-triceps portal is located 3 cm proximal to the tip of the olecranon in the midline posteriorly[6,16] (see Fig. 32-4). This portal allows visualization of the entire posterior compartment as well as the medial and lateral gutters.[17] The blunt trocar is advanced toward the olecranon fossa through the triceps tendon and posterior joint capsule. The medial gutter is evaluated initially along with the olecranon fossa, and any loose bodies noted in either of these are removed. The arthroscope is then continued into the lateral compartment, and a soft spot portal is established. In most cases of osteochondritis, a relatively large posterolateral plica will be noted, along with quite a bit of synovitis in this lateral compartment (Fig. 32-9). The soft spot portal is located in the center of the triangular area bordered by the olecranon, the lateral epicondyle, and the radial head. This portal is also known as the direct lateral portal or midlateral portal (see Fig. 32-4). The blunt trocar passes through the anconeus muscle and the posterior capsule and into the joint. This inflammatory

tissue is excised through a posterior soft spot portal. At this point, the 30-degree arthroscope is removed and a 70-degree arthroscope is substituted through the posterior central portal. Use of the 70-degree arthroscope allows complete evaluation of the osteochondritic lesion of the capitellum (Fig. 32-8). The shaver is placed through the soft spot portal, and any loose fragments of the osteochondritic area are débrided. The necrotic bone is then removed,

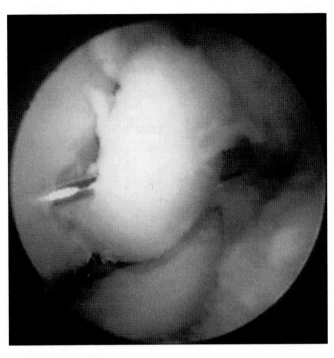

Figure 32-8 Arthroscopic management of a detached osteochondritic lesion of the capitellum viewed from the anteromedial portal. The loose fragment is temporarily stabilized with a spinal needle before excision with a grasper from the anterolateral portal.

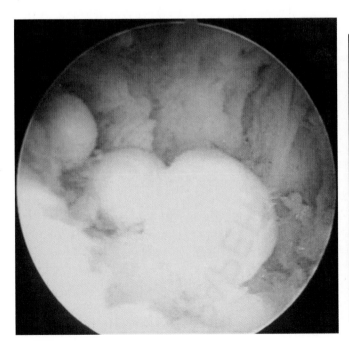

Figure 32-7 Loose bodies found in the anterior compartment of the elbow.

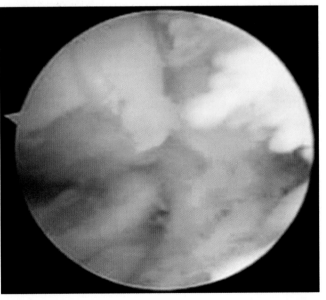

Figure 32-9 Posterolateral gutter of a patient with osteochondritis dissecans demonstrating the synovitis and inflamed posterolateral plica.

and in an attempt to stimulate blood flow, multiple drill holes are placed into the main body of the capitellum by use of either a drill or an awl (Fig. 32-10).

Arthroscopic fixation

Fixation of the fragment remains controversial. Several techniques, including Herbert screw fixation,[9] dynamic stapling,[12] Kirschner wires,[11] cancellous screws,[4] and bioabsorbable implants, have been described. Before reattachment, the débrided bone can be grafted to encourage healing. Although several studies have shown favorable results after reattachment of the fragment, none has clearly demonstrated marked improvement over excision and débridement alone.

Postoperative Considerations

Rehabilitation

Rehabilitation after surgery starts with the patient in a double-hinged elbow brace, and early motion is begun. As the swelling and pain subside, patients are allowed to resume athletic activities in the brace. The brace is gradually weaned 8 to 12 weeks postoperatively, as long as the patient remains free of significant pain or any mechanical symptoms.

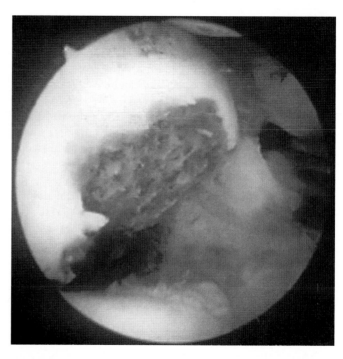

Figure 32-10 The subchondral base after excision of the fragment and débridement with a shaver.

Table 32-1 Results of Surgical Treatment of Osteochondritis Dissecans

Author	Type of Study	Patient Population	Type of Surgery	Follow-up Time	Results
Baumgarten et al[3] (1998)	Retrospective	16 adolescents 17 elbows	Arthroscopic abrasion chondroplasty and/or loose body removal	Average: 48 months; minimum: 24 months	Average flexion contracture decreased by 14 degrees, extension contracture by 6 degrees. All but 3 returned to preoperative level of activity
Byrd and Jones[6] (2002)	Retrospective	10 baseball players Average age: 13.8 years	Arthroscopic synovectomy, abrasion chondroplasty, and/or loose body removal	Average: 3.9 years	Excellent results in pain, swelling, mechanical symptoms, activity limitation, range of motion. Grade of lesion correlated poorly with outcome
Ruch et al[23] (1998)	Retrospective	12 adolescents Average age: 14.5 years	Arthroscopic débridement and/or loose body removal	Average: 3.2 years	11 patients reported excellent pain relief and no limitations of activities
Bauer et al[1] (1992)	Retrospective	7 children younger than 16 years 23 adults older than 16 years	23 loose body removal or removal of undisplaced lesion by open arthrotomy	Average: 23 years	Impaired motion and pain in half of elbows. Degenerative joint disease in more than half

Complications

Few complications associated with the treatment of osteochondritis dissecans have been documented. One patient in our series developed severe arthritic changes in the radial head that required an additional surgery. To date, we have had no neurologic complications associated with the treatment of osteochondritis of the capitellum.

Results

During the past 10 years, we have managed 23 elbows in 21 patients with osteochondritis dissecans of the capitellum. Approximately 76% of these patients (16 of 21) have been treated nonoperatively by a double-hinged offloading elbow brace with selective anti-inflammatory medications and physical therapy. Of the 16 patients, 3 (19%) failed bracing and underwent subsequent arthroscopic débridement and drilling of displaced lesions. The remaining patients were also treated with surgery. The surgically treated group was observed for a mean of 44.3 months, and the average range of motion at latest examination was −3.5 degrees of extension to 135 degrees of flexion. One patient maintained his valgus instability and two patients continued to have mild pain. Radiographic evidence of lesion healing was present in 7 of the 10 elbows. Seven patients responded with a return to normal activities, but at a decreased level. One patient failed the procedure and had a radial head resection for severe arthrosis.

Results of surgical treatment of osteochondritis dissecans are shown in Table 32-1.

32

References

1. Bauer M, Jonsson K, Josefsson PO, et al. Osteochondritis dissecans of the elbow: a long-term follow up study. Clin Orthop 1992; 284:156-160.
2. Baumgarten TE. Osteochondritis dissecans of the capitellum. Sports Med Arthr Rev 1995;3:219-223.
3. Baumgarten T, Andrews J, Satterwhite Y. The arthroscopic classification and treatment of osteochondritis dissecans of the capitellum. Am J Sports Med 1998;26:520-523.
4. Bradley J, Petrie R. Osteochondritis dissecans of the humeral capitellum: diagnosis and treatment. Clin Sports Med 2001;20:565-590.
5. Brown R, Blazina ME, Kerlan RK, et al. Osteochondritis of the capitellum. J Sports Med 1974;2:27-46.
6. Byrd T, Jones K. Arthroscopic surgery for isolated capitellar osteochondritis dissecans in adolescent baseball players: minimum three-year follow-up. Am J Sports Med 2002;30:474-478.
7. Chess D. Osteochondritis. In Savoie FH III, Field LD, eds. Arthroscopy of the Elbow. New York, Churchill Livingstone, 1996:77-86.
8. Fritz RC, Stoller DW. The elbow. In Stoller DW, ed. Magnetic Resonance Imaging in Orthopaedics and Sports Medicine, 2nd ed. Philadelphia, Lippincott-Raven, 1997:743-849.
9. Harada M, Ogino T, Takahara M, et al. Fragment fixation with a bone graft and dynamic staples for osteochondritis dissecans of the humeral capitellum. J Shoulder Elbow Surg 2002;11:368-372.
10. Holland P, Davies AM, Cassar-Pullicino VN. Computed tomographic arthrography in the assessment of osteochondritis dissecans of the elbow. Clin Radiol 1994;49:231-235.
11. Jackson DW, Silvino N, Reiman P. Osteochondritis in the female gymnast's elbow. Arthroscopy 1989;5:129-136.
12. Kiyoshige Y, Takagi M, Yuasa K. Closed-wedge osteotomy for osteochondritis dissecans of the capitellum: a 7- to 12-year follow-up. Am J Sports Med 2000;28:534-537.
13. Konig F. Über freie Korper in den Gelenken. Dtsch Zeitschr Chir 1887;27:90-109.
14. Kuwahata Y, Inoue G. Osteochondritis dissecans of the elbow managed by Herbert screw fixation. Orthopedics 1998;21:449-451.
15. McManama GB Jr, Micheli LJ, Berry MV, et al. The surgical treatment of osteochondritis of the capitellum. Am J Sports Med 1985; 13:11-21.
16. Menche DS, Vangsness CT Jr, Pitman M, et al. The treatment of isolated articular cartilage lesions in the young individual. Instr Course Lect 1998;47:505-515.
17. Mitsunaga MM, Adishian DA, Bianco AJ Jr. Osteochondritis dissecans of the capitellum. J Trauma 1982;22:53-55.
18. Nagura S. The so-called osteochondritis dissecans of Konig. Clin Orthop 1960;18:100-122.
19. Nakagawa Y, Matsusue Y, Ikeda N, et al. Osteochondral grafting and arthroplasty for end-stage osteochondritis dissecans of the capitellum: a case report and review of the literature. Am J Sports Med 2001;29:650-655.
20. Oka Y, Ikeda M. Treatment of severe osteochondritis dissecans of the elbow using osteochondral grafts from a rib. J Bone Joint Surg Br 2001;83:838-839.
21. Pappas AM. Osteochondritis dissecans. Clin Orthop 1981; 158:59-69.
22. Peterson RK, Savoie FH III, Field LD. Osteochondritis dissecans of the elbow. Instr Course Lect 1998;48:393-398.
23. Ruch D, Cory J, Poehling G. The arthroscopic management of osteochondritis dissecans of the adolescent elbow. Arthroscopy 1998; 14:797-803.
24. Schenck RC Jr, Goodnight JM. Osteochondritis dissecans. J Bone Joint Surg Am 1996;78:439-456.
25. Shaughnessy WJ. Osteochondritis dissecans. In Morrey BF, ed. The Elbow and Its Disorders, 3rd ed. Philadelphia, WB Saunders, 2000: 255-260.
26. Singer KM, Roy SP. Osteochondrosis of the humeral capitellum. Am J Sports Med 1984;12:351-360.
27. Takahara M, Ogino T, Sasaki I, et al. Long term outcome of osteochondritis dissecans of the humeral capitellum. Clin Orthop 1999; 363:108-115.
28. Takahara M, Shundo M, Kondo M, et al. Early detection of osteochondritis dissecans of the capitellum in young baseball players: report of three cases. J Bone Joint Surg Am 1998;80:892-897.
29. Takeda H, Watarai K, Matsushita T, et al. A surgical treatment for unstable osteochondritis dissecans lesions of the humeral capitellum in adolescent baseball players. Am J Sports Med 2002; 30:713-717.
30. Tivnon MC, Anzel SH, Waugh TR. Surgical management of osteochondritis dissecans of the capitellum. Am J Sports Med 1976; 4:121-128.
31. Woodward AH, Bianco AJ Jr. Osteochondritis dissecans of the elbow. Clin Orthop 1975;110:35-41.

CHAPTER 33

Arthroscopic Treatment of Elbow Stiffness

Jason Koh, MD

Alfred Cook, MD

Limitation of elbow motion can arise from a variety of causes, including acute or chronic trauma, heterotopic ossification, spasticity, burn scar contracture, and postoperative scarring. Inflammatory conditions as well as intra-articular lesions can cause decreased motion about the elbow. Examples of these lesions include osteophytes on the olecranon and coronoid processes, loose bodies, adhesions, synovitis, osteochondritis of the capitellum, and chondromalacia of the radial head.[6] Multiple techniques have been developed and employed to address these various pathologic processes. Several open techniques have been described to address elbow stiffness, such as a limited anterior capsulotomy with or without tenotomy as well as distraction arthroplasty, all of which have been effective.[3,8,15] These methods, however, tend to be technically demanding, and patients undergo significant morbidity and prolonged rehabilitation. Several authors have described and reported on arthroscopic techniques to address limited elbow motion. Authors have described arthroscopic release of the anterior capsule, removal of loose bodies, excision of osteophytes, and débridement of the olecranon fossa, either alone or in some combination.[4,6,9,12,14] The goal of all these techniques is to regain motion from 30 to 130 degrees. We focus on the arthroscopic management of the stiff elbow.

Preoperative Considerations

History

Patients present with complaints of limited range of motion and occasionally a history of trauma. It is commonly seen in men with a history of heavy use of the arm, weight lifters, and throwing athletes. These patients can present in the third to eighth decade, depending on the cause. Athletes and patients with osteochondritis dissecans present earlier. The history is characteristically one of mechanical impingement and pain at the extremes of motion (extension greater than flexion). The patient may complain of pain while carrying a briefcase secondary to the arm's being extended. A flexion contracture of 30 degrees is common.[9]

Physical Examination

It is important to inspect the skin for signs of obvious pathologic changes, such as burns. The patient's range of motion is documented and characterized. Is there a hard or soft endpoint? Is the arc of motion painful versus pain at the extremes of motion? Answers to these two questions can provide significant information concerning the etiology of the stiff elbow. When a soft endpoint is present, this probably represents a soft tissue constraint, whereas a hard endpoint is more consistent with bone impingement. Pain during the arc of motion represents an internal derangement from joint incongruity or degeneration. However, if there is pain at the extremes of motion, bone impingement is usually present.

A thorough neurovascular examination should be performed. Ulnar nerve function should be critically evaluated. Chronic contractures can damage the ulnar nerve and compromise function. In addition, the ulnar nerve is investigated for subluxation or dislocation anteriorly. This can occur in 16% of the population, and the ulnar nerve will be at risk for injury with anterior medial portal placement.[9]

Imaging

Combined with the history and physical examination, standard radiographs should be obtained. Anteroposterior and lateral views are usually sufficient (Fig. 33-1). The lateral view is especially helpful in delineating osteophyte involvement and appreciating any deformity in the olecranon or coronoid fossa. Radiographs also help identify loose bodies. A computed tomographic scan may offer information about the radiocapitellar and ulnar-trochlear articular surfaces.[9] We find magnetic resonance imaging helpful in visualizing the three-dimensional anatomy of the joint, in particular for the preoperative determination of planned amount of osteophyte resection and fossa deepening.

Indications

Indications for elbow arthroscopy include evaluation of the painful elbow, evaluation and treatment of osteochondritis dissecans of the capitellum, evaluation and treatment of osteochondral lesions of the radial head, and partial synovectomy. Specifically, treatment of early degenerative changes of the elbow that limit motion (i.e., olecranon and coronoid fossa osteophytes) with arthroscopy has been shown to be successful. With more advanced changes, an open approach is more appropriate because it is faster, technically easier, and more effective. In addition, contractures of the elbow and the removal of loose bodies can effectively be addressed with the use of arthroscopy.[12]

Contraindications

Contraindications to elbow arthroscopy are few but include an active infection in the region of planned surgery

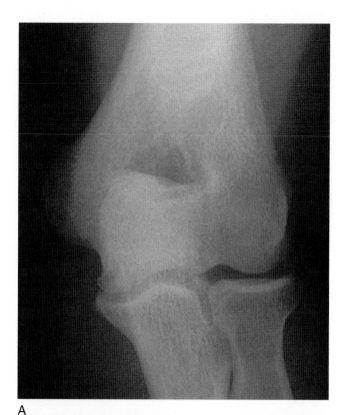

A

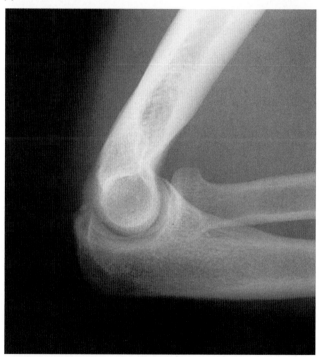

B

Figure 33-1 A, Preoperative anteroposterior radiograph demonstrating posteromedial olecranon osteophyte. **B,** Preoperative lateral radiograph demonstrating posterior olecranon osteophyte.

as well as bone ankylosis or severe fibrous ankylosis that prevents safe introduction of the arthroscope. Previous surgery that alters the normal anatomy, such as an ulnar nerve transposition, may limit portal selection. In addition, the intracapsular space is severely constricted in stiff elbows. Thus, the space in the anterior elbow is reduced. With this in mind, capsular distention is important to ensure that neurovascular structures are away from the operative area. Excessive distention of soft tissues will limit the time available for the operation. In severely stiff elbows, adequate distention may not be able to be achieved and the risk of neurovascular injury is too significant to proceed. An open procedure should be considered at that point.[2,9] Finally, arthroscopic capsular release is one of the most technically demanding and potentially risky of the arthroscopic procedures in the elbow, and the experience of the surgeon must guide the procedure.

Surgical Technique

Anesthesia and Positioning

Options for positioning of the patient include supine, prone, and lateral decubitus on a standard operating room table. A tourniquet is applied as high on the upper arm as possible to control bleeding. General anesthesia is usually administered because it allows complete muscle relaxation and eliminates intraoperative discomfort for the patient. Regional anesthesia can be given if the patient is supine; a major disadvantage is the inability to perform an accurate neurovascular examination after the operation. Local anesthesia is also an option and advantageous given that it allows the patient to communicate with the surgeon when instruments are placed near neurovascular structures. However, it does not allow the use of a tourniquet and should be avoided for longer arthroscopic procedures.[2]

When a supine position is used, the patient's arm is positioned so that it hangs free off the side of the table in a suspension device, with the shoulder in neutral rotation and 90 degrees of abduction and the elbow in 90 degrees of flexion. This position allows excellent access to both sides of the elbow and relaxes the neurovascular structures of the antecubital fossa. Standard arthroscopic portals can be employed.[2]

Although initially the preferred position for this procedure was supine, many surgeons prefer the lateral decubitus or prone position. Both positions offer similar convenience for the surgeon, with the prone position perhaps offering better access to the elbow. The prone position provides the added advantages of easier joint manipulation, improved access to the posterior aspect of the joint, and more complete viewing of the intra-articular structures. The patient is placed prone on chest rolls, and a tourniquet is applied to the proximal aspect of the arm.

An arm board is placed parallel to the operating room table. The shoulder and arm are then elevated on a sandbag that is placed on the arm board. The arm is then allowed to hang. No traction is needed. The arm is positioned so that the shoulder is in neutral rotation and 90 degrees of abduction. The elbow is flexed to 90 degrees with the hand pointing toward the floor. After positioning, the arm is prepared and draped in the normal sterile fashion, and bone landmarks and portals are outlined. Laterally, the lateral epicondyle and radial head are outlined; medially, the medial epicondyle is marked; and posteriorly, the olecranon tip is identified. The portals can then be defined.[2]

The lateral decubitus position was developed as a modification to the prone position. This position allows easy access to the posterior compartment and permits excellent management of the airway by anesthesia. The patient is held in this position with a beanbag and kidney rests. A tourniquet is applied, and the arm is placed over a bolster. The bolster should let the arm hang with the elbow in 90 degrees of flexion and provide unobstructed access to the anterior and posterior portals.[2]

Surgical Landmarks, Incisions, and Portals

The most commonly used portals for elbow arthroscopy are the direct lateral, proximal medial, anterolateral, anteromedial, posterolateral, and straight posterior portals (Fig. 33-2). The direct lateral (midlateral) portal is located at the "soft spot," which is formed by the triangle between the lateral epicondyle, olecranon, and radial head. This site is used for distention of the elbow. It can also be used as a working portal for access to the posterior chamber of the elbow when the patient is prone. This portal also allows access to the posterior aspect of the capitellum as well as the radiocapitellar and radioulnar joints. The posterior antebrachial cutaneous nerve is most at risk with this portal. It passes within an average of 7 mm of the portal.[1,9]

The proximal medial (superomedial) portal has also been described. It is located approximately 2 cm proximal to the medial humeral epicondyle and just anterior to the intermuscular septum. The arthroscopic sheath is introduced anterior to the intermuscular septum while contact is maintained with the anterior aspect of the humerus. The trocar is then directed toward the radial head. This portal provides excellent visualization of the anterior compartment of the elbow including the radiocapitellar joint. The median nerve is potentially at risk when this portal is established. However, this portal is potentially safer than the anteromedial portal because the more proximal portal permits the cannula to be directed distally. This allows the cannula to be directed almost parallel to the median nerve in the anteroposterior plane.[1,9]

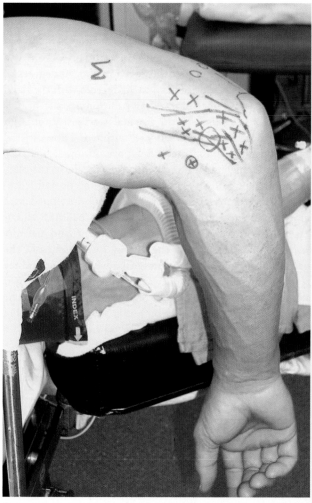

A

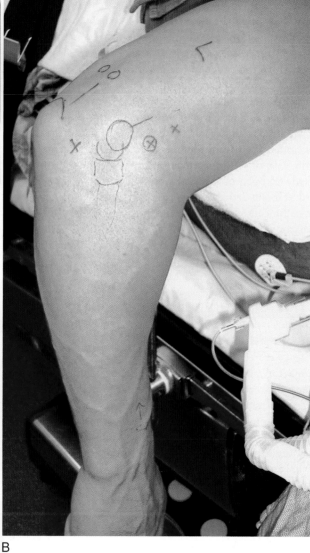

B

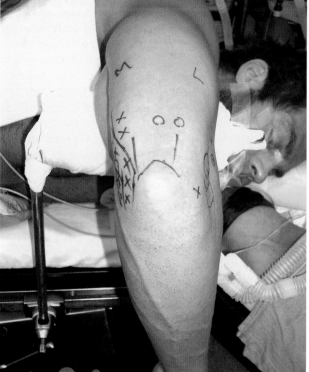

C

Figure 33-2 Medial, lateral, and posterior views of arthroscopic portals.
A, Medial elbow portals. In this patient, the ulnar nerve subluxates anterior, so the path of the nerve is indicated as it goes on top of the medial epicondyle.
B, Lateral portals. Note X for soft spot portal, circled x for lateral portal.
C, Posterior view. Note subluxating ulnar nerve, medial and lateral markings, direct posterior and posterolateral portal. The patient is in the lateral decubitus position with the arm over a padded bolster.

Several lateral portals have been described, with the safer portals located more proximally to avoid the radial nerve. The anterolateral portal is 3 cm distal and 2 cm anterior to the lateral humeral epicondyle and lies in the sulcus between the radial head and capitellum anteriorly. This portal provides excellent visualization of the medial plica, coronoid process, trochlea, coronoid fossa, and medial capsule. Superficially, the posterior antebrachial cutaneous nerve is at risk and lies approximately 2 mm from the cannula. The radial nerve is also at significant risk. It can lie as close as 3 mm from the cannula.[1,9] Stothers et al[13] compared a proximal lateral portal established 1 to 2 cm proximal to the lateral epicondyle with the standard distal anterolateral portal in cadaveric specimens and found that this proximal portal was safer and provided improved visualization, especially of the radiohumeral joint. We recommend the use of this portal instead of the anterolateral portal.

The anteromedial portal is made 2 cm distal and 2 cm anterior to the medial humeral epicondyle and passes through the common flexor origin. The anterior branch of the medial antebrachial cutaneous nerve and the median nerve are at risk. When the cannula is placed, the elbow should be flexed. In this position, the brachialis acts to protect the nerve. This portal provides excellent visualization of the radiocapitellar and humeroulnar joints, the coronoid fossa, the capitellum, and the superior capsule.[1,9]

The posterolateral portal is located 2 to 3 cm proximal to the tip of the olecranon at the lateral border of the triceps tendon. The trocar is directed toward the olecranon fossa. This portal provides excellent visualization of the olecranon tip, olecranon fossa, and posterior trochlea, but the posterior capitellum is not well seen. The medial and posterior antebrachial cutaneous nerves are the two structures at risk, passing an average of 25 mm from the portal. The ulnar nerve is at risk if the cannula is placed too far medial. The nerve is approximately 25 mm from the portal.[1,9]

The direct posterior portal is located 1 to 2 cm directly proximal to the tip of the olecranon, through the triceps. The trocar is directed to the olecranon fossa. The ulnar nerve is at risk if the cannula is placed too far medially.

Specific Steps (Box 33-1; authors' preference)

For the pathologic changes that occur with degenerative or post-traumatic elbow contractures to be adequately addressed, the anterolateral, anteromedial, and posterior portals are used. Before the patient is positioned, an examination under anesthesia is performed. The range of elbow motion is documented. The patient is placed in the lateral decubitus position with the operative extremity over a

Box 33-1 Surgical Steps

1. Anterior compartment adhesion release
2. Loose body removal
3. Incision or resection of anterior capsule from lateral to medial with an arthroscopic basket to visualize brachialis fibers
4. Posterior compartment débridement
5. Posterior capsule and medial and lateral gutter débridement or release

33

bolster or in an arm holder. A tourniquet is applied and is used at the surgeon's discretion. The arm is prepared and draped with an Ace wrap on the hand and forearm. Bone landmarks as well as the course of the ulnar nerve are outlined. Preoperatively, the ulnar nerve should be assessed for subluxation. The full range of excursion of the nerve should be marked out and avoided during surgery. Alternatively, the nerve can be dissected and protected through an open approach before arthroscopic releases are performed.

The elbow is distended by injection of fluid into the joint through the posterolateral soft spot. The elbow should extend slightly as the capsule is distended. Free fluid return through the needle should also be observed. We typically start with the anteromedial portal as described before, using a spinal needle directed toward the radiocapitellar articulation. The free flow of fluid should be observed from the spinal needle if the location of the needle is intra-articular. The spinal needle indicates the correct angle for trocar placement. The skin is then incised, and a small clamp is used to separate the subcutaneous tissues. A blunt trocar and cannula are introduced into the elbow, following the angle established by the spinal needle. Again, free flow of fluid should be observed from the trocar if it is intra-articular. If the joint capsule is adherent to the anterior humerus, a gentle sweeping motion with the trocar can elevate the anterior capsule and make a larger working space. The proximal lateral portal is used to enter the joint, with a spinal needle as a finder. Diagnostic arthroscopy is performed. Loose bodies are removed, and osteophytes are removed by a bur or shaver with minimal or no suction. It is helpful to preserve the capsule initially during removal of osteophytes to maintain distention and to protect anterior neurovascular structures. Loose bodies are often found at the proximal capsule attachment to the humerus or adjacent to the radiocapitellar joint.

If the anterior capsule is contracted, it is released from medial to lateral near the proximal anterior attachment, where the brachialis protects the neurovascular structures (Fig. 33-3). Because the radial nerve may lie almost directly on the distal lateral capsule, this area should be avoided. Capsulotomy can be performed by a

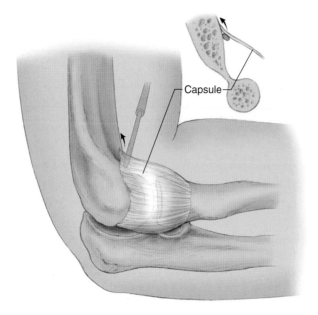

Figure 33-3 Demonstration of anterior capsular stripping.

basket or a duckbill hand instrument turned so that the tissue is visualized within the jaws of the instrument. This allows precise control of the tissue being divided. We prefer this to mechanical shavers or radiofrequency devices. On occasion, we use a blunt probe through an accessory portal to retract anterior tissues.

After the anterior procedures, the posterior ulnohumeral joint is carefully evaluated for a mechanical block. If a block is noted, posterolateral and direct posterior portals are established, and the olecranon fossa and tip of the olecranon are débrided with a mechanical shaver or bur to remove any osteophytes or excessive bone. Medially, the ulnar nerve is at risk, and great care must be taken in resecting tissue in this area, with use of minimal or no suction. A ⅛-inch osteotome can be introduced through the posterior portal to resect the olecranon tip. Extending the elbow can deliver the tip of the olecranon to the resection instrument and can evaluate adequacy of resection. Loose bodies can often be found in the posteromedial and posterolateral gutters.

In cases of severe motion restriction, particularly loss of pronation and supination, partial or complete arthroscopic radial head resection can be performed. The radiocapitellar joint can be visualized through the anteromedial portal and resected through the proximal lateral portal. Malunions may also involve the posterior portion of the radial head, which can be visualized through a well-placed posterior or posterolateral portal with the elbow in some extension and resected through the posterior soft spot portal. On occasion, the scope can be placed in the soft spot portal. A switching stick is used to place the visualization cannula in the correct position.

The final range of motion is evaluated, and the portals are sutured closed to avoid prolonged drainage or sinus formation. A compressive dressing is placed on the elbow, and the Ace bandage is removed.

Postoperative Considerations

The patient is instructed to start elbow motion as tolerated. The patient is also instructed to keep the elbow elevated to minimize swelling. If a synovectomy or débridement was performed, or if postoperative bleeding is expected, the limb can be splinted in full extension in a padded Jones dressing with an anterior slab of plaster and suspended vertically for 36 hours to minimize bleeding and edema. This position leaves the least volume of space available for swelling to occur. Another option is to use continuous passive motion postoperatively.[9] Gates et al[3] investigated the use of continuous passive motion after performing an anterior capsulotomy without tenotomy of the biceps tendon or myotomy of the brachialis muscle for post-traumatic flexion contracture. The patients were divided into two groups (one with continuous passive motion and one without). They found that although the postoperative use of continuous passive motion did not significantly improve mean active extension, it did improve active flexion and the total arc of motion. Postoperatively, we place these patients in a soft bulky dressing for 1 or 2 days, followed by an aggressive physical therapy protocol designed to promote range of motion.

Complications

Most complications of elbow arthroscopy are neurovascular in nature. Many authors have reported various neurovascular injuries secondary to multiple causes, including overdistention of the capsule, direct injury by instruments, and injury during portal placement.[1,7,10] Kelly et al[5] retrospectively reviewed 414 elbow arthroscopies that had been performed for osteoarthritis, loose bodies, and rheumatoid or inflammatory arthritis. Procedures performed during these arthroscopies included synovectomy, débridement of articular surfaces or adhesions, excision of osteophytes, diagnostic arthroscopy, loose body removal, and capsular procedures (such as capsulotomy, capsulectomy, and capsular release). Serious complications such as joint space infection occurred in four patients (0.8%). Minor complications occurred in 50 (11%) of the procedures. These complications included prolonged drainage, persistent minor contracture of 20 degrees or less, and 12 transient nerve palsies. The most significant risk factors for the development of a temporary nerve palsy were an underlying diagnosis of rheumatoid arthritis and a contracture. There were no permanent nerve injuries, hematomas, or compartment syndromes. All minor complications, with the exception of residual contractures, resolved without sequelae.[10]

PEARLS AND PITFALLS

Anterior Compartment

- It is always safer to start more proximal rather than distal.

- If there are joint capsule contractures, strip the anterior capsule off the humerus proximally to increase the working space.

- Exercise extreme caution on the anterior lateral side because of the proximity of the radial nerve.

- Use of a duckbill basket for capsulotomy allows the surgeon to precisely visualize the tissue being resected.

- Loose bodies will sometimes be found proximally at the anterior humerus or within the radiocapitellar joint.

Posterior Compartment

- Gentle blunt dissection in the olecranon fossa with the tip of a blunt trocar or switching stick can improve visualization.

- Starting with a 2.7- or 4.5-mm scope in the posterior soft spot portal directed into the olecranon fossa will often allow good visualization of the olecranon tip.

- Use extreme caution on the posterior medial side, with minimal suction.

- Always direct the shaver or bur blade away from the ulnar nerve.

- Loose bodies are sometimes found in the posterolateral gutter.

33

Table 33-1 Clinical Results of Arthroscopic Management of the Stiff Elbow

Author	Follow-up	Outcome
Timmerman and Andrews[14] (1994)	Average: 29 months	79% good–excellent results with arthroscopic débridement
Phillips and Strasburger[12] (1998)	Average: 18 months	All 25 patients showed statistically significant increases in motion and decreased pain
Koh et al[7] (1999)	Average: 25 months	88% good–excellent results with arthroscopic débridement
Kim et al[6] (1995)	Average: 25 months	92% of patients satisfied with arthroscopic débridement with increased range of motion and improved elbow scores
Jones and Savoie[4] (1993)	Average: 22 months	All patients were satisfied with their results and demonstrated decreased pain and improvement in range of motion
Ogilvie-Harris et al[11] (1995)	Average: 35 months	All 21 patients demonstrated good–excellent results. Pain, strength, motion, stability, and function improved significantly with arthroscopic treatment

Results

Results of arthroscopic approaches to elbow stiffness have rivaled those of open approaches (Table 33-1). In addition, arthroscopic treatment has the added benefit of less morbidity and earlier rehabilitation.[14] Phillips and Strasburger[12] treated 25 patients with limited range of motion, 10 secondary to degenerative arthritis and 15 secondary to post-traumatic arthrofibrosis. They performed a capsular release, removal of loose bodies, débridement of fibrotic tissue, and removal of osteophytes limiting motion. The patients obtained a significant increase in their range of motion. Koh et al[7] treated 17 patients with elbow stiffness secondary to post-traumatic contractures, osteoarthritis, and hemophiliac arthropathy. These patients underwent an arthroscopic débridement, capsular release, and removal of loose bodies. All patients demonstrated improved elbow motion postoperatively, and 15 had improved arc of motion postoperatively. Overall good to excellent results were achieved in 88% of patients. There were no neurovascular complications.

An arthroscopic approach to the stiff elbow provides reliable improvement in a patient's elbow range of motion. It is associated with less morbidity for the patient and earlier postoperative rehabilitation. Although damage to neurovascular structures is of concern, an arthroscopic approach is a safe and effective surgery to address the stiff elbow.

References

1. Baker CL, Jones GL. Arthroscopy of the elbow. Current concepts. Am J Sports Med 1999;27:251-264.
2. Canale ST, Phillips BB. In Canale ST, ed. Campbell's Operative Orthopaedics, 10th ed. St. Louis, Mosby, 2003:2613-2665.
3. Gates HS III, Sullivan FL, Urbaniak JR. Anterior capsulotomy and continuous passive motion in the treatment of post-traumatic flexion contracture of the elbow. J Bone Joint Surg Am 1992;74:1229-1234.

4. Jones GS, Savoie FH III. Arthroscopic capsular release of flexion contractures (arthrofibrosis) of the elbow. Arthroscopy 1993;9: 277-283.

5. Kelly EW, Morrey BF, O'Driscoll SW. Complications of elbow arthroscopy. J Bone Joint Surg Am 2001;83:25-34.

6. Kim SJ, Kim HK, Lee JW. Arthroscopy for limitation of motion of the elbow. Arthroscopy 1995;11:680-683.

7. Koh J, Parsons B, Hotchkiss RN, Altchek DW. Arthroscopic débridement and capsulotomy for restricted elbow motion. Presented at the 26th annual meeting of the American Orthopaedic Society for Sports Medicine, 1999.

8. Morrey BF. Post-traumatic contracture of the elbow. Operative treatment, including distraction arthroplasty. J Bone Joint Surg Am 1990;72:601-618.

9. O'Driscoll SW. Arthroscopic treatment for osteoarthritis of the elbow. Orthop Clin North Am 1995;26:691-706.

10. O'Driscoll SW, Morrey BF. Arthroscopy of the elbow. Diagnostic and therapeutic benefits and hazards. J Bone Joint Surg Am 1992; 74:84-94.

11. Ogilvie-Harris DJ, Gordon R, MacKay M. Arthroscopic treatment for posterior impingement in degenerative arthritis of the elbow. Arthroscopy 1995;11:437-443.

12. Phillips BB, Strasburger S. Arthroscopic treatment of arthrofibrosis of the elbow joint. Arthroscopy 1998;14:38-44.

13. Stothers K, Day B, Regan WR. Arthroscopy of the elbow: anatomy, portal sites, and a description of the proximal lateral portal. Arthroscopy 1995;11:449-457.

14. Timmerman L, Andrews JR. Arthroscopic treatment of posttraumatic elbow pain and stiffness. Am J Sports Med 1994;22: 230-235.

15. Urbaniak JR, Hansen PE, Beissinger SF, Aitken MS. Correction of post-traumatic flexion contracture of the elbow by anterior capsulotomy. J Bone Joint Surg Am 1985;67:1160-1164.

CHAPTER 34

Elbow Synovitis, Loose Bodies, and Posteromedial Impingement

Matthew A. Kippe, MD
Kyle Anderson, MD

Athletic activities can lead to elbow inflammation and synovitis, joint degeneration, and formation of spurs and loose bodies. In fact, loose body removal represents the most common indication for elbow arthroscopy in this population.[23] Because of the high demand an athlete places on the elbow and other joints, even relatively small but newly acquired deficits in range of motion for a competitive athlete can be extremely disabling. Chronic motion loss, however, may be more easily accommodated. The necessary range of motion varies with the type of sport, the position played, and the individual mechanics necessary to remain competitive. Certainly, loose bodies and osteophytes adherent to the joint capsule can create mechanical blocks to motion, resulting in pain as well as decreased performance. Posteromedial impingement is often the result of the tremendous strain an athlete places on the elbow. The repetitive valgus forces generated during the acceleration and follow-through phases of pitching as the elbow goes into extension can result in osteochondral changes of the olecranon and distal humerus.[10,24] A significant osteophyte forms on the posteromedial aspect of the olecranon process and impinges on the medial articular wall of the olecranon fossa. Over time, the osteophytes can fragment and form loose bodies.

Synovial disorders can also be the source of pain and mechanical symptoms equally disabling to an athlete. Diseases such as synovial chondromatosis, pigmented villonodular synovitis, and inflamed synovial plica can produce mechanical symptoms that can alter the normal mechanics of elbow motion.[8,14,19] The symptoms experienced may or may not be related to the activity. These conditions can sometimes be easily overlooked by assuming that the elbow symptoms are a result of the sports activity. The clinician should maintain a broad differential diagnosis. In this population, elbow arthroscopy can be an effective tool for the removal of inflamed synovial tissue, osteophytes, and loose bodies, returning an athlete to the previous level of competition.

Preoperative Considerations

History

A carefully performed history often provides the most important information. Symptoms are usually activity related. Patients often describe mechanical symptoms, such as catching, locking, and popping. The specific timing of pain can be important in determining the type of pathologic changes present.

Typical History

- Insidious and progressive posterior elbow pain and limited elbow extension result from impinging posterior osteophytes; popping, locking, or catching suggests loose bodies.

- Symptoms are usually most prominent during the involved activity; the patient is often asymptomatic at rest.

- Specific timing of pain exacerbation during the activity can be telling. Pain in late innings during pitching can indicate ligamentous disease often unmasked after forearm muscles fatigue, whereas arthrosis presents more as pain and stiffness early in the morning or early in the activity.

- Specific timing of pain during the throwing motion itself can help differentiate between ligamentous injury (often most symptomatic during early acceleration) and impingement (which typically produces pain at ball release or follow-through).[15,23]
- The patient may complain of intermittent swelling after activity.
- Paresthesias may result from ulnar nerve irritation either by impinging spurs or traction during throwing.

Physical Examination

- A brief examination of the cervical spine, shoulder, and wrist is always performed before the physical examination focuses on the elbow. Several conditions of the cervical spine and shoulder may present as elbow pain.
- Range of motion, loss of extension: posterior olecranon spur, posterior compartment loose bodies, bridging osteophyte across olecranon fossa, anterior capsule contracture, collateral ligament contracture with or without ossification
- Range of motion, loss of flexion: coronoid spur, anterior compartment loose bodies, coronoid fossa spur, posterior capsule contracture or triceps adhesions, collateral ligament contracture
- Palpation: with or without joint effusion, warmth, or crepitation; posteromedial tenderness with valgus hyperextension and posteromedial impingement[24] or posterolateral tenderness in cases of lateral synovial plicae[8,14]
- Ligamentous stability: medial collateral ligament insufficiency can lead to posteromedial fragmentation with formation of loose bodies or loss of extension; valgus testing is performed with the elbow in pronation at 30 and 90 degrees of elbow flexion.[7,10,24]
- Valgus extension overload test: combined valgus and gentle terminal extension[24]
- Neurovascular: palpate ulnar nerve during flexion and extension to assess for subluxation and assess for Tinel sign.
- Intra-articular injections can sometimes be helpful in assessing intra-articular versus extra-articular pathologic processes.

Imaging

Radiography

- Standard anteroposterior and lateral views are obtained (Fig. 34-1).

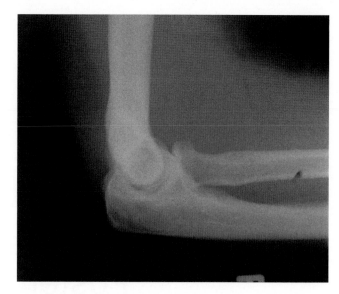

Figure 34-1 Lateral radiograph of a professional baseball player with pain and limited extension.

- The hyperflexion and external rotation view can increase visualization of the posteromedial olecranon out of its fossa (Fig. 34-2).
- When radiocapitellar disease is suspected, the external rotation view is obtained with the anterior elbow surface oriented at 40 degrees oblique relative to the cassette.

Other Modalities

- Computed tomographic scanning and magnetic resonance imaging without contrast enhancement can provide additional information and details about synovial disease, particularly loose bodies, osteophytes filling the olecranon and coronoid fossa, capsular thickening, and chondral thinning, as well as useful information about the integrity of the collateral ligaments (Fig. 34-3).
- Ultrasonography can also be an inexpensive modality that can provide additional information, especially in assessing collateral ligaments both statically and dynamically.
- The authors prefer magnetic resonance imaging to assess the structural integrity of the ulnar collateral ligament and to evaluate for intra-articular disease; dynamic ultrasonography is performed for functional assessment. The performance of dynamic ultrasonography requires education and skill of the radiologist in applying a valgus stress to the elbow.

Indications and Contraindications

In general, there are few absolute indications for surgery in dealing with an athlete. The primary indication is failure

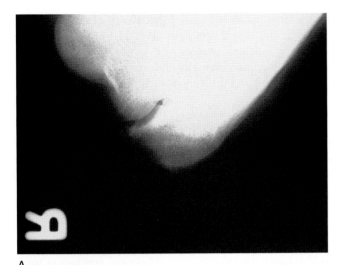

A

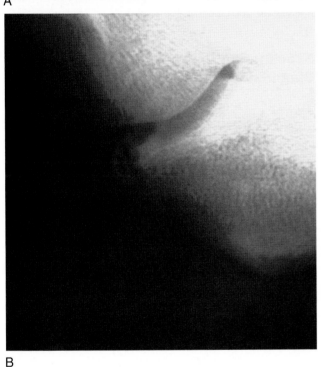

B

Figure 34-2 A, Hyperflexion and external rotation view of the same professional baseball player as in Figure 34-1 demonstrating posteromedial spur. **B,** Close-up view of the posteromedial fragment.

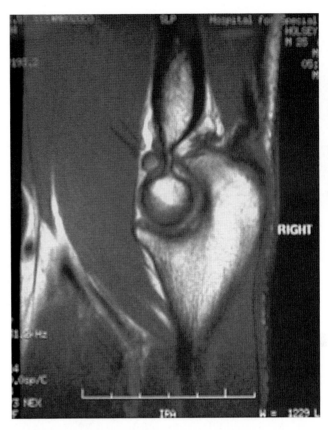

Figure 34-3 Magnetic resonance image demonstrating the position of a loose body within the elbow capsule at the coronoid fossa.

34

to return to competition after nonsurgical management. The most common indications for elbow arthroscopy in this population are removal of a loose body that is closely correlated with mechanical symptoms and loss of motion. The simple appearance of a loose body on radiographs may not necessarily produce symptoms. Most patients complain of locking, catching, or pain toward the extremes of motion.

In addition to osteophyte and loose body removal, arthroscopy is indicated for the treatment of synovial diseases, such as pigmented villonodular synovitis, synovial

chondromatosis, and synovial plicae, which often produce debilitating pain, mechanical symptoms, and effusion.

Surgical Technique

Anesthesia and Positioning

The procedure can be performed under general anesthesia, regional anesthesia, or a combination thereof, depending on the preferences of the surgeon, anesthesiologist, and patient. Most surgeons prefer a general anesthetic because it provides total muscle relaxation as well as allowing immediate postoperative neurologic assessment. The patient is positioned supine if arthroscopy is planned in combination with a reconstructive procedure. The supine position (Fig. 34-4) permits a smoother transition to an open procedure, such as collateral ligament reconstruction. Alternatively, arthroscopy can be performed in the prone position or the lateral decubitus position if a padded arm holder is available. Both of these positions can provide excellent arthroscopic exposure, but conversion to an open procedure can be more difficult.

After the patient is properly positioned and landmarks are identified, the elbow is flexed to 90 degrees and

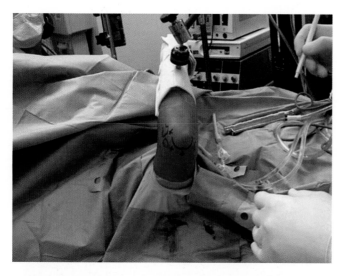

Figure 34-4 Arthroscopy in the supine position facilitates conversion to open procedures, such as a ligament reconstruction.

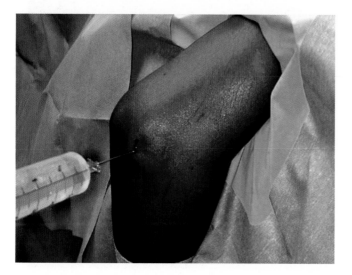

Figure 34-5 Before the surgeon establishes the first portal, the joint is distended with a saline injection through the midlateral soft spot.

the joint is distended with 20 to 40 mL of normal saline through the lateral soft spot (Fig. 34-5). This has been shown in cadaveric studies to help protect neurovascular structures by increasing the distance between neurovascular structures and the portals by up to 1 cm.[17]

Surgical Landmarks, Incisions, and Portals

The number and placement of portals may differ, depending on the condition being treated. Most surgeons use two anterior portals and two or three posterior portals. Several studies have suggested different initial portal sites, and there continues to be considerable controversy about the safest initial portal.[1,2,4,5,11,17,21] The most commonly used portals are described in Table 34-1.

Examination Under Anesthesia and Diagnostic Arthroscopy

Before the patient is positioned for arthroscopy, an examination under anesthesia is performed to evaluate range of motion as well as ligamentous stability. After the patient is positioned properly, the diagnostic arthroscopy is performed. The capsule and synovium may be thickened and inflamed, making introduction of the initial cannula difficult. In addition to a thorough inspection of both the anterior and posterior compartments, ligament integrity can be assessed with provocative testing under direct intra-articular visualization.[10,12] A negative valgus stress does not, however, exclude significant partial tears of the ligament.[16]

Table 34-1 Commonly Used Portals

Portal	Description	Nearest Neurovascular Structure
Midlateral	"Soft spot"—center of triangle between olecranon, radial head, capitellum	7 mm (posterior antebrachial cutaneous nerve)
Proximal lateral[1]	2 cm proximal, 1 cm anterior to lateral epicondyle	7.9 mm extended, 13.7 mm flexed (radial nerve)
Anterolateral[2]	3 cm distal, 1 cm anterior to lateral epicondyle	1.4 mm extended, 4.9 mm flexed (radial nerve)
Proximal medial[21]	2 cm proximal, just anterior to medial epicondyle	12-23 mm (median nerve)
Anteromedial[2]	2 cm distal, 2 cm anterior to medial epicondyle	2 mm extended, 7 mm flexed (median nerve); 4 mm (median nerve)
Posterolateral[5]	Proximal to olecranon, lateral edge of triceps	>15-20 mm
Posterocentral[2] (trans-triceps)	Proximal to olecranon, through triceps tendon	>15-20 mm

Specific Steps (Box 34-1)

1. Establishment of Portals

Whether a lateral or medial portal is established first is a matter of the surgeon's preference. It is more important that the surgeon develop a routine that is thorough and can be performed consistently. A secondary portal can be established under direct visualization with spinal needle localization if loose bodies are present. Surgeons who advocate establishing a medial portal first and then a lateral portal under direct visualization argue that this is safer because the average distance between the medial portals and the median nerve is greater than the distance between the lateral portals and the radial or posterior interosseous nerve.[4] We prefer to establish a proximal lateral portal as described by Field and Altchek,[10] which is on average 13.7 mm from the radial nerve in a flexed elbow (Fig. 34-6). This portal allows broad visualization of the anterior compartment.

2. Anterior Compartment Assessment and Débridement

When the procedure is started from the lateral portal, examination of the medial gutter is performed first, followed by a search for loose bodies across the entire ante-

Box 34-1 Surgical Steps

1. Establishment of portals
2. Anterior compartment assessment and débridement
3. Posterior compartment assessment and débridement
4. Closure

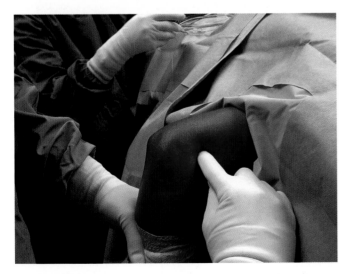

Figure 34-6 Photograph demonstrating the proximal lateral portal. The portal is placed just anterior to the humerus where the supracondylar ridge meets the lateral epicondyle.

rior compartment from medial to lateral. All fragments should be removed as they are encountered because visualization can change and loose bodies can move to a less accessible area during the procedure. An arthroscopic grasper or shaver is used for smaller fragments or fragments adherent to the capsule. A spinal needle can also be used to stabilize the fragment and prevent it from migrating into a recess. Fluid flow should be well controlled, especially once a loose body has been localized. Allowing outflow at the cannula can help bring the loose body toward the arthroscopic grasper. Very large loose bodies may need to be broken into smaller pieces to be removed through the cannula. This can also be accomplished by removal of the fragment and the cannula in one maneuver after the portal skin incision is extended and the portal carefully dilated with a spreading clamp (Fig. 34-7). The camera can also assist in pushing the fragment out through the portal while pulling with the grasper. Sometimes, the plica may be more easily resected by getting a rough edge started with either a bovie or a retractable hook blade. It may be necessary to switch portals and view from the medial side to resect all pathologic tissue completely from the lateral compartment.

An arthroscopic valgus instability test can be performed during viewing from the proximal lateral or anterolateral portal. The medial aspect of the ulnohumeral joint is observed for any gap formation (Fig. 34-8). Any gap greater than 2 mm is considered abnormal.[10]

3. Posterior Compartment Assessment and Débridement

After completion of the anterior compartment, a cannula is left in place to maintain joint distention while the transition is made to the posterior compartment. Next, a posterolateral portal is established, which is located just radial to the triceps tendon at the level of the tip of the olecranon. This is the primary viewing portal for work to be done in the posterior compartment. Careful inspection will reveal loose bodies, spurs, chondromalacia, and fibrous debris. Débridement and loose body removal can be accomplished through a posterocentral (trans-triceps) portal (Fig. 34-9). The olecranon should be probed because fibrous tissue can often hide fragmentation that may be a source of persistent pain. Extreme caution must be used in operating the motorized shaver, especially while suction is used, because of the proximity of the ulnar nerve along the posteromedial olecranon. The scope can be advanced into the midlateral viewing area to assess the radial gutter and to remove any remaining pathologic tissue along the posterior aspect of the radial head and capitellum. This can also be accomplished by use of a midlateral portal or a 70-degree scope to improve visualization of this small compartment. Most plicae are posterolateral and are best removed by viewing from posterolateral and working from the midlateral portal (Fig. 34-10). The plicae can be resected with a motorized shaver.

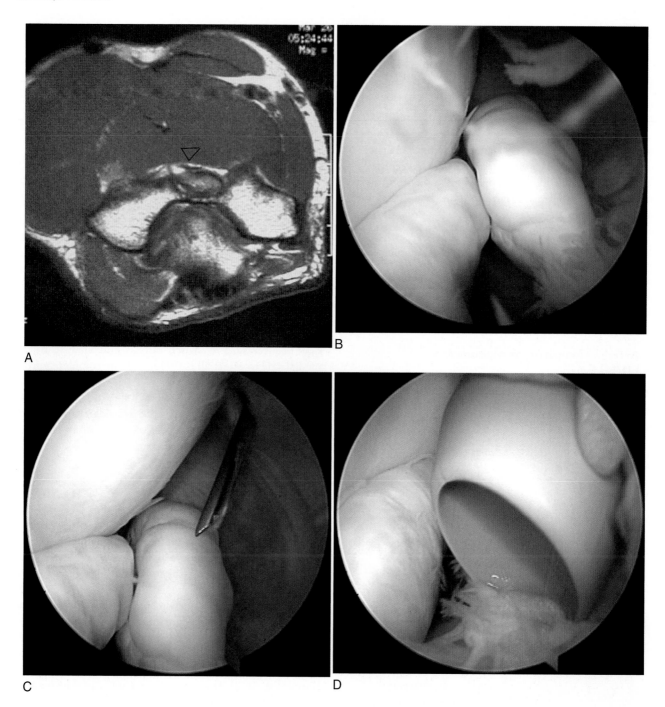

Figure 34-7 Loose body removal. **A,** Axial magnetic resonance image of a loose body in the coronoid fossa of the humerus causing mechanical symptoms. **B,** During arthroscopy, the loose body is visualized through the proximal lateral portal. **C,** A spinal needle is used to make an anteromedial portal under direct visualization as well as to prevent movement of the loose body. **D,** A cannula is placed in a proximal medial portal, through which the loose body was removed from the elbow joint.

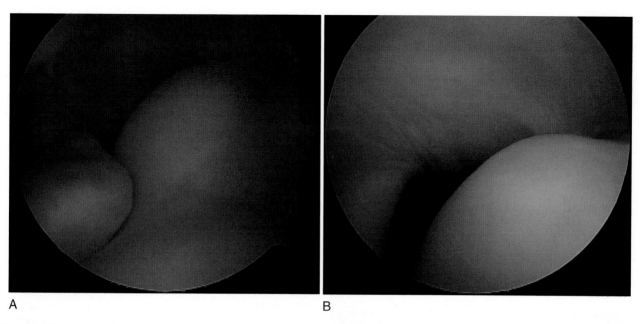

Figure 34-8 During diagnostic arthroscopy, ligamentous stability is assessed under direct visualization. **A,** Arthroscopic photograph of ulnohumeral joint without valgus stress applied. **B,** Arthroscopic photograph of medial opening of ulnohumeral joint with valgus stress.

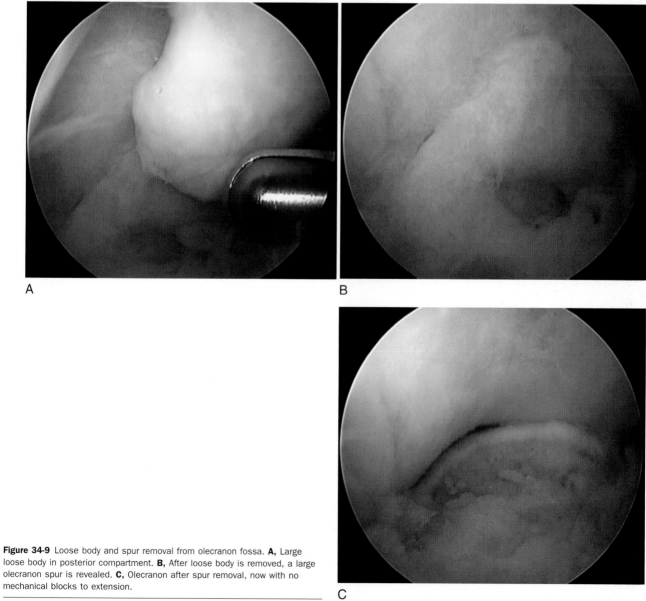

Figure 34-9 Loose body and spur removal from olecranon fossa. **A,** Large loose body in posterior compartment. **B,** After loose body is removed, a large olecranon spur is revealed. **C,** Olecranon after spur removal, now with no mechanical blocks to extension.

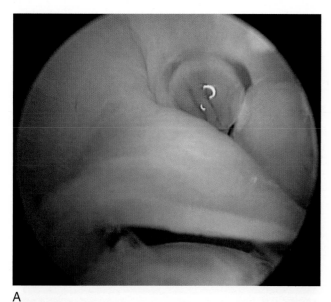

A

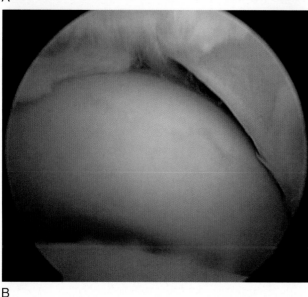

B

Figure 34-10 Lateral synovial plicae in a golfer causing pain and mechanical symptoms. **A,** Symptomatic lateral synovial plicae viewed from posterolateral portal. **B,** Radiocapitellar joint after removal of the lateral synovial plicae.

4. Closure

Portal incisions are closed with 4-0 nylon sutures in a simple interrupted fashion. Sterile dressings are applied, and the arm is placed in a sling for comfort.

Postoperative Considerations

Rehabilitation

- Reduce inflammation in the immediate postoperative period with ice, elevation, and anti-inflammatory medication.

- Passive range of motion is begun in the early postoperative period (phase 1: 3 to 6 weeks).
- In the second phase of rehabilitation (6 to 10 weeks), motion restoration is continued with the addition of strengthening.
- In the third phase, the focus is on advanced strengthening, resistive exercises, and sport-specific training, such as a graduated throwing program.
- General overall condition is emphasized throughout rehabilitation, including strengthening of adjacent joints, core strengthening, and cardiovascular conditioning.

PEARLS AND PITFALLS

- Keep the elbow flexed at 90 degrees and distended with saline before initial portal placement to help protect neurovascular structures.
- Fluid inflow can be achieved through an 18-gauge needle, which may improve distention for joint entry.
- A spinal needle can help stabilize loose fragments and prevent migration during removal.
- Loose bodies can be brought toward the cannula by allowing fluid outflow from a side port.
- Large loose bodies can be removed in one motion along with the cannula.
- Maintain low suction on the shaver while working in the proximity of the capsule.
- The posterolateral cannula can be advanced into the radial gutter to facilitate placement of a midlateral portal.
- Minimize joint entry without the use of a cannula.
- Do not rely on the brachialis muscle for neurovascular protection.

Complications

Elbow arthroscopy for the removal of loose bodies, débridement, and synovectomy is generally a safe procedure. Complications are uncommon and usually minor. The major concern is for the potential of neurovascular injury. The following complications have been reported[13,18]:

- Direct nerve laceration
- Nerve compression due to suboptimal portal placement and levering of instruments
- Postoperative stiffness
- Potential for further loose body formation
- Portal drainage
- Infection

Results

Arthroscopy for the treatment of posteromedial impingement and elbow joint synovitis and for loose body removal

Table 34-2 Clinical Results of Elbow Arthroscopy for Loose Body and Synovial Plicae Removal

Author	Follow-up	Outcome
Wilson et al[24] (1983)	12 months	5/5 pitchers returned for at least one full season of maximum effectiveness
Andrews and Timmerman[3] (1995)	42 months mean (minimum: 24 months)	47/59 professional baseball players returned for at least one season (however, 33% reoperation rate, and 25% required ulnar collateral ligament reconstruction)
Bradley[6] (1995)	24 months	6/6 excellent and good objective and subjective results
Reddy et al[22] (2000)	42.3 months mean (range: 7-115 months)	47/55 baseball players returned to competition
Kim et al[14] (2006)	33.8 months (range: 24-65.5 months)	11/12 athletes reported excellent outcome and returned to competition

34

in athletes can reduce pain and improve function. Most athletes are able to return to the same level of their sport after arthroscopic elbow surgery, particularly if no associated instability exists.[3,6,9,14,20,22,23] However, in certain athletes, depending on the type of sport and position played, reoperation rates are high, and return to the previous level of competition is less reliable.[3] Table 34-2 summarizes clinical results after elbow arthroscopy for posteromedial impingement, loose body removal, and treatment of common synovial diseases.

References

1. Adolfsson L. Arthroscopy of the elbow joint: a cadaveric study of portal placement. J Shoulder Elbow Surg 1994;3:53-61.
2. Andrews JR, Carson WG. Arthroscopy of the elbow. Arthroscopy 1985;1:97-107.
3. Andrews JR, Timmerman LA. Outcome of elbow surgery in professional baseball players. Am J Sports Med 1995;23:407-413.
4. Baker CL, Jones GL. Arthroscopy of the elbow. Am J Sports Med 1999;27:251-264.
5. Burman MS. Arthroscopy of the elbow joint: a cadaveric. J Bone Joint Surg 1932;14:349-350.
6. Bradley JP. Arthroscopic treatment of posterior impingement of the elbow in NFL lineman [abstract]. J Shoulder Elbow Surg 1995;2:S119.
7. Callaway GH, Field LD, Deng XH, et al. Biomechanical evaluation of the medial collateral ligament of the elbow. J Bone Joint Surg Am 1997;79:1223-1230.
8. Clarke RP. Symptomatic, lateral synovial fringe (plica) of the elbow joint. Arthroscopy 1988;4:112-116.
9. Fideler BM, Kvitne RS, Jordan S, et al. Posterior impingement of the elbow in professional baseball players: results of arthroscopic treatment [abstract]. J Shoulder Elbow Surg 1997;6:169-170.
10. Field LD, Altchek DW. Evaluation of the arthroscopic valgus instability test of the elbow. Am J Sports Med 1996;24:177-183.
11. Field LD, Altchek DW, Warren RF, et al. Arthroscopic anatomy of the lateral elbow: a comparison of three portals. Arthroscopy 1994;10:602-607.
12. Field LD, Callaway GH, O'Brien SJ, et al. Arthroscopic assessment of the medial collateral ligament complex of the elbow. Am J Sports Med 1995;23:396-400.
13. Kelly EW, Morrey BF, O'Driscoll SW. Complications of elbow arthroscopy. J Bone Joint Surg Am 2001;83:25-34.
14. Kim DH, Gambardella RA, ElAttrache NS, et al. Arthroscopic treatment of posterolateral elbow impingement from lateral synovial plicae in throwing athletes and golfers. Am J Sports Med 2006;34:1-7.
15. King JW, Brelsford HJ, Tullos HS. Analysis of the pitching arm of the professional baseball pitcher. Clin Orthop 1969;67:116-123.
16. Kooima CL, Anderson K, Craig JV, et al. Evidence of subclinical medial collateral ligament injury and posteromedial impingement in professional baseball players. Am J Sports Med 2004;32:1602-1606.
17. Lynch GH, Meyers JF, Whipple TL, et al. Neurovascular anatomy and elbow arthroscopy: inherent risks. Arthroscopy 1986;2:191-197.
18. Marshall PD, Faircloth JA, Johnson SR, et al. Avoiding nerve damage during elbow arthroscopy. J Bone Joint Surg Am 1993;74:129-131.
19. Ofluoglu O. Pigmented villonodular synovitis. Orthop Clin North Am 2006;37:23-33.
20. Ogilvie-Harris DJ, Schemitsch E. Arthroscopy of the elbow for removal of loose bodies. Arthroscopy 1993;9:5-8.
21. Poehling GG, Whipple TL, Sisco L, et al. Elbow arthroscopy. A new technique. Arthroscopy 1989;5:222-224.
22. Reddy AS, Kvitne RS, Yocum LA, et al. Arthroscopy of the elbow: a long term clinical review. Arthroscopy 2000;16:588-594.
23. Ward WG, Anderson TE. Elbow arthroscopy in a mostly athletic population. J Hand Surg Am 1993;18:220-224.
24. Wilson FD, Andrews JR, Blackburn TA, et al. Valgus extension overload in the pitching elbow. Am J Sports Med 1983;11:83-88.

CHAPTER 35

Elbow Arthroscopy for the Arthritic Elbow

Justin P. Strickland, MD
Scott P. Steinmann, MD

The indications for and thus the number of procedures that can be performed by arthroscopy of the elbow joint have increased recently. Initially used for loose body removal or examination of a painful joint, arthroscopy is performed to treat many of the pathologic changes encountered with osteoarthritis, inflammatory arthritis, and post-traumatic conditions.[11,12]

Elbow arthroscopy is technically challenging because of the small working space and the exclusive anatomy of the multiple articulations that make up the elbow. Potential advantages include improved articular visualization, decreased postoperative pain, and faster postoperative recovery. The immediacy of the major neurovascular structures is the greatest concern of most orthopedic surgeons.

The goal of this chapter is to introduce the common findings of arthritic conditions of the elbow while providing the technical steps and pearls for treatment of the unique aspects of these conditions.

Preoperative Considerations

History

Post-traumatic arthritis, osteoarthritis, and rheumatoid arthritis may affect the elbow joint. Pain is the most common complaint; however, patients may also complain of stiffness, weakness, instability, or cosmetic deformity.[7] A subjective description of the amount of motion loss and pain is an important part of the history. It is imperative to elucidate a history of trauma from patients. The most common injury that may cause post-traumatic arthritis is a comminuted intra-articular distal humerus fracture resulting in articular incongruity.[7] Post-traumatic contractures solely due to capsular fibrosis are secondary to hemarthrosis from various traumatic causes. The patient should be asked whether he or she had physical therapy, whether it was painful or relatively benign, and whether splints had been used for short- or long-term sessions.

Osteoarthritis involving the elbow is most commonly seen in men with a history of heavy labor using the arm, weight lifters, and throwing athletes.[7] They commonly present in the third to eighth decades. Patients typically complain of pain at extremes of motion with loss of terminal extension more than loss of flexion. Patients with osteoarthritis primarily do not have pain in the mid-arc of motion. Rheumatoid arthritis affects the elbow less commonly than other joints but can be quite debilitating when it does occur. Both elbows are commonly involved. Patients initially present with pain and swelling due to synovitis and effusion. Rheumatoid arthritis predominantly involves the ulnohumeral articulation. More severe involvement with loss of bone stock and failure of the soft tissues around the elbow joint may cause instability, which may increase articular destruction as a result of subluxation or malalignment.

Physical Examination

On examination, patients will have pain at the endpoints of motion. A flexion contracture of 30 degrees is common along with loss of flexion. Crepitus may also be present. It is important to record the passive and active ranges of motion. This aids in quantifying the functional deficits while determining the success of treatment. Although difficult, it may be useful to differentiate between a "soft" and "hard" endpoint as this may lead the examiner to determine the cause of stiffness. A complete neurovascular examination should always be performed. The physical examination findings are then correlated with the radiographic findings.

Imaging

Anteroposterior, lateral, and oblique views of the elbow should be obtained. On radiographic examination, osteophytes may be seen on the olecranon and coronoid processes and also in the olecranon and coronoid fossae. Most patients have loose bodies as a result of progressive degenerative arthritis. The presence of a loose body on an elbow radiograph is in most instances the sign of underlying degenerative arthritis.

Computed tomography, particularly three-dimensional reformatting, may be helpful for visualizing impinging osteophytes and malunions.

Indications

Surgery in an elbow with arthritis is indicated for patients with functional loss of motion and pain accompanied by osteophyte formation, loose bodies, and capsular contraction.

Surgical Technique

Anesthesia and Positioning

We prefer to use general anesthesia. This allows full muscle relaxation and permits the patient to be placed in either a prone or a lateral decubitus position, which might not be tolerated by an awake patient. Regional anesthetic blocks can be administered for elbow arthroscopy, but when these blocks are used, the patient should be in the supine position for comfort.

Placement of the patient in the lateral decubitus position allows excellent access to the elbow joint (Fig. 35-1). The arm is placed in a padded arm holder that is attached to the side of the table. A low-profile elbow arm

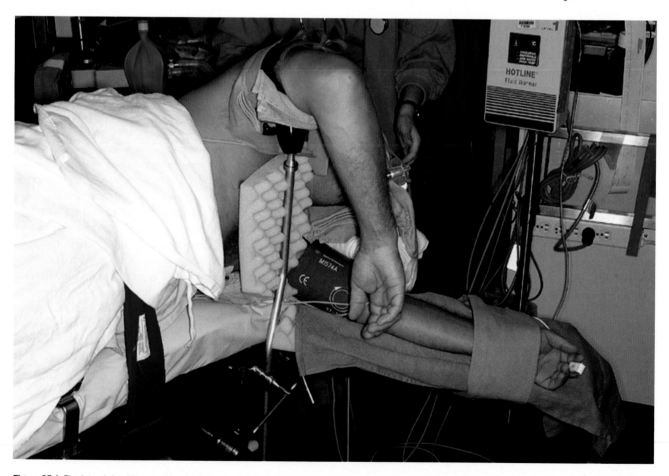

Figure 35-1 The lateral decubitus position for elbow arthroscopy. The arm is placed into a specially designed elbow arm holder with a nonsterile tourniquet. The arm is strapped into the arm holder to secure it during arthroscopic manipulation. The opposite arm is draped out on an arm board.

holder specifically designed for this purpose usually functions best.

A nonsterile tourniquet is then placed on the arm at the level of the arm holder, and the arm is firmly secured to the arm holder. This facilitates the arthroscopy by keeping the arm stable, just as a knee holder maintains stability during knee arthroscopy. The elbow should be positioned slightly higher than the shoulder. This allows 360-degree exposure of the elbow joint, eliminating the potential for impingement of the arthroscope or other instruments against the side of the body (Fig. 35-2).

Surgical Landmarks, Incisions, and Portals

All portal sites are marked before surgery, when the elbow is not distended or edematous and palpation of osseous landmarks is more precise (Fig. 35-3). Surface landmarks that should be marked with a pen on all patients are the lateral epicondyle, medial epicondyle, radial head, capitellum, and olecranon. The ulnar nerve is then palpated to be sure of its location and to check that it does not subluxate

from the cubital tunnel. The location of the ulnar nerve is then marked.

An 18-gauge needle is placed through the planned anterolateral portal. The elbow is then distended with 20 to 30 mL of saline solution. When the joint is distended, the major neurovascular structures are positioned farther away from the starting portal site, and entry into the joint is easier and potentially safer. Attempting to enter a nondistended elbow joint accurately with a trocar is considerably difficult.

Initial portal entry can be performed safely from either the medial or the lateral side, depending on the preference of the operating surgeon. All portals are made with a No. 11 blade, which is drawn across the skin to ensure that only the skin, and not the underlying soft tissue, is divided. The neurovascular structure that is at greatest risk of injury from a lateral portal is the radial nerve. There are two techniques to reduce the risk of injury to that nerve. The first is to establish an anterolateral portal as soon as the joint is distended, before fluid extravasation makes it difficult to see and to feel the anatomic landmarks. The anterolateral portal should be established just anterior to the sulcus between the capitellum and the

35

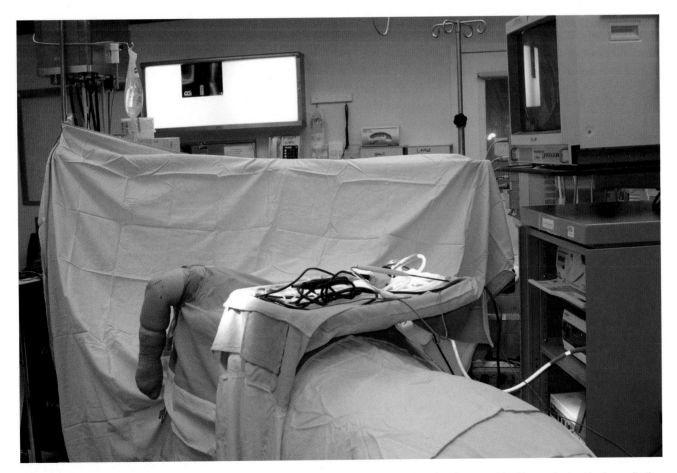

Figure 35-2 Overview of the operating room before elbow arthroscopy is begun. The patient is in lateral decubitus position. The monitor is placed opposite the surgeon for ease of viewing.

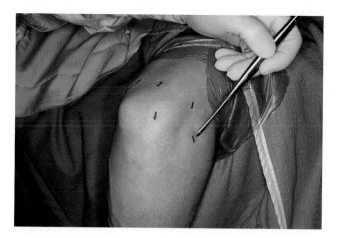

Figure 35-3 Intraoperative view of portal placement. The retractor is demonstrating the standard anterolateral portal.

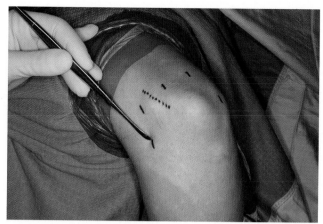

Figure 35-4 Medial view of intraoperative portal placement demonstrating the anteromedial portal with the retractor. The dotted line represents the ulnar nerve.

radial head. The other technique is to establish an antero-medial portal first. This portal is a safe distance away from the median and ulnar nerves. Then, under direct visualization with the arthroscope inside the joint, an anterolateral portal is established by placing a spinal needle into the joint and next placing a trocar and cannula. This can be a safe technique in experienced hands, but simply observing from inside of the joint, as is done with this technique, does not guarantee that the spinal needle and trocar are not being passed through the radial nerve.

Once the arthroscope (4-mm, 30-degree) has been placed into the joint, visualization is maintained by pressure distention of the capsule or mechanical retraction. Both methods work, but pressure distention leads to fluid extravasation during the course of a long arthroscopic procedure. The retractors can be simple lever retractors such as Howarth elevator or large Steinmann pins. They are placed into the elbow joint through an accessory portal, which is typically 2 to 3 cm proximal to the arthroscopic viewing portal. With the capsule and overlying soft tissue held away from the bone with the retractors, adequate visualization can be achieved with a high-flow, low-pressure system.

Direct Lateral or Midlateral Portal

The direct lateral or midlateral portal is located at the center of the triangle bounded by the olecranon, lateral epicondyle, and radial head. It is difficult to visualize the anterior aspect of the joint from this portal; however, it provides the best view of the posterior aspect of the capitellum, radial head, and radioulnar articulation. This is helpful, especially when one is examining a patient with osteochondritis dissecans of the capitellum. Because of the shallow nature of this portal and the limited space in which to work, it can be helpful to use a 2.7-mm arthroscope.

Anteromedial Portal

The anteromedial portal is placed 2 cm distal and 2 cm anterior to the medial epicondyle (Fig. 35-4). Instruments placed through this portal tend to penetrate the common flexor origin and the brachialis before entering the joint. Before any medial portals are placed, the ulnar nerve should be palpated and checked for any tendency to subluxate from the cubital tunnel. The medial antebrachial cutaneous nerve is most at risk with this portal. The median nerve is farther away, an average of 7 mm from the portal.

Posterior Portals

Two portals are necessary to visualize the posterior aspect of the elbow joint. The fat pad normally occupies a large portion of the potential space. A second portal is usually established simultaneously with the first since débridement with an arthroscopic shaver will be needed immediately to obtain a visible working space. The location of the ulnar nerve is confirmed before the first portal is established. Unlike the anterior portals, where palpation of the median or radial nerve is not possible, posterior portals can be established safely, once the ulnar nerve is identified.

The posterolateral portal is excellent for initial viewing of the posterior aspect of the elbow. It is made level with the tip of the olecranon, with the elbow flexed 90 degrees, at the lateral joint line. The trocar should be aimed at the center of the olecranon fossa. The direct posterior portal is established to 3 cm proximal to the tip of the olecranon, at the proximal margin of the olecranon fossa. The triceps is thick at this point, and a knife blade will be needed to penetrate directly into the elbow joint. After this portal is made, a shaver or radiofrequency probe can be placed into the joint and débridement can be performed. Loose bodies and osteophytes on the entire olecranon fossa can be removed through this portal while the surgeon views through the posterolateral portal. The arthroscope and the shaver can be switched back and forth to complete the débridement. Because of the frequent switching between portals and the relative safety of the portal location, it is not necessary to use a cannula in the posterior aspect of the elbow joint. However, an outflow cannula should be maintained in the anterior aspect of the elbow joint to limit fluid extravasation.

A good location for an initial posterior retractor portal is 2 cm proximal to the directly posterior portal. A Howarth elevator or similar type of retractor can be used to elevate the joint capsule out of view while not interfering with the working instruments. This can help with visualization of the medial and lateral gutters and also the release of a tight posterior aspect of the capsule in a stiff elbow.

Specific Steps

Arthroscopic débridement of an osteoarthritic elbow begins in the posterior aspect of the joint when the patient predominantly lacks flexion and in the anterior aspect of the joint when the patient predominantly lacks extension (Box 35-1). For greater flexion to be achieved at surgery, the posterior aspect of the capsule needs to be released. This is safest and easiest to perform early in the procedure, before any swelling or fluid extravasation has occurred. In particular, release of the posteromedial aspect of the capsule requires identification of the ulnar nerve so that the nerve will not be injured (Fig. 35-5). If the greatest limitation of motion is in extension, the procedure should begin in the anterior compartment.

The posterior compartment is visualized well from the posterolateral portal, and the directly posterior portal can be used as a working portal. Osteophytes develop both

Box 35-1 Surgical Steps

1. Mark all portal sites and surface anatomy
2. Elbow distention
3. Establish portals
4. Begin work in posterior compartment
5. Capsular release (posterior capsule first if patient lacks flexion)
6. Remove osteophytes along olecranon and olecranon fossa
7. Move to anterior compartment
8. Remove all obvious loose bodies; remove radial and coronoid osteophytes
9. Anterior capsulectomy off of humerus (lateral viewing portal)
10. Viewing from the medial portal, perform capsulectomy from radial head and capitellum

on the tip of the olecranon and along the medial and lateral sides of the ulna. It is important to check for osteophytes on the sides of the olecranon; often, they are overlooked, and only the one on the tip of the olecranon is addressed. In addition, the olecranon fossa should be checked for osteophytes along the rim on the posterior aspect of the humerus. These osteophytes often match arthritic osseous formation on the olecranon, and both sites of bone formation need to be excised to restore normal joint motion.

After initial joint inspection from an anterior portal and removal of obvious loose bodies, all work on bone is performed (Fig. 35-6). A shaver or bur can be used to remove osteophytes from the radial and coronoid fossae of the humerus. Often, these osteophytes are neglected, and only the tip of the coronoid is excised (Fig. 35-7). The medial aspect of the coronoid should also be examined for osteophytes, which may be missed if they are not specifically sought. Use of motorized instruments without a suction device attached allows adequate tissue removal and reduces the risk of inadvertent neurovascular injury.

Once all osteophytes have been excised, the anterior aspect of the capsule can be removed. It helps initially to take the capsule off of the humerus. This tends also to increase the working space in the anterior compartment. While viewing from the lateral side, the surgeon excises the anterior aspect of the capsule with a shaver or punch. The median nerve is the closest important structure, but it is behind the brachialis muscle. After the capsule is excised to the midline of the joint, the viewing portal is changed to the medial side, and the shaver is placed through the lateral portal. Care must be taken when the capsule is excised just anterior to the radial head and the capitellum. The radial nerve is at great risk for injury at this location. Often, a small fat pad can be visualized in this area. The radial nerve lies just anterior to this fat pad.

At the end of the procedure, the maximum range of motion of the elbow is evaluated and documented (Fig. 35-8). The elbow should then be placed in an extended position with a circumferential compressive dressing. The extended position limits the amount of swelling and accumulation of intra-articular fluid. The elbow should not be placed in flexion because this position allows the maximal amount of fluid to collect in the elbow joint. Patients are examined immediately after the surgical procedure, when they are awake in the recovery room, to confirm that the neurovascular status is stable postoperatively.

Postoperative Considerations

Rehabilitation

Elevation of the arm into a "Statue of Liberty" position overnight helps limit postoperative swelling. Motion can be delayed for 24 hours to allow edema to resolve.

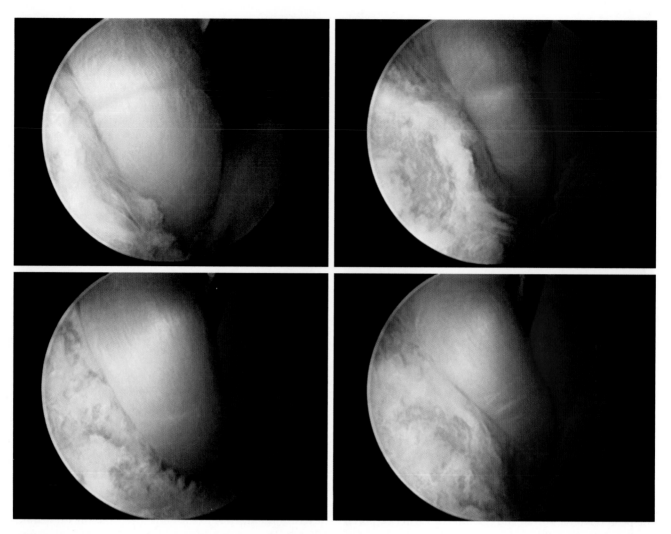

Figure 35-5 Arthroscopic views of the ulnar nerve after posteromedial capsular release.

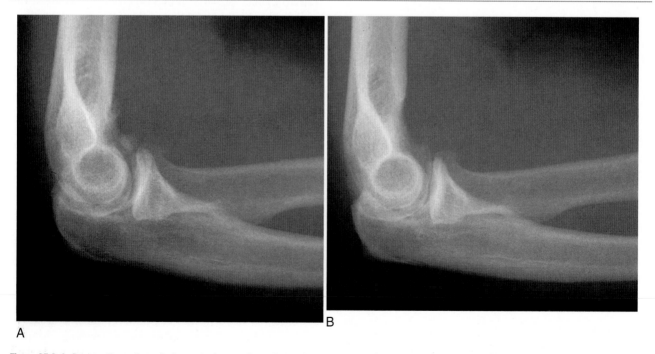

A

B

Figure 35-6 A, Preoperative radiograph demonstrating anterior and posterior osteophytes. **B,** Postoperative radiograph demonstrating osteophyte excision around the elbow joint.

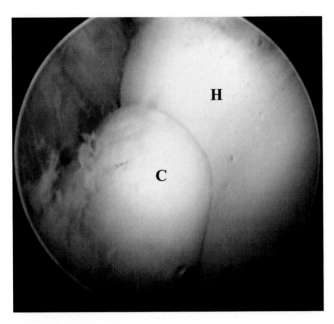

Figure 35-7 Arthroscopic view of the tip of the coronoid (C) and distal humerus (H).

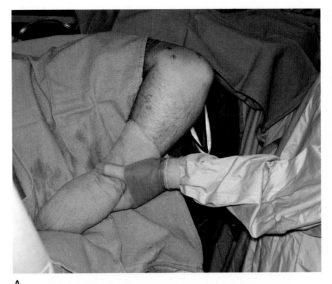

A

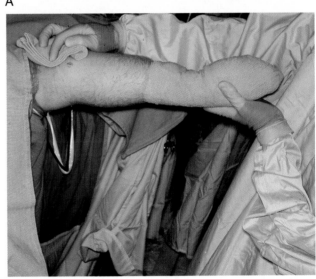

B

Figure 35-8 A, Intraoperative view demonstrating full flexion after arthroscopic release. **B,** Intraoperative view demonstrating full extension after arthroscopic débridement and release.

Continuous passive motion or splinting can then be started to help maintain the arc of motion achieved in the operating room. Continuous passive motion is often prescribed for patients who had the most restricted motion preoperatively. It is often not needed for those with a minimal loss of motion. However, there is little evidence to confirm that continuous passive motion restores motion better than splints alone or physical therapy. If continuous passive motion is used, it is typically applied for 23 hours a day, with breaks for cleaning and eating. The motion setting is started at the same maximum motion achieved in the operating room. We do not start with a gentle range of motion and "work up" to the range of motion restored in the operating room. Continuous passive motion can be used with an indwelling axillary block for paralysis and pain control for the first 24 hours, or intravenous narcotics can be used for pain control. We are not aware of any reports on the use of intra-articular catheters to deliver lidocaine or narcotics. Continuous passive motion is often used for the first 3 or 4 weeks after surgery.

Splinting is also an effective option, and it typically involves alternating periods of extension and flexion. Splinting is almost always used for patients who had the least amount of motion loss preoperatively. A static splint is thought to be the best type of splint. The patient is taught to alternate periods of flexion and extension, typically for an hour at each end of the range of motion achieved at surgery. The neurovascular status, in particular, the ulnar nerve, should be evaluated at regular intervals during postoperative rehabilitation, especially in patients in whom a significant amount of motion has been restored. An ulnar neuropathy has been noted after arthroscopic or open release in some patients who had 90 degrees or less of flexion preoperatively and in whom surgery restored substantially greater flexion.[2,5,15]

Complications

Complications of elbow arthroscopy include compartment syndrome, septic arthritis, and nerve injury. In a report of 473 elbow arthroscopies performed by experienced elbow arthroscopists, four types of minor complications, including infection, nerve injury, prolonged drainage, and contracture, were identified in 50 cases.[5] The most common complication was persistent portal drainage, and the most serious was deep infection. Neurologic complications were limited to transient nerve palsies; there were no permanent nerve injuries. Savoie and Field[10] reported a 3% prevalence of neurologic complications in a review of the results of 465 arthroscopy procedures presented in the literature. The rate of permanent neurologic injury appears to be higher in the elbow than in the knee or shoulder, and the risk of nerve injury at the elbow is higher in patients with rheumatoid arthritis or in those undergoing a capsular release.[5] Substantial injury involving the radial, median, and ulnar nerves has been reported during elbow arthroscopy.[4,8,14] The use of retractors for greater visualization and to facilitate exposure is probably the most important factor in preventing nerve injury.[5] In some cases, arthroscopic identification of nerves allows safe capsulectomy. This is particularly true with regard to the ulnar nerve.

PEARLS AND PITFALLS

- Although plain radiographs are adequate for preoperative planning, three-dimensional computed tomographic scanning is helpful for fully evaluating areas of osteophyte formation.

- Block anesthesia can be used for elbow arthroscopy; however, if the lateral or prone position is used, it can be difficult for the patient. In addition, if block anesthesia is used, the surgeon will be unable to evaluate for a potential nerve injury until many hours postoperatively.

- An arm holder made specifically for elbow arthroscopy makes positioning easier and helps eliminate instrument impingement.

- If the lateral decubitus position is used, the elbow should be positioned high in the operative field. This helps eliminate impingement of the arthroscope and instruments against the patient's body or surgical drapes.

- If the patient is tilted slightly to the surgeon, this helps prevent the arm holder from impinging on the antecubital fossa. This area must be kept free to allow saline distention of the anterior joint.

- Any portal can be used as an initial starting portal. However, the anterolateral portal is closest to a major nerve (radial nerve) and should be established either first, before any swelling has begun and bone landmarks can be palpated, or early in the procedure.

- Do not use suction on the shaver in the anterior aspect of the joint. This may inadvertently pull a nerve or vital structure into the shaver or bur.

- Attempt to do all bone work first in the elbow joint before removing capsule. This helps limit edema and potentially protects vital structures.

- Heterotopic bone can form even after an arthroscopic procedure on the elbow. To potentially limit this process, use the shaver after the bur to remove as many bone fragments as possible.

- Elevation of the patient's arm overhead in a fully extended Statue of Liberty position overnight can help quickly remove postoperative swelling to allow early active motion.

Results

Few reports of arthroscopic débridement for treatment of osteoarthritis of the elbow are available (Table 35-1). The current literature has shown satisfactory results with increases in range of motion and improvement of pain. These studies suggest that arthroscopic débridement of the arthritic elbow is a reasonable option in the arthritic patient.

Table 35-1 Results of Arthroscopic Débridement of the Arthritic Elbow

Author	Results
Cohen et al[3] (2000)	26 patients with excellent pain relief, no major complications
Savoie et al[11] (1999)	24 patients; all had decrease in pain, 81-degree increase in arc of motion
Phillips and Strasburger[9] (1998)	Satisfactory results in 25 patients with an increase of 41 degrees in total arc of motion
Kim and Shin[6] (2000)	30 patients with 92% improvement in the range of motion, from a mean of 81 degrees preoperatively to a mean of 121 degrees postoperatively
Adams and Steinmann[1] (2007)	41 patients with 81% good–excellent results; postoperative range of motion, 8.4 to 131.6 degrees

References

1. Adams JE, Wolff LH III, Merten SM, Steinmann SP: Osteoarthritis of the elbow: results of arthroscopic osteophyte resection and capsulectomy. Podium Presentation, Twenty-Third Annual Open Meeting of the American Shoulder and Elbow Surgeons, February 17, 2007, San Diego, California.

2. Aldridge JM 3rd, Atkins TA, Gunneson EE, Urbaniak JR. Anterior release of the elbow for extension loss. J Bone Joint Surg Am 2004;86:1955-1960.

3. Cohen AP, Redden JF, Stanley D. Treatment of osteoarthritis of the elbow: a comparison of open and arthroscopic débridement. Arthroscopy 2000;16:701-706.

4. Hahn M, Grossman JA. Ulnar nerve laceration as a result of elbow arthroscopy. J Hand Surg Br 1998;23:109.

5. Kelly EW, Morrey BF, O'Driscoll SW. Complications of elbow arthroscopy. J Bone Joint Surg Am 2001;83:25-34.

6. Kim SJ, Shin SJ. Arthroscopic treatment for limitation of motion of the elbow. Clin Orthop 2000;375:140-148.

7. O'Driscoll SW. Elbow arthritis. J Am Acad Orthop Surg 1993; 1:106-116.

8. Papilion JD, Neff RS, Shall LM. Compression neuropathy of the radial nerve as a complication of elbow arthroscopy: a case report and review of the literature. Arthroscopy 1998;4:284-286.

9. Phillips BB, Strasburger S. Arthroscopic treatment of arthrofibrosis of the elbow joint. Arthroscopy 1998;14:38-44.

10. Savoie F, Field LD. Complications of elbow arthroscopy. In Savoie F, Field LD, eds. Arthroscopy of the Elbow. New York, Churchill Livingstone, 1996:151-156.

11. Savoie F, Nunley PD, Field LD. Arthroscopic management of the arthritic elbow: indications, technique, and results. J Shoulder Elbow Surg 1999;8:214-219.

12. Steinmann SP. Elbow arthroscopy. J Am Soc Surg Hand 2003; 3:199-207.

13. Steinmann SP, King G, Savoie F. Arthroscopic treatment of the arthritic elbow. J Bone Joint Surg Am 2005;87:2113-2121.

14. Thomas MA, Fast A, Shapiro D. Radial nerve damage as a complication of elbow arthroscopy. Clin Orthop 1987;215:130-131.

15. Wright TW, Glowczewskie F Jr, Cowin D, Wheeler DL. Ulnar nerve excursion and strain at the elbow and wrist associated with upper extremity motion. J Hand Surg Am 2001;26:655-662.

35

Arthroscopic Treatment of Lateral Epicondylitis

Christian Lattermann, MD
Anthony A. Romeo, MD
Brian J. Cole, MD, MBA

Lateral epicondylitis is a well-known musculoskeletal phenomenon that can occur after minor trauma or chronic overuse. In general, lateral epicondylitis responds well to nonoperative management, including activity modification, counterforce bracing, physical therapy, and corticosteroid injections. A relatively small number of patients, however, present with refractory symptoms. In those cases, an operative procedure may be warranted. Many different operative techniques have been developed for the treatment of lateral epicondylitis. The goal of this chapter is to describe a more recent technique—arthroscopic extensor carpi radialis brevis (ECRB) release. We believe that this technique is advantageous because it offers direct visualization of the pathologic process, enables the surgeon to concomitantly address intra-articular disease, and is minimally invasive in nature and thus well tolerated by the patient.

Preoperative Considerations

History

Typical History

- Traumatic onset (usually minor trauma) aggravated by repetitive motion
- Insidious onset, chronic repetitive wrist and elbow motion at work or recreationally
- Tenderness directly over the origin of the ECRB on the lateral epicondyle
- Aggravation of symptoms with active resisted wrist extension and passive wrist flexion
- Often previously treated with nonoperative measures
- Pain with range of motion of the elbow and clicking may point to associated joint disease

Physical Examination

Factors Affecting Surgical Indication

- Range of motion: should be normal
- Clicking with range of motion (synovial plica)
- Effusion (intra-articular disease)

Factors Affecting Surgical Planning

- Previous ulnar nerve transposition
- Ulnohumeral or radiocapitellar arthritis
- Previous distal humerus or olecranon fracture

It is important to perform a thorough neurovascular examination to rule out entrapment of the posterior interosseous nerve, subluxation of the ulnar nerve, or degenerative changes in the radiocapitellar joint.

Imaging

Radiography

- Anteroposterior view of the elbow in full extension
- Lateral view of the elbow in 90 degrees of flexion

    Optionally:

- Axial view to outline the olecranon and its articulations
- Radial head view

Other Modalities

- Magnetic resonance imaging with or without the administration of gadolinium

Magnetic resonance imaging will demonstrate degenerative changes in the origin of the ECRB; it may show a synovial plica in the radiocapitellar joint when it is performed with the administration of contrast material. Visualization of loose bodies is generally better with magnetic resonance images than with plain radiographs, which will display loose bodies in only 25% of the cases.

Indications and Contraindications

The ideal patient has localized symptoms directly anterior and inferior to the lateral epicondyle at the origin of the ECRB and has full range of motion. Conservative treatment options have failed.

Contraindications are those generally associated with elbow arthroscopy. These include significant alterations of the normal bone anatomy, previous placement of hardware, ankylosis of the elbow joint, acute or chronic soft tissue infections, and osteomyelitis of the elbow.

Surgical Technique

Anesthesia and Positioning

The patient is placed in either the supine or prone position, according to the surgeon's preference for elbow arthroscopy (we prefer the prone position). The procedure can be performed under general anesthesia or regional block with simple sedation. However, some patients may not tolerate the prone position under sedation alone because of unrelated issues, such as shoulder pain in the ipsilateral or contralateral shoulder.

The patient is positioned prone with the arm hanging over the side in 90 degrees of abduction and neutral rotation (Fig. 36-1). Care needs to be taken that the arm is not abducted more than 90 degrees and that the shoulder is not hyperextended to minimize the risk of neurovascular

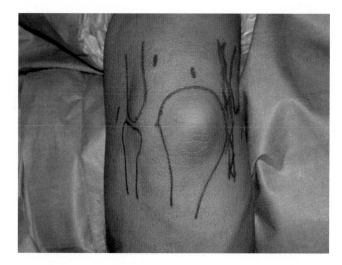

Figure 36-1 Patient in the prone position. Note that the arm is hanging down, thus avoiding hyperextension of the shoulder.

complications. A nonsterile tourniquet is used with inflation pressures between 200 and 250 mm Hg according to the size of the arm and systolic blood pressure. The procedure can be performed with the surgeon either standing or seated, and the operating table is adjusted accordingly.

Surgical Landmarks, Incisions, and Portals

Landmarks

- Tip of olecranon process
- Lateral epicondyle
- Medial epicondyle
- Ulnar nerve (test for subluxation)
- Radial head and radiocapitellar joint

Portals and Approaches

- Insufflation of joint with 30 mL of saline by use of a spinal needle
- Proximal medial viewing portal
- Proximal lateral portal
- Posterior superior portal (optional if there is posterior synovitis)
- Direct lateral (soft spot) portal (optional if there is radial head or capitellar disease)

Structures at Risk

- Proximal medial portal: ulnar nerve
- Proximal lateral portal: lateral antebrachial cutaneous nerve
- Excessive release: lateral ulnar collateral ligament, posterior interosseous nerve

Examination Under Anesthesia and Diagnostic Arthroscopy

Examination under anesthesia should evaluate range of motion and ligamentous stability. Diagnostic arthroscopy is useful to evaluate other intra-articular disease, such as loose bodies, ligamentous deficiency, or chondral defects.

Specific Steps (Box 36-1)

1. Portal Placement

Before any portals are placed, a thorough manual palpation of the olecranon tip, the radiocapitellar joint, the lateral medial epicondyle, and the ulnar nerve is performed. Particular attention is needed to determine whether the patient has ulnar nerve subluxation. The landmarks are marked clearly (Fig. 36-2). A sterile or nonsterile tourniquet is necessary and should be inflated before any portals are placed.

Then 30 mL of saline solution is instilled into the soft spot of the triangle formed between the tip of the olecranon, the lateral epicondyle, and the radial head. Visible distention of the joint and backflow through the injection needle (18-gauge) confirm intra-articular instillation.

Box 36-1 Surgical Steps

1. Portal placement

2. Diagnostic arthroscopy

3. Débridement of ECRB origin and release of ECRB

4. Closure

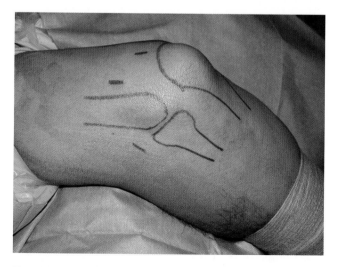

Figure 36-2 The portals and landmarks are clearly marked. The elbow can be accessed freely from medial, lateral, and posterior.

To establish the proximal medial viewing portal, the medial epicondyle and the medial intermuscular septum are directly palpated. At approximately 2 cm proximal to the medial epicondyle and 1 cm anterior to the medial intermuscular septum, a small skin incision is made with a No. 15 blade. A small hemostat is used to spread carefully down to the capsule, thus avoiding injury to the cutaneous sensory nerves. With the elbow maintained in 90 degrees of flexion and neutral rotation, the cannula with a blunt trocar is then introduced by sliding along the anterior surface of the distal humerus, aiming toward the radiocapitellar joint. Subsequently, the proximal lateral portal is established approximately 2 cm proximal and 2 cm anterior to the lateral epicondyle. The correct position of the portal is verified under direct vision by use of a spinal needle. Once the position is verified, the "nick and spread" technique is again used, and a blunt Wissinger rod is positioned to serve as a guide for a small 5-mm threaded arthroscopic cannula. An additional superior lateral portal can be helpful if the anterior capsule is capacious. A small key elevator can be inserted through this accessory portal and used to elevate the anterolateral capsule, greatly enhancing visualization from the medial portal.

2. Diagnostic Arthroscopy

A routine diagnostic arthroscopy is performed. If any pathologic process is suspected in the ulnohumeral joint, a posterior portal is established to evaluate the ulnar and radial recesses. The radiocapitellar joint is evaluated for, among other entities, a soft tissue band or plica overriding the radius with pronation and supination, because this can be a cause of impingement. The lateral joint capsule and the insertion of the ECRB are assessed under direct vision. We prefer to grade ECRB involvement according to the grading suggested by Baker et al.[1]

3. Débridement of ECRB Origin and Release of ECRB

A thorough appreciation of the anatomy of the elbow, and of the ECRB in particular, is paramount to mastering this arthroscopic technique. The ECRB origin is extra-articular, thus requiring the resection of the capsule adjacent to the capitellum to visualize the ECRB origin. We prefer to perform the resection sequentially in four steps, resulting in a diamond-shaped resection zone (Fig. 36-3).[2,7]

Step1: To visualize the ECRB, the overlying anterolateral capsule has to be removed, although in some patients, the capsule will already be torn, revealing the origin. The margins of the resection extend superiorly from the top of the capitellum to distally at the level of the midline of the radiocapitellar joint. If the resection extends farther distal than the midline of the radiocapitellar joint, the lateral collateral ligament is at risk.

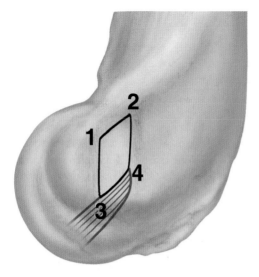

Figure 36-3 A diamond-shaped resection zone on the lateral epicondyle is débrided to perform a full resection of the ECRB origin. The lateral border is taken down to but not into the lateral collateral ligament. Steps 1 to 4 mark the sequence of the débridement zone.

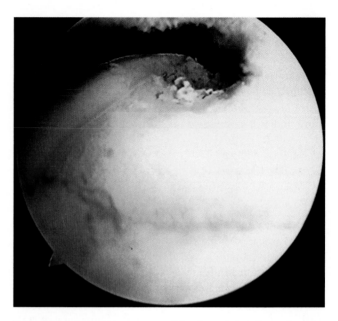

Figure 36-4 Arthroscopic appearance of the diamond-shaped resection zone after débridement.

Step 2: After adequate exposure has been obtained, we now turn our attention to resection of the ECRB origin. We start at the superior aspect of the capitellum, which represents the proximal and anterior margin of the resection. In a probing motion using a monopolar or bipolar radiofrequency probe, we resect the tendinous bands that represent the ECRB origin until we expose the red muscle fibers of the extensor carpi radialis longus.

Step 3: We then continue the resection anteroinferiorly. The posteroinferior border of the resection is marked by the lateral collateral ligament. One has to be careful to visualize the lateral collateral ligament. This is often easier once the semicircular fibers that cross from the lateral collateral to the annular radial ligament are visualized. Gravity inflow or the pump pressure can help with joint distention that separates the tendon from the lateral collateral ligament. The resection is performed under direct vision with the scope in the anteromedial portal (Fig. 36-4).

Step 4: The posterior aspect of the diamond-shaped resection zone is formed by the tendon of the extensor digitorum communis. The resection is carried up to the extensor digitorum communis tendon but not past it. There is a distinct fibrous band curving over top of the ECRB that constitutes the extensor aponeurosis. This band must not be cut because this could result in a subcutaneous fistula. The final portion of this step includes a decortication of the diamond-shaped débridement zone to create a biologic healing response. The capsule is not repaired.

4. Closure

Standard closure of the portals is performed.

Postoperative Considerations

Rehabilitation

- Sling for comfort
- Finger, wrist, and elbow motion as tolerated
- No lifting or gripping activities until follow-up (7 to 10 days)
- Continue with range-of-motion and very light gripping exercises at 10 days
- No resistive exercises until after 3 or 4 weeks, if pain free
- Full use of the arm without restrictions at 6 to 12 weeks

Complications

Complications are those of elbow arthroscopy:

- Ulnar or lateral antebrachial cutaneous nerve damage due to portal placement
- Posterior interosseous nerve or collateral ligament damage due to excessive release
- Infection
- Synovial fistula

Table 36-1 Clinical Results of Arthroscopic Treatment of Lateral Epicondylitis

Author	Follow-up	Outcome
Baker et al[1] (2000)	2.8 years	42 patients VAS: 0.9/10 for pain Grip strength: 96% Return to work at 2.2 weeks
Peart et al[6] (2004)	2 years	33 patients treated arthroscopically 72% good and excellent results compared with 69% by open treatment Earlier return to work for arthroscopically treated patients
Owens et al[5] (2001)	2 years	16 patients VAS: 0.59/10 for pain Average return to work at 6 days

VAS, visual analogue scale.

PEARLS AND PITFALLS

Visualization

- In case of a capacious anterior capsule that tends to obstruct viewing from the medial portal, a small key elevator can be inserted through a high anterolateral accessory portal to elevate the anterolateral capsule, greatly enhancing visualization from the medial portal.

Débridement

- The resection of the capsule and the ECRB should not extend farther distal than the midline of the radiocapitellar joint. Resection past this landmark puts the lateral collateral ligament at risk.

- Once the débridement of the ECRB has been performed, do not débride the extensor digitorum communis. Débridement of the extensor digitorum communis and extensor aponeurosis can result in a synovial fistula.

Results

After débridement for lateral epicondylitis, good to excellent results are achieved in 85% to 90% of cases. The results of arthroscopic débridement are certainly comparable, and the arthroscopic approach has the additional benefit of being able to address concomitant disease that does exist in approximately 30% of cases.[1,3,4] Patients often are immediately pain free and can return to work between 1 and 3 weeks, depending on their physical category of work (Table 36-1).

References

1. Baker CL Jr, Murphy KP, Gottlob CA, Curd DT. Arthroscopic classification and treatment of lateral epicondylitis: two-year clinical results. J Shoulder Elbow Surg 2000;9:475-482.
2. Cohen M, Romeo AA. Lateral epicondylitis: open and arthroscopic treatment. J Am Soc Surg Hand 2001;3:172-176.
3. Kuklo TR, Taylor KF, Murphy KP, et al. Arthroscopic release for lateral epicondylitis: a cadaveric model. Arthroscopy 1999;15:259-264.
4. Mullett H, Sprague M, Brown G, Hausman M. Arthroscopic treatment of lateral epicondylitis: clinical and cadaveric studies. Clin Orthop 2005;439:123-128.
5. Owens BD, Murphy KP, Kuklo TR. Arthroscopic release for lateral epicondylitis. Arthroscopy 2001;17:582-587.
6. Peart RE, Strickler SS, Schweitzer KM Jr. Lateral epicondylitis: a comparative study of open and arthroscopic lateral release. Am J Orthop 2004;33:565-567.
7. Romeo AA, Fox JA. Arthroscopic treatment of lateral epicondylitis—the 4-step technique. Available at: www.orthopedictechreview.com/issues/sepoct02/pg26.htm.

36

Ulnar Collateral Ligament Reconstruction

Champ L. Baker, Jr., MD
Champ L. Baker III, MD

Injury to the medial side of the elbow is common in overhead athletes, such as baseball pitchers, tennis players, and javelin throwers. The overhead throwing motion places a tremendous amount of valgus stress on the elbow that is resisted by the medial structures. The anterior bundle of the ulnar collateral ligament (UCL) has been demonstrated to be the primary restraint to valgus stress about the elbow.[6] Repeated high valgus stresses imparted from the repetitive act of throwing can result in chronic attenuation or acute rupture of the UCL. In the throwing athlete, UCL insufficiency can be manifested as disabling elbow pain with the inability to compete effectively. Since the first description of UCL reconstruction in the landmark work of Jobe et al,[8] there have been several modifications to the original technique. These modifications have attempted to reduce the amount of soft tissue dissection and the incidence of ulnar nerve complications and to provide more consistent and secure fixation. Constants in all described techniques include accurate diagnosis, appropriate selection of patients, anatomic reconstruction of the anterior bundle of the UCL, and maintenance of a specific rehabilitation program to allow the athlete to return successfully to sport.

Preoperative Considerations

History

The typical history in a throwing athlete with UCL injury is episodic medial elbow pain that prevents him or her from competing effectively. Pain is usually elicited in the early acceleration phase of throwing. Affected pitchers complain of loss of velocity or accuracy. On occasion, the athlete will sustain an acute injury with sudden onset of medial pain accompanied by a "pop" followed by an inability to continue throwing. Symptoms of ulnar nerve irritability, such as paresthesias, in the little and ring fingers may also be present.

Physical Examination

A thorough physical examination of the throwing athlete includes the following:

- Evaluation of the neck and entire upper extremity
- Direct assessment of the ulnar nerve for subluxation, irritability (presence of Tinel sign), and integrity of distal motor and sensory function in the hand
- Tenderness may be elicited over the UCL ligament slightly distal and posterior to the flexor-pronator muscle origin.

Several tests have been described to evaluate the integrity of the UCL:

- Manual valgus stress test performed at 30 degrees of elbow flexion
- "Milking maneuver"[16]
- Moving valgus stress test[10]

These tests may elicit medial elbow pain with valgus stress, or the examiner may appreciate medial joint line opening with stress especially in comparison with the contralateral elbow. Consideration of concurrent posteromedial impingement in the thrower's elbow can be evaluated with the valgus extension overload test.[2] If reconstruction of the UCL is considered, the presence of an ipsilateral or contralateral palmaris longus should be assessed.

Imaging

Radiography

- Anteroposterior, lateral, and axial views of the elbow

Plain radiographs are inspected for loose bodies, evidence of degenerative changes such as posteromedial osteophytes of the olecranon, medial joint line spurring, and possible calcifications in the UCL indicative of a chronic injury.

Other Modalities

- Computed tomographic arthrography
- Magnetic resonance imaging

The senior author prefers magnetic resonance imaging as the imaging modality of choice for detailed characterization of the integrity of the UCL and evaluation of other soft tissue structures (Fig. 37-1).

Indications and Contraindications

The indication for UCL reconstruction in a throwing athlete is medial elbow pain associated with UCL insuffi-

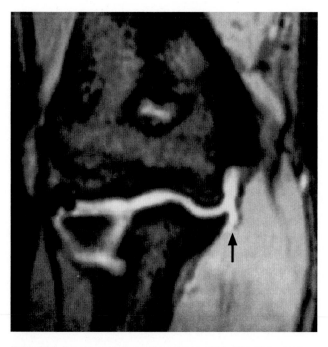

Figure 37-1 Coronal magnetic resonance image of this right elbow shows disruption of the ulnar collateral ligament (arrow).

ciency that prevents the athlete from competing effectively. Nonoperative treatment for elite throwing athletes is usually unsuccessful.[12] Athletes who do not plan on returning to sport and those who are able to return to sport after rehabilitation and do not subject their elbows to repeated valgus stress are not generally considered candidates for reconstruction.[4]

Surgical Planning

Concomitant procedures include ulnar nerve transposition based on preoperative symptoms suggestive of nerve irritability or subluxation. Findings of loose bodies, spurs, and posteromedial impingement can be addressed either arthroscopically or through an arthrotomy at the time of the reconstruction.

The initial graft choice is an ipsilateral palmaris longus tendon. If the tendon is not present in the patient, other choices are the contralateral palmaris longus tendon if it is present, gracilis or semitendinosus tendons, toe extensor, and allograft.

Surgical Technique

Anesthesia and Positioning

We prefer to perform the procedure under axillary block anesthesia, although on the basis of the surgeon's, patient's, and anesthesiologist's preferences, general anesthesia or a combination of general and regional anesthesia can be used. The patient is placed supine on the operating table with the affected extremity abducted and placed on an attached hand table. A sterile or nonsterile pneumatic tourniquet is placed about the arm as proximal as possible for exposure. The arm is then prepared and draped in the usual sterile fashion.

Specific Steps (Box 37-1)

1. Exposure

The limb is exsanguinated, and the tourniquet is inflated. The medial epicondyle is identified, and an approximately 8- to 10-cm curvilinear incision is made centered over the medial epicondyle. During the exposure, care is taken to identify and to protect the branches of the medial antebrachial cutaneous nerve that cross the operative field. Injury to these nerves can result in either sensory loss along the medial aspect of the forearm or a painful neuroma. Dissection is carried down to the level of the forearm fascia and the flexor-pronator aponeurosis

Box 37-1 Surgical Steps

1. Exposure

2. Harvest of palmaris longus graft

3. Preparation of ulnar tunnels

4. Preparation of humeral tunnels

5. Passage and tensioning of the graft

6. Closure

37

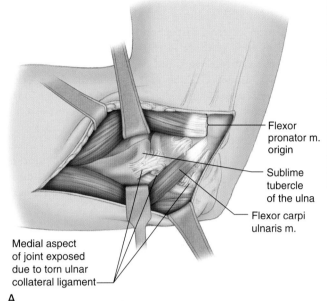

Flexor pronator m. origin

Sublime tubercle of the ulna

Flexor carpi ulnaris m.

Medial aspect of joint exposed due to torn ulnar collateral ligament

A

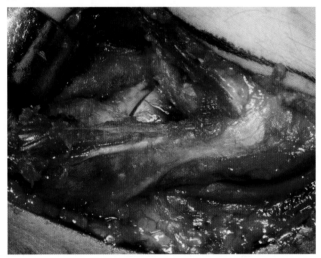

B

Figure 37-3 Drawing **(A)** and photograph **(B)** show approach to the ulnar collateral ligament. Application of valgus stress demonstrates medial joint line opening.

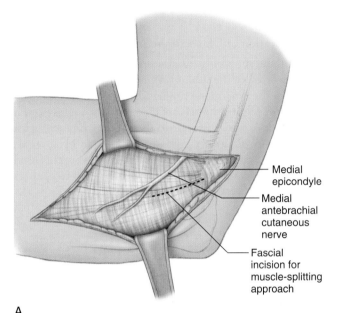

Medial epicondyle

Medial antebrachial cutaneous nerve

Fascial incision for muscle-splitting approach

A

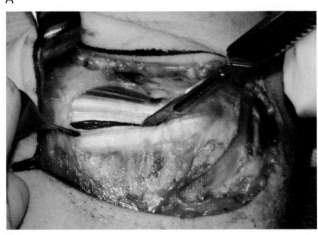

B

Figure 37-2 Drawing **(A)** and photograph **(B)** show muscle-splitting incision through fascia to expose the ulnar collateral ligament.

(Fig. 37-2). We prefer the muscle-splitting approach[14] for exposure of the UCL. A fascial raphe can usually be identified in the flexor-pronator mass at the junction of the anterior two thirds and posterior third of the muscle group. This raphe represents an internervous plane between the median nerve–innervated palmaris longus and deeper flexor digitorum superficialis and the ulnar nerve–innervated flexor carpi ulnaris. The fascia is split through the raphe from the medial epicondyle to a point approximately 1 cm distal to the sublime tubercle. The sublime tubercle can be palpated deep under the flexor mass. More distal dissection risks denervation of the surrounding musculature from crossing nerve branches. The muscle is then bluntly divided down to the level of the underlying UCL (Fig. 37-3). Care is taken during the split and division of the muscle because the ulnar nerve lies just posterior to the approach. A blunt self-retainer is used to retract the musculature, and a small periosteal elevator can be used to clean any remaining muscle fibers from the

UCL. Application of a valgus stress should reveal excessive medial joint line opening consistent with UCL insufficiency. After external inspection of the ligament, a longitudinal incision is made in the direction of its fibers to assess undersurface tears and degeneration. As much of the native, intact UCL is preserved as possible. Also through this incision, the joint can be inspected for loose bodies and other intra-articular disease.

2. Graft Harvest

If it is present, the ipsilateral palmaris longus tendon is harvested as the preferred graft (Fig. 37-4). The tendon is identified at the level of the proximal wrist flexion crease

as it inserts into the palmar fascia. A small 1- to 2-cm transverse incision is made directly over the tendon. A small hemostat is used to dissect the tendon, with care taken to protect the underlying median nerve. Tension is applied to the tendon with the hemostat, and two additional transverse incisions are made proximally over the tendon and myotendinous junction approximately 8 cm apart. The tendon graft is then incised proximally and distally and delivered out of the wound (Fig. 37-5). Ideally, the graft length is 12 to 15 cm. The graft is cleaned of muscle, and a running whipstitch is placed in both ends of the graft with No. 2 FiberWire (Arthrex, Inc., Naples, Fla).

3. Preparation of Ulnar Tunnels

With careful subperiosteal dissection, the medial aspect of the ulna distal to the sublime tubercle is exposed in preparation for the ulnar bone tunnels. By use of a 3.2-mm drill bit, two converging tunnels are made at right angles to each other anterior and posterior to the sublime tubercle, with care taken to maintain a good bone bridge of approximately 6 to 8 mm (Fig. 37-6). A small curved curet is used to clean the tunnel entrance of bone debris and to connect the tunnels.

4. Preparation of Humeral Tunnels

The insertion of the UCL is traced back to its origin on the medial epicondyle. The insertion is located on the anteroinferior surface of the epicondyle, usually in the middle two thirds of the epicondyle in the coronal plane.[9] A 3.2-mm drill bit is used to make a bone tunnel starting at the insertion and through the back of the medial epicondyle (Fig. 37-7). The ulnar nerve is carefully protected during this portion to avoid iatrogenic injury from the drill. Next, a minimal release is performed to allow safe retraction of the nerve. The proximal portion of the epicondyle anterior to the medial intermuscular septum is

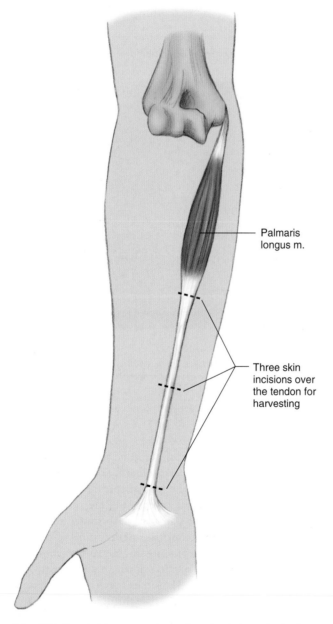

Figure 37-4 Three incisions are made over the palmaris longus tendon in preparation for harvesting of the graft.

Palmaris longus m.

Three skin incisions over the tendon for harvesting

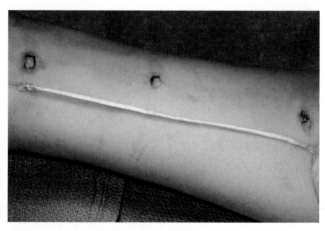

Figure 37-5 The graft is prepared by placement of a running whipstitch in both ends of the harvested palmaris longus tendon.

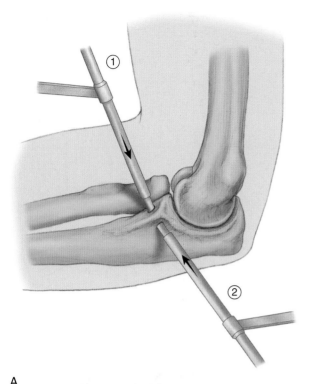

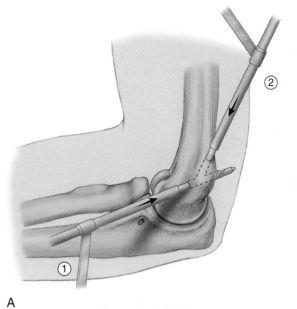

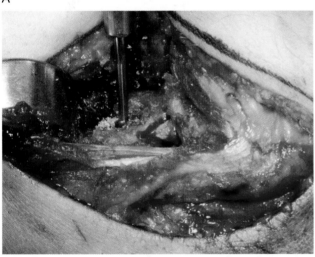

A

B

Figure 37-6 Drawing **(A)** and photograph **(B)** show placement of convergent drill holes in the ulna anterior and posterior to the sublime tubercle to develop the tunnel for the graft. (Note: labels 1 and 2 adjacent to drill bits indicate order in which holes are made to develop the tunnel.)

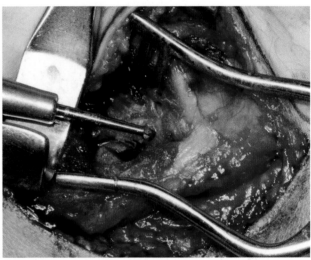

A

B

Figure 37-7 Drawing **(A)** and photograph **(B)** show placement of divergent drill holes in the medial epicondyle of the humerus to develop a tunnel for the graft. (Note: labels 1 and 2 adjacent to drill bits indicate order in which tunnels are made.)

then carefully exposed subperiostally. A 3.2-mm drill bit is used to make a second bone tunnel starting anterior to the medial intermuscular septum and aiming distally to approximately the middle portion of the previously drilled tunnel. Care is taken to maintain an adequate bone bridge of at least 5 mm between the tunnels and the trochlear articular surface. A small curved curet is then used to clean the tunnels of bone debris.

5. Passage and Tensioning of the Graft

The prepared graft is then passed from anterior to posterior in the ulnar tunnel with the help of a Hewson suture passer (Fig. 37-8). The graft is passed through the humeral tunnels in a figure-of-eight fashion with a three-ply reconstruction (Fig. 37-9). The elbow joint is then reduced with the application of a varus stress, and the elbow is flexed to approximately 45 degrees as tension is applied across the graft. The graft is then sutured to itself with No. 2 Fiber-Wire in a mattress fashion (Fig. 37-10). The native UCL is also sutured to itself and to the graft to reinforce the reconstruction.

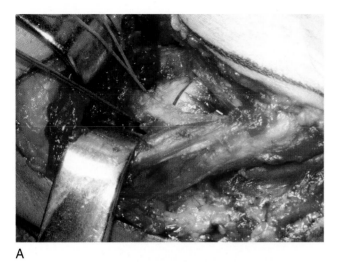

A

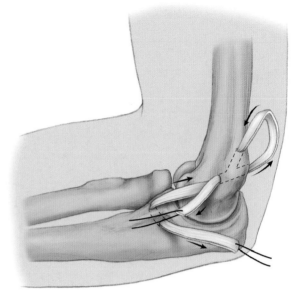

Figure 37-9 One limb of graft is passed through humeral tunnels to form figure-of-eight.

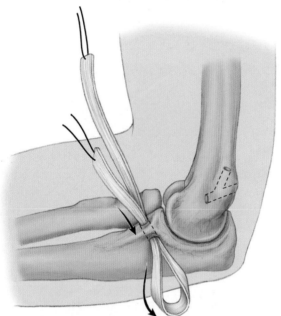

B

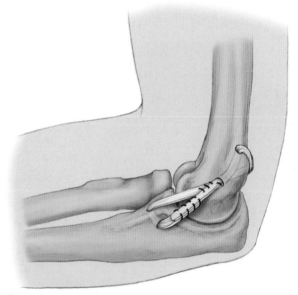

A

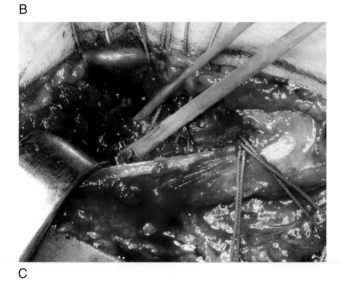

C

Figure 37-8 A, Photograph shows passage of graft through ulnar tunnel. **B,** Drawing shows sutures pulling one limb of graft through ulnar tunnel. **C,** Photograph shows passage of both limbs through tunnel.

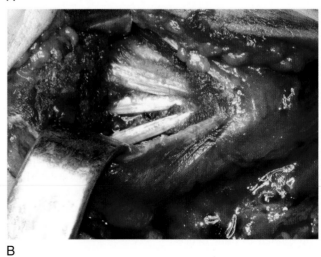

B

Figure 37-10 Drawing **(A)** and photograph **(B)** show both limbs of the graft sutured together and reinforced with whipstitches.

6. Closure

The tourniquet is deflated, and meticulous hemostasis is obtained to prevent a postoperative hematoma. The wound is thoroughly irrigated before closure. The flexor-pronator mass is closed with No. 0 Vicryl suture, followed by routine skin closure. A sterile dressing is applied, and the arm is splinted in approximately 90 degrees of flexion with the forearm in neutral rotation.

Postoperative Considerations

Follow-up

One week after surgery, the sutures are removed and a hinged elbow brace is applied.

Rehabilitation

A specific rehabilitation protocol is crucial to successful return to athletic competition.

- Motion is initially allowed only from 45 to 90 degrees and is gradually progressed in the brace so that full motion is obtained at approximately 6 weeks after surgery.
- Physical therapy is begun at 6 weeks with gradual strengthening of the shoulder and forearm musculature and correction of any losses of motion. Begin manual resisted exercises. Internal rotation exercises below shoulder level may begin.
- The brace is removed at 6 weeks after surgery, and wrist, elbow, and shoulder exercises are begun.
- At approximately 12 weeks, increased strength training is begun with a sport-specific rehabilitation program.
- Week 14: Begin modified throwing program on knees. Additional activities and exercises can be added.
- Weeks 15-28: For throwers, return to activity is initiated at approximately 15 weeks after surgery. Emphasis is placed on warm-up and a conditioning program. Phase 1 consists of an interval throwing program that is gradually progressed through week 28. The program begins with throws of 45 feet and progresses to long tossing up to 180 feet. Athletes throw every other day, with progress to the next phase allowed if they are free of pain. Pitchers perform the long-toss program to 120 feet before beginning interval throwing from off the mound. At week 28, pitchers can throw from the mound. Throwers ultimately return to competitive play at approximately week 52 or at the completion of their throwing program.

Complications

- Ulnar nerve irritation is the most common postoperative complication with a reported incidence of up to 21%.[7]
- Trauma to the medial antebrachial cutaneous nerve
- Hematoma
- Superficial or deep infection
- Fracture of the humeral or ulnar tunnels from an insufficient bone bridge

PEARLS AND PITFALLS

Pearls

- The primary indication for surgery is the patient's inability to throw without pain after rehabilitation. The decision for surgical treatment is not based on magnetic resonance imaging findings. The moving valgus stress test and the milking test are good prognosticators of injury to the ulnar collateral ligament.
- If the examination reveals pain in the posterior compartment as it comes into terminal extension, the posterior osteophyte should be addressed.
- The native ulnar collateral ligament should be repaired to itself first before the transferred tendon is sewn into the ligament to prevent extravasation of fluid from the joint and irritation of the tendon with flexion and extension.
- In the absence of preoperative ulnar nerve symptoms, transfer of the nerve is not necessary. However, it should be identified during dissection so that it can be retracted during drilling of the humeral epicondyle.

Pitfalls

- In drilling the holes for the sublime tubercle of the ulna, take care to maintain a significant bone bridge to prevent fracture. When the curet is used, do not elevate it anteriorly because it could fracture the bone.
- To avoid compressing the ulnar nerve when the flexor muscle tendon split is performed, do not use a retractor against the bone inferiorly.
- The final repair should be performed with the elbow flexed, supinated, and in varus to ensure tightness of the transferred tendon.
- During rehabilitation, the patient should be warned to avoid excessive valgus loading for 4 months after surgery.

Results

The results of UCL reconstruction are best measured by the athlete's return to sport. Successful return to elite throwing is a far more stringent outcome measure than is objective testing of valgus laxity.[13] Since the original description of the technique by Jobe, there have been several modifications to the technique to attempt to decrease morbidity and postoperative complications while allowing the athlete to safely return to sport (Table 37-1).

Table 37-1 Results of Ulnar Collateral Ligament Reconstruction

Author	Technique	Results
Jobe et al[8] (1986)	Original "Tommy John" method Flexor-pronator mass detached Figure-of-eight graft Submuscular ulnar nerve transposition	10/16 (63%) throwing athletes returned to same level
Conway et al[7] (1992)	Original method Flexor-pronator mass detached Figure-of-eight graft Submuscular ulnar nerve transposition	38/56 (68%) athletes returned to same level 12/56 (21%) postoperative ulnar nerve irritability Reconstruction better than repair
Azar et al[3] (2000)	Andrews modification of original Jobe technique Flexor mass divided with partial detachment of flexor carpi ulnaris Figure-of-eight graft Subcutaneous ulnar nerve transposition	78 UCL reconstructions; 41% professional 79% of athletes returned to same or higher level Average return: 9.8 months
Thompson et al[15] (2001)	Modified Jobe technique Muscle-splitting approach Figure-of-eight graft No ulnar nerve transposition	83 UCL reconstructions; 65% professional 100% of athletes returned to sport 82% returned to same or higher level 5% transient ulnar nerve irritability
Rohrbough et al[13] (2002)	Docking procedure modification Routine arthroscopic assessment Muscle-splitting approach Two tendon ends of graft docked into single humeral tunnel Selective subcutaneous ulnar nerve transposition	36 UCL reconstructions 33/36 (92%) returned to same or higher level Average 3.3-year follow-up
Cain et al[5] (2002)	Andrews modification of original Jobe technique	342 UCL reconstructions with minimum 2-year follow-up 96% baseball players; 45% professional, 45% collegiate, 10% high-school 83% returned to same or higher level Average return: 11.4 months
Paletta and Wright[11] (2002)	Docking procedure 4-strand technique reconstruction	25 UCL reconstructions in professional or collegiate throwing athletes; 2-year minimum follow-up 23/25 (92%) returned to same or higher level Average return: 12.5 months

Current techniques allow the competitive throwing athlete to return successfully to the same or higher level of sport approximately 79% to 92% of the time. Successful return also depends on completion of a dedicated prolonged rehabilitation protocol. Continued advances in technology, such as interference screw fixation[1] and hybrid techniques, may allow an even greater chance of success in the future, but clinical validation is pending.

References

1. Ahmad CS, Lee TQ, ElAttrache NS. Biomechanical evaluation of a new ulnar collateral ligament reconstruction technique with interference screw fixation. Am J Sports Med 2003;31:332-337.
2. Andrews JR, Whiteside JA, Buettner CM. Clinical evaluation of the elbow in throwers. Oper Tech Sports Med 1996;4:77-83.
3. Azar FM, Andrews JR, Wilk KE, Groh D. Operative treatment of ulnar collateral ligament injuries of the elbow in athletes. Am J Sports Med 2000;28:16-23.
4. Breazeale NM, Altchek DW. Ulnar collateral ligament injuries. In Baker CL, Plancher KD, eds. Operative Treatment of Elbow Injuries. New York, Springer-Verlag, 2002:89-100.

5. Cain EL, Andrews JR, Dugas JR, et al. Outcome of ulnar collateral ligament reconstruction of the elbow: minimum two-year follow-up. Transactions of the annual meeting of the American Orthopaedic Society for Sports Medicine, 2002:173.

6. Callaway GH, Field LD, Deng XH, et al. Biomechanical evaluation of the medial collateral ligament of the elbow. J Bone Joint Surg Am 1997;79:1223-1231.

7. Conway JE, Jobe FW, Glousman RE, Pink M. Medial instability of the elbow in throwing athletes: treatment by repair or reconstruction of the ulnar collateral ligament. J Bone Joint Surg Am 1992; 74:67-83.

8. Jobe FW, Stark H, Lombardo SJ. Reconstruction of the ulnar collateral ligament in athletes. J Bone Joint Surg Am 1986;68:1158-1163.

9. O'Driscoll SW, Jaloszynski R, Morrey BF, An KN. Origin of the medial ulnar collateral ligament. J Hand Surg Am 1992;17:164-168.

10. O'Driscoll SW, Lawton RL, Smith AM. The "moving valgus stress test" for medial collateral ligament tears of the elbow. Am J Sports Med 2005;33:231-239.

11. Paletta GA Jr, Wright RW. The docking procedure of elbow MCL reconstruction: two year follow up in elite throwers. Transactions of the annual meeting of the American Orthopaedic Society for Sports Medicine, 2002:172.

12. Rettig AC, Sherrill C, Snead DS, et al. Nonoperative treatment of ulnar collateral ligament injuries in throwing athletes. Am J Sports Med 2001;29:15-17.

13. Rohrbough JT, Altchek DW, Hyman J, et al. Medial collateral ligament reconstruction of the elbow using the docking technique. Am J Sports Med 2002;30:541-548.

14. Smith GR, Altchek DW, Pagnani MJ, Keeley JR. A muscle splitting approach to the ulnar collateral ligament of the elbow: neuroanatomy and operative technique. Am J Sports Med 1996;24:575-580.

15. Thompson WH, Jobe FW, Yocum LA, Pink M. Ulnar collateral ligament reconstruction in athletes: muscle splitting approach without transposition of the ulnar nerve. J Shoulder Elbow Surg 2001; 10:152-157.

16. Veltri DM, O'Brien SJ, Field LD, et al. The milking maneuver: a new test to evaluate the MCL of the elbow in the throwing athlete. J Shoulder Elbow Surg 1995;4:S10, 22.

37

CHAPTER 38

Surgical Treatment of Posterolateral Instability of the Elbow

Eric Rightmire, MD

Marc Safran, MD

Although the term *posterolateral rotatory instability* was coined by and credited to O'Driscoll on the basis of his publication in 1991,[10] it was probably first described in 1966 by Osborne and Cotterill.[14] Elbow stability is maintained by bone anatomy as well as by the ligamentous attachments and balanced muscle forces. The integrity of the bone structures as well as of the medial and lateral ligamentous complexes is essential to elbow stability.

The ulnohumeral, radiohumeral, and radioulnar joints are the three articulations that compose the bone anatomy of the elbow joint. Each contributes to the stability of the elbow, which is one of the most stable, constrained joints in the body. The lateral and medial sides of the elbow have distinct ligamentous complexes. The medial or ulnar collateral ligament complex has three components: the anterior oblique ligament, also known as the anterior bundle; the posterior oblique ligament, also known as the posterior bundle; and the transverse ligament, also known as Cooper ligament. The anterior oblique ligament is functionally subdivided into anterior and posterior bands; it is widely considered to be the primary restraint to valgus stress. The lateral or radial side, known as the lateral collateral ligament complex, has four components: the lateral (or radial) ulnar collateral ligament, the radial collateral ligament, the annular ligament, and the accessory lateral collateral ligament. Deficiency of the lateral ulnar collateral ligament (LUCL) is widely believed to be the primary component in posterolateral rotatory instability as demonstrated by O'Driscoll.[11] Studies have questioned whether the LUCL is the essential lesion in posterolateral rotatory instability or if injuries to the radial

collateral ligament and lateral capsule also contribute.[3] The lateral ligamentous injury that results in posterolateral rotatory instability usually occurs at the lateral epicondyle with at least some degree of tearing of the remainder of the lateral collateral ligament complex (namely, the radial collateral ligament). Furthermore, some cadaveric studies have been unable to produce posterolateral rotatory instability when the LUCL alone is cut.[18]

The LUCL attaches proximally to the lateral epicondyle of the humerus and distally to the tubercle of the supinator crest of the ulna. The humeral attachment is the isometric point on the lateral side of the elbow. The distal attachment is a broad fan-shaped thickening of the capsule that blends with and arches superficial and distal to the annular ligament to insert onto the ulna.[2] Besides acting as a stabilizer to varus stress of the elbow, it also serves as a posterior buttress to prevent posterior subluxation of the radial head. Posterolateral rotatory instability is defined as posterior radial head subluxation relative to the humerus while the normal proximal radioulnar relationship is maintained.

Preoperative Considerations

History

Patients present with symptoms of pain, locking, snapping, clicking, or recurrent instability usually preceded by trauma to the elbow (50% to 75%) or, less commonly, a history of previous elbow surgery.[4] A history of elbow dislocation is common, although some present with recurrent elbow sprains. Ligamentous laxity and childhood elbow fracture with a resultant cubitus varus deformity have also been reported to be predisposing factors.[12]

Disruption of the lateral ligaments with resultant posterolateral rotatory instability can occur iatrogenically from lateral elbow surgical approaches and arthroscopic elbow procedures. In the case of traumatic injury, the mechanism usually involves axial compression, hyperextension, and external rotation (supination) of the elbow (Fig. 38-1). Direct varus stress injuries are a less common cause. In general, injury to the lateral ligamentous structures is considered the initial stage in a continuum of instability[12] (Fig. 38-2). This begins with injury to the LUCL followed by injury to the entire lateral collateral ligament complex, the anterior and posterior capsule, and finally the posterior and anterior bands of the ulnar collateral ligament complex, leading to frank dislocation. O'Driscoll has also shown, however, that frank dislocation can occur before rupture of the ulnar collateral ligament.

Physical Examination

Clinical examination is usually unremarkable except for the posterolateral rotatory instability test (lateral pivot shift test), which is easiest to perform with the patient in a supine position (Fig. 38-3). With the shoulder forward elevated, the forearm is placed in full supination and extension. The elbow is then gently flexed while the examiner

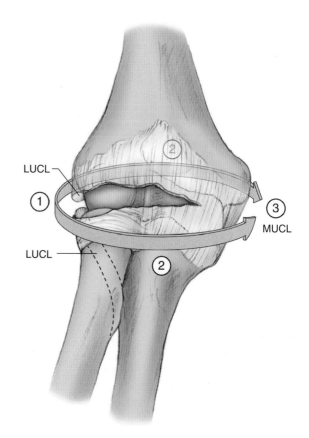

Figure 38-2 Continuum of instability.

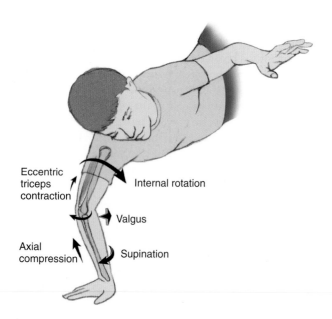

Figure 38-1 Axial compression, hyperextension, and external rotation (supination) mechanism of injury.

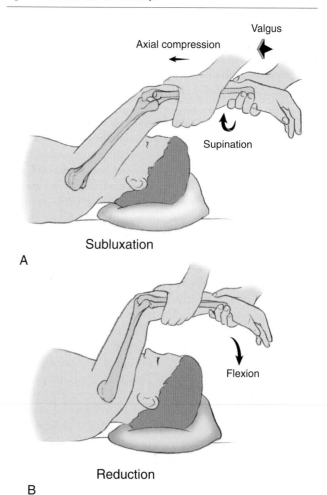

A

B

Figure 38-3 Posterolateral rotatory instability test.

applies a slight valgus force and axial load. The radial head is subluxated in this starting position. A rotatory subluxation of the ulnohumeral joint with posterior subluxation of the radial head can be palpated as a posterior prominence and dimple in the skin just proximal to the radial head. With further flexion beyond 40 degrees, the radial head spontaneously reduces with a "clunk" as the triceps becomes taut, reproducing the patient's symptoms and apprehension. With more significant injury and laxity, the clunk of reduction occurs in greater degrees of elbow flexion. This may be difficult to do in an awake patient, and thus guarding and apprehension alone are suggestive of a positive test result. Because of guarding, demonstration of the pivot shift may require local (intra-articular) or general anesthesia or fluoroscopy.

Other tests are the posterolateral drawer test, the prone pushup test, and the armchair pushup test.[16] The posterolateral drawer test is analogous to the rotatory version of the drawer or Lachman test of the knee. The prone pushup test is performed by asking the patient to attempt to push up from a prone position, first with the forearms maximally pronated and the thumbs pointed toward each other and then with the thumbs pointed outward and the forearms maximally supinated. The test result is positive if symptoms occur when the forearms are supinated but not when they are pronated. The chair pushup is performed by asking the patient to stand from a sitting position by pushing off of a chair with the hands grasping the armrests with palms facing inward (forearm supination). Pain on this maneuver is a positive test result. Reproducible symptoms of pain during the prone and chair pushup tests are positive results for posterolateral rotatory instability.

When a patient with chronic posterolateral rotatory instability is examined, evaluation for the presence of a palmaris longus tendon in either forearm or both forearms is important to determine whether the patient has this potential graft source.

Imaging

Although posterolateral rotatory instability is primarily a clinical diagnosis, radiologic evaluation can be helpful. Studies include the posterolateral rotatory instability pivot shift test with fluoroscopic control or with stress radiographs to demonstrate radial head subluxation and ulnohumeral joint widening. Plain films can show bone avulsions or subtle signs of subluxation. Magnetic resonance imaging has been shown to be useful in identifying components of the lateral collateral complex with the appropriate thin-cut pulse sequences and an experienced radiology staff.[15] Arthroscopy is a useful adjunct to help identify radial head subluxation or lateral joint widening with stress testing and to assess any intra-articular disease.

Indications and Contraindications

Acute injuries after an initial subluxation or dislocation event are best treated nonsurgically with a splint or brace, keeping the forearm in pronation to allow the lateral ligaments to heal. However, if a bone avulsion exists, primary surgical repair may provide good results and prevent chronic disability. Chronic injuries do not respond well to conservative therapy and usually require surgery. Surgery is indicated for patients with the symptoms stated before, including recurrent instability of the elbow and evidence of posterolateral rotatory instability. Braces for chronic injuries are usually cumbersome and not well tolerated by the patients. Prolonged bracing can result in stiffness.

Relative contraindications to surgery are open physes, elbow arthritis, generalized ligamentous laxity, and voluntary dislocators. No absolute contraindications exist.

Surgical Technique

General anesthesia with the patient in the supine position is preferred.

Examination under anesthesia is carried out to include medial and lateral stability testing and posterolateral rotatory stability testing. The upper extremity is prepared and draped in the usual fashion, and a sterile tourniquet is applied to the upper arm. The graft of choice is the palmaris longus, with ipsilateral being the first choice and contralateral the second. If no palmaris longus is present, a lower extremity is prepared and draped for semitendinosus harvesting. Also, an allograft can be used.

Specific Steps (Box 38-1)

An 8- to 10-cm lateral (Kocher) incision is made beginning approximately 3 cm proximal to the lateral epicondyle and

Box 38-1 Surgical Steps

1. Lateral (Kocher) incision 3 cm proximal to the lateral epicondyle and extending over the lateral epicondyle and along the anterior border of the anconeus distally

2. Primary repair: reattachment of the intact ligament to the inferior posterior portion of the lateral epicondyle

3. Reconstruction of the deficient LUCL with a free ligamentous autograft

4. Tensioning and suturing of the graft

5. Plication of the capsule over the graft

6. Final tensioning of the graft

extending over the lateral epicondyle and along the anterior border of the anconeus distally (Fig. 38-4). The interval between the anconeus and the extensor carpi ulnaris is developed. The proximal anconeus and distal triceps can be reflected from the lateral supracondylar ridge and the lateral epicondyle to improve exposure. The extensor carpi ulnaris is elevated off the annular ligament and the common extensor tendon—extensor carpi radialis brevis is elevated off the anterior aspect of the lateral epicondyle to expose the lateral ligamentous complex. Care must be taken to preserve the anterior capsule and LUCL remnant. This is best accomplished by beginning the dissection distally in the interval. Use of a periosteal or Freer elevator rather than a knife may facilitate dissection while reducing the risk of injury to the underlying lateral collateral ligament complex. The posterolateral rotatory instability pivot test can be performed again at this time to identify ligament and capsular deficiencies. The LUCL is examined and assessed for primary repair. If adequate tissue is not available, a ligamentous graft reconstruction is indicated.

Primary repair is performed by reattachment of the intact ligament to the inferior posterior portion of the lateral epicondyle with suture anchors or transosseous sutures with or without anterior and posterior capsular plication. Two drill holes are placed in the midportion of the lateral epicondyle at the anatomic origin of the LUCL. A nonabsorbable suture is placed through a drill hole, and a running locked stitch is placed down the ligament remnant and back up the contralateral side. The suture is then tied over the bone bridge. Alternatively, a suture anchor is placed at the origin of the LUCL, and a locked running suture is placed in the LUCL remnant for the primary repair. The forearm is pronated and splinted at 60 to 90 degrees of flexion.

Reconstruction of the deficient LUCL is performed with a free ligamentous autograft, such as the palmaris longus tendon or semitendinosus. Required graft length is approximately 20 cm. The palmaris longus can be harvested through a 1-cm incision at the distal volar wrist crease with a standard tendon stripper. A capsular incision is made anterior to the lateral ligamentous complex for joint inspection and later imbrication. Two 3.5-mm drill holes are placed in the ulna, one into the supinator tubercle just distal to the lateral attachment of the capsule and the other approximately 1 to 1.5 cm posterior in a perpendicular line to the axis of the LUCL. The underlying bone is channeled with a curved awl connecting the two holes (Fig. 38-5).

A suture is passed through the drill holes, and a hemostat is attached to help identify the isometric attachment of the lateral collateral ligament complex on the

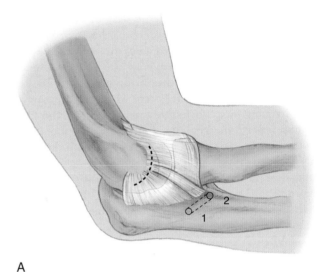

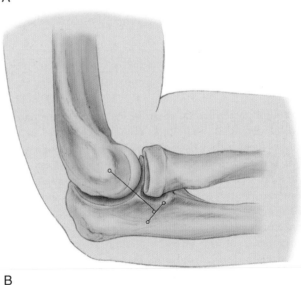

A

B

Figure 38-5 Two drill holes in ulna in supinator tubercle and 1 to 1.5 cm posterior and perpendicular to axis of LUCL.

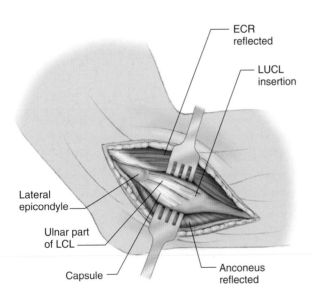

Figure 38-4 Surgical approach (Kocher).

ECR reflected

LUCL insertion

Lateral epicondyle

Ulnar part of LCL

Capsule

Anconeus reflected

lateral epicondyle. The hemostat is placed on the lateral epicondyle, and the elbow is flexed and extended to identify the isometric point at which both limbs of the suture remain taut (Fig. 38-6). This point should correspond to the middle of the capitellum on a lateral radiograph.

A 4.5-mm drill hole is placed at the isometric point angled medially and proximally toward the supracondylar ridge and burred to a size of 5 or 6 mm. This hole should tend anterior and proximal to the established isometric point, especially during enlargement, to ensure that the graft is tight in extension. A second hole is made just posterior to the supracondylar ridge, about 1.5 cm proximally, and a tunnel is developed between the two. A second tunnel is made from the same isometric entry point by drilling a third hole 1 to 1.5 cm distal to the second hole so that a bridge of bone remains between it and the first tunnel (Fig. 38-7).

The graft is passed through the ulnar tunnel from anterior to posterior. One end of the graft is passed into the isometric hole in the humerus, out the proximal tunnel, along the posterior humeral cortex, and back in the distal tunnel, emerging through the isometric hole (Fig. 38-8).

The graft is tensioned with the arm maximally pronated in 30 to 40 degrees of flexion and sutured to itself in a figure-of-eight configuration (Figs. 38-9 and 38-10).

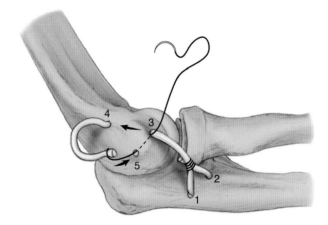

Figure 38-8 Passing of the graft.

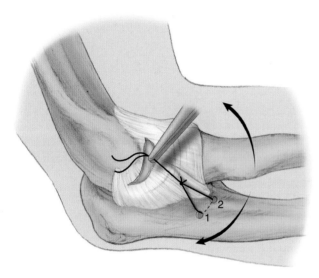

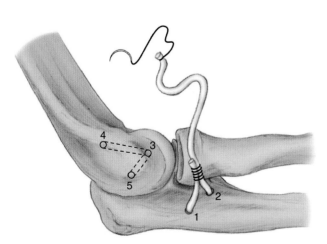

Figure 38-6 Determination of the isometric point.

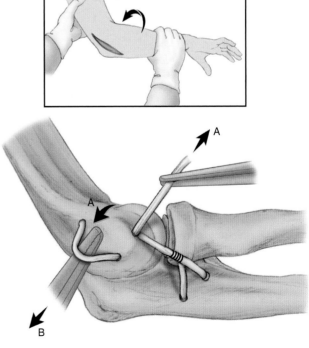

Figure 38-7 Drilling of the humeral tunnels.

Figure 38-9 Tensioning of the graft.

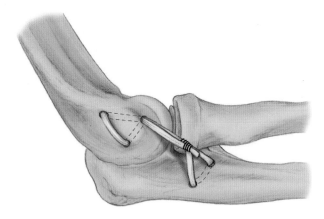

Figure 38-10 Tensioning and suturing of the graft.

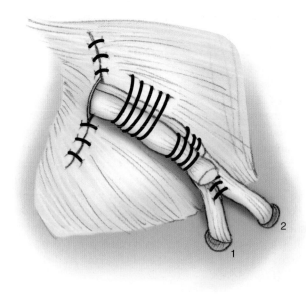

Figure 38-12 Final tensioning of the graft.

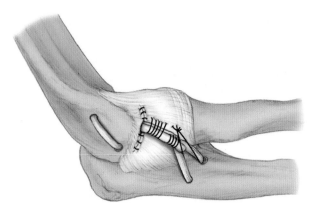

Figure 38-11 Plication of the capsule over the graft.

Alternatively, some surgeons make a single, blind-ended tunnel in the lateral epicondyle at the isometric point and fix the graft, after appropriate measurement, with an interference screw. This eliminates the need for three holes and two tunnels in the lateral epicondyle. The resultant graft is double-stranded instead of a three-ply reconstruction with the figure-of-eight graft originally described. Another variation uses a single blind-ended tunnel at the supinator crest with an interference screw. The interference screw technique can be used on either end or on both ends (humeral and ulnar) for fixation. The capsule is closed beneath the graft and plicated as necessary (Fig. 38-11).

The graft is tensioned further by pulling it anteriorly and suturing it to the capsule and by closing the distal loop of the figure-of-eight construct (Fig. 38-12). The overlying soft tissues are closed in layers in the standard fashion.

Postoperative Considerations

Rehabilitation

An above-elbow splint is placed postoperatively with the forearm in pronation and the elbow at 90 degrees of flexion. It is removed at 1 week, and a 30-degree extension block splint or hinged brace is applied for 6 weeks. Full range of motion in a hinged elbow brace is initiated at 6 weeks. Bracing is usually discontinued after 3 months, at which point the patient begins a strengthening program within pain-free limits. This can be variable on the basis of the patient's compliance and the strength of the repair. Full recovery is expected after 6 to 9 months.

Complications

Potential complications include cutaneous nerve damage (from incision or tendon harvesting), persistent flexion contracture, and persistent instability. Care is required to prevent fracturing through bone bridges. Persistent instability can often be attributed to a posteriorly placed tunnel on the humerus that leaves the graft lax in extension, where posterolateral rotatory instability tends to occur. Persistent flexion contracture (<10 degrees) can be protective as posterolateral rotatory instability occurs most frequently in extension.

Table 38-1 Results After Reconstruction of the Lateral Ulnar Collateral Ligament

Author	Follow-up (Mean)	Outcome
Sanchez-Sotelo et al (2005)	6 years	40 of 45 (89%) stable 38 of 45 (86%) satisfied
Olsen and Sojbjerg[13] (2003)	44 months	14 of 18 (78%) stable 17 of 18 (94%) satisfied
*Nestor et al[9] (1992)	42 months	10 of 11 (91%) stable 7 of 11 (64%) excellent
*Lee and Teo[6] (2003)	24 months	10 of 10 (100%) stable 10 of 10 (100%) satisfied

*Study group included direct repair and ligament reconstruction.

38

PEARLS AND PITFALLS

- The pivot shift maneuver will be met with apprehension in the clinic. It is uncommon to have a positive result of the pivot shift examination in the clinic, so if the patient has apprehension, one should consider examination under anesthesia to confirm the diagnosis.

- When the tunnels are drilled, after the first hole is made, hand position a small drill bit in that hole. Then, when the second hole is drilled to connect with the first, you will know you have connected the two holes to form a tunnel when the hand-placed drill bit moves as you drill the second tunnel, ensuring that the holes are connected to make a tunnel.

- To make the tunnels, one can use a 4-mm bur or 3.2-mm drill. To enlarge the tunnels, especially the tunnel at the apex of the lateral epicondyle, a curet may be used.

- An angled curet may be used to enlarge and connect the holes to make the tunnel.

- When the ulnar tunnel is drilled, make the tunnel perpendicular to the line of the graft—this makes for easier tensioning and less graft motion.

- To pass the sutures into the tunnels, it is sometimes easier to use a curved 22-gauge wire to pass your suture to check for isometry and for graft passage.

- On the humeral side, if one is to err on the isometric point of the tunnel, it is important to make the tunnel superior and anterior. Avoid making the tunnel posterior and distal.

- The humeral holes are made 1 cm apart to reduce the risk of fracture of the epicondyle. Further, one of the proximal humeral holes posterior to the epicondyle provides stronger bone to reduce fracture risk.

- The authors suture the graft arms to each other when possible, including the entry site into the tunnels and areas of overlap of the arms of the graft, to reduce slippage and to secure the graft.

- Suturing of the graft to itself just distal to the distal humeral tunnel can allow tensioning of the graft.

- Whereas the palmaris longus is the graft of choice, gracilis tendon may be used with excellent results.

- By use of the docking technique proximally, it is easier to tension the graft if the graft is substantive, such as the gracilis or a large palmaris longus.

Results

Primary repair of the LUCL, when possible, has excellent results. Osborne and Cotterill[14] reported excellent results in eight patients with transosseous repair, and Nestor et al[9] reported excellent results in three patients. Ligamentous reconstruction results have been mixed (Table 38-1). O'Driscoll and Morrey reported a 90% success rate in restoring stability in the absence of arthritis or radial head fracture; 60% of patients experienced excellent results, whereas 40% continued to have pain or some loss of motion.

References

1. Ball CM, Galatz LM, Yamaguchi K. Elbow instability: treatment strategies and emerging concepts. Instr Course Lect 2002;51:53-61.
2. Cohen MS, Hastings H II. Rotatory instability of the elbow: the anatomy and role of the lateral elbow stabilizers. J Bone Joint Surg Am 1997;79:225-233.
3. Dunning CE, Zarzour ZD, Patterson SD, et al. Ligamentous stabilizers against posterolateral rotatory instability of the elbow. J Bone Joint Surg Am 2001;83:1823-1828.
4. Hall JA, McKee MD. Posterolateral rotatory instability of the elbow following radial head resection. J Bone Joint Surg Am 2005;87:1571-1579.
5. King GJ, Dunning CE, Zarzour ZD, et al. Single-strand reconstruction of the lateral ulnar collateral ligament restores varus and posterolateral rotatory instability of the elbow. J Shoulder Elbow Surg 2002;11:60-64.
6. Lee BP, Teo LH. Surgical reconstruction for posterolateral instability of the elbow. J Shoulder Elbow Surg 2003;12:476-479.
7. Mehta JA, Bain GI. Posterolateral rotatory instability of the elbow. J Am Acad Orthop Surg 2004;12:405-415.
8. Morrey BF, O'Driscoll SW. Surgical reconstruction of the lateral collateral ligament. In Morrey BF. The Elbow, 2nd ed. Master Techniques in Orthopaedic Surgery. Philadelphia, Lippincott Williams & Wilkins, 2002:249-265.

9. Nestor BJ, O'Driscoll SW, Morrey BF. Ligamentous reconstruction for posterolateral rotatory instability of the elbow. J Bone Joint Surg Am 1992;74:1235-1241.

10. O'Driscoll SW, Bell DF, Morrey BF. Posterolateral rotatory instability of the elbow. J Bone Joint Surg Am 1991;73:440-446.

11. O'Driscoll SW, Morrey BF, Korinek S, An KN. Elbow subluxation and dislocation. A spectrum of instability. Clin Orthop 1992;280:186-197.

12. O'Driscoll SW, Spinner RJ, McKee MD, et al. Tardy posterolateral rotatory instability of the elbow due to cubitus varus. J Bone Joint Surg Am 2001;83:1358-1369.

13. Olsen BS, Sojbjerg JO. The treatment of recurrent posterolateral instability of the elbow. J Bone Joint Surg Br 2003;85:342-346.

14. Osborne G, Cotterill P. Recurrent dislocation of the elbow. J Bone Joint Surg Br 1966;48:340-346.

15. Potter HG, Weiland AJ, Schatz JA, et al. Posterolateral rotatory instability of the elbow: usefulness of MR imaging in diagnosis. Radiology 1997;204:185-189.

16. Regan WD, Korinek SL, Morrey BF, An KN. Biomechanical study of ligaments around the elbow joint. Clin Orthop 1991;271:170-179.

17. Sanchez-Sotelo J, Morrey BF, O'Driscoll SW. Ligamentous repair and reconstruction for posterolateral rotatory instability of the elbow. J Bone Joint Surg Br 2005;87:54-61.

18. Seki A, Olsen BS, Jensen SL, et al. Functional anatomy of the lateral collateral ligament complex of the elbow: configuration of Y and its role. J Shoulder Elbow Surg 2002;11:53-59.

19. Singleton SB, Conway JE. PLRI: posterolateral instability of the elbow. Clin Sports Med 2004;23:629-642.

20. Smith JP 3rd, Savoie FH 3rd, Field LD. Posterolateral rotatory instability of the elbow. Clin Sports Med 2001;20:47-58.

21. Yadao MA, Savoie FH 3rd, Field LD. Posterolateral rotatory instability of the elbow. Instr Course Lect 2004;23:629-642.

CHAPTER 39

Open Elbow Contracture Release

David Ring, MD, PhD
Diego Fernandez, MD, PD

Elbow motion can be restricted by contracture of the skin, capsule, and muscles; heterotopic ossification, osteophytes, or implants; articular incongruity or damage; and malunion or nonunion.[21] Ulnar neuropathy is commonly associated with elbow contracture and can be precipitated or exacerbated by surgeries that increase mobility.[2] The best candidate for an arthroscopic elbow contracture release is a patient with capsular contracture with or without osteophytes. Most patients with pure capsular contractures after trauma can achieve functional motion with time and exercises (including static progressive or dynamic elbow splinting).[5,8] Primary elbow arthritis is uncommon. Patients with less than 100 degrees of flexion or preexisting ulnar neuropathy merit ulnar nerve decompression.[2] Once the ulnar nerve is released, it is straightforward to perform a capsular excision from the medial side.[13] Arthroscopic elbow contracture release is more difficult and more dangerous than open contracture release, particularly because elbow arthroscopy is an uncommon procedure at which most of us are not well practiced.[3,9,14,16,24] For all of these reasons, operative treatment of elbow stiffness is best performed with an open procedure in most patients.

Preoperative Considerations

History

It is helpful to be aware of the details of prior trauma, burn, or central nervous system injury, prior surgeries in particular. In patients with prior central nervous system injury, one must determine the ability of the patient to participate in a postoperative rehabilitation protocol.[34] A painful contracture suggests arthritis or ulnar neuropathy. Numbness and dexterity problems suggest ulnar neuropathy.

Physical Examination

The quality of the skin is important, particularly in postburn contractures.[28] The status of the skin with respect to prior injury and operative treatment will influence the operative tactics. When planning operative treatment of a post-traumatic contracture, we prefer to wait until the skin and scar are mobile and soft and no longer edematous or adherent. A complete motor and sensory examination of the ulnar nerve is performed along with evaluation for Tinel sign and an elbow flexion test.

Imaging

Standard anteroposterior and lateral radiographs of the elbow are usually sufficient to identify and to characterize arthritis, heterotopic ossification, and nonunions, but computed tomography is occasionally of use. In more complex cases, the computed tomographic scan can help with preoperative planning.[34] Three-dimensional reconstructions are particularly easy to interpret. Computed tomographic scans may be particularly useful for characterizing malunion of the articular surface of the distal humerus.[20]

Neurophysiologic testing should be considered when there is any possibility of preoperative ulnar neuropathy.

Indications and Contraindications

Morrey et al[23] found that 15 daily activities could be accomplished with an arc of ulnohumeral motion between 30 and 130 degrees of flexion and an arc of forearm rotation from 50 degrees of pronation to 50 degrees of supination. However, these numbers should not be used to decide when to operate on elbow stiffness. Patients can adapt to and function well with much less motion,[6] perhaps more so when the stiffness is in the nondominant elbow. Therefore, the indication for operative contracture release is a combination of diminished elbow motion and disability directly related to stiffness.

Simple capsular contracture (no heterotopic bone, no malunion or nonunion, no implants blocking motion, no ulnar neuropathy) usually responds to reassurance and encouragement of exercises, time, and static progressive or dynamic elbow splinting.[5] Therefore, one should never rush into operative treatment of capsular contracture; patience and frequent visits for reassurance and encouragement are worthwhile.

Obvious hindrances to motion, including heterotopic bone, malunion, nonunion, prominent implants, and ulnar neuropathy, merit immediate operative treatment. Heterotopic ossification can be resected within 4 months of injury (when it is radiographically mature and the skin is mobile with little or no edema) regardless of activity on bone scans.[15,28,33,34] Stiffness associated with advanced arthrosis or unsalvageable nonunion or malunion should be treated by interpositional or prosthetic elbow arthroplasty.[21,22]

Surgical Planning

Elbow capsulectomy can be performed simultaneously with débridement of a deep infection. It also forms an integral part of the treatment of malunion,[20] nonunion,[11] and instability.[26] Unstable skin can be treated with either prior or concomitant procedures to improve soft tissue coverage.[28]

Patients with capsular contracture who desire extension can be treated with lateral capsulectomy (Fig. 39-1).[4,19] Patients with concomitant ulnar neuropathy or limitation of elbow flexion are best treated with medial capsulectomy (Fig. 39-2).[13,36] Patients with heterotopic bone, prominent implants, or complex contracture that cannot be adequately released from medial or lateral alone may benefit from a combined release.[13,28] Preoperative (within 24 hours) radiation therapy (a single 7-Gy dose) is administered to patients with heterotopic bone to be excised.

Direct anterior release[32] is rarely necessary because the anterior capsule can be more safely excised from medial or lateral. A posterior release with splitting of the triceps and fenestration of the olecranon fossa for access to the anterior elbow is used primarily for débridement of primary elbow arthrosis.[2]

This chapter describes elbow capsulectomy through lateral (Fig. 39-1) and medial (Fig. 39-2) intervals.

Surgical Technique

Open elbow contracture release can be performed under general anesthesia or brachial plexus block. The patient is supine, and the arm is supported on a hand table. A sterile tourniquet is applied to the upper arm.

The skin incision can be straight and directly over the muscle interval to be used or posterior with a skin flap elevated to expose the muscle interval (Fig. 39-1C). If both medial and lateral intervals are to be used, a single posterior incision or both medial and lateral incisions can be made. In the unusual case of a direct anterior release, a direct anterior skin incision that crosses the flexion creases obliquely is made.

Specific Steps

Lateral Elbow Capsulectomy (Box 39-1)

1. Lateral Approach and Posterior Dissection

Release of elbow stiffness from the lateral side preserves the common wrist and digit extensors overlying the lateral collateral ligament. The skin is mobilized off the fascia to help identify the appropriate deep muscle interval (Fig. 39-1D). Deep dissection begins by identification of the supracondylar ridge, dividing the overlying fascia and exposing the ridge (Fig. 39-1E). The triceps is elevated off the posterior humerus and elbow capsule (Fig. 39-1F). The posterior dissection continues distally in the interval between the anconeus and extensor carpi ulnaris. The anconeus is elevated off the capsule, the humerus, and the ulna (Fig. 39-1G). Care is taken to preserve the lateral collateral ligament complex while the posterior elbow capsule is excised. The olecranon fossa is cleared out and even burred to deepen it if necessary (Fig. 39-1H). Loose bodies are identified and removed (Fig. 39-1I). The tip of the olecranon can also be excised (Fig. 39-1J and K).

2. Anterior Dissection

The origin of the extensor carpi radialis and part of the origin of the brachioradialis are released and elevated along with the brachialis off the anterior humerus and elbow capsule (Fig. 39-1L and M). Distally, an interval is developed just anterior to the midportion of the capitel-

Text continued on p. 386.

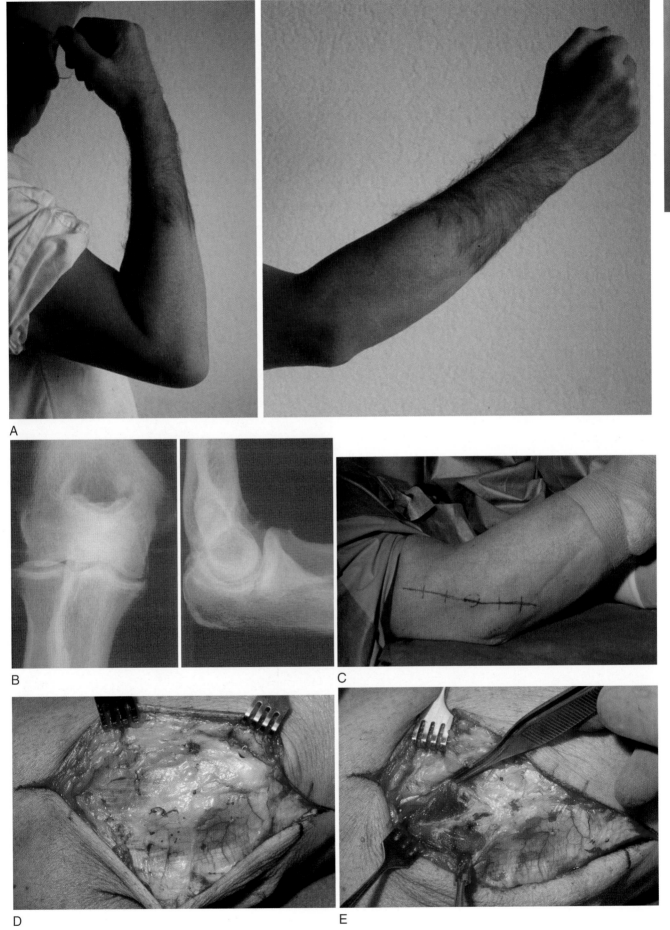

Figure 39-1 A, A man with a substantial flexion contracture and no ulnar neuropathy after trauma. **B,** Radiographs show mild osteoarthritis. **C,** A lateral skin incision is made. **D,** Full-thickness skin flaps are elevated. **E,** The supracondylar ridge is identified, and the origins of the radial wrist extensors are incised and elevated from the anterior humerus.

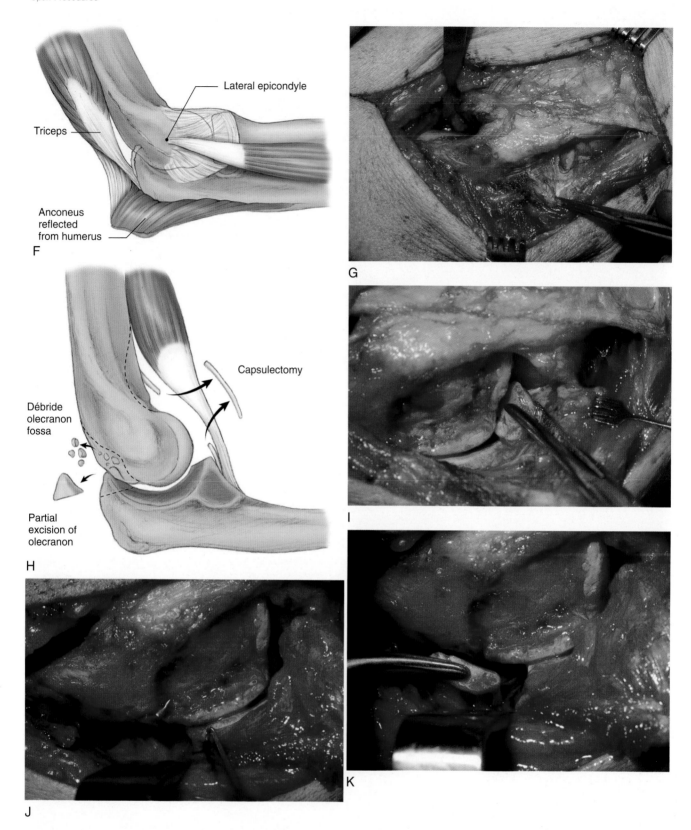

Figure 39-1, cont'd F, The anconeus and the triceps are elevated from the posterior aspect of the humerus and elbow articulation. **G,** The posterolateral capsule *(forceps)* is excised. **H,** Osteophytes are removed from the tip of the olecranon, and the olecranon fossa is cleared. **I,** Loose bodies *(forceps)* are often found in the posterolateral gutter. **J,** An osteotome is poised to cut the olecranon tip. **K,** Removal of the olecranon tip.

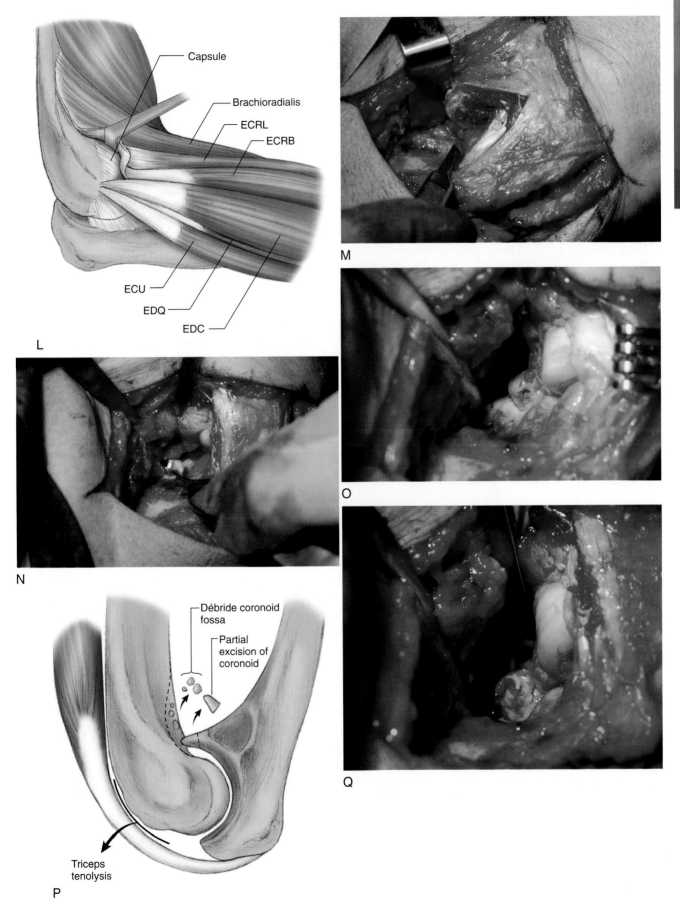

Figure 39-1, cont'd L, Anteriorly, the interval between the extensor carpi radialis brevis (ECRB) and the extensor digitorum communis (EDC) is developed to better expose the anterior elbow capsule. ECRL, extensor carpi radialis longus; ECU, extensor carpi ulnaris; EDQ, extensor digiti quinti. **M,** The anterior elbow capsule is excised. **N,** A loose body *(forceps)* was also found in the anterior part of the joint. **O,** The elbow after excision of the anterior capsule. **P,** At this point, the coronoid tip is excised and the coronoid fossa is cleared out. **Q,** An osteotome is poised to cut the coronoid tip.

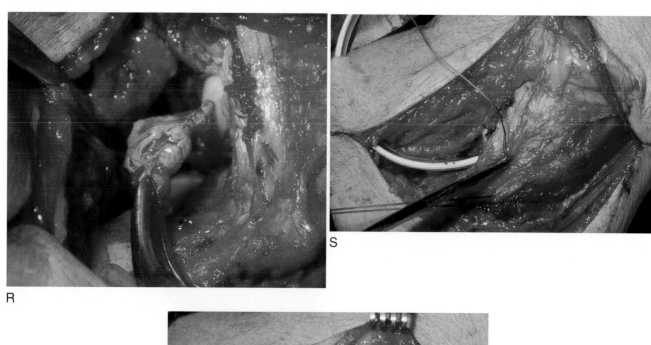

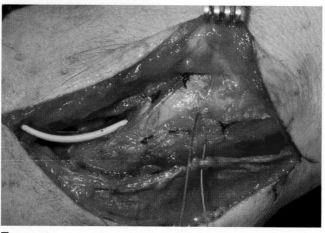

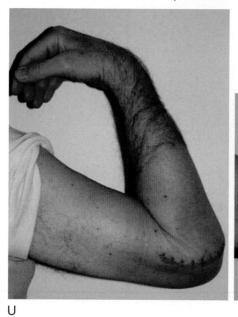

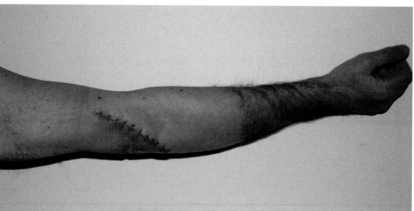

Figure 39-1, cont'd R, Removal of the olecranon tip *(forceps)*. **S,** The anterior interval is closed, in this case over a suction drain. **T,** Closure of the posterior interval. **U,** Final motion was excellent.

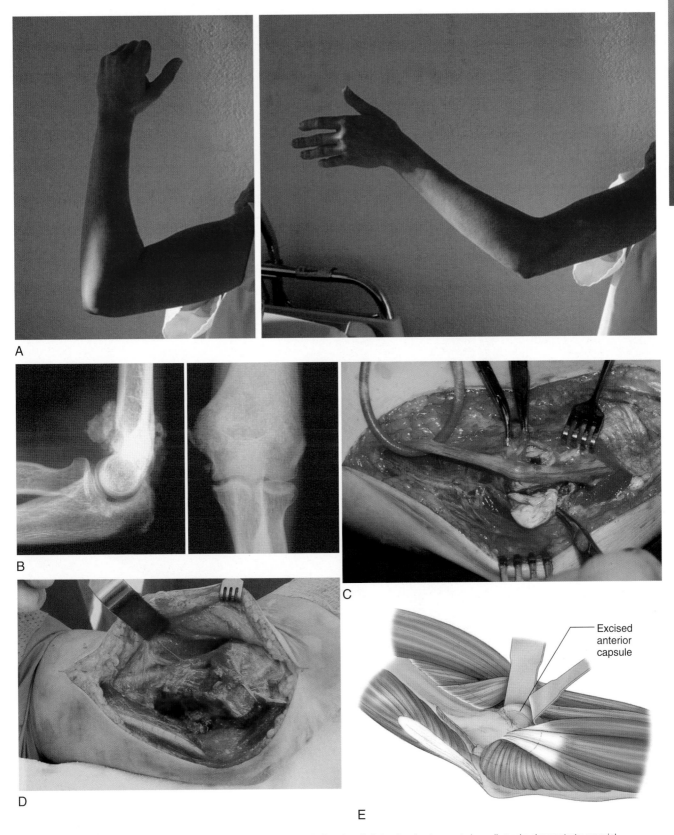

Figure 39-2 A, A patient with severe elbow contracture and ulnar nerve dysfunction. **B,** Lateral and anteroposterior radiographs demonstrate synovial chondromatosis. **C,** A complete release of the ulnar nerve is performed. The nerve is transposed anteriorly in the subcutaneous tissues at the end of the surgery. **D,** The flexor-pronator mass is split, and the anterior half is elevated off the anterior humerus and capsule along with the brachialis. **E,** A schematic drawing of the muscle interval and exposure of the anterior capsule.

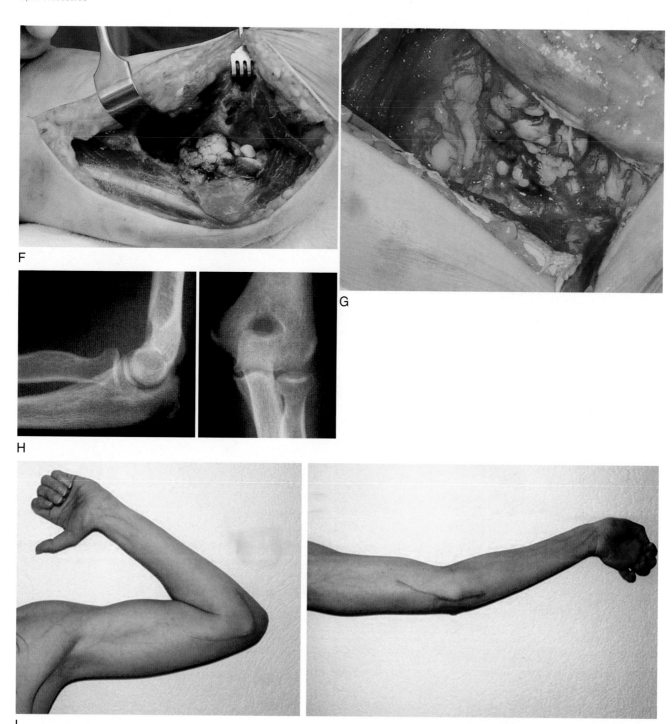

Figure 39-2, cont'd F, After capsular excision, the synovial chondromatosis is apparent. **G,** More synovial chondromatosis is seen after elevation of the triceps off the distal humerus and posterior capsule and excision of the posterior capsule. **H,** Final lateral and anteroposterior radiographs demonstrate resection of the synovial chondromatosis. **I,** Flexion and extension were improved.

Box 39-1 Surgical Steps for Lateral Capsulectomy

1. Lateral approach and posterior dissection

2. Anterior dissection

3. Medial dissection

lum, roughly corresponding to the split between the extensor carpi radialis brevis and the extensor digitorum communis, although in practice the interval is not precise (Fig. 39-1L, N, and O). Keeping the dissection over the anterior half of the radiocapitellar joint will protect the lateral collateral ligament complex. The anterior elbow capsule is excised (Fig. 39-1N).

3. Medial Dissection

At the medial side of the elbow, the capsulectomy may transition to a capsulotomy for safety, depending on visualization (Fig. 39-1O). The radial and coronoid fossae can be cleared out and deepened as needed (Fig. 39-1P). The tip of the coronoid can be excised (Fig. 39-1Q and R). Resection of a deformed radial head may also be helpful in some patients.

Both the anterior and the posterior muscle intervals are sutured (Fig. 39-1S and T). Drains are used at the discretion of the surgeon. The skin is closed according to the surgeon's preference.

Medial Elbow Capsulectomy

After skin incision, the ulnar nerve is identified on the medial border of the triceps. A complete release of the nerve through the arcade of Struthers, Osborne ligament, and flexor-pronator aponeurosis is then performed, along with neurolysis of the ulnar nerve if there is extensive scarring (Fig. 39-2C). Skin flaps can be safely elevated once the ulnar nerve is identified and protected.

The flexor-pronator mass is identified and split in half between the interval where the ulnar nerve runs and the anterior margin of the muscle mass. The anterior half of the flexor-pronator mass and the brachialis muscle are elevated off the anterior humerus and elbow capsule (Fig. 39-2D to F). The triceps is elevated off the distal humerus and the posterior elbow capsule (Fig. 39-2G). Capsular excision, fossae deepening, and coronoid and olecranon tip excision are as described for lateral capsulectomy.

Heterotopic Bone Excision and Other Factors

Heterotopic bone is excised piecemeal, with care taken to identify and to protect native bone and articulation. Bleeding bone surfaces are covered with bone wax. Implants are removed after capsulectomy and elbow manipulation to limit the risk of fracture. Malunion and nonunion are addressed as necessary.

Postoperative Considerations

Rehabilitation

Gravity-assisted and active-assisted range of motion exercises are initiated the morning after surgery. Static progressive or dynamic splints are used in patients who have

Table 39-1 Published Case Series Reporting the Results of Open Elbow Contracture Release

Author	No. of Patients	Diagnosis	Operative Technique	Preoperative Arc (degrees)	Postoperative Arc (degrees)
Tosun et al[31] (2006)	22	Post-traumatic	Combined lateral and medial	35	86
Ring et al[25] (2006)	46	Post-traumatic	Patient-specific, variable	45	103
Tan et al[30] (2006)	52	Post-traumatic	Patient-specific, variable	57	116
Ring et al[27] (2005)	42	Post-traumatic	Patient-specific, variable; 23 had hinged external fixation	21	105
Aldridge et al[1] (2004)	77	Post-traumatic	Anterior; most with continuous passive motion postoperatively	59	97
Gosling et al[7] (2004; Epub May 30, 2003)	59	Post-traumatic	Patient-specific, variable	68	101
Wu[37] (2003)	20	Post-traumatic	Patient-specific, variable	47	118
Heirweg and De Smet[10] (2003)	16	Post-traumatic	Patient-specific, variable	47	87
Stans et al[29] (2002)	37	Mixed; age younger than 21 years	Patient-specific, variable	66	94
Wada et al[35] (2000)	13	Post-traumatic	Medial	46	110
Kraushaar et al[17] (1999)	12	Post-traumatic	Lateral	70	117
Mansat and Morrey[19] (1998)	37	Mixed	Lateral	49	94
Cohen and Hastings[4] (1998)	22	Post-traumatic	Lateral	74	129
Hertel et al[12] (1997)	26	Mixed	Patient-specific, variable	66	100

trouble maintaining motion obtained in surgery. These splints are initiated as soon as the wound is stable.

Complications

Complications include recurrent stiffness and ulnar neuropathy (due to restoration of flexion or to handling of the nerve).

PEARLS AND PITFALLS

- Release of a flexion contracture, especially in patients with primary osteoarthritis, can result in ulnar neuropathy.

- The lateral collateral ligament can be protected by limiting the dissection to the anterior half of the radiocapitellar joint.

Results

The majority of published case series reporting the results of open elbow contracture release describe a single technique used to treat patients with a variety of diagnoses (Table 39-1). The results of various techniques seem comparable, although few data are available about the use of a medial exposure for post-traumatic contractures.[25,36] In general, about 75% regain at least an 80-degree arc of flexion.[25] Patients with limited flexion—particularly due to primary osteoarthritis—may be susceptible to ulnar neuropathy after release.[2] The results of excision of subtotal heterotopic ossification may be superior to the results of capsular contracture release alone,[18] but the results of excision of complete bone ankylosis, although generally rewarding, are less predictable.[28]

References

1. Aldridge JM 3rd, Atkins TA, Gunneson EE, Urbaniak JR. Anterior release of the elbow for extension loss. J Bone Joint Surg Am 2004;86:1955-1960.

2. Antuna SA, Morrey BF, Adams RA, O'Driscoll SW. Ulnohumeral arthroplasty for primary degenerative arthritis of the elbow: long-term outcome and complications. J Bone Joint Surg Am 2002; 84:2168-2173.

3. Ball CM, Meunier M, Galatz LM, et al. Arthroscopic treatment of post-traumatic elbow contracture. J Shoulder Elbow Surg 2002;11: 624-629.

4. Cohen MS, Hastings H. Post-traumatic contracture of the elbow: operative release using a lateral collateral ligament sparing approach. J Bone Joint Surg Br 1998;80:805-812.

5. Doornberg JN, Ring D, Jupiter JB. Static progressive splinting for posttraumatic elbow stiffness. J Orthop Trauma 2006;20:400-404.

6. Doornberg JN, Ring D, Fabian LM, et al. Pain dominates measurements of elbow function and health status. J Bone Joint Surg Am 2005;87:1725-1731.

7. Gosling T, Blauth M, Lange T, et al. Outcome assessment after arthrolysis of the elbow. Arch Orthop Trauma Surg 2004;124:232-236. Epub May 30, 2003.

8. Green DP, McCoy H. Turnbuckle orthotic correction of elbow-flexion contractures after acute injuries. J Bone Joint Surg Am 1979;61:1092-1095.

9. Haapaniemi T, Berggren M, Adolfsson L. Complete transection of the median and radial nerves during arthroscopic release of post-traumatic elbow contracture. Arthroscopy 1999;15:784-787.

10. Heirweg S, De Smet L. Operative treatment of elbow stiffness: evaluation and outcome. Acta Orthop Belg 2003;69:18-22.

11. Helfet DL, Kloen P, Anand N, Rosen HS. Open reduction and internal fixation of delayed unions and nonunions of fractures of the distal part of the humerus. J Bone Joint Surg Am 2003;85:33-40.

12. Hertel R, Pisan M, Lambert S, Ballmer F. Operative management of the stiff elbow: sequential arthrolysis based on a transhumeral approach. J Shoulder Elbow Surg 1997;6:82-88.

13. Hotchkiss RN. Elbow contracture. In Green DP, Hotchkiss RN, Pederson WC, eds. Green's Operative Hand Surgery. Philadelphia, Churchill Livingstone, 1999:667-682.

14. Jones GS, Savoie FH 3rd. Arthroscopic capsular release of flexion contractures (arthrofibrosis) of the elbow. Arthroscopy 1993;9: 277-283.

15. Jupiter JB, Ring D. Operative treatment of post-traumatic proximal radioulnar synostosis. J Bone Joint Surg Am 1998;80:248-257.

16. Kim SJ, Kim HK, Lee JW. Arthroscopy for limitation of motion of the elbow. Arthroscopy 1995;11:680-683.

17. Kraushaar BS, Nirschl RP, Cox W. A modified lateral approach for release of posttraumatic elbow flexion contracture. J Shoulder Elbow Surg 1999;8:476-480.

18. Lindenhovius AL, Linzel DS, Doornberg JN, et al. Comparison of elbow contracture release in elbows with and without heterotopic ossification restricting motion. J Shoulder Elbow Surg (in press).

19. Mansat P, Morrey BF. The column procedure: a limited lateral approach for extrinsic contracture of the elbow. J Bone Joint Surg Am 1998;80:1603-1615.

20. McKee MD, Jupiter JB, Toh CL, et al. Reconstruction after malunion and nonunion of intra-articular fractures of the distal humerus. J Bone Joint Surg Br 1994;76:614-621.

21. Morrey BF. Post-traumatic contracture of the elbow. Operative treatment, including distraction arthroplasty. J Bone Joint Surg Am 1990;72:601-618.

22. Morrey BF, Adams RA, Bryan RS. Total elbow replacement for post-traumatic arthritis of the elbow. J Bone Joint Surg Br 1991;73: 607-612.

23. Morrey BF, Askew LJ, Chao EY. A biomechanical study of normal functional elbow motion. J Bone Joint Surg Am 1981;63:872-880.

24. Phillips BB, Strasburger S. Arthroscopic treatment of arthrofibrosis of the elbow joint. Arthroscopy 1998;14:38-44.

25. Ring D, Adey L, Zurakowski D, Jupiter JB. Elbow capsulectomy for posttraumatic elbow stiffness. J Hand Surg Am 2006;31:1264-1271.

26. Ring D, Hannouche D, Jupiter JB. Surgical treatment of persistent dislocation or subluxation of the ulnohumeral joint after fracture-dislocation of the elbow. J Hand Surg Am 2004;29:470-480.

27. Ring D, Hotchkiss RN, Guss D, Jupiter JB. Hinged elbow external fixation for severe elbow contracture. J Bone Joint Surg Am 2005; 87:1293-1296.

28. Ring D, Jupiter J. The operative release of complete ankylosis of the elbow due to heterotopic bone in patients without severe injury of the central nervous system. J Bone Joint Surg Am 2003;85: 849-857.

29. Stans AA, Maritz NG, O'Driscoll SW, Morrey BF. Operative treatment of elbow contracture in patients twenty-one years of age or younger. J Bone Joint Surg Am 2002;84:382-387.

30. Tan V, Daluiski A, Simic P, Hotchkiss RN. Outcome of open release for post-traumatic elbow stiffness. J Trauma 2006;61:673-678.

31. Tosun B, Gundes H, Buluc L, Sarlak AY. The use of combined lateral and medial releases in the treatment of post-traumatic contracture of the elbow. Int Orthop 2006;Oct 12 [Epub ahead of print].

32. Urbaniak JR, Hansen PE, Beissinger SF, Aitken MS. Correction of post-traumatic flexion contracture of the elbow by anterior capsulotomy. J Bone Joint Surg Am1985;67:1160-1164.

33. Viola RW, Hanel DP. Early "simple" release of posttraumatic elbow contracture associated with heterotopic ossification. J Hand Surg Am 1999;24:370-380.

34. Viola RW, Hastings H. Treatment of ectopic ossification about the elbow. Clin Orthop 2000;370:65-86.

35. Wada T, Ishii S, Usui M, Miyano S. The medial approach for operative release of post-traumatic contracture of the elbow. J Bone Joint Surg Br 2000;82:68-73.

36. Wada T, Isogai S, Ishii S, Yamashita T. Débridement arthroplasty for primary osteoarthritis of the elbow. Surgical technique. J Bone Joint Surg Am 2005;87(suppl 1, pt 1):95-105.

37. Wu CC. Posttraumatic contracture of elbow treated with intraarticular technique. Arch Orthop Trauma Surg 2003;123:494-500.

CHAPTER 40

Open Treatment of Lateral and Medial Epicondylitis

Shervondalonn R. Brown, MD
Robert J. Goitz, MD

Lateral Epicondylitis

Elbow injuries in the athlete are common entities. Most of these injuries are secondary to repetitive or overuse activities. The sports-related variety of lateral epicondylitis is usually associated with racket sports. It occurs four to five times more frequently in men than in women and more frequently in the dominant arm. In this group of patients, abnormal stresses are placed across the wrist extensor origin and are thought to lead to pathologic changes within the muscle and tendon. Most commonly, the pathologic change associated with lateral epicondylitis arises in the region of the extensor carpi radialis brevis (ECRB). The pain is thought to originate from tendon degeneration and incomplete healing.

Numerous studies have reported 75% to 90% cure rates with a sufficient trial of nonoperative therapy. Initial treatment of lateral epicondylitis begins with activity modification. Patients are instructed to avoid lifting with the wrist extended and to lift objects with the elbow in flexion as close to the body as possible with the hand in supination or neutral position to avoid applying stresses to the wrist extensor muscles. Patients who actively participate in racket sports should consider rackets with better shock absorption and consult with their instructor on optimal mechanics to minimize persistent problems. Conservative treatment also includes physical therapy focusing initially on stretching and progressive light strengthening of the forearm wrist extensors. Orthotics, such as the counterforce brace (tennis elbow strap), and nighttime wrist extension splinting have proved to be supportive, especially in controlling pain. If a combination of physical therapy and bracing is unsuccessful, a local cortisone injection may be attempted. However, if nonoperative treatment for a period of 6 to 12 months fails, operative treatment is indicated for persistent pain and disability.

Many techniques have been described for release of the ECRB, including open, percutaneous, and arthroscopic approaches. Recent research has shown no significant difference in outcomes between open release and arthroscopic release. The authors prefer open excision of the pathologic portion of the ECRB tendon, stimulation of bleeding bone, and repair of the defect, given the reproducibility of the postoperative results and relative straightforwardness of the procedure.

Preoperative Considerations

History and Physical Examination

Evaluation of the athlete with lateral elbow pain begins with a thorough history. The history focuses on types of racket sports as well as any recent changes in equipment. A history of repetitive activity or overuse can often be elicited.

Athletes typically present with lateral elbow pain and decreased grip strength. The pain may extend into the dorsal forearm. Symptoms are exacerbated by activities involving wrist extension against gravity. During the physical examination, pain is elicited with palpation over the lateral epicondyle or slightly distal and anterior to the epicondyle. Pain is exacerbated with resisted wrist extension and long finger extension because of the ECRB origin from the base of the middle finger metacarpal.

Key Physical Findings

- Pain at the lateral elbow
- Exacerbation of pain with resisted wrist extension
- Pain localized to the anterior portion of the lateral epicondyle, which is the ECRB origin
- Decreased grip strength with elbow fully extended compared with elbow flexed
- Pain occasionally radiates along dorsum of forearm

Radiography

- Standard radiographs of elbow (anteroposterior, lateral, oblique)

Evaluate for calcifications, osteochondral defect, exostosis, and degenerative changes of the radiocapitellar joint.

Indications

The best candidate for operative intervention has had 6 to 12 months of conservative treatment, including bracing, physical therapy, and cortisone injections. Other causes of lateral elbow pain, such as radial tunnel syndrome, should be excluded. Results after surgical intervention reveal that 85% to 90% of patients who undergo débridement of the ECRB and repair technique return to full activity without pain.

Key Indications

- Cases that have failed conservative treatment for 6 to 12 months
- Highly competitive athletes
- Multiple cortisone injections (two or more)
- Lateral epicondylar bone exostosis or calcification of common extensor tendon
- Pain (constant) without activity

Surgical Technique

Several surgical techniques have been described for the treatment of lateral epicondylitis. Surgical treatment ranges from resection of the epicondyle to percutaneous or open division of the common extensor origin to tendon lengthening techniques. The most common technique involves identification and excision of the abnormal ECRB

origin with creation of a vascular bone bed to promote healing.

The authors prefer open excision of the pathologic portion of the ECRB tendon, stimulation of bleeding bone, and repair of the defect for initial surgical management. Retrospective results have revealed high success rates, with 80% to 90% of patients having good and excellent results.

Anesthesia and Positioning

On the basis of the surgeon's and anesthesiologist's preferences, the procedure can be performed under regional axillary block, Bier block, or local with sedation. However, tourniquet pain may become difficult for the patient to tolerate if the procedure takes more than 10 or 15 minutes. The patient is positioned supine on the operating room table with the arm on a standard hand table. A nonsterile tourniquet is placed around the upper arm.

Surgical Landmarks and Incisions

Landmarks

- Lateral epicondyle
- Radial head
- Olecranon

Skin Incision

- Centered slightly anterior to lateral epicondyle
- Extend 1 cm above the lateral epicondyle to 2 or 3 cm distally toward the radial head

Specific Steps (Box 40-1)

The skin incision is marked slightly anterior to the lateral epicondyle (Fig. 40-1) in a curvilinear pattern. Important landmarks to be outlined are the lateral epicondyle, radial head, and olecranon. Thick skin flaps are developed sharply down to the fascial layer. Typically, no significant cutane-

Box 40-1 Surgical Steps

1. Exposure
2. Identification of ECRB
3. Débridement of ECRB
4. Decortication of lateral epicondyle
5. Capsular and fascial closure
6. Skin closure

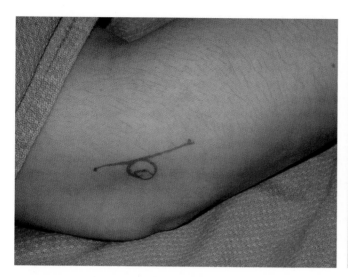

Figure 40-1 Curvilinear skin incision slightly anterior to the lateral epicondyle.

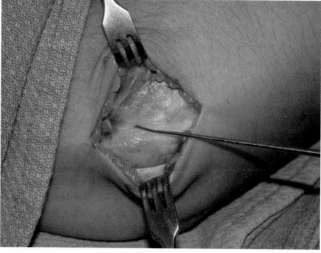

Figure 40-3 Fascial interval between the extensor carpi radialis longus and extensor digitorum communis aponeurosis.

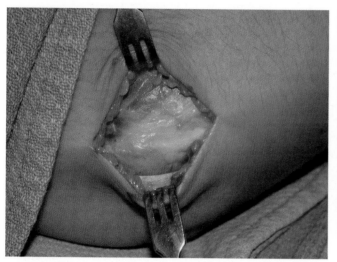

Figure 40-2 Thick skin flaps are developed down to the layer of the extensor carpi radialis longus and extensor digitorum communis aponeurosis.

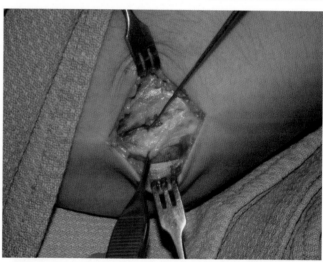

Figure 40-4 Forceps retracting extensor digitorum communis to reveal degenerated ECRS tendon.

ous nerves are present in this area because it is a watershed region between the posterior antebrachial cutaneous nerve and the lateral antebrachial cutaneous nerve (Fig. 40-2).

The ECRB is identified by locating the interval between the muscle and tendon at the lateral epicondyle. The tendinous edge marks the overlapping extensor digitorum communis and underlying ECRB (Fig. 40-3). Sharply incise the fascia between the extensor carpi radialis longus and extensor digitorum communis aponeurosis. Expose the ECRB origin below the extensor digitorum communis. The ECRB is often friable and amorphic, lacking the longitudinal fibers of the normal adjacent tendon.

The degenerated tendon is identified and then sharply débrided (Figs. 40-4 to 40-6). To avoid injury to

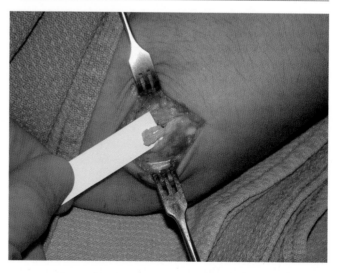

Figure 40-5 The friable and amorphic ECRB tendon is identified.

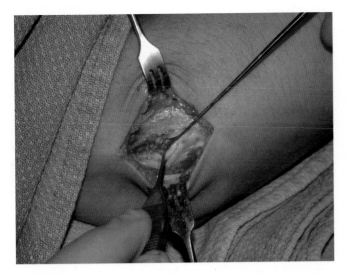

Figure 40-6 After débridement of the ECRB, forceps grasping more normal tendon striations of extensor origin.

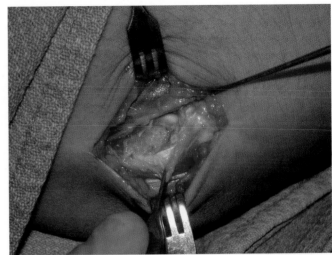

Figure 40-8 Radiocapitellar joint after adequate débridement of the ECRB.

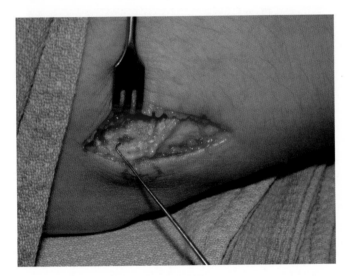

Figure 40-7 Lateral epicondyle decorticated.

PEARLS AND PITFALLS

Lateral Epicondylitis

- Differentiate lateral epicondylitis from radial tunnel syndrome, which usually presents as pain in the distal forearm that is not localized to the lateral epicondyle.
- Identify the exact area of pathologic change by palpation preoperatively.
- Complete release or excision of diseased tissue.
- If the joint is exposed, repair the capsule to prevent formation of a fistula.
- Avoid excessive resection to minimize injury of the lateral collateral ligament.

Postoperative Considerations

Follow-up

At 10 to 14 days postoperatively, the soft dressing is taken down and the wound is checked.

Rehabilitation

- 2 weeks: Active range-of-motion exercises are begun for the elbow, wrist, and forearm; progressive passive range of motion is instituted as necessary.
- 6 weeks: Gentle strengthening begins with light repetition. Gentle strokes are allowed for racket athletes.
- 3 months: Increased strengthening exercises are initiated. Return to competitive sports is permitted once strength has returned to 85% that of the contralateral upper extremity.

the lateral collateral ligament, stay anterior to the epicondyle. The lateral collateral ligament originates on the distal portion of the epicondyle. Once the tendon is adequately débrided, a rongeur or curet is used to decorticate the lateral epicondyle and enhance blood supply to the tendon (Fig. 40-7).

After adequate débridement, the capitellum may be partially visible (Fig. 40-8). Close the capsule to prevent fistula formation. A side-to-side repair of the extensor mechanism is achieved with interrupted 2-0 absorbable sutures.

The wound is copiously irrigated with antibiotic solution. The tourniquet is released, and adequate hemostasis is achieved. The subcutaneous tissues are closed with an absorbable suture, and the skin is closed with a 4-0 subcuticular stitch. The patient's elbow is then placed into a soft dressing.

Table 40-1 Results of Surgical Treatment of Lateral Epicondylitis

Author	Follow-up	Outcome
Nirschl and Pettrone[5] (1979)	6 years	85% complete relief of symptoms and no activity restrictions
Goldberg et al[3] (1988)	4 years	91% good and excellent results
Organ et al[6] (1997)	64 months	83% good to excellent results
Rosenberg and Henderson[7] (2002)	2 years	95% satisfactory results
Dunkow et al[2] (2004)	12 months	92% very pleased or satisfied (open technique) 100% very pleased or satisfied (percutaneous technique)
Coleman and Matheson[1] (2005)	9.8 years	97% good to excellent results

40

Complications

- Elbow instability secondary to excessive resection of lateral collateral ligament
- Joint fistula formation

Results

The results of surgical treatment of lateral epicondylitis are shown in Table 40-1.

Medial Epicondylitis

Medial epicondylitis is much less frequent than lateral epicondylitis. Medial epicondylitis is also associated with sports overuse activities. This disorder is an injury affecting many athletes at all levels, especially throwing athletes. Medial epicondylitis is also known as golfer's elbow and pitcher's elbow. The primary etiology of medial epicondylitis is an overuse syndrome of the flexor-pronator mass. The pronator teres and flexor carpi radialis are most commonly involved. The pathophysiologic process of medial epicondylitis represents a microtearing of the medial tendon and ligaments. Pain is the main presenting symptom; however, the athlete may also present with ulnar nerve symptoms of numbness and tingling in the small and ring fingers. The pain is localized to the medial aspect of the elbow. On occasion, pain may be distal to the medial epicondyle and radiate into the flexor-pronator mass. Activities that require pronation and flexion of the elbow and wrist exacerbate symptoms.

Nonoperative treatment begins with activity modification. Some racket athletes may need to adjust their racket grip, often to a larger size. Athletes are encouraged to avoid constant activities that require pushing the hand with the forearm in pronation. Athletes are also educated in proper warm-up technique and conditioning. Anti-inflammatories, stretching, and counterforce bracing may also be helpful. Anti-inflammatory medication is administered for a period of 10 to 14 days. Local steroid injections are indicated in refractory cases of medial epicondylitis. The steroid is injected deep to the flexor-pronator mass to minimize subcutaneous atrophy and hypopigmentation. When the athlete does not respond to conservative treatment for a period of 6 to 12 months, operative intervention is discussed. Open surgical release of the flexor-pronator origin remains the mainstay of operative treatment.

Preoperative Considerations

History and Physical Examination

The diagnosis of medial epicondylitis requires a thorough history and physical examination. Athletes present with tenderness over the medial epicondyle and pain with resisted pronation or wrist flexion. On occasion, the pain may radiate into the forearm. Athletes usually will present with a full range of motion at the elbow; however, they should be monitored for development of a flexion contracture. The findings on neurovascular examination are usually normal.

It is important to differentiate between ulnar neuropathy (cubital tunnel syndrome), ulnar collateral ligament instability, and medial epicondylitis. Ulnar neuropathy usually presents with a Tinel sign or positive elbow flexion test result on physical examination, which produces numbness and tingling in the ring and small fingers. Ulnar collateral ligament instability is confirmed with a positive result of the valgus stress test at 30 degrees of elbow flexion.

Radiographs are usually normal but should be obtained to check for calcification of the flexor-pronator mass or evidence of previous injury to the medial epicondyle, such as an avulsion. Calcification may suggest a previous injury to the ulnar collateral ligament.

Key Physical Findings

- Point tenderness at medial epicondyle
- Pain exacerbated with resisted wrist flexion and pronation
- Tinel sign and compression test at elbow
- Evaluate for ulnar nerve subluxation

Radiography

- Standard radiographs of elbow (anteroposterior, lateral, oblique)

Evaluate for medial ulnohumeral osteophytes, medial collateral ligament calcification, and evidence of previous injury to the medial epicondyle, such as a malunited avulsion fracture.

Indications

- Cases that have failed nonoperative treatment for 6 to 12 months
- Exclusion of other pathologic causes of medial-sided elbow pain
- Temporary relief after steroid injection

Surgical Technique

Surgical treatment of medial epicondylitis is not as well understood as that of lateral epicondylitis. Procedures for medial epicondylitis range from percutaneous epicondylar release to epicondylectomy. Most have agreed that standard surgical treatment of medial epicondylitis involves excision of the pathologic portion of the tendon and repair of the defect, similar to treatment of lateral epicondylitis.

Anesthesia and Positioning

- Regional axillary or Bier block anesthesia
- Patient supine on operating room table with upper arm on a hand table
- Nonsterile upper arm tourniquet

Surgical Landmarks and Incisions

Landmarks

- Medial epicondyle
- Flexor-pronator mass
- Ulnar nerve

Skin Incision

- Gently curved 3- to 4-cm incision along medial epicondyle

Specific Steps (Box 40-2)

The patient is placed supine on a standard operating room table with the arm on an arm board. A nonsterile tourniquet is placed on the upper arm. The arm is exsanguinated with an Esmarch band, and the tourniquet is inflated. A 3- to 4-cm oblique skin incision is made just anterior to the medial epicondyle, and the dissection is carried down through the subcutaneous tissue (Fig. 40-9).

Thick skin flaps are developed down to the flexor-pronator origin. Branches of the medial antebrachial cutaneous nerve, which are typically 1 inch distal to the medial epicondyle, should be identified and protected during this part of the surgical exposure (Fig. 40-10).

Box 40-2 Surgical Steps

1. Exposure
2. Identification of flexor-pronator mass
3. Identification and protection of ulnar nerve
4. Incision of common flexor origin fascial interval
5. Débridement of degenerative tissue on undersurface of flexor-pronator mass
6. Decortication of medial epicondyle
7. Repair of flexor-pronator mass
8. Skin closure

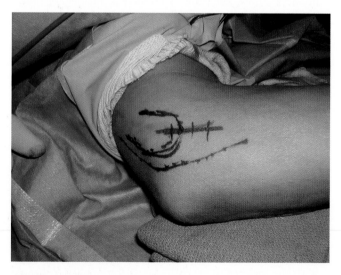

Figure 40-9 Medial epicondyle skin incision.

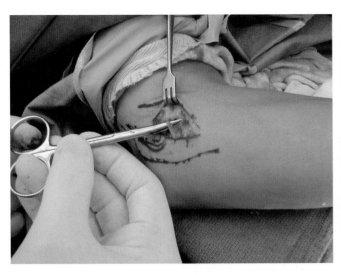

Figure 40-10 Skin incision and branch of the medial antebrachial cutaneous nerve.

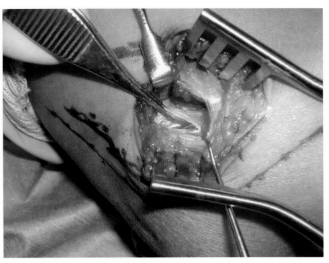

Figure 40-12 Degenerative tissue on the undersurface of the flexor-pronator mass débrided.

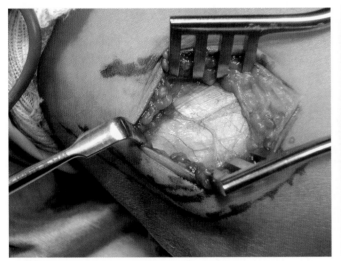

Figure 40-11 Fascial interval between the flexor carpi radialis and pronator teres.

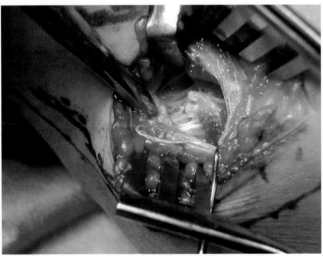

Figure 40-13 Rongeur used to decorticate the medial epicondyle.

The anterior skin flap is mobilized, and the flexor-pronator mass is identified. The ulnar nerve is identified and protected throughout the case. Once the common flexor origin is identified, the fascial interval between the flexor carpi radialis and pronator teres is sharply incised (Fig. 40-11).

The degenerative tissue on the undersurface of the flexor-pronator mass is identified and débrided (Fig. 40-12). Deep to the flexor-pronator mass lies the ulnar collateral ligament. Special attention should be given to protection of the medial collateral ligament during débridement. A rongeur or rasp is used to decorticate the medial epicondyle and create a vascular bed (Fig. 40-13).

The common flexor-pronator mass is repaired with an absorbable 2-0 suture (Fig. 40-14). The subcutaneous tissues are closed with 4-0 absorbable suture, and skin is closed with a 4-0 subcuticular suture. The patient is placed

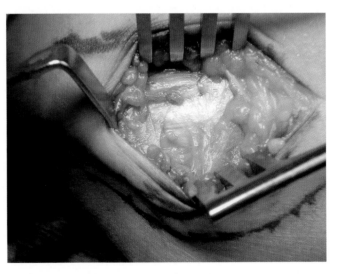

Figure 40-14 Common flexor-pronator mass repaired.

into a well-padded sterile dressing. A posterior splint may be used if the patient was particularly uncomfortable preoperatively.

Postoperative Considerations

Follow-up

The dressings are removed 10 to 14 days postoperatively.

Rehabilitation

- Days 10-14: Gentle active range-of-motion exercises are begun for the elbow as well as for the wrist and

hand, followed by progressive passive range of motion. A stretching program is resumed.

- 4-6 weeks: Strengthening program starts.
- 12 weeks: Return to play is permitted once strength is 85% that of the contralateral extremity.

Complications

- Residual pain
- Valgus instability
- Unaddressed cubital tunnel syndrome
- Hypoesthesia along proximal forearm
- Medial antebrachial cutaneous neuroma

Results

The results of operative treatment of medial epicondylitis are shown in Table 40-2.

Table 40-2 Results of Operative Treatment of Medial Epicondylitis

Author	Follow-up	Results
Vangsness and Jobe[8] (1991)	6 years	97% good to excellent results
Wittenberg et al[9] (1992)	4 years, 9 months	82% good to excellent results
Gable and Morrey[3] (1995)	7 years	87% good to excellent results

References

1. Coleman B, Matheson J. Surgical treatment of resistant lateral epicondylitis: a long-term follow-up. J Bone Joint Surg Br 2005;87(suppl III):335-336.
2. Dunkow PD, Jatti M, Muddu BN. A comparison of open and percutaneous techniques in the surgical treatment of tennis elbow. J Bone Joint Surg Br 2004;86:701-704.
3. Gabel GT, Morrey BF. Operative treatment of medial epicondylitis: the influence of concomitant ulnar neuropathy at the elbow. J Bone Joint Surg Am 1995;77:1065-1069.
4. Goldberg EJ, Abraham E, Siegel I. The surgical treatment of chronic lateral humeral epicondylitis by common extensor release. Clin Orthop 1988;233:208-212.
5. Nirschl RP, Pettrone FA. Tennis elbow: the surgical treatment of lateral epicondylitis. J Bone Joint Surg Am 1979;61:832-839.
6. Organ SW, Nirschl RP, Kraushaar BS, et al. Salvage surgery for lateral tennis elbow. Am J Sports Med 1997;25:746-750.
7. Rosenberg N, Henderson I. Surgical treatment of resistant lateral epicondylitis. Follow-up study of 19 patients after excision, release and repair of proximal common extensor tendon origin. Arch Orthop Trauma Surg 2002;122:514-517.
8. Vangsness C, Jobe FW. Surgical treatment of medial epicondylitis: results in 35 elbows. J Bone Joint Surg Br 1991;73:409-411.
9. Wittenberg RH, Schaal S, Muhr G. Surgical treatment of persistent elbow epicondylitis. Clin Orthop 1992;278:73-80.

Suggested Reading

Barrington J, Hage WD. Lateral epicondylitis (tennis elbow): nonoperative, open or arthroscopic treatment? Curr Opin Orthop 2003;14:291-295.

Baumgard SH, Schwartz DR. Percutaneous release of epicondylar muscles for humeral epicondylitis. Am J Sports Med 1982;10:233-236.

Ciccotti MG, Ramani MN. Medial epicondylitis. Tech Hand Up Extrem Surg 2003;7:190-196.

Cohen MS, Romeo AA. Lateral epicondylitis: open and arthroscopic treatment. J Am Soc Surg Hand 2001;1:172-176.

Jobe FW, Ciccotti MG. Lateral and medial epicondylitis of the elbow. J Am Acad Orthop Surg 1994;2:1-8.

Kaminsky SB, Baker CL. Lateral epicondylitis of the elbow. Tech Hand Up Extrem Surg 2003;7:179-189.

Peart RE, Strickler SS, Schweitzer KM. Lateral epicondylitis: a comparative study of open and arthroscopic lateral release. Am J Orthop 2004;33:565-567.

40

CHAPTER 41

Distal Biceps Repair

Robert W. Wysocki, MD

Nikhil N. Verma, MD

Rupture of the distal insertion of the biceps tendon is a relatively rare injury. The majority of ruptures occur proximally; distal ruptures represent only 3% of all biceps tendon ruptures, with an incidence of 1.2 of 100,000 persons per year. Despite being rare, this is an injury that usually occurs in highly functioning middle-aged men, often laborers; left untreated, it is associated with a significant functional and, often, financial loss. In contrast to proximal ruptures, untreated distal rupture more often results in chronic arm pain and weakness in elbow flexion and forearm supination.

Direct anatomic repair of the biceps to its insertion on the radial tuberosity has been shown to restore flexion and supination strength and lead to excellent functional outcomes.[3,13] Numerous repair techniques have been described for acute rupture, including the classic two-incision technique with transosseous suture fixation of Boyd and Anderson. This technique was introduced in an attempt to decrease the incidence of radial nerve injury seen with a similar procedure performed through a single anterior incision.[6] However, because of reports of radioulnar synostosis after the two-incision technique,[11,13] a muscle-splitting posterior approach[5] as well as anterior single-incision techniques with use of suture anchors[4] and more recently the EndoButton[2,9] (Acufex; Smith & Nephew, Inc., Andover, Mass) have been developed. Delayed operative treatment of chronic ruptures may require supplemental soft tissue tendon grafts for restoration of length to the retracted and scarred biceps tendon.[10]

Preoperative Considerations

History

Rupture of the distal biceps tendon is most common in the dominant extremity in middle-aged men. The mechanism of injury is an eccentric load with a sudden extension force being applied to the flexed arm. Often, the patient may report a painful tearing sensation or a "pop" in the antecubital fossa that progresses to a dull ache during a few hours. Variable swelling and ecchymosis may be present, although the lack of these findings does not rule out complete rupture. Chronically, this injury may manifest as activity-related pain and subjective weakness in flexion and supination.[14]

Partial rupture of the distal biceps has been reported.[5] Partial ruptures may present with mild antecubital swelling, decreased range of motion in flexion and supination, and more poorly defined time of onset. In patients without a palpable defect, alternative diagnoses such as cubital bursitis and bicipital tendinosis without rupture must be considered. In general, the diagnosis of partial rupture requires specific imaging modalities (i.e., magnetic resonance imaging).

Physical Examination

Physical examination may demonstrate swelling and ecchymosis in the antecubital fossa as well as loss of the normal contour of the arm with retraction of the biceps muscle belly (Fig. 41-1). In the case of a complete rupture, a defect may be palpable in the antecubital fossa, which is more difficult to appreciate if the bicipital aponeurosis is intact.[14] The defect may also be the only initial clinical sign as to whether a rupture is complete or partial[5]; objective weakness in flexion and supination is common with both and may be exaggerated by pain in the acute setting.

A squeeze test similar to the Thompson test for Achilles tendon rupture has been described[15] and has been shown to be highly effective in diagnosis of biceps rupture.

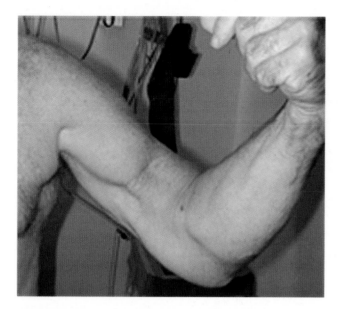

Figure 41-1 Left upper extremity in a patient with chronic distal biceps rupture demonstrating proximal retraction of the muscle belly and resultant "Popeye" sign.

With the patient's forearm rested on the lap, the elbow is held at 60 to 80 degrees to relax the brachialis and in slight pronation to tension the biceps. The examiner firmly squeezes with one hand at the myotendinous junction and the other hand over the biceps muscle belly. An intact biceps should elicit supination of the forearm, and lack of supination is a positive test result.

Similarly, passive forearm supination and pronation should result in myotendinous junction motion with an intact tendon. To test this, the elbow is placed in a 90-degree flexed position. The examiner's fingers are placed over the musculotendinous junction of the biceps, and the forearm is passively rotated. Lack of palpable motion at the musculotendinous junction indicates distal rupture.

Imaging

Although radiographs are typically normal, an anteroposterior, a lateral, and two oblique views are obtained. On occasion, avulsions of the tuberosity have been demonstrated in the acute setting. In the chronic setting, hypertrophic changes of the tuberosity may be noted.[14]

If the physical examination is conclusive, further imaging is not required; but magnetic resonance imaging can help confirm the diagnosis if the physical examination findings are unclear. Magnetic resonance imaging may also help identify the extent and location of injury, which may aid in surgical planning. For example, rupture at the myotendinous junction, although rare, can present difficulty when a standard surgical technique is attempted. In complete ruptures, findings include absence of the tendon distally, fluid-filled tendon sheath, muscle edema, and atrophy (Fig. 41-2).[8] For partial rupture, magnetic resonance

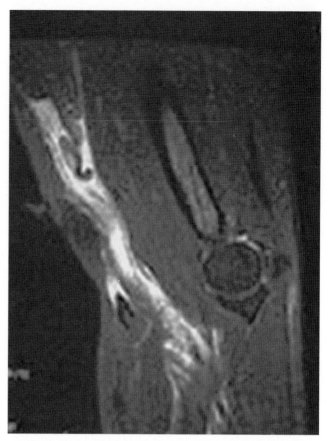

Figure 41-2 Sagittal T2-weighted magnetic resonance image demonstrating complete rupture of distal biceps tendon with proximal retraction and significant fluid within biceps sheath distally.

imaging can reveal high signal and fluid within the tendon or surrounding the tendon as it approaches the tuberosity, but one should be able to appreciate tendon all the way to the insertion on the tuberosity.

Other possible diagnoses, including cubital bursitis, biceps tendinosis, biceps hematoma, and brachialis contusion, can also be evaluated and differentiated on magnetic resonance imaging.[8] Ultrasonography has also been shown to be an inexpensive and reliable method to confirm diagnosis of biceps rupture, although this technique requires a skilled ultrasonographer for accurate interpretation.

Indications and Contraindications

Long-term functional deficits with loss of both supination and flexion strength after complete rupture have been clearly demonstrated.[13] Therefore, most healthy, active individuals should be strongly considered for operative repair. Nonoperative management should be considered ideally for elderly or sedentary patients with relatively low functional demand or those with comorbidities resulting in considerable increased risk with surgery.

In preoperative planning, it is important to identify the chronicity of the injury as well as whether the bicipital aponeurosis is intact. Delayed presentation secondary to missed diagnosis, the patient's neglect, or failure of conservative treatment is not uncommon. Because of poor tissue quality, altered anatomy, and retraction of the tendon with scarring of the biceps to the brachialis, delayed surgery is often difficult and may require allograft or autograft tendon reconstruction, especially if the bicipital aponeurosis is not intact.[14]

Treatment of partial ruptures initially consists of a trial of nonoperative management. Treatment modalities include anti-inflammatories, splinting, and physical therapy. Although formal outcomes of nonoperative management have not been reported, our experience with conservative management of partial tears is associated with limited improvement. If it is indicated, surgical management should include tendon release and reattachment to the radial tuberosity, yielding primarily excellent results.[5]

Surgical Technique

Anesthesia and Positioning

Our preferred anesthesia is a regional block, most commonly axillary or supraclavicular, which may minimize anesthetic morbidity and provide improved postoperative pain control. The patient is positioned supine with the arm on an arm board.

Surgical Landmarks, Incisions, and Portals

Our preferred incision for the EndoButton technique described below is a hockey stick–type incision along the medial border of the brachioradialis curving medially over the antecubital fossa in the elbow crease (Fig. 41-3). Alternative incisions are a transverse skin incision just distal to the elbow skin crease and a longitudinal incision as in a standard anterior Henry approach.

Specific Steps (Box 41-1)

EndoButton Technique[2,9]

1. Approach

The lateral antebrachial cutaneous nerve is identified and protected, and dissection is carried down toward the radial tuberosity (Fig. 41-4). The brachioradialis is retracted laterally, and the biceps tendon sheath is identified. Multiple recurrent branches of the radial artery may be encountered and should be ligated with endovascular clips. An inflammatory bursa at the former site of the tendon attachment may be encountered. Division of the lacertus fibrosus

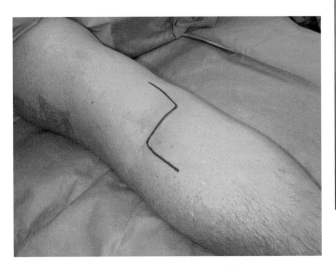

Figure 41-3 Typical anterior incision for the single-incision approach to chronic biceps tendon rupture. In acute cases, a smaller approach eliminating the proximal arm of the Z can be used.

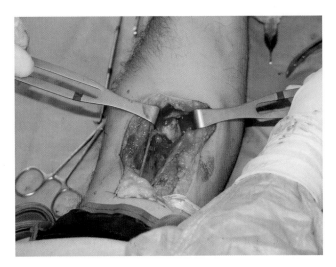

Figure 41-4 Dissection carried down to expose the radial tuberosity.

Box 41-1 Surgical Steps

1. Approach
2. Tuberosity preparation
3. Tendon preparation
4. Fixation
5. Closure

may be necessary for full access to the retracted biceps tendon.

During dissection, the elbow should be maintained in a supinated position. This allows improved access to the bicipital tuberosity and moves the posterior interosseus nerve laterally to improve the margin of safety. Care must

41

be taken to avoid vigorous retraction on the lateral side because the radial nerve is at risk. The tuberosity may be partially covered by the superior aspect of the supinator muscle, which can be retracted distally by blunt dissection.

2. Tuberosity Preparation

Once the tuberosity is sufficiently exposed, the tunnel for the EndoButton-tendon construct is prepared (Fig. 41-5). The tunnel should be located as medially in the radial tuberosity as possible with the forearm supinated to re-create the most anatomic location for the tendon. Our preferred technique is to establish a cortical window for the tendon on the anterior surface of the tuberosity by use of a high-speed bur. Next, a guide pin for the EndoButton cannulated drill is placed through the anterior tunnel through the posterior cortex to exit the skin posteriorly. This is then overdrilled with the EndoButton drill. Alternatively, the guide wire can be placed first and the anterior cortical tunnel made with a 6- or 7-mm cannulated acorn reamer.

3. Tendon Preparation

Next, the tendon stump is prepared. After the distal end of the biceps tendon is completely freed and the degenerated or necrotic portion is resected, a running locking type of suture is placed with a strong, braided No. 2 or No. 5 equivalent nonabsorbable suture. The starting point, and thus the location of the knot, should be about 2 to 3 cm proximal to the distal end of the tendon, allowing for adjustment of the knot later if needed (Fig. 41-6). Each suture passage must be tensioned in the tendon to prevent later elongation. The suture is advanced proximally on the tendon for about 2 cm and then distally exits the tendon end. The suture limb is then passed through the button before reentering the tendon to complete the loop. The knot should be tied leaving a maximum 2- to 3-mm gap between the button and the free tendon end to allow the button to be manipulated and "flipped" over the dorsal cortex.

4. Fixation

The two outer holes of the EndoButton are then each threaded with a different color suture to identify the sutures as they draw the EndoButton into the socket and onto the posterior cortex (Fig. 41-7). A Beath pin is advanced through the hole at the base of the tuberosity socket from anterior to posterior; the four suture ends (two ends of two sutures of different colors) are threaded through the eyelet, and the pin is withdrawn out the skin of the posterior forearm with the elbow in 90 degrees of flexion (Fig. 41-8). The two sutures are separated (with two strands each), and one is used to pull the EndoButton into and through the socket and drill hole in the posterior cortex (Fig. 41-9). Once the button clears the posterior cortex, the other suture is tensioned to flip the button onto the posterior cortex (Fig. 41-10). This process of button passage can be facilitated with fluoroscopic guidance. The sutures are carefully removed by pulling them out through the posterior stab wound.

5. Closure

After thorough irrigation, the skin is closed with interrupted 2-0 absorbable subcutaneous sutures and a running 3-0 absorbable subcuticular stitch. The arm is placed in a posterior splint with the elbow in 90 degrees of flexion and neutral rotation.

PEARLS AND PITFALLS

- The lateral antebrachial cutaneous nerve must be identified and protected throughout the case.
- Maintain the forearm in supination while working around the radial tuberosity to move the posterior interosseous nerve radially for increased protection.
- In placing the tendon suture, the first pass into the tendon should begin about 2 to 3 cm proximal to the tendon's edge. There should be no more than a 2- to 3-mm distance between the EndoButton and the tendon edge to achieve the maximal amount of tendon in the tunnel yet still allow the EndoButton to flip on the dorsal cortex.
- Use a FluoroScan to confirm that the EndoButton is properly flipped along the posterior radial cortex.

Postoperative Considerations

Follow-up

Patients are seen in the office between 7 and 10 days postoperatively for suture removal.

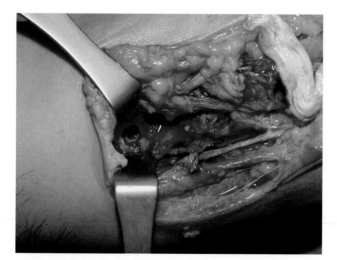

Figure 41-5 The prepared EndoButton tunnel in the radial tuberosity.

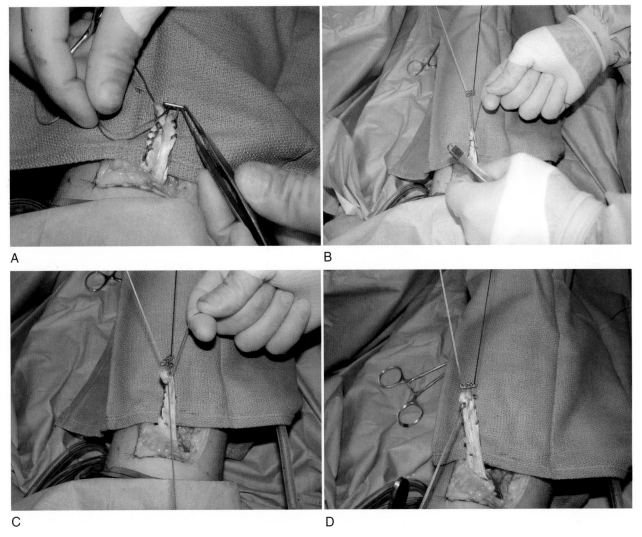

Figure 41-6 Preparation of the tendon. After the running suture finishes 2 to 3 cm proximal to the distal edge and is looped through the button **(A)**, the two ends are held and tensioned **(B)** so that the button is brought to within 2 to 3 mm of the tendon end **(C)**, and the knot is tied **(D)**.

Rehabilitation

- Splint in 90 degrees of flexion and neutral rotation until first postoperative visit at 7 to 10 days.
- A hinged elbow brace or removable posterior mold at 90 degrees of flexion is placed at the first postoperative visit.
- Initiate passive and active-assisted range of motion from 30 degrees to full flexion and increase to full extension by 6 weeks postoperatively.
- Unrestricted motion is permitted and strengthening is initiated at 6 weeks postoperatively.
- Return to unrestricted activities is allowed at 16 to 20 weeks postoperatively.

Alternative Techniques

Modified Two-Incision Technique

The original Boyd-Anderson technique describes a primary incision in the antecubital fossa and a secondary incision in the posterolateral forearm.[6] This technique, although effective, was found to be complicated by radioulnar synostosis attributed to aggressive elevation of the anconeus off the proximal ulna, with damage to the proximal interosseous membrane.[11,13] Agins[1] modified the original procedure first by a smaller anterior transverse incision and use of a small osteotome through a small posterior incision rather than a bur to form a trough for reattachment of the biceps tendon.

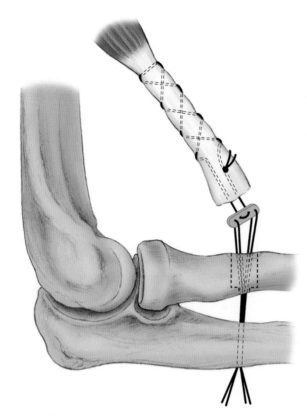

Figure 41-7 Diagram depicting single-incision EndoButton technique. The EndoButton is secured to the tendon, and passing sutures are placed through the posterior cortical tunnel ready for tendon passage. (Redrawn with permission from Greenberg JA, Fernandez JJ, Wang T, Turner C. EndoButton-assisted repair of distal biceps tendon ruptures. J Shoulder Elbow Surg 2003;12:484-490.)

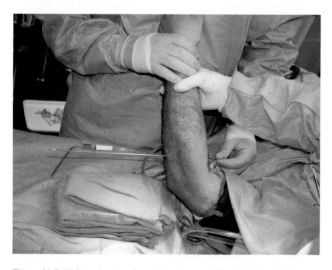

Figure 41-8 All four strands of passing suture are threaded through the eyelet of the guide wire and passed through the tuberosity tunnel and out the posterior skin.

Bourne and Morrey[5] suggested passing a blunt hemostat through the usual path of the biceps tendon until it is palpable on the posterior skin, then making the posterior incision over the instrument's tip. Rather than taking the supinator off the ulna, this technique allows the

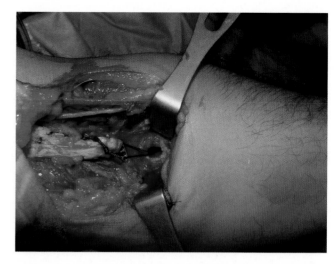

Figure 41-9 The tendon with EndoButton, prepared to be pulled through the tunnel by use of the passing sutures as kite strings.

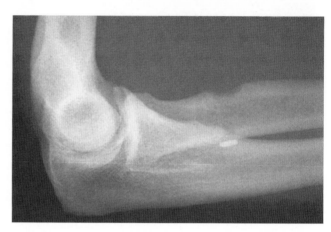

Figure 41-10 Lateral postoperative radiograph. Note the anterior cortical tunnel and the EndoButton securely seated in a horizontal fashion directly against the posterior cortex. (Reproduced with permission from Greenberg JA, Fernandez JJ, Wang T, Turner C. EndoButton-assisted repair of distal biceps tendon ruptures. J Shoulder Elbow Surg 2003;12:484-490.)

radial tuberosity to be exposed from the posterior incision by splitting the supinator and common extensor, requiring no muscle to be taken off the ulna and theoretically decreasing the risk of radioulnar synostosis (Fig. 41-11). During this posterior approach, the forearm is pronated to bring the tuberosity into view and to protect the posterior interosseous nerve.

Currently the most common technique is either a transverse or longitudinal (Henry) 3- to 5-cm incision anteriorly over the antecubital fossa to retrieve and débride the biceps tendon. As mentioned before, Bunnell-type or other running grasping sutures are used to secure the distal end of the tendon. With the forearm supinated, a hemostat is advanced along the medial border of the radial tuberosity to the dorsolateral forearm as described by Bourne and Morrey,[5] and an incision is made over the instrument's tip. One must be careful not to violate the

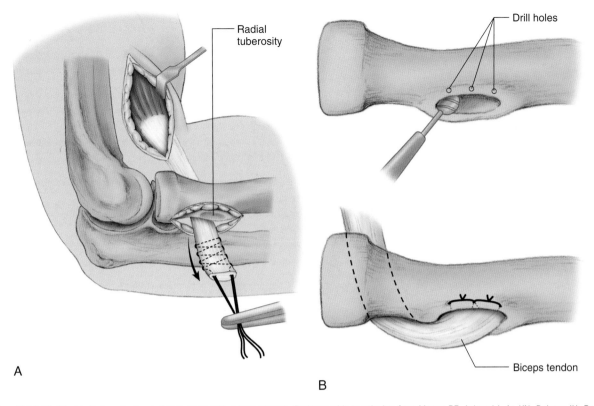

Radial
tuberosity

Drill holes

Biceps tendon

A

B

Figure 41-11 Modified technique for two-incision repair with a bone tunnel. (Redrawn with permission from Morrey BF, Askew LJ, An KN, Dobyns JH. Rupture of the distal tendon of the biceps brachii. A biomechanical study. J Bone Joint Surg Am 1985;67:418-421.)

periosteum of the ulna. With the forearm in maximal pronation, this posterior incision is carried down to the radial tuberosity by splitting the extensor muscle mass and supinator in line with their fibers. A bur or osteotome is then used to make a cavitary opening in the tuberosity large enough to pass the tendon through. Small drill holes are then made along the margin of the cavitary opening unicortically, one for each Bunnell strand. Once the biceps tendon is passed into the tunnel, the suture ends are passed back up through the drill holes and tied over a bone bridge. Rehabilitation is similar to that for the single-incision technique.

Delayed Treatment with Hamstring Allograft

Delayed treatment of distal biceps rupture is not uncommon and is complicated by tendon retraction, scarring to the brachialis, distorted anatomy, and poor-quality tissue. Especially in cases in which the bicipital aponeurosis is torn, the tendon may be retracted to the degree that a primary repair to the radial tuberosity either is impossible or would leave the patient with an unacceptable flexion contracture. In these cases, supplementary grafts are often needed, and grafting with fascia lata, palmaris longus,

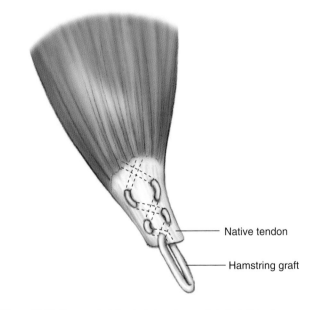

Native tendon

Hamstring graft

Figure 41-12 Diagram depicting technique for weaving allograft tendon through the native biceps muscle in cases of delayed reconstruction. (Redrawn with permission from Hallam P, Bain GI. Repair of chronic distal biceps tendon ruptures using autologous hamstring graft and the Endobutton. J Shoulder Elbow Surg 2004;13:648-651.)

Table 41-1 Results of Various Surgical Repair Techniques

Author	Methodology	Results
Bain et al[2] (2000)	12 patients EndoButton technique	All patients satisfied with result, returned to normal activities of daily living, and had subjective 5/5 strength when rehabilitated
Baker and Bierwagen[3] (1985)	13 patients 3 nonoperative treatments vs. 10 two-incision repairs Both groups compared with controls	Nonoperative: 55% weaker in flexion and 86% less supination endurance than control; 40% weaker in flexion and 79% less supination endurance than Boyd Two-incision: repair of dominant arm equal to nondominant in strength and endurance
El-Hawary et al[7] (2003)	Direct comparison of 9 one-incision repairs with two suture anchors vs. 10 modified two-incision repairs	Strength: no difference at 1 year, but slower recovery in one-incision group Range of motion: greater flexion in one-incision group at 1 year SF-36 scores: no difference Complications: more with one incision, especially lateral antebrachial cutaneous nerve injury
Greenberg et al[9] (2003)	14 patients, EndoButton, 20-month follow-up Cadaveric pullout strength in Boyd bone tunnel vs. one suture anchor vs. EndoButton	97% flexion and 82% supination strength compared with uninjured arm EndoButton pullout strength 3 times greater than Boyd, 2 times greater than single suture anchor
Karunakar et al[11] (1999)	21 patients, average 44-month follow-up Two-incision technique	100% good–excellent results 48% had supination weakness, 14% had flexion weakness Endurance decreased 38% in supination, 33% in flexion compared with uninjured arm Complications: 15% heterotopic ossification, one radioulnar synostosis
McKee et al[12] (2005)	53 patients One-incision technique with two suture anchors	DASH questionnaire: no difference from control in functional scores Strength: 96% flexion, 93% supination compared with uninjured side No repeated rupture, synostosis, or difference in range of motion

DASH, Disabilities of the Arm, Shoulder, and Hand; SF-36, short form 36 health survey.

Achilles tendon, and flexor carpi radialis has been described.

Our preferred grafting technique uses either allograft or autologous semitendinosus tendon for reconstruction. This technique combines the EndoButton principle with hamstring allograft for late reconstruction.[10] The initial stages are as described earlier for the EndoButton technique to prepare the tuberosity. The autograft tendon is then weaved through the distal biceps tendon (Fig. 41-12) with the free ends proximal so that they can be tensioned and shortened for appropriate graft length. Once the appropriate length is confirmed, the free ends are sutured together with nonabsorbable braided suture. Similar suture is passed through the two center holes of the Endo-Button and sutured in a running fashion to the medial and lateral arms of the graft to provide fixation of the biceps-graft complex to the button. As previously described for

acute rupture, the graft complex with the EndoButton is then passed through the radial tuberosity and flipped over the posterior cortex.

Results

Good to excellent results with regard to both elimination of pain and recovery of strength and function have been reported after single-incision and two-incision techniques for distal biceps tendon repair (Table 41-1). Potential complications include radioulnar synostosis with the two-incision technique and injury to the lateral antebrachial cutaneous nerve or radial nerve with the single-incision techniques. With either technique, repeated rupture is a rare but possible occurrence.

References

1. Agins HJ, Chess JL, Hoekstra DV, Teitge RA. Rupture of the distal insertion of the biceps brachii tendon. Clin Orthop 1988;234: 34-38.

2. Bain GI, Prem H, Heptinstall RJ, et al. Repair of distal biceps tendon rupture: a new technique using the Endobutton. J Shoulder Elbow Surg 2000;9:120-126.

3. Baker BE, Bierwagen D. Rupture of the distal tendon of the biceps brachii. Operative versus nonoperative treatment. J Bone Joint Surg Am 1985;67:414-417.

4. Barnes SJ, Coleman SG, Gilpin D. Repair of avulsed insertion of biceps. A new technique in four cases. J Bone Joint Surg Br 1993;75:938-939.

5. Bourne MH, Morrey BF. Partial rupture of the distal biceps tendon. Clin Orthop 1991;271:143-148.

6. Boyd HB, Anderson LD. A method for reinsertion of the distal biceps brachii tendon. J Bone Joint Surg Am 1961;43:1041-1043.

7. El-Hawary R, Macdermid JC, Faber KJ, et al. Distal biceps tendon repair: comparison of surgical techniques. J Hand Surg Am 2003;28:496-502.

8. Falchook FS, Zlatkin MB, Erbacher GE, et al. Rupture of the distal biceps tendon: evaluation with MR imaging. Radiology 1994;190: 659-663.

9. Greenberg JA, Fernandez JJ, Wang T, Turner C. EndoButton-assisted repair of distal biceps tendon ruptures. J Shoulder Elbow Surg 2003;12:484-490.

10. Hallam P, Bain GI. Repair of chronic distal biceps tendon ruptures using autologous hamstring graft and the EndoButton. J Shoulder Elbow Surg 2004;13:648-651.

11. Karunakar MA, Cha P, Stern PJ. Distal biceps ruptures. A follow-up of Boyd and Anderson repair. Clin Orthop 1999;363:100-107.

12. McKee MD, Hirji R, Schemitsch EH, et al. Patient-oriented functional outcome after repair of distal biceps tendon ruptures using a single-incision technique. J Shoulder Elbow Surg 2005;14:302-306.

13. Morrey BF, Askew LJ, An KN, Dobyns JH. Rupture of the distal tendon of the biceps brachii. A biomechanical study. J Bone Joint Surg Am 1985;67:418-421.

14. Ramsey ML. Distal biceps tendon injuries: diagnosis and management. J Am Acad Orthop Surg 1999;7:199-207.

15. Ruland RT, Dunbar SR, Bowen JD. The biceps squeeze test for diagnosis of distal biceps tendon ruptures. Clin Orthop 2005;437:128-131.

41

PART 3

The Knee

CHAPTER **42**

Patient Positioning, Portal Placement, and Normal Arthroscopic Anatomy

Melissa D. Koenig, MD
Robin V. West, MD

Identification

The Joint Commission on Accreditation of Healthcare Organizations adopted a protocol in 2004 to prevent wrong site surgery. The American Academy of Orthopaedic Surgeons has been working on this same issue since 1997. Implementation varies from hospital to hospital, but in general, the surgeon or a "credentialed provider" on the surgical team places his or her initials on the operative site in indelible ink before administration of anesthesia. No other marking, such as an X, is recommended because it may be misinterpreted. The initials should be located in a region that remains visible after preparation and draping. Finally, during a "time-out" with the surgical team and operating room nurse, the site is confirmed again with the surgeon and the consent before an incision is made.

Anesthesia

Several factors contribute to the decision of which type of anesthesia is most appropriate for a given patient. The decision to use local, regional, or general anesthesia depends on the planned procedure, the general health of the patient, and the preference of the patient, anesthesiologist, and surgeon.

Local Anesthesia

Before knee arthroscopy is performed by use of local anesthetic with or without intravenous sedation, several factors are considered. The anesthesia team may need to convert to an alternative form of anesthesia if airway management becomes difficult. With this technique, patients generally do not tolerate use of a tourniquet. In some cases, patients may experience discomfort during manipulation of the leg and introduction of instruments into the knee. For these reasons, short procedures that do not require excess manipulation or bone work are best suited for local anesthesia. Suitable procedures include diagnostic arthroscopy, synovial biopsy, removal of loose body, and partial meniscectomy. Advantages of this technique are low morbidity, low cost, and ease of recovery. A combination of lidocaine and bupivacaine (Marcaine) is typically used to provide short-term and long-term pain relief. Epinephrine can be used in combination with the anesthetic to aid in hemostasis.

Regional Anesthesia

Regional anesthetic options include spinal, epidural, and femoral nerve anesthesia. For patients whose medical issues put them at increased risk with general anesthesia, regional anesthesia provides satisfactory anesthesia for most arthroscopic knee procedures. Tourniquet use is generally well tolerated with these techniques. Possible complications are spinal puncture and spinal headache.

General Anesthesia

Newer anesthetic agents continue to make general anesthesia safer with easier recovery. Complete muscle relaxation with general anesthesia allows better visualization of the joint. Tourniquet and bone work are tolerated by the patient. Patients may have throat irritation with the use of an endotracheal tube.

Patient Positioning

The patient is positioned supine on a standard operating table. If a tourniquet is used, a layer of padding is placed on the thigh before its application. In our institution, we rarely use a tourniquet, relying instead on the epinephrine in the local anesthetic and pump pressure to ensure adequate visualization during the procedure. We prefer not to use a tourniquet because of data that show an adverse effect on quadriceps function postoperatively when it is used.

On the basis of the surgeon's preferences, one of two set-ups is used at our hospital. In the first, the patient lies supine on the table with the feet just short of the end of the table. The nonoperative leg is protected with foam padding. The operative leg is flexed to 90 degrees. A sandbag is taped to the table for the foot to rest on when the knee is flexed. A lateral post is attached to the table at the level of the distal thigh. The post helps stabilize the leg when a valgus force is applied to visualize the medial compartment. This method allows easy access to all aspects of the knee. However, an assistant is generally required to manipulate the leg during the case.

The other option entails placement of the thigh in a leg holder and flexion of the foot of the table. On the table, the patient's operative knee must be just distal to the level of the break in the bed. The operative leg is placed into a leg holder. The opposite leg is placed into a well-leg holder and protected with foam under the knee. The operative leg is manipulated by placing it on the surgeon's pelvis or thigh and applying a varus or valgus stress at the knee. If the leg holder is too tight, it can act as a venous tourniquet and cause bleeding during surgery. Whereas this method eliminates the need for an assistant, there is no support for the leg when it is in extension. Also, larger thighs may not fit well in the leg holder.

Examination Under Anesthesia

After the administration of anesthesia, a thorough examination is performed, including range of motion, patellar glide, instability tests, and documentation of an effusion. The contralateral knee is used as a comparison. Certain tests, such as a pivot shift, are better tolerated when the patient is completely relaxed. The findings of the examination are documented in the operative report. The surgeon also correlates the examination with the arthroscopic findings.

Arthroscopic Equipment

Arthroscopic equipment has continually improved in the years since its introduction. Better optical systems and the introduction of new instruments have broadened the number of ailments that can be treated arthroscopically. The scope of this chapter does not allow a comprehensive overview of all possible equipment.

Arthroscopes are described by their angle of inclination. A 0-degree scope looks straight-ahead; a 30-degree scope views at a 30-degree angle from the axis of the arthroscope. Rotation of the arthroscope increases the field of view compared with the straight-ahead view from a 0-degree scope. The 30-degree scope is used most commonly; a 70-degree scope is used for added visualization in tight spaces.

A surgeon uses the arthroscopic probe as an extension of his or her finger. The probe palpates various structures and provides tactile assessment of their condition. The probe can also be used as a measuring device for lesions in the joint. Most probe tips are calibrated to a known length, typically 3 mm. Besides assessing the menisci, articular cartilage, and ligaments, a probe can maneuver loose bodies into positions that facilitate their retrieval.

Arthroscopic biters are used to remove soft tissues, such as a torn meniscus or an anterior cruciate stump. These instruments come in a variety of shapes and sizes. The heads are angled in different directions to facilitate removal from areas that are difficult to reach. Use of an angled up-biter in the medial compartment helps the surgeon to reach the posterior meniscus by taking advantage of the convex nature of the medial tibial plateau.

Other instruments include graspers, scissors, motorized shavers and burs, and electrocautery devices. Various procedure-specific guides have been developed to assist in surgeries such as ligament reconstruction. The surgeon should take some time to become familiar with the instruments available from the hospital and various companies.

Arthroscopy Portals

Inferolateral Portal

The inferolateral portal, also called the anterolateral portal, is traditionally used as the viewing portal through which the camera is inserted. The portal is made in the palpable soft spot just off the lateral border of the patellar tendon at the level of the inferior border of the patella. We prefer to keep this portal "high and tight" to avoid entry through the fat pad. The anterior portion of the lateral meniscus is also at risk with inferior placement of this portal. Excessive medial placement of the portal risks damage to the patellar tendon.

Inferomedial Portal

The inferomedial (or anteromedial) portal is used primarily as a working portal. The incision is made in the medial soft spot, just medial to the patellar tendon approximately 1 cm below the inferior border of the patella. To prevent injury to the medial meniscus when the portal is established, it can be made under direct visualization after localization with a spinal needle.

Superomedial Portal

Historically, this portal was used for inflow or outflow of arthroscopy fluid. The portal is made 2 cm proximal to the superomedial border of the patella. The incision should be next to but not through the quadriceps tendon. During insertion, the trocar is angled into the suprapatellar pouch to avoid damage to the articular cartilage of the patella. If multiple passes are made through the soft tissues during insertion, fluid leak may occur and prevent adequate joint distention. To avoid trauma to the vastus medialis obliquus muscle, we do not routinely use this portal. Instead, we prefer to use a double-port cannula that allows inflow and outflow through the inferolateral portal. Studies have shown that use of the superomedial portal results in longer return of quadriceps strength and less total strength than with a standard two-portal technique.

Superolateral Portal (Fig. 42-1)

The superolateral portal allows visualization of the patellofemoral articulation, use for inflow or outflow, and removal of loose bodies from the suprapatellar pouch. This portal is made 2 cm proximal to the superolateral border of the patella. Entry through the interval between the vastus lateralis and the iliotibial band avoids injury to these structures. Use of the 70-degree arthroscope through the superolateral portal gives an excellent view of the patellofemoral articulation (Fig. 42-1).

Posterolateral Portal

Although it is rarely used, knowledge of this portal can facilitate repair of the posterior horn of the lateral

42

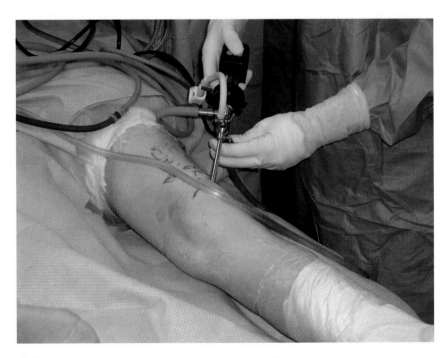

Figure 42-1 The arthroscope in the superolateral portal, viewing the patellofemoral articulation.

meniscus, removal of loose bodies, and synovectomy. The portal is made posterior to the lateral collateral ligament and anterior to the biceps tendon and the common peroneal nerve.

Posteromedial Portal (Fig. 42-3)

The posteromedial portal is established to view and to access the posterior portion of the medial compartment.

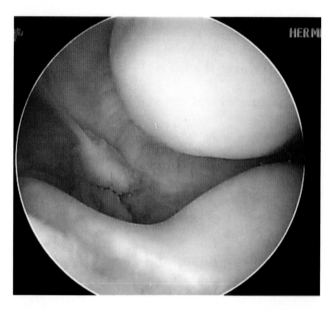

Figure 42-2 The patellofemoral view as seen from the superolateral portal with use of the 70-degree arthroscope.

This portal provides access to the tibial insertion of the posterior cruciate ligament and the posterior horn of the medial meniscus. The portal is marked preoperatively before the joint distends. The portal lies 2 cm above the joint line, 1 to 2 cm posterior to the medial femoral epicondyle. As establishment of this portal has a high risk of chondral or meniscal damage, we recommend use of a spinal needle under direct visualization to ensure accurate placement.

Transpatellar Tendon Portal

To establish this portal, a vertical slit is made in the central portion of the patellar tendon. This portal provides direct access to the intracondylar notch for either visualization or interference screw placement. Because of the risks of tendon irritation or rupture, this portal is rarely used.

Arthroscopic Evaluation

Each surgeon needs to develop a systematic, reproducible method of examining the intra-articular structures of the knee. Multiple pictures are taken throughout the examination to document the findings of the procedure. Our systematic approach is described.

As the knee is extended, the blunt trocar is introduced into the suprapatellar pouch through the inferolateral portal. The pouch is inspected for loose bodies and adhesions from previous surgery. The camera is slowly

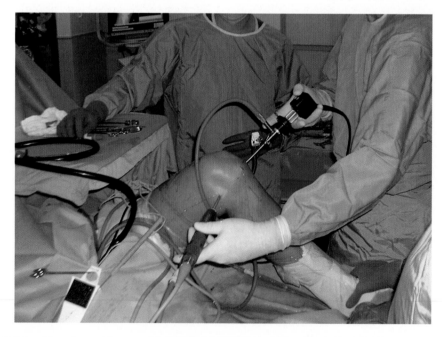

Figure 42-3 The posteromedial portal can be used to access the posterior compartment to aid in removal of loose bodies, to view the posterior horn of the medial meniscus, or to perform a posterior cruciate ligament reconstruction.

pulled back until the undersurface of the patella comes into view. Cartilage damage or osteophyte formation is evaluated. The camera is rotated to view the trochlea. Cartilage damage is noted, and patellar tracking in the trochlear groove is assessed (Fig. 42-4). The superolateral portal provides the best view of the patellofemoral joint. The 70-degree arthroscope aids in visualization from this portal.

The lateral and medial gutters are visualized by passing the arthroscope across each condyle. The gutters are visualized all the way down to the joint line. On the lateral side, loose bodies may settle in the popliteal hiatus, so this area must be inspected.

The medial compartment is entered by following the trochlea down into the intercondylar notch. A veil of tissue, the ligamentum mucosum, often covers the cruciate ligaments (Fig. 42-5). This tissue is either pulled aside with a probe or removed with a motorized shaver. The substance of the cruciates and their visible insertions are carefully inspected. Again, a probe is valuable in assessing the tension of the ligaments.

To enter the lateral compartment, a triangular space formed by the lateral border of the anterior cruciate ligament, the anterior horn of the lateral meniscus, and the lateral femoral condyle is identified. The arthroscope is directed into this space as the leg is placed into a figure-of-four position. An assistant can apply a varus stress by placing pressure on the medial aspect of the knee to open the joint further. The lateral meniscus is inspected and probed (Fig. 42-6). The popliteal tendon is seen passing through the popliteal hiatus. The leg is fully extended and flexed to assess the articular cartilage of the lateral compartment. If the scope is backed into the intercondylar notch with the knee in the figure-of-four position, the

posterolateral bundle of the anterior cruciate ligament can be well visualized (Fig. 42-7).

The medial compartment is then entered (Fig. 42-8). With varying degrees of flexion and valgus, the majority of the medial meniscus is clearly visualized. The camera is rotated to see the posterior horn more clearly. A probe is used to further assess the meniscus. The cartilage of the medial femoral condyle and the medial tibial plateau is examined for degeneration. The knee is flexed and extended to fully visualize the condyle.

In certain procedures, the posteromedial compartment needs to be assessed. Either the posteromedial portal or the Gilchrist view can be used to assess the posterior compartment. By the Gilchrist view, the posterior compartment can be viewed with the arthroscope in the

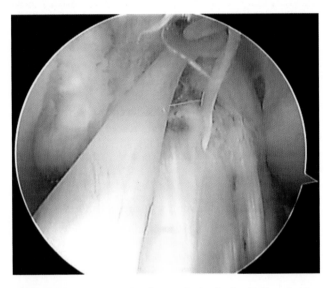

Figure 42-5 The anterior cruciate ligament is visualized under the veil of the ligamentum mucosum.

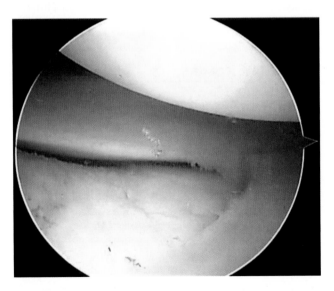

Figure 42-6 The lateral compartment.

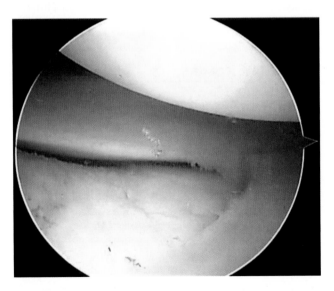

Figure 42-4 The patellofemoral joint as seen from the anterolateral portal with the 30-degree arthroscope.

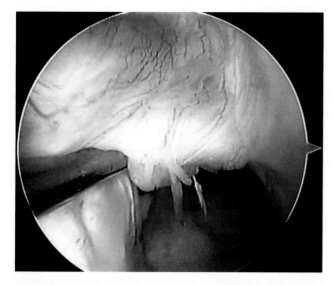

Figure 42-7 Viewing the posterolateral bundle of the anterior cruciate ligament in the figure-of-four position.

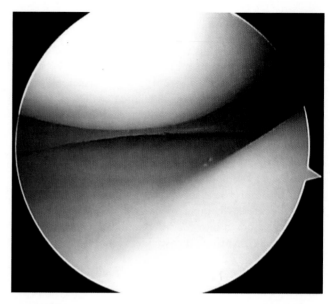

Figure 42-8 The medial compartment.

anterolateral portal. The knee is flexed to 90 degrees and held in position against a sandbag placed preoperatively. A 70-degree arthroscope is carefully advanced between the medial femoral condyle and the posterior cruciate ligament. Rotation of the arthroscope downward brings the posterior horn of the meniscus into view. This view also locates loose bodies in the posterior compartment and shows the tibial insertion of the posterior cruciate ligament.

Postoperative Course

The portals can be closed with either a nonabsorbable or an absorbable monofilament suture. An ice machine is used to help provide postoperative hemostasis and to decrease inflammation. Exercises, including quadriceps sets, straight-leg raises, heel slides, and calf pumps, are started immediately after surgery. Crutches are used initially until the quadriceps function returns (typically a few days). Physical therapy is generally started the week after surgery. Narcotic pain medication is prescribed and selected on the basis of the procedure, the patient's allergies, and the surgeon's preference. An anti-inflammatory can be used for the first week to potentiate the narcotic medication. Preoperative intravenous antibiotics are routinely administered at our institution, and postoperative oral antibiotics are prescribed only for longer arthroscopic procedures (i.e., multiple ligament reconstruction).

Suggested Reading

Brophy RH, Dunn WR, Wickiewicz TL. Arthroscopic portal placement. Tech Knee Surg 2004;3:2-7.

Iossifidis A. Knee arthroscopy under local anesthesia: results and evaluation of patients' satisfaction. Injury 1996;27:43-44.

Joint Commission on the Accreditation of Healthcare Organizations. Universal Protocol for Preventing Wrong Site, Wrong Procedure, Wrong Person Surgery, 2003.

Kim SJ, Kim HJ. High portal: practical philosophy for positioning portals in knee arthroscopy. Arthroscopy 2001;17:333-337.

Ochi M, Adachi N, Sumen Y, et al. A new guide system for posteromedial portal in arthroscopic knee surgery. Arch Orthop Trauma Surg 1998;118:25-28.

Ogilvie-Harris DJ, Biggs DJ, Mackay M, Weisleder L. Posterior portal for arthroscopic surgery of the knee. Arthroscopy 1994;10:608-613.

Ong BC, Shen FH, Musahl V, et al. Knee: patient positioning, portal placement, and normal arthroscopic anatomy. In Miller MD, Cole BJ, eds. Textbook of Arthroscopy. Philadelphia, Elsevier, 2004:463-469.

Stetson WB, Templin K. Two- versus three-portal technique for routine knee arthroscopy. Am J Sports Med 2002;30:108-111.

Wu WH, Richmond JC. Arthroscopy of the knee: basic setup and technique. In McGinty JB, Burkhart SS, Jackson RW, et al, eds. Operative Arthroscopy. Philadelphia, Lippincott Williams & Wilkins, 2003:211-217.

Arthroscopic Meniscectomy

David C. Flanigan, MD
Christopher Kaeding, MD

Tears of the meniscus have been known to cause pain and mechanical symptoms of the knee. Historically, open meniscectomy has been shown to lead to the development of progressive radiographic signs (Fairbank changes) of osteoarthritis in the meniscus-deficient compartment. With the advent of arthroscopy, partial, subtotal, or total meniscectomy can be performed with minimal incisions and on an outpatient basis. In fact, arthroscopic meniscectomy is the most commonly performed orthopedic procedure in the United States. Despite the minimally invasive nature of arthroscopy and its faster recovery, radiographic changes can still be seen with partial meniscectomies because of the increased articular contact pressures. The goal of arthroscopic meniscectomy today is to remove as little meniscal tissue as possible to achieve a pain-free, stable meniscus.

Preoperative Considerations

History

Patients typically recall an acute sudden twisting mechanism that caused the onset of pain. Degenerative tears may be more subacute in nature and subtle in onset with underlying arthritic or baseline pain that has now become localized and sharp. A detailed history of previous knee pain, previous surgeries in the knee, and other injuries (ligament injury, fracture) should be elicited.

Symptoms

- Medial or lateral compartment pain, often posteriorly
- Pain with deep knee bending, walking, twisting mechanisms, activity
- Sensation of "giving way"
- Mechanical symptoms: catching, locking, clicking
- Continuous or recurrent effusions

Physical Examination

A thorough knee examination is crucial because meniscal tears are commonly associated with other injuries, such as anterior cruciate ligament injuries and tibial plateau fractures. A detailed knee examination has been consistently shown to be reliable in diagnosis of a meniscal tear.

Specific findings for meniscal tears may include the following:

- Antalgic gait
- Pain with squatting
- Loss of motion
- Locked knee
- Effusion
- Joint line tenderness
- Pain with hyperflexion or hyperextension
- Positive result of McMurray test
- Perimeniscal cysts or Baker cyst

Imaging

Baseline plain radiography is of limited importance for diagnosis of meniscal disorders but is necessary to rule out other pathologic processes, such as stress fracture, avascular necrosis, tumor, and arthritis, that may mimic meniscal signs and symptoms. Standard radiographs include a 45-degree flexed posteroanterior view, weight-bearing anteroposterior view, lateral view, and Merchant view.

Magnetic resonance imaging is not a substitute for a good examination, but it can be a useful tool to confirm the diagnosis or to differentiate pathologic changes in difficult cases. Meniscal tears on magnetic resonance imaging are described as abnormal meniscal signal that extends to the articular surface of the meniscus (grade 3 meniscal signal). Numerous studies have shown that the accuracy of magnetic resonance imaging is 95% or greater for meniscal tears.

Classification

Arthroscopic evaluation has aided in the classification of meniscal tears. Meniscal tears can be classified by vascular zone or tear patterns. Both classifications are often used in determining whether a tear is favorable for repair.

Arnoczky and Warren[2] reported on the vascularity of the meniscus, which is divided into three zones: red-red (peripheral 25% to 33%) , red-white, and white-white (central 33%). Healing has been found to be more favorable in the vascular zones (i.e., red-red and red-white).

Meniscal tears are commonly described by tear pattern. Examples of common tear patterns are illustrated in Figure 43-1.

Indications and Contraindications

Meniscectomy is indicated for any symptomatic meniscal tear that is abnormally mobile or not conducive to repair and has failed conservative measures.

Contraindications are active septic arthritis and significant medical comorbidities.

Instruments

Multiple manufacturers have produced meniscal baskets, biters, graspers, scissors, and arthroscopic shavers. Common instruments needed for arthroscopic meniscectomy are illustrated in Figure 43-2. These include the following:

- Meniscal biters or baskets: straight, up-going, 90-degree right and left, backbiting
- Meniscal scissors
- Meniscal grasper
- Arthroscopic shaver: 3.5- to 4.5-mm full radius

Surgical Technique

Anesthesia and Positioning

The operative leg is marked in the holding area, and preoperative antibiotics are administered 30 minutes before the case is begun. The procedure can be performed under general, regional, spinal, or, in some cases, local anesthesia. The patient is positioned supine with all bone prominences well padded; a tourniquet is placed high on the operative thigh, and the leg is positioned in a standard leg holder. The nonoperative leg is placed in the lithotomy position, well padded. The foot of the table is then flexed down, allowing full flexion of the operative leg. The leg is prepared and draped in a standard fashion (Fig. 43-3). The tourniquet can be inflated per the surgeon's preference.

Portals (Fig. 43-4)

- Inferomedial portal: just medial to the patellar tendon at the joint line
- Inferolateral portal: just lateral to the patellar tendon at the joint line
- Superomedial or superolateral portal: for inflow or outflow as needed, placed approximately 1 cm proximal to the superior pole of the patella, entering just posterior to the quadriceps tendon

Arthroscopic Evaluation

A thorough arthroscopic evaluation of the knee is performed. The meniscus should be visually inspected and probed to determine the zone of the tear, the pattern of the tear, the length of the tear, and whether it is stable or unstable. Flipped meniscal segments or bucket-handle tears should be reduced for meniscal evaluation.

At times, placement of the scope through the notch is necessary to determine the extent of the tear at its posterior horn or to visualize any flipped segment or loose piece posteriorly (Fig. 43-5).

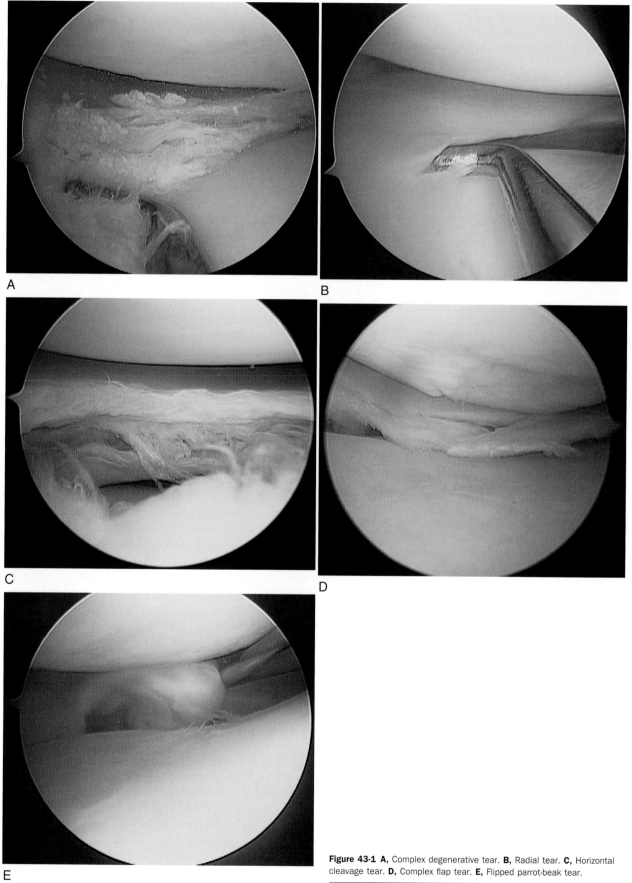

Figure 43-1 A, Complex degenerative tear. **B,** Radial tear. **C,** Horizontal cleavage tear. **D,** Complex flap tear. **E,** Flipped parrot-beak tear.

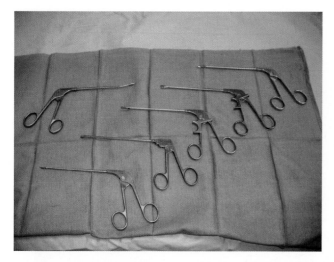

Figure 43-2 Standard arthroscopic meniscectomy instruments.

Arthroscopic Meniscectomy (Box 43-1)

Radial Tears

The goal is to saucerize the tear from the native meniscus. With use of the meniscal scissors or basket, gradually start to remove normal meniscal tissue and taper it toward the apex of the tear. It is important to move arthroscopic instruments in a controlled fashion to minimize iatrogenic cartilage damage. Care should be taken to keep the meniscal basket in contact with the meniscus at all times to allow consistency of meniscal tissue removal. To ensure a smooth transition, the anterior aspect of the tear may require resection with a 90-degree basket if the ipsilateral portal is used or a straight basket if the contralateral portal is used. An arthroscopic shaver can smooth any edges.

Bucket-Handle Tears

Bucket-handle tears that are irreparable because of tissue quality, deformation, or zone of injury should first be reduced to assess the length of the tear. Visualization of the extent of the posterior aspect of the tear may be improved by assessing the meniscus through the notch. Appropriate planning to truncate the posterior attachment without leaving an abrupt edge is needed. This may require rotation of the meniscal basket or scissors more centrally and posteriorly to make a proper transition to the tear. It is typically easier to remove most of the posterior attachment first, leaving just a few strands of tissue that can easily be torn by rotating the meniscus for removal. This will prevent the meniscus from becoming a loose body when the anterior aspect is removed. The anterior aspect of the tear can then be addressed through the ipsilateral or contralateral portal as discussed before. After the

ipsilateral portal is enlarged with a hemostat, a grasper can be used to firmly grab the meniscus. Enlargement of the portal by several millimeters is often needed to ensure that the resected fragment is not dislodged from the grasper during extraction. Rotation of the meniscus should avulse the remaining strands of the posterior meniscus, and the meniscus can be removed en bloc through the portal. Care must be taken not to allow the resected fragment to become a loose body. A meniscal shaver can smooth any edges as necessary. Alternatively, for small bucket-handle tears, the anterior edge can be removed as detailed before, and the meniscal shaver can débride the meniscus to its posterior base.

Horizontal Cleavage Tears

Controversy still exists about how to properly approach a horizontal cleavage tear. Options include removal of the most unstable leaf (superior or inferior) and removal of both leaves of the tear. Cleavage tears often make a flap on one of the leaflets that causes pain and mechanical symptoms. Although horizontal cleavage tears typically extend to the peripheral margin, it is not necessary to remove all of the meniscal tissue to make a stable tear and smooth transition.

Our bias is to remove the most unstable leaf, retaining part of the meniscus for function. The approach is similar to removal of a bucket-handle tear. The majority of the posterior attachment is removed through the ipsilateral portal, then the anterior attachment is removed through the contralateral portal. Finally, by use of a basket or meniscal scissors, the peripheral attachment is resected, leaving some pericapsular meniscal tissue. The leaf is removed either en bloc with the grasper or piecemeal with a shaver. The arthroscopic shaver is used to smooth any edges, but care must be taken with the thinned meniscus as the shaver may aggressively remove the tissue that is to be preserved.

Meniscal Cysts

Meniscal cysts are common findings that typically indicate intra-articular disease. Meniscal tears commonly make a rent in the capsular tissue and a one-way valve occurs, allowing synovial fluid to collect extra-articularly. Lateral meniscal cysts are located off the lateral joint line associated with a midportion lateral meniscus tear. Posterior medial cysts (Baker cyst) commonly associated with a posterior medial meniscus tear dissect between the medial head of the gastrocnemius and the semimembranosus. The meniscal cyst is often decompressed with treatment of the intra-articular meniscal tear. Commonly, with a lateral meniscal cyst, a spinal needle can be entered percutaneously at the lateral joint line level through the meniscal tear to aid in its decompression.

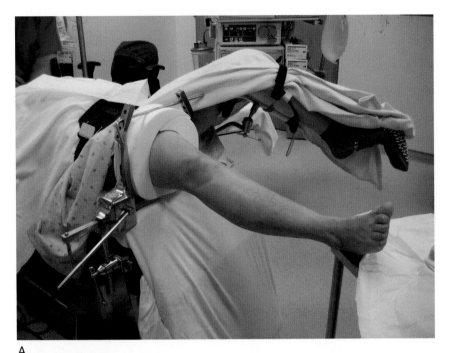

A

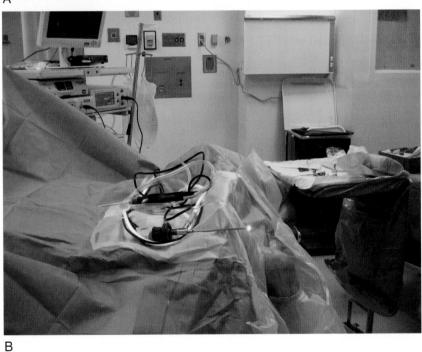

B

Figure 43-3 A, Patient positioning with a leg holder. **B,** Knee arthroscopy set-up after sterile preparation and draping.

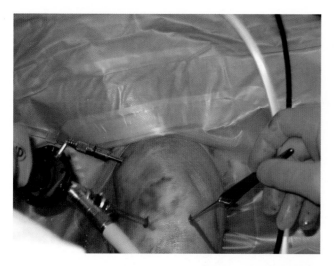

Figure 43-4 Standard arthroscopic portals. In this case, a superolateral portal was used for inflow, the inferolateral portal for the arthroscope, and the inferomedial portal for instrumentation.

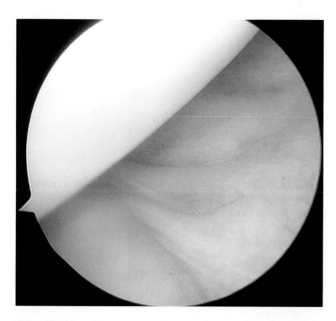

Figure 43-5 View of the posteromedial compartment by placement of the arthroscope through the notch just medial to the posterior cruciate ligament.

Postoperative Considerations

Follow-up

Patients are seen at 1 week postoperatively for wound check and suture removal. Subsequent follow-up is scheduled for 1 month postoperatively for evaluation of knee symptoms, range of motion, and strength.

Box 43-1 Key Principles of Arthroscopic Meniscectomy

- Repair of meniscus, if possible
- Resection of any abnormal mobile meniscal fragments
- Smooth transition without abrupt edges
- Preservation of the meniscocapsular junction
- Conservative resection of meniscal tissue
- Minimization of trauma to chondral surfaces

Rehabilitation

Goals are to reduce pain, inflammation, and swelling and to restore motion and strength. This can typically be accomplished with a home exercise program. Formal physical therapy can assist older patients. A standard protocol consists of the following:

- Crutches for 24 to 72 hours, as needed
- Ice for 20 minutes, three to six times a day
- Immediate progression of unrestricted range-of-motion exercises (passive, active-assisted, and active), quadriceps exercises, straight-leg raises
- No impact activities for 4 weeks
- Return to play with no inflammation, full motion, and 80% of strength of contralateral extremity

Complications

- Infection
- Deep venous thrombosis
- Arthrofibrosis
- Portal herniation or fistula
- Neuroma at portal site
- Retained meniscal fragment (loose body)
- Repeated tear of meniscus
- Continued pain in the compartment (chondral erosions)

Results

Results of studies of arthroscopic meniscectomy are shown in Table 43-1.

Table 43-1 Results of Studies of Arthroscopic Meniscectomy

Author	Medial or Lateral	Type of Tear	Follow-up (Years)	Results	Symptoms	Radiographic Changes	Notes
Chatain et al[7] (2003)	Both	Mix	10	95% satisfied	14% medial 20% lateral	22% medial 38% lateral	Better prognosis with medial tears, age <35 years, vertical tear, no cartilage damage, intact peripheral rim
Hulet et al[10] (2004)	Lateral with cyst	Mix (57% horizontal cleavage)	5	87% good–excellent		9%	
Pearse et al[15] (2003)	Both	Mix (degenerative)	1	65% improvement		Preexisting severe OA	At 4 years, 32% with further surgery
Bonneux and Vandekerckhove[5] (2002)	Lateral	Mix	8	64.5% good–excellent		93%	Amount or resection correlates with results
Menetrey et al[14] (2002)	Medial	Mix	3-7	90% NDM 20% DM			NDM, DM
Andersson-Molina et al[1] (2002)	Both	Mix	14	70%	14%	33% partial meniscectomy 72% total meniscectomy	
Scheller et al[16] (2001)	Lateral	Mix	10	77%		78%	Results decrease over time
Crevoisier et al[8] (2001)	Both	Degenerative, mix	4	80% satisfied 55% satisfied		Grade 0-2 OA Grade 3-4 OA	Age >70 years
Hoser et al[9] (2001)	Lateral	Mix	10	58% good–excellent		95%	29% reoperation
Hulet et al[11] (2001)	Medial	95% vertical 5% complex	12	95% very satisfied–satisfied		16%	
Kruger-Franke et al[12] (1999)	Medial	Mix	7	96%		33%	Women at greater risk of degenerative changes
Barrett et al[3] (1998)	Lateral	Mix	3	94%, 80% improvement		Grade 0-2 Grade 3-4	14% failure
Schimmer et al[17] (1998)	Both	Mix	4, 12	92%, 78% good–excellent	Worse at 5 years if cartilage damage		Underlying cartilage damage faired worse
Burks et al[6] (1997)	78% medial 19% lateral	Mix	14	88% good–excellent			No difference medial vs. lateral; ACL-deficient and female patients did worse
Matsusue and Thomson[13] (1996)	Medial	Mix	7.8	83% good–excellent			Worse outcomes with grade 3-4 OA
Bonamo et al[4] (1992)	Both	Mix	3	83% satisfied		Preexisting grade 3-4	Worse outcomes with women, age >60 years, grade 4 changes

ACL, anterior cruciate ligament; DM, degenerative meniscus; NDM, nondegenerative meniscus; OA, osteoarthritis.

References

1. Andersson-Molina H, Karlsson H, Rockborn P. Arthroscopic partial and total meniscectomy: a long-term follow-up study with matched controls. Arthroscopy 2002;18:183-189.

2. Arnoczky SP, Warren RF. Microvasculature of the human meniscus. Am J Sports Med 1982;10:90-95.

3. Barrett GR, Treacy SH, Ruff CG. The effect of partial lateral meniscectomy in patients ≥60 years. Orthopedics 1998;21:251-257.

4. Bonamo JJ, Kessler KJ, Noah J. Arthroscopic meniscectomy in patients over the age of 40. Am J Sports Med 1992;20:422-428; discussion 428-429.

5. Bonneux I, Vandekerckhove B. Arthroscopic partial lateral meniscectomy long-term results in athletes. Acta Orthop Belg 2002;68:356-361.

6. Burks RT, Metcalf MH, Metcalf RW. Fifteen-year follow-up of arthroscopic partial meniscectomy. Arthroscopy 1997;13:673-679.

7. Chatain F, Adeleine P, Chambat P, Neyret P. A comparative study of medial versus lateral arthroscopic partial meniscectomy on stable knees: 10-year minimum follow-up. Arthroscopy 2003;19:842-849.

8. Crevoisier X, Munzinger U, Drobny T. Arthroscopic partial meniscectomy in patients over 70 years of age. Arthroscopy 2001;17:732-736.

9. Hoser C, Fink C, Brown C, et al. Long-term results of arthroscopic partial lateral meniscectomy in knees without associated damage. J Bone Joint Surg Br 2001;83:513-516.

10. Hulet C, Souquet D, Alexandre P, et al. Arthroscopic treatment of 105 lateral meniscal cysts with 5-year average follow-up. Arthroscopy 2004;20:831-836.

11. Hulet CH, Locker BG, Schiltz D, et al. Arthroscopic medial meniscectomy on stable knees. J Bone Joint Surg Br 2001;83:29-32.

12. Kruger-Franke M, Siebert CH, Kugler A, et al. Late results after arthroscopic partial medial meniscectomy. Knee Surg Sports Traumatol Arthrosc 1999;7:81-84.

13. Matsusue Y, Thomson NL. Arthroscopic partial medial meniscectomy in patients over 40 years old: a 5- to 11-year follow-up study. Arthroscopy 1996;12:39-44.

14. Menetrey J, Siegrist O, Fritschy D. Medial meniscectomy in patients over the age of fifty: a six year follow-up study. Swiss Surg 2002;8:113-119.

15. Pearse EO, Craig DM. Partial meniscectomy in the presence of severe osteoarthritis does not hasten the symptomatic progression of osteoarthritis. Arthroscopy 2003;19:963-968.

16. Scheller G, Sobau C, Bulow JU. Arthroscopic partial lateral meniscectomy in an otherwise normal knee: clinical, functional, and radiographic results of a long-term follow-up study. Arthroscopy 2001;17:946-952.

17. Schimmer RC, Brulhart KB, Duff C, Glinz W. Arthroscopic partial meniscectomy: a 12-year follow-up and two-step evaluation of the long-term course. Arthroscopy 1998;14:136-142.

CHAPTER 44

Arthroscopic Meniscus Repair: Inside-Out Technique

Riley J. Williams III, MD

Warren R. Kadrmas, MD

The meniscus functions to evenly distribute and transmit loads within the knee and provides secondary stability to tibial translation on the femur. Although Annandale[2] reported the first meniscus repair in 1885, it was nearly a century later that the practice of meniscal preservation became the standard. Fairbank[10] was the first to indirectly question the practice of complete meniscectomy and described the degenerative changes that result from its functional loss. Open repair, as popularized by DeHaven,[7,8] was initially developed in an attempt to preserve meniscal function. The introduction of arthroscopic surgery soon led Henning[15] to advocate a combined arthroscopic and open technique, which involves small posteromedial and posterolateral incisions to receive sutures that are placed from within the joint. Many additional techniques have been described to repair the meniscus.[5,16] However, the inside-out arthroscopically assisted technique is widely held as the standard with which other repair techniques are compared.

Preoperative Considerations

History

It is critical to obtain a detailed history, including the mechanism of injury, associated injuries, date of injury, and previous treatments that may have been rendered. The patient's presenting symptoms and expectations of outcome should be addressed at the initial visit. If surgical intervention has been attempted previously, it is important to obtain the operative reports as well as intraoperative photographs if they are available.

Typical History

- Acute noncontact twisting injury to the knee is often described.
- Effusion usually develops immediately after injury as well as subsequent activity-related swelling.
- Mechanical symptoms, such as locking and clicking, may be present.
- Occasional episodes of giving way are often reported.
- Joint line or posterior knee pain is commonly reported.

Physical Examination

- Gait is usually normal, although there may be a flexed knee or antalgic gait if the patient is presenting acutely or with a locked meniscal tear.
- Effusion is frequently present.
- Range of motion is usually limited if the patient is presenting early with an effusion or with a locked meniscal tear. Range of motion may be normal if the patient is presenting late or after an initial course of physical therapy.
- Joint line tenderness or popliteal fossa fullness may be noted.

- Ligamentous stability is examined for associated pathologic changes (i.e., anterior cruciate ligament tear).
- Mild quadriceps atrophy may be present.

Imaging

Radiography

- Weight-bearing anteroposterior radiograph in full extension
- Weight-bearing posteroanterior 45-degree flexion radiograph
- Non–weight-bearing 45-degree flexion lateral radiograph
- Patella sunrise radiograph

Other Modalities

Magnetic resonance imaging allows the determination of the location and orientation of the tear as well as full evaluation of associated ligamentous and chondral injury.

Indications and Contraindications

Many factors contribute to the success of meniscal repair. The ideal candidate is a young (younger than 45 years), active patient with a traumatic vertical tear at the meniscosynovial junction. Location of the tear has been shown to be the most important predictor of success.[9,17] Historically, repair has been indicated for tears in the peripheral, vascular portion of the meniscus as described by Arnoczky and Warren.[4] However, reports have documented successful repair of tears in the avascular zone in young patients.[13,14] Complex and chronic tears have a lower success rate after repair.[9,17] Meniscal tears that are not suitable for repair are degenerative in nature and involve moderate to severe damage to the meniscal body fragment. Repair is generally not recommended in elderly, less active individuals or in those unable to comply with the postoperative rehabilitation regimen.

Surgical Technique

Anesthesia and Positioning

Meniscal repair may be performed by general, regional, or spinal anesthesia on the basis of the patient's, anesthesiologist's, and surgeon's preferences. The patient is placed supine on a standard operating room table, and a thigh tourniquet is applied. The patient should be positioned with the knee distal to the break in the bed to allow full flexion of the knee, and a leg holder or lateral post is applied. Circumferential access to the knee is required for posterolateral or posteromedial approaches for meniscal suturing.

Surgical Landmarks, Incisions, and Portals

Landmarks

- Patellar tendon
- Tibial plateau
- Fibular head
- Medial-lateral joint line

Portals

- Inferomedial portal
- Inferolateral portal
- Additional outflow portal as needed (superolateral or superomedial)

Approaches

- Posterolateral approach
- Posteromedial approach

Examination Under Anesthesia and Diagnostic Arthroscopy

Examination under anesthesia is performed to evaluate range of motion as well as associated ligamentous stability. Complete diagnostic arthroscopy is always performed before any meniscal pathologic process is addressed. Injuries to the chondral surfaces or intra-articular ligaments may need to be addressed in conjunction with the meniscal repair.

Specific Steps (Box 44-1)

1. Diagnostic Arthroscopy

The diagnostic arthroscopy portion of any case is always the same. The patient is placed supine on the operating table, and a tourniquet is applied to the upper thigh. Arthroscopy is performed with a lateral post or a leg holder on the basis of the surgeon's preference. An initial inferolateral portal is made adjacent to the patellar tendon, and the arthroscope is inserted. A complete arthroscopy is performed to visualize the knee and to identify any pathologic change that has not been found on plain film or magnetic resonance imaging. This also provides direct examination of the menisci and allows final assessment of the reparability of the tear. Additional pathologic changes

Box 44-1 Surgical Steps

1. Diagnostic arthroscopy
2. Meniscal preparation

3. Exposure
   a. Posteromedial
   b. Posterolateral

4. Suture placement
5. Suture tying
6. Closure

44

within the knee may need to be addressed in conjunction with the meniscal repair.

    Correct placement of the inferomedial portal is critical in addressing a meniscal tear. The location of the portal can be visualized directly by insertion of a spinal needle medial to the patellar tendon. The spinal needle should enter the medial compartment superior to the medial meniscus and parallel to the tibial plateau. The location of the portal needs to be customized on the basis of the location of the tear. To have access to the posterior horn of the lateral meniscus, for example, the portal may need to be placed slightly more proximal and immediately adjacent to the patellar tendon for access to be gained above the tibial spines. An arthroscopic probe is then placed within the working portal, and the meniscal tear is evaluated for its reparability.

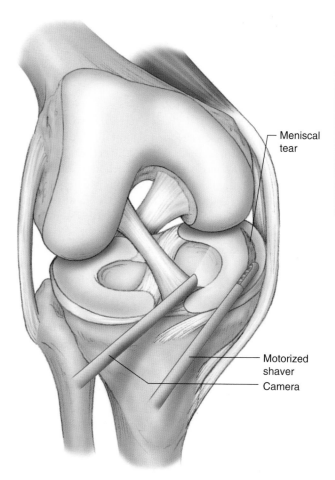

Figure 44-1 The meniscal tear is prepared with a motorized shaver to stimulate bleeding within the tear.

2. Meniscal Preparation

Once the tear has been deemed appropriate for repair, it is prepared with a hand-held rasp or mechanical shaver to stimulate bleeding within the tear (Fig. 44-1). An arthroscopic probe may be pressed against the capsule at the junction of the middle and posterior portions of the meniscus to facilitate accurate placement of the posteromedial or posterolateral incision. The tip of the probe can usually be palpated at the posterior aspect of the joint line before an incision is made.

3a. Exposure: Posteromedial

A vertical 3- to 4-cm incision is made over the posteromedial joint line centered over the palpated arthroscopic probe with the knee flexed 60 to 90 degrees. The incision is carried through the skin, and Metzenbaum scissors are used to dissect the subcutaneous tissues. Care must be taken to protect the greater saphenous nerve, which generally lies posterior to the skin incision. Dissection continues to the level of the pes fascia, which can be identified by its obliquely oriented fibers. The fascia is incised sharply with a scalpel at the superior margin of the sartorius, and blunt dissection is performed with the surgeon's finger (Fig. 44-2). The posteromedial capsule can easily be

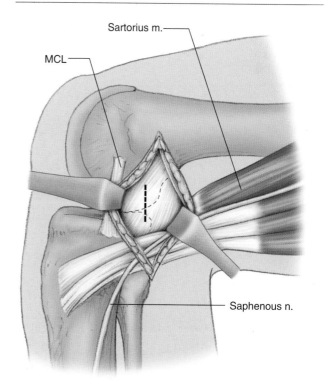

Figure 44-2 Posteromedial exposure. MCL, medial collateral ligament.

palpated at the depth of the incision and a popliteal retractor placed at its posterior margin. The popliteal retractor separates the posteromedial capsule laterally from the saphenous nerve and pes tendons medially.

3b. Exposure: Posterolateral

With the knee flexed 90 degrees, a vertical 3- to 4-cm incision is made over the posterolateral joint line centered over the palpated arthroscopic probe. Dissection is carried through the skin, and Metzenbaum scissors are used to dissect the subcutaneous tissues. The interval between the iliotibial band and the biceps tendon is identified and sharply incised with a scalpel. The biceps tendon is retracted posteriorly and serves to protect the peroneal nerve. Blunt dissection with the surgeon's finger allows direct palpation of the posterolateral capsule and the lateral head of the gastrocnemius at the depth of the incision (Fig. 44-3). A popliteal retractor is placed at the posterior margin of the capsule and separates the posterolateral capsule medially from the lateral head of the gastrocnemius laterally. The remainder of the lateral meniscal repair is usually performed in the figure-of-four position.

4. Suture Placement

The meniscal body fragment is reduced with a probe in preparation for suture repair. We prefer to use a curved, zone-specific cannula system, although many varieties of suture repair systems are widely available. The arthroscope remains in the ipsilateral portal for viewing; the contralateral portal is used for suture placement in the anterior and central horns of the meniscus during repair. Viewing and working portals may need to be switched for placement of posterior horn sutures. Suture placement begins at the posterior extent of the identified tear and gradually extends to the anterior margin. Double-arm meniscal repair needles are delivered into the joint and guided into position with the zone-specific cannula system. The curve of the cannula should be directed medially for a medial meniscus tear and laterally for a lateral meniscus tear to facilitate exit into the popliteal retractor. A single limb of the suture is initially passed through the meniscus and retrieved by a surgical assistant as it exits within the popliteal retractor (Fig. 44-4). The remaining limb of the suture is placed in a similar manner to form a mattress stitch, and the pair are held with a clamp to facilitate suture management (Fig. 44-5). Sutures are placed sequentially from posterior to anterior until the full extent of the tear is addressed (Fig. 44-6). Sutures are placed at 3- to 5-mm intervals and

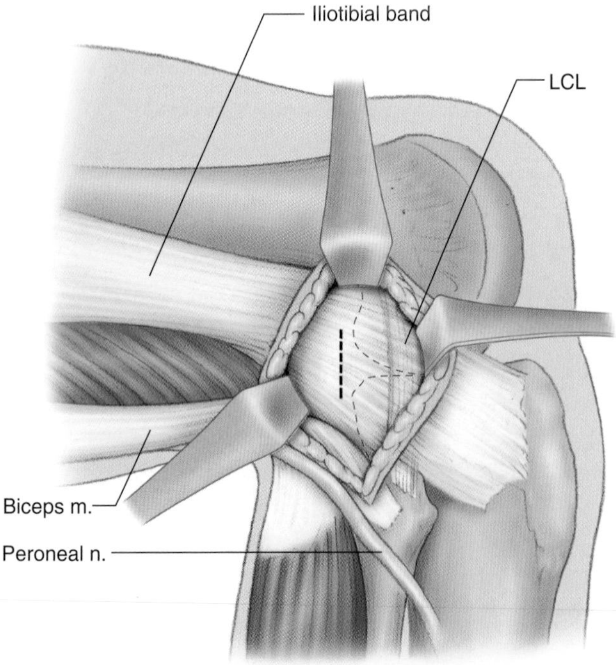

Figure 44-3 Posterolateral exposure. LCL, lateral collateral ligament.

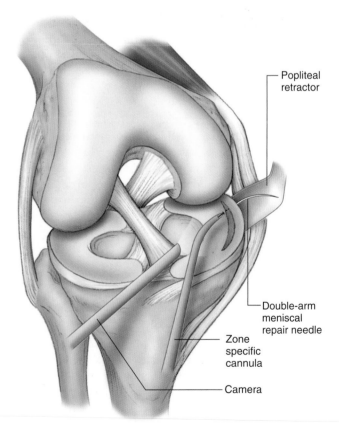

Figure 44-4 A single limb of the double-arm meniscal repair suture is passed through the posterior aspect of the meniscal tear and retrieved within the popliteal retractor by a surgical assistant.

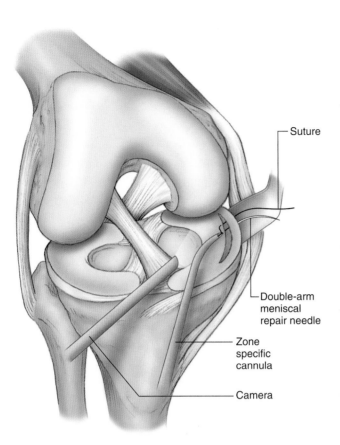

Figure 44-5 The remaining limb of the double-arm meniscal repair suture is passed to form a mattress stitch.

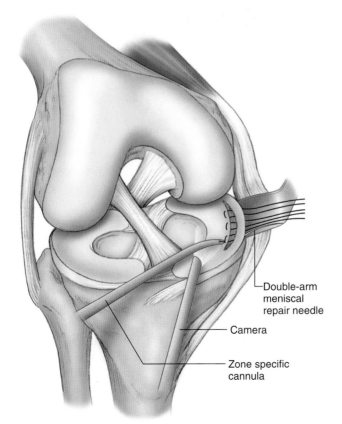

Figure 44-6 Sutures are placed from posterior to anterior at 3- to 5-mm intervals until the full extent of the tear is addressed.

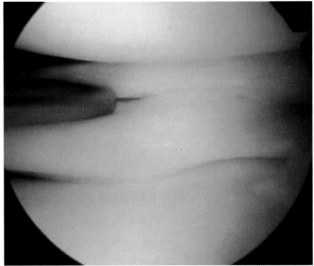

A

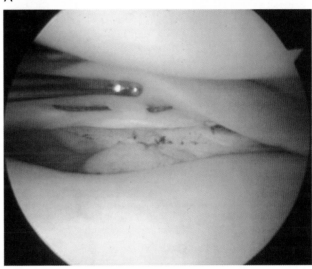

B

Figure 44-7 Sutures may be alternated on the superior **(A)** and inferior **(B)** aspect of the meniscus to provide a stable repair.

may alternate on the superior and inferior surface of the meniscus (Fig. 44-7).

5. Suture Tying

The sutures are serially tied from posterior to anterior against the capsule with care not to overtighten or to deform the meniscal body (Fig. 44-8). A fibrin clot may be placed within the meniscal tear, particularly for those tears that extend to the avascular zone (e.g., complete radial tear in a young patient), before the sutures are tied. The knee is taken through a full range of motion and visualized for gap formation or suture breakage.

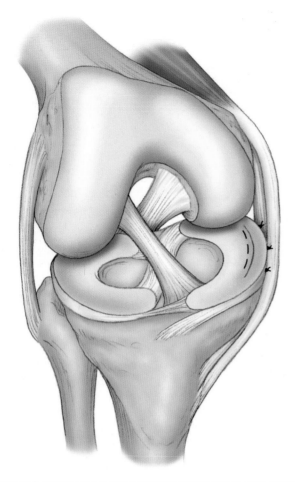

Figure 44-8 Sutures are tied from posterior to anterior over the joint capsule to complete the repair.

6. Closure

The arthroscopic portals are closed in the standard fashion, and the accessory wound is closed in layers.

Postoperative Considerations

Rehabilitation

- Immediate toe-touch weight bearing is allowed in a hinged knee brace with range of motion limited to 0 to 90 degrees of flexion.
- Straight-leg raises are begun immediately postoperatively.
- Full weight bearing and gradual strengthening exercises are instituted at 6 weeks postoperatively.
- In-line running is permitted after 4 months.

- Return to full, unrestricted activity is permitted after 6 months if the patient is asymptomatic.

Complications

- Infection
- Arthrofibrosis
- Failure of meniscus to heal
- Nerve injury (saphenous medially, peroneal laterally)
- Vascular injury (popliteal fossa)

PEARLS AND PITFALLS

- The authors recommend the use of braided polyester suture for most meniscal repair procedures.
- The posterior capsular incision should be made such that the length of the incision starts at the level of the joint line. Placement of the incision here facilitates capture of the flexible needles during suture passage.
- Beware of the infrapatellar branch of the saphenous nerve during medial meniscal repairs. This nerve typically lies within the surgical field just superficial to the semimembranosus expansion and can be retracted inferiorly. Entrapment of this nerve is possible during tying of the passed sutures. Such nerve entrapment is a possible cause of acute postoperative pain at the surgical site. Failure to recognize this complication can result in the formation of a neuroma.
- Beware of the peroneal nerve during lateral repairs. This nerve lies posterior and lateral to the lateral head of the gastrocnemius muscle and biceps femoris tendon. This nerve can be entrapped by meniscal sutures if the deep retractor is not placed *deep* to the gastrocnemius. One must confirm that the retractor sits directly behind the capsule before suture passage. The posterior capsule should be directly visualized before sutures are tied laterally.
- Once the sutures have been passed, each suture should be sequentially tied (central to peripheral) with the leg in *extension*. This maneuver prevents the tethering of the posterior capsule by the meniscal sutures and decreases the likelihood of a postoperative flexion contracture.
- A soup spoon or vaginal speculum can be used as a deep retractor in inside-out meniscal repair procedures.

Results

After meniscal repair, good to excellent results can be expected in approximately 85% of patients (Table 44-1). Results are greatest for traumatic vertical tears in young patients who undergo concomitant anterior cruciate ligament reconstruction. However, excellent results have also been reported for isolated meniscal repairs as well as for complex tears extending to the avascular portion of the meniscus.

Table 44-1 Results of Inside-Out Meniscal Repair

Author	No. of Repairs	Criteria	Follow-up	Concomitant ACL Tear	Results
Johnson et al[11] (1999)	38	Clinical	10 years, 9 months (average)	None	76% successful
Cannon and Vittori[6] (1992)	90	Arthroscopy or arthrography	7 months (mean): isolated repairs 10 months (mean): concurrent ACL reconstructions	68 ACL tears (76%) All reconstructed	93% success with ACL reconstruction 50% success of isolated repair
Miller[12] (1988)	79	Arthroscopy or arthrography	3.25 years (mean)	68 reconstructions 22 stable ACL	93% healed with ACL reconstruction 84% healed with isolated meniscal repair
Tenuta and Arciero[17] (1994)	54	Clinical and arthroscopy	11 months (mean)	40 reconstructions 14 stable ACL	Arthroscopy 90% healed with ACL reconstruction 57% healed with isolated meniscal repair Better with rim width <4 mm, age <30 years
Rubman et al[14] (1998)	198	Clinical ± arthroscopy	Clinical examination: 42 months (23-116) 180 meniscal repairs (91%) in 160 patients Arthroscopy: 18 months (2-81) 91 meniscal repairs (46%) in 79 patients	128 ACL tears (72%) 126 reconstructed 96 concurrent 30 delayed	80% asymptomatic (clinically) 20% (39) repeated arthroscopy for symptoms 2 (5%) healed 13 (33%) partially healed 24 (62%) failed Arthroscopy (91 repairs) 23 (25%) completely healed 35 (38%) partially healed 33 (36%) failed
Eggli et al[9] (1995)	54	Clinical ± magnetic resonance imaging	7.5 years (average)	None	73% success 64% of failures in first 6 months Better with acute injury (<8 weeks), age <30 years, tear length <2.5 cm Worse with rim width >3 mm, absorbable sutures
Albrecht-Olsen and Bak[1] (1993)	27	3 clinical	3 years (median)	None	63% success

ACL, anterior cruciate ligament.

References

1. Albrecht-Olsen PM, Bak K. Arthroscopic repair of the bucket-handle meniscus: 10 failures in 27 stable knees followed for 3 years. Acta Orthop Scand 1993;64:446-448.
2. Annandale T. An operation for displaced semilunar cartilage. Br Med J 1885;1:779.
3. Arciero RA, Taylor DC. Inside-outside and all-inside meniscus repair: indications, techniques and results. Oper Tech Orthop 1995;5:58-69.
4. Arnoczky SP, Warren RF. Microvasculature of the human meniscus. Am J Sports Med 1982;10:90-95.

5. Bottoni CR, Arciero RA. Conventional meniscal repair techniques. Oper Tech Orthop 2000;10:194-208.

6. Cannon WD Jr, Vittori JM. The incidence of healing in arthroscopic meniscal repairs in anterior cruciate ligament–reconstructed knees versus stable knees. Am J Sports Med 1992;20:176-181.

7. DeHaven KE, Hales W. Peripheral meniscus repair: an alternative to meniscectomy. Orthop Trans 1981;5:399-400.

8. DeHaven KE, Black KP, Griffiths HJ. Open meniscus repair technique and two to nine year results. Am J Sports Med 1989;17:788-795.

9. Eggli S, Wegmuller H, Kosina J, et al. Long-term results of arthroscopic meniscal repair: an analysis of isolated tears. Am J Sports Med 1995;23:715-720.

10. Fairbank TJ. Knee joint changes after meniscectomy. J Bone Joint Surg Br 1948;30:664-670.

11. Johnson MJ, Lucas GL, Dusek JK, et al. Isolated arthroscopic meniscal repair: a long-term outcome study (more than 10 years). Am J Sports Med 1999;27:44-49.

12. Miller DB Jr. Arthroscopic meniscus repair. Am J Sports Med 1988;16:315-320.

13. Noyes FR, Barber-Westin SD. Arthroscopic repair of meniscal tears extending into the avascular zone in patients younger than twenty years of age. Am J Sports Med 2002;30:589-600.

14. Rubman MH, Noyes FR, Barber-Westin SD. Arthroscopic repair of meniscal tears that extend into the avascular zone: a review of 198 single and complex tears. Am J Sports Med 1998;26:87-95.

15. Scott GA, Jolly BL, Henning CE. Combined posterior incision and arthroscopic intra-articular repair of the meniscus. J Bone Joint Surg Am 1986;68:847-861.

16. Sgaglione NA, Steadman J, Shaffer B, et al. Current concepts in meniscus surgery: resection to replacement. Arthroscopy 2003;19:161-188.

17. Tenuta JJ, Arciero RA. Arthroscopic evaluation of meniscal repairs. Factors that affect healing. Am J Sports Med 1994;22:797-802.

CHAPTER 45

Arthroscopic Meniscal Repair: Outside-In Technique

Fintan J. Shannon, FRCS (Tr & Orth)

Scott A. Rodeo, MD

The anatomy, structure, blood supply, and function of the menisci are well understood. There is now strong evidence supporting the preservation of viable meniscal tissue in an otherwise intact knee.

All-inside, inside-out, and outside-in techniques are useful options for repair of meniscal tears. The outside-in technique was first described by Warren[14] as a method to decrease the risk of peroneal nerve injury during lateral meniscal repair. The choice of which technique is used is predominantly affected by the surgeon's experience and the morphologic features of the tear. However, not all tears should be repaired, and surgical outcome for these repairs is determined by careful meniscal and patient selection.

Preoperative Considerations

History

Acute tears typically present with focal pain and mild swelling. Unstable meniscal tears may present with catching or locking. The patient usually recalls a twisting injury or deep flexion event. A longer history or history of antecedent pain, locking, swelling, or instability may indicate chronic meniscal disease.

Details of previous treatments and operative reports are helpful. Other factors to be considered are the age of the patient, the expected compliance of the patient with rehabilitation, and the patient's physical ability to be non–weight bearing postoperatively.

Physical Examination

Nonspecific important observations:

- Alignment: neutral, varus, or valgus
- Gait: is it antalgic?
- Loss of end range of motion: deep flexion and full extension
- Focal pain
- Painful clicking

Signs supportive of meniscal tear:

- Effusion
- Soft block to extension: suggests displaced fragment (bounce test)
- Pain on passive deep flexion
- Focal tenderness along joint line
- Pain with meniscal compression: McMurray and Apley tests

Imaging

Radiography

- Weight-bearing views: anteroposterior in full extension and posteroanterior in 45 degrees of flexion
- Non–weight-bearing lateral view in 45 degrees of flexion
- Merchant view of patellofemoral joint
- Long-cassette mechanical axis view to evaluate alignment

Other Modalities

- Magnetic resonance imaging

Evaluate meniscal tear location (inner, middle, or outer third) and amount of abnormal meniscus, intrameniscal signal, articular cartilage, and cruciate ligament integrity. Increased intrameniscal signal indicates poorer healing potential.

Indications and Contraindications

When the history and preoperative imaging suggest that a meniscal tear may be amenable to repair, careful preoperative counseling of the patient is essential. The patient must be aware that postoperative restrictions are significant, and the patient's compliance is key to a successful outcome.

The ideal candidate for an outside-in repair is a young, compliant patient with a short history of pain, a stable knee, and a vertical longitudinal tear in the red-red zone of a meniscus. Other specific indications include suturing of a meniscal replacement (allograft or replacement device, such as a collagen meniscus implant) and suturing of a Wrisberg-type discoid lateral meniscus in a small knee. Specific advantages are precise needle placement with reduced risk of chondral injury and relative ease of technique for anterior horn tears.

Relative contraindications for meniscal repair in general include degenerative flap or horizontal cleavage tears, partial-thickness tears, stable tears (<2 cm), tears in the white-white zone, and patients with an unstable or anterior cruciate ligament (ACL)–deficient knee.[5,10] Radial tears, particularly in the posterior horn, are reparable where there is a rich blood supply. Better healing has been demonstrated with lateral meniscal tears, and therefore indications for lateral meniscal repair are broader. Small, vertical, longitudinal tears posterior to the popliteus tendon and small avulsion tears of the posterior horn in the setting of injury to the ACL may be observed.[3]

Other contraindications include far posterior tears (difficult to place sutures perpendicular to tear; use inside-out technique or all-inside), complex tears, older patients (older than 50 years), and chronic tears with deformation of the meniscus.

Surgical Technique

Anesthesia and Positioning

The decision regarding type of anesthesia is generally made between the anesthesiologist and the patient. Spinal anesthesia is effective for outpatient knee arthroscopy surgery and meniscal repair work. Femoral nerve blocks, although helpful, can potentially delay rehabilitation and return of quadriceps function.

Standard set-up includes a thigh tourniquet and a lateral post. The limb should be placed on the operating table in such a position that when the end of the table is flexed, the end of the thigh protrudes over the table break. This provides access to the posteromedial and posterolateral corners of the knee.

Specific Knee Positions

- 10 degrees of flexion with valgus stress for medial meniscal repair. The saphenous nerve and vein lie anterior to the palpable semitendinosus tendon; therefore, you work posterior to them. This position is good for posterior and middle-third tears.
- 50 to 60 degrees of flexion for anterior horn of medial meniscus. Work anterior to pes anserinus tendons and saphenous nerve branches.
- 90 degrees of flexion for lateral meniscal repair: figure-of-four position. The needle must remain anterior to the biceps tendon to avoid peroneal nerve injury.

Surgical Landmarks, Incisions, and Portals

Landmarks

- Patella
- Patellar tendon
- Joint line–plateau: mark with surgical marker
- Fibular head, biceps tendon

Incisions and Portals

Use a standard anterolateral portal for initial arthroscopy. Determine the best anteromedial portal after spinal needle confirmation of correct height and location. Portal location is less important in this type of repair, whereas instrument trajectory is crucial in all-inside and inside-out repairs. For the lateral meniscus, use the high anteromedial portal.

The large posterior incisions are not necessary in performing the outside-in repair. However, it is difficult to place perpendicular sutures for far posterior tears, and oblique suture orientation compromises fixation stability.[13] In performing the dissection down to capsule for needles introduced posteromedially or posterolaterally, consider underlying superficial structures:

- Posteromedial: saphenous nerve, medial collateral ligament
- Posterolateral: peroneal nerve, lateral collateral ligament

Examination Under Anesthesia

Examination of range of motion and stability is performed before sterile preparation and draping of the lower extremity.

Diagnostic Arthroscopy

- Joint surfaces
- ACL
- Location, orientation, and stability of tear. Visualization of the posterior horn of the medial meniscus is facilitated by inserting the arthroscope through the anterolateral portal and passing it between the posterior cruciate ligament and the medial femoral condyle.
- Abrade surfaces of tear to make a bleeding bed with a rasp or 3.5-mm full-radius resector.[2] Consider the posteromedial portal for this purpose. Flex knee, palpate pes anserinus tendons, and introduce spinal needle anterior to these. The portal incision is posterior and proximal to the medial joint line.
- Abrade synovial membrane adjacent to tear to stimulate additional vascularity.[9]

Specific Steps (Box 45-1)

Equipment

- 18-gauge spinal needles
- Arthroscopic grasper
- Suture: rigid, monofilament; No. 0 polydioxanone (PDS)

1. Prepare Meniscus

Prepare the meniscus by gentle débridement or abrasion of the edges of the tear and the synovial fringe that appears on the superior and inferior surface of the capsule. Use a rasp or 3.5-mm full-radius resector.

Box 45-1 Surgical Steps

1. Prepare meniscus
2. Locate skin surface over meniscal tear
3. Pass one spinal needle
4. Make small skin incision around needle
5. Pass second spinal needle
6. Secure sutures

2. Locate Skin Surface over Meniscal Tear

Locate the skin surface over the meniscal tear by use of topographic landmarks, palpation, and transillumination. Transillumination minimizes injury to cutaneous nerves and vessels.

3. Pass One Spinal Needle

Pass one spinal needle through the skin, subcutaneous tissue, capsule, and outer edge of the meniscus across the tear and through the inner meniscus (Fig. 45-1). The needle can exit either the superior (femoral) or inferior (tibial) surface of the meniscus. A probe or small loop curet may be used to control needle position or to provide counterpressure on the meniscus while the needle is being passed. Do not pass through the inner rim of the meniscus; this is thin tissue that will tear or fold when sutures are tensioned. Consider curved needles for posterior tears.

4. Make Small Skin Incision Around Needle

Make a small skin incision around the needle and spread the subcutaneous tissue down to the capsule (Fig. 45-2). Be careful to consider the saphenous nerve on the medial side.

5. Pass Second Spinal Needle

Pass the second spinal needle through this incision from outside-in, emerging from the meniscus adjacent to (~5 mm) the first needle (Fig. 45-3). Needle placement dictates suture orientation (vertical or horizontal mattress). The vertical mattress configuration shows the least displacement under load.[8] Consider alternating femoral and tibial surface sutures.

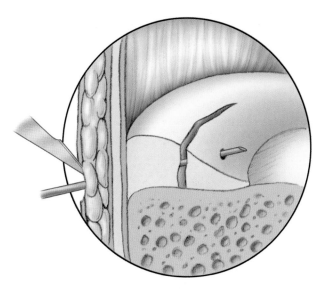

Figure 45-1 Once you are satisfied with needle position, make a small skin incision.

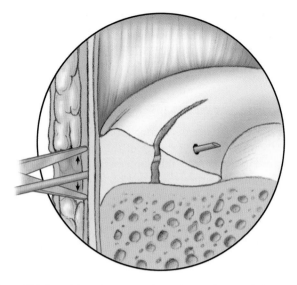

Figure 45-2 Spread the subcutaneous tissue down to the capsule by use of a hemostat.

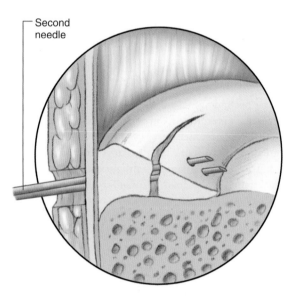

Second needle

Figure 45-3 A second needle is introduced through this skin incision and across the tear.

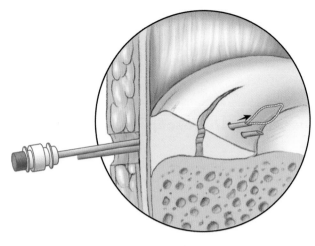

Figure 45-4 Pass the cable loop through one needle.

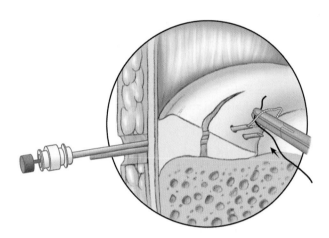

Figure 45-5 Place an absorbable suture with the grasper through the anterior portal into the wire loop.

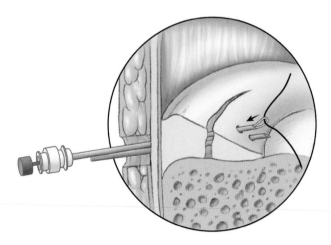

Figure 45-6 The cable loop is withdrawn out the needle with the suture.

6. Secure Sutures

Use a working cannula through the anteromedial portal. Most graspers and instruments can be used through a 7-mm portal. Four options for securing sutures are as follows.

1. Cable Loop Pull-Through Technique (Johnson[4])

Pass cable loop through one needle (Fig. 45-4). Place absorbable suture with grasper through anterior portal into wire loop (Fig. 45-5). Pull suture through meniscus (Fig. 45-6). Repeat steps with other end of suture and other needle (Fig. 45-7). Withdraw needles and tie the single suture subcutaneously over the capsule (Fig. 45-8).

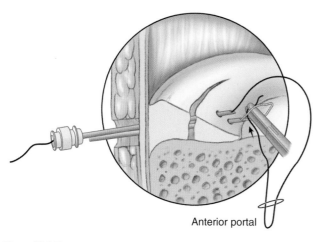

Figure 45-7 The procedure is repeated for the second needle, feeding the other end of the suture through the cable loop.

If a cable loop is not available, the No. 0 PDS suture can be passed through the spinal needle out through the anteromedial portal, where a permanent suture can be tied to the PDS. The knot is then pulled through the meniscus. The process is repeated, resulting in a mattress suture.[16]

2. Cable Loop Capture Technique (Cooper[1])

Place suture through one needle. Pass wire cable loop through other needle and capture end of suture material in joint (Fig. 45-9). Pull suture end out through meniscus and tie subcutaneously over capsule.

3. Mulberry Knot Technique (Warren[15])

Pass suture (No. 0 PDS) into needle, grasp inside joint, and pull out through anterior portal. Pass second suture (No. 0 PDS) into adjacent needle and repeat procedure.

45

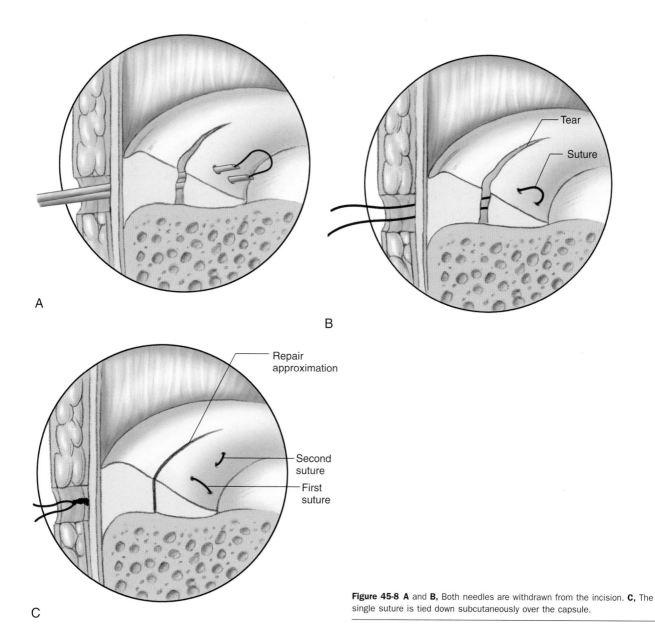

Figure 45-8 A and **B**, Both needles are withdrawn from the incision. **C**, The single suture is tied down subcutaneously over the capsule.

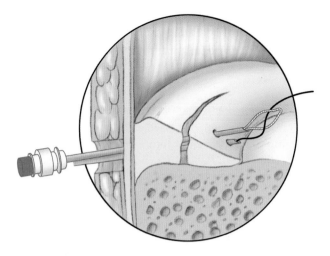

Figure 45-9 The cable loop capture technique. See text.

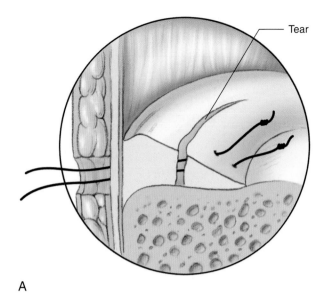

A

Tear

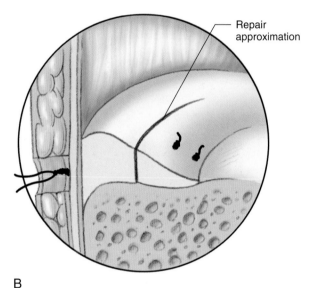

Repair approximation

B

Figure 45-10 A and **B,** The mulberry knot technique. See text.

Tie a knot (three or four throws) in the end of each suture, then pull knot back into joint so that knots lie against meniscus and maintain tear in reduced position. Use a cannula in the anterior portal to avoid entrapment of the knot in soft tissues. Tie adjacent sutures together over capsule (Fig. 45-10).

4. Dilator Knot Technique (Cooper[1])

Pass suture (No. 0 PDS) into needle, grasp inside joint, and pull out through anterior portal. Pass second suture (No. 0 PDS) into adjacent needle and repeat procedure. Use a cannula in the anterior portal to avoid entrapment of soft tissues between the sutures.

Tie a small knot (two throws) in one suture. Then tie adjacent sutures together outside portal. Pull suture with smaller knot (dilator knot) through meniscus (inside-out) ahead of the knot holding the two sutures together (Fig. 45-11). Now you can tie the single suture subcutaneously over the capsule.

Supplementary Options

Supplementary options to provide access to marrow-derived cells or factors are fibrin clot insertion[12] and microfracture in the notch.

Technical Considerations and Complications

- Stay anterior to biceps tendon on lateral side to avoid injury to peroneal nerve.
- Beware of posterior capsular entrapment, especially on medial side. Avoid excessive flexion during medial repairs. Use absorbable suture. For posterior horn tears of medial meniscus, tie suture with knee extended. This helps reduce meniscal tear to capsule and prevents entrapment of posterior capsule.
- Absorbable sutures should be used if suture placement requires penetration of the medial collateral ligament, semimembranosus, or popliteal tendon.

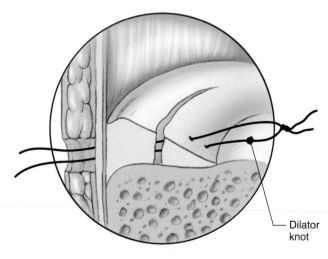

Dilator knot

Figure 45-11 The dilator knot technique. See text.

- The strength of vertical mattress repairs is ultimately limited by the strength of the suture material. Therefore, in tears with marginal healing ability (i.e., complex type, marginal vascularity, chronic tear), a nonabsorbable suture in vertical mattress orientation may enhance the likelihood of a successful repair.

Postoperative Considerations

Rehabilitation

Clinical studies demonstrate good results with accelerated rehabilitation[6]; however, few studies have used objective evaluation of meniscus healing (arthroscopy, magnetic resonance imaging). It is known that a tear may be only partially healed yet asymptomatic.[13] The long-term fate of such tears is unknown. Consider tailoring the postoperative protocol on the basis of the type of meniscal tear.

Authors' Protocol

- A hinged double-upright brace is applied.
- Early range-of-motion exercise is prescribed.
- Flexion is limited to 90 degrees during the first 4 weeks to protect posterior horn repairs.
- Full weight bearing with the brace locked in full extension is allowed for bucket-handle and vertical longitudinal tears.
- For radial and complex tears (such as double longitudinal tears), only toe-touch weight bearing is recommended for the first 3 weeks and flexion is limited to 90 degrees during the first 4 weeks.
- Closed kinetic chain strengthening exercises are begun in the second week.
- Open the brace 0 to 40 degrees at 4 weeks.
- Weight bearing out of the brace is permitted at 4 to 6 weeks.
- Sport-specific activities are initiated at 6 to 8 weeks for further development of strength and proprioception.
- Running is allowed at 4 months.
- Return to full athletic participation is permitted by 5 months.
- Squatting and hyperflexion are avoided for up to 6 months.
- Concomitant ACL reconstruction: follow routine ACL rehabilitation protocol. Limit flexion and consider delayed weight bearing for radial and complex tears. No flexion limitations have occurred with use of this protocol.

Other Considerations

- Consider a less aggressive rehabilitation protocol if there is axial malalignment of the limb (e.g., repair of a medial meniscus in a varus knee) because the meniscus may be under higher loads.
- Consider the use of an "unloader" brace, which serves to shift the weight-bearing stresses to the opposite tibiofemoral compartment.

Complications

Neurovascular Injury

- Use transillumination
- Blunt dissection down to capsule

Failure of Meniscal Repair

- Poor selection
- Poor technique
- Oblique suture orientation
- Inadequate protection of repair
- Instability of knee
- Reinjury

45

PEARLS AND PITFALLS

- Preoperative counseling of the patient is important because compliance with rehabilitation is essential.
- The indications for lateral meniscal tears are broader because of better healing rates.
- Posterior horn tears of the medial meniscus are best considered unsuitable for outside-in repair owing to difficulty in achieving perpendicular needle placement across a far posterior tear.
- Position the patient such that the thigh protrudes over the table break if the table is flexed. This aids access to the posteromedial and posterolateral corners of the knee.
- To avoid nerve injury, stay anterior to the biceps tendon on the lateral side. On the medial side, work anterior to hamstrings for anterior third and posterior for middle third.
- A high anteromedial portal will help in visualization and repair of the lateral meniscus.
- Abrade surfaces of the meniscal tear and synovium adjacent to the tear with a rasp or 3.5-mm full-radius resector. Consider microfracture in the notch to provide access to marrow-derived mesenchymal cells.
- Transillumination minimizes injury to cutaneous nerves and vessels.
- Use a probe to apply counterpressure against the meniscus when needles are inserted.
- Use vertical mattress configuration.
- Prescribe early range of motion. Limit flexion and weight bearing for radial and complex tears.

Table 45-1 Results of Outside-In Meniscal Repair

Author	No. of Repairs	Evaluation	Follow-up	Outcome
Morgan et al[7] (1991)	74 (of 353 repaired menisci)	Second-look arthroscopy		84% successful outcome (62/74) 65% healed (48/74) 19% partially healed (14/74) 16% failure rate (12/74) Increased failure in ACL-deficient knees and posterior horn tears of medial meniscus
Rodeo and Warren[11] (1996)	90	Computed tomographic arthrography	Minimum of 2 years	86% successful outcome (partial or complete healing with minimum symptoms) Increased failure in unstable knees
van Trommel et al[13] (1998)	51	Arthroscopy, arthrography, magnetic resonance imaging, or combination	Average of 15 months (range: 3-80)	45% complete healing 32% partial healing 24% no healing Significantly lower healing for tears in posterior horn of medial meniscus

ACL, anterior cruciate ligament.

Results

Results of meniscal repair by the outside-in technique are shown in Table 45-1.

In the Hospital for Special Surgery experience,[11] an 86% successful outcome was reported: 67% asymptomatic with objective evidence for complete healing, 19% minimally symptomatic with objective evidence for partial healing, and 14% failure rate (significant symptoms or objective evidence of failure to heal). The failure rate was based on knee stability: stable knees, 15% (5 of 33); unstable knees, 38% (5 of 13); and concomitant ACL reconstruction, 5% (2 of 38). Fibrin clot was used in 17 repairs with a failure rate of 35% (6 of 17) due to unrepaired ACL insufficiency (3) and complex tears in the avascular zone of the meniscus (3). Complications (3%) included saphenous nerve entrapment (1), thrombophlebitis (1), and infection (1).

In the study of Morgan et al,[7] the majority of failures occurred in posterior horn tears of the medial meniscus (11 of 12 failures), and all failures occurred in ACL-deficient knees. Healing was complete with disappearance of the absorbable suture in approximately 4 months. These authors were among the first to point out that incompletely healed menisci can be clinically asymptomatic.

van Trommel et al[13] described different regional healing rates with the outside-in technique. A significantly lower healing rate was reported for tears in the posterior horn of the medial meniscus, which was thought to be due to the obliquity of the sutures in this region. It can be difficult to place the needles perpendicular to the tear in the far posterior zone of the meniscus, resulting in oblique suture placement. The inside-out or all-inside technique should be considered for repair of tears in the posterior horn of the medial meniscus.

References

1. Cooper DE. Arthroscopic meniscus repair: outside-in technique. Oper Tech Sports Med 1994;2:1997.
2. Cooper DE, Arnoczky SP, Warren RF. Meniscal repair. Clin Sports Med 1991;10:529-548.
3. Fitzgibbons RE, Shelbourne RD. "Aggressive" non-treatment of lateral meniscal tears seen during anterior cruciate ligament reconstruction. Am J Sports Med 1995;23:156-159.
4. Johnson LL. Meniscus repair: the outside-in technique. In Jackson DW, ed. Reconstructive Knee Surgery. Master Techniques in Orthopaedic Surgery. Philadelphia, Lippincott Williams & Wilkins, 2003:39.
5. Levy IM, Torzilli PA, Warren RF. The effect of medial meniscectomy on anterior-posterior motion of the knee. J Bone Joint Surg Am 1982;64:883-888.
6. Miriani PP, Santori N, Adriani E, et al. Accelerated rehabilitation after arthroscopic meniscal repair: a clinical and magnetic resonance imaging evaluation. Arthroscopy 1996;12:680-686.
7. Morgan CD, Wojtys EM, Casscells CD, Casscells SW. Arthroscopic meniscal repair evaluated by second-look arthroscopy. Am J Sports Med 1991;19:632-638.
8. Rankin CC, Lintner DM, Noble PC, et al. A biomechanical analysis of meniscal repair techniques. Am J Sports Med 2002;30:492-497.

9. Ritchie JR, Miller MD, Bents RT, et al. Meniscal repair in the goat model. The use of healing adjuncts on central tears and the role of magnetic resonance arthrography in repair evaluation. Am J Sports Med 1998;26:278-284.

10. Rodeo SA. Arthroscopic meniscal repair with use of the outside-in technique. Instr Course Lect 2000;49:195-206.

11. Rodeo SA, Warren RF. Meniscal repair using the outside-to-inside technique. Clin Sports Med 1996;15:469-481.

12. van Trommel MF, Simonian PT, Potter HG, Wickiewicz TL. Arthroscopic meniscal repair with fibrin clot of complete radial tears of the lateral meniscus in the avascular zone. Arthroscopy 1998;14:360-365.

13. van Trommel MF, Simonian PT, Potter HG, Wickiewicz TL. Differential regional healing rates with the outside-in technique for meniscal repair. Am J Sports Med 1998;26:446-452.

14. Warren RF. Arthroscopic meniscal repair. Arthroscopy 1985;1:170-172.

15. Warren RF. Chronic anterior cruciate ligament injury. In Parisien JS, ed. Arthroscopic Surgery. New York, McGraw-Hill, 1988:130.

16. Wolf BR, Cohen DB, Rodeo SA. Outside-in meniscal repair. Tech Knee Surg 2004;3:19-28.

45

CHAPTER 46

Arthroscopic Meniscus Repair: All-Inside Technique

Joshua Baumfeld, MD
David Diduch, MD

The all-inside technique for meniscal repair was first introduced in 1991. Since then, several generations of change have taken place with improvements in implant designs and technique. Inherent advantages of an all-inside technique are the avoidance of accessory incisions and their potential risks, the decrease in operative time, and the ease of insertion compared with other meniscal repair techniques.

The success of an all-inside repair is directly related to its ease of use and its ability to restore stability and to re-create normal anatomy. It must compare favorably with traditional arthroscopic methods of meniscal repair, such as suture repair by the inside-out technique. Potential complications, such as device breakage, pullout, and chondral damage, must be avoided.

This chapter briefly discusses the first three generations of all-inside meniscal repair and concentrates on the surgical techniques associated with the latest fourth-generation implants, specifically the FasT-Fix (Smith & Nephew, Inc., Andover, Mass) and the RapidLoc device (Mitek Worldwide, Westwood, Mass).

Preoperative Considerations

History

Meniscal injury commonly occurs with a twisting injury to the knee and, at times, in conjunction with knee ligamentous injury. There are usually joint line tenderness and mechanical symptoms that include catching, locking, and giving way. Swelling typically occurs overnight in the acute setting and on an intermittent, activity-related basis with a chronic tear.

Physical Examination

- Full knee evaluation bilaterally
- Rule out any hip, pelvic, or back disease that may be contributing to "knee" pain

    Key examination elements for meniscal tears include the following:

- Presence of an effusion
- Extension deficit (which may indicate a locked meniscal fragment)
- Joint line tenderness
- Positive results of McMurray test and Apley test

    Positive findings suggest a meniscal tear.

Imaging

Radiography

Plain radiographs are helpful in assessing for gonarthrosis as well as limb alignment.

- Standing anteroposterior and posteroanterior flexed views
- Lateral and sunrise views

Other Modalities

Magnetic resonance imaging can be more than 90% accurate in identifying meniscal lesions and may be used to help confirm their presence. However, it is not as helpful in predicting whether a tear is reparable. The decision for repair versus partial resection usually requires arthroscopic assessment.

Indications and Contraindications

Many factors play a role in meniscal treatment decision-making. Age of the patient, presence of meniscal degeneration, tear size, tear pattern, vascularity, associated instability, chronicity of the tear, and integrity of the meniscal body must be taken into account. Longitudinal, peripheral (vascular) tears are the most amenable to repair. If there is ligamentous instability, it should be addressed at the time of meniscus repair, if possible, or in the near future if the procedure must be staged. As with other forms of repair, the all-inside technique yields better results with acute, traumatic tears and in those knees undergoing concomitant anterior cruciate ligament (ACL) reconstruction. Tears that are stable with less than 3 mm of displacement with probing and that are less than 1 cm in length can be left unrepaired with predictable results.

Relative contraindications to an all-inside repair are tears that occur at the meniscocapsular junction and tears that extend to the anterior horn. There must be a meniscal rim intact for the anchoring mechanisms of these devices to work appropriately. The anterior horn is difficult to access through anterior portals with any of the available all-inside devices. These situations may be better served with a suture technique, such as the inside-out or outside-in technique.

Surgical Technique

Set-up and Positioning

For knee arthroscopy with meniscal repair, one may use a lateral post or a leg holder. The patient is placed supine. A tourniquet of the appropriate size is placed high on the thigh. When a lateral post is to be used, the leg of the bed need not be broken, although it may improve posterior access. With a leg holder, it is important to position the patient far enough down the bed to allow adequate knee flexion for the operation.

After standard arthroscopic portals are established, a complete diagnostic knee arthroscopy is performed. Meniscal disease is identified, and if it is amenable to repair, the meniscus is prepared with standard techniques as appropriate, such as gentle rasping of the torn surfaces

and more aggressive rasping of the adjacent synovium to stimulate proliferation. For isolated meniscal repair, one may consider biologic augmentation with a fibrin clot. Delivery to the tear can be facilitated by use of an absorbable suture. When an ACL reconstruction is performed simultaneously, fibrin clot occurs naturally.

The portal that affords the most perpendicular approach to the tear should be used to place the device. Typically, this will be the contralateral portal (i.e., introduce the device through the lateral portal for placement in the medial meniscal body). It is common to change portals for optimal access as devices are placed around the meniscal rim. If possible, leave sutures attached until all implants are placed so that they can be tensioned again for optimal compression.

Specific Steps

RapidLoc

Meniscal tear repair by the RapidLoc system is illustrated in Figure 46-1.

FasT-Fix

Meniscal tear repair by the FasT-Fix system is illustrated in Figure 46-2.

Meniscus Arrow and Other Barbed Implants

The implant is introduced into the joint with either a hand inserter or a gun (Fig. 46-3). The tip of the implant is used to reduce the meniscus, and the arrow is placed across the tear by hand or gun. It is nearly impossible to re-tension after the implant is placed.

Meniscal Root or Ossicle Repair

The meniscal ossicle is seen as calcification within the meniscus. Most often, it is found within the posterior root of the medial meniscus. Some believe these represent vestigial structures, whereas others believe that they are secondary to trauma. The same technique may be used for acute avulsion of the meniscal root with or without the presence of an ossicle.

The technique for repair of a meniscal root tear is illustrated in Figure 46-4.

First-Generation Repairs

Originally described in 1991, the first generation of all-inside meniscal repair used curved suture hooks to pass suture across tears from the back of the knee through additional portals, allowing retrieval of the suture followed by knot tying. Technical challenges associated with this technique along with potential risk to the neurovascular structures led to second-generation implants.

Text continued on p. 452.

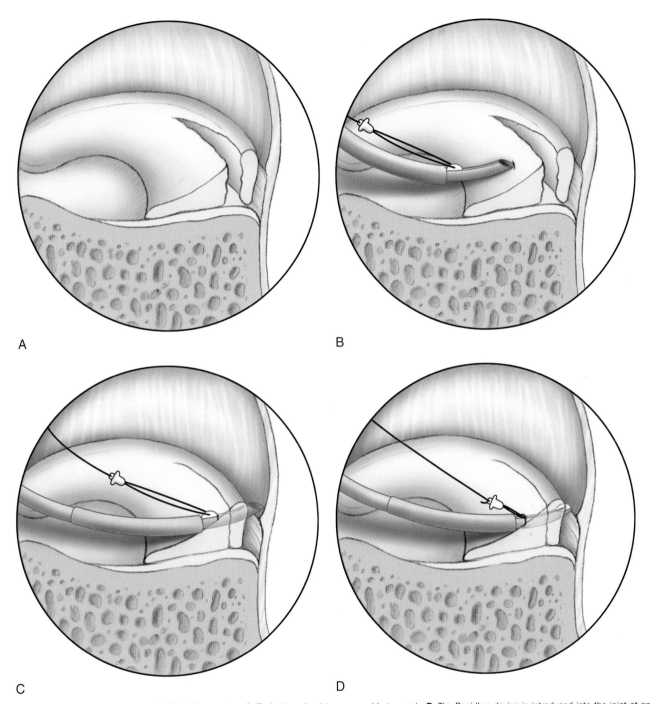

A

B

C

D

Figure 46-1 Meniscal tear repair by the RapidLoc system. **A,** Typical meniscal tear amenable to repair. **B,** The RapidLoc device is introduced into the joint at an angle perpendicular to the tear. The needle is advanced to the surface of the meniscus. **C,** The needle is placed across the meniscal tear and just through the meniscocapsular junction. The silicone sleeve acts as a depth limiter at 13 mm of needle penetration. **D,** The backstop is on the rim of the meniscal tissue.

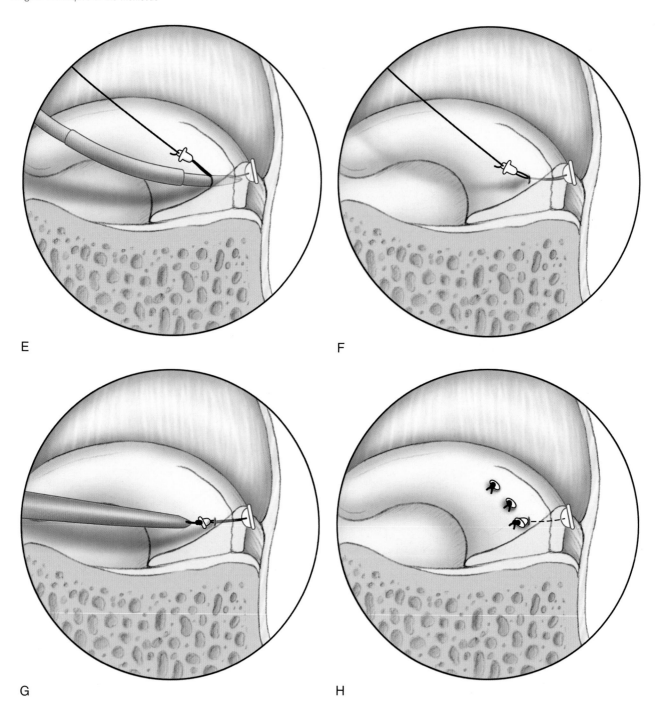

E

F

G

H

Figure 46-1, cont'd E, The needle is removed, leaving the backstop in place. **F,** The suture, with a pre-tied slip knot, is pulled to advance the top hat down to the meniscus. **G,** A knot pusher is used to adjust the compression across the tear. Once complete, the excess suture can be trimmed. **H,** Completed meniscal repair with three RapidLoc implants.

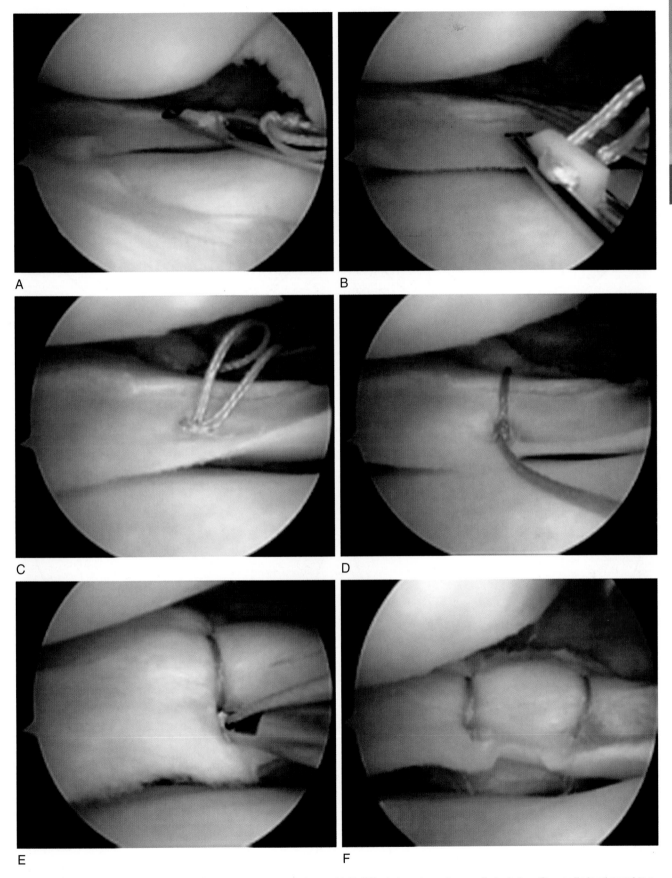

A

B

C

D

E

F

Figure 46-2 Meniscal tear repair by the FasT-Fix system. **A,** Longitudinal tear with FasT-Fix device advanced perpendicular to tear. The needle is advanced to a preset depth to safely engage the peripheral meniscal rim. The FasT-Fix needle is then pulled back while the device is left within the joint. A button on the handle adjacent to one's thumb is then advanced forward to advance the second FasT-Fix implant into place at the needle tip. **B,** The second implant may then be placed in either a horizontal or vertical mattress configuration. In this case, a vertical mattress orientation is chosen. The needle is again advanced to its preset stop. The entire device is withdrawn from the joint. **C,** The vertical mattress suture loop can be seen across the tear before tightening. **D,** The suture limb that exits the joint has a pre-tied slip knot that can be advanced into the joint by pulling on the free suture limb. Variable compression can be attained with the aid of a knot pusher. **E,** The excess suture is then cut. **F,** Final repair with two FasT-Fix sutures in place.

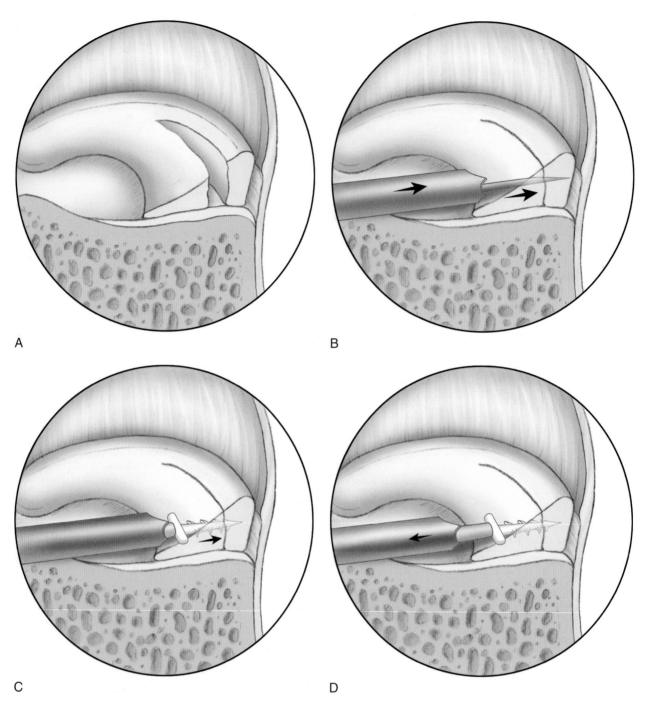

A

B

C

D

Figure 46-3 Meniscal tear repair by the meniscus arrow system.

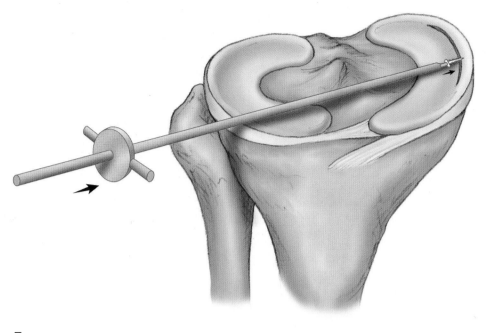

E

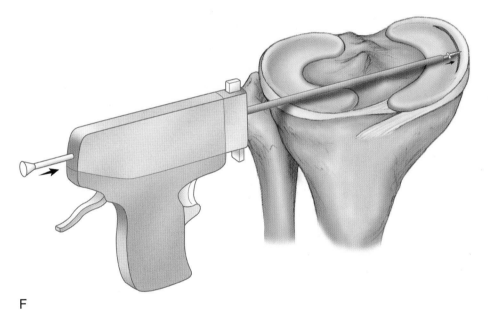

F

Figure 46-3, cont'd

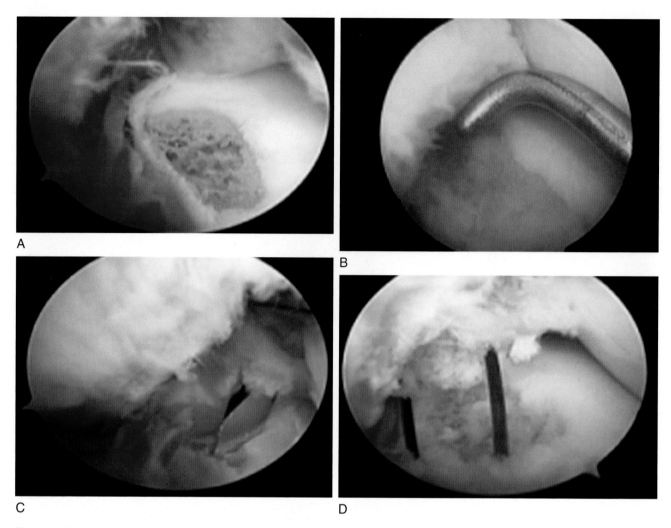

A

B

C

D

Figure 46-4 Technique for repair of a meniscal root tear. **A,** The meniscal ossicle is visualized as a firm, nodular portion of the posterior horn with a matching donor lesion on the tibia. To better visualize the ossicle and donor site, the scope can be driven through the notch to the posterior medial compartment. A limited débridement should be performed of the donor site as well as the posterior horn of the meniscus if there is any surrounding loose meniscal tissue. Débride the donor site and the displaced fragment (if it is an avulsion) back to bleeding bone. A posteromedial working portal is made under direct visualization at an angle amenable to the repair. A 6-mm cannula is placed under direct visualization for the posteromedial working portal. **B,** The probe is passed under the posterior cruciate ligament from the anteromedial portal to manipulate the ossicle. **C** and **E,** Once reduced, the root of the medial meniscus is pierced with a Beath needle through the posteromedial cannula and tensioned, after which the needle is drilled into the donor site and out through the anterolateral tibial cortex. A second pass with the Beath needle is performed 5 mm posterior to the first and also drilled through the tibia to make an inside-out mattress stitch with a No. 1 polydioxanone (PDS) or equivalent suture. **D** and **F,** The sutures are pulled through the tibia, tensioned, and tied over a 10-mm bone bridge on the subcutaneous anterolateral tibial cortex. The pins have to be directed anterior and proximal to avoid the muscles of the anterior compartment of the leg.

Second-Generation Repairs

Second-generation repairs began the evolution of placing devices across the tear by use of standard arthroscopic portals. The T-Fix (Smith & Nephew, Inc., Andover, Mass) had sutures connected to a polyethylene bar that was deployed through a needle to capture the peripheral meniscus or capsule. Pairs of sutures could be tied with a square knot that was pushed onto the meniscal surface, which presented a technical challenge to some. The inability to tension the knot provided another technical drawback. The preliminary results were encouraging with short-term success rates of 80% to 90%.[3,5,10] The T-Fix taught surgeons that an all-inside device could be safely delivered through anterior portals without undue neurovascular risk. However, the desire for a simpler device with more compression across the repair led to the development of third-generation devices.

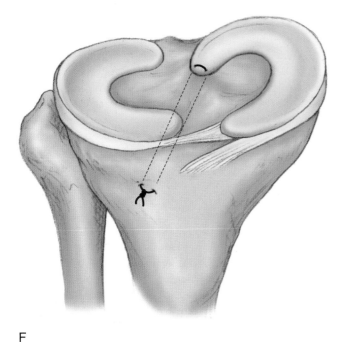

E

F

Figure 46-4, cont'd

Third-Generation Repairs

Many absorbable repair devices, including arrows, screws, darts, and staples, then became available. These capture the torn meniscus and anchor it to its peripheral portion or capsule. Common features of these devices include long-term absorbable material, such as polylactic acid, and a rigid design. The meniscal arrow (Linvatec, Largo, Fla) has achieved popularity secondary to its ease of use and early success rates. Our early experience with the arrow showed a 90.6% success rate with average 2-year follow-up in a population undergoing concurrent ACL reconstruction with the arrow.[12] However, when the same group was observed to 6.6 years, our success rate dropped to 71.4%.[17] This observation suggests that some tears partially heal and become symptomatic as the polylactic acid device dissolves at 2 to 3 years. In addition, longer follow-up may be needed to better determine true outcomes. We have since abandoned the use of the arrow.

Complications reported with these devices, especially the arrow, have included transient synovitis, inflammatory reaction, migration of devices, chondral damage, cyst formation, and device failure (Fig. 46-5).[2,7,14,19,21,22,24-26] A study with a 2-year minimum follow-up had a clinical failure rate of only 7% but had a local soft tissue complication rate of 31.6% with two devices that migrated through the skin.[15]

In a prospective randomized study of 68 patients, a comparison of the arrow and a horizontal mattress suture technique was evaluated. Unique to this study was that a second-look arthroscopy was performed in 96% of the participants at 3 to 4 months. The investigators reported 91% and 75% healing rates for the arrow versus suture,

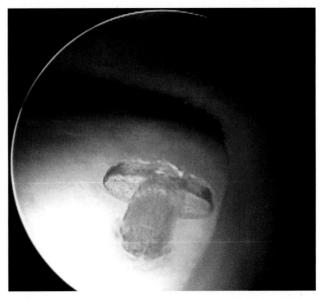

Figure 46-5 Arthroscopic picture of a prominent third-generation device used for repair of a meniscal tear.

respectively. The operative time for arrow insertion was half that of the suture technique. No complications were reported for either group.[1] However, another study comparing suture, arrows, and the T-Fix showed success rates of 78.6%, 56.5%, and 57.1%, respectively.[27] Laprell et al[16] reported on the Mitek meniscal repair system in 2002 in 37 menisci. They found a success rate of 86% at 1 year. In addition, 17 patients underwent second-look arthroscopy at 6 to 8 weeks, and there were five patients with a residual cleft and one with a chondral abrasion. However, all 17 menisci were still reduced. The findings of the long-term arrow study help point out the need for follow-up beyond the point at which these devices dissolve.

Some of these techniques remain popular when they are used in a hybrid fashion with a combination of suture in the body and anterior horn and third-generation implants for the posterior portion of tears. Placement of inside-out suture across the extreme posterior horn can be the most technically demanding and pose the greatest risk to the neurovascular structures. Use of one or two all-inside devices at the extreme posterior horn helps improve these issues.

The majority of the third-generation devices are rigid, increasing the potential for articular cartilage injury. In addition, the native meniscus moves and changes shape with activity. This may be impaired with the use of such rigid devices. Furthermore, once these devices are placed, it is nearly impossible to modify the position if more compression is needed across the tear or if the top of the implant is proud relative to the meniscal surface. The chondral risk and lack of adjustability have led to the fourth-generation devices.

Fourth-Generation Repairs

The fourth-generation devices are flexible and suture based and allow variable compression across the meniscal tear. Two systems are currently available, the FasT-Fix and the RapidLoc meniscal repair device. The FasT-Fix has an inserter with two implants loaded. Each implant consists of 5-mm suture bar anchors and braided No. 0 polyester suture. A needle inserter with an implant loaded at its tip is advanced across the tear, and the anchor is deployed. The needle inserter is withdrawn from the meniscal tissue while it remains within the joint. A button on the handle of the inserter is advanced to allow the second implant to be loaded at the tip of the needle inserter. This can then be advanced through the meniscus in a different location, leaving a suture bridge in either a horizontal or vertical mattress fashion across the tear. A pre-tied slip knot is then advanced to apply variable compression across the tear by use of the knot pusher or suture-cutting device (see Fig. 46-2).

In a prospective case study of 42 meniscal tears treated with the FasT-Fix with an average 2-year follow-up, the group with concurrent ACL reconstruction had a reported success rate of 91%; with isolated repair, that dropped to 80%. No complications were noted, including no chondral abrasion in eight follow-up arthroscopies. In fact, the authors stated that the healing response around the sutures made them barely visible or completely incorporated into the meniscus.[13]

The RapidLoc device is an absorbable anchor and suture device with a pre-tied slip knot to compress an absorbable top hat on the surface of the meniscus (see Fig. 46-1). The top hat is made from either PDS or polylactic acid; the suture options include Ethibond and slowly resorbing Panacryl. A single case applier is introduced with a 0-, 12-, or 27-degree needle with the device loaded. The needle is advanced across the tear, as perpendicular as possible, to its silicone hub, limiting insertion depth to 13 mm. The handle on the applier is fired, which advances and deploys the backstop. The applier is removed. A knot pusher advances the pre-tied slip knot with top hat to the meniscus surface and allows variable tensioning across the tear.

In a study of the RapidLoc, we reviewed 75 meniscal repairs in patients who had undergone concomitant ACL reconstruction with a mean follow-up of 35 months. There was a 90.7% clinical success rate, similar to the equivalent group in the FasT-Fix study. Univariate analysis suggested that negative prognostic factors included a bucket-handle configuration, multiplanar morphologic features, tear length greater than 2 cm, and more than 3 months from tear to repair. Second-look arthroscopy in a small group showed healing and incorporation of the top hat into the meniscal tissue and no chondral abrasion, similar to the FasT-Fix study (Fig. 46-6).[23]

Cadaveric studies of both the RapidLoc and FasT-Fix have been performed. Of the 48 RapidLoc anchors placed by two experienced surgeons, popliteus tendon and superficial medial collateral ligament entrapments by the backstops were the only potential complications encountered, an outcome common with suture techniques and of doubtful clinical importance. More than 80% were placed correctly, and no cartilage injury or vessel entrapment was noted.[20]

In a similar study of the FasT-Fix, 45 anchors were placed. Only 27 were thought to be in the correct position. The original 22-mm preset length was too long and led to penetration of the collateral ligaments, iliotibial tract, and skin. There was difficulty with suture tensioning and early deployment of the anchors. Since the time of this study, modifications to the system have been made, including a shorter insertion device and improvements in its tensioning and deployment characteristics. It is recommended that the optional depth limiter be trimmed to no longer than 15 mm to help avoid potential entrapments and neurovascular injury.

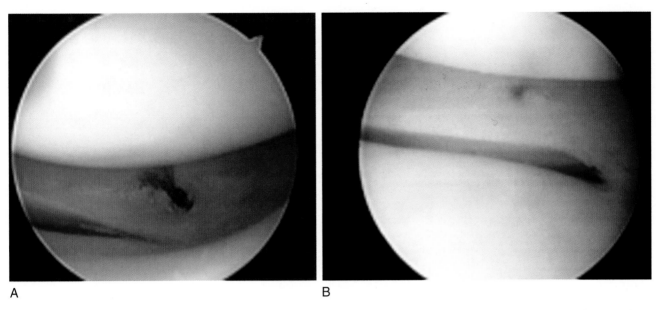

Figure 46-6 Arthroscopic images at the time of meniscal repair **(A)** and second-look arthroscopy **(B)** showing incorporation of the top hat into the meniscal tissue.

Biomechanics

Biomechanical characteristics are shown in Table 46-1.

PEARLS AND PITFALLS

- Use a portal that affords the most perpendicular approach to the tear.
- Change portals as necessary.
- Leave suture attached to implants until all implants are in to allow repeated tensioning.
- Newer, suture-based devices (i.e., RapidLoc, FasT-Fix) offer definite advantages over rigid devices (i.e., arrow), including adjustable tension, low profile, and less chondral risk.
- Do not attempt all-inside repairs on tears at the meniscocapsular junction or tears that affect the anterior horn.
- Isolated meniscus tear without ACL reconstruction may be best repaired with inside-out suture or hybrid techniques.
- With the FasT-Fix, trim the optional depth limiter to no longer than 15 mm to help avoid potential entrapments and neurovascular injury.

Postoperative Considerations

Follow-up

- 10 to 14 days for suture removal and wound check
- 6-week follow-up and progress check

Rehabilitation

For meniscal repair in conjunction with ACL reconstruction, the standard ACL protocol is used with the addition of the following:

- Postoperative hinged ACL brace for 6 weeks, 0 to 90 degrees of motion
- 50% weight bearing for 6 weeks

For isolated meniscal repair without ACL reconstruction, return to sports is permitted at 5 months.

Complications

Most complications are the same as in other types of meniscal repair. The complications specific to all-inside techniques are listed in Box 46-1.

Discussion

All-inside meniscal repair is an attractive option for surgeons. It is easier and can be done with fewer assistants than inside-out and outside-in techniques. Longer follow-up with third-generation rigid devices, such as the meniscal arrow, has shown decreased success rates from originally

Table 46-1 Biomechanics

Author		Vertical FasT-Fix	Horizontal FasT-Fix	Arrow	RapidLoc	Vertical Suture	Horizontal Suture
Barber et al[4] (2004)	Load to failure (N)	70.9	72.1		43.28	80.43	55.9
Fisher et al[11] (2002)	Load to failure (N)			45.89			107.65
Durselen et al[9] (2003)	Load to failure (N)			52			103
	Load to failure after cyclic load (N)			48			82
McDermott et al[18] (2003)	Load to failure (N)		49.1	34.2		72.7	
	Gap after cycling (mm)		3.47	2.18		3.29	
Dervin et al[8] (1997)	Load to failure (N)			29.6		58.3	
Zantop et al[28] (2005)	Load to failure (N)	94.1	80.8		30.3	71.3	50.2
	Gap after cycling (mm)	5.34	6.23		6.84	5.61	6.03
Borden et al[6] (2003)	Load to failure (N)		104	49		102	
	Gap after cycling (mm)		5.1	NA		6	
	Stiffness		7.7	6.1		7.7	

Box 46-1 Complications Specific to All-Inside Techniques

Third-generation rigid devices
- Transient synovitis
- Inflammatory reaction
- Migration of devices
- Chondral damage
- Cyst formation
- Device failure

Fourth-generation implants
- Popliteus entrapment
- Superficial medial collateral ligament entrapment
- Penetration of iliotibial band, collateral ligaments, skin, and, theoretically, the neurovascular structures

reported promising midterm results with various complications, including chondral abrasion. The newer fourth-generation devices are promising in that they are flexible and allow variable tensioning across the repair, characteristics that are more similar to the inside-out technique. The early 2- to 3-year follow-up studies of both the FasT-Fix and RapidLoc are promising, particularly in those patients with smaller tears undergoing concomitant ACL reconstruction, in which greater than 90% success rates have been seen. Second-look arthroscopies with both implants are promising in that there have been no reports

of chondral abrasion, and it appears that the meniscal tissue can grow over these devices.

Currently, we recommend use of these devices for meniscal repairs in conjunction with an ACL repair. On the basis of a critical analysis of our RapidLoc data, we think that to achieve results similar to those of the inside-out techniques, the optimal tear configuration for an all-inside repair includes tears less than 2 cm in length, acute tears (less than 3 months from injury), and those that are in a vertical, non–bucket-handle configuration (cannot be displaced into the notch).[23] It is important that a peripheral rim of meniscal tissue be present. Inside-out techniques should be used for meniscocapsular junction tears. Isolated tears without ACL reconstruction may be best repaired with inside-out or hybrid techniques (all-inside device posteriorly, inside-out suture for remaining posterior horn and body) until long-term follow-up studies are available for these new devices. Inside-out suture remains the "gold standard" against which all new devices must be measured.

Results

Results of studies of all-inside techniques are listed in Table 46-2.

Table 46-2 Results of Studies of All-Inside Techniques

Third-Generation Devices				
Author	**Device**	**Follow-up**	**Success Rate**	**Notes**
Gill and Diduch[12] (2002)	Arrow	2 years (average)	90.6%	
Lee and Diduch[17] (2005)	Arrow	6.6 years (average)	71.4%	Same population with longer follow-up
Albrecht-Olsen et al[1] (1999)	Arrow Suture	3-4 months	91% 75%	Second-look arthroscopy
Venkatachalam et al[27] (2001)	Arrow Suture FasT-Fix		78.6% 56.5% 57.1%	
Laprell et al[16] (2002)	Mitek repair system	1 year	86%	1/17 patients with second-look arthroscopy with chondral injury
Fourth-Generation Devices				
Author	**Device**	**Follow-up**	**Success Rate**	**Notes**
Hass et al[13] (2005)	FasT-Fix	2 years	91% 80%	With ACL reconstruction Isolated repair, no ACL
Quinby et al[23] (2005)	RapidLoc	35 months	90.7%	With ACL reconstruction

ACL, anterior cruciate ligament.

References

1. Albrecht-Olsen P, Kristensen G, Burgaard P, et al. The arrow versus horizontal suture in arthroscopic meniscus repair. A prospective randomized study with arthroscopic evaluation [see comment]. Knee Surg Sports Traumatol Arthrosc 1999;7:268-273.
2. Anderson K, Marx RG, Hannafin J, Warren RF. Chondral injury following meniscus repair with a biodegradable implant. Arthroscopy 2000;16:749-753.
3. Asik M, Sen C, Erginsu M. Arthroscopic meniscal repair using T-fix. Knee Surg Sports Traumatol Arthrosc 2002;10:284-288.
4. Barber FA, Herbert MA, Richards DP. Load to failure testing of new meniscal repair devices. Arthroscopy 2004;20:45-50.
5. Barrett GR, Treacy SH, Ruff CG. Preliminary results of the T-fix endoscopic meniscus repair technique in an anterior cruciate ligament reconstruction population. Arthroscopy 1997;13:218-223.
6. Borden P, Nyland J, Caborn DN, Pienkowski D. Biomechanical comparison of the FasT-Fix meniscal repair suture system with vertical mattress sutures and meniscus arrows. Am J Sports Med 2003;31:374-378.
7. Calder SJ, Myers PT. Broken arrow: a complication of meniscal repair. Arthroscopy 1999;15:651-652.
8. Dervin GF, Downing KJ, Keene GC, McBride DG. Failure strengths of suture versus biodegradable arrow for meniscal repair: an in vitro study. Arthroscopy 1997;13:296-300.
9. Durselen L, Schneider J, Galler M, et al. Cyclic joint loading can affect the initial stability of meniscal fixation implants. Clin Biomech 2003;18:44-49.
10. Escalas F, Quadras J, Caceres E, Benaddi J. T-Fix anchor sutures for arthroscopic meniscal repair. Knee Surg Sports Traumatol Arthrosc 1997;5:72-76.
11. Fisher SR, Markel DC, Koman JD, Atkinson TS. Pull-out and shear failure strengths of arthroscopic meniscal repair systems. Knee Surg Sports Traumatol Arthrosc 2002;10:294-299.
12. Gill SS, Diduch DR. Outcomes after meniscal repair using the meniscus arrow in knees undergoing concurrent anterior cruciate ligament reconstruction. Arthroscopy 2002;18:569-577.
13. Haas AL, Schepsis AA, Hornstein J, Edgar CM. Meniscal repair using the FasT-Fix all-inside meniscal repair device. Arthroscopy 2005;21:167-175.
14. Hechtman KS, Uribe JW. Cystic hematoma formation following use of a biodegradable arrow for meniscal repair. Arthroscopy 1999;15:207-210.
15. Jones HP, Lemos MJ, Wilk RM, et al. Two-year follow-up of meniscal repair using a bioabsorbable arrow. Arthroscopy 2002;18:64-69.
16. Laprell H, Stein V, Petersen W. Arthroscopic all-inside meniscus repair using a new refixation device: a prospective study. Arthroscopy 2002;18:387-393.
17. Lee GP, Diduch DR. Deteriorating outcomes after meniscal repair using the Meniscus Arrow in knees undergoing concurrent anterior cruciate ligament reconstruction: increased failure rate with long-term follow-up [see comment]. Am J Sports Med 2005;33:1138-1141.
18. McDermott ID, Richards SW, Hallam P, et al. A biomechanical study of four different meniscal repair systems, comparing pull-out strengths and gapping under cyclic loading [see comment]. Knee Surg Sports Traumatol Arthrosc 2003;11:23-29.
19. Menche DS, Phillips GI, Pitman MI, Steiner GC. Inflammatory foreign-body reaction to an arthroscopic bioabsorbable meniscal arrow repair. Arthroscopy 1999;15:770-772.
20. Miller MD, Blessey PB, Chhabra A, et al. Meniscal repair with the Rapid Loc device: a cadaveric study. J Knee Surg 2003;16:79-82.
21. Oliverson TJ, Lintner DM. Biofix arrow appearing as a subcutaneous foreign body. Arthroscopy 2000;16:652-655.
22. Otte S, Klinger HM, Beyer J, Baums MH. Complications after meniscal repair with bioabsorbable arrows: two cases and analysis of literature. Knee Surg Sports Traumatol Arthrosc 2002;10:250-253.

23. Quinby J, Hart JA, Golish R, Diduch DR. Meniscal repair using the RapidLoc in knees undergoing concurrent ACL reconstruction. Virginia Orthopedic Society 58th annual meeting; The Homestead, Hot Springs, Va; 2005.

24. Ross G, Grabill J, McDevitt E. Chondral injury after meniscal repair with bioabsorbable arrows. Arthroscopy 2000;16:754-756.

25. Song EK, Lee KB, Yoon TR. Aseptic synovitis after meniscal repair using the biodegradable meniscus arrow [see comment]. Arthroscopy 2001;17:77-80.

26. Tingstad EM, Teitz CC, Simonian PT. Complications associated with the use of meniscal arrows. Am J Sports Med 2001;29:96-98.

27. Venkatachalam S, Godsiff SP, Harding ML. Review of the clinical results of arthroscopic meniscal repair. Knee 2001;8:129-133.

28. Zantop T, Eggers AK, Musahl V, et al. Cyclic testing of flexible all-inside meniscus suture anchors: biomechanical analysis. Am J Sports Med 2005;33:388-394.

CHAPTER 47

Allograft Meniscus Transplantation: Bridge in Slot Technique

Andreas Gomoll, MD
Jack Farr, MD
Brian J. Cole, MD, MBA

It is generally believed that any significant meniscectomy alters the biomechanical and biologic environment of the normal knee, eventually resulting in pain, recurrent swelling, and effusions. Overt secondary osteoarthritis is often the endpoint.[1,2] Recognition of these consequences has led to a strong commitment within the orthopedic community to meniscus-sparing interventions. However, there are cases in which meniscal preservation is not possible. In carefully selected patients, meniscal allografts can restore nearly normal knee anatomy and biomechanics, providing excellent pain relief and improved function.[5]

Several techniques exist for allograft meniscus transplantation, including bone plugs, a keyhole technique, and a dovetail technique. The senior authors prefer the bridge in slot technique, as described previously,[6] because of its simplicity and secure bone fixation, the ability to more easily perform concomitant procedures such as osteotomy and ligament reconstruction, and the advantages of maintaining the relationship of the native anterior and posterior horns of the meniscus.

Preoperative Considerations

History

It is essential to elicit a thorough history, including the causative mechanism, associated injuries, and prior treatments. Operative reports are helpful to evaluate arthritic changes that could constitute a contraindication to meniscal transplantation.

Typical History

- Knee injury, often an acute traumatic event initiating meniscal treatment
- One or more meniscectomies, open or arthroscopically performed with initial improvement
- Subsequent development of ipsilateral joint line pain and activity-related swelling
- Giving way (occasionally reported)

Physical Examination

Factors Affecting Surgical Indication

- Range of motion: usually preserved
- Effusion
- Joint line or femoral condyle tenderness
- Objective evidence of joint space narrowing (magnetic resonance imaging, flexion weight-bearing radiographs), development of localized or diffuse chondral disease in the ipsilateral compartment

Factors Affecting Surgical Planning

- Preexisting incisions
- Limb malalignment (may require concomitant realignment procedure)

- Ligamentous instability (may require prior or concomitant reconstructive procedure)
- Chondral injury, typically involving the femoral condyle (may require concomitant cartilage repair procedure)

Imaging

Radiography

- Weight-bearing anteroposterior radiograph in full extension
- Weight-bearing posteroanterior 45-degree flexion radiograph
- Non–weight-bearing 45-degree flexion lateral view
- Axial view of the patellofemoral joint
- Long-cassette mechanical axis view to evaluate malalignment

Other Modalities

- Magnetic resonance imaging with or without the intra-articular administration of contrast material is performed to assess extent of meniscectomy, degree of articular cartilage damage, and presence of subchondral edema in the involved compartment.
- Technetium bone scan may indicate stress overload in the involved compartment or overt osteoarthritis.

Indications and Contraindications

The ideal candidate has a history of prior total or subtotal meniscectomy with persistent pain localized to the involved compartment, intact articular surfaces (ideally, grade I or II), normal alignment, and a stable joint. Associated pathologic findings, such as malalignment, discrete chondral defects, and ligamentous instability, are not contraindications in an otherwise appropriate candidate because they can be addressed in either staged or concomitant procedures.

In addition to uncorrected comorbidities (malalignment, ligament deficiency, uncorrected localized chondral damage in the involved compartment), contraindications are overt arthroscopic or radiographic arthritic changes (especially associated with femoral condyle or tibial flattening), history of inflammatory arthritis, marked obesity, and previous infection.

Surgical Planning

Concomitant Procedures

Significant limb malalignment, ligamentous instability, or discrete chondral defects can be addressed either before or concomitant with meniscus transplantation.

Allograft Sizing

Meniscal allografts are size and compartment specific. Preoperative measurements are obtained from anteroposterior and lateral radiographs with magnification markers placed on the skin at the level of the joint line. After radiographic magnification is accounted for, meniscal width is measured on the anteroposterior radiograph from the edge of the ipsilateral tibial spine to the edge of the tibial plateau. Meniscal length is calculated by multiplying the depth of the tibial plateau (as measured on lateral radiographs) by 0.8 for the medial meniscus and 0.7 for the lateral meniscus (Fig. 47-1).

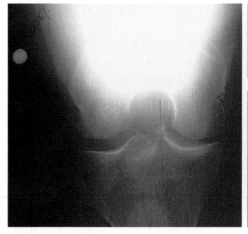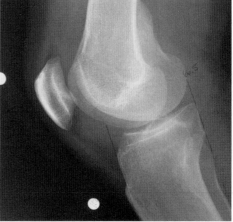

Figure 47-1 Graft sizing on anteroposterior and lateral radiographs.

Meniscal Graft Processing and Preservation

Meniscal allografts are harvested by sterile surgical technique, most commonly within 24 hours of donor asystole. Unlike with fresh osteochondral allografts, cell viability in meniscal allografts does not seem to improve the morphologic or biochemical characteristics of the grafts; thus, the most commonly implanted grafts are either fresh-frozen or cryopreserved. The risk of disease transmission is minimized through rigid donor screening, graft culturing, and polymerase chain reaction testing for human immunodeficiency virus. Several tissue banks are evaluating secondary sterilization techniques to further improve the safety of meniscal allograft tissue.

Surgical Technique

Anesthesia and Positioning

On the basis of the surgeon's, anesthesiologist's, and patient's preferences, the procedure can be performed under general, spinal, or regional anesthesia or a combination thereof. The patient is positioned supine on a standard operating room table, with a thigh tourniquet, and the extremity is placed in a standard leg holder allowing full knee flexion or hyperflexion (Fig. 47-2). The posteromedial or posterolateral corner must be freely accessible for inside-out meniscus suturing to be performed.

Surgical Landmarks, Incisions, and Portals

Landmarks

- Patella
- Patellar tendon
- Tibial plateau
- Fibular head

Portals and Approaches (Fig. 47-3)

- Inferomedial portal
- Inferolateral portal
- Additional outflow portals as needed
- Posteromedial or posterolateral approach
- Mini-arthrotomy through ipsilateral side of patellar tendon

Structures at Risk

- Posterolateral approach: peroneal nerve, lateral collateral ligament

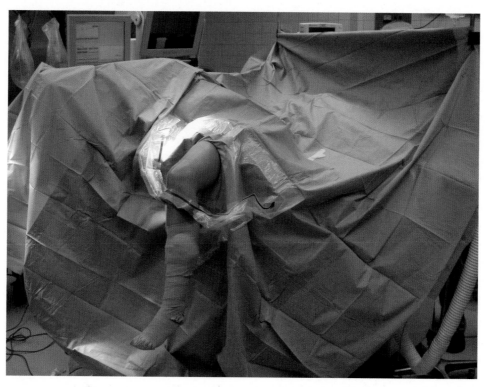

Figure 47-2 Patient positioning.

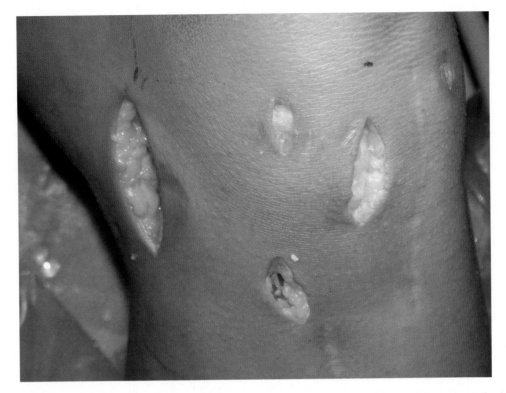

Figure 47-3 Incisions: accessory posteromedial incision (left); inferomedial and inferolateral arthroscopy portals, mini-arthrotomy for meniscal insertion (between portals); accessory incision for concomitant allograft anterior cruciate ligament reconstruction in this patient (inferior).

- Posteromedial approach: saphenous nerve, medial collateral ligament
- Mini-arthrotomy: patellar tendon

Examination Under Anesthesia and Diagnostic Arthroscopy

Examination under anesthesia should evaluate range of motion and ligamentous stability. Diagnostic arthroscopy is useful to evaluate for other intra-articular pathologic processes, such as loose bodies, ligamentous deficiency, and chondral defects.

Specific Steps (Box 47-1)

1. Arthroscopic Preparation

The initial steps for medial and lateral meniscus transplantation are similar. The remaining meniscus is débrided to a stable, 1- to 2-mm peripheral rim until punctate bleeding occurs (Fig. 47-4). The most anterior aspect of the meniscus can be excised under direct visualization by use of a No. 11 scalpel blade placed through the ipsilateral portal followed by the use of an aggressive arthroscopic shaver. The anterior and posterior horn insertion sites should be maintained because they are helpful markers during slot

Box 47-1 Surgical Steps

1. Arthroscopic preparation
2. Exposure
3. Slot preparation
4. Allograft preparation
5. Graft insertion and fixation
6. Closure

preparation. A limited notchplasty along the most inferior and posterior aspect of the ipsilateral femoral condyle allows improved visualization of the posterior horn and facilitates graft passage.

2. Exposure

A mini-arthrotomy is performed in line with the anterior and posterior horn insertion sites of the involved meniscus (see Fig. 47-3). This allows correct orientation of the slot and introduction of the graft. Depending on the surgeon's preference, the arthrotomy can be performed either directly adjacent to or through the patellar tendon in line with its fibers. An ipsilateral (either posteromedial or posterolateral) approach is required for meniscal repair (see Fig. 47-3). The incision should extend approximately one third

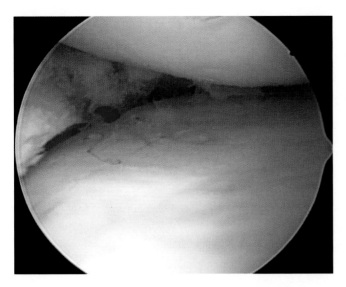

Figure 47-4 Meniscus débrided back to a stable and bleeding rim.

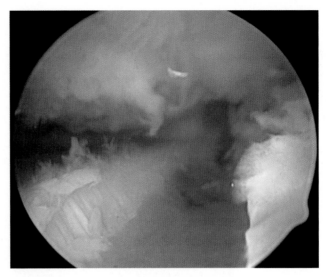

Figure 47-5 Reference slot prepared with a bur.

above and two thirds below the joint line and allow adequate exposure to protect the neurovascular structures during passage of the inside-out sutures. The ipsilateral gastrocnemius muscle–tendon junction is elevated off the posterior capsule, and a meniscal retractor is placed anterior to it. Elevation of either the iliotibial band–tensor fascia lata or sartorius fascia anteriorly allows suture tying beneath these structures to minimize the chances of capturing the knee due to soft tissue tethering.

3. Slot Preparation

Slot orientation follows the normal anatomy of the meniscus attachment sites. By use of electrocautery, the centers of the anterior and posterior horn attachment sites are connected with a line. With this line as a guide, a 4-mm bur is used to make a reference slot in the tibial plateau. Its height and width will equal the dimensions of the bur, and its alignment in the sagittal plane should parallel the slope of the tibial plateau (Fig. 47-5). Slot dimensions should be confirmed by placement of a depth gauge in the reference slot, which also measures the anteroposterior length of the tibial plateau (Fig. 47-6). With use of a drill guide, a guide pin is placed just distal and parallel to the reference slot (Fig. 47-7) and advanced to but not through the posterior cortex. The pin is subsequently overreamed with a 7- or 8-mm cannulated drill bit (Fig. 47-8), again with care taken to maintain the posterior cortex. A box cutter is then used to make a slot 7 to 8 mm wide by 10 mm deep (Fig. 47-9), which is smoothed and refined with a 7- to 8-mm rasp to ensure that the bone bridge will slide smoothly into the slot (Fig. 47-10).

4. Meniscal Allograft Preparation

This technique uses a bone bridge to secure the graft to the tibial plateau. The bone bridge is intentionally undersized by 1 mm to facilitate graft passage and to reduce the

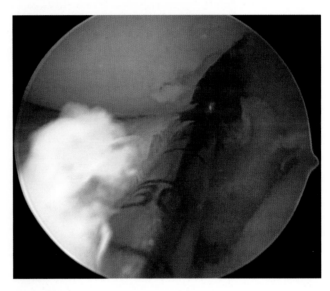

Figure 47-6 Guide probe in reference slot.

risk of inadvertent bridge fracture during insertion. The attachment sites of the meniscus are identified on the bone block, and the accessory attachments are débrided. Only the true attachment sites should remain, usually 5 to 6 mm wide. The bone bridge is then cut to a width of 7 mm and a height of 1 cm. Also, any bone extending beyond the posterior horn attachment site is removed; bone anterior to the attachment site of the anterior horn should be preserved to maintain graft integrity during insertion. A vertical mattress traction suture of No. 0 polydioxanone (PDS) is placed at the junction of the posterior and middle thirds of the meniscus (Fig. 47-11).

On occasion, the anterior horn attachment can be larger, up to 9 mm wide. If the anterior horn attachment site is wider than the intended width of the bone bridge,

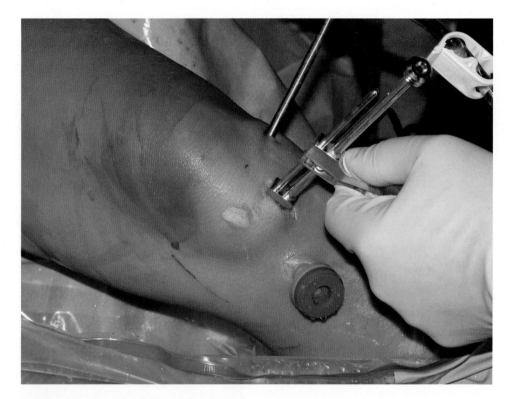

Figure 47-7 Guide pin placement.

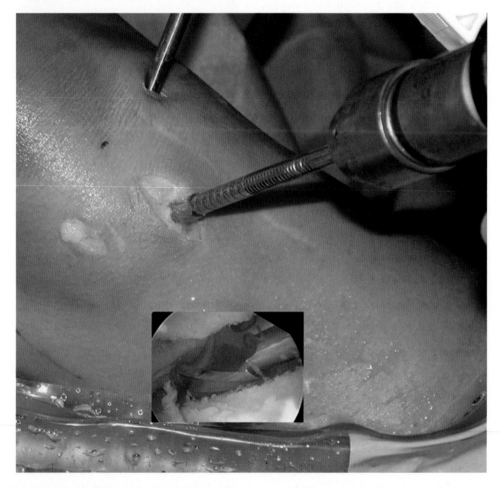

Figure 47-8 Overburring of guide pin to make the slot. *Inset:* arthroscopic view.

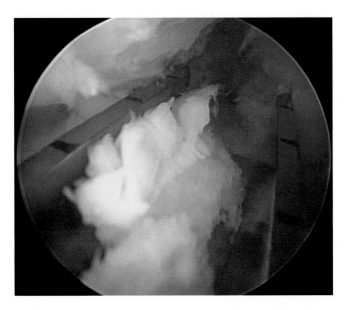

Figure 47-9 View of the box cutter connecting the superficial reference slot and deeper bur tunnel.

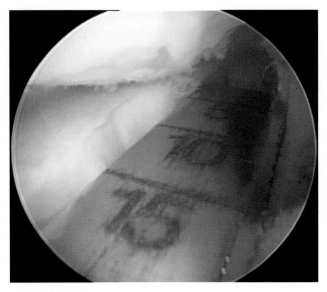

Figure 47-10 Rasping to smooth the slot.

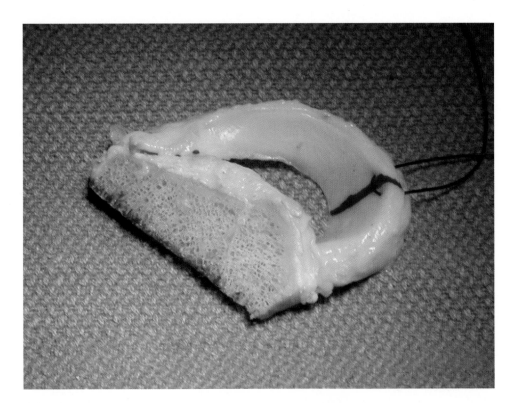

Figure 47-11 Prepared allograft with traction suture.

the attachment should be left intact, and the width of the bone bridge should be increased accordingly in the area of the anterior horn insertion only; the remainder of the bone bridge should be trimmed to 7 mm as intended. To accommodate the increased width, the corresponding area of the recipient slot should be widened accordingly.

5. Meniscus Insertion and Fixation

A single-barrel, zone-specific meniscal repair cannula placed through the contralateral portal on viewing through the ipsilateral portal is directed toward the capsular attachment site of the posterior and middle thirds of the meniscus. A long, flexible nitinol suture-passing pin is placed through the capsule to exit the accessory posteromedial or posterolateral incision. The proximal end of the nitinol pin is then withdrawn from the anterior arthrotomy site (Fig. 47-12), the allograft traction sutures are passed through the loop of the nitinol pin, and the pin and sutures are withdrawn through the accessory incision (Fig. 47-13). With the aid of the traction sutures, the meniscal allograft is pulled into the joint through the anterior arthrotomy while the bone bridge is advanced into the tibial slot, and the meniscus is manually reduced under the condyle with a finger placed through the arthrotomy (Fig. 47-14). Appropriate valgus or varus stress to open the ipsilateral compartment aids in graft introduction and reduction. Once the meniscus is reduced, the knee is cycled to ensure proper placement and capturing by the tibiofemoral articulation, and the bone bridge is secured within the tibial slot with a bioabsorbable cortical interference screw. Finally, the graft is attached to the capsule with standard inside-out vertical mattress sutures placed equally on the dorsal and ventral meniscal surfaces (Fig. 47-15). This fixation can be supplemented with appropriate all-inside fixation devices placed most posteriorly and outside-in suture placed most anteriorly.

6. Closure

Standard closure of the arthrotomy and accessory incisions is performed.

Combined Procedures

Anterior Cruciate Ligament Reconstruction and Medial Meniscus Allograft Transplantation

- Prepare the soft tissue graft (hamstring autograft or Achilles tendon, tibialis anterior, or hamstring allograft).
- Drill tibial tunnel for anterior cruciate ligament (ACL) as oblique as possible, entering lateral aspect of tibial footprint.
- Drill femoral tunnel for ACL.
- Prepare meniscal slot as usual.
- Pass and fix femoral side of ACL graft.
- Pass meniscus and reduce soft tissue and bone components.
- Fix tibial side of ACL graft.
- Place interference screw against meniscus bridge (between ACL and most lateral aspect of bridge).
- Repair meniscus.
- Note: notching bone bridge may reduce intersection pressure of ACL graft against bone bridge.

Tibial Osteotomy and Medial Meniscus Allograft Transplantation

- Perform all aspects of meniscus transplantation first.

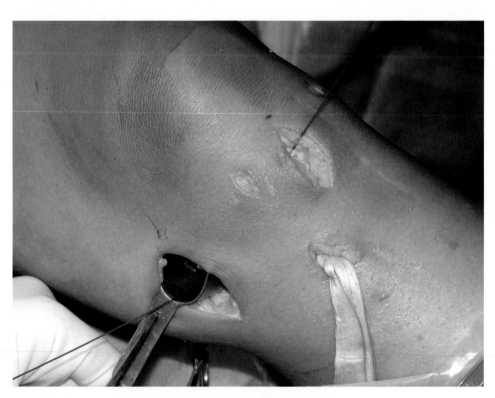

Figure 47-12 Nitinol wire in place. Also shown is an Achilles tendon allograft for anterior cruciate ligament reconstruction.

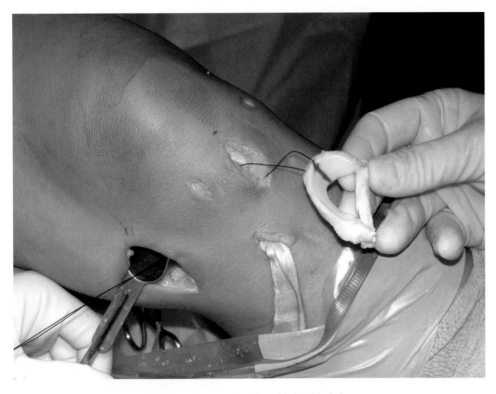

Figure 47-13 The traction sutures have been passed through the accessory incision with the nitinol pin.

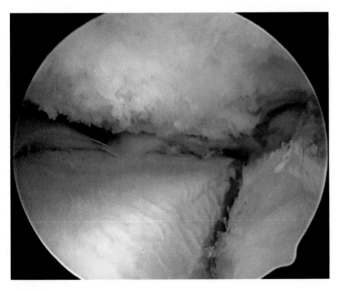

Figure 47-14 The reduced meniscus and bridge situated in the slot.

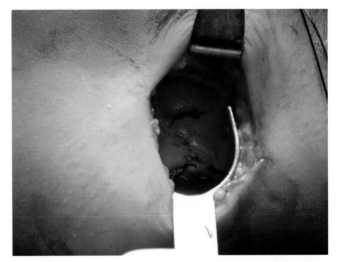

Figure 47-15 Capsular sutures for the meniscal repair as viewed through the posteromedial incision.

- Perform opening wedge osteotomy such that line of osteotomy passes at least 1.5 cm below bottom of tibial slot.

Postoperative Considerations

Follow-up

- At 7 to 10 days for suture removal and postoperative radiographs (Fig. 47-16)

Rehabilitation

- Immediate partial weight bearing is allowed in a hinged knee brace; range of motion is limited to 0 to 90 degrees of flexion.
- Non–weight-bearing flexion beyond 90 degrees is allowed immediately.
- Full weight-bearing and range-of-motion and gentle strengthening exercises are initiated at 4 weeks postoperatively.
- In-line running is permitted after 16 weeks.
- Return to full activities is permitted after 6 months, once strength has returned to more than 80% that of the contralateral leg.

Complications

Complications are those of meniscal repair:

- Incomplete healing of the meniscus repair
- Infection
- Arthrofibrosis

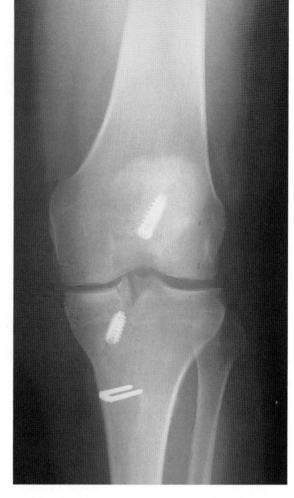

Figure 47-16 Postoperative radiograph (concomitant anterior cruciate ligament reconstruction).

- Neurovascular injury (saphenous nerve medially, peroneal nerve laterally)

Traumatic tears of the transplanted meniscus are treated with standard arthroscopic meniscal repair or partial meniscectomy as indicated.

PEARLS AND PITFALLS

- The posterior meniscal horn can be débrided more easily and more completely once the slot has been made.
- The anterior meniscal horn can be cut with a scalpel blade through the ipsilateral portal to improve débridement. Be careful not to break the blade (especially No. 11 blades).
- In making the superficial slot with the bur, sometimes the bur catches and pulls across the articular surface of the tibia. A secure hold on the bur, reversal of its direction, and strong downward pressure can minimize the risk of this occurrence.

With Concomitant ACL Reconstruction

- Achilles allograft has been helpful because it has no bone block in the tibia that would interfere with the slot for the meniscal allograft.

- Use a more vertical tibial tunnel that enters the joint more toward the contralateral side of the meniscal allograft.
- Pass the ACL graft and perform the femoral fixation, then pass the meniscus and seat the slot. Finally, fix the tibial ACL and place the interference screw adjacent to the meniscus bridge for final fixation.

With Concomitant Osteotomy

- Finish the meniscal transplantation before performing the osteotomy because introduction of the meniscus requires significant varus or valgus stress. This could jeopardize fixation if the osteotomy were to be performed first.
- In wedging open a high tibial osteotomy, a thin osteotome can be placed proximal to the wedges to support the tibial plateau; otherwise, the crack could propagate into the meniscal allograft slot, resulting in a tibial plateau fracture.

Table 47-1 Clinical Results of Meniscal Allograft Transplantation

Author	Follow-up	Outcome
Milachowski et al[10] (1989)	14-month mean	19 of 22 (86%) successful
Garrett[7] (1993)	2-7 years	35 of 43 (81%) successful
Noyes and Barber-Westin[11] (1995)	30-month mean (range: 22-58 months)	56 of 96 (58%) failed
van Arkel and de Boer[16] (1995)	2-5 years	20 of 23 (87%) successful
Goble et al[8] (1996)	2-year minimum	17 of 18 (94%) successful
Cameron and Saha[2] (1997)	31-month mean (range: 12-66 months)	58 of 63 (92%) successful
Carter[3] (1999)	48-month mean	45 of 51 (88%) successful
Rodeo[13] (2001)	2-year minimum	22 of 33 (67%) successful 14 of 16 (88%) with bone fixation 8 of 17 (47%) without bone fixation
Rath et al[12] (2001)	5.4-year mean (range: 2-8 years)	14 of 22 (64%) successful
Verdonk et al[17] (2005)	7.2-year mean (range: 0.5-14.5 years)	10 of 61 (16%) lateral transplants failed 11 of 39 (28%) medial transplants failed
Cole et al[4] (2006)	33.5-month mean (range: 24 to 57 months)	41 of 45 (91%) successful 85% of successful transplants would have surgery again

Results

After meniscal allograft transplantation, good to excellent results are achieved in nearly 85% of cases, and patients demonstrate a measurable decrease in pain and increase in activity level (Table 47-1). The risk of graft failure appears greatest with irradiated grafts, grade III to IV osteoarthritic changes, and residual malalignment or instability.

References

1. Alford W, Cole BJ. The indications and technique for meniscal transplant. Orthop Clin North Am 2005;36:469-484.
2. Cameron JC, Saha S. Meniscal allograft transplantation for unicompartmental arthritis of the knee. Clin Orthop 1997;337:164-171.
3. Carter TR. Meniscal allograft transplantation. Sports Med Arthrosc Rev 1999;7:51-62.
4. Cole BJ, Dennis MG, Lee SJ, et al. Prospective evaluation of allograft meniscus transplantation: a minimum 2-year follow-up. Am J Sports Med 2006;34:919-927.
5. Cole BJ, Rodeo S, Carter T. Allograft meniscus transplantation: indications, techniques, results. J Bone Joint Surg Am 2002;84:1236-1250.
6. Farr J, Meneghini RM, Cole BJ. Allograft interference screw fixation in meniscus transplantation. Arthroscopy 2004;20:322-327.
7. Garrett JC. Meniscal transplantation: a review of 43 cases with two to seven year follow-up. Sports Med Arthrosc Rev 1993;1:164-167.
8. Goble EM, Kane SM, Wilcox TR, Doucette SA. Meniscal allografts. In McGinty JB, Caspari RB, Jackson RW, Poehling GG, eds. Operative Arthroscopy. Philadelphia, Lippincott-Raven, 1996:317-331.
9. Graf KW, Sekiya JK, Wojtys EM. Long-term results following meniscal allograft transplantation: minimum eight and one half-year follow-up. Arthroscopy 2004;20:129-140.
10. Milachowski KA, Weismeir K, Wirth CJ. Homologous meniscus transplantation: experimental and clinical results. Int Orthop 1989; 13:1-11.
11. Noyes FR, Barber-Westin SD. Irradiated meniscus allografts in the human knee: a two to five year follow-up. Orthop Trans 1995; 19:417.
12. Rath E, Richmond J, Yassir W, et al. Meniscal allograft transplantation: two to eight year results. Am J Sports Med 2001;29:410-414.
13. Rodeo SA. Current concepts: meniscus allografts—where do we stand? Am J Sports Med 2001;29:246-261.
14. Sekiya JK, Giffin RJ, Irrgang JJ, et al. Clinical outcomes following combined meniscal allograft transplantation and anterior cruciate ligament reconstruction. Am J Sports Med 2003;31:896-906.
15. Sekiya JK, West RV, Groff YJ, et al. Clinical outcomes following isolated lateral meniscal allograft transplantation. Arthroscopy 2006;22:771-780.
16. van Arkel ERA, de Boer HH. Human meniscal transplantation: preliminary results at 2- to 5-year follow-up. J Bone Joint Surg Br 1995;77:589-595.
17. Verdonk PC, Demurie A, Almqvist KF, et al. Transplantation of viable meniscal allograft. Survivorship analysis and clinical outcome of one hundred cases. J Bone Joint Surg Am 2005;87:715-724.
18. Yoldas EA, Sekiya JK, Irrgang JJ, et al. Arthroscopically assisted meniscal allograft transplantation with and without combined anterior cruciate ligament reconstruction. Knee Surg Sports Traumatol Arthrosc 2003;11:173-182.

CHAPTER 48

Allograft Meniscus Transplantation: Dovetail Technique

Thomas R. Carter, MD

The meniscus provides many functions for the well-being of the knee, including load bearing, joint stability, and congruency. With so many roles in maintaining normal knee function, it is of little debate that excision results in an increased risk of arthritis. Unfortunately, the ideal replacement for the meniscus has yet to be discovered. At present, meniscal allografts have served as the most successful substitute. Whereas the durability and the ability to prevent or to delay arthritis are questioned, studies have shown that patients typically have less pain and improved function after meniscus implantation. However, the indications are narrow, and the procedure is technically challenging.

Many surgical methods have been described for meniscal allograft transplantation. They are typically classified into two broad categories on the basis of securing the meniscus at its attachments sites with bone or without bone. Although bone fixation techniques are more difficult, several basic science studies have shown that they more closely replicate normal meniscus stress force protection. With this fact, until clinical studies show otherwise, bone fixation methods are recommended.

Within the bone fixation category, several techniques are used. These include bone plugs, keyhole method, slot technique, and dovetail technique. Each has its pros and cons. I prefer the dovetail technique for lateral meniscus and bone plugs for medial meniscus. The rationale for the medial side takes into consideration that the distance between the anterior and posterior horns is several centimeters, with a highly variable anterior attachment site. By having the horns separate (i.e., two separate bone plugs), it enables placement of the bone plugs to match the native meniscus insertion sites. Because the anterior and posterior horns of the native lateral meniscus are close, maintaining a bone bridge between the horns is recommended. The dovetail method enables not only preparation of the channel under direct observation but also a press-fit fixation.

Preoperative Considerations

History

Although it is intuitive, the first item is confirmation that the meniscus has been excised. Intraoperative photographs, operative reports, and magnetic resonance imaging studies should be available. If any doubt remains, diagnostic arthroscopy should be performed.

Typical History

The typical history for appropriate candidates is as follows:

- Symptoms are localized to the involved compartment.
- Discomfort is commonly present with activities of daily living and enhanced activity.
- Joint effusions may occur and are commonly activity related.

Physical Examination

Appropriate candidates typically have minimal physical findings beyond joint line tenderness and, at most, mild joint effusions.

More often, patients have findings that may preclude surgical candidacy:

- Evidence of diffuse arthritis: palpable osteophytes, decreased range of motion, crepitus
- Ligamentous instability (needs to be corrected before or at the time of implantation)
- Limb alignment (if mechanical axis is through involved compartment, may need realignment)
- Morbid obesity
- Other limb or back abnormalities

Imaging

Radiography

Include a magnification marker for reference in graft sizing.

- Weight-bearing 45-degree posteroanterior view
- Weight-bearing anteroposterior view in full extension
- Non–weight-bearing 45-degree lateral view
- Axial view of the patellofemoral joint
- Full-length view of limb for mechanical axis evaluation

Other Modalities

Magnetic resonance imaging is performed if there is a question of degree of meniscectomy, associated pathologic change, to degree of stress reaction of bone.

A bone scan is obtained if there is a question of stress to the involved knee compartment. However, use has declined with advancement of magnetic resonance imaging techniques.

Indications and Contraindications

The ideal candidate is a patient who has had a prior meniscectomy in an otherwise normal knee and experiences pain localized to this compartment. The degree of articular cartilage damage is slight with no greater than Outerbridge grade II chondrosis in the involved compartment. Patients with grade III chondrosis may also be candidates, but not grade IV, unless it is a discrete defect that can be corrected before or at the time of meniscal implantation. Associated pathologic processes, such as ligament instability and limb malalignment, provided correction can be performed, do not exclude patients.

Contraindications are advanced arthrosis of the involved compartment and diffuse knee joint chondrosis. Comorbidities that are not correctable are exclusion criteria. Obesity, inflammatory arthropathy, and avascular necrosis are also contraindications. Unrealistic expectations of the patient should also be taken into consideration (the knee will not be returned to normal).

Surgical Planning

Concomitant Procedures

Ligament instability and contained chondral defects are addressed at the time of the meniscus implantation. Controversy exists as to whether limb realignment should be performed any time the mechanical axis passes through the involved compartment or only if there is a measurable difference between the two legs. Apart from this debate, limb realignment procedures are usually performed when the meniscus is implanted.

If both osteotomy and ligament reconstructions are necessary, it is common to stage the procedures because of the concern of tunnel or screw overlap and associated adequate fixation. My preference is to perform the osteotomy first and, after healing, then the meniscus and ligament reconstructions.

Allograft Sizing

Various methods have been used for sizing of meniscal allografts to match the host. Whereas magnetic resonance images and computed tomographic scans can be used, plain radiographs are the most common means. Anteroposterior and lateral views are obtained with a magnification marker placed at the level of the joint line. Any obliquity or rotation that may affect measurement of the tibial plateau is not acceptable. Tissue banks do not have uniform methods of sizing. Therefore, if any question is present, it is wise to verify the size match.

Meniscal Graft Processing and Preservation

Although the risk of disease transmission from meniscal allografts is minimal, it still exists. It is thus prudent to diminish risk of contamination even further by making certain the tissue bank is certified by the American Association of Tissue Banks. To obtain the certification, the bank must follow stringent methods of procurement and processing of the allograft tissue.

Grafts can be fresh, cryopreserved, or frozen. Fresh grafts are typically not used because of the increased risk of disease transmission. Whereas some degree of cell viability is able to be achieved with cryopreservation, the clinical benefit compared with frozen grafts, which are acellular, has not been answered. Lyophilization (i.e., freeze-drying) eliminates contamination, but it is not recommended because of the deleterious effect it has on the structural integrity of the meniscal allograft.

Surgical Technique

Anesthesia and Positioning

The procedure is typically performed under general anesthesia. The patient's position and set-up are the same as the surgeon's preference in performing a meniscus repair.

Surgical Landmarks, Incisions, and Portals

Landmarks

- Patella
- Patellar tendon
- Tibial plateau
- Fibular head (lateral meniscus)

Portals and Approaches

- Anteromedial: border of patellar tendon
- Anterolateral: border of patellar tendon
- Outflow portal as desired
- Posteromedial or posterolateral: ipsilateral of graft for suturing
- Mini-arthrotomy: extend ipsilateral portal for graft insertion

Structures at Risk

- Posteromedial approach: saphenous nerve
- Posterolateral approach: peroneal nerve, popliteal tendon

Examination Under Anesthesia and Diagnostic Arthroscopy

The meniscal allograft should not be opened before a complete physical examination of the knee and diagnostic arthroscopy are performed. Their significance is to confirm that the patient is a candidate for a meniscal allograft.

Specific Steps (Box 48-1)

1. Arthroscopic Host Site Preparation

The initial arthroscopic portal should be established on the side opposite the graft, immediately adjacent to the patellar tendon border. This enables passage of the scope through the notch and visualization of the posterior horn attachment. Before the graft-side portal is made, a spinal needle is used to confirm that the portal site is directly in line with the horn attachments. Any obliquity in the skin incision to the horn attachments can cause difficulty in the proper orientation when the bone channel is prepared. Once the portals are made, the meniscal remnant is débrided to approximately a 2-mm vascular rim (Figs. 48-1 and 48-2). The anterior portion of the meniscus can be addressed after the arthrotomy is made. To ensure proper channel height and alignment, a burr is used to remove the tibial spine to a height that is equal to the level of the tibial plateau articular cartilage and straight in line with the attachment sites. If there is still any difficulty in full visualization of the posterior horn attachment, a limited notchplasty should be performed. Likewise, the entire anterior attachment needs to be seen to be used as a reference for initial placement of the osteotome. Although a tourniquet can be inflated at any time, it is typically not

Box 48-1 Surgical Steps

1. Arthroscopic host site preparation
2. Meniscal allograft preparation
3. Arthrotomy with graft insertion
4. Securing of graft
5. Closure

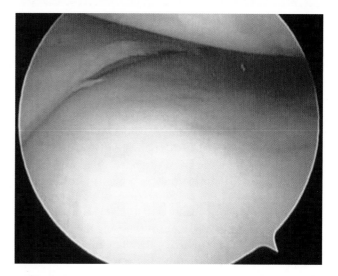

Figure 48-1 Lateral compartment showing complete meniscectomy.

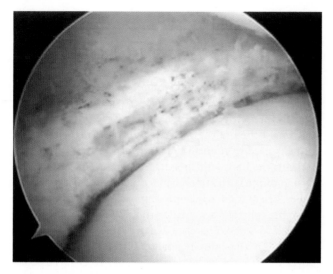

Figure 48-2 Remnant débrided to a bleeding border.

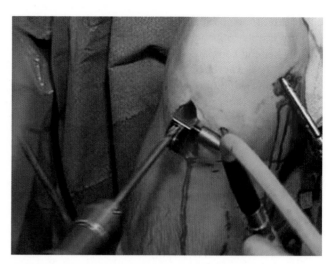

Figure 48-4 Drill guide attached to the osteotome and used to prepare the channel.

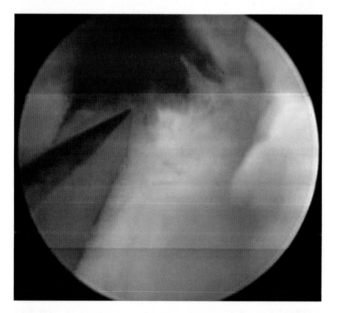

Figure 48-3 Osteotome used as reference parallel to horn attachments with a depth line for reference in drilling.

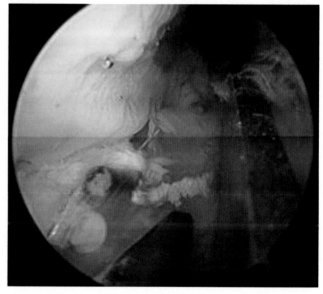

Figure 48-5 Second drill used to deepen the channel.

done so until this point. By waiting, it allows confirmation of a vascular rim and conserves tourniquet time. Higher pressure and inflow rates are often needed to limit bleeding during bone channel preparation, which is why the tourniquet may be required at this point in the case.

The ipsilateral portal is extended to approximately 3 cm in length. The osteotome is brought into the knee and used as a guide for further channel preparation. It follows the initial trough and is placed at the most central aspect of the knee near the notch (hugging the tibial anterior cruciate ligament insertion) to allow room for proper drill placement. A guideline on the osteotome is followed to ensure the proper depth in the tibial plateau at all times (Fig. 48-3). The osteotome should be inserted to 1 or

2 mm just short of the back of the plateau to maintain a back wall and prevent overinsertion of the graft. The initial osteotome attachment guide is placed and allows a 6-mm drill to initiate the channel under direct visualization (Fig. 48-4). The second osteotome attachment is used for a 7-mm drill placement just beneath the level of the first drill (Fig. 48-5). A rasp and tamp finish the dovetail slot by expanding the channel and compressing the cancellous bone at it borders (Figs. 48-6 and 48-7).

2. Meniscal Allograft Preparation

One of the main benefits of the dovetail method is the use of cutting guides to prepare the graft, rather than preparation of the graft by a free-hand technique. As a result, it not only saves time but, more important, decreases the

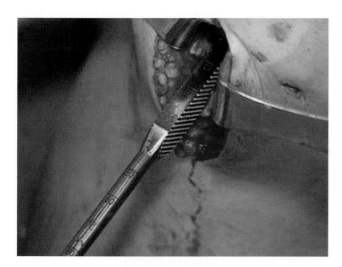

Figure 48-6 Rasp inserted to complete channel.

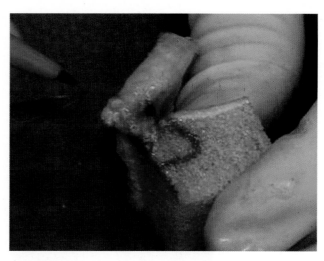

Figure 48-8 Graft marked with the dovetail template.

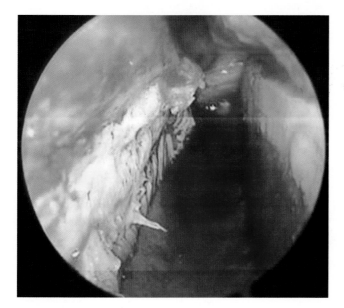

Figure 48-7 Appearance of completed dovetail slot.

chance of an improper match between the recipient channel and graft. The graft is initially sawed so that the horn attachments are flush with the ends of the allograft bone, and the graft is marked with the dovetail template (Fig. 48-8). It is then inserted upside-down into the graft station and secured with the side attachments. The three cutting guides are then used in sequential order to cut the bone, resulting in a dovetail design (Fig. 48-9).

The dovetail graft sizer is used to confirm that the allograft will slide through the channel, but with a snug fit so that it will maintain a press fit (Fig. 48-10). Any minor adjustments should be made at this time rather than attempted during insertion of the graft.

3. Arthrotomy with Graft Insertion

As with a standard meniscus repair by inside-out technique, a posteromedial or posterolateral incision is made to retrieve the meniscal sutures. A "reduction" suture is placed through the graft at the 10- or 2-o'clock position, passed into the joint, and retrieved. Proper placement of the reduction suture is important. When it is placed in the middle of the graft, it has a tendency to not bring the graft fully into the joint. With the suture retrieved, the meniscus is inserted into the channel and gently pushed inward while carefully pulling on the suture (Fig. 48-11). Extreme force should not be used because the sutures can be pulled through the graft and the bone bridge either fractured or inserted too far into the channel. Provided the channel and the graft bone are of proper size, a tamp can be used to assist in insertion. Care must be taken on insertion of the graft, for too forceful insertion may break out the posterior wall. Gentle tension on the reduction suture and application of an appropriate amount of varus or valgus stress on the knee aid in reduction of the meniscus (Fig. 48-12).

Once the graft is reduced, there is a tendency first to repair the anterior aspect of the graft under direct visualization before the arthrotomy is closed. However, to ensure anatomic position, the graft is initially secured with sutures in the posterior third and then the middle third of the graft. By proceeding in this manner, the anterior aspect is more forgiving in making adjustments in the graft position when the meniscus does not match perfectly.

4. Securing of Graft

Numerous methods can be used to secure the graft, but inside-out vertical mattress sutures are preferred because of greater strength. Either absorbable or nonabsorbable sutures can be used, for healing of the graft to the host readily occurs. Eight sutures are typically all that is needed (Fig. 48-13).

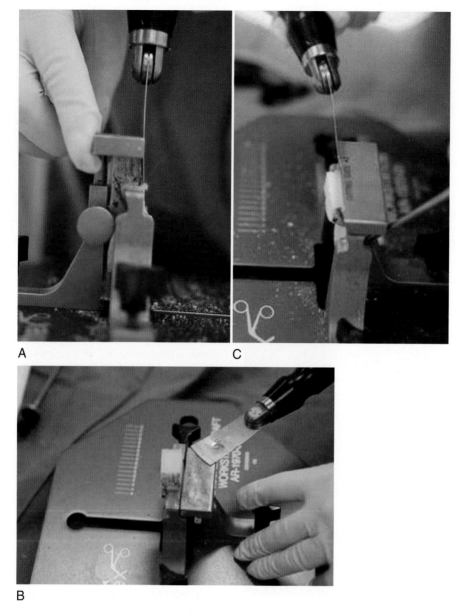

A

C

B

Figure 48-9 Three cutting guides complete the graft preparation.

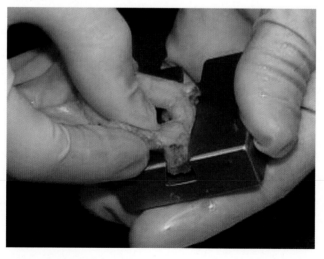

Figure 48-10 Graft sizer used to confirm press fit capability.

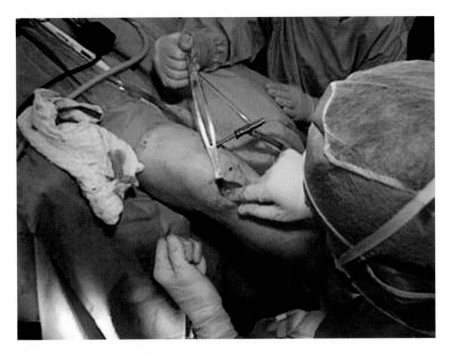

Figure 48-11 Graft brought into the knee with traction as aid.

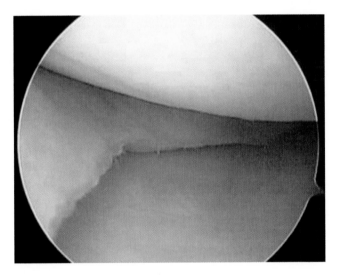

Figure 48-12 Graft reduced into the channel and ready for suturing.

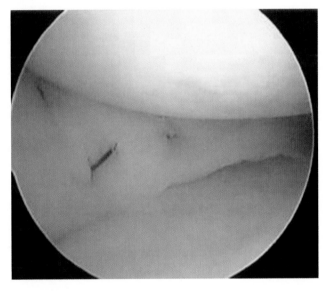

Figure 48-13 Completed meniscal allograft.

5. Closure

The wounds are closed, and dressing is applied by the treating surgeon's preference. A postoperative brace is applied and initially locked in full extension.

Combined Procedures

Anterior Cruciate Ligament Reconstruction and Meniscal Allograft Transplantation

- Arthroscopic preparation for both is performed first.
- The meniscus is placed and sutured.
- The anterior cruciate ligament (ACL) is then reconstructed.
- Proper tunnel and channel placements should not result in overlap.
- Meniscus is completed first to decrease difficulty in meniscus insertion.

Tibial Osteotomy and Meniscal Allograft Transplantation

- Meniscus implantation is completed first.
- Osteotomy is performed second to avoid possible fluid extravasation during the meniscus insertion.
- Perform osteotomy line as low as possible to avoid disruption of dovetail bone.

Tibial Osteotomy, Anterior Cruciate Ligament Reconstruction, and Meniscal Allograft Transplantation

- These procedures are typically staged owing to concern for overlap of channel, tunnels, and screws and poor fixation.
- Osteotomy is performed first, then ACL reconstruction and meniscus implantation.

PEARLS AND PITFALLS

- Proper placement of the arthroscopic portals has a major effect on ensuring that the channel is a straight line between the two meniscus attachments and enables complete visibility of the posterior horn. The contralateral portal is made first and hugs the patellar tendon. Ipsilateral portal placement can be ensured by use of a spinal needle before the incision is made. Any obliquity on the ipsilateral side can result in improper channel alignment.
- On occasion, the graft has a tendency to be pulled outward when it is sutured. Placement of the initial few sutures in horizontal fashion on the superior aspect of the meniscus can aid in maintaining proper position.

With Concomitant ACL Reconstruction

If a soft tissue graft is used for the ACL reconstruction, wait until meniscus implantation is completed before passage of the ACL graft. If there is any channel or tunnel overlap, a small portion of the meniscus bone can be removed without detriment. When the ACL is reconstructed in conjunction with the meniscus, the knee is prepared as a standard ACL reconstruction, except the tunnels are not drilled until the meniscus is completed. By waiting to drill the tunnels, fluid extravasation is avoided. In addition, delay of ACL graft passage and fixation enables ease in opening of the knee for meniscus insertion and suturing. If the tunnels and channel are properly prepared, overlay within the bone should not occur.

Postoperative Care

Follow-up

- The initial postoperative visit is at 7 to 10 days with anteroposterior and lateral radiographs also obtained.

- Monthly visits are common until a stationary point is attained.

Rehabilitation

- A brace is applied in full extension after the procedure. Range of motion is permitted once the patient is able to straight-leg raise.
- Partial weight bearing with the postoperative brace set at 0 to 90 degrees is permitted during the initial 4 weeks.
- Full weight bearing and unrestricted range of motion are permitted after 4 weeks.
- Progressive strengthening and functional training similar to ACL protocols are followed.
- Running is permitted at 12 weeks.
- Return to full activities is permitted at 4 months if strength is 80% or greater compared with the contralateral limb with normal functional testing. However, most patients do not achieve these goals until 5 to 6 months postoperatively.

Complications

- Infection
- Arthrofibrosis
- Neurovascular injury during implantation
- Meniscus tear or incomplete healing
- Graft extrusion due to improper placement or size
- Loss of bone fixation or fracture

Results

Many studies have evaluated the use of meniscal allografts, with the initial group finding various outcomes. However, as the indications and surgical techniques have evolved, so has the rate of success. At present, most studies that follow the appropriate indications and operative methods report a success rate of 80% to 90%.

The number of published series regarding meniscal allografts are too numerous to list. Table 48-1 summarizes several exemplary studies that have contributed to the progression of our current guidelines.

Table 48-1 Results of Studies of Meniscal Allografts

Study	Follow-up (Mean)	Study Size	Clinical Results	Information Gained
Garrett[3] (1993)	2-7 years (unknown)	43 patients 44 grafts	35 of 43 (81%) successful 20 of 28 intact at second-look arthroscopy 8 failures related to arthrosis	Grafts can reliably heal Advanced arthrosis results in failure
Noyes and Barber-Westin[4] (1995)	22-58 months (30 months)	82 patients 96 grafts	58% of failed grafts were lyophilized, and majority of patients had advanced arthrosis	Arthritic knees and lyophilized grafts have high failure rates
Carter[1] (1999)	24-73 months (35 months)	46 patients 46 grafts	45 patients had improvement in pain 38 grafts were healed at second-look arthroscopy	Successful outcome with stringent patient selection Excellent healing to host
Rodeo[5] (2001)	Range unknown (2-year minimum)	33 patients 33 grafts	22 of 33 successful: 14 of 16 with bone fixation, 8 of 17 without bone	Bone fixation results are more favorable than when horns are not secured with bone
Wirth et al[9] (2002)	12-15 years (14 years)	22 patients 23 grafts	Magnetic resonance imaging evaluation: 6 deep-frozen, similar to normal meniscus; 17 lyophilized, similar to meniscectomy	Arthritis progression slowed with use of frozen grafts
van Arkel and de Boer[7] (2002)	4-126 months (60 months)	57 patients 63 grafts	Cumulative survival rate of 76%, 50%, and 67% for lateral, medial, and combined, respectively	Results deteriorate over time
Ryu et al[6] (2002)	12-72 months (33 months)	17 patients 25 grafts	14/18 with grade III or lower: good–excellent 3/7 grade IV: good–excellent	Results deteriorate as the grade of arthrosis is increased
Verdonk et al[8] (2005)	7.2 years (5-14.5 years)	100 grafts 96 patients	Cumulative survival of 74% medial and 70% lateral at 10 years	Results deteriorate with time Graft shrinkage can occur
Cole et al[2] (2006)	33.5 months (24-57 months)	45 patients	41 of 45 (91%) successful	High rate of success with strict indications

References

1. Carter TR. Meniscal allograft transplantation. Sports Med Arthrosc Rev 1999;7:51-62.
2. Cole BJ, Dennis MG, Lee SJ, et al. Prospective evaluation of allograft meniscus transplantation: a minimum 2-year follow-up. Am J Sports Med 2006;34:919-927.
3. Garrett JC. Meniscal transplantation: a review of 43 cases with two to seven year follow-up. Sports Med Arthrosc Rev 1993;2:164-167.
4. Noyes FR, Barber-Westin SD. Irradiated meniscus allografts in the human knee: a two to five year follow-up. Orthop Trans 1995;19: 417.
5. Rodeo SA. Meniscal allografts—where do we stand? Am J Sports Med 2001;29:246-261.
6. Ryu RK, Dunbar WH, Morse GG. Meniscal allograft replacement: a 1-year to 6-year experience. Arthroscopy 2002;18:989-994.
7. van Arkel ER, de Boer HH. Survival analysis of human meniscal transplantations. J Bone Joint Surg Br 2002;84:227-231.
8. Verdonk PC, Demurie A, Almqvist KF, et al. Transplantation of viable meniscal allograft. Survivorship analysis and clinical outcome of one hundred cases. J Bone Joint Surg Am 2005;87:715-724.
9. Wirth CJ, Peters G, Milachowski KA, et al. Long-term results of meniscal allograft transplantation. Am J Sports Med 2002;30: 174-181.

Suggested Reading

Alhalki MM, Howell SM, Hull ML. How three methods for fixing a medial meniscal autograft affect tibial contact mechanics. Am J Sports Med 1999;27:320-328.

Arnoczky SP, McDevitt CA. The meniscus: structure, function, repair and replacement. In Buckwalter JA, Einhorn TA, Simon SR, eds. Orthopaedic Basic Science: Biology and Biomechanics of the Musculoskeletal System, 2nd ed. Rosemont, Ill, American Academy of Orthopaedic Surgeons, 2000:531-545.

Berlet GC, Fowler PJ. The anterior horn of the medial meniscus: an anatomic study of its insertion. Am J Sports Med 1998;26:540-543.

Cameron JC, Saha S. Meniscal allograft transplantation for unicompartmental arthritis of the knee. Clin Orthop 1997;337:164-171.

Chen MI, Branch TP, Hutton WC. Is it important to secure the horns during lateral meniscal transplantation? A cadaveric study. Arthroscopy 1996;12:174-181.

Cole B, Carter T, Rodeo S. Allograft meniscal transplantation: background, techniques, and results. J Bone Joint Surg Am 2002;84:1236-1250.

Fritz JM, Irrang JJ, Harner CD. Rehabilitation following allograft meniscal transplantation: a review of the literature and case study. J Orthop Sports Phys Ther 1996;24:98-106.

Graf KW, Sekiya JK, Wojtys EM. Long-term results after combined medial meniscal allograft transplantation and anterior cruciate ligament reconstruction: minimum 8.5 year follow-up study. Arthroscopy 2004;20:129-140.

Hommen JP, Applegate GR, Del Pizzo W: Meniscus allograft transplantation: ten-year results of cryopreserved allografts. Arthroscopy 2007;23:388–393.

Jackson DW, Whelan J, Simon TM. Cell survival after transplantation of fresh meniscal allografts. DNA probe analysis in a goat model. Am J Sports Med 1993;21:540-550.

Johnson DL, Swenson TM, Livesay GA, et al. Insertion site anatomy of the human menisci: gross, arthroscopic and topographical anatomy as a basis for meniscal transplantation. Arthroscopy 1995;11:386-394.

Kohn D, Moreno B. Meniscus insertion anatomy as a basis for meniscus replacement: a morphological cadaveric study. Arthroscopy 1995;11:96-103.

Milachowski KA, Weismeler K, Wirth CJ. Homologous meniscus transplantation. Experimental and clinical results. Int Orthop 1989;13:1-11.

Noyes FR, Barber-Westin SD, Butler DL, et al. The role of allografts in repair and reconstruction of knee joint ligaments and menisci. Instr Course Lect 1998;47:379-396.

Noyes FR, Barber-Westin SD, Rankin M. Meniscal transplantation in symptomatic patients less than fifty years old. J Bone Joint Surg Am 2004;86:1392-1404.

Paletta GA, Manning T, Snell E, et al. The effects of allograft meniscal replacement on intra-articular contact area and pressures in the human knee: a biomechanic study. Am J Sports Med 1997;25:692-698.

Pollard ME, Kang Q, Berg EE. Radiographic sizing for meniscal transplantation. Arthroscopy 1995;11:684-687.

Potter HG, Rodeo SA, Wickiewicz TL, et al. MR imaging of meniscal allografts: correlation with clinical and arthroscopic outcomes. Radiology 1996;198:509-514.

Rath E, Richmond JC, Yassir W, et al. Meniscal allograft transplantation. Two- to eight-year results. Am J Sports Med 2001;29:410-414.

Rijk PC. Meniscal allograft transplantation—part I: background, results, graft selection and preservation, and surgical considerations. Arthroscopy 2004;20:728-743.

Rijk PC. Meniscal allograft transplantation—part II: alternative treatments, effects on articular cartilage, and future directions. Arthroscopy 2004;20:851-859.

Sekiya JK, Giffin JR, Irrang JJ, et al. Clinical outcomes after combined meniscal allograft transplantation and anterior cruciate ligament reconstruction. Am J Sports Med 2003;31:896-906.

Stollsteimer GT, Shelton WR, Dukes A, et al. Meniscal allograft transplantation: a 1 to 5 year follow-up of 22 patients. Arthroscopy 2000;16:343-347.

Szomor ZL, Martin TE, Bonar F, et al. The protective effects of meniscal transplantation on cartilage: an experimental study in sheep. J Bone Joint Surg Am 2000;82:80-88.

van Arkel ER, de Boer HH. Human meniscal transplantation: preliminary results at two to five year follow-up. J Bone Joint Surg Br 1995;77:589-595.

Verdonk R. Alternative treatments for meniscal injuries. J Bone Joint Surg Br 1997;79:866-873.

CHAPTER 49

Arthroscopic Meniscus Transplantation: Bone Plug

Kent R. Jackson, MD

Thomas L. Wickiewicz, MD

The intact meniscus serves a number of functions in the knee; it increases the tibiofemoral contact area, decreases tibiofemoral contact pressures, provides shock absorption, and aids in joint stability, all of which are beneficial to the underlying articular cartilage. With this improved understanding of the importance of the meniscus, there has been an increased emphasis on the repair of meniscal tears, with indications extending to complex tears and tears in avascular regions. Even with these advanced techniques, there are tears not amenable to repair, for which total or subtotal meniscectomy may be required for symptomatic relief. For these patients, there are few options to slow the known progression of articular cartilage degeneration.[3] First reported in 1881, meniscal allograft transplantation is one option.[14] Several studies have shown that for the ideally suited meniscus-deficient patient, with pain localized to the tibiofemoral compartment and no evidence of advanced degenerative changes, a predictable reduction of pain and improved function can result.[5,6,15]

Preoperative Considerations

History

A thorough history and physical examination are critical to the appropriate selection of meniscal allograft transplantation candidates. A pertinent history focuses on the location, character, duration, and quality of pain and any associated swelling or mechanical symptoms. Antecedent trauma or any exacerbating events, such as instability episodes, should be documented along with any history of prior surgery. Prior operative reports, including a detailed description of the procedures performed and comments on the status or quality of the articular cartilage, can be helpful in the surgical decision-making process. It is also imperative to rule out other potential sources of pain, including complex regional pain syndrome, in the patient who has likely had multiple operations. Classic signs and symptoms of meniscus-deficient patients include tibiofemoral joint pain, joint effusion, and a history of prior surgery with total or subtotal meniscectomy.

Routine knee physical examination includes inspection of gait and axial alignment; assessment of range of motion; and evaluation for effusion, joint line tenderness to palpation, and crepitus. Healed incisions should correspond with prior surgeries as gleaned from the surgical history, most notably prior meniscal surgery. Instability examination should be performed to evaluate the cruciates, collaterals, and posterolateral corner. Instability that is detected can be addressed with either staged or combined reconstructive procedures.

Imaging

Radiography

Plain radiographic evaluation includes standing postero-anterior, flexion standing posteroanterior, flexion lateral,

Merchant, and standing hip-to-ankle radiographs. Standing views are critical for the evaluation of the remaining tibiofemoral joint space; standing flexion views specifically examine the posterior weight-bearing portions of the femur. Degenerative changes on plain radiographs include a decreased joint space, osteophytes, flattening of the posterior femoral condyles, and increased concavity of the tibial plateau. Hip-to-ankle views are important for assessing the mechanical axis of the lower extremity for possible staged or combined corrective osteotomies.

Other Modalities

High-resolution magnetic resonance imaging with the appropriate cartilage-specific sequences is useful in the assessment of the meniscus and, more important, in the assessment of the articular cartilage. Magnetic resonance imaging is sensitive and can be used to detect early changes in the articular cartilage manifested as subchondral marrow edema, subchondral remodeling, softening, and fibrillation. These sequences can be useful in deciding whether the patient will be a realistic candidate for transplantation.

Bone scan has also been described for the evaluation of the articular cartilage. Increased uptake is indicative of early degenerative changes in the compartment that are often not manifested on plain film or at the time of arthroscopy.

Preoperative Sizing

Preoperative sizing of the meniscal allograft for transplantation is critical for its optimal mechanical function. Plain radiographs, computed tomographic scans, and magnetic resonance images have all been used for preoperative sizing, with no real agreement in the literature as to the best method.[12] Our current method is to use plain radiographs (with an appropriate-size marker) and magnetic resonance images to determine tibial plateau dimensions and then to obtain a matching plateau with an attached meniscus for transplantation.

Indications and Contraindications

Meniscal transplantation is indicated for a meniscus-deficient patient with symptoms of pain in the tibiofemoral compartment and no evidence of advanced degenerative changes on imaging.

Contraindications for meniscal transplantation are advanced degenerative changes, prior joint infection, and axial malalignment or joint instability for which the patient refuses to undergo combined or staged osteotomy or ligament reconstruction. We have not used age criteria as a strict contraindication; however, the likelihood of an older patient's satisfying all of the criteria is significantly decreased.

Surgical Technique

Anesthesia and Positioning

There are numerous techniques for meniscal allograft transplantation. Here we describe the arthroscopic plug technique, which we think is ideally suited for the medial meniscus. On the lateral side, we prefer some of the other techniques using a bone bridge because of the proximity of the anterior and posterior horns. These anatomic considerations are important because of the close apposition of the tunnels required on the lateral side and also the increased potential for problems when an additional tunnel for anterior cruciate ligament reconstruction is added.

Before the induction of anesthesia, the graft is thawed and inspected. Potential problems at this time include a damaged graft and the incorrect side, which would result in cancellation of the case before the patient receives an anesthetic. We use only fresh-frozen nonirradiated grafts from a certified and trusted tissue bank.

With a satisfactory, appropriately sized graft in the room, anesthesia is then induced with a regional or general agent. The patient is then placed in the supine position on the operating room table. A well-padded nonsterile tourniquet is placed on the upper thigh in addition to a well-padded thigh post for the application of valgus stress.

Specific Steps (Box 49-1)

The room set-up is important with appropriate positioning of the patient, camera equipment, and anesthesia staff to maximize efficiency and to minimize the risk of contamination. A separate table for graft preparation should be set up with the appropriate equipment, including oscillating saw, drill, and additional instruments for graft preparation.

The extremity is prepared from the tourniquet distally with povidone-iodine (Betadine) and draped with a nonimpervious stockinette, half sheets, and an extremity drape. After a standard examination under anesthesia, any combined corrective osteotomies are performed first, followed by a standard diagnostic arthroscopy. Arthroscopy is performed by use of the standard anterolateral viewing portal, anteromedial instrumentation portal, and superomedial or superolateral outflow portal. Diagnostic arthroscopy is useful for confirming the diagnosis and also assessing the status of the articular cartilage. At our institution, the status of the cartilage is assessed preoperatively by cartilage-sensitive magnetic resonance imaging. Without these special sequences, it may be important to counsel the patient that the decision to proceed with meniscal transplantation is contingent on the suitability of the articular cartilage. After completion of the diagnostic arthroscopy,

Box 49-1 Surgical Steps

1. The meniscal bed is prepared.

2. Notchplasty is performed on the medial femoral condyle.

3. The graft is trimmed to the appropriate-sized bone plugs.

4. No. 5 nonabsorbable Ethibond suture is passed with straight needles through the bone plugs.

5. The guide wire is placed and the tunnel drilled with use of the anterior cruciate ligament guide for the posterior horn of the meniscal allograft.

6. A wire is passed through the tibial tunnel in a retrograde fashion and retrieved by a grasper in preparation for eventual graft passage.

7. The graft is passed through the arthrotomy by traction on the tibial bone plug and meniscal body sutures.

8. The guide wire is overreamed with a 10-mm reamer for the anterior tibial tunnel through the anterior arthrotomy.

9. The allograft is repaired to the capsule–meniscal remnant by a standard inside-out technique.

10. The allograft is seated and secured.

11. The bone plug sutures are tied over a bone bridge.

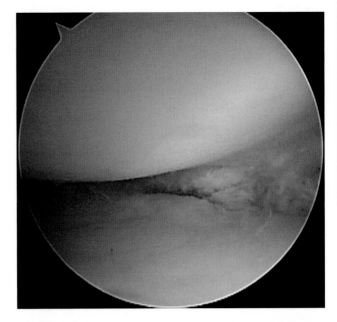

Figure 49-1 The meniscal bed has been prepared with arthroscopic baskets and shavers, leaving 2 to 3 mm of peripheral meniscus as a substrate for reattachment.

the meniscal remnant is débrided with a combination of arthroscopic baskets and motorized shavers, ideally leaving a cuff of 2 to 3 mm of native meniscus as a substrate for firm reattachment of the meniscal allograft (Fig. 49-1). The adjacent capsule and meniscal remnant are then rasped to stimulate bleeding for the reparative response. Notchplasty is then performed on the medial femoral condyle with a 4.5-mm motorized shaver, making sure that there is adequate arthroscopic access to the posterior horn of the meniscus for visualization and anatomic placement of the meniscal allograft (Fig. 49-2). Any indicated concomitant cartilage resurfacing procedures are performed at this time. Similarly, with a combined ligamentous reconstruction, bone tunnels are drilled at this time.

After it is determined that the patient is a reasonable candidate, an appropriately sized allograft can be prepared. The superior surface of the graft is marked with an *A* adjacent to the anterior horn and a *P* adjacent to the posterior horn to avoid any confusion at implantation in regard to orientation. By use of an oscillating saw, the plateau is trimmed to bone plugs attached to the anterior and posterior horns of the meniscus (Fig. 49-3). The anterior horn bone plug should be fashioned to a size of 10 mm in diameter and 15 mm in length. The posterior bone plug should be fashioned to a size of 8 mm in diameter and 15 mm in length. With use of a 2-mm drill bit, two drill holes are made in each bone plug. One No. 5 nonabsorbable Ethibond (Ethicon, Inc., Somerville, NJ) suture is

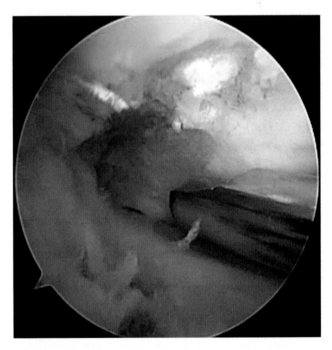

Figure 49-2 Notchplasty is performed on the medial femoral condyle with use of a 4.5-mm shaver until adequate visualization and access to the posterior horn have been established for eventual graft passage.

passed in a retrograde and then antegrade fashion through each bone plug in addition to one No. 5 Ethibond locking suture in the meniscus adjacent to the bone plugs for tibial tunnel fixation (Figs. 49-4 and 49-5). It is important that the bone plug sutures exit at the inferior surface of the

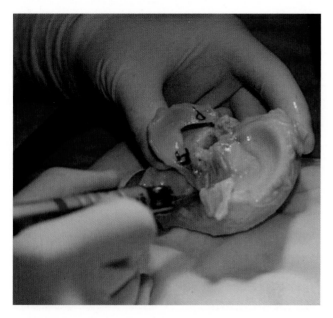

Figure 49-3 The superior surface of the allograft has been marked with an *A* and a *P* adjacent to the anterior and posterior horns, respectively. By use of an oscillating saw, the graft is trimmed to the appropriate-sized bone plugs.

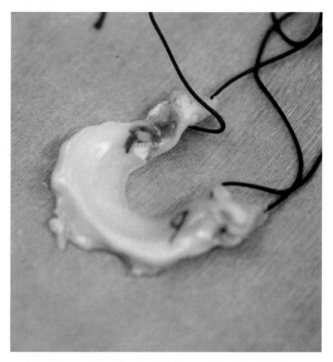

Figure 49-5 The completed meniscal allograft before placement of the meniscal body suture.

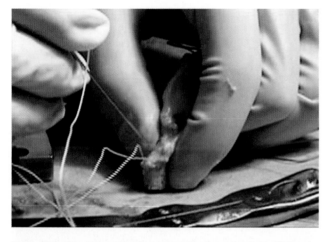

Figure 49-4 After drilling of the bone plugs, No. 5 nonabsorbable Ethibond suture is passed with straight needles through the bone plugs.

bone plug to help guide the nose of the bone plug into the tibial tunnel during graft passage.

After completion of the meniscal bed preparation and notchplasty, the leg is exsanguinated and the tourniquet is adjusted to an appropriate pressure. A 5-cm anteromedial arthrotomy is made for graft passage, and a standard posterior medial approach for inside-out suture passage is made. The anteromedial arthrotomy should include the anteromedial portal and also incorporate the intended bone tunnel sites. With use of an anterior cruciate ligament guide set at the appropriate angle, a pin is inserted from adjacent to the tibial tubercle to the anatomic insertion site of the posterior horn of the medial meniscus

under direct visualization (Fig. 49-6). The guide wire is then overreamed with a 10-mm reamer, and the tunnel edges are chamfered with a curved 4.5-mm shaver. A looped 20-gauge wire is advanced in the tibial tunnel in a retrograde fashion and retrieved out of the arthrotomy with a grasper (Fig. 49-7). The sutures in the posterior bone plug are then passed through the wire loop and retrieved through the tunnel. The graft is then passed through the arthrotomy and into the knee with the knee in 15 to 20 degrees of flexion and under a maximum valgus stress (Fig. 49-8). The meniscus is then reduced into position with direct pressure by use of a probe, a technique similar to the reduction of a bucket-handle meniscal tear. In some instances, this may require release of the superficial fibers of the medial collateral ligament for adequate clearance in the medial compartment. Once the meniscus is reduced, the posterior bone plug is seated in the tunnel with the aid of a probe and traction on the plug sutures. The posterior bone plug is purposely undersized by 2 mm for ease of passage at this stage. A snap is placed on the posterior bone plug suture limbs as they exit the distal tibial tunnel to maintain tension until the rest of the meniscus can be secured.

Next, the ideal location for the anterior bone plug is determined on the basis of the native anatomy and after the knee is ranged from full flexion to extension. Through the arthrotomy, with retractors in place, a reamer guide wire is drilled perpendicular to the articular surface in the appropriate position to a depth of 20 mm under direct

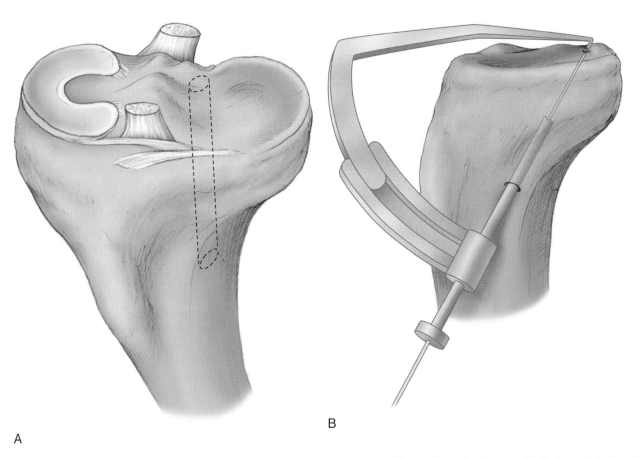

A

B

Figure 49-6 Drawing depicts the placement of the guide wire and drilling of the tunnel with use of the anterior cruciate ligament guide for the posterior horn of the meniscal allograft. The starting point for the tunnel is adjacent to the tibial tubercle, with the exiting point at the anatomic attachment of the posterior horn of the meniscus.

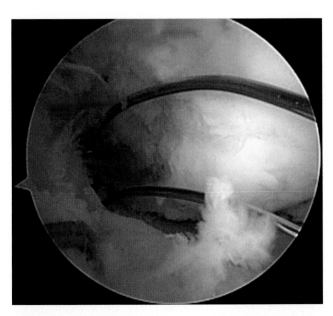

Figure 49-7 A passing wire has been passed through the tibial tunnel in a retrograde fashion and retrieved by a grasper in preparation for eventual graft passage.

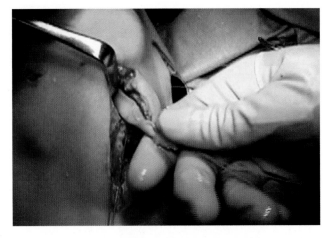

Figure 49-8 The graft is passed through the arthrotomy by traction on the tibial bone plug and meniscal body sutures.

vision (Fig. 49-9). Care is taken to provide enough room anteriorly to leave a rim of anterior cortex after reaming. This guide wire is then overreamed with a 10-mm reamer to a depth of 15 mm. Drill holes in the anterior cortex of the tibia are made with a 2-mm drill bit communicating with the anterior tunnel. Suture limbs from the anterior bone plug are then retrieved through these drill holes by use of a suture shuttle device, and the anterior bone plug is seated with gentle traction under direct vision. The suture limbs are snapped to maintain tension on the anterior bone plug. With the arthroscope in the anterolateral portal, a standard inside-out meniscal repair with zone-specific cannulas is performed with 2-0 nonabsorbable Ethibond suture in a vertical fashion at approximately 8- to 10-mm intervals (Fig. 49-10). Each suture is placed and secured and tied over the capsule while the apposition of the meniscus to the capsule is observed (Fig. 49-11). As you proceed anteriorly, repair can be difficult arthroscopically but can easily be performed under direct vision through the arthrotomy with 2-0 nonabsorbable Ethibond suture. An alternative technique is to perform a standard outside-in repair for the anterior horn if visualization is poor or in trying to minimize the incision. After completion of the meniscal reapproximation, the bone plug suture limbs are tied under appropriate tension over the bone bridge to each other or individually to a Teflon button, making sure not to recess the bone plugs below the level of the articular surface (Fig. 49-12). The meniscus is then probed for stability and its position re-evaluated through a full range of motion and rotation. It is important to make sure that the bone plugs are not overrotated or recessed in the tunnels. If the position is acceptable, the tourniquet is let down, hemostasis is achieved with electrocautery, and the wounds are closed in a standard fashion. Sterile dressings are applied, and the patient's leg is wrapped loosely with an elastic bandage. The patient is then placed in a double upright brace with the knee locked in extension.

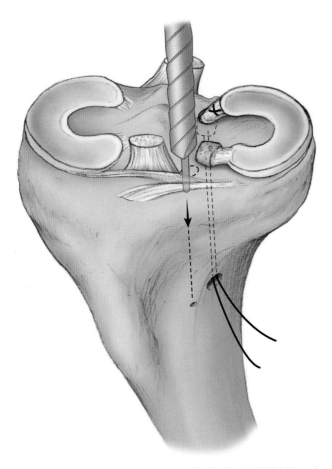

Figure 49-9 An appropriately placed guide wire for the anterior tibial tunnel is overreamed with a 10-mm reamer through the anterior arthrotomy.

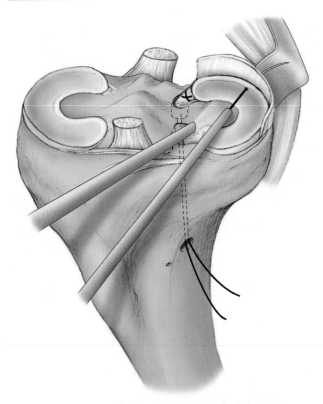

Figure 49-10 With the meniscus reduced, the allograft is repaired to the capsule–meniscal remnant by a standard inside-out technique with zone-specific cannulas through a standard posteromedial approach. (Redrawn from Noyes FR, Barber-Westin SD, Rankin M. Meniscal transplantation in symptomatic patients less than fifty years old. J Bone Joint Surg Am 2005;87:149-165.)

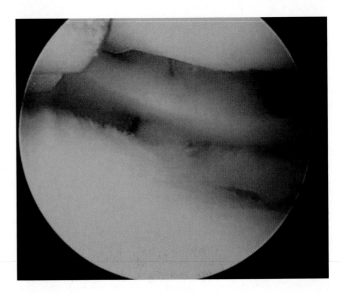

Figure 49-11 The meniscal allograft after reapproximation to the meniscal remnant and capsule with an inside-out repair.

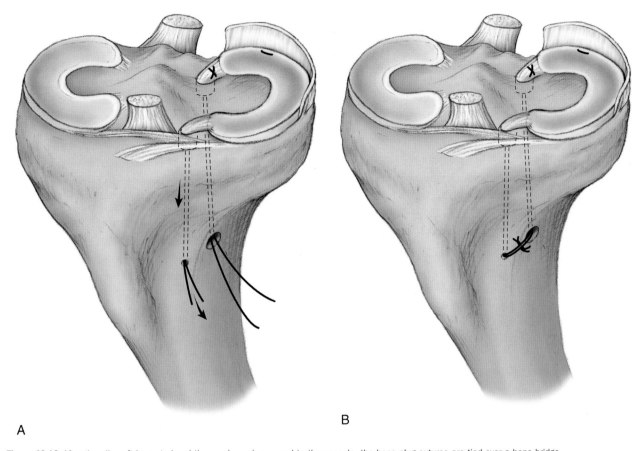

A B

Figure 49-12 After the allograft is seated and the meniscus is secured to the capsule, the bone plug sutures are tied over a bone bridge.

Postoperative Considerations

Rehabilitation

The patient is maintained in a double upright, hinged knee brace for the first 6 weeks. The orders are non weight bearing with the knee locked in extension for the first 4 weeks, partial weight bearing for weeks 5 and 6, and then full weight bearing after 6 weeks with an unloader brace for an additional 6 weeks. Range-of-motion exercises are started immediately, including full extension with flexion limited to 90 degrees to avoid increased stress on the meniscus. Closed-kinetic-chain strengthening exercises are started in the third week while observing the flexion limits. Light, sports-specific exercises are begun at 4 months, with return to straight-line running at 6 months. Squatting or hyperflexion activities are discouraged for 6 months. Return to high-load activities, including jumping, cutting, and pivoting, in the current state of meniscal transplantation is not recommended. In addition, as part of our protocol, magnetic resonance imaging is repeated at 6 to 12 months for all patients to evaluate the graft for healing, position, and possible extrusion or tearing. These protocols should serve as guidelines and would obviously be modified as a result of concomitant procedures performed.

PEARLS AND PITFALLS

Patient Selection

- Contraindications: advanced arthrosis, history of infection, other ligamentous or alignment disease that the patient refuses to have corrected.
- Appropriate radiographs include hip-knee-ankle films. Consider cartilage-sensitive magnetic resonance imaging.
- Plan surgery to address all of the patient's issues, including potential ligamentous and alignment problems.

Graft Preparation

- Before induction of anesthesia, the graft should be checked for appropriateness to continue with the planned case.
- The graft should be marked appropriately for orientation to include the anterior and posterior horns in addition to the superior and inferior surfaces.
- The posterior bone plug is undersized by 2 mm to ease the graft's passage.

Surgery Technical Points

- A thorough diagnostic arthroscopy should be performed. The decision to proceed with meniscal transplantation is predicated on articular cartilage of suitable quality.
- An adequate notchplasty should be performed to visualize the anatomic location of the posterior horn of the medial meniscus.
- A looped 20-gauge wire is used for suture passage of the posterior horn bone plug.
- Graft passage can be facilitated with release of the superficial fibers of the medial collateral ligament and valgus stress.
- The graft is tentatively reduced and brought through a full range of motion to mark the anatomic site of the anterior horn for tunnel drilling.

Complications

Potential complications include persistent pain, infection, loss of range of motion, and neurovascular complications. Specific to this procedure, graft failure is the most concerning complication and can be due to a number of factors. Repeated tearing or failure of the meniscal allograft most often occurs in the setting of coexisting osteoarthritis with advanced changes in the articular cartilage and remodeling of the femoral condyles.[5,6] Technical considerations include anatomic placement of the anterior and posterior horns of the meniscus and proper graft sizing. Proper placement of the horns of the meniscus restores the meniscal functions, including load transmission and shock absorption.[1,7] The type of fixation is also important, and it has been shown that secure anatomic fixation of bone plugs is required to best restore normal contact mechanics.[7] Improper sizing can result in an abnormal distribution of loads; undersized grafts show increased loads due to poor conformity, and oversized grafts are likely to extrude and not transmit any tibiofemoral forces.[1,7] Partial tears of the graft can be treated with partial meniscectomy, whereas worsening of symptoms or graft failure may require graft removal.

Results

In evaluating the literature, the results of meniscal allograft transplantation are difficult to assess because of a number of factors. Most studies have small numbers with limited follow-up. Methods of graft sizing and tissue processing are varied. Different surgical techniques include techniques with bone plugs, dovetail, slot, and soft tissue fixation only. A large number of patients had concomitant procedures that were performed in either a staged or combined fashion, including corrective osteotomy, ligament reconstruction, and cartilage procedures. Another confounding variable is the degree and extent of articular cartilage degeneration that is present in these patients. Because of the number of confounding variables and lack of objective findings, we think it is difficult to draw any definitive conclusions from the literature. A summary of the current literature is seen in Table 49-1.

We do believe that for the appropriately selected meniscus-deficient patient, a well-performed meniscal allograft transplantation can provide a predictable result of improved pain relief and increased function. With future

Table 49-1 Summary of Literature on Meniscal Allograft Transplantation

Study	No. of Grafts	Mean Follow-up	Concomitant Procedures	Clinical Results	Comments
Garret[4] (1993)	43	2-7 years	24 ACL reconstructions 13 osteotomies 11 osteochondral allografts		Failures related to grade III-IV chondromalacia
Cameron and Saha[2] (1997)	67	31 months	5 ACL reconstructions 28 tibial osteotomies 6 femoral osteotomies 7 ACL reconstructions and tibial osteotomies	87% good–excellent 13% poor–fair	No shrinkage in 67 gamma-irradiated deep-frozen allografts
Wirth et al[16] (2002)	22	14 years	22 ACL reconstructions 19 femoral advancements of MCL	Deterioration during follow-up 100% lyophilized with abnormal MRI signal 100% deep-frozen with normal MRI signal	Frozen grafts better than lyophilized
Noyes et al[5] (2004)	40	40 months	7 ACL reconstructions 1 PCL reconstruction 1 MCL reconstruction 16 osteochondral autografts	89% rated knee improved 59% increase in number of patients who participated in light sports 68% had no tibiofemoral pain	Concomitant cartilage and ligament procedures improved knee function and did not increase the rate of complications
Verdonk et al[15] (2005)	100	7.2 years	3 ACL reconstructions 4 osteochondral autografts 3 microfractures 15 tibial osteotomies 2 femoral osteotomies	79% success rate Mean cumulative survival: 11.6 years	Survival analysis: beneficial effect remained in about 70% of patients at 10 years

ACL, anterior cruciate ligament; MCL, medial collateral ligament; MRI, magnetic resonance imaging; PCL, posterior cruciate ligament.

studies, we hope to answer the question of whether these known improvements in symptoms and function correlate to delayed progression or arrest of articular cartilage degeneration.

References

1. Alhalki MM, Hull ML, Howell SM. Contact mechanics of the medial tibial plateau after implantation of a medial meniscal allograft: a human cadaveric study. Am J Sports Med 2000;28:370-376.

2. Cameron JC, Saha S. Meniscal allograft transplantation for unicompartmental arthritis of the knee. Clin Orthop 1997;337:164-171.

3. Fairbanks TJ. Knee joint changes after meniscectomy. J Bone Joint Surg Br 1948;30:664-670.

4. Garrett JC. Meniscal transplantation: a review of 43 cases with two to seven year follow-up. Sports Med Arthrosc Rev 1993;2:164-167.

5. Noyes FR, Barber-Westin SD, Rankin M. Meniscal transplantation in symptomatic patients less than fifty years old. J Bone Joint Surg Am 2004;86:1392-1404.

6. Noyes FR, Barber-Westin SD, Rankin M. Meniscal transplantation in symptomatic patients less than fifty years old. J Bone Joint Surg Am 2005;87:149-165.

7. Paletta GA, Manning T, Snell E, et al. The effect of allograft meniscal replacement on intra-articular contact area and pressures in the human knee. A biomechanical study. Am J Sports Med 1997;25: 692-698.

8. Potter HG, Rodeo SA, Wickiewicz TL, Warren RF. MR imaging of meniscal allografts: correlation with clinical and arthroscopic outcomes. Radiology 1996;198:509-514.

9. Rath E, Richmond JC, Yassir W, et al. Meniscal allograft transplantation. Two- to eight-year results. Am J Sports Med 2001;29:410-414.

10. Rodeo SA. Meniscal allografts—where do we stand? Am J Sports Med 2001;29:246-261.

11. Sekiya JK, Giffin JR, Irrgang JJ, et al. Clinical outcomes after combined meniscal allograft transplantation and anterior cruciate ligament reconstruction. Am J Sports Med 2003;31:896-906.

12. Shaffer B, Kennedy S, Klimkiewicz J, Yao L. Preoperative sizing of meniscal allografts in meniscus transplantation. Am J Sports Med 2000;28:524-533.

13. Stollsteimer GT, Shelton WR, Dukes A, Bomboy AL. Meniscal allograft transplantation: a 1-to 5-year follow-up of 22 patients. Arthroscopy 2000;16:343-347.

14. Vangsness CT, Garcia IA, Mills RC, et al. Allograft transplantation in the knee: tissue regulation, procurement, processing, and sterilization. Am J Sports Med 2003;31:474-481.

15. Verdonk P, Demurie A, Almqvist KF, et al. Transplantation of viable meniscal allograft. Survivorship analysis and clinical outcome of one hundred cases. J Bone Joint Surg Am 2005;87:715-724.

16. Wirth CJ, Peters G, Milachowski KA, et al. Long-term results of meniscal allograft transplantation. Am J Sports Med 2002;30: 174-181.

CHAPTER 50

Combined Anterior Cruciate Ligament and Meniscal Allograft Transplantation

Fotios P. Tjoumakaris, MD

Jon K. Sekiya, MD

The menisci play a vital role in maintaining normal knee function. Shock absorption, stabilization, lubrication of the knee joint, proprioception, and load sharing are important functions of these cartilaginous structures. It has been demonstrated that significant joint changes follow complete or subtotal meniscectomies, and for this reason, many techniques to repair the menisci have been devised. Unfortunately, preservation of the meniscus cannot always be accomplished, and partial or total meniscectomy may be required.

The medial meniscus is an important secondary stabilizer to anterior-posterior knee translation. In the anterior cruciate ligament (ACL)–deficient knee, the medial meniscus takes on an even larger role in preventing excessive laxity. Results after ACL reconstruction in patients with deficient medial menisci are usually worse than when the meniscus is intact. Given these findings, meniscal allograft transplantation with concomitant ACL reconstruction has been performed to provide patients with a more stable knee as well as a mechanism to delay the arthritic process. This chapter outlines the senior author's preferred technique for meniscal transplantation and concomitant ACL reconstruction in patients with combined deficiencies.

Preoperative Considerations

History

It is paramount to elicit a complete history. This includes any initial injury that may have occurred, prior treatments

for the injury, activity restrictions imposed by the injury, and the patient's expectations of treatment. Any previous arthroscopic pictures or operative reports that may be available are helpful and may obviate the need for a staging diagnostic arthroscopy.

Typical History

- Previous acute knee injury requiring arthroscopic (or open) meniscectomy
- Subsequent injury with "giving way" episode
- Pain in the affected compartment
- Activity-related effusions or generalized swelling
- Continued, symptomatic instability
- Failed previous ACL surgery

Physical Examination

A comprehensive physical examination is undertaken to evaluate the patient's stance, gait pattern, and ability to squat. The overall lower extremity alignment is observed and compared with the contralateral extremity. Joint line palpation, results of the McMurray test, range of motion, and degree of quadriceps atrophy are documented. The presence of an effusion is assessed, and the ligamentous evaluation is performed to evaluate the integrity of the ACL (Lachman, pivot shift, and anterior drawer tests). An anterior drawer examination with as much anterior translation as in the Lachman test is suggestive of the loss of secondary stabilization from the posterior horn of the medial meniscus and is indicative of symptomatic medial meniscus deficiency that is compounding ACL laxity. Any prior surgical incisions are documented because these may affect surgical planning.

Typical Findings

- Joint line pain; pain with squatting
- Effusion
- Full, symmetric knee range of motion
- 2+ Lachman test score, 2+ pivot shift test score, 2+ anterior drawer test score

Imaging

Radiography

- 45-degree flexion posteroanterior weight-bearing radiographs (both knees)
- Non–weight-bearing flexion lateral radiograph of the affected knee
- Merchant views of both knees
- Long-cassette anteroposterior radiographs for mechanical axis alignment

Magnetic Resonance Imaging (with or without Contrast Enhancement)

- T2-weighted sequences are obtained to evaluate the subchondral bone and presence of any chondral defects.
- T1- and T2-weighted sagittal images are obtained to evaluate the integrity of the ACL.
- T1-weighted coronal and sagittal images are obtained to evaluate the dimensions of the remaining meniscus.

Other Modalities

Other imaging modalities, such as computed tomography and technetium bone scans, may be used to assess rotational alignment (computed tomography) or any degenerative changes not visualized on initial screening radiographs (bone scan).

Indications and Contraindications

The ideal candidate undergoing concomitant ACL reconstruction and meniscal transplantation is a young patient with meniscus deficiency and full knee range of motion, pain localized to the affected joint compartment, symptoms of persistent instability, prior failed ACL surgery (particularly with medial meniscus deficiency), cartilage surfaces that are relatively intact (grade I-II, preferably confined to the meniscal weight-bearing region), and no evidence of malalignment on long-cassette radiographs. If patients are found to have malalignment (weight-bearing

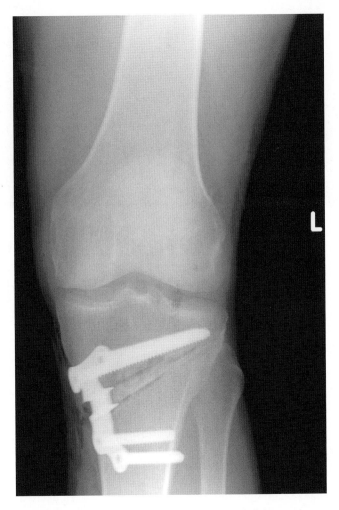

Figure 50-1 Example of a patient with medial meniscus deficiency and malalignment who required a staged reconstruction after medial opening wedge high tibial osteotomy.

line falls through the affected compartment), we prefer an osteotomy to realign the weight-bearing axis through the unaffected compartment and perform a staged reconstruction (Fig. 50-1).

Contraindications to the performance of this procedure are inflammatory arthritis, history of previous infection, evidence of severe degenerative changes (either arthroscopic or radiographic), body mass index above 35, and unwillingness of the patient to cooperate with a comprehensive rehabilitation program.

Surgical Planning

Meniscus Allograft

Correct sizing of the meniscal allograft is critical for healing. We obtain measurements from the preoperative posteroanterior and lateral radiographs after they have been corrected for magnification. This sizing technique is similar to that of Pollard and colleagues.[10] This size is then given to the tissue bank, and an isotropic graft (graft matched for right or left knee and for medial or lateral compartment) is obtained. All meniscal allografts are sterilely harvested and fresh-frozen. None of the grafts are irradiated before transplantation.

Anterior Cruciate Ligament Allograft

For ACL reconstruction with concomitant meniscal transplantation, we prefer to use a bone–patellar tendon–bone allograft. All of our bone–patellar tendon–bone allografts are fresh-frozen and irradiated before use. We have found that use of an allograft in this setting minimizes postoperative donor site pain and can hasten the recovery of the quadriceps after surgery. Another outstanding allograft option is a tibialis anterior tendon.

Surgical Technique

Anesthesia and Positioning

Our preferred technique uses a lower extremity sciatic and femoral nerve block to assist with postoperative analgesia. Typically, the patient is also given general anesthesia (or regional if general is contraindicated) and positioned supine on a regular operating room table. A thigh tourniquet is applied as well as a lateral post just below the level of the greater trochanter. A bump is taped to the bed that will position the leg at approximately 70 degrees of knee flexion. The table is lowered to its lowest level, and once the extremity is sterilely prepared, a bump is placed between the lateral post and the thigh with the knee flexed 70 degrees on the table.

Surgical Landmarks, Incisions, and Portals

Landmarks
- Borders of the patellar tendon
- Medial-lateral joint line
- Fibular head
- Tibial tubercle and proximal medial border of the tibia

Portals and Incisions
- Anterolateral portal (converted to arthrotomy for later passage of lateral meniscus graft)
- Anteromedial portal (converted to arthrotomy for later passage of medial meniscus graft)

- Proximal medial tibial incision (ACL tibial tunnel)
- Posterior medial approach over joint line (for fixation of medial meniscus)
- Posterior lateral approach over joint line (for fixation of lateral meniscus)

Structures at Risk
- Lateral collateral ligament, peroneal nerve (lateral approach)
- Medial collateral ligament, saphenous nerve (medial approach)

Examination Under Anesthesia and Diagnostic Arthroscopy

A thorough examination under anesthesia is performed to document anteromedial rotatory instability (in cases of medial meniscus deficiency) as well as anterior laxity (pivot shift test, Lachman test, anterior drawer test).

Diagnostic arthroscopy is performed to evaluate for other intra-articular disease as well as to critically assess the remaining meniscal rim available for placement of sutures.

Specific Steps (Box 50-1)

1. Preparation of Allografts

Once the diagnosis is confirmed, the allografts are thawed and washed with antibiotic solution according to the vendor's guidelines. The patellar tendon allograft is prepared so that each bone plug measures 10 mm in diameter and 30 mm in length. All loose tissue is débrided from the tendon, and two drill holes are placed within each plug, through which No. 5 braided, nonabsorbable sutures are placed to assist with graft passage. With the meniscus allograft, a rim of the outer portion is trimmed to provide

Box 50-1 Surgical Steps

1. Preparation of allografts
2. Preparation of meniscal rim
3. Tunnel drilling for the ACL
4. Slot preparation (lateral meniscus) or bone plug preparation (medial meniscus)
5. ACL insertion
6. Meniscal graft insertion
7. Fixation
8. Closure

a fresh surface for repair and subsequent healing. An 8- to 9-mm diameter (5-mm length) bone plug (medial meniscus) for the anterior horn is prepared and secured with No. 5 braided, nonabsorbable suture. The posterior horn bone plug is then prepared and secured in a similar fashion. In the posteromedial corner of the medial meniscus allograft, one No. 2 braided, nonabsorbable suture is placed within the rim to assist with graft passage and fixa-tion to the posteromedial capsule and posterior oblique ligament. For the lateral meniscus, we use a bone bridge (8 or 9 mm) secured with two No. 5 braided, nonabsorbable sutures through drill holes corresponding to the lengths made within the trough. In the posterolateral corner of the meniscus, we place a No. 2 braided, nonabsorbable suture through the rim to assist with graft passage (Figs. 50-2 and 50-3).

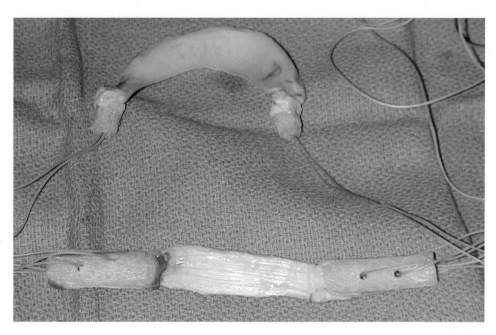

Figure 50-2 Preparation of the medial meniscus allograft with 8-mm bone plugs and the bone–patellar tendon–bone allograft with 10 × 30-mm bone plugs is performed on the back table.

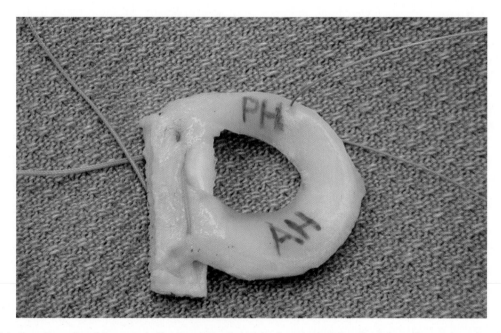

Figure 50-3 The lateral meniscus allograft is prepared with a bone bridge that retains the natural relationships between the anterior and posterior horns.

2. Preparation of Meniscal Rim

The involved posterior horns of the native menisci are trimmed to provide a bleeding surface that will support allograft healing. We prefer a 1- to 2-mm rim because this gives the sutures a more stable platform to fix the allograft. The anterior and posterior horn attachments are identified and marked. Care should be taken to maintain these anatomic landmarks (when available) because they help configure tunnel placement (Fig. 50-4).

3. Tunnel Drilling for the ACL

A notchplasty is usually not necessary in our experience. For tibial guide pin placement, the tibial insertion of the ACL is identified at the intersection of the posterior border of the anterior horn of the lateral meniscus and the posterior third of the ACL stump. The ACL guide is set to 50 to 55 degrees and drilled to 10 mm. The dilators can be used to assess for the presence of any graft impingement when it is viewed arthroscopically. Extreme caution must be taken with this tibial ACL tunnel in conjunction with the trough used for lateral meniscus transplantation; these often communicate with each other, and so care must be taken in passing and securing either graft in place.

Next, attention is directed to preparation of the femoral ACL tunnel. The over-the-top position is identified at the 10-o'clock position (right knee). A 30-degree Steadman awl brought through the medial portal can be used to mark the insertion site (approximately 6 mm from the back wall, providing a 1-mm back wall after tunnel drilling; Fig. 50-5). We prefer drilling transtibially through the tunnel if we are able to get down the face of the femur to 10-o'clock and posterior. If we are unable to do this, with the knee flexed to approximately 115 degrees, a pin

is tapped into place at the femoral insertion site through the medial portal. A 10-mm acorn drill bit is then run over the pin to a depth of 40 mm, if possible. This allows us to pull the bone-tendon-bone allograft deeper into the femoral tunnel if the tibial bone plug is too long and protruding from the tibial tunnel.

4. Slot Preparation (Lateral Meniscus) or Bone Plug Preparation (Medial Meniscus)

Once attention is turned to preparation of the meniscus, a femoral distractor is placed on the extremity. The joint is slightly distended so that the surgery can easily be accomplished at 70 degrees of knee flexion (Fig. 50-6).

For the lateral meniscus, we prefer a bridge and slot technique. A trough is first made in the medial aspect of the lateral tibial plateau to accept the allograft bone bridge (Fig. 50-7). A ¼-inch curved osteotome is brought through the medial portal with the curve facing medially, hugging the lateral aspect of the tibial insertion of the ACL. A cut is made, making sure to keep the trough in the sagittal plane. A second cut is then made with the osteotome, lateral and parallel to the first cut. The bridging bone is then removed, and prefabricated gouges are used to finish the trough (total diameter of 8 to 9 mm). An ACL drill guide is then used to make two holes in the trough, spaced approximately 10 mm apart on the tibial surface for later fixation of the meniscal allograft. Two Hewson suture passers are placed within these holes to facilitate later graft passage.

For the medial meniscus, we prefer a bone plug technique for anterior and posterior horn fixation. The anterior tunnel for the anterior bone plug is drilled with the assistance of an ACL guide at the anatomic insertion of

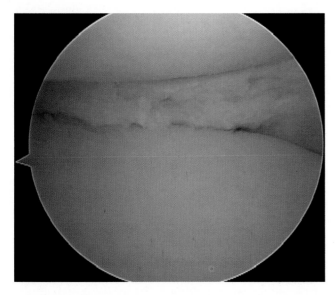

Figure 50-4 Example of a meniscus rim remnant in a patient undergoing transplantation. This was débrided until punctuate bleeding was visualized.

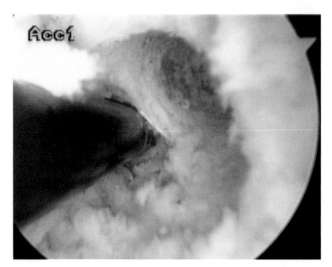

Figure 50-5 The ACL femoral tunnel is prepared with a 1-mm back wall at the 2-o'clock position (left knee) on the lateral femoral condyle.

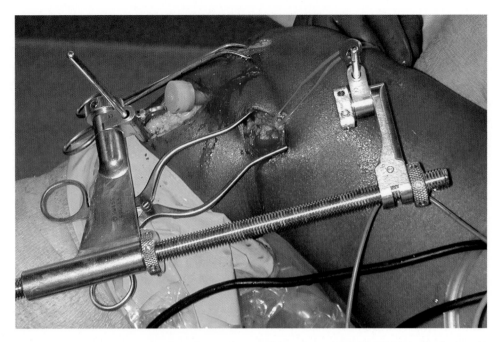

Figure 50-6 A femoral distractor is placed on the medial aspect of the knee that allows surgery to be performed easily at 90 degrees of knee flexion.

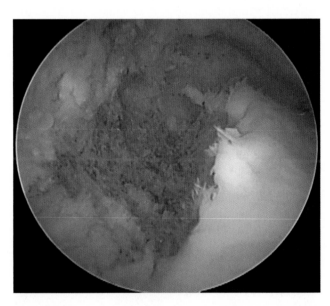

Figure 50-7 Preparation of the bone trough in the lateral tibial plateau with the use of prefabricated gouges.

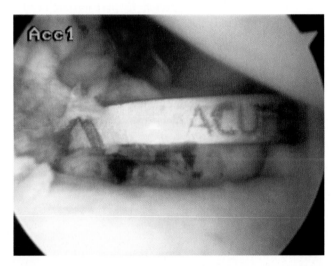

Figure 50-8 An ACL guide is used to drill the posterior horn bone tunnel for the medial meniscus bone plug.

the anterior horn of the medial meniscus. Visualization is greatly aided with the use of the femoral distractor. The guide is brought through the lateral portal, and a guide pin is placed in the anatomic posterior horn of the medial meniscus and then overdrilled by 1 mm of whatever the bone plug diameter is with an acorn reamer (Fig. 50-8). The anterior horn can usually be made through the antero-medial arthrotomy; a blind tunnel is drilled in the anatomic insertion of the anterior horn, which is then connected to the anteromedial tibial metaphysis with a 2.0

drill. Special care needs to be taken to avoid communication of the meniscus horn tunnels and the tibial ACL tunnel during preparation.

5. ACL Insertion

Before the passage and fixation of the meniscal allograft, the ACL is passed in a retrograde fashion with the assistance of a Beath pin and suture loop. If the medial portal technique is used for femoral tunnel preparation, the Beath pin is first sent through the medial portal, up the femoral tunnel, and exits the lateral aspect of the thigh. The suture loop attached to the Beath pin is brought into the joint, and a suture grasper is used to grab it from the tibial tunnel. The sutures attached to the allograft bone plugs are then shuttled through the tibial and femoral tunnels, and the graft is secured in place. The femoral side of the graft is then fixed with a metal interference screw. The tibial bone plug is not fixed until the meniscus transplantation is completed.

6. Meniscal Graft Insertion

Lateral meniscus: A small lateral parapatellar arthrotomy is made in line with the previous lateral portal. Four No. 0 braided, nonabsorbable sutures are then placed in the anterior rim of the lateral meniscal remnant for later use in fixation of the anterior horn. A small posterolateral incision is made, centered over the posterior border of the lateral collateral ligament. The interval between the iliotibial band and the biceps is incised toward Gerdy's tubercle. The posterolateral joint capsule is then exposed between the interval consisting of the lateral collateral ligament anteriorly and the gastrocnemius posteriorly. The anterior and posterior sutures of the bone bridge are threaded through the Hewson suture passers and pulled into the tunnels. The posterolateral passing suture is shuttled through the posterolateral incision and the meniscus allograft is brought into the joint, with care taken not to tangle the sutures (Fig. 50-9). Arthroscopic visualization then confirms that the bone bridge is in correct position, and the sutures are tied down on the medial aspect of the tibia over a 10-mm cortical bridge.

Medial meniscus: A small medial parapatellar arthrotomy is made in line with the medial portal. As for the lateral meniscus insertion, four nonabsorbable sutures are placed within the anterior horn remnant. A small posteromedial incision is then made, centered over the posterior border of the medial collateral ligament. The sartorius fascia is incised, and the interval between the semimembranosus and the medial gastrocnemius is developed, exposing the posteromedial joint capsule. This exposure will be used for inside-out meniscus repair suture techniques.

The posterior horn of the meniscus allograft is delivered through the anteromedial arthrotomy and pulled into the posterior horn tunnel. The posteromedial traction suture is used to reduce the posterior horn into the medial compartment. The posterior bone plug and sutures are pulled into their drill holes by a similar technique, and the allograft is reduced into the medial compartment (Fig. 50-10). Once reduction has been achieved, the sutures are tied on the lateral tibial metaphysis over a cortical bridge.

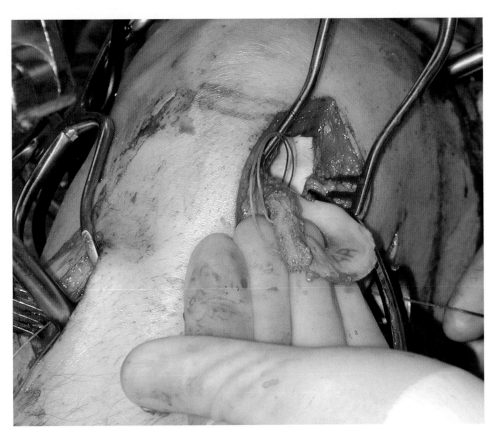

Figure 50-9 The lateral meniscus, with preparation completed and all sutures passed, is ready to be reduced into the lateral compartment.

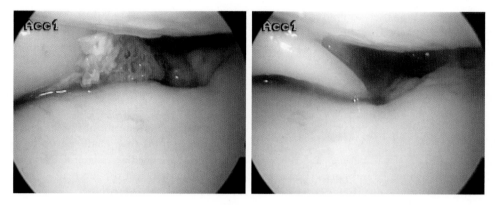

Figure 50-10 Arthroscopic view of the posterior bone plug and posterior horn being reduced into the bone tunnel.

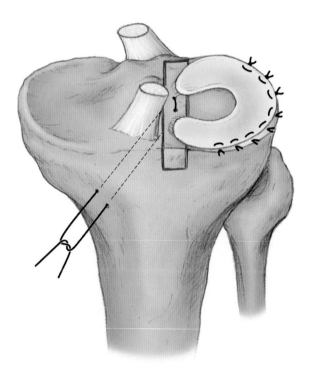

Figure 50-11 Diagram depicting final fixation of the lateral meniscus allograft.

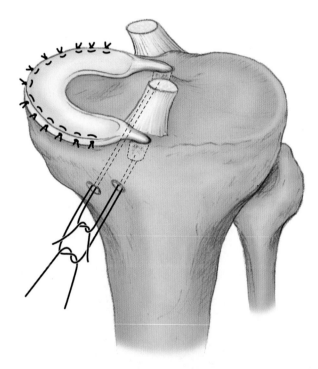

Figure 50-12 Diagram depicting fixation of medial meniscus allograft.

7. Fixation

Lateral meniscus: The meniscal allograft is secured by arthroscopic inside-out techniques through the lateral incision. Care is taken to not fix the popliteus tendon to the meniscus during fixation. Once all of the posterior horn and body sutures have been passed, the anterior horn is secured with the nonabsorbable sutures that had been placed in the meniscal remnant. This is achieved at 70 degrees of knee flexion. Fixation of the remaining sutures is performed at 30 degrees of knee flexion after the ACL has been fixed on the tibial side (Fig. 50-11).

Medial meniscus: The meniscal allograft is secured by arthroscopic inside-out techniques through the postero-medial incision. The anterior horn is secured in a fashion similar to that of the lateral meniscus, and the remaining meniscus is fixed by arthroscopic inside-out techniques. Final fixation of the sutures is performed at 30 degrees of knee flexion after the ACL has been fixed on the tibial side (Fig. 50-12).

ACL: The ACL is fixed on the tibial surface with a metal interference screw as the knee is slightly flexed (15 degrees) and a slight posterior drawer force is applied.

8. Closure

Standard closure is performed for the arthrotomy and all accessory incisions.

Postoperative Considerations

The patient is admitted for an overnight stay in the hospital and returns to the office 6 to 8 days after the procedure for radiographs and wound observation.

Rehabilitation

- Patients are partial weight bearing on the affected extremity in a hinged knee brace and progress to weight bearing as tolerated during 4 weeks.
- Continuous passive motion is begun 24 hours after surgery, as are quadriceps sets, heel slides, and straight-leg raises.

- Range-of-motion goals: full extension within 1 week; 90 degrees of flexion in 4 to 6 weeks.
- Crutches are discontinued after 4 weeks.
- Rehabilitation continues for 2 to 3 months with an emphasis on restoration of full knee motion, stability, and strength.
- Low-impact aerobic activity is permitted at 8 weeks.
- Running is permitted after 5 to 6 months
- Light and moderate sports begin at 6 to 9 months.
- Strenuous sport is not recommended indefinitely.

Complications

- Infection
- Arthrofibrosis
- Incomplete healing or recurrent tears of the implanted meniscus
- Neurovascular injury (saphenous or peroneal nerve)

PEARLS AND PITFALLS

Pearls

- When bone plugs are used on the medial transplant, it is important to follow these steps:
  Keep the bone plugs short, particularly the posterior plug; this allows easier passage into the respective tunnels.
  Do not use a diameter smaller than 8 mm. Plugs smaller than this are easily broken.
  Attach the bone plug suture to the meniscus soft tissues as well for extra-secure fixation.
  Use adequate force with the femoral distractor to ensure sufficient space for bone plug passage. The femoral distractor is an invaluable tool for three phases of this technique: tunnel or trough placement, graft passage, and graft fixation.
- Leave the native meniscus rim intact, if possible. This provides a secure area to which to repair the meniscus transplant and maintains some of the patient's native circumferential hoop stresses.

- Use bone fixation for medial and lateral meniscus transplants for additional stability, better load transmission biomechanics, and improved bone-to-bone healing.

Pitfalls

- Be cautious in using a bone bridge for medial transplantation. To avoid compromising the ACL, the tendency is to medialize the medial meniscus attachment sites. Our preference is to use bone plugs for the medial transplant.
- Make sure to place meniscus transplant attachment sites in the anatomic origins of the native meniscus. Studies have shown that deviations as small as 5 mm have profound biomechanical consequences.
- Make sure to put the knee through a full range of motion while visualizing the meniscus transplant. This is to ensure that full motion has been obtained and the fixation is stable.

Results

After combined ACL and meniscal transplantation surgery, good results are achieved in nearly 85% of patients (Fig. 50-13). The senior author's results are presented in Table 50-1. Other authors' results of meniscus transplantation are presented elsewhere in this book and referenced.

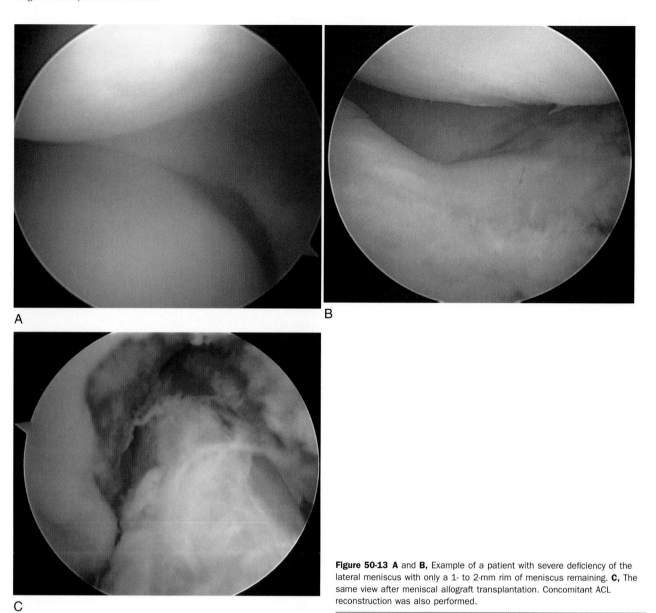

Figure 50-13 A and **B,** Example of a patient with severe deficiency of the lateral meniscus with only a 1- to 2-mm rim of meniscus remaining. **C,** The same view after meniscal allograft transplantation. Concomitant ACL reconstruction was also performed.

Table 50-1 The Pittsburgh-Michigan Experience with Meniscus Transplantation ± ACL Surgery

Author	Study	Follow-up	Outcome
Sekiya et al[16] (2006)	Lateral meniscus transplantation	3.3 years	79% normal IKDC score
Graf et al[6] (2004)	ACL–medial meniscus transplantation	8.5 years	7/8 normal IKDC score
Sekiya et al[15] (2003)	ACL–meniscus transplantation	2.8 years	86%-90% normal IKDC score
Yoldas et al[21] (2003)	ACL–meniscus transplantation	2.2 years	95% normal IKDC score

ACL, anterior cruciate ligament; IKDC, International Knee Documentation Committee.

References

1. Cameron JC, Saha S. Meniscal allograft transplantation for unicompartmental arthritis of the knee. Clin Orthop 1997;337:164-171.

2. Carter TR. Meniscal allograft transplantation. Sports Med Arthrosc Rev 1999;7:51-62.

3. Cole BJ, Dennis MG, Lee SJ, et al. Prospective evaluation of allograft meniscus transplantation: a minimum 2-year follow-up. Am J Sports Med 2006;34:919-927.

4. Cole BJ, Rodeo S, Carter T. Allograft meniscus transplantation: indications, techniques, results. J Bone Joint Surg Am 2002;84:1236-1250.

5. Garrett JC. Meniscal transplantation: a review of 43 cases with two to seven year follow-up. Sports Med Arthrosc Rev 1993;2:164-167.

6. Graf KW, Sekiya JK, Wojtys EM. Long-term results following meniscal allograft transplantation: minimum 8.5-year follow-up. Arthroscopy 2004;20:129-140.

7. Kurtz CA, Bonner KF, Sekiya JK. Meniscus transplantation utilizing the femoral distractor. Arthroscopy 2006;22:568.e1-3.

8. Milachowski KA, Weismeir K, Wirth CJ. Homologous meniscus transplantation: experimental and clinical results. Int Orthop 1989;13:1-11.

9. Noyes FR, Barber-Westin SD, Rankin M. Meniscal transplantation in symptomatic patients less than fifty years old. J Bone Joint Surg Am 2004;86:1392-1404.

10. Pollard ME, Kang Q, Berg EE: Radiographic sizing for meniscal transplantation. Arthroscopy 1995;11:684–687.

11. Rath E, Richmond JC, Yassir W, et al. Meniscal allograft transplantation. Two- to eight-year results. Am J Sports Med 2001;29:410-414.

12. Ryu RK, Dunbar WH, Morse GG. Meniscal allograft replacement: a 1-year to 6-year experience. Arthroscopy 2002;18:989-994.

13. Sekiya JK, Elkousy HA, Harner CD. Meniscal transplant combined with anterior cruciate ligament reconstruction. Oper Tech Sports Med 2002;10:157-164.

14. Sekiya JK, Ellingson CI. Meniscal allograft transplantation. J Am Acad Orthop Surg 2006;14:164-174.

15. Sekiya JK, Giffin RJ, Irrgang JJ, et al. Clinical outcomes following combined meniscal allograft transplantation and anterior cruciate ligament reconstruction. Am J Sports Med 2003;31:896-906.

16. Sekiya JK, West RV, Groff Y, et al. Clinical outcomes following isolated lateral meniscal allograft transplantation. Arthroscopy 2006;22:771-780.

17. Stollsteimer GT, Shelton WR, Dukes A, et al. Meniscal allograft transplantation: a 1 to 5 year follow-up of 22 patients. Arthroscopy 2000;16:343-347.

18. van Arkel ER, de Boer HH. Human meniscal transplantation: preliminary results at two to five year follow-up. J Bone Joint Surg Br 1995;77:589-595.

19. Verdonk PC, Demurie A, Almqvist KF, et al. Transplantation of viable meniscal allograft. Survivorship analysis and clinical outcome of one hundred cases. J Bone Joint Surg Am 2005;87:715-724.

20. Wirth CJ, Peters G, Milachowski KA, et al. Long-term results of meniscal allograft transplantation. Am J Sports Med 2002;30:174-181.

21. Yoldas EA, Sekiya JK, Irrgang JJ, et al. Arthroscopically assisted meniscal allograft transplantation with and without combined anterior cruciate ligament reconstruction. Knee Surg Sports Traumatol Arthrosc 2003;11:173-182.

50

Débridement of Articular Cartilage in the Knee

Ryan Aukerman, MD

Shawn Wynn, MD

Lee Kaplan, MD

Articular cartilage injuries in the knee are a relatively common problem in today's population. In fact, an estimated 900,000 Americans suffer cartilage injuries each year.[8] The integrity of a normally structured articular cartilage envelope is essential for proper joint function.[5] Curl et al[6] evaluated 31,516 arthroscopies and found 53,569 hyaline cartilage lesions during a 4-year period. Whereas articular cartilage injuries are common, injured cartilage has a limited ability to heal itself.[6]

The pain experienced with chondral lesions is believed to stem from the nerve endings in the exposed subchondral bone and knee effusions caused by articular debris.[20,23] Studies have shown that loose articular cartilage flaps and exposed subchondral bone cause significant disability in the knee joint.[11] One study injecting cartilage fragments into rat knees resulted in joint effusions, articular cartilage friability, pitting, discoloration, and inflammatory arthritis.[8]

Once it is damaged, articular cartilage has a severe limitation for self-repair. Our knowledge of the pathophysiologic mechanisms of damage and repair of articular cartilage is currently in its infancy. This lack of complete understanding has stimulated a great deal of interest as well as research in this area. Multiple techniques ranging from mechanical débridement to surgical repair and cartilage transplantation exist for the treatment of articular cartilage defects.

Arthroscopic mechanical débridement with abrasion arthroplasty was first described by Johnson[14,15] in the 1980s. Mechanical débridement of articular cartilage can remove unstable flaps, remove loose particles, and ultimately improve pain and function of the knee.

Preoperative Considerations

History

Articular cartilage defects can often be difficult to diagnose, with or without imaging. It is important to determine the possible cause of the cartilage defect. Any traumatic event in the past may be important; this may have been the inciting event that disrupted the integrity of the delicate articular cartilage. The degree of injury may be variable as well. A patient who suffered a severe knee dislocation may have larger or more extensive cartilage defects than a patient with the insidious onset of knee pain and no major trauma. An accurate history, including the duration and severity of symptoms, may be of great benefit when treatment options are considered. Associated ligamentous or meniscal injuries will also be important factors in compiling a treatment plan.

Signs and Symptoms

Patients with articular cartilage lesions often present with intermittent knee pain. The pain is commonly accompanied by intermittent effusions. In fact, effusions can occur in up to 70% of patients with articular cartilage lesions.[17] The presence of an effusion at the actual time of examination can be variable. Regardless, the presence of a knee effusion should not be overlooked. Patients may or may not remember a specific event or injury that is related to their symptoms. Pain, however, is the most common complaint. It may be reproduced at certain degrees of flexion or with certain positions or activities. Mechanical symptoms, such as popping, catching, and even locking, can be experienced as well.

Physical Examination

Visual inspection, palpation, range-of-motion evaluation, joint line palpation, and ligament testing are performed in examination of the knee. A Lachman examination, pivot shift test, and anterior and posterior drawer tests are conducted, as is varus and valgus testing for lateral collateral ligament and medial collateral ligament stability. Ambulation and gait are observed. Strength testing and neurovascular examination are performed. Examination of the patellofemoral joint with squat testing, apprehension, and load testing is an important aspect as well. Specific to this type of lesion, the patient may be tender to palpation directly over the femoral condyles, in the location of the lesion. Palpation of the lesion often will produce a sharp pain in this region. Joint effusion is common and should be evaluated. Crepitation can also be felt while the knee is moved through a range of motion.

Imaging

Radiography

Radiographs should always be obtained in symptomatic patients but may be of limited use in narrowing the diagnosis to a cartilage lesion. Radiographs are important to eliminate other possible causes of pain. Weight-bearing anteroposterior, lateral, sunrise, 45-degree flexion posteroanterior, and alignment views are usually obtained and can help rule out degenerative joint disease, loose bodies, and fractures.

Magnetic Resonance Imaging

Magnetic resonance imaging (MRI) is the most useful imaging modality for the diagnosis of chondral lesions (Fig. 51-1); however, this is controversial. One study has shown the sensitivity of MRI for evaluation of chondral lesions to be as low as 21%.[18] Disler et al,[7] however, found a 93% sensitivity and 94% specificity for detection of cartilage lesions by three-dimensional spoiled gradient-echo MRI. The sensitivity and specificity of MRI depend on the imaging sequence as well as the grade of the cartilage lesion.[4] Ligament and meniscal pathologic processes are seen very well on MRI, as is soft tissue disease. Cartilage defects are more difficult to assess. The development of

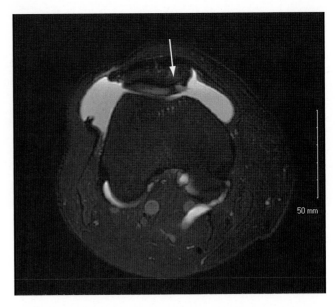

Figure 51-1 A magnetic resonance image with a chondral flap on the medial facet of the patella in a patient who had a history of a direct fall onto the knee and was complaining of patellofemoral pain.

improved MRI machines, as well as new imaging sequences, may improve the sensitivity of MRI for identification of chondral lesions in the future.

Indications and Contraindications

Nonoperative treatment is typically the first line of treatment with these types of injuries. The duration of nonoperative treatment is surgeon and patient dependent. Treatment modalities include physical therapy, anti-inflammatory drugs, ice, rest, and closed chain muscle strengthening. Weight loss is also an important consideration. Compressive wraps or neoprene sleeves can be used to control and to minimize intermittent joint effusions.

Operative treatment is reserved for those whose course of nonoperative treatment has failed. This is often after 8 to 12 weeks of treatment but can be variable. The primary indication for operative treatment is mechanical symptoms. The goals of treatment are to stabilize loose articular cartilage, to decrease pain, and to improve function.

Mechanical débridement may be contraindicated in elderly patients with advanced degenerative changes, as the procedure may be of little benefit in advanced degenerative disease.

Surgical Technique

Anesthesia and Positioning

The choice of anesthesia is based on the preferences of the surgeon, the anesthesiologist, the patient, and the patient's general medical condition. General endotracheal, spinal, and regional anesthesia with sedation are viable anesthetic options.

A proper time-out is performed to identify the patient, limb of surgery, and surgical procedure in the operating room. The patient is then placed in a supine position on a standard operating table. A side thigh post is used, and the foot of the bed is not dropped. Once adequate anesthesia is obtained, the patient is given preoperative prophylactic antibiotics, and a well-padded tourniquet is applied to the upper thigh. The tourniquet is placed but not inflated. The arthroscopy portal sites are preinjected with lidocaine and epinephrine.

Examination Under Anesthesia

After the patient has obtained adequate anesthesia, a standard ligamentous knee examination is performed. Range of motion, anterior cruciate ligament, posterior cruciate ligament, lateral collateral ligament, and medial collateral ligament are examined in standard fashion.

Surgical Landmarks, Incisions, and Portals

Standard arthroscopy portals are used. Landmarks include the medial and lateral joint lines, patella, and patellar tendon.

A superomedial portal is made for the inflow cannula. Next, an inferolateral camera portal is placed. An inferomedial portal is also made under direct visualization.

Specific Steps (Box 51-1)

A diagnostic arthroscopy is performed first. Special focus is placed on evaluation of the entire articular surface of the

Box 51-1 Surgical Steps

1. Perform diagnostic arthroscopy and evaluate the entire articular surface of the patella, trochlear groove, medial and lateral femoral condyles, and tibial plateaus.

2. Identify the chondral lesion; palpate the defect and its borders with a blunt probe to expose loose flaps and any areas of delamination.

3. Identify areas where the cartilage is softened; if the cartilage has an intact surface, it should not be débrided.

4. Place a 4.5-mm aggressive shaver for mechanical removal of the loose flaps and debris until stable borders are obtained.

5. Probe the débrided area to assess stability of the remaining cartilage.

patella, trochlear groove, medial and lateral femoral condyles, and tibial plateaus. The inferomedial portal is placed under direct visualization.

The chondral lesion is identified (Fig. 51-2), and the defect and its borders are carefully and systematically palpated with a blunt probe. This will expose loose flaps and any areas of delamination. It is also important to identify areas where the cartilage is softened (Fig. 51-3); but if the cartilage has an intact surface, it should not be débrided. Once loose flaps of cartilage are identified, a 4.5-mm aggressive shaver is placed, and the loose flaps and debris are mechanically removed until stable borders are obtained (Figs. 51-4 and 51-5). A whisker-type shaver may also be

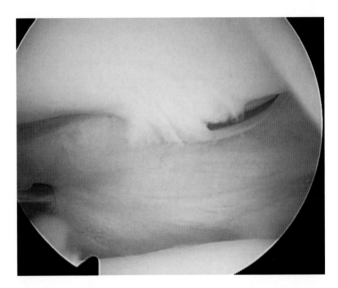

Figure 51-2 The chondral lesion is identified, and the defect and its borders are carefully and systematically palpated with a blunt probe to expose loose flaps and any areas of delamination.

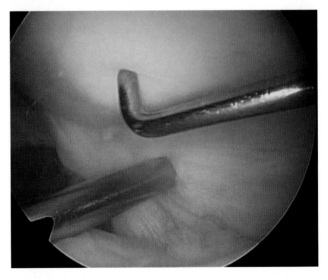

Figure 51-3 It is also important to identify areas where the cartilage is softened, but the cartilage should not be débrided if it has an intact surface.

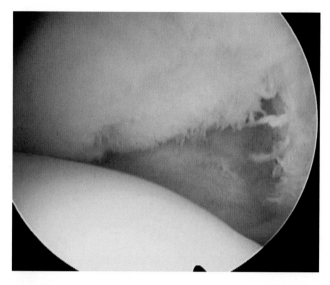

Figures 51-4 Once loose flaps of cartilage are identified, a 4.5-mm aggressive shaver is placed. The loose flaps and debris are mechanically removed until stable borders are obtained.

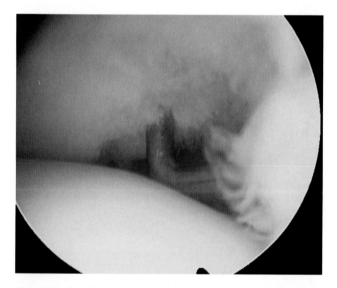

Figure 51-5 The débrided area is probed to assess stability of the remaining cartilage.

used for less aggressive débridement. Care must be taken not to peel off the articular cartilage but only to remove the unstable borders. The posteromedial and posterolateral gutters are also visualized to evaluate for intraarticular loose bodies. The blunt arthroscopy obturator is placed through the notch into the posterolateral and posteromedial recess of the knee under direct visualization. Once it is in position, the camera is then placed into the obturator sleeve, and the posterolateral and posteromedial notch recesses are visualized.

It is helpful to document the size and location of the lesion in the operative report. On the patella, the description should include the facet on which the lesion is located

as well as the flexion angle at which the lesion comes in contact with the trochlea. On the trochlea, describe whether the lesion is medial, lateral, or centrally located. If the lesion involves the medial or lateral femoral condyles, documentation of the flexion angle of the knee where the lesion becomes weight bearing is helpful for reference.

PEARLS AND PITFALLS

- Use a probe to frequently check the cartilage lesion for stable borders.
- For complete evaluation, the patellofemoral joint may need to be viewed from the superomedial or superolateral portal.
- Measure lesions before and after shaving and débridement.
- Use a mechanical shaver for most débridement; a pituitary instrument may be used for the edges of the lesion.
- A whisker-type shaver is useful for less aggressive débridement.
- Do not débride softened but intact cartilage.
- Document the location of lesions as well as size; note facet location on patella and location on trochlea.
- Document the flexion angle at which the lesion becomes weight bearing on the medial and lateral femoral condyles.
- Inspect posteromedial and posterolateral compartments for loose bodies (70-degree arthroscope may be needed).
- Accessory posteromedial and posterolateral portals may be necessary for removal of loose bodies.

Postoperative Considerations

Follow-up

Sutures are removed in 7 to 10 days. Close attention is paid to obtaining postoperative range of motion. Also, postoperative effusions and any activity-related effusions are worrisome and should be addressed with repeat examination and possible MRI.

Rehabilitation

Patients are allowed to bear weight postoperatively as tolerated. Crutches are prescribed to assist with ambulation, and patients may be weaned from postoperative crutches when they no longer demonstrate a limp. Once the incisions are healed, pool therapy can also be of significant benefit.

Complications

Complications can include infection, continued pain, advancement to degenerative arthritis, and possible arthrofibrosis.

Results

The results of treatment of chondral lesions with mechanical débridement are variable (Table 51-1). These are complex and often frustrating problems. Mechanical symptoms, such as catching and popping, are often alleviated with mechanical débridement. Hunt et al[12] believe that improved pain relief and longer duration of pain relief are achieved in patients who have acute onset of pain, mechanical symptoms, normal lower extremity alignment, and minimal degenerative changes on radiographic examination. Kruger et al[16] found that after an average follow-up of 40 months, patients with severe articular cartilage lesions who had undergone articular lavage alone showed significantly poorer results than did those treated with mechanical débridement.

Table 51-1 Clinical Results of Débridement and Abrasion Arthroplasty of Articular Cartilage

Author	Study Design	Technique	No. of Patients	Indications	Follow-up	Outcomes
Moseley et al[21] (2002)	Prospective, randomized, controlled trial	3 groups (lavage, débridement, placebo)	165	Degenerative arthritis	2 years	No difference between the 3 groups
Jackson et al[13] (1986)	Prospective, randomized	Lavage ± débridement	202 total 65 lavage 137 lavage + débridement	Degenerative arthritis	3 years	Lavage: 45% improved Lavage + débridement: 68% improved
Livesley et al[19] (1991)	Prospective, controlled trial	Physiotherapy ± lavage	61 total 37 physiotherapy + lavage 24 physiotherapy alone	Degenerative arthritis	1 year	Better pain relief in lavage group, more effective in earlier stages of osteoarthritis
Aichroth et al[1] (1991)	Prospective review	Débridement	254	Degenerative arthritis	44 months (mean)	75% good–excellent 85% satisfied
Kruger et al[16] (2000)	Retrospective	Abrasion arthroplasty	161	Degenerative arthritis	40 months (mean)	29.2% improved 54.7% unchanged 16.1% worse
Rand[22] (1991)	Retrospective	Abrasion arthroplasty	28	Degenerative arthritis	3.8 years (mean)	39% good–excellent 29% fair 32% poor
Baumgaertner et al[2] (1990)	Retrospective	Abrasion arthroplasty	46 (41 knees)	Degenerative arthritis	33 months (mean)	52% improved 39% no change 9% temporary improvement
Bert and Maschka[3] (1989)	Retrospective	Abrasion arthroplasty	59	Degenerative arthritis	60 months (mean)	51% good–excellent 16% fair 33% poor
Bert and Maschka[3] (1989)	Retrospective	Débridement	67	Degenerative arthritis	60 months (mean)	66% good–excellent 13% fair 21% poor
Johnson[14] (1986)	Retrospective	Abrasion arthroplasty	104	Degenerative arthritis	2 year	78% subjective improvement 15% no change 7% worse
Friedman et al[9] (1984)	Retrospective	Abrasion arthroplasty	73	Degenerative arthritis	>6 months (mean)	60% good–excellent 34% fair 6% poor

51

References

1. Aichroth PM, Patel DV, Moyes ST. A prospective review of arthroscopic débridement for degenerative joint disease of the knee. Int Orthop 1991;15:351-355.

2. Baumgaertner MP, Cannon WD Jr, Vittori JM, et al. Arthroscopic débridement of the arthritic knee. Clin Orthop 1990;253:197-202.

3. Bert J, Maschka K. The arthroscopic treatment of unicompartmental gonarthrosis: a five-year follow-up study of abrasion arthroplasty plus arthroscopic débridement and arthroscopic débridement alone. Arthroscopy 1989;5:25-32.

4. Bredella MA, Tirman PF, Peterfy CG, et al. Accuracy of T2-weighted fast spin-echo MR imaging with fat saturation in detecting cartilage defects in the knee: comparison with arthroscopy in 130 patients. AJR Am J Roentgenol 1999;172:1073-1080.

5. Buckwalter JA, Mow VC. Basic science and injury of articular cartilage, menisci, and bone. In DeLee JC, Drez D, Miller MD, eds. Orthopaedic Sports Medicine: Principles and Practice, 2nd ed. Philadelphia, WB Saunders, 2003:67-87.

6. Curl WW, Krome J, Gordon ES, et al. Cartilage injuries: a review of 31,516 knee arthroscopies. Arthroscopy 1997;13:456-460.

7. Disler DG, McCauley TR, Wirth CR, Fuchs MD. Detection of knee hyaline cartilage defects using fat-suppressed three-dimensional spoiled gradient-echo MR imaging: comparison with standard MR imaging and correlation with arthroscopy. AJR Am J Roentgenol 1995;165:377-382.

8. Evans CH, Mazzocchi RA, Nelson DD, Rubash HE. Experimental arthritis induced by intraarticular injection of allogenic cartilaginous particles into rabbit knees. Arthritis Rheum 1984;27:200-207.

9. Friedman M, Beraso D, Fox J. Preliminary results with abrasion arthroplasty in the osteoarthritic knee. Clin Orthop 1984;182:200-205.

10. Genzyme. Cartilage repair symposium. American Academy of Orthopaedic Surgeons annual meeting; San Francisco, Calif; 1995.

11. Hoover NW. Injuries of the popliteal artery associated with fractures and dislocations. Surg Clin North Am 1961;41:1099-1124.

12. Hunt SA, Jazrawi LM, Sherman OH. Arthroscopic management of osteoarthritis of the knee. J Am Acad Orthop Surg 2003;11:290.

13. Jackson RW, Silver R, Marans H. Arthroscopic treatment of degenerative joint disease [abstract]. Arthroscopy 1986;2:114.

14. Johnson LL. Arthroscopic abrasion arthroplasty historical and pathologic perspective: present status. Arthroscopy 1986;2:54-69.

15. Johnson LL. Arthroscopic abrasion arthroplasty. In McGinty JB, Caspari RB, Jackson RW, Poehling GG, eds. Operative Arthroscopy, 2nd ed. Philadelphia, Lippincott-Raven, 1996:427-446.

16. Kruger T, Wohlrab D, Birke A, Hein W. Results of arthroscopic joint débridement in different stages of chondromalacia of the knee joint. Arch Orthop Trauma Surg 2000;120:338-342.

17. Levy AL, Goltz DH. Articular cartilage. In Garrett WE, Speer KP, Kirkendall DT, eds. Principles and Practice of Orthopaedic Sports Medicine. Philadelphia, Lippincott Williams & Wilkins, 2000: 787-804.

18. Levy AS, Lohnes J, Sculley S, et al. Chondral delamination of the knee in soccer players. Am J Sports Med 1995;24:634-639.

19. Livesley PJ, Doherty M, Needhoff M, Moulton A. Arthroscopic lavage of osteoarthritic knees. J Bone Joint Surg Br 1991;73:922-926.

20. Mayer G, Seidlein H. Chondral and osteochondral fractures of the knee joint—treatment and results. Arch Orthop Trauma Surg 1988;107:154-157.

21. Moseley JB, O'Malley K, Peterson NJ, et al. A controlled trial of arthroscopic surgery for osteoarthritis of the knee. N Engl J Med 2002;347:81-88.

22. Rand J. Role of arthroscopy in osteoarthritis of the knee. Arthroscopy 1991;7:358-361.

23. Zamber RW, Teitz CC, McGuire DA, et al. Articular cartilage lesions of the knee. Arthroscopy 1989;5:258-268.

CHAPTER 52

Microfracture Technique in the Knee

J. Richard Steadman, MD

William G. Rodkey, DVM

Karen K. Briggs, MPH

Full-thickness chondral defects in the knee are common and present in a variety of clinical settings and at different ages. The shearing forces of the femur on the tibia as a single event may result in trauma to the articular cartilage, causing the cartilage to fracture, lacerate, and separate from the underlying subchondral bone or to separate with a piece of the subchondral bone. Chronic repetitive loading in excess of normal physiologic levels also may result in the fatigue and failure of the chondral surface. The single events are usually found in younger groups, whereas chronic degenerative lesions are more common in the middle-aged and older groups. Articular cartilage defects that extend full thickness to subchondral bone rarely heal without intervention.[7-12] Techniques to treat chondral defects include abrasion, drilling, osteochondral autografts, osteochondral allografts, and autologous cell transplantation.[11] The senior author (J. R. S.) developed the microfracture technique to enhance chondral resurfacing by providing a suitable environment for new tissue formation and taking advantage of the body's own healing potential,[7-12] and the clinical experience now includes more than 3000 patients in whom microfracture has been done.

We have documented that arthroscopic débridement accompanied by microfracture of subchondral bone is a reliable and repeatable procedure to stimulate biologic repair of cartilage defects of the knee in patients in whom nonoperative treatment has failed or in whom acute lesions are encountered during arthroscopy. More invasive procedures, such as osteotomy, cartilage grafting, and unicompartmental arthroplasty, thus might be avoided or at least delayed for several years. Specifically, the goals of this procedure are to alleviate the pain and disabilities that can result from the chondral lesions and further to prevent late degenerative changes in the joint by restoring the joint surface.[7,9-12]

Preoperative Considerations

Physical Examination

Patients who present with knee pain undergo a thorough physical and orthopedic examination. The cartilage lesions can be on the joint surfaces of the femur, tibia, or patella. At times, the physical diagnosis can be difficult and elusive, especially if only an isolated chondral defect is present. Identification of point tenderness over a femoral condyle or tibial plateau is a useful finding but in itself is not diagnostic. If compression of the patella elicits pain, this finding might be indicative of a patellar or trochlear lesion.

Indications and Contraindications

The microfracture technique is most commonly indicated for full-thickness loss of articular cartilage either in a weight-bearing area between the femur and tibia or in an area of contact between the patella and trochlear groove.[7-12] Unstable cartilage that overlies the subchondral bone is also an indication for microfracture. If a partial-thickness lesion is probed and the cartilage simply scrapes off down to bone, we consider this to be a full-thickness lesion. Degenerative joint disease in a knee that has proper axial alignment is another common indication for microfracture (Table 52-1).

Patients with acute chondral injuries are treated as soon as practical after the diagnosis is made, especially if the knee is being treated concurrently for meniscus or anterior cruciate ligament disease. Patients with chronic or degenerative chondral lesions often are treated nonoperatively (conservatively) for at least 12 weeks after a suspected chondral lesion is diagnosed. This treatment regimen includes activity modification, physical therapy, nonsteroidal anti-inflammatory drugs, viscosupplement injections, and perhaps dietary supplements that may have cartilage-stimulating properties. If nonoperative treatment is not successful, surgical treatment is considered.[7-12]

No limitations are placed on how large an acute lesion can be and still be considered suitable for microfracture.[7-9,11] We have observed that even very large acute lesions respond well to microfracture.[7-9,11] Treatment of chronic degenerative lesions is not specifically limited by size, but more emphasis is placed on proper axial alignment and the presence of global degenerative changes throughout the knee.[6,9,13] General considerations for use of the microfracture procedure include the patient's age, acceptable biomechanical alignment of the knee, the patient's activity level, and the patient's expectations.[6,9,11,13]

Specific contraindications to microfracture are axial malalignment, unwillingness or inability of the patient to follow the required strict and rigorous rehabilitation protocol, partial-thickness defects, and inability of the patient to use the opposite leg for weight bearing during the minimal or non–weight-bearing time (see Table 52-1).[9-11] Other specific contraindications include any systemic immune-mediated disease, disease-induced arthritis, and cartilage disease. A relative contraindication is for patients older than 65 years because the authors have observed that some patients older than 65 years experience difficulty with crutch walking and the required rigorous rehabilitation.[9-11] Microfracture is also contraindicated with global degenerative osteoarthrosis or if the cartilage surrounding the lesion is too thin for a perpendicular rim to be established to hold the marrow clot.[6,9-11] In these advanced

degenerative cases, axial malalignment is also a confounding factor.[6,9-11,13]

Imaging

For diagnostic imaging, we use long standing radiographs to observe for angular deformity and for joint space narrowing that is often indicative of loss of articular cartilage. We also obtain standard anteroposterior and lateral radiographs of both knees as well as weight-bearing views with the knees flexed to 30 to 45 degrees. Patellar views are also useful to evaluate the patellofemoral joint.

Magnetic resonance imaging that employs newer diagnostic sequences specific for articular cartilage has become a mainstay of our diagnostic work-up of patients with suspected chondral lesions.

Surgical Technique

Specific Steps (Box 52-1)

Standard arthroscopic portals can be used for microfracture (Fig. 52-1). We make three portals: a superior and medially placed inflow portal and medial and lateral parapatellar portals (Fig. 52-2). Accessory portals are occasionally made as needed for lesions in difficult locations. We typically do not use a tourniquet during the microfracture procedure; rather, we vary the arthroscopic fluid pump pressure to control bleeding. An initial thorough diagnostic examination of the knee should be done. We carefully inspect all geographic areas of the knee including the suprapatellar pouch, the medial and lateral gutters, the patellofemoral joint, the intercondylar notch and its contents, and the medial and lateral compartments including the posterior horns of both menisci. We do all other intra-articular procedures before completing microfracture, with the exception of ligament reconstruction. This sequence helps prevent loss of visualization when the fat droplets and blood enter the knee from the microfracture holes. This technique also decreases the amount of time that the microfractured bone is exposed to the elevated intra-articular pressures and fluid flow, which can decrease the

Table 52-1 Indications for and Contraindications to Microfracture

Indications	Contraindications
Full-thickness defect (grade IV), acute or chronic	Partial-thickness defects
Unstable full-thickness lesion	Uncorrected axial malalignment
Degenerative joint disease lesion (requires proper knee alignment)	Inability of patient to commit to rehabilitation protocol
Acceptance by patient of rehabilitation protocol	Global degenerative osteoarthrosis

Box 52-1 Surgical Steps

1. Complete a thorough arthroscopic diagnostic examination, inspecting all geographic areas of the knee. Perform all other intra-articular procedures before completing microfracture, with the exception of ligament reconstruction.

2. Assess the chondral lesion, and then débride all loose or marginally attached cartilage down to exposed bone.

3. Thoroughly and completely remove the calcified cartilage layer with a hand-held curet, but do not penetrate the subchondral bone.

4. Use a microfracture awl to make microfracture holes in the subchondral bone, working first all the way around the periphery and then into the center of the lesion.

5. Microfracture holes should be about 3 to 4 mm apart so that one does not break into another, and they should penetrate approximately 2 to 4 mm deep to access the marrow elements.

6. Reduce the irrigation pump pressure (or tourniquet) and observe for marrow element flow from all holes.

7. Remove all instruments and evacuate the joint. Do *not* use a drain in the joint.

8. Wound closure is routine.

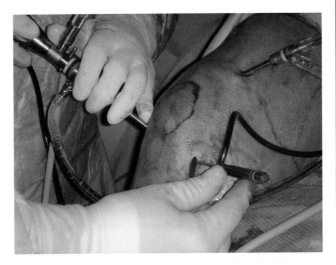

Figure 52-2 The medial and lateral parapatellar portals allow access with the arthroscope and working instruments for a thorough joint inspection and all necessary procedures.

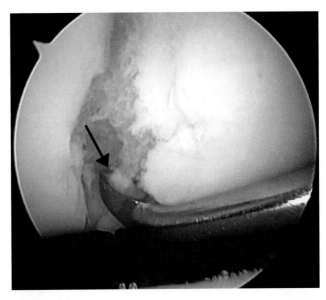

Figure 52-3 A curet is used to remove all damaged and unstable cartilage until a stable perpendicular rim is established around the entire full-thickness defect. Care is taken to remove the calcified cartilage layer completely *(arrow)*.

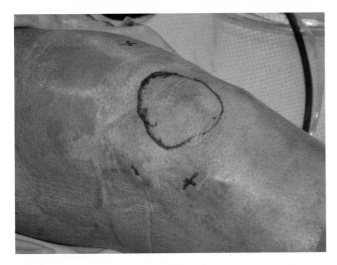

Figure 52-1 Standard arthroscopic portals are used for the microfracture procedure. These include a superior and medially placed inflow portal as well as medial and lateral parapatellar portals.

formation of the clot that is critical to success. We pay particular attention to soft tissues, such as plicae and the lateral retinaculum, which potentially could produce increased compression between cartilage surfaces.[7-12]

After careful assessment of the full-thickness articular cartilage lesion, we débride the exposed bone of all remaining unstable cartilage. We use a hand-held, curved curet and a full-radius resector to débride the cartilage. It is critical to débride all loose or marginally attached cartilage from the surrounding rim of the lesion (Fig. 52-3). Establishment of a stable full-thickness border of cartilage surrounding a central lesion is optimal for microfracture because it provides some degree of protection to the regenerating tissue that is forming in the treated lesion. The calcified cartilage layer that remains as a cap to many lesions must be removed, preferably by use of a curet (see Fig. 52-3). Thorough and complete removal of the calcified cartilage layer is extremely important on the basis of animal studies we have completed.[1,2] Care should be taken to maintain the integrity of the subchondral plate by not débriding too deeply; otherwise, the joint shape and geometry might be negatively altered. This prepared lesion, with a stable perpendicular edge of healthy, well-attached viable cartilage surrounding the defect, provides a pool that helps hold the marrow clot ("super clot," as we have termed it) as it forms.[9,11]

After preparation of the lesion, we use an arthroscopic awl to make multiple holes, or microfractures, in the exposed subchondral bone plate. We use an awl with an angle that permits the tip to be approximately perpendicular to the bone as it is advanced, typically 30 or 45 degrees (Fig. 52-4). There also is a 90-degree awl that should be used only on the patella or other soft bone. The 90-degree awl should be advanced only manually, not with a mallet. The holes are made as close together as possible, but not so close that one breaks into another, thus damaging the subchondral plate between them and potentially altering the joint shape. This technique usually results in microfracture holes that are approximately 3 to 4 mm apart. When fat droplets can be seen coming from the marrow cavity, the appropriate depth (approximately 2 to 4 mm) has been reached (Fig. 52-5). The arthroscopic awls produce essentially no thermal necrosis of the bone compared with hand-driven or motorized drills. We make microfracture holes around the periphery of the defect first, immediately adjacent to the healthy stable cartilage rim (see Figs. 52-4 and 52-5); then we complete the process by making the microfracture holes toward the center of the defect (Fig. 52-6). We assess the treated lesion at the conclusion of the microfracture to ensure that a sufficient number of holes has been made before reducing the

arthroscopic irrigation fluid flow (Fig. 52-7). After the arthroscopic irrigation fluid pump pressure is reduced, under direct visualization we are able to observe the flow of marrow fat droplets and blood from the microfracture holes into the prepared lesion (Fig. 52-8). The quantity of marrow contents flowing into the joint is judged to be adequate when we observe marrow elements emanating from all microfracture holes (Fig. 52-9). We then remove

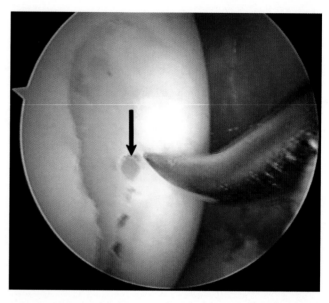

Figure 52-5 The presence of a fat droplet *(arrow)* from the marrow cavity indicates adequate penetration of the subchondral bone by the microfracture awl.

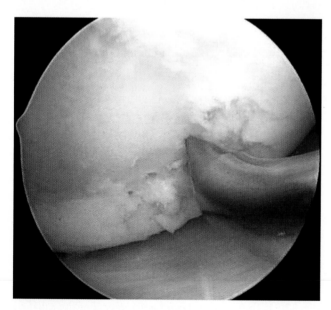

Figure 52-4 After preparation of the lesion, the microfracture holes are begun at the periphery of the lesion adjacent to the stable cartilage rim.

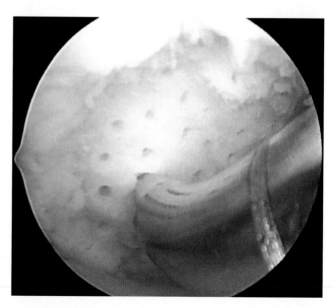

Figure 52-6 After starting at the periphery, the microfracture holes are continued into the center of the prepared lesion. The microfracture awl penetrates the subchondral bone to a depth of approximately 2 to 4 mm.

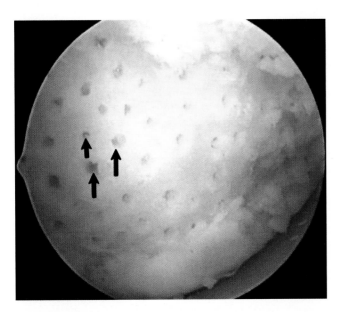

Figure 52-7 When the microfracture procedure has been completed, the proximity of the holes is about 3 to 4 mm apart as noted by the arrows.

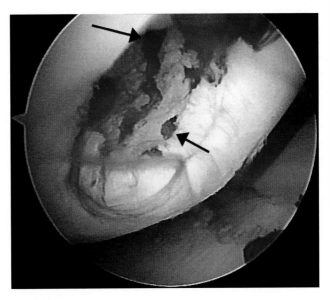

Figure 52-9 Once the arthroscopic irrigation fluid pressure is reduced completely, the blood and fat droplets flow readily from the marrow cavity through the microfracture holes (arrows) into the lesion.

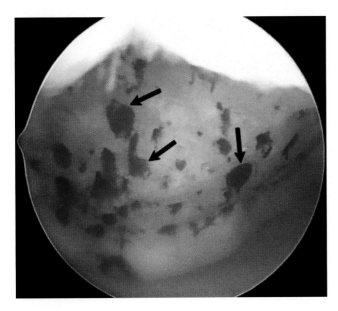

Figure 52-8 Just as the arthroscopic irrigation fluid pressure is reduced, as indicated by the arrows, marrow elements can be seen near the surface of the subchondral bone. Note that the marrow elements can be seen at essentially all of the microfracture holes.

all instruments from the knee and evacuate the joint of fluid.[9-11] Intra-articular drains should not be used because the goal is for the surgically induced marrow clot rich in marrow elements to form and to stabilize while covering the lesion.[1,2]

Chronic degenerative chondral lesions commonly have extensive eburnated bone and bone sclerosis with thickening of the subchondral plate,[6] thus making it diffi-

cult to do an adequate microfracture procedure. In these instances and when the axial alignment and other indications for microfracture are met, we first make a few microfracture holes with the awls in various locations of the lesion to assess the thickness of the eburnated bone. We often use a motorized bur to remove the sclerotic bone until punctate bleeding is seen. After the bleeding appears uniformly over the surface of the lesion, a microfracture procedure can be performed as previously described.[6,9-11] We have observed noticeably improved results for these patients with chronic chondral lesions since we began using this technique. However, if the surrounding cartilage is too thin for a perpendicular rim to be established to hold and protect the marrow clot, we probably would not do a microfracture procedure in patients with such advanced degenerative lesions.[6,9-11]

The microfracture awl produces a rough surface in the subchondral bone to which the marrow clot can adhere more easily, yet the integrity of the subchondral plate is maintained for joint surface shape and geometry (see Fig. 52-7). The microfracture procedure virtually eliminates thermal necrosis and provides a roughened surface for blood clot adherence, and the different angles of arthroscopic awls available provide easier access to areas of the knee that are difficult to reach. The awls provide not only perpendicular holes but also improved control of depth penetration compared with drilling. We believe that the key to the entire procedure is to establish the marrow clot to provide the optimal environment for the body's pluripotential marrow cells (mesenchymal stem cells or progenitor cells) to differentiate into stable tissue within the lesion.[1,2]

Postoperative Considerations

Rehabilitation

The rehabilitation program after microfracture for treatment of chondral defects in the knee is crucial to optimize the results of the surgery.[7,11] The rehabilitation promotes the optimal physical environment for the mesenchymal stem cells to differentiate and to produce new extracellular matrix that eventually matures into a durable repair tissue (Fig. 52-10). The surgically induced marrow clot provides the basis for the most ideal chemical environment to complement the physical environment.[1,2] This newly proliferated repair cartilage then fills the original defect. The rehabilitation protocol varies on the basis of anatomic location. The protocols for femorotibial lesions and for patellofemoral lesions are summarized in the Key Rehabilitation Points.

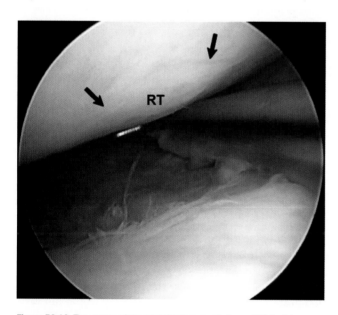

Figure 52-10 The status of the microfracture repair tissue (RT) in this second-look photograph is about 7 years after microfracture. The interface between the repair tissue and the normal articular cartilage is barely discernible (arrows).

KEY REHABILITATION POINTS

Femorotibial Lesions

- Immediate continuous passive motion, 8 hours daily for 8 weeks; 1 cycle/min, largest range of motion tolerated
- No brace
- Touch-down (20% to 30%) crutch walking for 8 weeks
- Cycling (light resistance): start 1 to 2 weeks postoperatively
- Deep-water exercise: start 1 to 2 weeks postoperatively
- After 8 weeks, full weight bearing and active range of motion
- No cutting, turning, or jumping for at least 4 months or until good quadriceps muscle tone
- May be longer for competitive or "heavy" patients

Patellofemoral Lesions

- Immediate continuous passive motion, 8 hours daily for 8 weeks at 0 to 50 degrees ROM
- Brace locked at 0 to 20 degrees; full weight bearing after 1 week
- Stationary bike (light resistance): start 1 to 2 weeks postoperatively
- Water program (no impact): start 1 to 2 weeks postoperatively
- After 8 weeks, begin walking without brace
- Treadmill at 7-degree incline starting 12 weeks postoperatively
- Intense biking and water program 8 to 12 weeks postoperatively
- Sport cord (elastic resistance) program with 0- to 30-degree knee bends starting 12 weeks postoperatively

Results

Patients are focused on their abilities to regain knee function over time and to return to their desired level of activities, especially athletics.[4] We advise patients that they may not reach their maximum level of improvement for at least 2 years after undergoing the microfracture procedure.[7] However, the repair tissue appears to be durable (see Fig. 52-10) and permits return of knee function and increased activity levels.

Functional[5] and activity level[14] scores that appear in published reports on microfracture are summarized in Table 52-2.

Table 52-2 Average Functional and Activity Scores of All Patients after Microfracture

Author	Focus	Follow-up (Range)	Age Range of Patients	Lysholm Function	Tegner Activity
Steadman et al[7] (2003)	Traumatic lesions	Average of 11.3 years (7 to 17)	13-45 years	89	6
Knutsen et al[3] (2004)	Traumatic lesions	Average of 2 years	18-45 years	76	4
Steadman et al[8] (2003)	NFL players	Average of 4.5 years (2 to 13)	22-36 years	90	9
Miller et al[6] (2004)	Degenerative knees	Average of 2.6 years (2 to 5)	40-70 years	83	4.5
Sterett and Steadman[13] (2004)	High tibial osteotomy and microfracture	Average of 3.8 years (2 to 7)	34-79 years	78	5

References

1. Frisbie DD, Oxford JT, Southwood L, et al. Early events in cartilage repair after subchondral bone microfracture. Clin Orthop 2003;407: 215-227.

2. Frisbie DD, Trotter GW, Powers BE, et al. Arthroscopic subchondral bone plate microfracture technique augments healing of large osteochondral defects in the radial carpal bone and medial femoral condyle of horses. J Vet Surg 1999;28:242-255.

3. Knutsen G, Engebretsen L, Ludvigsen TC, et al. Autologous chondrocyte implantation compared with microfracture in the knee. J Bone Joint Surg Am 2004;86:455-464.

4. Kocher MS, Steadman JR, Briggs KK, et al. Reliability, validity, and responsiveness of the Lysholm knee scale for various chondral disorders of the knee. J Bone Joint Surg Am 2004;86:1139-1145.

5. Lysholm J, Gillquist J. Evaluation of knee ligament surgery with special emphasis on use of a scoring scale. Am J Sports Med 1982;10:150-154.

6. Miller BS, Steadman JR, Briggs KK, et al. Patient satisfaction and outcome after microfracture of the degenerative knee. J Knee Surg 2004;17:13-17.

7. Steadman JR, Briggs KK, Rodrigo JJ, et al. Outcomes of microfracture for traumatic chondral defects of the knee: average 11-year follow-up. Arthroscopy 2003;19:477-484.

8. Steadman JR, Miller BS, Karas SG, et al. The microfracture technique in the treatment of full-thickness chondral lesions of the knee in National Football League players. J Knee Surg 2003; 16:83-86.

9. Steadman JR, Rodkey WG, Briggs KK. Microfracture chondroplasty: indications, techniques, and outcomes. Sports Med Arthrosc Rev 2003;11:236-244.

10. Steadman JR, Rodkey WG, Briggs KK. Microfracture to treat full-thickness chondral defects. J Knee Surg 2002;15:170-176.

11. Steadman JR, Rodkey WG, Briggs KK, Rodrigo JJ. Débridement and microfracture for full-thickness articular cartilage defects. In Scott WN, ed. Insall & Scott Surgery of the Knee. Philadelphia, Churchill Livingstone, 2006:359-366.

12. Steadman JR, Rodkey WG, Rodrigo JJ. Microfracture: surgical technique and rehabilitation to treat chondral defects. Clin Orthop 2001;391(suppl):S362-S369.

13. Sterett WI, Steadman JR. Chondral resurfacing and high tibial osteotomy in the varus knee. Am J Sports Med 2004;32: 1243-1249.

14. Tegner Y, Lysholm J. Rating systems in the evaluation of knee ligament injuries. Clin Orthop 1985;198:43-49.

52

CHAPTER 53

Primary Repair of Osteochondritis Dissecans in the Knee

L. Pearce McCarty III, MD

Osteochondritis dissecans is a rare pathologic process affecting subchondral bone and overlying articular cartilage. It probably represents a common end point for multiple possible pathways of injury, including traumatic, ischemic, endocrine, and genetic predisposition. With respect to the knee, the lateral posterior portion of the medial femoral condyle is most commonly affected, representing 70% of occurrences, and has been referred to as the classic lesion.[1] Overall, an estimated 80% of lesions arise in the medial femoral condyle, 15% in the lateral femoral condyle (inferocentral), up to 5% in the inferomedial portion of the patella, and 1% to 2% within the femoral trochlea.[1,3]

Regardless of etiology or location, however, the essential lesion in osteochondritis dissecans remains injury to the subchondral plate with resultant destabilization of overlying articular cartilage and increased susceptibility to stress and shear. Eventual fragmentation and loss of articular integrity can occur, leading to early degenerative changes and loss of function in the affected compartment. Because this process is *osteochondral* rather than purely *chondral* in nature, primary repair by rigid, compressive fixation of unstable lesions offers an attractive and, as the literature suggests, effective means of treatment.

Preoperative Considerations

One must ascertain the degree of fragment stability as accurately as possible before being able to select the appropriate treatment. Modalities tend to fall into one of two categories. On the one hand, strategies such as nonoperative activity modification, trans-lesion marrow stimulation, and primary repair through fragment reduction and rigid, compressive fixation attempt to *restore* native subchondral bone to a healthy state, thereby preserving native articular cartilage. On the other hand, strategies such as autologous cultured chondrocyte implantation, autologous osteochondral transfer, and allogeneic osteochondral grafting attempt to *replace* an osteochondral defect with hyaline or hyaline-like articular cartilage, thereby reestablishing articular congruity. The latter techniques can be viewed as salvage procedures, however, as in these cases a decision has been made that the native articular surface cannot be preserved.

History

Typical History

- Up to 60% of patients provide an account of a minor traumatic incident involving the affected knee.
- Pain and swelling with activity are reported.
- Mechanical symptoms, such as clicking, popping, and locking, suggest the presence of a loose body produced by an unstable, displaced lesion.

Physical Examination

Typical Findings

- Antalgic gait pattern
- Wilson sign: ambulation with the affected leg maintained in a position of relative external rotation

to avoid discomfort caused by impingement of the medial tibial eminence on a classic lesion[17]

- Wilson test: reproduction of pain through internal rotation of the tibia between 30 and 90 degrees of flexion and relief with subsequent external rotation. This test has low sensitivity, but if the result is positive initially, it reliably becomes negative with healing of the lesion.[4,17]
- Effusion
- Limited range of motion
- Quadriceps atrophy: indicative of duration of symptoms
- Focal tenderness to palpation at the site of the lesion (Axhausen sign): suggestive of subchondral instability. This has also been recommended as a simple means of monitoring resolution of the condition.

Imaging

Radiography

Plain film radiography remains an important first step in imaging of osteochondritis dissecans lesions. The following views are recommended:[13]

- Weight-bearing anteroposterior radiograph in full extension
- Weight-bearing posteroanterior radiograph in 30 degrees of flexion (tunnel view): particularly useful for visualizing classic lesions along the lateral posterior aspect of the medial femoral condyle (Fig. 53-1)
- Non–weight-bearing 45-degree flexed lateral view
- Axial view of the patellofemoral joint

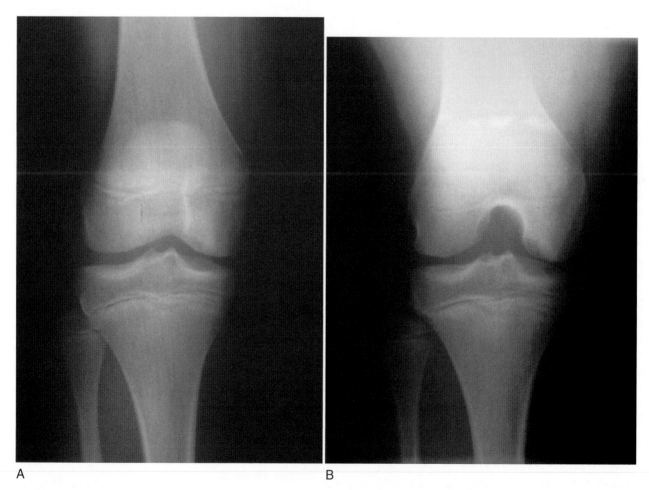

A   B

Figure 53-1 A, Weight-bearing anteroposterior radiograph of right knee in a skeletally immature patient depicting a classic osteochondritis dissecans lesion. **B,** Weight-bearing, 30-degree flexed posteroanterior radiograph, or tunnel view, in the same patient. The osteochondritis dissecans lesion is visualized much more readily with this view.

Magnetic Resonance Imaging

Standard (nonarthrographic) magnetic resonance imaging is the most informative imaging modality in the preoperative work-up. It reliably indicates lesion location, size, depth, and, most important, stability. The presence of one or more of the following four magnetic resonance criteria has been shown to offer up to 97% sensitivity and 100% specificity in predicting lesion stability. High signal is defined as signal intensity equal to that of fluid and greater than the signal intensity of adjacent fat.[6-8]

- Thin, ill-defined or well-defined line of high signal intensity 5 mm or more in length at the interface between the osteochondritis dissecans lesion and the underlying bone (Fig. 53-2)
- Discrete, round area of homogeneous high signal intensity 5 mm or more in diameter beneath the lesion (i.e., cyst)
- Focal defect with a width of 5 mm or more in the articular surface of the lesion (i.e., articular gap)
- High signal intensity line traversing the articular cartilage and subchondral bone plate into the lesion (i.e., discrete break in articular surface extending into the lesion)

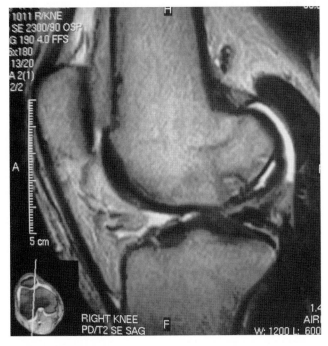

Figure 53-2 Proton density, T2-weighted sagittal magnetic resonance image through the lateral femoral condyle. A high signal intensity interface between the osteochondritis dissecans lesion and underlying bone suggests instability.

Indications and Contraindications

Careful attention must be given to the presenting symptoms, size, location, and stability of a juvenile osteochondritis dissecans lesion in weighing nonoperative versus operative treatment options. Nonoperative treatment consisting of close observation, activity modification, and a variable period of restricted weight bearing serves as an appropriate first line of treatment in many cases of juvenile osteochondritis dissecans. The patient and parents should understand that 12 to 18 months of activity modification may be required for complete healing of the lesion. Furthermore, certain sites have been observed to have a much lower rate of spontaneous resolution than others. Lesions in the classic location have proved to be particularly problematic, with spontaneous resolution rates as low as 30%, versus those in inferocentral medial or lateral sites, for which 88% to 100% healing rates have been reported with nonoperative treatment. Results have been uniformly poor with nonoperative treatment of symptomatic adult osteochondritis dissecans, however, and one should therefore follow a more aggressive, operative tactic in approaching symptomatic lesions in this population.

The ideal osteochondritis dissecans lesion for primary repair is the unstable lesion in situ in an active, symptomatic patient who acknowledges and is willing to comply with postoperative weight-bearing and activity restrictions and who understands the need for a second procedure for implant removal. In addition, patients who fail to demonstrate symptomatic or radiographic improvement after 6 months of appropriate nonoperative therapy should also be considered for surgical treatment. Primary repair is not recommended in the case of grossly unstable lesions that have produced a loose body with less than 3 mm of subchondral bone remaining on the fragment. These cases may be treated with excision of the loose body and either marrow stimulation or one of a variety of secondary salvage cartilage restoration techniques (e.g., osteochondral autograft transfer, osteochondral allograft, autologous chondrocyte implantation), depending on the size and depth of the lesion.

Surgical Technique

With a congruent reduction of the osteochondral flap, primary repair of an osteochondritis dissecans lesion may be performed either arthroscopically or with use of a small parapatellar arthrotomy. A noncongruent reduction with articular step-off, however, typically requires open technique to permit autogenous bone grafting at the base of the lesion. Reduction and fixation of suitable fragments that are detached and loose inside the joint also generally require open technique, permitting the fragment to be recontoured and fixed appropriately.

Anesthesia and Positioning

Depending on the preferences of the patient, surgeon and anesthesiologist, one of several anesthesia options can be used: general, spinal, regional, or a combination thereof. The patient is positioned supine on a standard operating-room table with a padded thigh tourniquet, and the affected extremity is secured in a standard leg holder placed around the proximal thigh to permit broad access to the knee. The contralateral extremity may be positioned in an obstetric-type leg holder. When this type of device is used, care should be taken to provide adequate padding around the common peroneal nerve, as the leg has a tendency to externally rotate, putting pressure on the region around the fibular head. The bed is placed in 15 to 20 degrees of reflex to take the lumbar spine out of extension. The foot of the operating room table is dropped completely. An additional advantage of this type of positioning is ease of access should one wish to confirm the placement of implants by intraoperative fluoroscopy.

Surgical Landmarks, Incisions, and Portals

Landmarks
- Joint line
- Patella
- Patellar tendon
- Tibial tubercle

Portals (Arthroscopic Technique)
- Inferomedial portal
- Inferolateral portal
- Superomedial or superolateral outflow portal
- Accessory instrumentation portal for placement of fixation. This portal should be established by standard spinal needle localization such that fixation can be orthogonal to the plane of the lesion.

Approaches (Open Technique)
- Midline utility skin incision (may be adjusted slightly medial or lateral of midline, depending on location of lesion)
- Medial or lateral parapatellar arthrotomy. Patellar lesions treated in open fashion require a larger arthrotomy to permit partial or complete eversion and exposure of the lesion. For standard condylar lesions, a mini-arthrotomy, extending from the joint line to mid-patellar level, typically suffices.

Structures at Risk
- Meniscus (during open approach)
- Patellar tendon (during open approach)
- Infrapatellar branches of the saphenous nerve

Examination Under Anesthesia

A standard examination under anesthesia documents range of motion and ligamentous stability.

Specific Steps (Box 53-1)

Key surgical steps for primary repair remain essentially the same whether the lesion is approached in open or arthroscopic fashion.

1. Diagnostic Arthroscopy

A complete, systematic arthroscopic evaluation of each compartment and its structures is performed to identify any additional sources of intra-articular disease.

2. Identification and Assessment of Lesion Stability

With use of the elbow of a standard arthroscopic probe, the boundaries and stability of the lesion are assessed. In many cases, the borders of the lesion are obvious, with fissuring, fibrillation, and even gross gapping in the articular surface (Fig. 53-3). However, definition of the lesion can be more subtle in some cases. Nevertheless, even without obvious visual clues, a distinct transition from firm to soft or the ballottement of a segment of articular cartilage can typically be appreciated as one moves the elbow of the probe from normal cartilage to that overlying an osteochondritis dissecans lesion. The tactile feedback received is that of the elbow of the probe falling into a small crevasse as the lesion boundary is crossed (Fig. 53-4). In the rare case that the lesion cannot be identified through visualization and tactile feedback, intraoperative fluoroscopy can confirm the lesion's location.

Box 53-1 Surgical Steps

1. Diagnostic arthroscopy
2. Identification and assessment of lesion stability
3. Débridement of lesion bed and undersurface of the fragment
4. Microfracture of lesion bed with further débridement as needed and assessment of fragment reduction
5. Fixation of lesion
6. Implant removal (for nonabsorbable implants, 3 to 4 months after fixation)

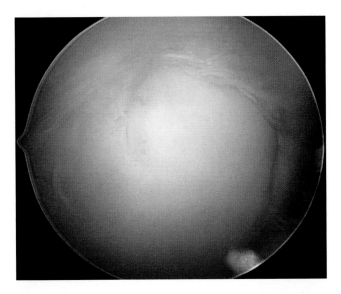

Figure 53-3 Large osteochondritis dissecans lesion of the medial femoral condyle bordering the intercondylar notch. Cartilage fissuring and fibrillation demarcate lesion borders.

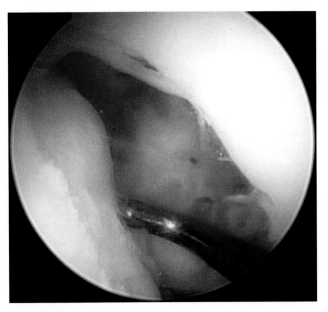

Figure 53-5 The lesion is opened on an intact fibrocartilaginous hinge that borders the intercondylar notch.

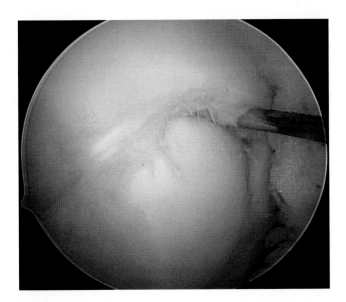

Figure 53-4 Further definition of lesion borders and arthroscopic assessment of lesion stability are carried out with a standard arthroscopic probe.

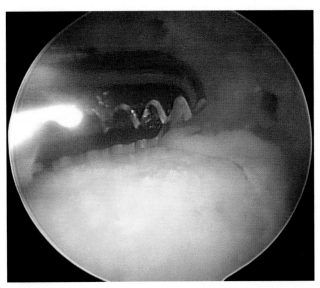

Figure 53-6 A mechanized shaver or bur is used to débride the base of the lesion and undersurface of the fragment.

3. Débridement of Lesion Bed and Undersurface of the Fragment

Any disruption in the articular surface or observation of ballottement with palpation confirms instability and indicates a need to expose and to débride the lesion. Careful manipulation of the lesion boundary with a probe will typically reveal a tendency for the lesion flap to hinge open in one particular direction (Fig. 53-5). For those lesions bordering on the intercondylar notch, the general tendency is for the lesion to hinge on the intercondylar side. A 15-degree arthroscopic Bankart elevator can be useful in opening the lesion. Once the osteochondral flap has been opened, a curet is used to débride the base of the lesion of any granulation tissue or sclerotic bone, and then an aggressive mechanized shaver or spherical bur (4 to 4.5 mm; angled may be useful and should be available) to "freshen" the undersurface of the osteochondral flap and further débride the base of the lesion (Fig. 53-6).

4. Microfracture of Lesion Bed with Further Débridement as Needed and Assessment of Fragment Reduction

A standard set of microfracture awls is used to penetrate the base of the lesion at 5-mm intervals. Inflow should be shut off after microfracture to confirm efflux of marrow elements from the base of the lesion (Fig. 53-7). If the process of microfracture generates an uneven surface that may impede congruent reduction, a small bur may be used to smooth the lesion bed. The osteochondral fragment is then reduced and held firmly in place with the elbow of a probe. Attention is given to the congruency of the reduction. Any step-off greater than 1 mm suggests the need for autogenous bone grafting to the bed of the lesion.

5. Fixation of Lesion

By spinal needle localization technique, a line orthogonal to the plane of the lesion is established and an accessory portal made (Fig. 53-8). This is an extremely important step; application of compressive force along a nonorthogonal vector can produce shear and nonanatomic reduction of the osteochondral fragment.

A variety of implants can be used for fixation. I currently prefer a nonabsorbable, cannulated, headless, variable-pitch compression screw because of the rigidity of fixation provided and compatibility with arthroscopic technique. Cannulated implants are recommended for open technique as well, however, as the placement of implant guide wires helps maintain reduction during fixation. Although success has been reported with bioabsorbable implants, they must be viewed with caution owing to their potential to generate sterile effusions, to be absorbed and dissociate at the shaft-head junction

(producing intra-articular loose bodies), and to loosen and back out (causing injury to the opposing articular surface).[10,15]

With use of an ipsilateral viewing portal, a guide wire is introduced through the accessory instrumentation portal and drilled into the lesion (Fig. 53-9). A second guide wire is then placed to provide countertorque during drilling and placement of the first screw (Fig. 53-10). Small lesions may permit use of a single screw for adequate fixation, but larger lesions may require two or even three screws, and careful consideration should be given to the

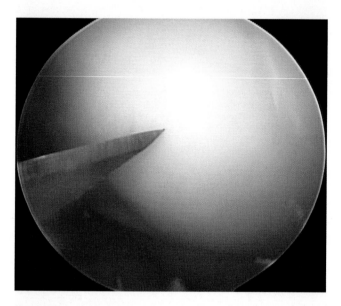

Figure 53-8 An accessory instrumentation portal is established orthogonal to the plane of the lesion.

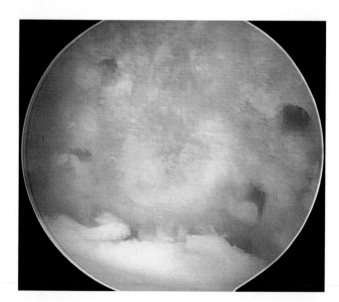

Figure 53-7 Microfracture is performed on the base of the lesion. Appropriate depth of penetration is confirmed by visualization of marrow efflux from perforations.

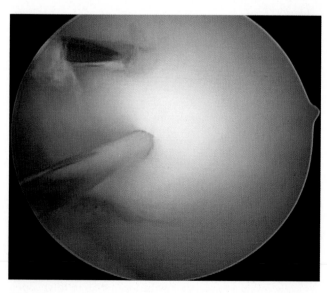

Figure 53-9 Two guide wires are placed to control rotation during fixation with cannulated implants.

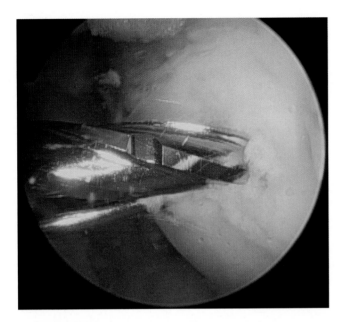

Figure 53-10 A cannulated drill bit is introduced and drilled to the appropriate depth.

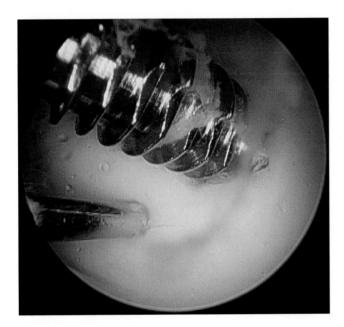

Figure 53-11 Rigid, compressive fixation is obtained with a cannulated, headless, variable-pitch compression screw.

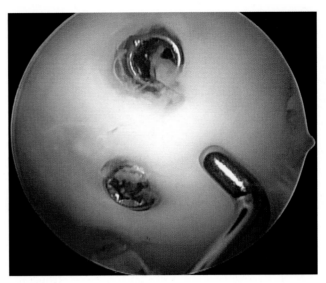

Figure 53-12 After fixation, the lesion is probed for stability.

spacing of implants to avoid crowding and fracture of the osteochondral flap. As these lesions occur in a younger population with excellent bone quality, implants will typically obtain tremendous purchase and can easily generate excessive compression at the lesion site, fracturing the osteochondral flap if overtightening is allowed (Fig. 53-11). Slight overdrilling is necessary at times to avoid overtightening. When cannulated implants are used, it is helpful to remove the guide wire once the screw has been seated two thirds of the way and to finish seating the screw with a noncannulated screwdriver. This avoids difficulty in

removing the guide wire and eliminates the fracture risk to a cannulated screwdriver tip by the torque generated by the compression screw. Implants are countersunk to permit range of motion without risk of injury to the opposing articular surface. After fixation, the lesion is probed for stability and observed through several cycles of flexion-extension for flap motion (Fig. 53-12).

For lesions requiring autogenous bone grafting, adequate cancellous graft can be obtained from Gerdy's tubercle with minimal additional morbidity. If it is available, an 8-mm diameter harvesting trocar for osteochondral autograft transfer can be used to harvest the bone graft in a minimally invasive fashion. A 1-cm vertical incision is made overlying Gerdy's tubercle. A subperiosteal flap is elevated, and the harvesting trocar is introduced with slight distal and medial angulation. Depending on the size of the lesion, one or two plugs will provide sufficient graft. Alternatively, a slightly longer incision can be made over Gerdy's tubercle, a 1-cm cortical window made with an osteotome, and a curet used to remove cancellous autograft. The cortical flap is then replaced, and the incision is irrigated and closed in layers. Cancellous autograft is then tamped into the base of the lesion until a congruent reduction can be obtained. Fixation is applied as described.

6. Implant Removal (for Nonabsorbable Implants, 3 to 4 Months after Fixation)

Use of nonabsorbable fixation typically requires a second procedure for implant removal. Implant removal can almost always be accomplished arthroscopically, regardless of whether initial fixation was obtained by open or arthroscopic technique. A diagnostic arthroscopy is performed to re-evaluate the joint and to assess healing of the lesion by arthroscopic visualization and palpation. Spinal needle localization is used to establish the appropriate vector for implant removal (Fig. 53-13). A noncannulated

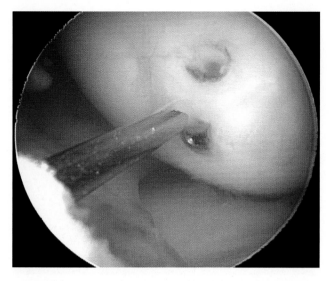

Figure 53-13 The accessory instrumentation portal is re-established at the appropriate angle for removal of implants.

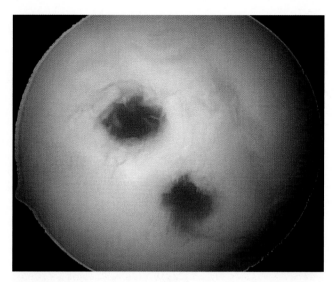

Figure 53-15 Lesion stability is reassessed after removal of fixation.

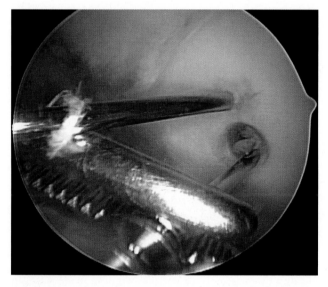

Figure 53-14 The tip of a hemostat is clamped on the guide wire distal to the tip of the screw being removed to prevent loss of the screw in the joint, fat pad, or extra-articular soft tissue.

screwdriver is used to initiate screw removal because a sufficient amount of torque may be applied during this process to fracture the tip of a cannulated screwdriver. Once the screw has been backed out over several turns, a guide wire is threaded down the shaft of the screw and a cannulated screwdriver completes removal. Once the tip of the screw has been disengaged from the articular surface, the guide wire is clamped with a hemostat at a point distal to the tip of the screw to prevent loss of the screw in the joint or extra-articular soft tissue (Fig. 53-14). The lesion should then be probed for stability and the knee brought through a cycle of flexion-extension (Fig. 53-15).

Postoperative Considerations

Follow-up

- At 7 to10 days for suture removal and postoperative non–weight-bearing anteroposterior and lateral radiographs

Radiographs should be repeated at regular 4- to 6-week intervals until healing of the lesion is observed.

Rehabilitation

- Patients treated with nonabsorbable implants are kept non–weight bearing until implant removal.
- Continuous passive motion is prescribed for 4 to 6 weeks, followed by active range of motion.
- Heel slides, quadriceps sets, straight-leg raises, and ankle pumps are initiated immediately postoperatively.
- Repeat films every 4 to 6 weeks until consolidation is evident.

Complications

- Failure of the lesion to heal
- Injury to opposing articular surface by implants used for fixation
- Synovitis from bioabsorbable implants
- Infection

Table 53-1 Clinical Results of Primary Repair of Osteochondritis Dissecans of the Knee

Author	Mean Follow-up	Lesion Location (No. of Knees)	Implant	Outcome
Nakagawa et al[14] (2005)	5 years	MFC (4), LFC (1), T (3)	PLLA (7), bone peg (1)	Healing in 7 of 8 knees
Larsen et al[11] (2005)	2.6 years	MFC (7)	PGA-PLLA copolymer	Healing in 6 of 7 knees
Makino et al[12] (2005)	4.2 years	MFC (14), LFC (1)	Metallic VPCCS	Healing in 14 of 15 knees; 13 of 15 knees "normal" by IKDC score
Dervin et al[9] (1998)	2.75 years	MFC (9)	PLLA	Healing in 8 of 9 knees
Zuniga et al[18] (1993)	1.3 years	MFC (11)	Metallic VPCCS	Healing in 8 of 11 knees
Cugat et al[5] (1993)	3.5 years	MFC (14), T (1)	Metallic CCS	Healing in 15 of 15 knees
Anderson et al[2] (1990)	6 years	MFC (17)	Threaded Kirschner wire	Healing in 16 of 17 knees

CCS, cannulated compression screw; IKDC, International Knee Documentation Committee; LFC, lateral femoral condyle; MFC, medial femoral condyle; PGA, polyglycolic acid; PLLA, poly-L-lactic acid; T, trochlea; VPCCS, variable pitch cannulated compression screw.

53

- Iatrogenic fracture of the osteochondral flap during implant placement
- Implant complications (e.g., fracture of cannulated screwdriver tip during implant removal, shearing off of guide wire during drilling process)

Results

Results after primary repair of appropriately selected osteochondritis dissecans lesions in the knee have typically been reported as excellent, with fragment union reported in 72% to 100% of cases (Table 53-1).[2,5,9,11,12,14,16,18]

PEARLS AND PITFALLS

- Excision of a portion of the anterior fat pad can improve visualization of the lesion and greatly facilitate insertion of cannulated implants during arthroscopic treatment.

- In the arthroscopic treatment of medial femoral condyle lesions, particularly classic lesions that abut the intercondylar notch, it is often easiest to hinge the lesion open along its intercondylar edge.

- The guide wires provided for headless, variable-pitch screw systems are fragile and easily sheared by the accompanying cannulated drill bit. It is imperative that there is no change in hand or knee position during the drilling process to minimize the risk of this complication.

- To facilitate removal of headless, variable-pitch screws, once the screw has been removed from bone over the guide wire, and with the guide wire still in place, the tip of a hemostat is clamped distal to the tip of the screw. The hemostat can then be used both to prevent loss of the screw into the joint space or extra-articular soft tissue and to apply outward pressure to facilitate removal of the screw.

- In removing headless, variable-pitch screws, a noncannulated screwdriver should be used to initiate removal. The torque required to initiate unscrewing of a well-seated screw is sufficient to cause the tip of a cannulated screwdriver to break. Once approximately two thirds of the screw has been unscrewed, a guide wire should be inserted and the cannulated screwdriver used to complete the removal.

- Treatment of osteochondritis dissecans lesions should be thought of as fracture fixation. Compression should be generated along a vector orthogonal to the fracture site to optimize healing.

References

1. Aichroth P. Osteochondritis dissecans of the knee. A clinical survey. J Bone Joint Surg Br 1971;53:440-447.
2. Anderson AF, Lipscomb AB, Coulam C. Antegrade curettement, bone grafting and pinning of osteochondritis dissecans in the skeletally mature knee. Am J Sports Med 1990;18:254-261.
3. Cahill BR, Phillips MR, Navarro R. The results of conservative management of juvenile osteochondritis dissecans using joint scintigraphy. A prospective study. Am J Sports Med 1989;17:601-605; discussion 605-606.
4. Conrad JM, Stanitski CL. Osteochondritis dissecans: Wilson's sign revisited. Am J Sports Med 2003;31:777-778.
5. Cugat R, Garcia M, Cusco X, et al. Osteochondritis dissecans: a historical review and its treatment with cannulated screws. Arthroscopy 1993;9:675-684.
6. De Smet AA, Fisher DR, Graf BK, Lange RH. Osteochondritis dissecans of the knee: value of MR imaging in determining lesion stability and the presence of articular cartilage defects. AJR Am J Roentgenol 1990;155:549-553.
7. De Smet AA, Ilahi OA, Graf BK. Reassessment of the MR criteria for stability of osteochondritis dissecans in the knee and ankle. Skeletal Radiol 1996;25:159-163.
8. De Smet AA, Ilahi OA, Graf BK. Untreated osteochondritis dissecans of the femoral condyles: prediction of patient outcome using radiographic and MR findings. Skeletal Radiol 1997;26:463-467.
9. Dervin GF, Keene GC, Chissell HR. Biodegradable rods in adult osteochondritis dissecans of the knee. Clin Orthop 1998;356:213-221.

10. Friederichs MG, Greis PE, Burks RT. Pitfalls associated with fixation of osteochondritis dissecans fragments using bioabsorbable screws. Arthroscopy 2001;17:542-545.
11. Larsen MW, Pietrzak WS, DeLee JC. Fixation of osteochondritis dissecans lesions using poly(l-lactic acid)/poly(glycolic acid) copolymer bioabsorbable screws. Am J Sports Med 2005;33:68-76.
12. Makino A, Muscolo DL, Puigdevall M, et al. Arthroscopic fixation of osteochondritis dissecans of the knee: clinical, magnetic resonance imaging, and arthroscopic follow-up. Am J Sports Med 2005;33: 1499-1504.
13. Milgram JW. Radiological and pathological manifestations of osteochondritis dissecans of the distal femur. A study of 50 cases. Radiology 1978;126:305-311.
14. Nakagawa T, Kurosawa H, Ikeda H, et al. Internal fixation for osteochondritis dissecans of the knee. Knee Surg Sports Traumatol Arthrosc 2005;13:317-322.
15. Scioscia TN, Giffin JR, Allen CR, Harner CD. Potential complication of bioabsorbable screw fixation for osteochondritis dissecans of the knee. Arthroscopy 2001;17:E7.
16. Thomson NL. Osteochondritis dissecans and osteochondral fragments managed by Herbert compression screw fixation. Clin Orthop 1987;224:71-78.
17. Wilson JN. A diagnostic sign in osteochondritis dissecans of the knee. J Bone Joint Surg Am 1967;49:477-480.
18. Zuniga JJR, Sagastibelza J, Blasco JJL, Grande MM. Arthroscopic use of the Herbert screw in osteochondritis dissecans of the knee. Arthroscopy 1993;9:668-670.

CHAPTER 54

Osteonecrosis of the Knee

Michael B. Boyd, DO
William D. Bugbee, MD

Osteonecrosis of the knee is a difficult clinical entity. Three general categories include idiopathic or spontaneous osteonecrosis (also known as Ahlbäck disease), secondary or atraumatic osteonecrosis, and traumatic osteonecrosis. The diagnosis of osteonecrosis can be arduous. A common error is to misdiagnose degenerative subchondral bone cysts of osteoarthritis as spontaneous osteonecrosis. There are several theories of the etiology of spontaneous osteonecrosis and atraumatic osteonecrosis, but in general, these premises are not well understood. Traumatic osteonecrosis hypothetically occurs after fracture or surgery. This chapter focuses on the unique presentations and various treatment options of spontaneous osteonecrosis and atraumatic osteonecrosis.

Preoperative Considerations

History

A thorough history may simplify the diagnosis of osteonecrosis. Risk factors for atraumatic osteonecrosis include corticosteroid use, alcohol consumption, Gaucher disease, sickle cell disease, caisson disease, coagulopathy, and systemic lupus erythematosus. The typical patient with spontaneous osteonecrosis is an obese woman older than 55 years. Spontaneous osteonecrosis is usually unilateral and typically affects just one condyle. Atraumatic osteonecrosis often presents bilaterally and can affect multiple condyles or plateaus. In addition, it is frequently seen in other joints.

Signs and Symptoms

Spontaneous Osteonecrosis

- Sudden pain usually over the medial aspect of the knee (may be initiated by a minor injury)
- Increased pain at night and with activity

Atraumatic Osteonecrosis

- Long-standing insidious pain (note: some patients may be asymptomatic)
- Pain may be difficult to localize

Physical Examination

Typical Findings

Spontaneous Osteonecrosis

- Range of motion may be decreased secondary to pain, muscle spasm, or subchondral collapse
- High sensitivity to touch over the lesion (usually, the medial femoral condyle)
- Swelling (±), effusion (±)
- Ligaments: stable

Atraumatic Osteonecrosis

- Range of motion may be decreased secondary to pain, muscle spasm, or subchondral collapse
- Nonspecific knee pain (especially with multiple lesions)
- No swelling, no effusion
- Ligaments: stable

Imaging

Radiography

- Weight-bearing anteroposterior radiograph of knee in full extension with a radiopaque magnification marker (Fig. 54-1A)
- Non–weight-bearing 90-degree-flexion lateral view of knee (Fig. 54-1B)
- Notch (Fig. 54-1C) or Rosenberg view of knee

Optional

- Merchant view of patellofemoral joint
- Long-leg anteroposterior mechanical axis view to evaluate for malalignment

Other Modalities

Magnetic resonance imaging can help confirm the diagnosis and the extent of the lesion (Fig. 54-2)

Technetium Tc 99 m bone scan is generally unreliable but may assist in diagnosis when radiographs are

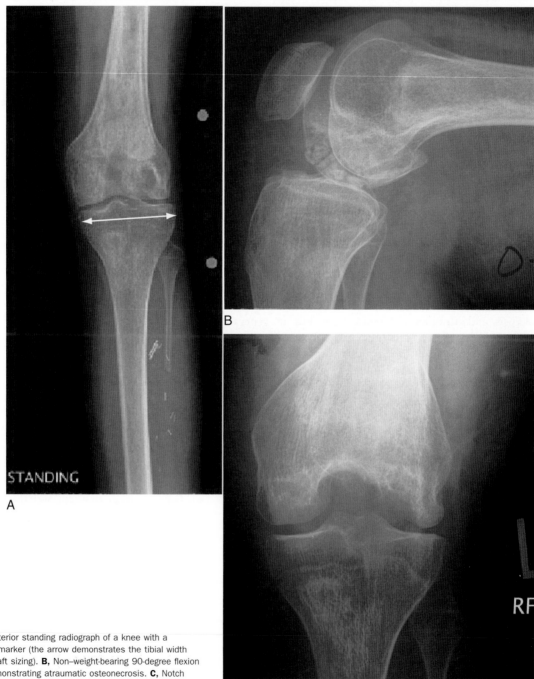

Figure 54-1 A, Anteroposterior standing radiograph of a knee with a radiopaque magnification marker (the arrow demonstrates the tibial width dimension used for allograft sizing). **B,** Non–weight-bearing 90-degree flexion lateral view of a knee demonstrating atraumatic osteonecrosis. **C,** Notch view of a knee depicting atraumatic osteonecrosis.

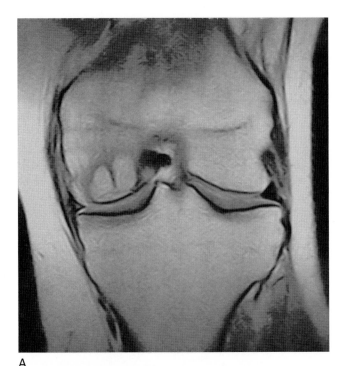

A

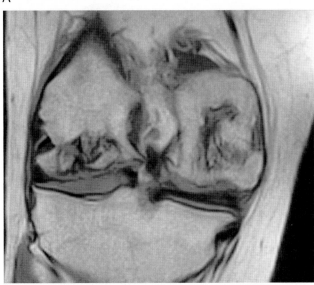

B

Figure 54-2 Magnetic resonance images of a knee exhibiting spontaneous osteonecrosis **(A)** and atraumatic osteonecrosis **(B)**.

Box 54-1 Aglietti Classification for Spontaneous Osteonecrosis (Modified Koshino)

Stage I	Normal radiographs; magnetic resonance imaging abnormalities
Stage II	Some flattening of the weight-bearing portion of the condyle
Stage III	Subchondral radiolucency with surrounding sclerosis without sequestration
Stage IV	↑ Sclerosis with subchondral collapse and sequestration; visible as a calcium plate
Stage V	Secondary degenerative changes (narrowing of joint space, osteophyte formation, subchondral sclerosis) associated with some erosions

Box 54-2 Mont and Hungerford Classification for Atraumatic Osteonecrosis (Modified Ficat-Arlet)

Stage I	Normal radiographs, magnetic resonance imaging abnormalities
Stage II	Cysts and sclerosis present
Stage III	Subchondral collapse is seen as the crescent sign
Stage IV	Secondary degenerative changes (narrowing of joint space, osteophyte formation) on both sides of joint

Staging

The Aglietti classification for spontaneous osteonecrosis (modified Koshino) and the Mont and Hungerford classification for atraumatic osteonecrosis (modified Ficat-Arlet) are described in Boxes 54-1 and 54-2.

Treatment

Nonoperative

- Anti-inflammatory medicines (? benefit)
- Analgesics
- Pharmacologic treatment based on underlying disease process
- Activity modifications, protective weight bearing
- Closed-chain quadriceps exercises
- Unloader knee brace

Operative

- Arthroscopy ± débridement
- Core decompression by extra-articular drilling ± bone grafting

normal. Bipolar uptake is more indicative of osteoarthritis, except in the *late* stages of osteonecrosis. Conversely, simultaneous atraumatic osteonecrosis of the ipsilateral tibial plateau and femoral condyle is certainly possible during *any* stage and usually presents with more intense uptake than with osteoarthritis.

54

- Osteochondral allograft for large lesions versus osteochondral autograft for small lesions
- Realignment procedure: high tibial osteotomy for genu varum versus distal femoral osteotomy for genu valgum
- Unicompartmental knee arthroplasty versus total knee arthroplasty

Because of the heterogeneous nature of osteonecrosis of the knee in both etiology and stage, no single technique is always preferred. Treatment should be individualized. Core decompression and allografting with or without realignment are our preferred treatments for the younger population of patients and are further discussed in this chapter. Our general treatment algorithm is presented in Figure 54-3.

Core Decompression

Brief Description

Extra-articular drilling is recommended in the treatment of symptomatic osteonecrosis of the knee in pre–subchondral collapse stages. Core decompression can be done in conjunction with knee arthroscopy. A small incision is made just proximal to the metaphyseal flare for femoral lesions and adjacent to the tubercle for tibial lesions. With fluoroscopic guidance, a 3- to 6-mm trephine is advanced to within 3 mm of the subchondral bone. The surgeon may elect to lightly pack autologous iliac crest bone graft inside the lesion. Postoperatively, the patient is restricted to 50% partial weight bearing for 4 to 6 weeks.

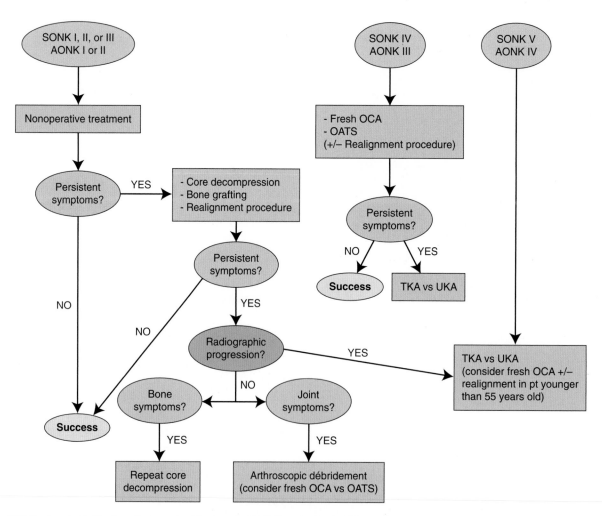

Figure 54-3 Treatment algorithm for osteonecrosis of the knee (modified Mont algorithm). SONK, spontaneous osteonecrosis; AONK, atraumatic osteonecrosis; OATS, osteochondral autograft; OCA, osteochondral allograft; TKA, total knee arthroplasty; UKA, unicompartmental knee arthroplasty.

Fresh Osteochondral Allografting for Osteonecrosis of the Knee

Indications and Contraindications

Fresh osteochondral allografting can be used as a salvage procedure in patients for whom other treatments of osteonecrosis have failed, including nonoperative care, arthroscopy, and core decompression. Allografts are used as an alternative to arthroplasty in the young population. Typically, the lesions should be more than 2 cm (approximately) in diameter. Osteochondral autografting is an excellent alternative for smaller lesions with compromised articular cartilage.

Relative contraindications to fresh osteochondral allografting include uncorrected limb malalignment and joint instability. The senior author has not found steroid dependency to be a contraindication to fresh osteochondral allografts, as previously reported in the literature.[7a] Allografting should not be considered an alternative to total knee arthroplasty or unicompartmental knee arthroplasty in a patient with symptoms, age, and activity level appropriate for prosthetic replacement. Finally, fresh osteochondral allografting should not be performed in the individual with advanced multicompartmental knee arthrosis.

Surgical Planning

Concomitant Procedures

Significant limb malalignment, ligamentous instability, or meniscal disease can be addressed either before or concomitant with fresh osteochondral allograft transplantation. Concomitant distal femoral osteotomy or femoral condyle osteochondral allografting is not recommended and should be staged because of the increased fear of nonunion.

Allograft Sizing

A measurement of the width of the tibia, a few millimeters inferior to the plateau, is made from a standing anteroposterior knee radiograph with a radiopaque magnification marker (see Fig. 54-1A). The measurement is corrected for magnification and sent to the tissue bank for a matched donor.

Surgical Technique: Fresh Osteochondral Allografting

Anesthesia and Positioning

Anesthesia

- General
- Epidural
- Spinal
- Regional (±)

Positioning

- Supine on a standard operating room table
- Padded thigh tourniquet
- Leg holder to position knee between 70 and 100 degrees of flexion for access to the lesion

Surgical Landmarks, Incisions, and Portals

Landmarks

Patella

Patellar tendon

Joint line

Tibial tubercle

Approaches

- Mini medial parapatellar arthrotomy
- Mini lateral parapatellar arthrotomy
- Standard medial parapatellar arthrotomy for bicondylar lesions

Structures at Risk

- Medial parapatellar approach: anterior horn of medial meniscus, patellar tendon
- Lateral parapatellar approach: anterior horn of lateral meniscus, patellar tendon

Examination Under Anesthesia and Diagnostic Arthroscopy

Examine the knee's range of motion and stability under anesthesia. Perform a diagnostic arthroscopy before the allografting procedure if questions about the meniscus or articular cartilage exist.

54

Specific Steps (Box 54-3)

1. Exposure

A standard midline incision is made from approximately the center of the patella to the tip of the tibial tubercle (Fig. 54-4). A medial or lateral parapatellar arthrotomy is then made extending from the superomedial or superolateral aspect of the patella down to the distal end of the incision. The incision can be extended for bicondylar lesions. Care is taken to preserve the anterior horn of the meniscus after incision through the infrapatellar fat pad. For access to deep posterior femoral condyle lesions, the meniscus may need to be taken down, leaving a cuff of tissue for later repair. Retractors are placed medially and laterally to better expose the condyle. One of these retractors is carefully placed in the notch, retracting the patella and protecting the cruciate ligaments. The knee is then flexed to the appropriate level to deliver the lesion to the arthrotomy. If additional mobilization of the patella is necessary, the fat pad can be released further, staying anterior to the anterior horn of the opposite meniscus.

2. Recipient Site Preparation

Two techniques are used for osteochondral allografting, the dowel and the shell techniques. When possible, a dowel or plug (generally 20 mm or larger) is the preferred technique as the instrumentation facilitates the procedure (Fig. 54-5). This is the typical scenario for spontaneous osteonecrosis. Often, however, the disease is too extensive for a dowel or multiple dowels, and a freehand shell technique is performed (typical for atraumatic osteonecrosis lesions).

With the dowel technique, the lesion is inspected and probed to assess its margins. A guide wire is then drilled perpendicular to the curvature of the articular surface into the center of the lesion. The graft is sized with cannulated dowels. A cannulated cutting reamer is used to penetrate the remaining articular cartilage. Next, 3 to 4 mm of subchondral bone is removed with the appropriately sized cannulated bone reamer. If it is indicated, more necrotic bone can be reamed down to bleeding margins, not to exceed 6 to 10 mm. The guide wire is then removed (Fig. 54-6). The depth of the lesion is measured in four

Box 54-3 Surgical Steps

| 1. Exposure |
| 2. Recipient site preparation |
| 3. Fresh osteochondral allograft preparation |
| 4. Graft insertion and fixation |
| 5. Closure |

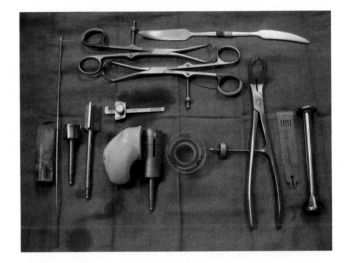

Figure 54-5 Dowel technique instrumentation and fresh hemicondylar femoral allograft.

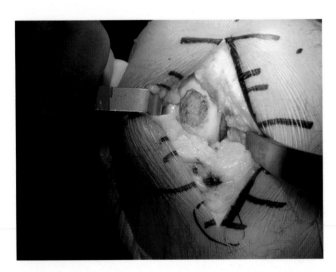

Figure 54-4 Standard midline incision, medial parapatellar approach.

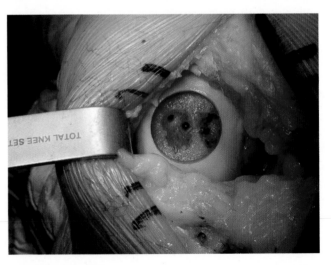

Figure 54-6 Dowel technique—lesion reamed down to bleeding bone.

quadrants (Fig. 54-7). If necessary, multiple small drill holes can be made to decompress the lesion. Curettage and autologous bone grafting (i.e., iliac crest bone graft) can be performed for extensive bone deficiency. At times, a second graft is necessary to cover the entire lesion. In this case, the dowel technique is repeated, overlapping the grafts (Fig. 54-8).

Alternatively, the entire condyle might be involved, rendering it difficult to graft with simple dowels (Fig. 54-9A). In this situation, the recipient site is prepared by a freehand technique with osteotomes and burs. The goal is to produce a simple geometric pattern (Fig. 54-9B). This often incorporates the entire hemicondyle. The dimensions and position of the prepared site are measured and transferred to the allograft.

3. Fresh Osteochondral Allograft Preparation

With the dowel technique, the matching anatomic location on the donor graft is identified. The graft is held securely by an assistant with a large tenaculum bone clamp. A saw guide is placed perpendicular to the articular surface. The appropriately sized tube saw is placed over the guide and used to core the graft (Fig. 54-10). The graft is then amputated from the condyle with a cut at its base by an oscillating saw. The previously measured recipient site depths are marked at the four corresponding quadrants of the graft. The graft is placed in a special bone holder, and the oscillating saw is used to make the final cut at the marks. Fine adjustments can be made with a bone rasp. To reduce its immunogenicity, the graft is then copiously irrigated with bacitracin solution by the jet lavage system to remove any remaining bone marrow elements (Fig. 54-11).

With the shell technique, the cuts are made freehand, forming a geometric match of the recipient site (Fig. 54-12). Repeated trial fittings are performed. The graft is

54

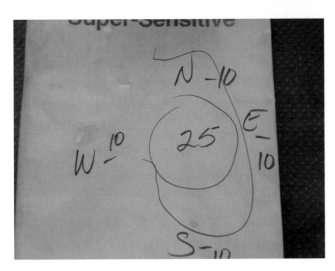

Figure 54-7 Depth measurements of a dowel in four quadrants.

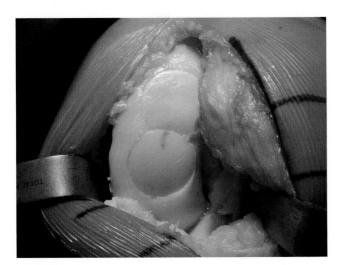

Figure 54-8 Overlapping dowel technique.

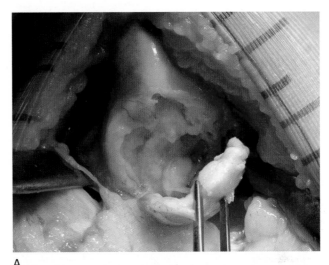

A

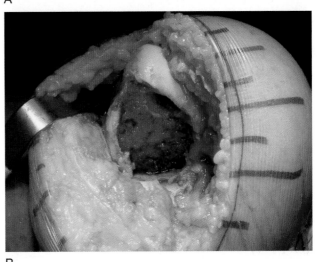

B

Figure 54-9 A, Severe atraumatic osteonecrosis lesion of the lateral femoral hemicondyle requiring a shell technique. **B,** Lesion after débridement into simple geometric configuration.

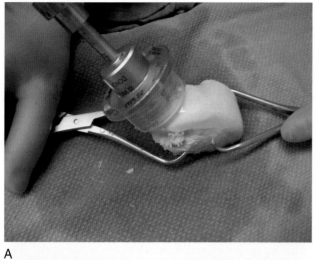

A

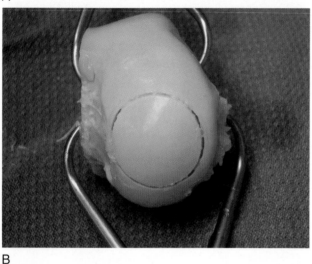

B

Figure 54-10 A, Preparation of dowel allograft with a reamer. **B,** View of dowel allograft before amputation.

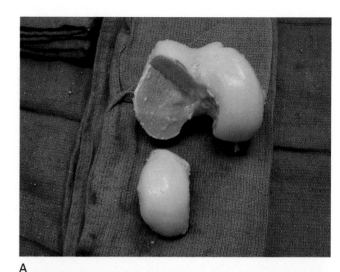

A

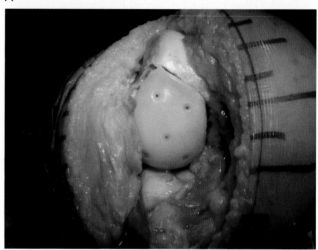

B

Figure 54-12 A, Example of shell allograft. **B,** Shell allograft implanted in lesion seen in Figure 54-9.

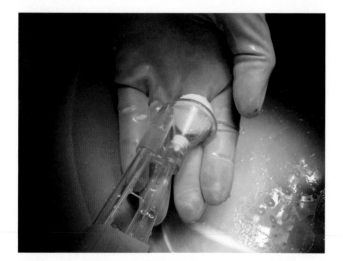

Figure 54-11 The allograft is washed thoroughly with a jet lavage system to remove bone marrow elements.

modified accordingly until the articular geometry is restored.

4. Graft Insertion and Fixation

With the appropriate orientation, the allograft dowel is manually inserted and gently tapped in place until flush. If necessary, the recipient site can be opened up farther with an oversized dilator. Fine adjustments to the allograft are made. An excellent press fit is typically noted (Fig. 54-13); however, the graft can be secured further with bioabsorbable pins. With a shell graft, fixation is obtained with a combination of bioabsorbable pins and small titanium screws. The knee is then put through a range of motion to assess for graft stability and possible impingement, especially at the notch.

5. Closure

Standard layered closure of the arthrotomy is performed over a ⅛-inch drain.

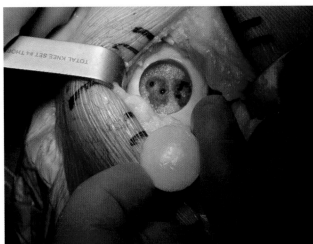

A

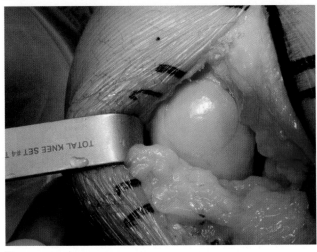

B

Figure 54-13 A, Example of dowel graft adjacent to recipient site. **B,** Excellent press fit of dowel graft.

- With meniscal detachment or repair and large posterior grafts, flexion is limited to 60 degrees for 4 to 6 weeks.
- Progressive weight-bearing begins at 6 to 12 weeks.
- Sports and recreation are resumed at 6 months.

Complications

- Delayed union or nonunion of the allograft
- Infection
- Arthrofibrosis

54

PEARLS AND PITFALLS

General

- Degenerative subchondral bone cysts (usually large, isolated defects about the medial femoral condyle) are commonly misdiagnosed as osteonecrosis but are rather a variant presentation of early osteoarthritis.
- Defining the stage and lesion size (volume and surface area) is key to sound application of our treatment algorithm.
- Subchondral fracture or collapse drastically alters prognosis and limits treatment options.

Surgical

- Concomitant distal femoral osteotomy or femoral condyle osteochondral allografting is not recommended and should be staged because of fear of nonunion.
- For access to deep posterior femoral condyle lesions, the meniscus may need to be taken down, leaving a cuff of tissue for later repair.
- If mobilization of the patella is necessary, the fat pad can be released, staying anterior to the anterior horn of the opposite meniscus.

Postoperative Considerations

Hospital Course

- Hospital admission for 23 to 48 hours
- Intravenous antibiotics for 24 hours
- Drain removed on postoperative day 1

Rehabilitation

- Immediate touch-down weight bearing is permitted with unlimited range of motion and quadriceps strengthening for 6 to 12 weeks.
- Stationary bicycling is started at 4 weeks.

Results

Core decompression can be an effective way to treat osteonecrosis of the knee, especially before the development of subchondral collapse. Recent data have shown a 94% success rate with fresh osteochondral allografting with or without realignment in steroid-induced osteonecrosis of the knee in the young patient. Unicompartmental knee arthroplasty has been shown to be successful for the treatment of end-stage spontaneous osteonecrosis. Total knee arthroplasty is an excellent treatment for all end-stage osteonecroses. The use of cemented stems during total knee arthroplasty improves the long-term results in patients with mutifocal osteonecrosis. Uncemented total knee arthroplasty is no longer recommended in the treatment of osteonecrosis. These results are summarized in Table 54-1.

Table 54-1 Clinical Results of Various Treatment Options of Osteonecrosis

Procedure	Osteonecrosis Type	Author	Mean Follow-up	Miscellaneous Notes	Outcome
High tibial osteotomy	Spontaneous	Koshino[9] (1982)	5.1 years	23 knees with concomitant core decompression or bone grafting	35 of 37 (95%) successful
Unicompartmental knee arthroplasty, total knee arthroplasty	Spontaneous	Aglietti et al[1] (1983)	4.4 years	35 total, 2 unicompartmental; all stages included	35 of 37 (95%) successful
Fresh osteochondral allograft, débridement, high tibial osteotomy, core decompression	Atraumatic, spontaneous, traumatic	Bayne et al[2] (1985)	4.8 years	3 of 3 patients with steroid-induced osteonecrosis treated with only fresh osteochondral allograft failed after 18 months	6 of 13 (46%) spontaneous successful; 4 of 7 (57%) atraumatic successful
Core decompression	Atraumatic	Jacobs et al[8] (1989)	4.5 years	16 of 18 patients with steroid-induced osteonecrotic lesions	7 of 7 (100%) stage I-II successful; 11 of 21 (52%) stage III successful
Total knee arthroplasty	Atraumatic, spontaneous	Bergman and Rand[3] (1991)	4 years	Only a 68% 5-year predicted implant survivorship by revision due to pain as end point	33 of 38 (87%) successful
Unicompartmental knee arthroplasty	Spontaneous	Marmor[10] (1993)	5.5 years	2 of 4 failures due to subsequent osteonecrosis of opposite femoral condyle	30 of 34 (88%) successful
Fresh-frozen osteochondral allograft	Atraumatic, spontaneous, traumatic	Flynn et al[5] (1994)	4.2 years	Young patient group, 2 patients with steroid-induced osteonecrosis converted to total knee arthroplasty	12 of 17 (71%) successful
Nonoperative treatment	Atraumatic	Mont et al[11] (1997)	11 years	Mean asymptomatic period, 11 months; all but 6 required total knee arthroplasty by 6 years	26 of 32 (81%) unsuccessful
Core decompression	Spontaneous	Forst et al[6] (1998)	3 years	No late stages	16 of 16 (100%) successful
Total knee arthroplasty	Atraumatic	Seldes et al[14] (1999)	5.3 years	5 patients required revision (3, aseptic loosening; 2, sepsis)	26 of 31 (84%) successful
Core decompression	Atraumatic	Mont et al[12] (2000)	7 years	No late stages; 15 successful knees needed repeated surgery	72 of 91 (79%) successful
Total knee arthroplasty	Atraumatic, spontaneous	Mont et al[13] (2002)	9 years	Improved results attributed to use of cement in all patients and stems as warranted	31 of 32 (97%) successful
Iliac crest autograft with periosteum	Atraumatic	Fukui et al[7] (2002)	6.6 years	Young patient group with large steroid-induced osteonecrotic lesions	9 of 10 (90%) successful
Fresh osteochondral allograft	Atraumatic	Bugbee et al[4] (2004)	5.3 years	Young patient group with large steroid-induced osteonecrotic lesions	17 of 18 (94%) successful

References

1. Aglietti P, Insall JN, Buzzi R. Idiopathic osteonecrosis of the knee. Aetiology, prognosis and treatment. J Bone Joint Surg Br 1983;65:588-597.
2. Bayne O, Langer F, Pritzker KP, et al. Osteochondral allografts in the treatment of osteonecrosis of the knee. Orthop Clin North Am 1985;16:727-740.
3. Bergman NR, Rand JA. Total knee arthroplasty in osteonecrosis. Clin Orthop 1991;273:77-82.
4. Bugbee WD, Khadivi B, Jamali A. Fresh osteochondral allografting in the treatment of osteonecrosis of the knee [paper No. 108]. American Academy of Orthopaedic Surgeons annual meeting; San Francisco, Calif; 2004.
5. Flynn JM, Springfield DS, Mankin HJ. Osteoarticular allografts to treat distal femoral osteonecrosis. Clin Orthop 1994;303:38-43.
6. Forst J, Forst R, Heller KD, Adam G. Spontaneous osteonecrosis of the femoral condyle: casual treatment by early core decompression. Arch Orthop Trauma Surg 1998;117:18-22.
7. Fukui N, Kurosawa H, Kawakami A, et al. Iliac bone graft for steroid-associated osteonecrosis of the femoral condyle. Clin Orthop 2002;401:185-193.
7a. Gross AF, McKee NH, Pritzker KP, et al. Reconstruction of skeletal deficits of the knee: a comprehensive osteochondral transplant program. Clin Orthop 1983;174:96-106.
8. Jacobs MA, Loeb PE, Hungerford DS. Core decompression of the distal femur for avascular necrosis of the knee. J Bone Joint Surg Br 1989;71:583-587.
9. Koshino T. The treatment of spontaneous osteonecrosis of the knee by high tibial osteotomy with and without bone-grafting or drilling of the lesion. J Bone Joint Surg Am 1982;64:47-58.
10. Marmor L. Unicompartmental arthroplasty for osteonecrosis of the knee joint. Clin Orthop 1993;294:247-253.
11. Mont MA, Tomek IM, Hungerford DS. Core decompression for avascular necrosis of the distal femur—long term followup. Clin Orthop 1997;334:124-130.
12. Mont MA, Baumgarten KM, Rifai A, et al. Atraumatic osteonecrosis of the knee. J Bone Joint Surg Am 2000;82:1279-1290.
13. Mont MA, Rifai A, Baumgarten KM, et al. Total knee arthroplasty for osteonecrosis. J Bone Joint Surg Am 2002;84:599-603.
14. Seldes RM, Tan V, Duffy G, et al. Total knee arthroplasty for steroid-induced osteonecrosis. J Arthroplasty 1999;14:533-537.

54

CHAPTER 55

Osteochondral Autograft for Cartilage Lesions of the Knee

R. David Rabalais, MD

Kenneth G. Swan, Jr., MD

Eric McCarty, MD

Articular cartilage is arguably the most precious body tissue to the orthopedic surgeon and his or her patients. Be it orthopedic trauma or sports medicine, the management goal is often similar: restoration or maintenance of the articular cartilage. Isolated cartilage defects can occur secondary to acute trauma or be atraumatic in nature. The atraumatic defect is often in the form of osteochondritis dissecans, the etiology of which is not fully understood, and can be found in juveniles or adults. The distinction here is important because patients with open physes have a much better prognosis with nonoperative treatment.[5]

Patients with symptomatic focal cartilage defects are candidates for operative treatment to relieve symptoms and also potentially to prevent subsequent arthritic changes.[15] Of the treatment possibilities available, none of which is ideal, osteochondral autograft transplant surgery may be the best option in appropriately selected cases. Several different transplant systems are available, but the concept remains the same: the transplantation of full-thickness osteochondral bone plugs from an area of the knee that is non–weight bearing or with low contact pressures to the osteochondral defect of the ipsilateral knee.

Preoperative Considerations

History

Patients with focal osteochondral lesions typically present with pain and swelling that is intermittent in nature. The history may mimic that of meniscal disease.

Typical History

- Age of the patient may vary from adolescence to middle age
- Intermittent pain
- Pain elicited by low- or high-impact activities (tibiofemoral disease) or stair climbing and prolonged sitting (patellofemoral disease)
- Recurrent swelling
- Frequently a history of acute or distant trauma, including patellar dislocation
- Mechanical symptoms common

Physical Examination

Typical Findings

- Effusion
- Relatively preserved range of motion
- Joint line tenderness (±)
- Patellar instability, apprehension (±)

Factors Affecting Surgical Planning

- Limb malalignment (may compromise repair, require realignment procedure)
- Concomitant ligamentous injury (may require prior or concomitant reconstruction)

Imaging

Radiography

- Standard anteroposterior and lateral knee views
- Sunrise patellofemoral view to visualize patellar and trochlear lesions
- Notch view may be best to visualize lateral aspect of medial femoral condyle (typical location of osteochondritis dissecans)[17]
- Mechanical axis view if malalignment is suspected

Other Modalities

- Magnetic resonance imaging is necessary to best evaluate location and size of articular cartilage lesions. It is also important for evaluation of menisci, ligaments, and the remainder of the articular cartilage.
- Bone scans, computed tomography, and tomography are not as useful as magnetic resonance imaging for evaluation of osteochondritis dissecans lesions and the remainder of the knee.
- Contrast arthrography (intra-articular or intravenous) may prove to be more sensitive than magnetic resonance imaging alone, which can have a high false-negative rate.[23]
- Arthroscopy remains the "gold standard" for evaluation of articular cartilage lesions.

Indications and Contraindications

Indications

The indications for osteochondral autograft transplant surgery are narrow. The patient generally has a small, isolated lesion in an otherwise healthy knee. However, concomitant ligament, meniscus, or alignment disease may be present and can be addressed simultaneously or with a staged procedure.

Typically, during concomitant procedures, the surgeon performs autologous osteochondral grafting and anterior cruciate ligament reconstruction or high tibial osteotomy. During anterior cruciate ligament reconstruction, the osteochondral grafting should proceed after meniscal or cartilage disease is addressed and notchplasty has been performed but before anterior cruciate ligament graft fixation. Similarly, the osteochondral grafting should be done before the high tibial osteotomy is performed. If the procedures are staged, the osteochondral grafting surgery should be done first.

We prefer to use single-plug autograft transplants on defects 1 cm^2 in diameter or smaller; allograft transplants are used for larger defects. However, some authors perform autograft transplantation on defects as large as 4 cm^2, with good results[8] with use of multiple plugs.

Contraindications

- Generalized arthritis
- Inflammatory arthritis
- Lesions >1 cm^2 for single plugs
- Lesion >3 cm^2 for multiple plugs
- Uncorrected malalignment or knee instability

Surgical Planning

Osteochondral defects are frequently diagnosed in the office after the history, physical examination, and interpretation of radiographs and magnetic resonance imaging scans. The patient and surgeon might then plan for single-stage surgery with arthroscopic examination of the knee to assess the defect. If it is applicable, autograft transplantation with single or multiple plugs can be performed. The number and size of osteochondral plugs required cannot be determined until the defect is thoroughly examined by arthroscopy. Defects that are discovered to be excessively large may require allograft transplantation, which must be anticipated and planned for. This is typically performed as a second procedure.

At times, osteochondritis dissecans lesions are not appreciated preoperatively and are discovered during routine knee arthroscopy. The morbidity of the procedure and its rehabilitation process are different from those of a standard knee arthroscopy. These patients usually require a second procedure for definitive treatment at a later date unless the surgeon and patient have discussed this possibility preoperatively.

Surgical Technique

Short Surgical Steps

The short surgical steps for osteochondral autograft transfer are listed in Box 55-1.

Expanded Surgical Technique

Three different systems are commercially available in the United States. All three are similar but differ in the available graft sizes and minor variations of technique. This is shown in Table 55-1. An example of the necessary equipment is shown in Figure 55-1.

Positioning

The patient is placed in the supine position with a lateral post, and a sandbag is taped to the bed to facilitate a fixed

90-degree flexion of the knee. The surgeon should be able to flex the knee to 120 degrees with ease. A sliding footstep may be used to allow different angles of knee flexion. Alternatively, an arthroscopic leg holder may be used per the surgeon's preference. We typically do not drop the foot of the bed. A tourniquet is applied but not elevated, and the operative site is prepared and draped. The tourniquet may be inflated if arthroscopic visualization becomes difficult from intra-articular bleeding.

Arthroscopy

The surgeon performs a diagnostic arthroscopy of the knee. Portal sites can be varied to maximize perpendicular access to the donor and recipient sites. This can be performed with spinal needles before the portals are made. A

central patellar tendon portal can provide good access to the medial surfaces of the medial and lateral femoral condyles.[11] The defect site is identified, and loose debris, cartilage flaps, and superficial fibrocartilage are removed with a mechanized resector. A thorough evaluation of the patellofemoral joint is performed with consideration for donor site grafting ramifications. The knee is carefully inspected for loose bodies, with examination of the lateral and medial gutters and posterior medial and lateral recesses.[20] Examination of the condyles in full flexion is performed to identify any other defects of the weight-bearing surface. The defect is measured by use of measurement probes or size-specific cannulas that vary with the particular system (Fig. 55-2). The surgeon at this time should evaluate the curvature of the surrounding articular cartilage and plan the number and size of grafts to be used. We routinely use an all-arthroscopic technique, but depending on the defect's size and the surgeon's preference, a mini-arthrotomy (1 to 2 cm) may be used for both harvest and implantation. We routinely do not inflate the tourniquet throughout the procedure.

Box 55-1 Surgical Steps

1. Perform diagnostic arthroscopy to débride and to measure the defect; plan number, size, and placement of specific grafts. *The remainder of the procedure can be performed as a mini-open repair, if desired.*

2. Place donor harvester perpendicular to donor site and tamp harvester to required depth. *View measurement on outside of harvester.*

3. Disengage graft from local bed. *Method for disengagement of the graft varies with the system.*

4. Remove graft donor assembly from knee with autograft plug and measure depth of plug.

5. Tamp recipient harvester into defect to desired depth (1 to 2 mm deeper than plug). *Keep recipient harvesting tools perpendicular to articular surface.*

6. Insert graft under direct visualization through optional clear tube. *Be careful to keep tube on articular surface during implantation.*

7. Remove clear tube and gently seat graft with plastic tamp until the graft is flush with the articular surface.

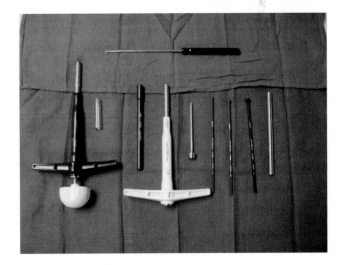

Figure 55-1 Arthrex Osteochondral Autograft Transfer System (OATS).

Table 55-1 Specific Aspects of the Commercially Available Osteochondral Autograft Systems

System	Graft Sizes (Diameter)	Specific Technical Differences	Comments
Single-use OATS (Arthrex, Inc., Naples, Fla)	6-, 8-, and 10-mm plugs	Disengagement of graft from bed requires 90-degree rotation from starting position	Must "lever" graft from donor bed
COR repair system (DePuy-Mitek, Norwood, Mass)	4-, 6-, and 8-mm plugs	Disengagement of donor grafts from bed requires two complete turns with T-handle	"Toothed" harvester allows undercutting of donor graft from donor bed
MosaicPlasty systems (Smith & Nephew, Inc., Andover, Mass)	2.7-, 3.5-, 4.5-, 6.5-, and 8.5-mm plugs	"Toggle" graft to remove from donor bed	Dilator used in recipient site to compact surrounding bone; smaller grafts available

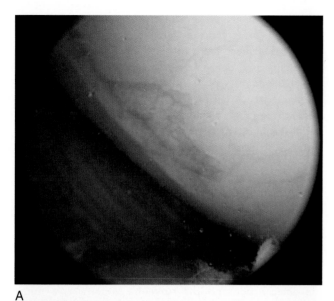

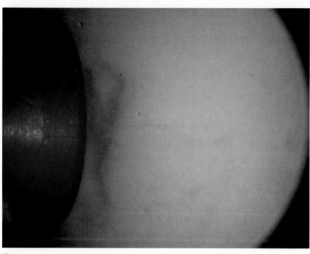

Figure 55-2 A, Femoral condyle defect. **B,** The 8-mm defect sizer.

Graft Harvesting

Available donor sites include the lateral femoral condyle above the sulcus terminalis, the peripheral aspect of the medial femoral condyle, and the lateral superior aspect of the intercondylar notch. The medial aspect of the medial femoral condyle can be easier to access during graft harvest because the intra-articular distention can push the patella laterally.[11] Contact pressures may be lower in donor sites from the distal medial trochlea.[1,7] The central condylar notch is routinely removed during notchplasty (roofplasty) in anterior cruciate ligament reconstruction, but the curvature is generally concave and has poorer congruity with typical recipient sites on the lateral and medial femoral condyles.[3] We routinely use the superior medial aspect of the medial femoral condyle as a donor site. The largest size amenable to single-plug harvest is 1 cm^2 in diameter, as discussed before. Multiple plugs should be harvested for defects between 1 and 3 cm^2 in diameter.

Each system has a T-handle instrument that must be assembled at the back table and varies with the graft diameter that is to be used. This donor harvester is then inserted into the knee perpendicular to the articular surface and held firmly against the cartilage during the extraction. Holding the donor harvester firmly against the surface ensures that a cylindrical (not "crooked") graft is harvested and helps prevent loss of the graft in the joint during extraction. The donor harvester is impacted with a mallet to the desired depth of penetration, usually 15 mm. The different systems then recommend different techniques to extract the graft from the surrounding bed. The Osteochondral Autograft Transfer System (OATS) employs a 90-degree rotation both clockwise and counterclockwise from the starting position. The COR system has a "tooth" at the distal aspect of the harvester; when the desired depth is achieved, the T-handle is rotated two full revolutions to undercut the graft, minimizing leverage against the native bone. The MosaicPlasty system recommends "gentle toggling" to break the deep subchondral bone before graft removal (Fig. 55-3).

Measure the graft length after removal to plan defect drilling. This is performed either through reference lines on the exterior of a clear sheath holding the graft or by placing the graft on the back table in a moist sponge, depending on the system used. Reinsertion of the plunger into the donor site defect can also assist with measurement of the depth (Fig. 55-4).

Recipient Site Preparation

At this point, the surgeon should have a clear plan for number of grafts, placement of specific graft plugs, and depth of each plug. The knee can now be further flexed if needed to ensure perpendicular drilling of the defect. The diameter of the reamer used should correspond to the diameter of the graft taken. The appropriately sized reamer can now be used to drill the recipient hole. Each recipient hole should be separated from adjacent holes with at least a 1- to 2-mm bridge. The depth of each recipient hole should be 1 to 2 mm deeper than the measured plug. This reduces resultant force during impaction[24] and can minimize intraosseous pressure. The MosaicPlasty system recommends dilation of the recipient hole before insertion. All loose cartilage and bone fragments can be safely removed with a small curet (Fig. 55-5).

Graft Implantation

At this time, the graft should be in the delivery tube. The delivery tube is seated perpendicular to the reamed hole of matching size and held firmly against the surface. Graft implantation is achieved by gentle tapping of the impactor (plunger) with a mallet. The use of excessive force and large blows should be avoided.[24] Once the graft is almost fully seated and stable in the hole, the delivery tube is removed (Fig. 55-6). Care should be taken not to shear off the cartilage cap of the graft when the insertion tube is

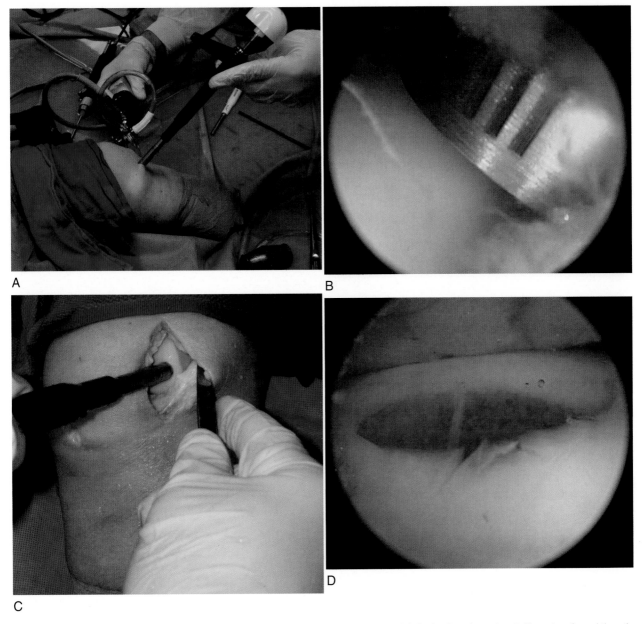

A

B

C

D

Figure 55-3 A and **B,** Arthroscopic graft harvest from the medial aspect of the medial femoral condyle by the donor harvester. **C,** Harvest performed through a mini-arthrotomy. **D,** Donor site after harvest as seen arthroscopically.

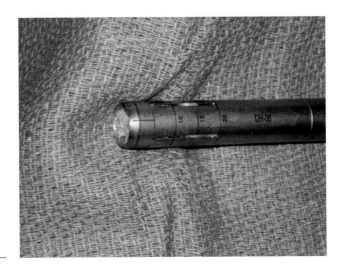

Figure 55-4 The 8 × 15-mm osteochondral plug within the 8-mm harvester.

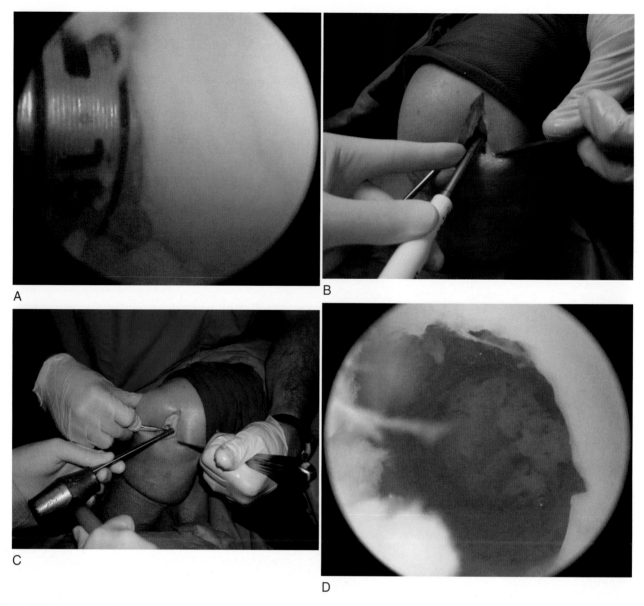

Figure 55-5 The osteochondral recipient site is prepared to appropriate depth by use of the recipient harvester through an arthroscopic **(A)** or mini-open **(B)** technique. **C,** A graduated alignment rod refines the depth and angle of the recipient site, in this case through an open technique. **D,** Recipient site as seen arthroscopically.

removed.[20] Gentle impaction with a plastic rod or impactor is performed until the surface of the graft is flush with the level of surrounding articular cartilage. The graft should not be left proud. This can result in increased contact pressures[25] or increased gap formation at the graft-tunnel junction with perigraft fissuring, fibroplasia, and subchondral cavitations.[19] If the graft is accidentally impacted deeper than the surrounding surface, the surgeon may drill an adjacent small recipient hole and elevate the graft with an arthroscopic probe to the desired level.[11]

Large Defects

Several pitfalls are encountered in addressing large defects. First, achieving good surface congruity is more difficult.

The surgeon should ream recipient sites perpendicular to the surface in the central areas while increasing obliquity 10 to 15 degrees inward toward the periphery.[20] In addition, care must also be taken not to violate adjacent recipient holes during reaming. The sequence of graft harvest, reaming, and implantation should be performed for each individual hole in a step-by-step manner until the defect is covered.[11] The spacing of 1 to 2 mm between grafts in the recipient site should be similar to the spacing of grafts in smaller defects. The surgeon should not obtain all grafts and then ream all recipient holes.

Wound Closure

The knee is cleared of all debris and irrigated. Standard wound closure is performed over suction drains.

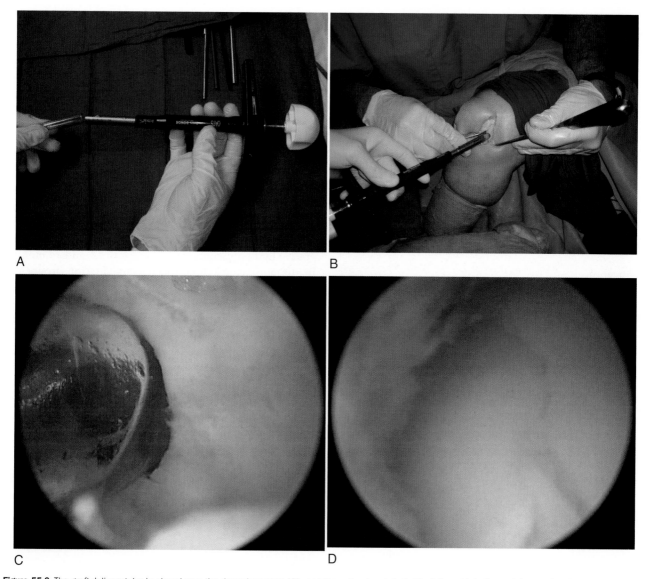

A

B

C

D

Figure 55-6 The graft-delivery tube is placed over the donor harvester **(A)**, and the osteochondral plug is delivered into the recipient socket through a mini-arthrotomy **(B)** or arthroscopic **(C)** technique. The osteochondral plug is made flush with the native chondral surface **(D)**.

PEARLS AND PITFALLS

Pearls

- Full-length alignment films should be considered in all patients.

- Guide pin insertion at the recipient site must be in a perpendicular fashion and in the center of the lesion. The donor graft must be harvested in the same perpendicular plane.

- The recipient bed should be drilled with a small 1.6-mm drill bit to enhance the vascular healing response.

- Bone edges of the donor plug should be rounded ("bulletized") with a rongeur to aid insertion.

- The donor site may be left as is or "backfilled" with one of several marketed biosynthetic scaffold materials. Alternatively, the recipient defect may be plugged back into the donor site and then fixed into place

- The surgeon may choose for the patient to avoid nonsteroidal anti-inflammatory drugs so as not to diminish the healing response.

Pitfalls

- Malalignment must be corrected before or during the OATS procedure; otherwise, the OATS outcome will be suboptimal.

- Mismatch positioning between recipient and donor will risk early failure of the graft.

- Plan minimal drilling to avoid fracture of subchondral bone.

- Noncontoured plug may be difficult to insert and require excessive force on chondrocytes during impaction.

- Backfilling of the donor defect can potentially result in a source of additional symptoms or a loose body if it is not done appropriately.

Postoperative Considerations

- The patient is observed in postoperative recovery.
- Drains are removed before discharge.
- The operative dressing is changed at 48 hours.
- Perioperative antibiotics are instituted at the surgeon's preference.
- Continuous passive motion is begun on the first postoperative day.

Complications

- Infection
- Hematoma formation
- Poor motion
- Thromboembolic events
- Reflex sympathetic dystrophy
- Loose body formation
- Dislodgement or loosening of the graft
- Donor site morbidity
- Progression of osteoarthritis
- Continued symptoms from the affected region

Rehabilitation

- Non–weight bearing is maintained for 6 weeks.
- Toe-touch weight bearing is continued until 8 to 12 weeks to ensure full graft maturation.
- Continuous passive motion is prescribed for 4 to 6 weeks, 4 hours per day.
- Active and passive range of motion is instituted as the patient can tolerate motion.
- High-impact activities are avoided until 16 to 20 weeks.

Results

The results in the literature are generally good for patients with small defects. The results in the literature are difficult to interpret because of differences in operative technique, defect size, and donor site location. In addition, the majority of published reports are less than optimal in that they are of level IV evidence. Results are summarized in Table 55-2. Three of the more significant studies are described here.

Hangody and Fules[10] reported the most extensive experience in the literature, with 831 patients with autologous osteochondral transplantation (mosaicplasty) at 10 years, with 92% good to excellent results for femoral condyle implantations. The results significantly decreased for tibial plateau defects (87%) and patella-trochlea defects (79%); donor site disturbances were identified in 3% of the patients.

Horas et al[12] reported a prospective, randomized study comparing 40 patients who underwent either autologous chondrocyte implantation (20) or OATS (20) for lesions 3.2 to 5.6 cm^2 at 2 years of follow-up. The postoperative Lysholm scores were lower at 6, 12, and 24 months in the autologous chondrocyte–implantation group; the Meyers and Tegner scoring systems were equal in the two groups at 24 months.

Gudas et al[8] published a prospective randomized study comparing arthroscopic mosaic osteochondral autologous transplantation (28) with microfracture (29) in 57 femoral condyle lesions smaller than 4 cm^2 at 37.1 months. The authors reported 96% good to excellent results in the osteochondral autologous transplantation group compared with 52% for the microfracture group with the Hospital for Special Surgery and International Cartilage Repair Society scoring systems.

Conclusion

There are several options for the orthopedic surgeon in addressing the patient with a focal cartilage defect of the knee. Osteochondral autografting with either single or multiple plugs provides the surgeon with a viable solution to the defect smaller than 3 cm^2. Single plugs are appropriate for defects smaller than 1 cm^2, whereas multiple plugs are appropriate for defects smaller than 3 cm^2. This technique can be used in combination with other knee procedures, such as anterior cruciate ligament reconstruction and high tibial osteotomy. The procedure is straightforward and supported by the published literature to be as good as if not superior to other techniques, such as microfracture and autologous chondrocyte implantation, for defects in this size range. Further research must be explored to better define its place in cartilage restoration surgery. We recommend that the articular cartilage surgeon become familiar with all available techniques to provide the best care to the patient.

Table 55-2 Brief Overview of Results of OATS in the Literature

Author	Number	Follow-up	Results	Scoring System	Type of Study	Level of Evidence
Hangody and Fules[10] (2003)	831	10 years	92% good–excellent (femoral condyles)	Bandi	Case series Mosaicplasty	IV
Horas et al[12] (2003)	40 (20 OATS vs. 20 ACI)	24 months	Lysholm lower at 6, 12, 24 months for ACI Tegner equal at 24 months	Lysholm Tegner	Prospective, randomized OATS (multiple plugs) vs. ACI	II
Gudas et al[8] (2005)	57 (28 OATS vs. 29 microfracture)	37.1 months	96% good–excellent with OATS 52% good–excellent with microfracture	HSS ICRS	Prospective, randomized OATS (multiple plugs) vs. microfracture	II
Chow et al[6] (2004)	30	45.1 months	83% good–excellent, Lysholm 87% "normal knee," IKDC	Lysholm IKDC	Case series Multiple plugs	IV
Koualis et al[13] (2004)	18	27.2 months	12 "normal" 6 "near normal"	ICRS	Case series Mosaicplasty	IV
Andres et al[2] (2003)	19 (22 knees)	24 months	88% of mosaicplasty with osteoarthritis "improved"	WOMAC SF-36 VAS	Comparative case series Mosaicplasty in osteoarthritis	III
Outerbridge et al[18] (2000)	16 (18 knees)	7.6 years	83% good	Cincinnati	Case series with patella donor graft, single graft	IV
Laprell and Petersen[14] (2001)	29	8.1 years	26/29 "normal" or "nearly normal"	ICRS	Case series (one or two plugs)	IV
Ma et al[16] (2004)	18	42 months	89% good–excellent	Lysholm Tegner	Case series (multiple plugs)	IV
Bobic[4] (1996)	10	2 years	"Promising results"		Case series OATS (multiple plugs) + ACL reconstruction	IV
Sharpe et al[22] (2005)	13	3 years	10/13 with "significant improvement"	KSS	Case series OATS (multiple plugs) + ACL	IV
Sanders et al[21] (2001)	21	22 months	Maximum signal intensity of grafts at 4-6 weeks		Case series of magnetic resonance imaging results, multiple plugs	IV

ACI, autologous chondrocyte implantation; ACL, anterior cruciate ligament; HSS, Hospital for Special Surgery; ICRS, International Cartilage Repair Society; IKDC, International Knee Documentation Committee; KSS, Knee Society Score; SF-36, short form 36 health survey; VAS, visual analogue scale; WOMAC, Western Ontario and McMaster Universities Osteoarthritis Index.

References

1. Ahmad CS, Cohen ZA, Levine WN, et al. Biomechanical and topographic considerations for autologous osteochondral grafting in the knee. Am J Sports Med 2001;29:201-206.
2. Andres BM, Mears SC, Somel DS, et al. Treatment of osteoarthritic cartilage lesions with osteochondral autograft transplantation. Orthopedics 2003;26:1121-1126.
3. Bartz RL, Kamaric E, Noble PC, et al. Topographic matching of selected donor and recipient sites for osteochondral autografting of the articular surface of the femoral condyles. Am J Sports Med 2001;29:207-212.
4. Bobic V. Arthroscopic osteochondral autograft transplantation in anterior cruciate ligament reconstruction: a preliminary

55

clinical study. Knee Surg Sports Traumatol Arthrosc 1996;3: 262-264.

5. Cahill BR. Osteochondritis dissecans of the knee: treatment of juvenile and adult forms. J Am Acad Orthop Surg 1995;3:237-247.

6. Chow JC, Hantes ME, Houle JB, Zalavras CG. Arthroscopic autogenous osteochondral transplantation for treating knee cartilage defects: a 2- to 5-year follow-up study. Arthroscopy 2004;20: 681-690.

7. Garretson RB 3rd, Katolik LI, Verma N, et al. Contact pressure at osteochondral donor sites in the patellofemoral joint. Am J Sports Med 2004;32:967-974.

8. Gudas R, Kalesinskas RJ, Kimtys V, et al. A prospective randomized clinical study of mosaic osteochondral autologous transplantation versus microfracture for the treatment of osteochondral defects in the knee joint in young athletes. Arthroscopy 2005;21:1066-1075.

9. Hangody L. The mosaicplasty technique for osteochondral lesions of the talus. Foot Ankle Clin 2003;8:259-273.

10. Hangody L, Fules P. Autologous osteochondral mosaicplasty for the treatment of full-thickness defects of weight-bearing joints: ten years of experimental and clinical experience. J Bone Joint Surg Am 2003;85(suppl 2):25-32.

11. Hangody L, Rathonyi GK, Duska Z, et al. Autologous osteochondral mosaicplasty. Surgical technique. J Bone Joint Surg Am 2004;86(suppl 1):65-72.

12. Horas U, Pelinkovic D, Herr G, et al. Autologous chondrocyte implantation and osteochondral cylinder transplantation in cartilage repair of the knee joint. A prospective, comparative trial. J Bone Joint Surg Am 2003;85:185-192.

13. Koulalis D, Schultz W, Heyden M, Konig F. Autologous osteochondral grafts in the treatment of cartilage defects of the knee joint. Knee Surg Sports Traumatol Arthrosc 2004;12:329-334.

14. Laprell H, Petersen W. Autologous osteochondral transplantation using the diamond bone-cutting system (DBCS): 6-12 years' follow-up of 35 patients with osteochondral defects at the knee joint. Arch Orthop Trauma Surg 2001;121:248-253.

15. Linden B. Osteochondritis dissecans of the femoral condyle: a long term follow-up study. J Bone Joint Surg Am 1977;59:769-776.

16. Ma HL, Hung SC, Wang ST, et al. Osteochondral autografts transfer for post-traumatic osteochondral defect of the knee—2 to 5 years follow-up. Injury 2004;35:1286-1292.

17. Milgram JW. Radiological and pathological manifestations of osteochondritis dissecans of the distal femur. A study of 50 cases. Radiology 1978;126:305-311.

18. Outerbridge HK, Outerbridge RE, Smith DE. Osteochondral defects in the knee. A treatment using lateral patella autografts. Clin Orthop 2000;377:145-151.

19. Pearce SG, Hurtig MB, Clarnette R, et al. An investigation of 2 techniques for optimizing joint surface congruency using multiple cylindrical osteochondral autografts. Arthroscopy 2001;17:50-55.

20. Poelstra KA, Neff ES, Miller MD. Osteochondral autologous plug transfer in the knee. In Miller MD. Textbook of Arthroscopy. Philadelphia, WB Saunders, 2004.

21. Sanders TG, Mentzer KD, Miller MD, et al. Autogenous osteochondral "plug" transfer for the treatment of focal chondral defects: postoperative MR appearance with clinical correlation. Skeletal Radiol 2001;30:570-578.

22. Sharpe JR, Ahmed SU, Fleetcroft JP, Martin R. The treatment of osteochondral lesions using a combination of autologous chondrocyte implantation and autograft: three-year follow-up. J Bone Joint Surg Br 2005;87:730-735.

23. Stanitski CL. Correlation of arthroscopic and clinical examinations with magnetic resonance imaging findings of injured knees in children and adolescents. Am J Sports Med 1998;26:2-6.

24. Whiteside RA, Jakob RP, Wyss UP, Mainil-Varlet P. Impact loading of articular cartilage during transplantation of osteochondral autograft. J Bone Joint Surg Br 2005;87:1285-1291.

25. Wu JZ, Herzog W, Hasler EM. Inadequate placement of osteochondral plugs may induce abnormal stress-strain distributions in articular cartilage—finite element simulations. Med Eng Phys 2002; 24:85-97.

CHAPTER 56

Osteochondral Allografting in the Knee

Richard W. Kang, MS, MD

Andreas H. Gomoll, MD

Brian J. Cole, MD, MBA

Osteochondral allografting in the knee has been used for more than 20 years to reconstruct osteochondral defects resulting from trauma, malignant disease, and developmental disorders. In current practice, osteochondral allografts are most commonly used for the treatment of symptomatic osteochondritis dissecans and other chondral lesions that have failed primary treatment, such as internal fixation of osteochondritis dissecans fragments, marrow stimulation, mosaicplasty, and autologous chondrocyte implantation. Increasingly, allografts are now also being used as the primary treatment in situations in which other restorative procedures have demonstrated limited success, such as in the very large or uncontained defect and in the older population of patients. Initially limited by the low number of available grafts, fresh allograft tissue is becoming increasingly available as a result of improved harvesting and storage protocols, but the supply is still outpaced by a rapidly increasing demand.

Preoperative Considerations

History

Osteochondral allografting is indicated in two distinctive populations: those with a history of osteochondritis dissecans and those with chondral defects of other, often traumatic causes. Patients with osteochondritis dissecans often report a history of failure of other treatment modalities, such as immobilization, open reduction and fixation of the fragment, and simple excision. The onset of symptoms is mostly insidious, with no distinctive trauma. Con-

versely, chondral defects often result from athletic injuries that lead to tears of the anterior cruciate ligament or the meniscus, which in turn result in acute or secondary damage to the articular surface.

Typical History

- Prior knee injury or surgery
- Activity-related knee pain and swelling
- Mechanical symptoms, such as locking, catching, and giving way

Physical Examination

- Variable amounts of effusion
- Varus alignment in large medial femoral condyle lesions
- Pain to deep palpation of the affected compartment
- Usually intact range of motion, but can be limited in the presence of loose bodies
- Quadriceps atrophy correlates with duration of symptoms
- Catching or crepitation in the involved compartment

Imaging

Radiography (Fig. 56-1)

- Standing anteroposterior view with knee in full extension

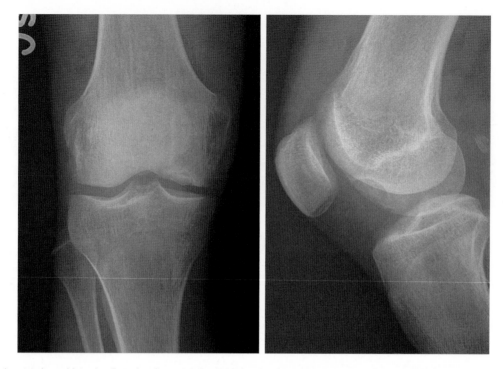

Figure 56-1 Anterior-posterior and lateral radiographs of an osteochondral (osteochondritis dissecans) lesion of the femoral condyle.

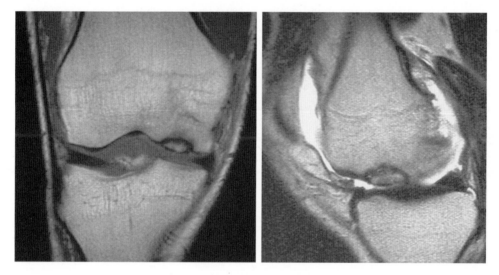

Figure 56-2 Coronal and sagittal magnetic resonance images show osteochondritis dissecans lesion.

- Standing posteroanterior view with knee in 30 to 60 degrees of flexion (notch or tunnel view)
- Lateral view
- Patellar sunrise view
- Bilateral long-leg alignment views

Magnetic Resonance Imaging

Magnetic resonance imaging is the "gold standard" for osteochondral lesions (Fig. 56-2). Fluid or edema behind the lesion is suggestive of an unstable fragment.

Evaluate the extent and depth of osseous involvement. Beware of high sensitivity for subchondral edema, which leads to false positives for osseous disease.

Indications and Contraindications

The typical candidate for osteochondral allografting presents with a large full-thickness chondral defect; prior procedures, such as the repair of an unstable osteochondritis dissecans lesion, microfracture, osteochondral autograft transfer, and autologous chondrocyte implantation, have failed. Some lesions preclude the use of other cartilage repair procedures because of their large size, specific location, or associated deep osseous defects. Localized unipolar lesions larger than 2 to 3 cm^2 provide an optimal environment for osteochondral grafting.

Comorbidities that must be addressed either before or at the time of the osteochondral allografting procedure include malalignment, ligament deficiency, and meniscal insufficiency. Bipolar lesions present a relative contraindication and result in less predictable outcomes. Both lesions should be treated concomitantly; the larger and deeper defect is commonly allografted, and the kissing lesion is often amenable to microfracture.

Surgical Technique

Anesthesia and Positioning

On the basis of the preferences of the surgeon, anesthesiologist, and patient, the procedure can be performed under general, spinal, or regional anesthesia or a combination thereof. Before induction of anesthesia, the surgeon must ensure that the fresh graft is size and side matched and of sufficient quality. The patient is positioned supine on a standard operating table with a thigh tourniquet. Especially in posterior lesions of the femoral condyle, a leg positioning device is helpful to stabilize the knee in hyperflexion.

Surgical Landmarks, Incisions, and Portals

Landmarks

- Patella
- Patellar tendon
- Tibial tubercle

Incisions

- Anterior midline or paramedian skin incision
- Medial or lateral peripatellar arthrotomy, subvastus or midvastus approach

Structures at Risk

- Infrapatellar branch of the saphenous nerve
- Articular surfaces (at risk during arthrotomy)
- Patellar tendon (risk of avulsion with vigorous retraction)
- Menisci

Examination Under Anesthesia and Diagnostic Arthroscopy

Examination under anesthesia should reveal stable ligaments and full range of motion. Although it is not mandatory, diagnostic arthroscopy as an initial staging procedure is helpful to better assess the extent of the chondral lesion as well as to rule out associated pathologic change, such as ligamentous or meniscal insufficiency.

Specific Steps (Box 56-1)

1. Exposure (Fig. 54-3)

Osteochondral allografting is an open procedure requiring the use of an arthrotomy sized to be consistent with the location and extent of the lesion. Most commonly, an anterior midline incision is made from the proximal pole of the patella to the tibial tubercle, but medial or lateral paramedian incisions can be used as well. The incision is carried down to the capsule; then full-thickness skin flaps are raised to make a mobile window. A medial or lateral peripatellar capsulotomy is performed from the superior pole of the patella to the tibial tubercle. More limited incisions, such as the subvastus and midvastus approaches, have recently gained popularity, and we think that these approaches allow accelerated postoperative quadriceps rehabilitation. The patella is retracted with either a Z or bent Hohman retractor placed into the notch. We have found it helpful to release the fat pad and to dissect the anterior meniscal horn from the capsule for better exposure, especially with small incisions.

The most commonly used technique is the press-fit plug technique; several proprietary systems have been developed to facilitate graft sizing and preparation (Fig. 56-4). For comprehensiveness, we also discuss the shell graft technique, which is technically more challenging but allows the treatment of very large and irregularly shaped defects not amenable to the plug technique.

Box 56-1 Surgical Steps

1. Exposure
Press-fit plug technique
2a. Defect preparation
2b. Allograft preparation
2c. Graft insertion and fixation
Shell technique
2a. Defect preparation
2b. Allograft preparation
2c. Graft insertion and fixation
3. Closure

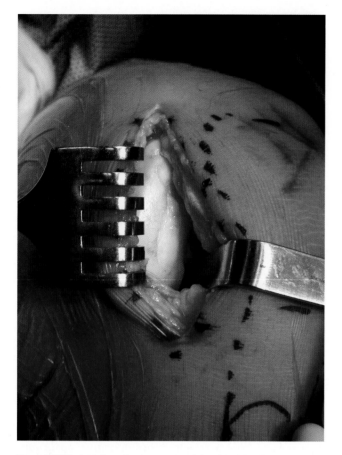

Figure 56-3 Peripatellar arthrotomy to reveal the chondral defect.

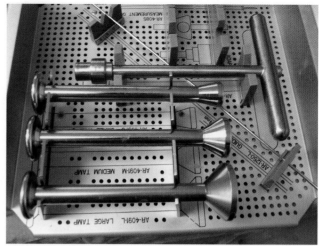

A

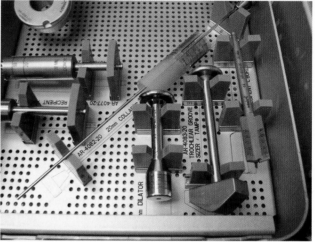

B

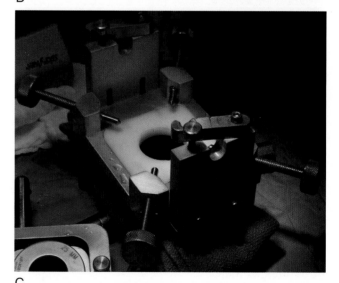

C

Figure 56-4 Osteochondral allograft OATS system (Arthrex, Inc., Naples, Fla). **A,** Tamps and measurement guides. **B,** Harvesters and dilator. **C,** Instrumentation workstation.

Press-Fit Plug Technique

2a. Preparation of the Recipient Site

Once the lesion is exposed, the abnormal cartilage is identified. It is of utmost importance to reconstruct the normal geometry of the articular surface with the donor graft.

The axis of the recipient hole is matched with the axis of the donor plug:

1. Place a cylindrical sizing guide over the defect to determine the optimal plug diameter (Fig. 56-5).
2. A circumferential mark is made around the guide, followed by a mark at the 12-o'clock position of the recipient cartilage.
3. A guide pin is placed into the defect to a depth of 2 to 3 cm.
4. A counterbore reamer is used to make a recipient socket with a depth of 6 to 8 mm (Fig. 56-6).
5. The depth of the cylindrical defect is measured in all four quadrants.

2b. Preparation of the Donor Graft

1. Identify and outline the appropriate donor site.
2. Secure the donor condyle in the allograft workstation.

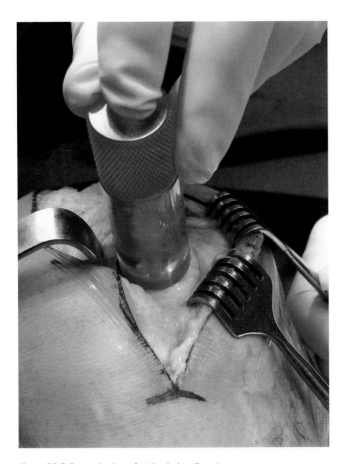

Figure 56-5 Determination of optimal plug diameter.

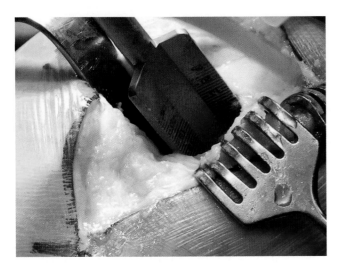

Figure 56-6 Counterbore used to drill to 6 to 8 mm or until bleeding bone is established.

3. The bushing with the appropriate graft size diameter is placed in the workstation over the marked allograft and set to the appropriate angle to match the contour of the recipient site (Fig. 56-7).

4. A donor harvester is passed through the proximal graft housing and used to drill through the entire depth of the donor condyle.

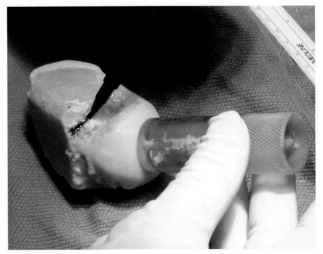

A

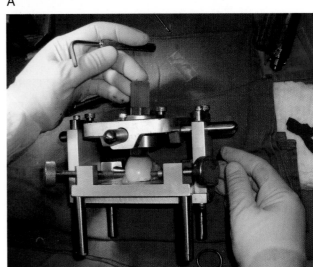

B

Figure 56-7 A and **B,** Matching the size and surface contour of the donor condyle with the recipient condyle.

5. After extraction of the graft from the donor harvester, the depth measurement guide is used to mark out the four quadrants of the graft to match the depths recorded from the recipient site (Fig. 56-8). The graft is also marked at the 12-o'clock position to match the one made at the recipient site.

6. The allograft is held with the allograft forceps and trimmed down with a saw.

2c. Graft Insertion and Fixation

1. An additional 0.5 mm of dilation is achieved by inserting a calibrated dilator into the recipient site.

2. The graft's corners may be beveled to assist insertion. It is generally preferable to trim the graft slightly and to use supplemental fixation, rather than to use excessive force to press fit the graft, which will lead to chondrocyte injury and death.

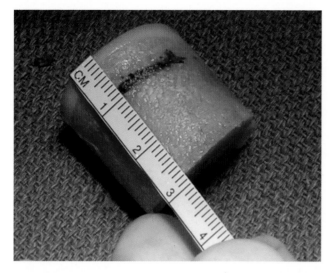

Figure 56-8 After removal of the plug, depth measurement markings are made on the graft to match the measurements taken from the recipient site.

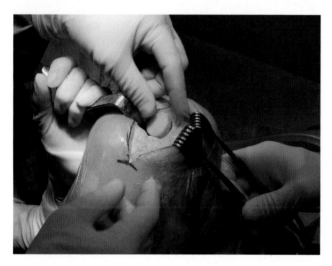

Figure 56-9 Press fitting of the graft by hand.

3. The graft is press fitted into the recipient defect while matching the markings made on both the graft and recipient site (Fig. 56-9)

4. An oversized tamp is then used to make the graft surface flush with the surrounding native cartilage. It is preferable to recess the graft rather than leaving it proud (Fig. 56-10).

5. If fixation is deemed necessary, absorbable polydioxanone pins may be used.

Shell Allograft Technique

2a. Preparation of the Recipient Site

1. The lesion is outlined with a surgical pen.

2. A No. 15 blade is then used to cut the borders of the lesion.

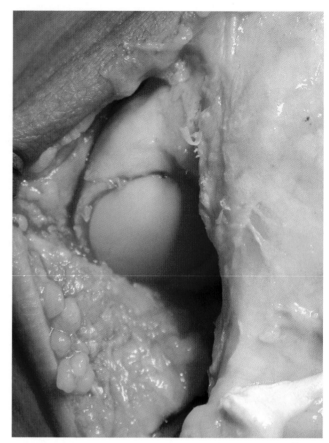

Figure 56-10 Graft is flush with recipient articular surface.

3. A 4-mm bur and sharp curets are used to débride the defect down to a depth of 4 to 5 mm.

2b. Preparation of the Allograft

1. The matched allograft is marked with a surgical pen to match the shape of the recipient site. The markings made on the allograft may be slightly larger than the ones made on the recipient site to facilitate multiple trial fittings.

2. A shell graft is cut out with 4 to 5 mm of subchondral bone.

2c. Graft Placement and Fixation

1. Place graft flush with articular surface of recipient site.

2. Fixation is established with bioabsorbable pins or compression screws.

3. Closure

The graft may be trimmed down if it causes impingement. The knee is taken through a full range of motion to ensure that the graft is stable and does not cause catching or obstruction. The arthrotomy is closed per the surgeon's preference with interrupted or running heavy suture. Skin closure is performed in several layers with subcuticular resorbable sutures or staples.

Postoperative Considerations

Rehabilitation

General rehabilitation guidelines are described in Table 56-1. The benefit of continuous passive motion after osteochondral allografting is less clear than after marrow-stimulating techniques or autologous chondrocyte implantation because fully formed cartilage is transplanted that does not require stimulation to enhance maturation. It may be useful, however, to improve range of motion and to reduce the risk of postoperative stiffness.

Full range of motion is allowed unless patients have had other concomitant procedures (i.e., meniscus transplantation, osteotomy, ligament repair) that would dictate otherwise. After the first postoperative visit at 1 week, patients start supervised physical therapy for range-of-motion exercises along with quad sets and patellar mobi-

lization. During this period, the patients remain non–weight bearing. At 6 weeks, weight-bearing status is gradually advanced to full weight bearing; brace use is discontinued once quad control is re-established, and closed chain strengthening exercises are added to the rehabilitation protocol. By 3 months, patients are expected to have regained full and pain-free range of motion with nearly normal quadriceps strength, and recreational sports may be resumed at 6 months postoperatively. However, the patient should avoid excessive impact loading of the allograft during the first year.

Complications

- Infection
- Disease transmission
- Graft nonunion, fragmentation, or collapse (months to years postoperatively)
- Immune response
- Stiffness
- Reflex sympathetic dystrophy

56

PEARLS AND PITFALLS

- Ensure that the graft has been received in acceptable condition and is the correct size before the patient is anesthetized.
- Adequate exposure is key to ensure perpendicular pin placement before overreaming.
- Take down of the meniscus can improve access; this is repaired during closing.
- A positioning device can be helpful to stabilize the extremity in hyperflexion for very posterior lesions.

- Grafts most commonly fail through the bone, not the cartilage; make sure to keep the plug thin (6 to 8 mm), so that only little bone has to be incorporated.
- Dilate the recipient site and bevel the graft edges to facilitate introduction with little force.
- It is preferable to recess the graft rather than to leave it proud.
- Avoid excessive impact activities during the first year. The subchondral bone is only slowly substituted and is at its weakest several months after the operation.

Table 56-1 Rehabilitation Protocol After Osteochondral Allografting

Modality	Time Frame
Continuous passive motion	6-8 weeks (optional but desirable)
Brace	6-12 weeks (patellofemoral or tibial-femoral grafts)
Weight-bearing status	Toe-touch weight bearing or non–weight bearing for 6-12 weeks (based on size of graft)
Closed chain exercises, straight-leg raises	Immediately postoperatively
Stationary cycling	Beginning at 4-8 weeks postoperatively
Light recreational sports	Consider at 4-6 months postoperatively
High-impact sports	Consider at 6 months postoperatively for smaller lesion; not recommended for larger lesions

Table 56-2 Results of Osteochondral Allografting

Author	No. of Patients	Mean Age	Location	Mean Follow-up	Results
Myers et al[12] (1989)	39	38 years	F, T, P	3.6 years	78% success 22% failure
Garrett[8] (1994)	17	20 years	F	3.5 years	94% success
Ghazavi[10] (1997)	123	35 years	F, T, P	7.5 years	85% success
Chu et al[6] (1999)	55	35 years	F, T, P	75 months	76% good–excellent 16% failure

F, femur; T, tibia; P, patella.

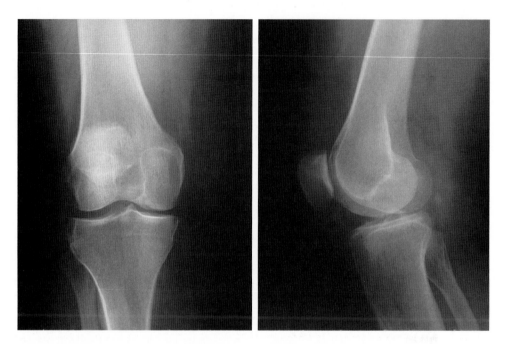

Figure 56-11 The 2-year follow-up radiograph shows well-incorporated graft and maintenance of the joint space.

Results

After osteochondral allograft transplantation, good to excellent results are achieved in nearly 85% of cases, and patients demonstrate a measurable decrease in pain and increase in activity level (Table 56-2). The degree of graft incorporation can be assessed on follow-up radiographs (Fig. 56-11).

References

1. Alford JW, Cole BJ. Cartilage restoration, part 2: techniques, outcomes, and future directions. Am J Sports Med 2005;33:443-460.
2. Aubin PP, Cheah HK, Davis AM, Gross AE. Long-term follow-up of fresh femoral osteochondral allografts for posttraumatic knee defects. Clin Orthop 2001;391:S318-S327.
3. Beaver RJ, Mahomed M, Backstein D, et al. Fresh osteochondral allografts for post-traumatic defects in the knee: a survivorship analysis. J Bone Joint Surg Br 1992;74:105-110.
4. Bugbee WD, Convery FR. Osteochondral allograft transplantation. Clin Sports Med 1999;18:67-75.
5. Bugbee WD. Fresh osteochondral allografts. J Knee Surg 2002; 15:191-195.
6. Chu CR, Convery FR, Akeson WH, et al. Articular cartilage transplantation. Clinical results in the knee. Clin Orthop 1999;360:159-168.
7. Fox JA, Freedman KB, Lee SJ, Cole BJ. Fresh osteochondral allograft transplantation for articular cartilage defects. Oper Tech Sports Med 2002;10:168-173.
8. Garrett J. Fresh osteochondral allografts for treatment of articular defects in osteochondritis dissecans of the lateral femoral condyle in adults. Clin Orthop 1994;303:33-37.

9. Garrett J, Wyman J. The operative technique of fresh osteochondral allografting of the knee. Oper Tech Orthop 2001;11:132-137.

10. Ghazavi MT, Pritzker KP, Davis AM, Gross AE. Fresh osteochondral allografts for post-traumatic osteochondral defects of the knee. J Bone Joint Surg Br 1997;79:1008-1013.

11. Gitelis S, Cole BJ. The use of allografts in orthopaedic surgery. Instr Course Lect 2002;51:507-520.

12. Meyers MH, Akeson W, Convery FR. Resurfacing of the knee with fresh osteochondral allograft. J Bone Joint Surg Am 1989;71:704-713.

13. Oakeshott RD, Farine I, Pritzker KP, et al. A clinical and histologic analysis of failed fresh osteochondral allografts. Clin Orthop 1988;233:283-294.

14. Shasha N, Krywulak S, Backstein D, et al. Long-term follow-up of fresh tibial osteochondral allografts for failed tibial plateau fractures. J Bone Joint Surg Am 2003;85(suppl 2):33-39.

15. Sirlin CB, Brossmann J, Boutin RD, et al. Shell osteochondral allografts of the knee: comparison of MR imaging findings and immunological responses. Radiology 2001;219:35-43.

16. Williams JM, Virdi AS, Pylawka TK, et al. Prolonged-fresh preservation of intact whole canine femoral condyles for the potential use as osteochondral allografts. J Orthop Res 2005;23: 831-837.

56

CHAPTER 57

Autologous Chondrocyte Implantation in the Knee

James B. Day, MD, PhD
Scott D. Gillogly, MD

Articular cartilage injury is extremely common, and until recently, methods for treatment of the cartilaginous lesions did not produce good long-term results. The technique of autologous chondrocyte implantation (ACI), first reported by Peterson, Brittberg, and colleagues in 1994, has gained a major role in the treatment of large full-thickness chondral injuries.[4] Results are now available with up to 12 years of follow-up, and more than 80% of the patients have had improvement with relatively minor complications.[1,15] In this technique, a small biopsy specimen of healthy chondral tissue obtained arthroscopically undergoes in vitro chondrocyte amplification in cell culture, returning autologous chondrocyte cells available for implantation into the defect at the second stage of the repair procedure. The goal in use of autologous chondrocytes is to produce a repair tissue that more closely resembles the morphologic characteristics of the type II hyaline cartilage (>90%), thus restoring the durability and natural function of the knee joint.[4,5]

Preoperative Considerations

History

The first step in determining the appropriate treatment of a suspected chondral defect is to obtain an adequate history. Even in the face of a known cartilage defect, it must be determined whether the symptoms are originating from the defect or arising from some as yet unrecog-

nized pathologic process that would not benefit from ACI. This is particularly relevant to patients who have undergone prior repair techniques, such as marrow stimulation, for the cartilage defect. Whether the symptoms are arising from the previously treated lesion, from a new source, or perhaps as a result of an incomplete rehabilitation program must be discerned.

Patients with condylar lesions typically have pain with weight bearing or increased loading, complaints of mechanical symptoms, swelling, or point tenderness in the area of the defect. The presence of a trochlear or patellar lesion will register similar complaints, but with exacerbation of symptoms by stairs or getting in and out of a chair or car and with anterior knee pain. Patellar subluxation symptoms are often present as well.

Finally, characteristics of the individual patient must be considered in the complete treatment and follow-up planning. Information is often available through previous operative reports and intraoperative photographs. Taking advantage of any available information will help in determining the suitability of the defect for ACI.

Physical Examination

Physical examination provides the critical step in evaluation and assessment of the patient's suitability for ACI. A thorough evaluation of the lower extremity, including observation of gait and a hip and possibly an ankle examination, is warranted, as is a complete evaluation of the knee. A knee ligamentous examination will establish stability. Should there be any question regarding the ligamentous examination, magnetic resonance imaging can *assist* in confirming the clinical findings. Evaluation on physical examination of meniscal function includes provocative meniscal tests, radiographic assessment, and possibly magnetic resonance imaging evaluation.

Imaging

For adequate evaluation of a patient for ACI, it is essential that weight-bearing anteroposterior and 45-degree posteroanterior and patellar alignment radiographs be obtained.[7,10] This allows evaluation of the alignment of the tibiofemoral and patellofemoral portions of the knee and gives an indication of any underlying bone involvement associated with the defect. A long-leg limb alignment radiograph view can assess the mechanical axis and determine the potential need for realignment. As mentioned, magnetic resonance imaging can then be used to assess both the ligament and the meniscal status as well as to define the degree of subchondral bone involvement. Increased signal and edema in the subchondral bone of a chronic nature may indicate persistent overload of the involved compartment, making realignment considerations more likely to be necessary in addition to ACI. Bone loss of more than 7 to 8 mm in depth requires bone grafting before or at the time of cell implantation. Whereas magnetic resonance imaging is helpful to evaluate subchondral bone loss and the soft tissues of the knee, it presently does not have adequate sensitivity or specificity, as performed in the community, to evaluate the extent of chondral injury or subtle chondromalacia changes.[10]

Indications and Contraindications

ACI is indicated for symptomatic, full-thickness chondral lesions and osteochondritis dissecans lesions of the femoral condyles and trochlear groove in physiologically young patients who can be compliant with the rehabilitation protocol. Results of treatment of chondral injuries of the patella and tibia with ACI have not been as consistently good as those of the femoral condyles and trochlea, although with realignment and appropriate patellar tracking, the results are more favorable. ACI is not indicated for treatment of advanced osteoarthritis or in the presence of bipolar sclerotic bone-on-bone lesions. ACI is also contraindicated in active inflammatory arthritis or infection.[10]

In summary, the prerequisites for a successful outcome with ACI (in addition to a focal chondral defect) include appropriate bone alignment, ligamentous stability, meniscal function, adequate motion and muscle strength, and compliance of the patient, without significant bone arthritic changes.

Surgical Planning

Good results with ACI, as with any method of cartilage repair, should not be expected if coexisting knee disease is not addressed. In the senior author's (S. D. G.) experience, performance of one additional procedure at the time of ACI is generally preferred; otherwise, staging is more prudent. Of the author's initial 285 patients undergoing ACI, 60.1% underwent a concomitant procedure. In order of decreasing frequency, these included anteromedialization of the tibial tubercle, high tibial osteotomy or distal femoral osteotomy, anterior cruciate ligament reconstruction, and meniscal transplantation. An additional 11.5% underwent a staged procedure, typically bone grafting of an osteochondral defect or hemicallotasis osteotomy.[7]

Surgical Technique

Anesthesia and Positioning

ACI is typically performed under general anesthesia. In general, we prefer to allow the patient and the anesthesiologist to decide on the specific technique. The patient is placed on the operating table in the supine position. The involved lower extremity is positioned so that the knee may be placed into maximum flexion, if necessary, and rests with the foot on a sandbag or other positioning device so the knee is at 90 degrees of flexion. Prophylactic antibiotics are routinely administered.

After preparation and draping, a midline incision is generally recommended, followed by a medial or lateral parapatellar arthrotomy, exposing the corresponding chondral injury for condyle defects. For patellar defects, the patella is generally reflected superiorly through a tibial tubercle osteotomy that is commonly done for purposes of patellofemoral realignment. As with any surgical procedure, good exposure is critical for performance of the intended technique and good outcome. The approach must allow the surgeon access to properly suture the periosteal patch to the chondral defect. The end result should never be compromised for the sake of an ill-advised concern to keep the approach small.

Surgical Landmarks, Incisions, and Portals

- Tibial tubercle
- Inferior, lateral, and medial poles of the patella
- Patellar tendon
- Lateral and medial femoral condyle
- Tibia plateau

Examination Under Anesthesia

An examination of the knee under general anesthesia is beneficial in revealing pathologic changes, such as ligamentous laxity, in the relaxed patient that may have previously gone undetected.

Specific Steps (Box 57-1)

ACI is a staged procedure. An arthroscopic chondral biopsy specimen is first obtained and sent for culture; then, in the second stage, the actual implantation of the cultured chondrocytes is performed. Whereas the first step is intended for the chondral biopsy, it also serves as a determination of the suitability of the chondral lesion for ACI. At this time, the size and location of the defect, the depth of the defect, the status of the surrounding articular cartilage and underlying bone, and the status of the opposing chondral surfaces are definitively evaluated. Containment of the defect is assessed, and other pathologic processes that might require treatment for optimal ACI results are determined. In general, the defects treated by this technique are larger than 2 cm^2; the average size in the authors' series has been well over 5.6 cm^2.[2,5,7,9]

Stage 1: Chondral Biopsy

1. Arthroscopic Evaluation

A standard arthroscopic approach to the knee is used. The knee must be thoroughly evaluated in all three compartments. Any coexisting pathologic process must be noted and addressed for optimal outcome. Examination under anesthesia again confirms previous clinical assessments.

2. Chondrocyte Biopsy

If a chondral lesion is considered appropriate for ACI, a biopsy specimen is obtained. The most common site is the superomedial edge of the medial femoral condyle or the superolateral edge of the lateral femoral condyle that is non–weight bearing and nonarticulating with the tibia or patella. The other area from which a biopsy specimen is frequently obtained is the lateral intercondylar notch of the medial femoral condyle, particularly if a notchplasty has been performed. An arthroscopic gouge or ring curet is used to obtain several slivers of full-thickness cartilage, each approximately the size of a pencil eraser (i.e., 5 mm by 10 mm). After the slivers are removed from the knee, they are placed in the biopsy medium or shipping vial in sterile fashion. Two or three slivers of cartilage will provide chondrocytes for culturing a 12-fold increase in autologous cells.

Stage 2: Chodrocyte Implantation

1. Arthrotomy

A standard medial or lateral parapatellar incision and arthrotomy are used for exposure. As with any surgical procedure, exposure is essential. If the lesion is on the central portion of the condyle, a mini-arthrotomy can be used. For larger, difficult to reach chondral injuries, a medial or lateral incision with a medial or lateral parapatellar arthrotomy and eversion of the patella may be necessary, especially when the lesion is on the posterior portion of the lateral condyle. We favor a subvastus approach rather than cutting the quadriceps tendon, when feasible.

2. Defect Preparation

During débridement of the defect, all damaged and unhealthy-appearing cartilage, calcified cartilage, and fibrocartilage must be removed. Any thinned, fissured, or damaged surrounding cartilage needs to be débrided to an edge leaving healthy, firm articular cartilage. Bleeding may introduce stem cells and fibroblasts into the defect and therefore must be controlled. The goal of adequate débridement of the defect is to have a dry bed with clean subchondral bone and a healthy, sharply demarcated cartilage border at the periphery. This is best accomplished by scoring the periphery of the defect with a No. 15 scalpel blade and using curets to remove the damaged tissue (Fig. 57-1). The best method for obtaining the correct size for

Box 57-1 Surgical Steps[5,6,9]

Stage 1: Chondral biopsy
1. Arthroscopic evaluation
2. Chondrocyte biopsy

Stage 2: Chodrocyte implantation
1. Arthrotomy
2. Defect preparation
3. Periosteal harvest
4. Periosteal fixation
5. Sealing the periosteal graft
6. Implantation of chondrocytes
7. Wound closure

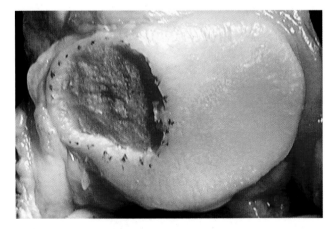

Figure 57-1 Prepared patellar defect.

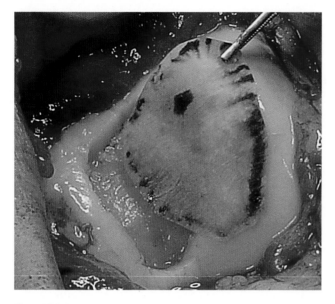

Figure 57-2 Paper template of the trochlear defect.

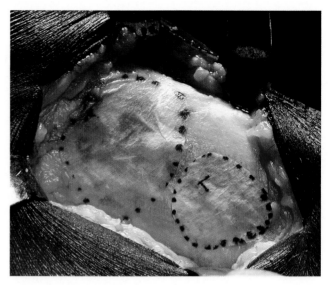

Figure 57-3 Layout of multiple periosteum graft templates.

the periosteal graft is to cut a template from sterile paper (glove wrapping). The template is oversized by 1 to 1.5 mm around the circumference because the harvested periosteum tends to contract (Fig. 57-2).

3. Periosteal Harvest

The periosteum harvest is from the proximal medial tibia, two fingerbreadths distal to the pes anserinus and medial collateral ligament insertion on the subcutaneous border. An incision is made just anterior to the posterior border of the tibia. All fat and fascia layers should be removed from the periosteum by both sharp and blunt dissection with a moist sponge. Leaving the thin fascia layer on the periosteum is one of the most common mistakes made with harvesting of the periosteal graft. The template is then placed over the exposed periosteum, and a scalpel (No. 15 blade) is used to sharply demarcate the periosteal graft (Fig. 57-3). A sharp curved periosteal elevator is used to gently elevate the periosteum off the bone.

4. Periosteal Fixation

The periosteal graft is then aligned over the defect in the orientation matching the template, with the cambium layer facing the defect. The periosteum is then sutured to the cartilage rim with multiple 6-0 Vicryl interrupted sutures spaced every 2 to 3 mm (Fig. 57-4). If the defect is uncontained—meaning that there is not a circumferential rim of healthy cartilage through which sutures can be passed—suture anchors may be used to attach the periosteal graft on the uncontained side (Fig. 57-5). The knots should be tied on the periosteal side, not over the surface of the cartilage, thus minimizing any friction or toggling that could cause loosening of the knots. Redundant periosteal graft can be trimmed as the graft is being secured, ensuring that even tension is maintained on the graft. A

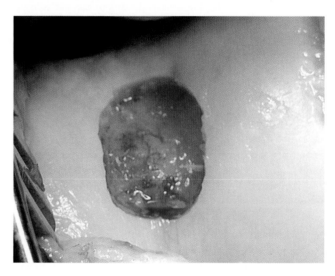

Figure 57-4 Contained trochlear defect.

small opening is maintained on one edge of the graft to allow injection of chondrocyte cells.

5. Sealing the Periosteal Graft

The watertight integrity of the secured graft can be tested by an 18-gauge catheter and a saline-filled tuberculin syringe placed deep to the periosteum through the small opening. Additional sutures can be placed as necessary to ensure a watertight seal. The suture line at the periosteal graft edge is then sealed with fibrin glue with one of the commercially available preparations (Fig. 57-6).

6. Implantation of Chondrocytes

The sterile cells are aspirated from the shipping vial into a tuberculin syringe by sterile technique. The autologous

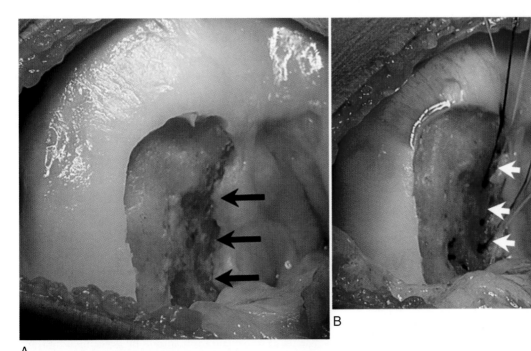

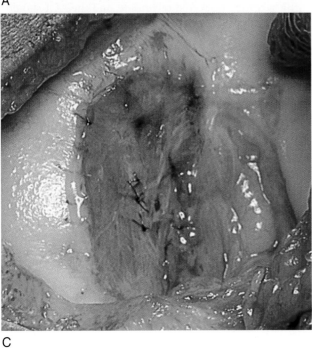

Figure 57-5 A, Medial femoral condyle defect uncontained medially. **B,** Uncontained defect with suture anchors. **C,** Uncontained defect with graft secured.

chondrocytes are then introduced through the tuberculin syringe with an 18-gauge plastic angiocatheter and injected under the periosteal graft. The injection site is then closed with one or two additional sutures and sealed with fibrin glue. No additional manipulation of the joint should follow the implantation (Fig. 57-7).

7. Wound Closure

The arthrotomy and wound are then closed in a layered fashion, and a soft sterile dressing and knee immobilizer are applied to the knee. A drain is not typically used so as not to place any suction on the graft. A subcutaneous drain may be placed after the joint is closed, if necessary.

Combined Procedures[7]

Tibiofemoral Malalignment

- Tibiofemoral malalignment is addressed at the time of ACI.

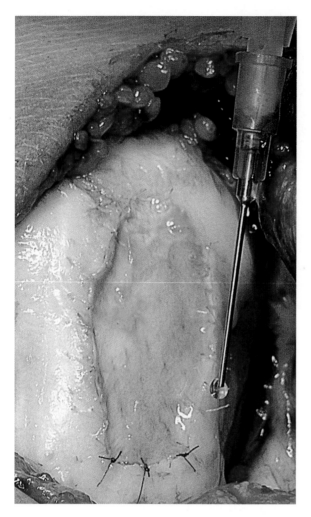

Figure 57-6 Fibrin glue applied to medial femoral condyle.

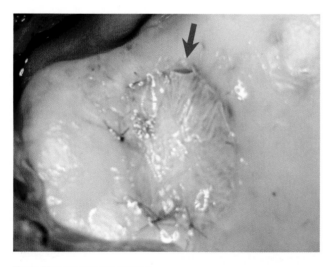

Figure 57-7 Injection site opening.

- Overcorrection is generally not required because off-loading is all that is desired.
- Suturing of the periosteum and implantation of the cells are completed after the osteotomy is fixed.

Ligamentous Insufficiency

- Ligament reconstruction should be done first; then proceed with the ACI (this protects the periosteal graft).
- ACI rehabilitation program is the overriding protocol postoperatively.

Meniscal Deficiency

- Meniscus reconstruction is considered in knees that have had a total meniscectomy performed in the same compartment as the chondral injury.
- Meniscal transplantation is performed in younger patients versus osteotomy in older patients with long-standing meniscectomy.
- Meniscal transplantation should be performed first, by the surgeon's preferred technique, and the ACI should follow to prevent disruption of the periosteal graft by any necessary manipulation.

Patellofemoral Malalignment

- Realignment may be performed at initial arthroscopy if ACI is not to be done in the patellofemoral joint; otherwise, perform realignment at the time of ACI as the defect is more readily approached when the patella and tendon are reflected upward.

Bone Deficiency

- Autologous bone graft is placed in débrided defect bed.
- ACI is performed 4 to 6 months after the bone graft.

Postoperative Considerations

Rehabilitation

- Continuous passive motion is started 6 to 12 hours after surgery.
- Initial touch-down weight bearing is usually progressed to full weight bearing after 4 to 6 weeks.
- Strengthening exercises are initiated after 3 months.
- Impact loading activities begin after 6 months.
- Patellar and trochlear defect repairs are protected from open-chain exercises and shear loading for at least the first 3 months.

Rehabilitation after ACI is based on the maturation process of the chondrocytes, the size of the defect, and the location of the defect.[7,9] The concept of a slow, gradual maturation of the repair tissue is crucial to understanding the rehabilitation after ACI.[9] The hyaline-like repair tissue must be both protected and stimulated to allow the maturation and remodeling of the tissue in the proper manner. In multiple procedures, ACI should remain the determining step in rehabilitation while the principles of early motion and progressive joint loading are maintained.

Complications[13]

- Arthrofibrosis (2%)
- Graft failure or delamination (1.4%)
- Periosteal overgrowth (1.3%-17%)
- Mechanical symptoms (1%)
- Infection

PEARLS AND PITFALLS

Pearls

- Consider ACI in defects larger than 2.0 cm².
- Tie the knot on the periosteum side of the graft, cambium layer toward the defect.
- Perform complete radiographic evaluation of the joint to include alignment radiographs.
- Ensure that other knee pathologic changes (alignment, stability) are addressed; consider staging of the procedures.
- Include the physical therapist in early postoperative planning to ensure a complete understanding of the rehabilitation protocols.

Pitfalls

- Failure to recognize the underlying cause and pathologic changes of the cartilage defect
- ACI in arthritic knees
- ACI in unstable or malaligned knees without correction of these issues first
- ACI in patients who do not understand the nature of the procedure and rehabilitation process
- ACI on tibial plateaus

Results

See Table 57-1.

Discussion

Since the first 23 cases reported in 1994, ACI has been performed in more than 8000 patients throughout the world with more than 12 years of follow-up (Fig. 57-8).[1,5,12,15-17] These results show a significant trend toward objective and subjective satisfaction in patients and their treating physicians. The mechanical durability of ACI cartilage also appears to be significantly greater compared with fibrocartilage regeneration techniques as evaluated by

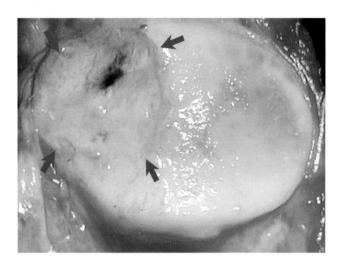

Figure 57-8 Patella, lateral facet. Arrows define ACI.

Table 57-1 Follow-up Results

Author	Follow-up	Outcome
Peterson et al[16] (2000)	2 to 9 years	23 of 25 simple condyle defects: successful 16 of 18 (89%) patients with osteochondritis dissecans: good–excellent
Bahuaud et al[2] (1998)	2 years	84% good–excellent
Minas et al[14] (1998)	6 years	87% of 235 with good results
Bentley et al[3] (2003)	19 months	88% good results for ACI versus 69% after mosaicplasty
Gillogly and Hamby[8] (2001)	5 years	91% of 112 with good–excellent results
Knutsen et al[11] (2002)	2 years	40 patients with ACI versus 40 patients with microfracture: similar results

ACI, autologous chondrocyte implantation.

second-look arthroscopy and duration of satisfactory results.[15,16] In all, ACI holds significant promise in the armamentarium of the orthopedic surgeon in treating cartilage injuries.

Peterson et al[15] have also published long-term biomechanical durability data, showing a 96% durability factor with the first 62 consecutive patients treated at 2 years and then again at 7.5 years.

References

1. Anderson AF, Browne JE, Erggelet C, et al. Cartilage Repair Registry, vol 7. Genzyme Biosurgery, a Division of Genzyme Corporation, 2001:1-7.
2. Bahuaud J, Maitrot RC, Bouvet R, et al. Autologous chondrocyte implantation for cartilage repair. Presentation of 24 cases. Chirurgie 1998;123:568-571.
3. Bentley G, Biant LC, Carrington M, et al. A prospective, randomised comparison of autologous chondrocyte implantation versus mosaicplasty for osteochondral defects in the knee. J Bone Joint Surg Br 2003;85:223-230.
4. Brittberg M. Autologous chondrocyte transplantation. Clin Orthop 1999;367S:S147-S155.
5. Brittberg M, Lindahl A, Nilsson A, et al. Treatment of deep cartilage defects in the knee with autologous chondrocyte transplantation. N Engl J Med 1994;331:889-895.
6. Cole BJ, D'Amato M. Autologous chondrocyte implantation. Oper Tech Orthop 2001;11:115-131.
7. Gillogly SD. Autologous chondrocyte implantation: complex defects and concomitant procedures. Oper Tech Sports Med 2002; 10:120-128.
8. Gillogly SD, Hamby TS. Clinical results of autologous chondrocyte implantation for large full-thickness chondral defects of the knee: five-year experience with 112 consecutive patients. American Orthopaedic Society for Sports Medicine annual meeting; Keystone, Colorado; June 28, 2001.
9. Gillogly SD, Voight M, Blackburn T. Treatment of articular cartilage defects of the knee with autologous chondrocyte implantation. J Orthop Sports Phys Ther 1998;28:241-251.
10. Hamby TS, Gillogly SD, Peterson L. Treatment of patellofemoral articular cartilage injuries with autologous chondrocyte implantation. Oper Tech Sports Med 2002;10:129-135.
11. Knutsen G, et al: Autologous chondrocyte implantation vs microfracture: a prospective randomized Norwegian multicenter trial. International Cartilage Repair Society meeting; Toronto, Canada; 2002.
12. Lohnert J. Regeneration of hyalin cartilage in the knee joint by treatment with autologous chondrocyte transplantation. Langenbecks Arch Chir Suppl Kongressbd 1998;115:1201-1207.
13. Micheli L, Browne JE, Erggelet C, et al: Autologous chondrocyte implantation of the knee: multicenter experience and minimum 3 year follow-up. Clin J Sport Med 2001;11:223-228.
14. Minas T. Autologous cultured chondrocyte implantation in the repair of focal chondral lesions of the knee: clinical indications and operative technique. J Sports Traumatol Rel Res 1998;20: 90-102.
15. Peterson L, Lindahl A, Brittberg M, Kiviranta Nilsson A. Autologous chondrocyte transplantation: biomechanics and long-term durability. Am J Sports Med 2002;30:2-12.
16. Peterson L, Minas T, Brittberg M, et al. Two- to 9-year outcome after autologous chondrocyte transplantation of the knee. Clin Orthop 2000;374:212-234.
17. Richardson J, Caterson B, Evans E, et al. Repair of human articular cartilage after implantation of autologous chondrocytes. J Bone Joint Surg Br 1999;81:1064-1068.

CHAPTER 58

High Tibial Osteotomy

Jeffrey T. Junko, MD
Annunziato Amendola, MD

High tibial osteotomy is a useful technique for altering lower limb alignment, thereby allowing the surgeon to adjust the biomechanical environment of the knee. Jackson and Waugh first described a dome osteotomy of the proximal tibia to treat osteoarthritic knees with either varus or valgus malalignment. Coventry later described the use of either medial or lateral closing wedge high tibial osteotomy for malaligned knees with early signs of degenerative arthritis. Subsequent experience and the improved longevity of total knee arthroplasty have narrowed the indications for high tibial osteotomy in patients with knee arthritis. High tibial osteotomy is now receiving renewed interest as it has become evident that coronal and sagittal plane correction of the knee can augment or in some cases supplant the function of certain structures within the knee. The development of meniscal transplantation and the treatment of femoral chondral defects have opened the need to use the high tibial osteotomy to offload these injury-prone areas. Increased or decreased proximal tibial slope has been shown to affect the function of the cruciates and can be a contributing factor to recurrent cruciate injury. High tibial osteotomy can be used to correct the aforementioned sagittal plane deformities of the proximal tibia. This chapter outlines the preoperative considerations and appropriate indications as well as describes the surgical techniques used by the authors in performing a high tibial osteotomy for a variety of conditions.

Preoperative Considerations

Several factors are involved in ensuring a successful outcome of high tibial osteotomy, but none is more important than proper selection of the patient. The selection of the proper patient begins with a detailed history and physical examination and is aided by appropriate radiographic imaging. These aspects are then combined to determine which patients will benefit from high tibial osteotomy and which are better served by other treatment modalities.

The history should cover aspects including age of the patient, activity level, occupation, possible comorbidities, and previous conservative or surgical interventions. A history of antecedent trauma or injury to the affected knee needs to be elucidated. One of the most important facts to gather is the activity level the patient hopes to resume after surgery. The area of pain distribution is vitally important, and every effort should be made to accurately identify the specific locus of the patient's knee pain. The presence or absence of mechanical symptoms, such as locking, catching, or episodes of instability, should be addressed as these may indicate underlying pathologic processes that may benefit from arthroscopic management at the time of high tibial osteotomy.

The physical examination notes the patient's overall body habitus as well as the overall level of conditioning. Both lower extremities should be fully visualized in both the coronal and sagittal planes, with attention given to areas of deformity and overall limb alignment. Rotational malalignment is also sought. The patient's gait is observed and evaluated for any thrusts in the direction of the deformity, which may reveal an underlying dynamic component. Deformities are assessed for potential to be corrected. The knee is inspected for previous surgical incisions or areas with suspect soft tissue that could alter standard surgical approaches. Range of motion is evaluated, as are any alterations in patellar tracking. Presence or absence of an effusion is noted. Palpation of the entire knee is carried out in an attempt to identify underlying mechanical sources of the patient's pain. A thorough ligamentous examination is carried out to look for collateral or cruciate laxity. The ability of a valgus force to decrease the patient's pain as the knee is put through a range of motion is assessed and may mimic the unloading effect of a proposed osteotomy. Other sites that can refer pain to the knee, such as the low back, hip, and ankle, are evaluated.

Imaging

In addition to a thorough history and physical examination, radiographic evaluation is an integral portion of the work-up for a high tibial osteotomy. Plain radiographs are essential for preoperative assessment and planning and consist of a series of five films. The series is made up of bilateral anteroposterior weight-bearing views at full extension, bilateral posteroanterior weight-bearing views at 45 degrees of flexion, a Merchant view, and a lateral view of the affected knee. In addition, a full-length alignment view in double limb stance is obtained. It is important that weight-bearing views be obtained because supine views tend to underestimate both joint line narrowing and soft tissue laxity. Controversy exists as to whether single limb stance or double leg stance should be used for operative planning; however, single limb stance tends to overestimate the soft tissue laxity component of the deformity and is therefore not used for this purpose at our institution.

Various measurements are made from the radiographs to assist in preoperative planning. Common measurements taken are the axis of weight bearing, the joint congruency angle, and the articular angles of the tibia and femur to aid in determination of the site of deformity. To determine the axis of weight bearing, a line is drawn on the full-length radiographs from the center of the femoral head to the center of the tibiotalar joint. Articular angles are determined along with determination of the axes of both the tibial and femoral shafts to uncover coronal plane deformities. In like fashion, the lateral radiograph is used to calculate tibial slope for the assessment of sagittal plane deformities.

Calculations of Corrections

Several methods have been reported for determining the required correction on preoperative radiographs. In general, the desired location of the weight-bearing line postoperatively is determined and the angular correction is then calculated to achieve this position. In practice, satisfactory results are achievable with overcorrection of medial compartment arthritis into slight valgus alignment and with correction to neutral alignment when operating for lateral compartment arthrosis. High tibial osteotomy is most commonly performed for genu varum with associated medial compartment arthrosis, and an example of the calculation for correction is presented here. Dugdale et al first described the current method of calculation used at our institution. Full-length standing anteroposterior radiographs of both lower extremities are used. The final position of the weight-bearing line should rest in the zone of 62% to 66% as described by Dugdale. A line is then drawn from the center of the femoral head through this point at the knee joint. A line is then drawn from the center of the ankle joint to the same point at the knee, bisecting and forming an angle with the femoral line. The angle formed by this intersection represents the amount of angular correction needed to place the weight-bearing line at the desired more lateral position. A line is then drawn over the proximal tibial metaphysis, simulating the proposed position of the tibial osteotomy. The osteotomy should run in a medial-distal to proximal-lateral direction, with care taken to leave at least 1 cm of intact bone superior to the lateral extent of the osteotomy to prevent fracture into the joint at the time of angular correction. This point is usually just at the superior extent of the proximal tibia-fibula joint. The length of this cut is then calculated. The length of the cut is then transposed over the angular correction line, and the length between the two bisector lines at this level is calculated. The length measured represents the height of the wedge needed to create the exact angular correction. Measuring wedge height facilitates intraoperative correction and alleviates the need for intraoperative angular measurement.

Indications

The main indication for a high tibial osteotomy is in a young patient with isolated medial compartment arthritis or overload and a malaligned limb or in the older patient who is active and in whom a unicompartmental or knee arthroplasty is likely to fail. High tibial osteotomy can be used in patients with concomitant anterior cruciate ligament laxity or failed cruciate reconstruction who have varus malalignment and medial compartment overload. Also in the patient with cruciate laxity due to variances in proximal tibial slope, adjustment of the tibial slope can partially compensate for the cruciate deficiency by decreasing tibial translation. An example is increasing posterior tibial slope to compensate for a posterior cruciate ligament–deficient knee with a posterior sag and instability. Osteochondral defects and avascular necrosis of the medial femoral condyle can be off-loaded with a high tibial osteotomy. Realignment after meniscal or cartilage transplantation is another area in which high tibial osteotomy has proved useful.

Contraindications

High tibial osteotomy is contraindicated in individuals with concomitant arthritis in the opposite tibiofemoral compartment. Arthritic changes in the patellofemoral compartment are to be considered and may be a relative contraindication or concern. Other contraindications are pain referable to other areas of the knee and the lack of a functional lateral meniscus. Poor bone quality at the osteotomy site or other factors that might inhibit healing need to be considered.

Surgical Technique

The technique most commonly used at this institution is the medial opening wedge osteotomy (Box 58-1). The following is our step-by-step approach for performing this technique. The patient is generally given both femoral and sciatic single shot nerve blocks and then given a general anesthetic. The patient is placed in a supine position at the edge of the table on the operative side to facilitate intraoperative fluoroscopic imaging. A tourniquet is used in all cases. The operative limb is prepared and draped free. The surface anatomy is palpated, and the following structures are drawn on the skin: medial edge of the tibial tubercle and patellar tendon, inferior joint line, and posterior medial border of the tibia (Fig. 58-1).

A 6-cm incision is made 1 cm distal to the joint line and halfway between the tibial tuberosity and the posteromedial border of the tibia. The subcutaneous tissue is dis-

sected sharply down to the level of the sartorius fascia. Starting at the medial edge of the tibial tubercle, the sartorius fascia is incised longitudinally. The sartorius fascia and the pes anserine are then elevated off the medial tibia to the level of the medial collateral ligament. The deep fibers of the medial collateral ligament are then raised from an anterolateral to posteromedial direction subperiosteally. A Homan retractor is then placed around the posteromedial corner of the tibia. The medial edge of the patellar tendon is then identified, and a longitudinal incision just medial to the tendon is made for a short distance in a superior direction. This allows placement of a second Homan retractor just superior to the tibial tuberosity and underneath the patellar tendon, thereby protecting it during the osteotomy cuts (Fig. 58-2). The medial proximal tibia is thus exposed. Two parallel guide pins are placed just proximal to the intended osteotomy line. The starting point for these pins is approximately 3 to 4 cm distal to the medial joint line. The pins are directed in an oblique fashion from an inferior-medial position to a

Box 58-1 Surgical Steps in Medial Opening Wedge Osteotomy

- Operative draping and surface anatomy references drawn on skin
- Exposure of proximal medial tibial cortex with retractor placement
- Guide pin placement just proximal to proposed osteotomy line
- Fluoroscopy to ensure integrity of the lateral tibial cortex
- Two Arthrex osteotomes for "stacking" technique to accomplish initial opening of osteotomy
- Screw jack technique for opening osteotomy
- Placement of graduated wedge to preoperatively calculated depth
- Placement of wedged Puddu plate anterior to single stem of the graduated wedge
- Puddu plate fixation as far posterior as possible to avoid iatrogenic changes in posterior tibial slope
- Corticocancellous wedge and morselized femoral head allograft
- Placement of correctly sized wedge anterior to Puddu plate for added stability

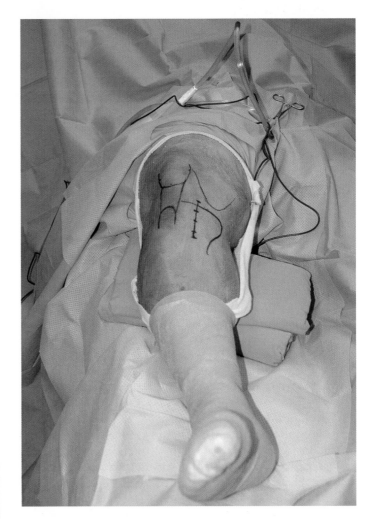

Figure 58-1 Operative draping and surface anatomy references drawn on skin.

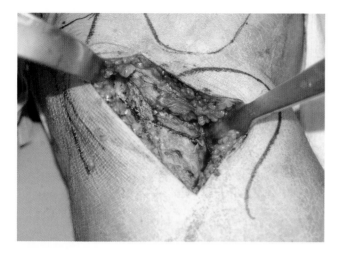

Figure 58-2 Exposure of proximal medial tibial cortex with retractor placement.

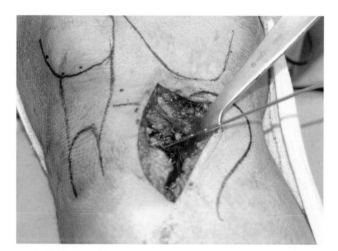

Figure 58-3 Guide pin placement just proximal to proposed osteotomy line.

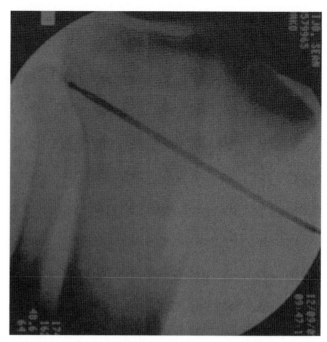

Figure 58-4 Fluoroscopic anteroposterior image of correct guide pin placement.

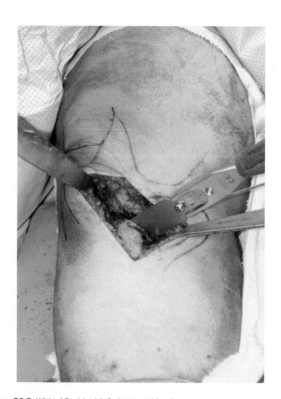

Figure 58-5 Wide AO chisel inferior to guide pin.

superior-lateral position (Figs. 58-3 and 58-4). Because the proximal tibia is sloped posteriorly, the osteotomy must be made in an oblique fashion to maintain an adequate bridge of bone along the posterior cortex of the tibia. The pins should be no less than 1 cm from the joint surface of the lateral tibial plateau. The pins guard against proximal migration of the osteotomy toward the joint. Distances less than 1 cm are more likely to fracture into the joint at the time of osteotomy correction. Absolute requirements for pin placement include osteotomy placed above the insertion of the patellar tendon, adequate distal starting point to allow proximal plate fixation, and osteotomy at least 1 cm distal to lateral tibial articular surface. A small sagittal saw is then used from anterior to posterior to initiate the osteotomy cut just below the two guide pins and parallel to them. Thin broad AO osteotomes are then used to complete the osteotomy. The use of thicker, more traditional osteotomes can lead to fracture into the joint. Fluoroscopic images are obtained throughout to ensure

that the lateral tibial cortex is not violated and to ensure parallelism between the guide pins and the osteotome (Figs. 58-5 and 58-6).

Once the osteotomy is complete, a second osteotome is placed under the first to begin to open the osteotomy. A

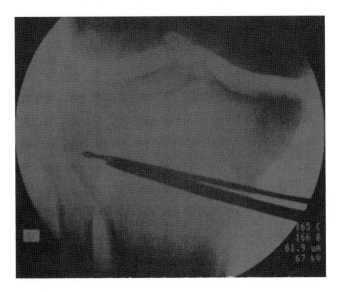

Figure 58-6 Fluoroscopic anteroposterior image of chisel just inferior to guide pin.

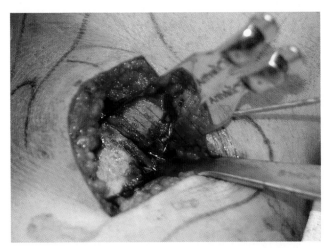

Figure 58-7 Two Arthrex osteotomes used for "stacking" technique to accomplish initial opening of osteotomy.

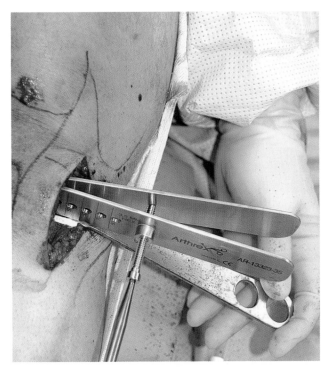

Figure 58-8 Screw jack technique for opening osteotomy.

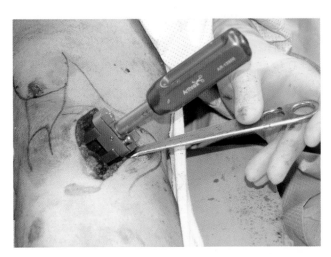

Figure 58-9 Placement of graduated wedge to depth calculated preoperatively.

third can also be added if the need arises. This stacking technique gradually opens the osteotomy, leaving the lateral tibial cortex intact. A gentle valgus stress can also be applied on the knee to assess mobility of the osteotomy (Fig. 58-7).

The medial aspect of the osteotomy can be opened further for larger corrections by inserting the screw jack into the osteotomy and gradually advancing the screw to apply a controlled opening force (Fig. 58-8). A graduated Puddu wedge is then inserted at the same angle as the osteotomy, creating the exact wedge height as had been calculated preoperatively. The graduated wedge should be advanced slowly (5 mm/min) to allow gradual opening of the osteotomy (Fig. 58-9). A wedged Puddu plate of the same size is then inserted (Fig. 58-10). The graduated

wedge is removed, and the plate is then placed in a more posterior position. A common mistake is to leave the plate in an anterior position, which leads to an unwanted increase in posterior tibial slope. The plate is then secured with two 6.5-mm cancellous screws superiorly and two 4.5-mm cortical screws inferiorly (Fig. 58-11). Femoral head allograft is then morselized and placed into the wedge defect. A corticocancellous wedge is then placed just anterior to the plate to help maintain the open wedge (Fig. 58-12 and 58-13). Autologous iliac crest can be used, but this can lead to donor site morbidity. Final images are

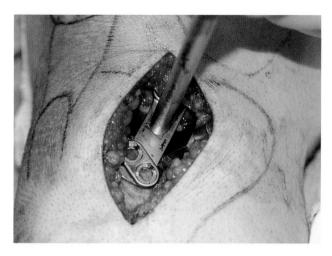

Figure 58-10 Placement of wedged Puddu plate anterior to single stem of the graduated wedge.

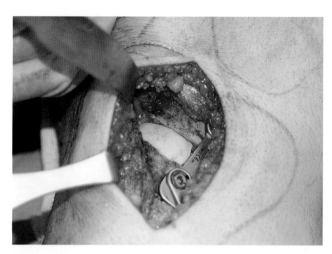

Figure 58-13 Placement of correctly sized wedge anterior to Puddu plate for added stability.

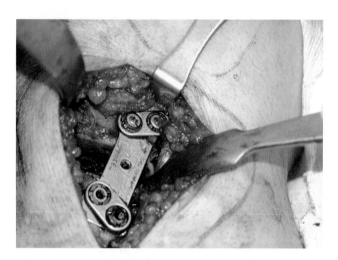

Figure 58-11 Puddu plate fixation as far posterior as possible to avoid iatrogenic changes in posterior tibial slope.

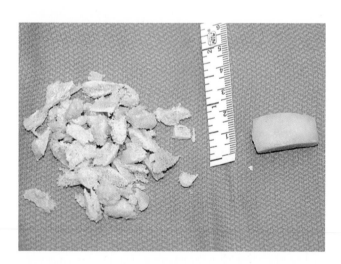

Figure 58-12 Corticocancellous wedge and morselized femoral head allograft.

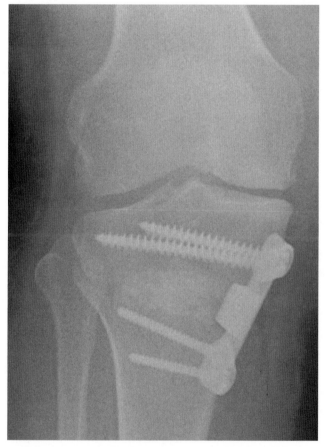

Figure 58-14 Final anteroposterior image. Note disruption of the lateral tibial cortex, indicating need for more prolonged period of protected weight bearing.

obtained to ensure proper hardware placement (Fig. 58-14). The wound is irrigated, and the pes anserine and sartorius fascia are repaired over the plate. The subcutaneous tissue is reapproximated, the skin is closed and a dressing applied.

Combined Procedures

Anterior Cruciate Ligament Reconstruction and High Tibial Osteotomy

The high tibial osteotomy is generally performed after harvesting of the hamstring tendons if autograft is being used. Once the high tibial osteotomy is complete, the anterior cruciate ligament reconstruction can be performed. The tibial tunnel should be placed just proximal to the proximal screws of the high tibial osteotomy.

58

Postoperative Management

The patient is placed in a hinged knee brace that allows motion from 0 to 90 degrees of flexion. The patient is kept overnight for pain control and to work with physical therapy. The patient is kept touch-down weight bearing in the hinged knee brace for 6 weeks. The patient is encouraged to work on range of motion from 0 to 90 degrees in the hinged knee brace during this time. Plain films are obtained at 6 weeks postoperatively, and if adequate healing is apparent, progressive weight bearing is initiated. If the lateral cortex was violated during the operative procedure, the weight-bearing protocol is adjusted to include a longer interval of protected weight bearing. Total time for recovery and resumption of normal activities generally averages 6 months.

Results

Longer term follow-up studies of high tibial osteotomy demonstrate a general decline in the therapeutic effects with time (Table 58-1). Studies have shown that high tibial osteotomy is more effective in the younger, more active patient with maintenance of knee range of motion. The higher demands placed on the knee by these more active individuals may make high tibial osteotomy a better alternative to knee arthroplasty. High tibial osteotomy may be effective for 10 to 20 years in these well-selected patients. Factors that predict a poorer outcome include advanced age, severe arthrosis, joint instability, limited range of motion, operative overcorrection or undercorrection, and loss of correction.

Table 58-1 Longer Term Follow-Up Studies of High Tibial Osteotomy

Study	Length of Follow-Up	Results
Aglietti et al[1] (1983)	10-year minimum follow-up	88 of 139 (64%) excellent or good results
Ritter and Fechtman[6] (1988)	4.2-year average follow-up	6-year survival rate of 80%
Rudan and Imurda[7] (1990)	5.8-year average follow-up	63 of 79 (80%) excellent or good results
Berman et al[2] (1991)	8.5-year average follow-up	22 of 35 (57%) good results
Yasuda et al[9] (1992)	6-year follow-up 10-year follow-up	49 of 56 (88%) satisfactory results 35 of 56 (63%) satisfactory results
Nagel et al[3] (1996)	8-year average follow-up	28 of 34 (82%) satisfied with surgical result
Rinonapoli et al[5] (1998)	15-year average follow-up	37 of 60 (55%) excellent or good results
Naudie et al[4] (1999)		10-year survivorship 51% 15-year survivorship 39%
Tang and Henderson[8] (2005)		10-year survivorship 74.7% 15- and 20-year survivorship 66.9%

References

1. Aglietti P, Rinonapoli E, Stringa G, Taviani A. Tibial osteotomy for the varus osteoarthritic knee. Clin Orthop 1983;176:239-251.

2. Berman AT, Bosacco SJ, Kirshner S, Avolio A Jr. Factors influencing long-term results in high tibial osteotomy. Clin Orthop 1991;272:192-198.

3. Nagel A, Insall JN, Scuderi GR. Proximal tibial osteotomy. A subjective outcome study. J Bone Joint Surg Am 1996;78:1353-1358.

4. Naudie D, Bourne RB, Rorabeck CH, Bourne TJ. The Insall award. Survivorship of the high tibial valgus osteotomy. A 10- to 22-year follow-up study. Clin Orthop 1999;367:18-27.

5. Rinonapoli E, Mancini GB, Corvaglia A, Musiello S. Tibial osteotomy for varus gonarthrosis. A 10- to 21-year follow-up study. Clin Orthop 1998;353:185-193.

6. Ritter MA, Fechtman RA. Proximal tibial osteotomy. A survivorship analysis. J Arthroplasty 1988;3:309-311.

7. Rudan JF, Imurda MA. High tibial osteotomy. A prospective clinical and roentgenographic review. Clin Orthop 1990;255:251-256.

8. Tang WC, Henderson IJ. High tibial osteotomy: long term survival analysis and patients' perspective. Knee 2005;12:410-413.

9. Yasuda K, Majima T, Tsuchida T, Kaneda K. A ten- to 15-year follow-up observation of high tibial osteotomy in medial compartment osteoarthrosis. Clin Orthop 1992;282:186-195.

Suggested Reading

Amendola A, Panarella L. High tibial osteotomy for the treatment of unicompartmental arthritis of the knee. Orthop Clin North Am 2005;36:497-504.

Coventry MB. Osteotomy of the upper portion of the tibia for degenerative arthritis of the knee. J Bone Joint Surg Am 1965;47:984-990.

Dugdale TW, Noyes FR, Styer D. Preoperative planning for high tibial osteotomy. The effect of lateral tibiofemoral separation and tibiofemoral length. Clin Orthop 1992;274:248-264.

Insall JN, Joseph DM, Msika C. High tibial osteotomy for varus gonarthrosis. A long-term follow-up study. J Bone Joint Surg Am 1984;66:1040-1048.

Jackson JP, Waugh WW. Tibial osteotomy for osteoarthritis of the knee. J Bone Joint Surg Br 1961;43:746-751.

Matthews LS, Goldstein SA, Malvitz TA, et al. Proximal tibial osteotomy. Factors that influence the duration of satisfactory function. Clin Orthop 1988;229:193-200.

CHAPTER 59

Distal Femoral Osteotomy

Fred Flandry, MD
Declan J. Bowler, MD, FRCSI (Tr & Orth)

Malalignment affects the articular surfaces of the knee more than any joint of the lower extremity. Deformity of the distal femur can arise as a genetically determined morphologic characteristic; from congenital disorders; from metabolic disorders, such as rickets; from developmental causes, such as asymmetric growth arrest; or as a result of traumatic or infectious sequelae. With so broad a range of etiologic factors, no two deformities are alike, and a "cookbook" approach to distal femoral osteotomy should be avoided. Further, it is not uncommon for vectors causing deformity in the distal femur to affect other metaphyseal and diaphyseal segments of the lower extremity. For this reason, the surgeon should be keenly aware of the mechanical alignment and joint orientations of the entire limb and not just those of the knee.

Box 59-1 outlines our approach to planning and performing distal femoral osteotomies.

Preoperative Considerations: Define the Deformity

History

The history should elicit an approximate, if not specific, time of onset of symptoms and when the deformity was first noted. A cause, if possible, is determined. The location, character, and exacerbating and relieving aspects of pain are documented. It is not uncommon for the patient with lateral gonarthrosis, the most common indication for distal femoral osteotomy, to present with pain symptoms lagging far behind those expected from the radiographic

appearance of the joint. Crepitation, a sign of chronic synovial inflammation, may be a more constant sign of the chronic arthritic changes.

The presence of clicks, pops, catching, and locking may suggest internal derangement, such as meniscal tears, chondral lesions, or synovial plicae, that should be addressed, usually arthroscopically, at the time of the osteotomy.

Physical Examination

During the physical examination, visual inspection of the standing patient should be carried out from the coronal and sagittal perspectives. If the pelvis is not level, leveling blocks are placed under the short limb until a level pelvis is achieved, and the height of those blocks is noted. The examination should include a Trendelenburg test, and the gait pattern should be characterized (e.g., Duchenne, antalgic, selective motor weakness). With the patient supine, leg length and tibiofemoral angles are measured. Clinical measures for rotational deformity (femoral anteversion, thigh-foot angle, transmalleolar axis) are recorded. A comprehensive examination is conducted of the hip, knee, ankle, and hindfoot-midfoot joints, looking critically for instability, internal derangement, and arthritis. If ligament instability is diagnosed, stress radiographs as well as standard views should be ordered.

Imaging

Proper imaging protocols are necessary to facilitate preoperative planning. The most critical view is a coronal plane

- Assess the deformity
- Determine the location for the osteotomy
- Perform or stage intra-articular procedures
- Select a surgical approach
- Perform the osteotomy
- Provide appropriate rehabilitation

anteroposterior film showing the entire limb. This view is typically obtained with the patient standing and with blocks under the foot of a short side (if such exists) to level the pelvis. A 51-inch cassette or newer digital stitching technique is used to capture the image. The flexion axis of the knee should be oriented to lie in the plane of the film to allow accurate determination of the mechanical and anatomic axes and coronal plane joint orientation angles (Fig. 59-1). Supine anteroposterior and lateral images with the beam centered at the knee are obtained for specific osteotomy planning. A lateral film in extension encompassing at least the distal half of the femur and proximal half of the tibia is needed to determine if any sagittal planar deformity exists, which could indicate the need for biplane osteotomy techniques. If deformity or incongruity of the articular surface is suspected, it is best evaluated by computed tomographic coronal and sagittal plane reconstructions. Axial malalignment may be more precisely quantified with computed tomographic alignment studies (Fig. 59-2). If the clinical examination suggests ligament and meniscal disorders, they can be further characterized by magnetic resonance imaging.

Indications and Contraindications

A significant mechanical axis deviation, if left untreated, causes unicompartmental overload, meniscal damage, and arthritic deterioration.[7,14] Distal femoral osteotomy is indicated when a mechanical axis deviation is present and the deformity is determined to exist in the distal femur. If the deformity is elsewhere, a distal femoral osteotomy can cause malalignment of normal joint orientation. Distal femoral osteotomy can also be done as an adjunct to knee ligament surgery when medial ligament instability and valgus of the limb deformity coexist or if lateral ligament instability and varus deformity of the limb coexist. Again, the axis of the limb deformity must be in the distal femur. There is a relative contraindication for patients who are smokers or have vascular insufficiency, contracture at the knee, or advanced arthrosis.

Preoperative Planning: Determine the Location for the Osteotomy

The completion of an analytical and in-depth preoperative plan is as essential to a successful outcome as the surgical technique. Paley[12] and coworkers have developed a rational and comprehensive method for deformity correction planning, which consists of a malalignment test, joint orientation measurement, joint line congruence assessment, and determination of the proposed level of correction.

The malalignment test involves determination of mechanical axis deviation on a full-limb coronal plane image.

Step 1: A line is extended from the center of the femoral head to the center of the tibial plafond. This line should fall on the tibial spine. If it falls medial to the tibial spine, varus malalignment exists; and if it falls lateral to the tibial spine, valgus malalignment exists (Fig. 59-3). If no mechanical axis deviation can be demonstrated, the benefit of osteotomy should be questioned.

Step 2: The mechanical lateral distal femoral angle (mLDFA) or anatomic lateral distal femoral angle (aLDFA) is measured (Fig. 59-4). If it is found to be outside the range of normal, the deformity contributing to malalignment at least partly exists at the level of the distal femur. *For a distal femoral osteotomy to be indicated, there should be an abnormal mLDFA or aLDFA.*

Step 3: The medial proximal tibial angle is measured (see Fig. 59-4). If it is found to be outside the range of normal, the deformity contributing to malalignment at least partly exists at the level of the proximal tibia.

Step 4: The joint line congruence angle is measured. If it is greater than 2 degrees, some component of the malalignment is due to loss of joint cartilage, ligament laxity, or condylar malalignment, which should be determined and factored into the ultimate correction (Fig. 59-5).

It is also important to determine what malorientation, if any, exists at the hip and ankle. Malorientation of the hip may require a second, more proximal osteotomy or an adjustment of the osteotomy level on the femur to restore a normal mechanical axis (even if it results in a slightly nonanatomic diaphysis). More important, if a distal femoral osteotomy of any significant degree is performed, the degree to which it will change the plane of the ankle to the plane of the floor *must* be considered. If an oblique ankle joint plane is created as a result of a distal femoral (or proximal tibial) osteotomy, a second normalizing osteotomy to correct the ankle must be planned as well (Fig. 59-6).

Joint line congruence can affect mechanical axis deviation in several ways (see Fig. 59-5). Ligamentous laxity

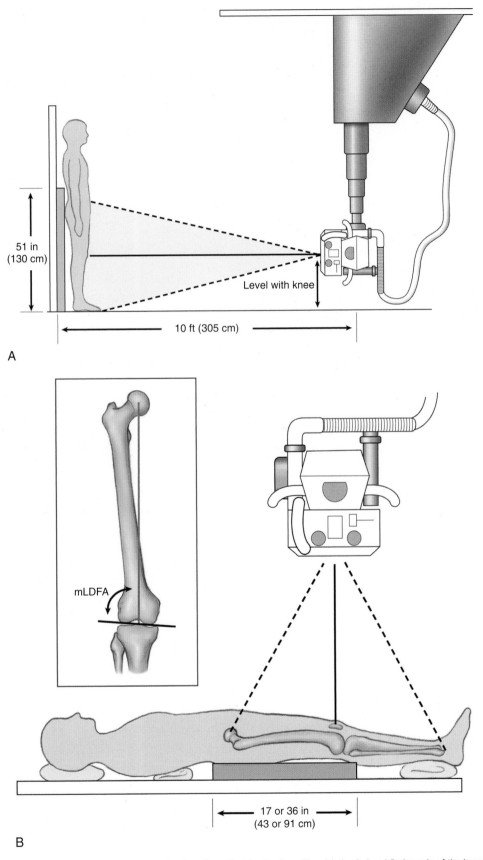

A

B

Figure 59-1 A, Technique for lower extremity coronal plane imaging; the patient is standing with pelvis leveled and flexion axis of the knee oriented to the coronal plane. The x-ray tube or digital sender is positioned 10 feet from and at the level of the knee. **B,** With the patient supine, anteroposterior and lateral views are obtained. If images are to be obtained of a single bone, the beam should be centered on the joint adjacent to the planned osteotomy. (After Paley.[12])

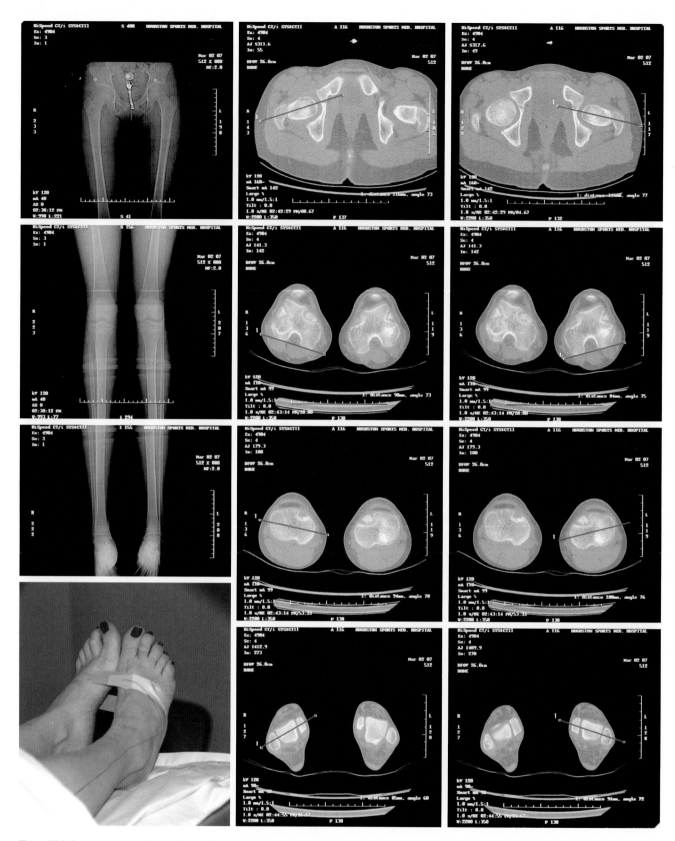

Figure 59-2 Computed tomography rotational alignment protocol used in our institution. The patient's feet are strapped together to normalize transmalleolar axis to the plane of the floor. Computed tomographic axial slices are obtained through the femoral neck, distal femur, proximal tibia, and ankle to allow more precise determination of the location and magnitude of any rotational deformity.

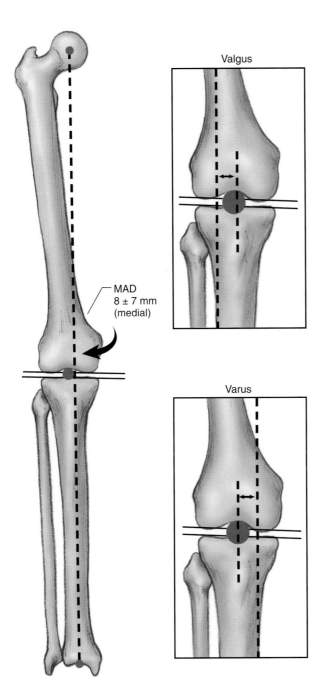

Valgus

Varus

MAD
8 ± 7 mm
(medial)

Figure 59-3 The malorientation test. Mechanical axis deviation (MAD) exists if a line extending from the center of the femoral head to the center of the tibial plafond passes medial to the tibial spine (varus malalignment) or lateral to the tibial spine (valgus malalignment). (After Paley.[12])

femoral). These lines should be collinear, and if they are not, the varus and valgus deformity and mechanical axis deviation result at least in part from the articular surface deformity.

An understanding of the terms *angular correction axis, center of rotation of angulation,* and *transverse bisector line* is important when the surgeon is planning an osteotomy. When an angular correction is performed, an axis line in space, that is, a hinge, is defined on which one bone segment rotates relative to the other. This axis is referred to as the angular correction axis. Any angular deformity of bone can be thought of as having one bone axis proximal to the deformity and another distal to the deformity. The point of intersection of the proximal and distal axes is the center of rotation of angulation. Finally, a line drawn through the center of rotation of angulation that bisects the medial and lateral angles subtended by the proximal and distal axis line intersections is referred to as the transverse bisector line (Fig. 59-7). The significance of the transverse bisector line is that if the angular correction axis is located anywhere along it, there will be collinear realignment of the axis. If a closing wedge osteotomy is to be performed, the angular correction axis is placed on the transverse bisector line where it intersects the concave cortex. For an opening wedge osteotomy, the angular correction axis should be located on the transverse bisector line where it intersects the convex cortex (Fig. 59-8).

Paley[12] described three rules governing osteotomy planning:

1. If the osteotomy and the angular correction axis pass through the center of rotation of angulation, collinear realignment of the axis of the bone segments occurs (Fig. 59-8).

2. When the angular correction axis is placed at the center of rotation of angulation and the osteotomy site is placed at a level away from the center of rotation of angulation, the axis realigns; but both angulation *and translation* occur at the osteotomy site (Fig. 59-9).

3. If the osteotomy *and* the angular correction axis are away from the center of rotation of angulation, *a secondary translational deformity will occur* (Fig. 59-10).

Ideally, the most straightforward osteotomy plan is to follow osteotomy rule 1; however, anatomic, fixation, or pathologic constraints may force the osteotomy to be positioned away from the center of rotation of angulation. The surgeon must realize that in this situation, if the angular correction axis (or hinge) is placed at the osteotomy and *not at the center of rotation of angulation,* a translational correction must be performed to correct the secondary translational deformity created. If this is not appreciated and not done, the mechanical axis deviation may not be corrected and joint overload may still exist even though

may not be apparent in a standing or static film, making a ligamentous examination of the knee an essential component of the initial evaluation. If it is suggested from the examination, stress radiographs should also be obtained. If the midpoints of the femoral and tibial condyles diverge by more than 3 mm, subluxation exists and is therefore at least a component of the mechanical axis deviation. Finally, condylar incongruity can be detected by extending lines across the medial and lateral hemicondyles (tibial and

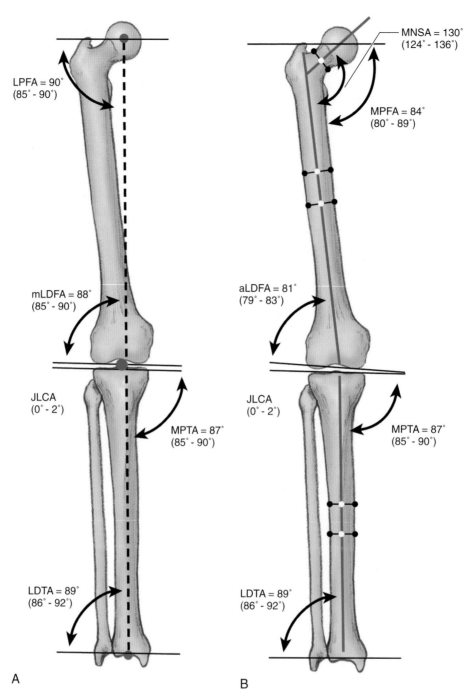

Figure 59-4 A, Mechanical joint orientation angles are based off the mechanical axis. The lateral proximal femoral angle (LPFA) is an angle subtended by the mechanical axis and a line extending from the tip of the greater trochanter to the center of the femoral head (normal, 90 degrees; range, 85 to 95 degrees). The mechanical lateral distal femoral angle (mLDFA) is an angle subtended by the mechanical axis and a line connecting the joint center points of the medial and lateral femoral condyles (normal, 88 degrees; range, 85 to 90 degrees). The medial proximal tibial angle (MPTA) is an angle subtended by the mechanical axis and a line connecting the joint center points of the medial and lateral tibial plateaus (normal, 87 degrees; range, 85 to 90 degrees). The joint line congruence angle (JLCA) is an angle, if any, subtended by the femoral and tibial joint lines as defined (normal, 0 to 2 degrees). The lateral distal tibial angle (LDTA) is an angle subtended by the mechanical axis and a line extending through the plane of the tibial plafond (normal, 89 degrees; range, 86 to 92 degrees). **B,** Anatomic joint orientation angles are derived from an extension of the mid-diaphyseal lines of the bones. The medial proximal femoral angle (MPFA) is an angle subtended by the femoral anatomic axis and a line extending from the tip of the greater trochanter to the center of the femoral head (normal, 84 degrees; range, 80 to 89 degrees). The anatomic lateral distal femoral angle (aLDFA) is an angle subtended by the femoral anatomic axis and the femoral condylar joint line, as defined in **A** (normal, 81 degrees; range, 79 to 83 degrees). The femoral anatomic and mechanical axis subtends an angle of 7 degrees. The anatomic and mechanical axes of the tibia are roughly parallel, so no joint orientation lines based on the tibial anatomic axis are defined. MNSA, mechanical neck shaft angle. (After Paley.[12])

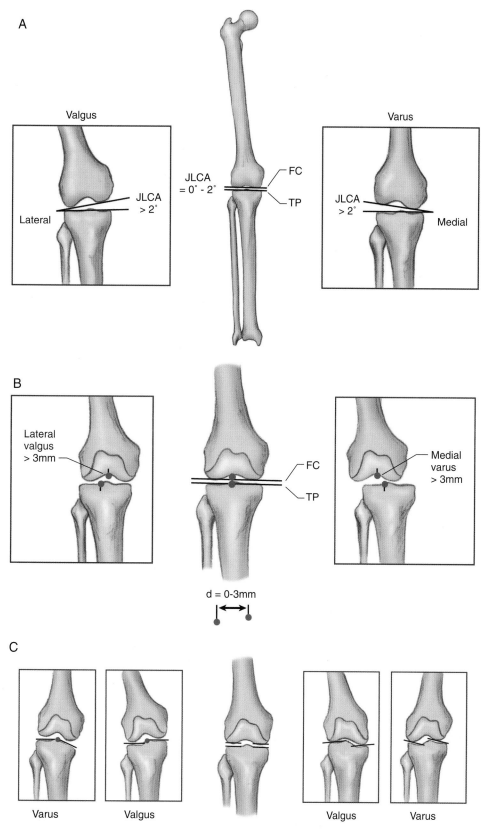

Figure 59-5 Joint line congruence can affect mechanical axis deviation in several ways. **A,** Ligamentous laxity can be unmasked with a standing stress radiograph that shows a joint line congruence angle (JLCA) greater than 2 degrees. **B,** A shift of the midpoints of the femoral and tibial condyles greater than 3 mm indicates subluxation. **C,** Lines extended across the hemicondyles that are not collinear indicate articular incongruity, such as deficient hemicondyles or post-traumatic deformity. FC, femoral condyle; TP, tibial plateau. (After Paley.[12])

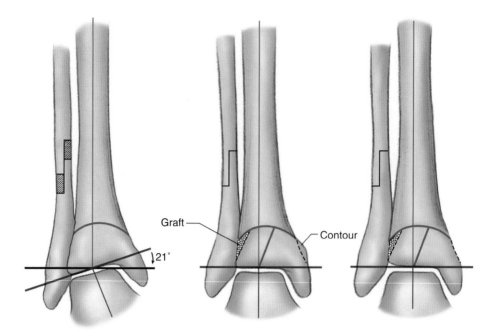

Figure 59-6 A preoperative plan for correction of varus ankle joint orientation. The ankle plane was parallel to the floor because a valgus deformity existed at the knee. If the ankle malorientation is ignored when a distal femoral osteotomy is performed, the plane of the ankle will be oblique (in this case, varus) to the plane of the floor. In this case, the center of rotation angle is at the level of the plafond; thus, a focal dome supramalleolar osteotomy corrects the varus without inducing a secondary translation (which would be the case if an opening or closing wedge were placed at the same level).

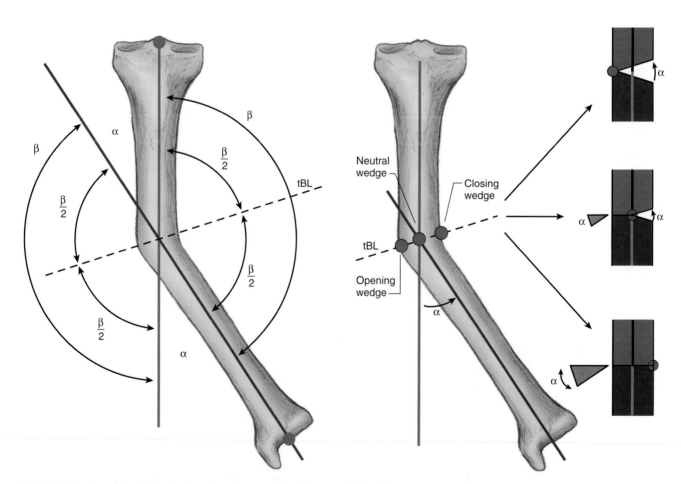

Figure 59-7 The intersection of axis lines (mechanical or anatomic) at the center of rotation angle subtends medial and lateral (ß) as well as proximal and distal (α) angles. A transverse bisector line (tBL) bisects the medial and lateral (ß) angles (ß/2). The α angle indicates the magnitude of correction angle. (After Paley.[12])

Figure 59-8 An angular correction axis placed on the center of rotation angle or anywhere along the transverse bisector line (tBL) results in collinear realignment of the proximal and distal bone segment (anatomic or mechanical) axis. The α angle indicates the magnitude of the correction angle. (After Paley.[12])

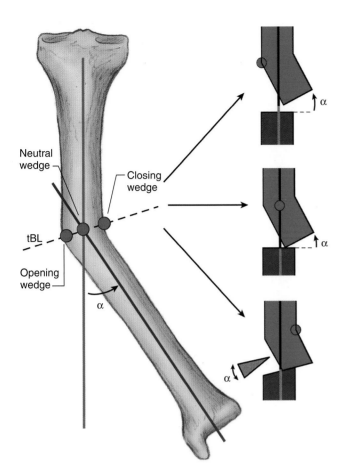

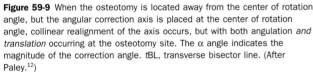

Figure 59-9 When the osteotomy is located away from the center of rotation angle, but the angular correction axis is placed at the center of rotation angle, collinear realignment of the axis occurs, but with both angulation *and translation* occurring at the osteotomy site. The α angle indicates the magnitude of the correction angle. *t*BL, transverse bisector line. (After Paley.[12])

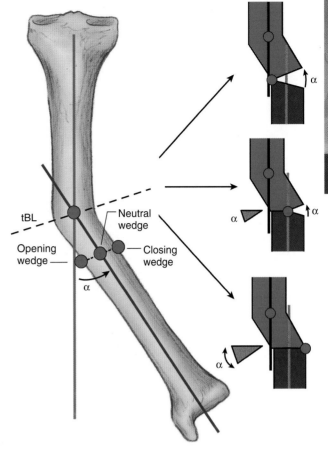

Figure 59-10 If the osteotomy and angular correction axis occur away from the center of rotation angle, a secondary translational deformity is created that may cause persistent mechanical axis deviation. The α angle indicates the magnitude of the correction angle. *t*BL, transverse bisector line. (After Paley.[12])

the limb may appear realigned. One subtle example of this occurs in the case of joint incongruity and a mechanical axis deviation with no other metaphyseal or diaphyseal deformity. In such a patient, the deformity is based entirely on the joint surface deformity, and the center of rotation of angulation will be at the joint line. Any osteotomy other than a focal dome invokes osteotomy rule 3, resulting in a secondary translation deformity, which requires a translation correction to resolve the secondary translation.

To plan a coronal plane distal femoral osteotomy:

- Obtain a standing anteroposterior pelvis to foot radiograph with the beam centered on the knee as shown in Figure 59-1A.

- Obtain supine anteroposterior and lateral films of the femur with the beam centered at the level of the knee as shown in Figure 59-1B.

- Perform the malalignment test by extending a line from the center of the hip to the center of the ankle and determine mechanical axis deviation (Figs. 59-11 and 59-12).

- Determine the mLDFA or aLDFA. *It must be abnormal for a distal femoral osteotomy to be indicated* (see Figs. 59-11 and 59-12).

- Determine medial proximal tibial angle and other joint orientations. If they are also abnormal, multifocal osteotomies may be required (see Figs. 59-11 and 59-12).

- Analyze the joint line congruence angle for ligamentous laxity, subluxation, and joint surface incongruency (see Fig. 59-8).

- Plot the mechanical and anatomic axes of the femur (see Figs. 59-11 and 59-12).

- Extend a normal mLDFA or aLDFA from the plane of the femoral condyles (see Figs. 59-11 and 59-12).

- The intersection of these two lines determines the center of rotation of angulation (see Figs. 59-11 and 59-12).

- From the location of the center of rotation of angulation and anatomic considerations, determine the

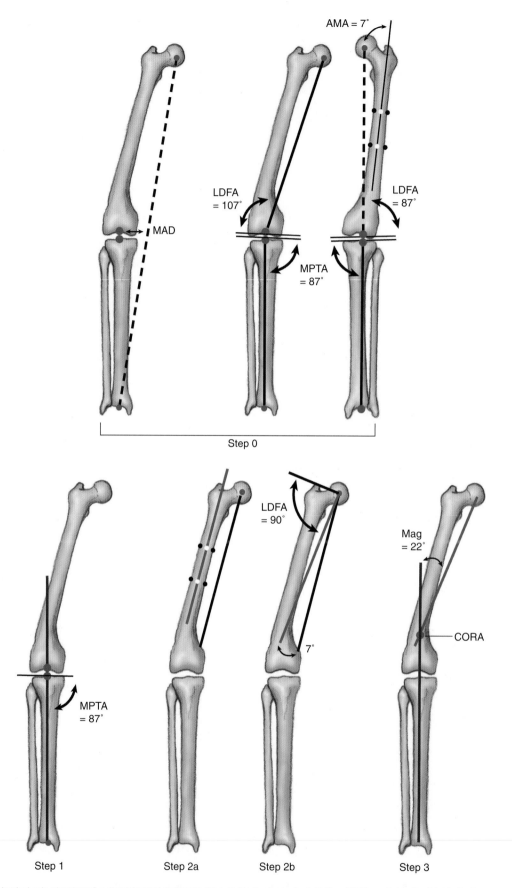

Step 0

Step 1   Step 2a   Step 2b   Step 3

Figure 59-11 Mechanical axis planning of a distal femoral deformity. Step 0: Mechanical axis deviation (MAD) medial to the joint indicates a severe varus deformity. A greater than normal mechanical lateral distal femoral angle (LDFA) indicates deformity on the femoral side. The anatomic-mechanical angle (AMA) is determined from the opposite side. Step 1: Normal medial proximal tibial angle (MPTA) indicates that no deformity exists on the tibial side, so this axis can be extended proximally to locate the center of rotation of angulation (CORA). Step 2: The AMA is used to construct the proximal femoral mechanical axis. Step 3: The intersection of these two lines locates the CORA in the distal femur. LDFA, lateral distal femoral angle; Mag, magnitude of correction. (After Paley.[12])

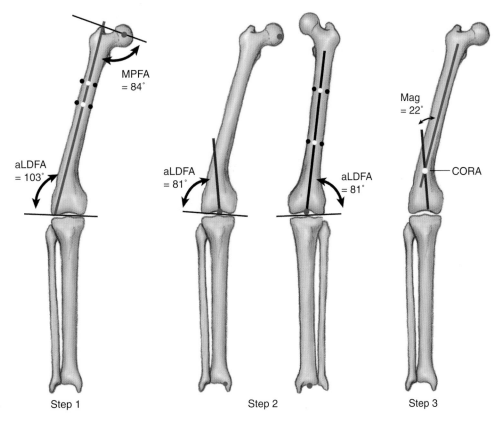

Figure 59-12 Anatomic axis planning of same deformity as shown in Figure 59-11. Step 1: The anatomic axis of the femur is drawn and an anatomic lateral distal femoral angle (aLDFA) determined. Step 2: From the normal side, the aLDFA is determined and drawn. Step 3: The intersection of these two lines indicates the center of correction angulation and the subtended α angle indicates the magnitude of correction (Mag). (After Paley.[12])

level of osteotomy, type of osteotomy, angular correction axis, and whether a compensatory translation will be required.

- Note that before the preceding step, deformity in the sagittal plane, axial malrotation, and length discrepancy must also be determined and factored into the correction.

In the foregoing description, we addressed only the most straightforward single-locus coronal plane deformity. However, the deformity can be sagittal as well as coronal; it can involve axial rotation, lengthening, or shortening; and it can occur at multiple loci on one bone or on both the femoral and tibial segments. The ultimate operative plan resolves all the vectors of deformity to restore normal limb mechanical alignment, joint orientation, and length.

Surgical Technique

Anesthesia, Room Set-up, and Positioning

We perform osteotomies of the lower extremity with the patient under general anesthesia unless medical comor-

bidities preclude such. The patient is positioned supine on an orthopedic table with a completely radiolucent top (Jackson table; OSI, Union City, Calif). We typically use the same preparation and draping for the arthroscopic procedure (if one is performed) and the osteotomy procedure. The limb is draped free from hemipelvis distally; traction is not used. Useful positioning devices include a lateral post on the upper thigh, a roll of sterile bath towels approximately 1 foot in diameter secured with a sterile elastic adhesive wrap bolster under the knee during surgical approaches, and a sandbag or gel cushion secured to the table with tape so the heel can rest on it to help maintain a desired degree of knee flexion (Fig. 59-13). The surgeon stands on the same side for lateral and anterior approaches and on the contralateral side for medial approaches. A C-arm image intensifier is positioned on the opposite side of the surgeon.

Perform or Stage Intra-articular Procedures

Some forms of correction, such as those that involve the use of ring external fixators, may preclude the ability to move the limb through an adequate range of motion to

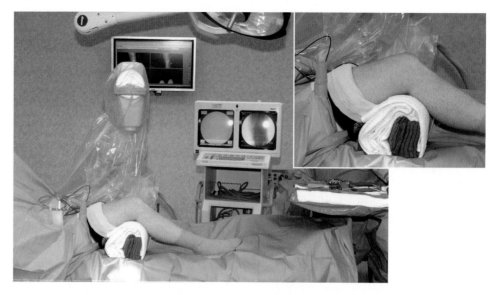

Figure 59-13 Surgical positioning. The patient is supine on a Jackson table with fully radiolucent top. A lateral post and bath towel roll aid in maintaining position for the approach and closure. A sterile tourniquet is used for exposure. A C-arm image intensifier is positioned on the opposite side of the table.

prevent adhesions or the ability to treat the patient with continuous passive motion. In such cases, the intra-articular reconstructions may be done before the osteotomy or at a later date. The latter has greater appeal if intra-articular adhesions have formed; the arthroscopy can be an adjunct to their removal.

Surgical Exposure: Select an Approach

The knee is flexed to 90 degrees and the hip to 45 degrees for exposure and closure to normalize anatomic relationships and to maintain an even skin tension. If a tourniquet is to be used, we use a sterile tourniquet and maintain its inflation only for the exposure. Closure for all approaches is in layers. A bulky dressing and elastic outer wrap minimize edema and effusion.

Lateral Approach

We use a lateral hockey-stick incision for lateral opening and closing wedge osteotomies (Fig. 59-14). The incision can be extended as far proximally as fixation demands. The skin incision is 2 cm anterior to the palpable posterior border of the iliotibial tract. Distally, this incision extends just dorsal and medial to the lateral tibial or Gerdy tubercle. The tract is split just anterior to the lateral intermuscular septum in the interval between the iliotibial tract and iliopatellar ligament fibers. The vastus lateralis muscle fibers of origin can be gently swept off the intermuscular septum with a sharp Cobb elevator. Some vascular perforators may be encountered as the dissection proceeds proximally; they must be cauterized or ligated. If dissection must extend distally to the condylar flare, the superolateral geniculate artery will be encountered and must be

ligated. Subperiosteal dissection can then be carried out just at the osteotomy site, maintaining an intact periosteal sleeve.

Medial Approach

We use a medial hockey stick incision for medial opening and closing wedge osteotomies (Fig. 59-15). The incision can be extended as needed with the caveat that Hunter canal and the femoral artery will be encountered above the distal third of the medial thigh; therefore, care must be exercised to prevent arterial direct or stretch injury. The skin incision is placed just anterior to the medial intermuscular septum and curves as it extends distally to course just medial to the patella and patellar tendon. The sartorial fascia is divided just on the anterior edge of the medial intermuscular septum. The origins of the vastus medialis oblique and vastus medialis muscles are elevated off the intermuscular septum. Again, vascular perforators, the superomedial geniculate artery (distally) and the femoral artery (proximally), may be encountered.

Anterior Approach

This approach is used primarily for a focal dome osteotomy. A full extensile approach, much like that used for total knee arthroplasty, is described here. However, the approach can be minimized by splitting it into a mini–medial arthrotomy (for insertion of a retrograde nail if retrograde nail fixation is used) and a minimal, or percutaneous, quadriceps tendon–splitting incision (for the osteotomy). The extensile skin incision closely parallels the medial border of the patellar tendon and patella, extending proximal to the knee in the anterior midline. The deeper arthrotomy incision divides the retinaculum on the medial border of the patella. The upper border of

59

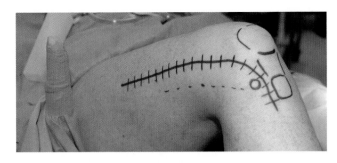

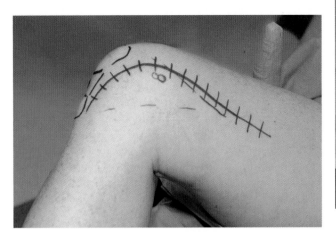

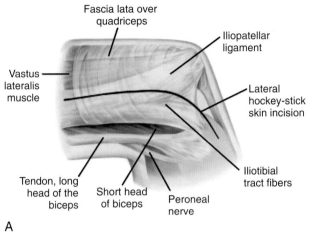

Fascia lata over quadriceps

Vastus lateralis muscle

Iliopatellar ligament

Lateral hockey-stick skin incision

Iliotibial tract fibers

Tendon, long head of the biceps

Short head of biceps

Peroneal nerve

A

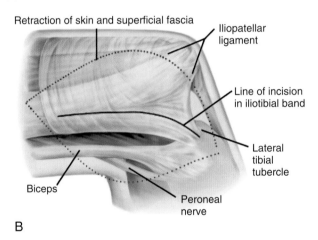

Retraction of skin and superficial fascia

Iliopatellar ligament

Line of incision in iliotibial band

Lateral tibial tubercle

Biceps

Peroneal nerve

B

Figure 59-14 Lateral approach for distal femoral osteotomy. **A,** The skin incision is made 2 cm anterior to the palpable posterior border of the iliotibial tract. **B,** The iliotibial band is split between the iliopatellar ligament and iliotibial tract fibers just on the anterior edge of the lateral intermuscular septum.

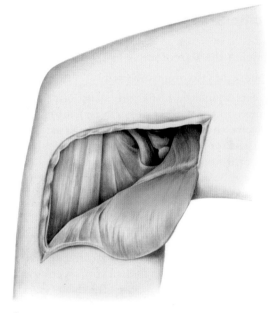

A

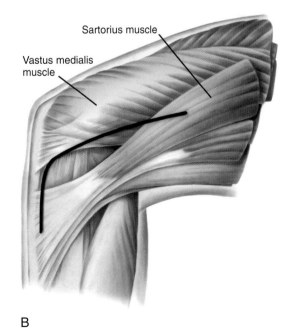

Sartorius muscle

Vastus medialis muscle

B

Figure 59-15 Medial approach for distal femoral osteotomy. The skin incision (**A**) and deeper dissection (**B**) are depicted. Distally, the sartorial fascia is divided along the posterior border of the vastus medialis muscle just anterior to the medial intermuscular septum. As dissection is extended proximally, an interval is developed between the sartorius and vastus medialis muscles.

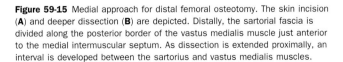

the fat pad may need to be incised. It is better to do so than to traumatize the fat pad, which can lead to fibrosis and secondary infrapatellar contracture. If a synovial plica is encountered, it can be spared or excised, but it should not be incised and repaired, which would lead to painful scarring. As the arthrotomy is extended proximally, it splits the quadriceps tendon along its medial border, leaving a thin cuff of tendon on the vastus medialis to facilitate closure. If the osteotomy is performed within the confines of the suprapatellar pouch, the synovial fatty layer over the periosteum should be incised sharply, protected, and repaired to minimize the possibility of adhesion of the quadriceps tendon to the femur.

Specific Steps (Box 59-2)

Performing the Osteotomy

1. Choose an Osteotomy Method

Bone cuts should be made with sharp blades or bits to minimize heat and thermal necrosis. Cutting technique can involve an oscillating saw cut, a Gigli saw cut (especially useful for metaphyseal percutaneous cuts), an osteotome corticotomy technique, and multiple drill holes (which can be a straight-line cut or involve use of guides such as focal dome guides).

2. Choose an Osteotomy Type

Closing wedge. With this classic corrective osteotomy type, a wedge corresponding to the angle of correction is removed in an attempt to maintain a small corticoperiosteal hinge at the angular correction axis. The bone is gradually deformed into closure by axial loading (Fig. 59-16). This osteotomy is usually stable and heals readily (6 to 10 weeks) when it is placed in metaphyseal bone. If the hinge fractures, it may be necessary to stabilize it as well. Once closed, an osteotomy in the metaphyseal segment will result in some degree of step-off, which increases with the magnitude of correction. Our general rule is to limit closing wedge osteotomies to a magnitude of correction resulting in a step-off no greater than 25% of the longer of the two osteotomy cuts. If a closing wedge is performed by other than osteotomy rule 1, a translation of the mechanical axis will occur unless the hinge is displaced.

Opening wedge. The execution of this osteotomy is simpler because it requires only a single cut and no bone

removal (Fig. 59-17). Again, preservation of a corticoperiosteal hinge at the angular correction axis is a goal, unless osteotomy rule 2 or rule 3 is being followed. The osteotomy is then angularly distracted by use of a variety of instruments, such as lamina spreaders, specialized osteotomy distractors, and temporary external fixators. Once it is open and stabilized, the defect is customarily grafted. We have had excellent success using a combination of a structural allograft (freeze-dried femoral head fashioned as a cortical wedge) with a center core filled with reamed autograft by the reamer-irrigator-aspirator system (Synthes USA, Paoli, Pa).

Biplane wedge. When an angular deformity occurs in both the coronal and sagittal planes, a variant of the closing and opening wedge osteotomies may be required. A biplane wedge can be cut (closing wedge type) or biplane distraction and fixation performed (opening wedge type) to achieve correction of the more complex deformity.

Focal dome. When the center of rotation of angulation exists at or extremely near the joint line, a focal dome osteotomy allows correction of the angular deformity without causing a secondary translation of the mechanical axis. For this type of osteotomy, a special focal dome guide is used (Fig. 59-18). Its axis of rotation is placed at the center of rotation of angulation, which will also become the angular correction axis. The osteotomy is usually performed with multiple drill holes and may even be accomplished through a minimal incision or percutaneous approach. The drill holes are connected with a narrow osteotome. The undulations of such a cut provide additional stability from derotation of the osteotomy once correction is achieved. They also act as gears for correction because the osteotome can be inserted into the osteotomy site and rotated, catching a drill hole edge and rotating the segment around the angular correction axis.

One method of focal dome correction, fixator-assisted nailing, involves the intraoperative application of a temporary monopolar external fixator to aid in achieving and holding a focal dome correction while a retrograde nail is passed (Fig. 59-19). This method ensures that the nail is channeled precisely through the distal segment to achieve the greatest stability. It also facilitates an almost percutaneous approach to performance and fixation of this osteotomy. The fixator is removed after the nail is locked.[12]

Callus distraction. Callus distraction, or Ilizarov-like procedures, are the method of choice for the following corrections: a severe magnitude; a deformity with a structure at risk, for example, a case in which an acute correction could result in neurovascular compromise; a significant translation; a leg length discrepancy as a component of the deformity; a severe rotational deformity; and a multiplane deformity that requires correction of angulation, translation, and rotation simultaneously. In these procedures, the frame is mounted to the limb segment, and a limited incision corticotomy is performed. For simpler angular correc-

Text continued on p. 593.

Box 59-2 Surgical Steps

1. Choose an osteotomy method
2. Choose an osteotomy type
3. Perform and assess correction intraoperatively
4. Select a fixation method

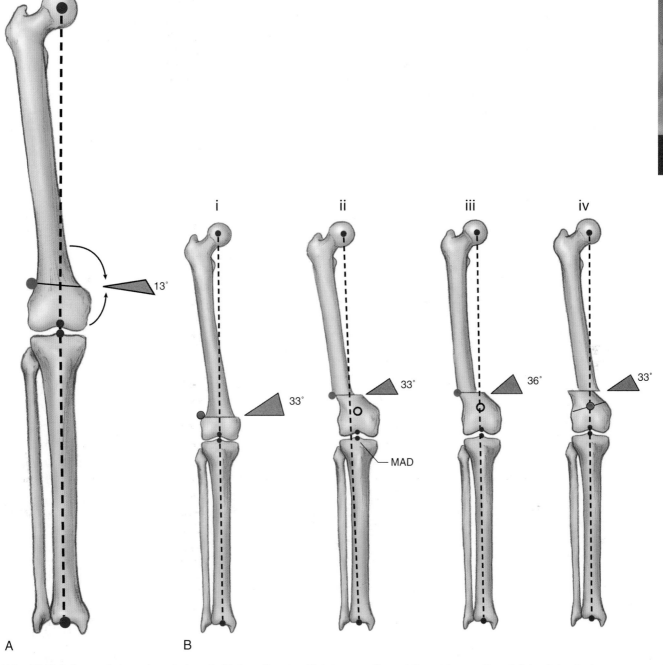

i ii iii iv

A B

Figure 59-16 A, A varus closing wedge osteotomy. In this knee, there is a 13-degree correction, and the angular correction axis is located on the transverse bisector line at the lateral cortex. **B,** The effect of location of the osteotomy. **i,** The osteotomy is near the center of rotation axis, and mechanical axis deviation is corrected without a secondary translation. **ii,** The angular correction axis and the osteotomy are at a different level from the center of rotation axis, and a translation has been created; mechanical axis deviation (MAD) may not be corrected unless a greater correction angle is chosen (**iii**) or a translation correction is performed as well (**iv**). (After Paley.[12])

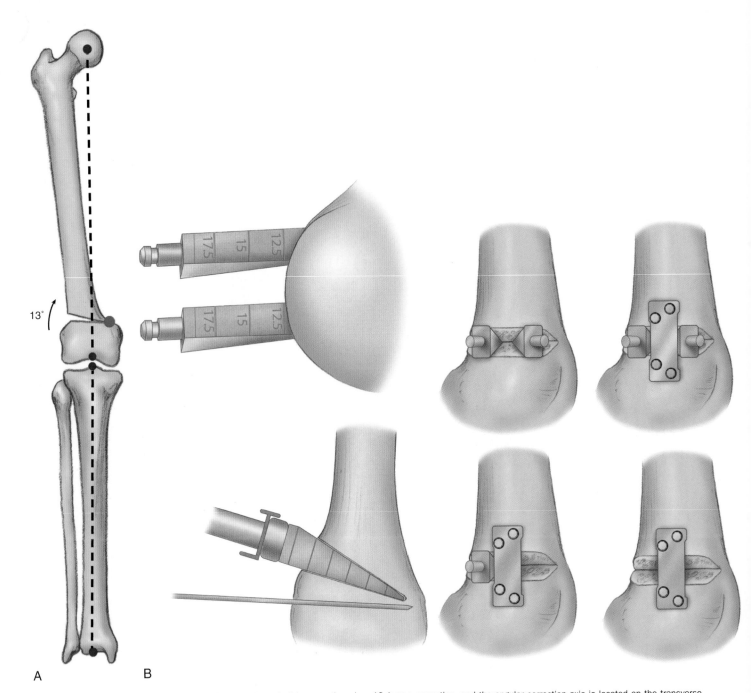

Figure 59-17 A, A varus opening wedge osteotomy. In this case, there is a 13-degree correction, and the angular correction axis is located on the transverse bisector line at the medial cortex. **B,** Wedge distractors designed by Puddu and Arthrex open the osteotomy to the desired correction and maintain that correction until fixation is secured. (After Paley.[12])

A

B

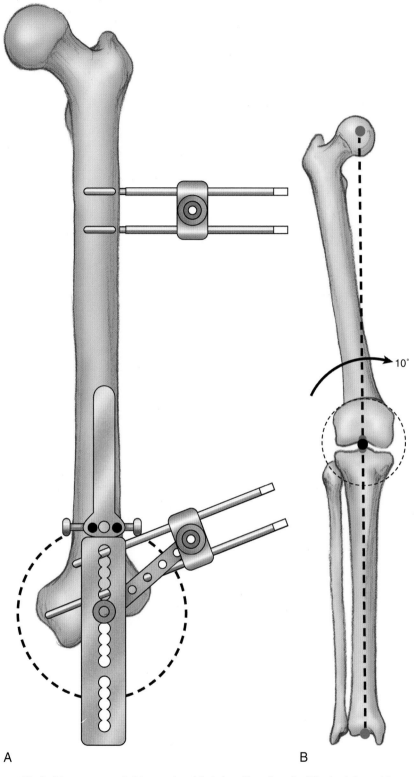

A   B

Figure 59-18 A, A focal dome guide (in this case, connected to an external fixator) positions the axis of the focal dome at the angular correction axis and center of rotation of angulation and guides placement of multiple drill holes in an arc of variable radius from the angular correction axis. **B,** A focal dome osteotomy with the angular correction axis and center of rotation of angulation at the joint line. Mechanical axis deviation is corrected without an induced translation. (After Paley.[12])

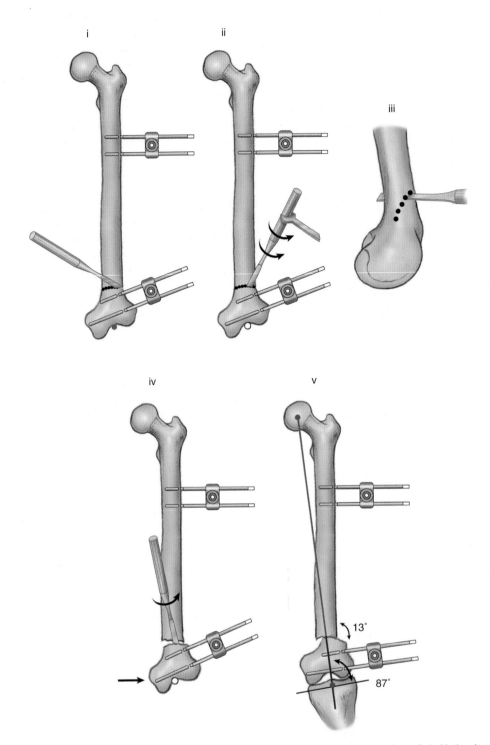

Figure 59-19 Fixator-assisted correction. **i,** A temporary monopolar external fixator with distal angulator pin clamp is applied with the pins eccentric so as not to occlude the intramedullary canal, and a focal dome osteotomy is performed. **ii** and **iii,** A narrow osteotome inserted in the osteotomy and gently rotated causes the osteotomy to rotate into correction, the drill holes acting as gears against the instrument. **iv,** The fixator and manipulation of the extremity aid in correction. The angular correction axis and center of rotation of angulation are on the joint line. **v,** With correction obtained and mechanical axis deviation eliminated, the fixator can be used to hold correction and even compress the osteotomy while definitive fixation, such as a retrograde intramedullary nail, is applied. The fixator is then removed. (After Paley.[12])

tions, the external fixator is applied so that the "hinge" of the fixator is placed on the angular correction axis or somewhere along the transverse bisector line. These more straightforward corrections can be accomplished with angulator-type monopolar fixators, such as the Heidelberg frame (Smith & Nephew, Memphis, Tenn). However, as the osteotomy nears the joint line, a ring with tensioned wires becomes necessary for adequate fixation of a short segment. The more complex deformities are best addressed with multiaxial frames, such as the Taylor Spatial Frame (Smith & Nephew, Memphis, Tenn), that allow correction of 6 degrees of freedom simultaneously. It is far beyond the scope of this chapter to discuss callus distraction techniques in detail, but many excellent resources exist for further training in these methods.

3. Perform and Assess Correction Intraoperatively

For single-stage osteotomies, correction is achieved by trying to maintain a corticoperiosteal hinge (for opening and closing wedge types) and intact periosteal sleeve. Closing wedge osteotomies are best corrected by gradual axial loading, deforming the hinge into closure. A variety of internal distractors or use of a temporary external fixator aids in achieving correction of opening wedge osteotomies. Focal dome osteotomies can be literally cranked into position by rotating a narrow osteotome inserted into the osteotomy site. Correction of the mechanical axis can be estimated intraoperatively by stretching a Bovie cord from the center of the femoral head to the center of the ankle (position verified by fluoroscopy and imaging of the knee to determine where the corrected mechanical axis falls; Fig. 59-20).

For callus distraction methods using external fixation and gradual correction, intraoperative assessment is obviously limited to ensuring that a complete corticotomy has been accomplished. The corticotomy is then compressed, and the external fixator position is locked.

4. Select a Fixation Method

A variety of fixation devices are available for stabilizing osteotomies of the distal femur.

Plate fixation. Probably the classic fixation of recent decades has been the fixed-angle blade plate. It affords excellent stability but is more technically demanding than other methods. The condylar screw plate offers the stability of a fixed-angle device but is technically easier to implant. This ease of insertion does, however, come at the expense of lesser rotational stability of the distal segment in the sagittal plane. Newer distal femoral locking plates function as a fixed-angle device with stability equivalent to a blade plate. They are less technically demanding than a blade plate or condylar screw plate, and many of these plates offer the ability to be implanted through a minimal incision. As the osteotomy level approaches the diaphyseal-metaphyseal junction, simple dynamic compression–like or locking plates may be adequate. A recent variant,

the strut buttress plate, such as the Puddu plate (Arthrex, Naples, Fla), has been developed specifically for stabilizing opening wedge osteotomies (see Fig. 59-17).

Intramedullary rod. The retrograde rod and fixator-assisted nailing are discussed earlier in the section on focal dome osteotomy. Retrograde rods are capable of stable fixation of very distal osteotomies, although some morbidity to the knee joint is associated with their insertion. As the osteotomy level moves proximally, conventional antegrade nails can also be used. It is important to stabilize the correction provisionally, as with the fixator-assisted nailing technique, and to centralize reaming in the distal segment to prevent recurrence of the deformity. Blocking screws remain an option to aid in stabilizing antegrade rods in short distal metaphyseal segments.

External fixation. These techniques and options are discussed earlier in the section on callus distraction. They include monopolar, monopolar angulator, ring, and spatial frames.

PEARLS AND PITFALLS

- Do not approach realignment osteotomy without a sound preoperative plan that determines all the elements (magnitude, angulation, translation, rotation) and locations of the deformity, the anatomic constraints, and the location and types of osteotomies with respective fixation.

- Osteotomy should not be approached as a "cookbook" procedure. Choose the osteotomy (or combination of osteotomies) that best addresses the deformity.

- Be aware of the effect of a distal femoral osteotomy on the joint orientation of the ankle.

- If the center of rotation of angulation is on the joint line, focal dome osteotomy alone will correct the angulation without requiring a secondary translation correction.

- Consider staging intra-articular procedures in cases of poor bone quality or any other situation in which rehabilitation of the intra-articular procedure may be compromised by the osteotomy or its fixation.

- Check the adequacy of correction intraoperatively (unless distraction techniques are to be used) by simulating the malalignment test with a cautery cord stretched from the hip center to ankle center.

- Limit closing wedge osteotomies to a magnitude of correction that will result in a step-off no greater than 25% of the longer of the two osteotomy cuts.

Postoperative Considerations

Rehabilitation

It is critical to begin joint mobilization immediately, particularly if intra-articular procedures such as arthroscopy, synovectomy, and chondroplasty have been a part of the surgical technique. We begin passive joint mobilization and active-assisted joint range-of-motion exercises on postoperative day 1. If articular surface reconstruction was

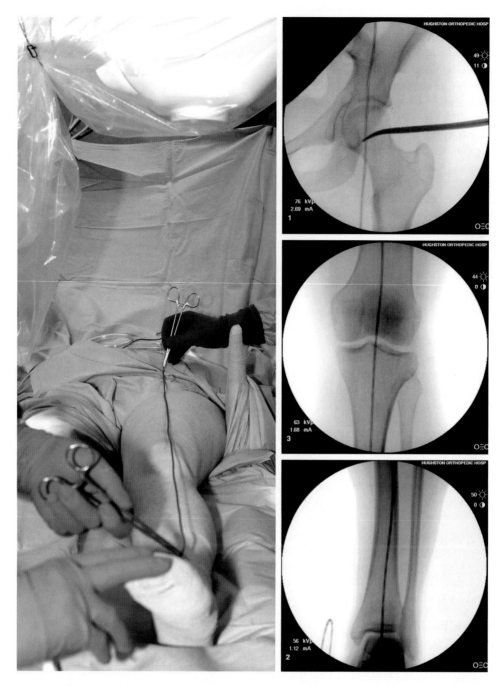

Figure 59-20 Determination of mechanical axis deviation correction intraoperatively. A cautery cord is stretched from the center of the femoral head to the center of the ankle plafond as determined fluoroscopically. Mechanical axis deviation can then be assessed from a fluoroscopic image of the knee.

performed, we awaken the patient secured on continuous passive motion (CPM). CPM is continued 10 hours a day for 3 to 4 weeks, depending on the magnitude of the procedure. For non-CPM patients, an exercise bicycle with minimal resistance is initiated early. CPM patients transition off CPM to the bicycle. If joint rehabilitation as outlined cannot be undertaken as a result of the stability or constraints of fixation, for example, with the use of ring fixators, articular procedures are best done before, or preferably, after the osteotomy.

Isometric muscle rehabilitation is begun immediately. Closed chain resistive exercise is started as quickly as the limb allows. Functional rehabilitation begins when the osteotomy is sufficiently healed and motion and strength are within 20% of normal.

The surgery to weight-bearing interval is governed by a number of variables, including type of osteotomy, stability of fixation, bone quality, complexity of the correction, and whether the correction is being accomplished by single-stage osteotomy or callus distraction techniques.

Complications

With proper planning and patient selection, good technique, and appropriate rehabilitation, complications should be minimal. In our institution, the most common cause of reoperation after osteotomy has been for planned hardware removal. Incomplete planning, inadequate execution, and poor compliance of the patient can lead to a failure of a complete correction. This is also true with regard to a delayed union or nonunion that is affected by poor bone quality, poor circulation, and smoking during the healing or callus-distraction phase. Lack of adequate rehabilitation or failure to stage a procedure when appropriate may lead to persistent joint pain and stiffness. *A failure to institute appropriate measures to identify risk and to provide adequate prophylaxis may lead to venous thrombosis.* Nerve or vascular injury, although always a concern, is more of a risk in patients who require severe magnitude corrections. Unless it is preexisting, infection can be minimized with aseptic intraoperative and perioperative technique. If external fixation is used, pin track sepsis can be minimized with proper pin placement and a structured postoperative pin-site care program.

Results of Distal Femoral Osteotomy (Table 59-1)

Lateral Osteoarthritis and the Valgus Knee, Closing Wedge with a Blade Plate

Healy et al[5] reported their results in a series of 23 distal femoral osteotomies with a follow-up of 4 years. The Hospital for Special Surgery knee score improved from an average of 65 points to 86 points postoperatively in patients with osteoarthritis. McDermott et al[10] reported a successful result in 22 of 24 patients, for whom the greatest improvement was found in the pain category. Miniaci et al[11] reported 86% good or excellent results in a series of 40 patients, with a mean follow-up of 5.5 years. Finkelstein et al,[2] in a study of 21 knees, demonstrated that the probability of survival at 10 years was 64%. In an analysis of 15 closing wedge varus femoral osteotomies, Marti et al[9] obtained 75% good results without any complications. Marin Morales et al[8] reported on 17 cases of osteoarthritis of the knee with valgus deformity in 17 patients, treated by femoral supracondylar varus osteotomy. The mean follow-up time was 6.5 years. The Hospital for Special Surgery score was used to evaluate the clinical results, and nearly 75% were excellent or good. Wang and Hsu[16] described 30 patients with a mean duration of follow-up of 99 months; 25 patients (83%) had a satisfactory result and two had a fair result according to the Hospital for Special Surgery rating system. The remaining three patients had conversion to a total knee arthroplasty. With conversion to total knee arthroplasty as the endpoint, the cumulative 10-year survival rate for all patients was 87%, and the results did not appear to be affected by the presence of patellofemoral arthritis.

Other Fixation

Stahelin et al[15] used an incomplete oblique osteotomy of the distal aspect of the femur in 21 knees and stabilized the osteotomy site with a malleable semitubular plate, which was bent to form an angled plate, and lag screws. The mean duration of follow-up was 5 years. The osteosynthesis failed in only one knee. The loss of correction in 18 knees, after bone healing, averaged 1.7 degrees.

Types of Fixation

Koval et al[6] performed a biomechanical cadaver study in which a distal femoral osteotomy was created, reduced, and stabilized under compression by random assignment to one of three methods of fixation: (1) six-hole 95-degree supracondylar plate, (2) retrograde inserted statically locked supracondylar intramedullary nail, and (3) antegrade inserted statically locked nail. The 95-degree plate provided significantly stiffer fixation than the supracondylar intramedullary nail or antegrade nail in both a compressed transverse and a gap distal femoral osteotomy model. The 95-degree plate and antegrade nail had greater loads to failure than the supracondylar intramedullary nail.

Table 59-1 Clinical Results of Distal Femoral Osteotomy

Author	Mean Follow-up	No. of Procedures	Outcome
Lateral Osteoarthritis, Valgus Knee, Closing Wedge with Blade Plate			
Healy et al[5] (1988)	4 years	23 in 21 patients	83% (19/23) good or excellent, 17% (4/23) fair or poor; mean HSS knee score improved 21 points
McDermott et al[10] (1988)	4 years	24 patients	22 successful
Miniaci et al[11] (1990)	5.5 years	40 patients	86% good or excellent
Finkelstein et al[2] (1996)	133 months	21 in 20 patients	64% 10-year survival rate
Marti et al[9] (2000)	Not reported	15	75% good results
Marin Morales et al[8] (2000)	6.5 years	17 in 17 patients	75% good or excellent HSS score
Wang and Hsu[16] (2005)	99 months	30 in 30 patients	87% 10-year survival rate
Lateral Osteoarthritis, Valgus Knee with Other Fixation			
Stahelin et al[15] (2000)	5 years	21 in 19 patients	17 successful; 3 prolonged crutch use of immobilization; 1 failure 18 loss of correction of 1.7 degrees
Lateral Osteoarthritis with Ligamentous Laxity			
Cameron and Saha[1] (1994)	Not reported	35	34 improved gait pattern
Paley et al[13] (1994)	1 year	23 in 17 patients	19 excellent; 2 fair; 2 poor
Focal Dome Osteotomy			
Gugenheim and Brinker[3] (2003)	33 months	14	12 had normal mechanical lateral femoral angle
Pediatric Torsional Deformity			
Handelsman et al[4] (2005)	Not reported	38 in 21 patients	Bone union occurred at an average of 10 weeks

HSS, Hospital for Special Surgery.

Ligamentous Laxity

Cameron and Saha[1] treated 35 patients with chronic medial collateral ligament instability with a distal femoral osteotomy. Improvement in gait pattern was achieved in 34 of 35 patients, but the medial collateral ligament usually remains lax even after the osteotomy. In another series, Paley et al[13] reported excellent results in 19 of 23 knees with medial collateral ligament laxity corrected by osteotomy and distraction osteogenesis, although most of the patients in the study had congenital or developmental dysplasia.

Focal Dome Osteotomy

Gugenheim and Brinker[3] reported a series of patients with 14 femora with abnormal mechanical lateral distal femoral angles. They used an external fixator–assisted retrograde intramedullary nail and a percutaneous distal femoral dome osteotomy. The mean duration of follow-up was 33 months, and the mean healing time was 13 weeks. The mechanical lateral distal femoral angle was normal in 12 of the 14 knees.

Pediatric Torsional Deformity

Supracondylar osteotomies were performed on 38 femora in 21 children with femoral torsional and angular deformities.[4] All osteotomies were maintained by an external fixator. Bone union occurred at an average of 10 weeks.

References

1. Cameron JC, Saha S. Management of medial collateral ligament laxity. Orthop Clin North Am 1994;25:527-532.

2. Finkelstein JA, Gross AE, Davis A. Varus osteotomy of the distal part of the femur. A survivorship analysis. J Bone Joint Surg Am 1996;78:1348-1352.

3. Gugenheim JJ Jr, Brinker MR. Bone realignment with use of temporary external fixation for distal femoral valgus and varus deformities. J Bone Joint Surg Am 2003;85:1229-1237.

4. Handelsman JE, Weinberg J, Friedman S. The role of the small AO external fixator in supracondylar rotational femoral osteotomies. J Pediatr Orthop B 2005;14:194-197.

5. Healy WL, Anglen JO, Wasilewski SA, et al. Distal femoral varus osteotomy. J Bone Joint Surg Am 1988;70:102-109.

6. Koval KJ, Kummer FJ, Bharam S, et al. Distal femoral fixation: a laboratory comparison of the 95 degrees plate, antegrade and retrograde inserted reamed intramedullary nails. J Orthop Trauma 1996;10:378-382.

7. Maquet PGJ. Biomechanics of the Knee: With Application to the Pathogenesis and Surgical Treatment of Osteoarthritis, 2nd ed. New York, Springer-Verlag, 1984.

8. Marin Morales LA, Gomez Navalon LA, Zorrilla Ribot P, et al. Treatment of osteoarthritis of the knee with valgus deformity by means of varus osteotomy. Acta Orthop Belg 2000;66:272-278.

9. Marti R, Schroder J, Witteveen A. The closed wedge varus supracondylar osteotomy. Oper Tech Sports Med 2000;8:48-55.

10. McDermott AG, Finklestein JA, Farine I, et al. Distal femoral varus osteotomy for valgus deformity of the knee. J Bone Joint Surg Am 1988;70:110-116.

11. Miniaci A, Grossman S, Jacob R. Supracondylar femoral varus osteotomy in the treatment of valgus knee deformity. Am J Knee Surg 1990;3:65-73.

12. Paley D. Principals of Deformity Correction. New York, Springer-Verlag, 2002.

13. Paley D, Bhatnagar J, Herzenberg JE, et al. New procedures for tightening knee collateral ligaments in conjunction with knee realignment osteotomy. Orthop Clin North Am 1994;25:533-555.

14. Pauwels F. Biomechanics of the Locomotor Apparatus. New York, Springer-Verlag, 1980.

15. Stahelin T, Hardegger F, Ward JC. Supracondylar osteotomy of the femur with use of compression. Osteosynthesis with a malleable implant. J Bone Joint Surg Am 2000;82:712-722.

16. Wang JW, Hsu CC. Distal femoral varus osteotomy for osteoarthritis of the knee. J Bone Joint Surg Am 2005;87:127-133.

59

Patellar Tendon Autograft for Anterior Cruciate Ligament Reconstruction

Joshua M. Alpert, MD
Charles A. Bush-Joseph, MD
Bernard R. Bach, Jr., MD

Anterior cruciate ligament (ACL) rupture commonly occurs among both professional and amateur athletes. As the ACL is the primary restraint to anterior displacement of the tibia on the femur and a secondary stabilizer to tibial rotation, an ACL-deficient knee can lead to meniscal injury, functional instability, and early-onset osteoarthritis.[3] These are potentially devastating consequences in certain populations of patients, especially in athletes who participate in cutting or pivoting activities. The ACL is the most frequently torn knee ligament requiring surgical repair, and there are more than 100,000 ACL reconstructions each year in the United States.[14]

There are a variety of treatment options in regard to surgical technique, graft source, and graft fixation for ACL reconstruction. Graft options may include autograft (bone–patellar tendon–bone, hamstring, and quadriceps tendon) or allograft (bone–patellar tendon–bone, Achilles tendon, and anterior tibialis tendon) tissue. The bone–patellar tendon–bone autograft is the most commonly used graft during the last 15 years and the graft of choice of physicians treating NCAA Division 1A and professional athletes.[2,6-8,12] This is due to the graft's ready accessibility, good mechanical strength, bone healing, and interference screw fixation. This chapter details the surgical technique for endoscopic ACL reconstruction with a bone–patellar tendon–bone autograft.

Preoperative Considerations

History

The diagnosis of ACL injury is often apparent from the characteristic history alone that is provided by the patient. Typical descriptions of the injury mechanism include the following:

- A noncontact injury that occurs during a change-of-direction maneuver, such as pivoting, cutting, or decelerating.
- The patient may note knee hyperextension during an awkward landing.
- A "pop" is heard or felt during the event.
- Acute onset of significant swelling often develops in minutes to hours.
- A sensation of instability limits one's ability to return to play.
- The patient complains of catching or locking (signifies meniscal disease, stump impingement, or loose bodies).
- The patient's age, history of anterior knee pain or patellar instability and other previous knee injury, and contralateral knee instability are critical to decision-making.

Physical Examination

The physical examination is essential in the diagnosis of ACL injury and the evaluation of associated pathologic changes, such as meniscal or chondral damage and associated ligamentous injury.

Assessment of the injured knee includes evaluation of gait, limb alignment, presence of an effusion, knee range of motion, patellar instability, anterior knee or joint line tenderness, and varus or valgus laxity. The Lachman and pivot shift tests remain the most specific examinations for the evaluation of ACL injury. A positive result of the posterior drawer test, posterior sag, or increased tibial external rotation at 30 or 90 degrees signals the presence of associated posterior cruciate ligament (PCL) or posterolateral corner injury. Instrumented knee arthrometry with anterior drawer testing at 30 degrees can be helpful in confirming ACL injury when the side-to-side difference is greater than 3 mm.

Imaging

Radiography

Despite recent trends, plain radiographic imaging remains critical in the initial evaluation of patients with suspected ACL injuries. Weight-bearing radiographs are essential to visualize joint space, notch architecture, and bone alignment. Lateral radiographs may reveal an avulsion of the tibial eminence or lateral capsule (Segond fracture). Radiographic views commonly used in evaluating patients with knee ligament injuries include the following:

- Weight-bearing anteroposterior radiograph in full extension
- Weight-bearing posteroanterior 45-degree flexion radiograph
- Non–weight-bearing 45-degree flexion lateral view
- Axial view of the patellofemoral joint (Merchant view)

Magnetic Resonance Imaging

Magnetic resonance imaging is performed to evaluate the ACL, PCL, medial collateral ligament, lateral collateral ligament, menisci, and associated articular cartilage injury.

Indications and Contraindications

The ideal candidate for an ACL reconstruction with bone–patellar tendon–bone autograft is a young, active patient with no effusion, full range of motion, and no patellar tendon disease. In addition, those patients with symptomatic intra-articular disease, such as meniscal injury or loose bodies, may benefit from earlier surgical intervention. Of note, it is vital to educate the patient concerning the risks and benefits of the various graft options for the patient to make the final informed decision. For example, patients with certain professions, such as roofers and carpet layers, should be counseled about the increased incidence of discomfort with kneeling.

ACL reconstruction with a bone–patellar tendon–bone autograft is relatively contraindicated in patients with degenerative joint disease, in patients with a history of patellar tendon disease, and in those patients who are sedentary, inactive, or elderly. In addition, patients who have limited motion preoperatively or who are unable to comply with a rigorous postoperative protocol are poor candidates as well. Patients with a history of anterior knee pain or pain with kneeling should be advised to choose a different graft option. Last, ACL reconstruction in the skeletally immature patient remains a challenge and requires extensive discussion of the risks and benefits involved. In patients with significant growth remaining, soft tissue grafts such as hamstring, rather than bone–patellar tendon–bone grafts, are thought to pose less risk of premature physeal closure.

Surgical Planning

Preoperative rehabilitation is essential to successful surgical outcomes. Before surgery, all patients undergo extensive physical therapy, focusing on closed-chain hamstring and quadriceps stretching and strengthening to regain full range of motion and a normal gait pattern.

Surgical Technique

Anesthesia and Positioning

After induction of general, spinal, or regional anesthesia, the patient is placed in the supine position on a standard operating room table. A thorough examination under anesthesia is performed.

Examination under anesthesia includes the Lachman test, anterior and posterior drawer tests, varus and valgus stress testing, and pivot shift test. Evaluation of external rotation at 30 and 90 degrees of flexion is important to assess the stability of the posterolateral corner. Comparison examination of the contralateral knee is done as well. If pivot shift testing demonstrates clear ACL insufficiency, the bone–patellar tendon–bone graft can be harvested before diagnostic arthroscopy.

At this time, a tourniquet is placed and the thigh secured in a leg holder for added stability. The contralateral leg is positioned in a well-padded foot holder with the knee and hip flexed to protect the peroneal nerve. The foot

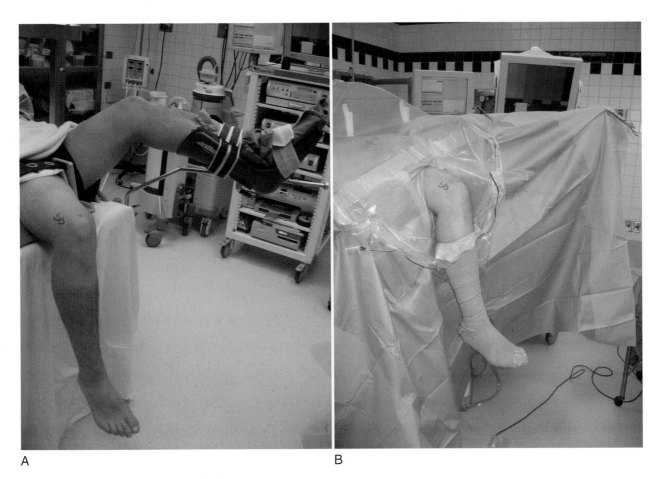

A   B

Figure 60-1 Positioning of the patient before (**A**) and after (**B**) draping.

of the operating room table is then dropped and the waist is flexed to diminish the amount of lumbar extension (Fig. 60-1). The leg is prepared and draped in sterile fashion as preoperative antibiotics are administered.

Surgical Landmarks, Incisions, and Portals

Landmarks

- Patella
- Patellar tendon
- Tibial tubercle
- Fibular head
- Gerdy tubercle

Incision

The longitudinal incision for the bone–patellar tendon–bone harvest starts at the most distal aspect of the patella, just medial to the midline, coursing distally to 2 cm below the tibial tubercle (Fig. 60-2).

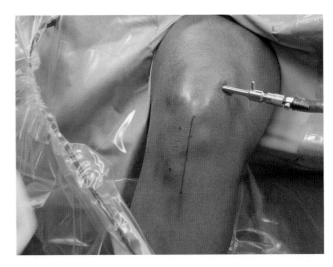

Figure 60-2 Surgical landmarks and skin incision.

Portals

- Superomedial portal
- Inferolateral portal
- Inferomedial portal (made through graft harvest site)

Examination Under Anesthesia and Diagnostic Arthroscopy

Examination under anesthesia is completed as previously described. Of note, if the examination under anesthesia is unclear regarding ACL rupture, diagnostic arthroscopy is performed before harvesting of the bone–patellar tendon–bone graft.[7]

Diagnostic arthroscopy evaluates the patellofemoral joint, medial and lateral gutters, suprapatellar pouch, and medial and lateral compartments to assess for any meniscal disease, loose bodies, and articular cartilage injury. The intercondylar notch is visualized as well to evaluate the PCL and ACL for injury.

Specific Steps (Box 60-1)

1. Bone–Patellar Tendon–Bone Graft Harvest

After the anatomic landmarks have been appropriately marked and the knee is flexed, a longitudinal incision, just medial to midline, is made from the distal tip of the patella to 2 cm distal to the tibial tubercle. This incision allows graft harvest and placement of the tibial tunnel through the same operative approach. This incision is carried directly down to the transverse fibers of the peritenon of the patellar tendon. After skin flaps are raised both medially and laterally, a No. 15 blade is used to incise the peritenon longitudinally at its midline. Metzenbaum scissors extend this cut proximally and distally as well as undermine the peritenon medially and laterally to fully expose the entire patellar tendon.

The patellar tendon's width is measured proximally and distally and marked with a marking pen. The bone–patellar tendon–bone autograft ideally is 10 mm wide with 10×25-mm bone plugs. Parallel longitudinal incisions spaced 10 mm apart are made in the patellar tendon, then the periosteum and soft tissues overlying the tibial and patellar bone cuts are outlined with the blade. The tendon incisions are performed with the knee flexed, thus keeping the patellar tendon on tension; extension of the knee aids in the transverse crosscuts at the patellar and tibial bone block edges.

Box 60-1 Surgical Steps

1. Graft harvest
2. Graft preparation
3. Notch preparation and notchplasty
4. Tibial tunnel placement
5. Femoral tunnel placement
6. Graft placement and fixation
7. Closure

At this point, an oscillating saw is used to make first the tibial, then the patellar bone plug. With use of the nondominant thumb to stabilize the saw and the index finger to protect the graft between the inner and outer portion of the graft (Fig.60-3), the tibial cortex is scored longitudinally on profile to remove an equilateral triangle of bone. This leaves a maximal amount of bone around the tibial tubercle and remaining patellar tendon to minimize the risk of postoperative complications, such as patellar tendon avulsion or tubercle fracture. The distal transverse tibial crosscut is made with the saw held at a 45-degree oblique angle to the cortex by use of the corner of the blade on each side of the plug, but the tibial bone plug is left in place at this time. The patellar tendon bone plug is then made in a trapezoid shape, with a depth not exceeding 6 to 7 mm to avoid damage to the articular surface. Once again, the proximal transverse crosscut is made at a 45-degree oblique angle to the cortex. The saw is then placed parallel to the medial and lateral edges to complete the patellar bone plug crosscuts. Half-inch and quarter-inch curved osteotomes are now used to carefully mobilize the bone plugs without levering. A lap sponge can be placed around the freed tibial plug to improve traction, and Metzenbaum scissors are used to carefully remove any remaining fat or soft tissues. Once it is freed, the graft is wrapped in a moist sponge and walked to the back table by the operative surgeon, where it is placed in a safe location known to all members of the surgical team.

2. Graft Preparation

Ideally, 10×25-mm bone plugs are sized. The first step involves measurement and documentation of the overall graft length, the length of the bone plugs, and the length of the tendinous portion of the graft. At this time, the bone plugs are sized with a small rongeur to remove excess bone and to contour the bone appropriately to fit the desired tunnel diameter, frequently 10 mm. Excess bone should be saved for grafting of the harvest sites. The longer bone plug can be placed on the femoral side, thus avoiding a length mismatch between the tibial tunnel and graft. If one bone plug is wider, we prefer to use it on the tibial side, where we usually drill an 11-mm tunnel.

Next, drill holes are made in the tibial and femoral bone blocks. Various configurations have been described. We prefer two holes in the tibial and one hole in the femoral bone block for heavy nonresorbable sutures (Fig. 60-4). These holes can be placed either through the cortex or parallel to it; the latter decreases the risk of cutting the sutures during interference screw placement but also decreases pullout strength from the bone block. If a "push-through" technique is used, the femoral bone plug does not require any holes or sutures and remains as is. A sterile pen is used to mark the cortical surface of the tibial bone plug to assist in graft orientation; the femoral bone plug is marked at the bone-tendon junction to better assess correct seating of the plug within the tunnel.

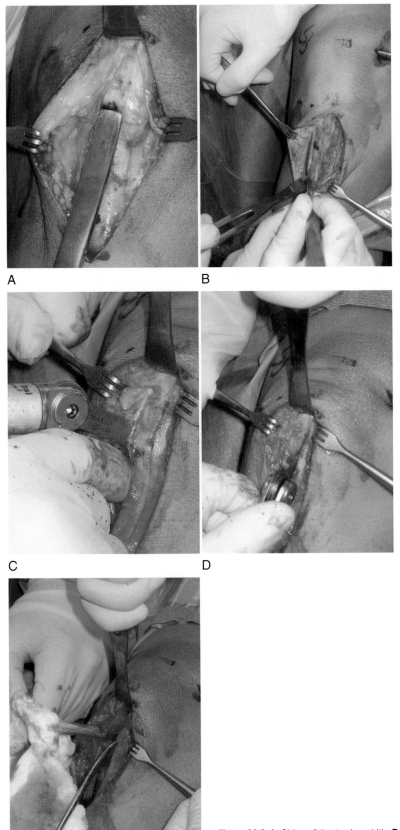

Figure 60-3 A, Sizing of the tendon width. **B,** Transverse tibial cut. **C,** Oscillating saw cut while the tendon is protected. **D,** Longitudinal bone cuts. **E,** Removal of the graft from the harvest site.

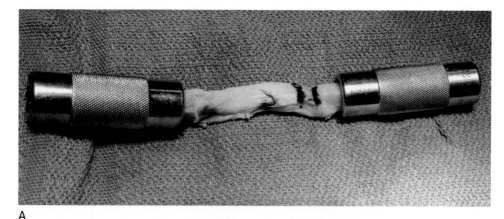

A

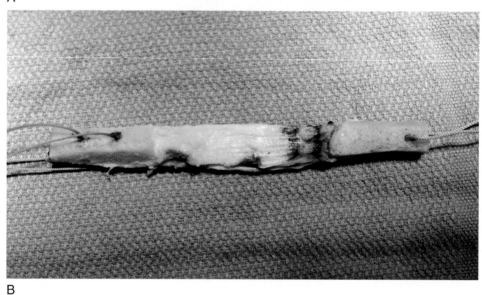

B

Figure 60-4 Graft preparation. **A,** The graft is sized to fit through a 10-mm tunnel. **B,** The finally prepared patellar tendon autograft with sutures passed through the femoral and tibial bone plugs.

3. Notch Preparation and Notchplasty

While the graft is being prepared on the back table, the intercondylar notch is prepared and notchplasty may be performed as needed. The ACL stump as well as residual soft tissue is removed from the lateral wall of the notch and the tibial footprint by arthroscopic instruments, the shaver, and electrocautery. A curet can also be a helpful and efficient tool to remove residual soft tissue from the posterior aspect of the lateral wall. Fat pad and ligamentum mucosum are removed as needed to improve visualization. Once all remaining soft tissue is removed from the notch, a notchplasty is performed if needed to avoid graft impingement, particularly in full knee extension (Fig. 60-5).

A notchplasty can also be necessary to improve visualization of the "over-the-top" position on the femur. A ¼-inch curved osteotome, placed through the inferomedial portal, is used to begin the notchplasty on the articular surface, and the arthroscopic grasper is used to remove the fragments. Next, with a 5.5-mm spherical bur, the notch is widened from posterior to anterior and apex to inferior.

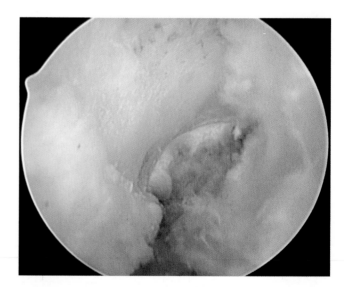

Figure 60-5 Notch preparation. The notch after soft tissue and bone débridement.

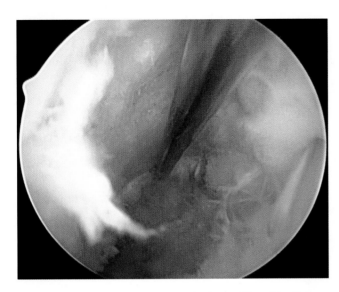

Figure 60-6 Confirmation of the true posterior extent of the notch with the probe in the over-the-top position.

Commonly, a vertical ridge is present approximately 1 cm anterior to the posterior edge, which can be misidentified as the posterior wall ("resident's ridge"). A probe must be able to hook under the over-the-top position, and it is used to confirm the sharp edge signifying the correct posterior aspect of the notch (Fig. 60-6). It is important to avoid excessive removal of bone along the lateral femoral condyle to prevent excessive lateralization of the isometric point.

4. Tibial Tunnel Placement

The tibial tunnel is placed through the same incision that was used for the graft harvest. The entrance for the tibial tunnel is approximately 1.5 cm medial to the tibial tubercle and 1 cm proximal to the pes anserine tendons. A 1-cm longitudinal periosteal incision is made parallel and just proximal to the hamstrings, and a medially based rectangular periosteal flap is elevated to expose cortical bone. Care is taken to avoid injury to the medial aspect of the patellar tendon, the superficial medial collateral ligament, or the pes anserine tendons. Orientation of the tibial tunnel is crucial because it determines the position of the femoral tunnel as the femoral guide is placed through the tibial tunnel.

A tibial guide aids in drilling and proper placement of the tibial tunnel. In general, the N + 7 rule helps determine the tibial guide angle. The rule adds 7 degrees to the length of the graft (e.g., 48-mm tendon, plus 7, yields a 55-degree angle); in a majority of cases, a 55-degree angle can be used. The guide is then introduced through the inferomedial portal. At times, an accessory portal inferior to the inferomedial portal can become necessary if the soft tissues would otherwise push up the aiming arm, which would result in a shortened tibial tunnel (Fig. 60-7).

The ideal placement of the guide pin is at the level of the posterior edge of the anterior horn of the lateral meniscus, or approximately 7 mm anterior to the PCL, and just lateral to the medial tibial spine. As there frequently is a large amount of soft tissue overlying the tibial plateau, where the pin appears to be entering the joint is actually posterior and lateral to the true entry point on the tibial plateau. Thus, it is advised that the pin enter the posterior aspect of the tibial footprint to avoid anterior tunnel placement.

The stylet is appropriately positioned intra-articularly, and the cannulated guide aimer is placed on the tibial cortex 1.5 cm medial to the tibial cortex and 1 cm proximal to the pes anserinus tendons. The guide pin is placed through the guide arm and drilled into the joint, and proper pin position is confirmed arthroscopically. The leg is then extended slowly to make certain that the pin is not impinging on the superior notch. After the knee is returned to a flexed position, the pin is advanced with a mallet until it contacts the intercondylar notch, thus stabilizing the pin during reaming.

The arthroscopy pump is turned off, the appropriately sized cannulated reamer (usually 10 or 11 mm) is placed over the guide pin, and the tibial tunnel is reamed. Bone chips can be collected with Owens gauze as the reamer is removed. At this time, the inflow pump is turned on; the ledge at the posterior aspect of the tibial tunnel is removed with a chamfer reamer and smoothed down with an arthroscopic hand rasp.

5. Femoral Tunnel Placement

The retrograde femoral tunnel offset guide is placed through the tibial tunnel. This guide courses through the joint and hooks the posterior aspect of the notch in the over-the-top position. Ideally, the tunnel originates at the 11-o'clock position in the right knee and the 1-o'clock position in the left knee (Fig. 60-8). The guide assists in avoiding posterior cortical wall blowout if it is positioned appropriately. A 10-mm-diameter tunnel is usually drilled in the posterior cortex with a 7-mm offset guide, resulting in a 2-mm posterior wall. On occasion, when the orientation of the tibial tunnel interferes with correct placement of the femoral tunnel, the femoral offset guide can be placed (with the knee hyperflexed) through an accessory inferomedial portal. The arthroscopic pump is turned off, the femoral guide is placed in the over-the-top position, and a probe is placed into the joint through the inferomedial portal to retract and protect the PCL.

A guide pin is drilled approximately 3 cm into the femur; in the pull-through technique, a Beath pin is used in place of the shorter guide pin and drilled through the femur and out the skin. A 10-mm reamer is placed over the guide pin, and the tunnel is reamed initially only to a depth of 1 cm. The reamer is then retracted, allowing verification of posterior wall integrity. Reaming is resumed to a depth of 5 to 7 mm greater than the length of the femoral bone plug to eliminate graft mismatch. As the reamer is removed, the pump inflow is turned on, and loose bone

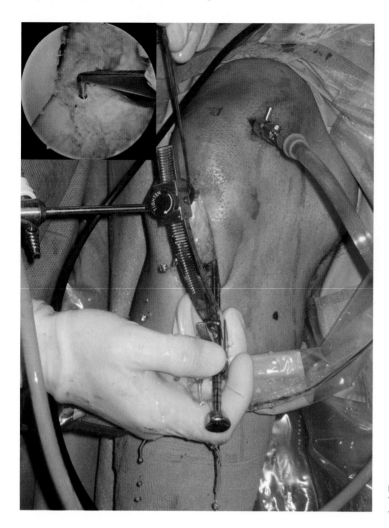

Figure 60-7 Tibial drill guide—sleeve is seated on the tibial cortex. The stylet points at the original ACL footprint *(inset)*.

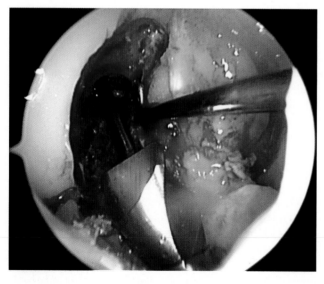

Figure 60-8 Reaming of the femoral tunnel with the PCL protected.

can once again be collected with Owens gauze.[7,8] Final tunnel integrity can be assessed by removal of the reamer and guide pin and placement of the arthroscopic camera through the tibial tunnel and directly into the femoral tunnel.

6. Graft Placement and Fixation

In the push-in technique, the graft is advanced through the tibial tunnel into the joint by use of a two-pronged pusher at the base of the femoral plug (Fig. 60-9A). A hemostat is placed through the inferomedial portal, grasping the femoral bone plug at the junction of the proximal and middle thirds. With the cortical surface of the femoral plug oriented posteriorly, the hemostat is used to guide the femoral plug into the femoral tunnel (Fig. 60-9B).

In the pull-through technique, the femoral bone plug suture is threaded through the eye of the Beath pin and retrieved proximally by pulling the Beath pin from its exit site in the thigh. The sutures of the femoral bone plug and the tibial bone plug are held taught as the graft is pulled through the knee. A probe or hemostat can be used to ensure proper orientation of the femoral bone plug as it enters the femoral tunnel.

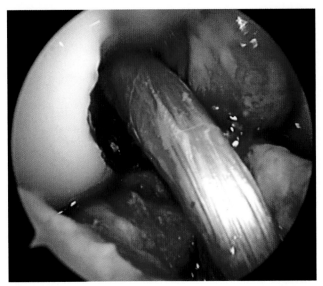

Figure 60-10 Final appearance of the ACL reconstruction.

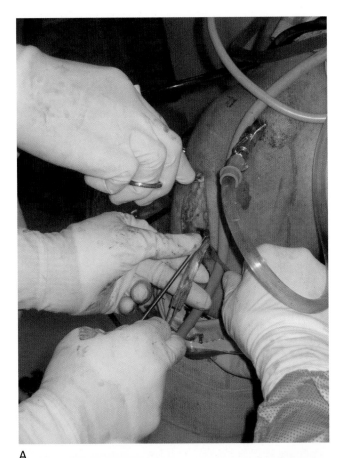

A

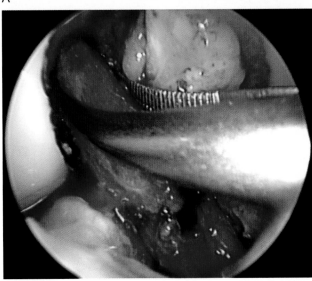

B

Figure 60-9 A and **B,** The push-through technique.

Once the femoral bone plug is completely seated in the femoral tunnel, a nitinol guide pin (Linvatec, Largo, Fla) is placed into the femoral tunnel at the 11-o'clock position of the graft. The knee is flexed to 110 to 120 degrees, allowing easier passage of the guide pin within the femoral tunnel. The pin should be introduced without resistance; otherwise pin divergence should be suspected.

A satellite pusher can be used to seat the femoral bone plug as needed. The tibial bone plug should be evaluated at this time for graft-tunnel mismatch. If the tibial plug is overhanging from the tibial tunnel, the graft can be removed and the femoral tunnel further recessed.

Femoral graft fixation is performed with an interference screw placed over the nitinol guide wire with the knee hyperflexed. The screw should be placed against the cancellous surface of the bone plug, away from the tendon insertion, to diminish the risk of graft injury or laceration. While tension is held on the tibial plug sutures, the knee is brought from 100 degrees to full extension to cycle the graft to ensure minimal graft motion as well as to assess impingement.

At this time, the tibial bone plug is externally rotated 180 degrees (toward the lateral side). This maneuver allows the tibial screw to be placed along the cortical surface and anterior. This screw placement avoids possible damage to the graft by a posteriorly placed screw with the knee in flexion as well as limits impingement that may occur with an anteriorized graft and a posteriorly placed screw.

The knee is placed in full extension, tension is held firmly on the tibial sutures, a nitinol wire is placed anterior to the tibial plug, and the interference screw is advanced and seated just below the cortical surface of the tibia. At this time, the arthroscope is placed into the knee, the ACL is visualized and probed to ensure proper tension, and a Lachman test and pivot shift test are performed (Fig. 60-10).

7. Closure

After irrigation with sterile saline, the knee is flexed to avoid excessive shortening. The patellar tendon defect is approximated with three or four simple interrupted No. 1 Vicryl sutures. The periosteal flap raised to drill the tibial tunnel is closed with No. 1 Vicryl as well. Bone graft from the reamings is placed in the patellar and tibial bone defects. The peritenon is closed with a running 2-0 Vicryl suture, and the incision is closed with interrupted 2-0 Vicryl for the subcutaneous tissues and a running 3-0 Prolene pullout stitch for the skin. The arthroscopy portals are closed with simple 3-0 Prolene stitches.

The wound and portals are injected with 0.5% bupivacaine (Marcaine) for postoperative analgesia. Steri-Strips and a sterile dressing are applied, followed by Kerlix, an ice cryotherapy device, and an elastic wrap. Finally, the leg is placed in a knee immobilizer or hinged knee brace locked in extension.

Postoperative Considerations

Follow-up

Patients are seen by a physical therapist the day of surgery before discharge home from the surgical center. On postoperative day 1, patients return to the office for evaluation of the wound and assessment for any effusion consistent with hemarthrosis. A sterile joint aspiration is recommended for decompression of any large postoperative hemarthrosis to accelerate rehabilitation.

Rehabilitation

Rehabilitation focuses on accelerated, closed-chain exercises with a goal of achieving full range of motion while maintaining stability and avoiding patellofemoral symptoms.

Postoperative Protocol

Immediate full weight bearing is permitted locked in extension.

- Week 1: Quad sets, straight-leg raises, and patellar mobilizations are initiated with the knee in extension.
- Weeks 2-4: Start closed chain extension exercises, hamstring curls, and stationary biking.
- Weeks 4-6: Start stair climbing machines. Goal range of motion: 120 degrees of flexion to full extension.
- Weeks 6-12: Begin advanced closed chain exercises, light jogging, and outdoor biking.
- Months 4-6: Start sports-specific exercises and plyometrics; initiate agility drills and gradual return to sports. The patient is discharged from supervised physical therapy to a home or health club program.

Complications

The reoperation rate after patellar tendon reconstruction with bone–patellar tendon–bone autograft ranges from

4% to 31%.[12] In a comprehensive literature review of arthroscopic ACL reconstruction with bone–patellar tendon–bone autografts, Nedeff detailed the mean rates of reoperation as 13%, arthrofibrosis as 7% (1% to 12%), and infection as 0.4% (0% to 4%).[12] Other complications include the following:

- Graft fracture
- Graft contamination
- Femoral tunnel posterior wall blowout
- Graft impingement
- Graft-tunnel mismatch
- Persistent instability secondary to graft malposition
- Failure of graft incorporation
- Patellar tendon rupture, patellar fracture, patellofemoral symptoms, kneeling pain
- Compartment syndrome, complex regional pain syndrome, deep venous thrombosis

---

PEARLS AND PITFALLS

- The initial 8-cm longitudinal incision is made in line with the medial border of the patellar tendon and should course from the distal pole of the patella to the tibial tubercle. This allows adequate visualization of the patellar tendon and permits the tibial tunnel to be made through the same incision.
- Harvest the bone–patellar tendon–bone autograft with the leg in flexion. Flexion of the knee keeps tension on the graft and aids the surgeon in making longitudinal cuts in the patellar tendon.
- Changing hands while the saw is used enhances visualization of the bone cuts.
- Make a triangular cut for the tibial bone plug and a trapezoidal cut for the patellar bone plug. The latter avoids penetration into the patellar articular surface.
- Avoid levering of the graft because it may damage the bone plug or result in an intraoperative patellar fracture.
- Ideally, 10×25-mm bone plugs are fashioned for an 11-mm tibial tunnel and a 10-mm femoral tunnel.
- The femoral tunnel posterior wall should be identified with a probe and hooked posteriorly to ensure the proper over-the-top position. This tunnel originates at the 11-o'clock position in the right knee and the 1-o'clock position in the left knee.
- After the graft is passed, the femoral interference screw is positioned against the cancellous surface of the bone plug, away from the tendon insertion. This decreases the risk of graft injury or laceration.
- The tibial bone plug is externally rotated 180 degrees (toward the lateral side), the knee is extended, and the tibial screw is placed anterior, along the cortical surface. This limits anterior migration of the graft, subsequent impingement, and laceration of the graft.

Results

The clinical results of ACL reconstruction with bone–patellar tendon–bone autograft are shown in Table 60-1.

Table 60-1 Clinical Results of ACL Reconstruction with Bone–Patellar Tendon–Bone Autograft

Author	Follow-up	Outcome—Subjective Assessment
Buss et al[4] (1993)	2-year minimum	59/68 (86%) excellent or good
Bach et al[2] (1998)	2-year minimum	96/103 (93%) mostly or completely satisfied
Kleipool et al[11] (1998)	4-year minimum	26/32 (70%) normal–nearly normal
Otto et al[13] (1998)	9-year minimum	52/68 (80%) normal–nearly normal
Webb et al[16] (1998)	2-year minimum	71/82 (86%) normal–nearly normal
Jomha et al[10] (1999)	7-year minimum	55/59 (93%) normal–nearly normal
Ao et al[1] (2000)	1-year minimum	18/20 (90%) excellent or good
Deehan et al[6] (2000)	5-year minimum	81/90 (90%) normal–nearly normal
Jager et al[9] (2003)	10-year minimum	62/74 (84%) normal
Chaudhary et al[5] (2005)	1-year minimum	68/78 (87%) excellent or good
Salmon et al[15] (2006)	13-year minimum	65/67 (96%) normal–nearly normal

60

References

1. Ao Y, Wang J, Yu J, et al. Arthroscopically assisted anterior screw [in Chinese]. Zhonghua Wai Ke Za Zhi 2000;38:250-252, 15.
2. Bach BR Jr, Levy ME, Bojchuk J, et al. Single-incision endoscopic anterior cruciate ligament reconstruction using patellar tendon autograft. Minimum two-year follow-up evaluation. Am J Sports Med 1998;26:30-40.
3. Beynnon BD, Johnson RJ, Abate JA, et al. Treatment of anterior cruciate ligament injuries, part I. Am J Sports Med 2005;33:1579-1602.
4. Buss DD, Warren RF, Wickiewicz TL, et al. Arthroscopically assisted reconstruction of the anterior cruciate ligament with use of autogenous patellar-ligament grafts. Results after twenty-four to forty-two months. J Bone Joint Surg Am 1993;75:1346-1355.
5. Chaudhary D, Monga P, Joshi D, et al. Arthroscopic reconstruction of the anterior cruciate ligament using bone–patellar tendon–bone autograft: experience of the first 100 cases. J Orthop Surg (Hong Kong) 2005;13:147-152.
6. Deehan DJ, Salmon LJ, Webb VJ, et al. Endoscopic reconstruction of the anterior cruciate ligament with an ipsilateral patellar tendon autograft. A prospective longitudinal five-year study. J Bone Joint Surg Br 2000;82:984-991.
7. Ferrari J, Bush-Joseph C, Bach BR Jr. Endoscopic anterior cruciate ligament reconstruction with patellar tendon autograft: surgical technique. Tech Orthop 1998;13:262-274.
8. Flik K, Bach BR Jr. Anterior cruciate ligament reconstruction using an endoscopic technique with patellar tendon autograft. Tech Orthop 2005;20:361-371.
9. Jager A, Welsch F, Braune C, et al. Ten year follow-up after single incision anterior cruciate ligament reconstruction using patellar tendon autograft [in German]. Z Orthop Ihre Grenzgeb 2003;141:42-47.
10. Jomha NM, Pinczewski LA, Clingeleffer A, Otto DD. Arthroscopic reconstruction of the anterior cruciate ligament with patellar-tendon autograft and interference screw fixation. The results at seven years. J Bone Joint Surg Br 1999;81:775-779.
11. Kleipool AE, Zijl JA, Willems WJ. Arthroscopic anterior cruciate ligament reconstruction with bone–patellar tendon–bone allograft or autograft. A prospective study with an average follow up of 4 years. Knee Surg Sports Traumatol Arthrosc 1998;6:224-230.
12. Nedeff DD, Bach BR Jr. Arthroscopic anterior cruciate ligament reconstruction using patellar tendon autografts: a comprehensive review of contemporary literature. Am J Knee Surg 2001;14:243-258.
13. Otto D, Pinczewski LA, Clingeleffer A, Odell R. Five-year results of single-incision arthroscopic anterior cruciate ligament reconstruction with patellar tendon autograft. Am J Sports Med 1998;26:181-188.
14. Owings MF, Kozak LJ. Ambulatory and inpatient procedures in the United States 1996. Vital Health Stat 13 1998;139:1-119.
15. Salmon LJ, Russell VJ, Refshauge K, et al. Long-term outcome of endoscopic anterior cruciate ligament reconstruction with patellar tendon autograft: minimum 13-year review. Am J Sports Med 2006;34:721-732.
16. Webb JM, Corry IS, Clingeleffer AJ, Pinczewski LA. Endoscopic reconstruction for isolated anterior cruciate ligament rupture. J Bone Joint Surg Br 1998;80:288-294.

CHAPTER 61

Patellar Tendon Allograft for Anterior Cruciate Ligament Reconstruction

Justin W. Chandler, MD
R. Alexander Creighton, MD

Anterior cruciate ligament (ACL) reconstruction is one of the most common procedures performed by orthopedic surgeons today. There are numerous graft choices, both autograft and allograft, and each has its advantages and disadvantages. The ideal graft should reproduce native anatomy of the ACL, ensure secure fixation with rapid biologic incorporation, and minimize morbidity to the patient. Bone–patellar tendon–bone autograft, one of the most common graft choices, provides excellent bone fixation, strength, and anatomic reconstruction. However, this graft choice has been criticized for donor site morbidity with postoperative patellofemoral pain in up to 55% of patients.[8]

Bone–patellar tendon–bone allografts have been used in revision procedures but are now being used increasingly in primary reconstructions because of elimination of donor site morbidity, smaller incision, decreased operative time, and decreased postoperative pain. Potential disadvantages include possible disease transmission, slower biologic remodeling time, possible low-level immune response, limited availability, and increased cost.[5]

Preoperative Considerations

History

A thorough history should be elicited. This includes mechanism of injury, associated injuries, prior level of activity, current symptoms of instability, any prior surgery, and any history of immune compromise that may preclude use of allograft tissue.

Typical History

- Often, low-energy injury during athletic activity
- Noncontact injury with sudden deceleration and rotational maneuvers, such as cutting-type running or jumping activities
- Direct blow with hyperextension or valgus stress
- Sensation of "popping" at time of injury may be recalled
- Sensation of instability or giving way

Physical Examination

Factors Affecting Surgical Indication

- Range of motion
- Effusion
- Lachman test for anterior translational instability
- Pivot shift test for rotational instability

Factors Affecting Surgical Planning

- Preexisting scars
- Overall alignment of knee
- Joint line tenderness for associated meniscal injury
- Varus, valgus, posterior drawer, and external rotation dial test for associated ligament injury
- Fat globules in joint aspirate (could indicate associated osteochondral injury)

Imaging

Radiography

- Lateral capsular Segond avulsion fracture
- Tibial eminence avulsion fracture
- Osteochondral injury or loose body
- Overall alignment of knee

Magnetic Resonance Imaging

- Discontinuity of ACL fibers
- Typical bone bruises on lateral femoral condyle and lateral tibial plateau
- Associated meniscal, chondral, and ligament injuries

Indications and Contraindications

There are several populations of patients in which allograft may be preferred to autograft in ACL reconstruction[11]:

- Patients older than 30 years, who may benefit from faster postoperative recovery time
- Skeletally immature patients for avoidance of growth plate disruption
- Patients with patellofemoral pain or previous patellar surgeries
- Laborers or athletes who require a kneeling position
- Patients undergoing revision or multiligament procedures

Autograft bone–patellar tendon–bone may be the better choice in a high-demand athlete who wishes to return to play as soon as possible, given the slower biologic remodeling time for allograft tissue. In addition, given the small risk of disease transmission, allograft may not be a good choice in an immunocompromised patient.

Surgical Technique

Allograft Selection

Once the decision has been made to proceed with allograft tissue, it is the surgeon's responsibility to ensure that there is an appropriate graft at the time of surgery. According to Bernard R. Bach, Jr., MD (personal communication), the length of a bone–patellar tendon–bone allograft can be estimated on the basis of the patient's height (Table 61-1). The information on the graft label is double-checked before the patient is brought to the operating room. It may be prudent to have a second graft specimen available in case any problems are encountered after thawing of the graft or in its preparation.

Table 61-1 Estimated Allograft Length Based on Patient's Height in Inches

Patient's Height	Estimated Graft Length
60 inches	35-37 mm
62 inches	38-40 mm
65 inches	40-42 mm
68 inches	42-44 mm
72 inches	45-47 mm
74 inches	48-50 mm
77 inches	>50 mm

Anesthesia and Positioning

The procedure can be performed under regional, spinal, or general anesthesia on the basis of the surgeon's, anesthesiologist's, and patient's preferences. A femoral nerve block may aid in immediate postoperative pain control. The patient is placed in the supine position on the operating table, and a thorough examination under anesthesia is performed. The operative leg is placed in a leg holder with a tourniquet on the upper thigh (Fig. 61-1). It is essential to be able to flex the knee to at least 110 degrees to facilitate femoral screw placement. The contralateral leg is placed in a padded foot holder with the hip and knee slightly flexed to prevent common peroneal nerve or femoral nerve palsy. The leg is then prepared and draped.

Surgical Landmarks, Incisions, and Portals

Landmarks

- Patella
- Patellar tendon
- Tibial plateau
- Tibial tubercle

Portals and Incisions (Fig. 61-2)

- Superomedial or superolateral outflow portal
- Inferomedial portal
- Inferolateral portal
- Tibial tunnel incision
- Accessory portal for femoral screw insertion

Examination Under Anesthesia and Diagnostic Arthroscopy

A thorough examination under anesthesia includes Lachman, anterior and posterior drawer, varus and valgus,

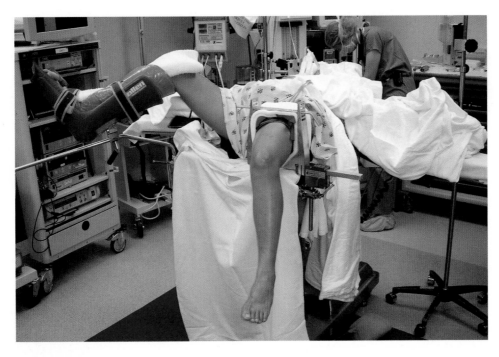

Figure 61-1 Positioning of the patient.

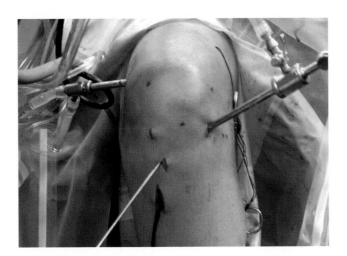

Figure 61-2 Incisions: superomedial outflow portal, inferomedial and inferolateral portals, accessory portal for femoral screw placement, and tibial tunnel incision.

Box 61-1 Surgical Steps

1. Notch preparation and notchplasty

2. Allograft preparation

3. Tibial tunnel

4. Femoral tunnel

5. Graft insertion and fixation

6. Closure

and pivot shift testing. External rotation and thigh-foot angles at 30 and 90 degrees are evaluated for assessment of posterolateral instability. Findings are compared with the contralateral knee.

Diagnostic arthroscopy is performed for assessment of associated chondral lesions, ligament injuries, and meniscal disease.

Specific Steps (Box 61-1)

1. Notch Preparation and Notchplasty

Remnant ACL and soft tissue are débrided from the lateral wall and roof by a combination of arthroscopic scissors, a 4.5-mm full-radius shaver, and a tissue ablator. The notchplasty is performed with a quarter-inch curved osteotome, arthroscopic grabber, and 5.5-mm spherical bur, moving from anterior to posterior and from apex to inferior, making sure to avoid misinterpretation of a vertical ridge two thirds posteriorly as the true posterior outlet. The goals of the notchplasty are to allow visualization of the entire lateral wall and over-the-top position and to prevent graft impingement with the knee in full extension. A probe is used to palpate the over-the-top position to confirm the appropriate position (Fig. 61-3).

2. Allograft Preparation

The allograft is thawed by soaking it in normal saline at room temperature (Fig. 61-4). Excess fat pad and soft tissue are removed from the graft. The graft construct length is measured, as the length of the soft tissue affects

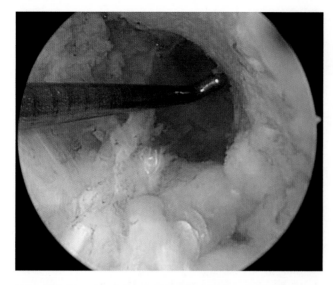

Figure 61-3 Adequate notchplasty with probe to hook over-the-top position.

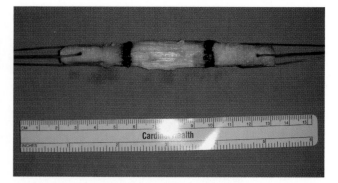

Figure 61-5 Prepared allograft.

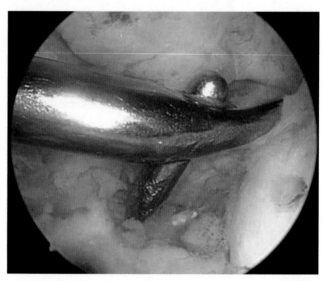

Figure 61-6 Tibial tunnel guide in center of ACL stump, offset from tibial posterior cruciate ligament insertion by 7 mm.

3. Tibial Tunnel

A variable-angle tibial guide is set on the basis of the N+10 measurement and placed in the inferomedial portal to determine the location of the incision for the tibial tunnel. This should be at least 25 mm below the joint line and superior to the insertion of the pes anserinus tendons. A 2-cm skin incision is made at this point, and skin flaps are elevated. A periosteal window is elevated with a Cobb elevator on the medial flare of the tibia. Intra-articularly, the guide is positioned in the sagittal plane by use of the posterior edge of the anterior horn of the lateral meniscus. The guide should be centrally placed to allow passage of the graft between the posterior cruciate ligament and the lateral wall of the notch. It should be approximately 7 mm anterior to the posterior cruciate ligament (Fig. 61-6). The guide pin is drilled through the guide, and it is arthroscopically verified that it is posterior (3 to 5 mm) to the intercondylar notch with the knee extended. The pin is then reamed with the appropriately sized reamer based on the size of graft bone plugs. The intra-articular edges of the tunnel are smoothed with a rasp (Fig. 61-7).

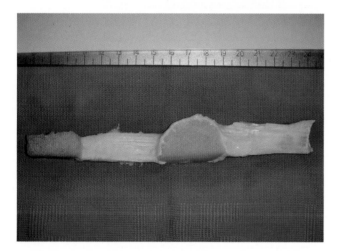

Figure 61-4 Thawed, unprepared bone–patellar tendon–bone allograft.

the angle selected on the tibial aiming device. N+10 mm is generally sufficient to reduce significant graft construct mismatch; this is a modification of Miller's N+7 mm rule whenever the tibial tunnel drill angle equals the length of the soft tissue component of the graft plus 10. For example, if the soft tissue measures 45 mm, the selected drill angle is 45+10 or 55 degrees. The bone plugs should be approximately 25 mm in length. The bone plugs are contoured to fit easily through a 10-mm sizer tube.

The femoral bone plug–tendon interface is marked on the cancellous surface with a sterile marking pen to ensure complete seating of the bone plug in the femoral tunnel during placement. Two 1.6-mm holes are drilled through the tibial and femoral bone plugs parallel and perpendicular to the cortical surfaces. A No. 5 braided polyester suture is passed through each hole (Fig. 61-5).

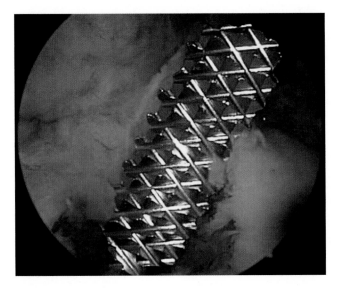

Figure 61-7 A rasp is used to smooth the intra-articular edges of the tibial tunnel.

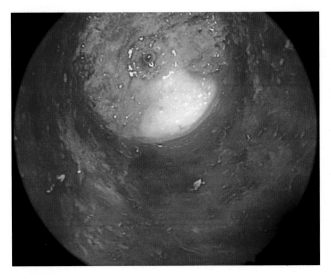

Figure 61-9 View with arthroscope in femoral tunnel showing intact posterior cortex.

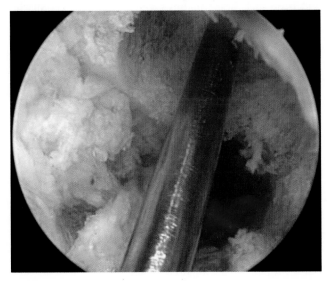

Figure 61-8 Guide pin in reamed femoral tunnel.

4. Femoral Tunnel

The goal of femoral tunnel preparation is to prepare a tunnel that originates at the 1- to 1:30-o'clock position in the left knee and the 10:30- to 11-o'clock position in the right knee. This provides a nearly anatomic-isometric position of the graft. With the pump turned off and the knee "dry," a 7-mm femoral offset guide is placed through the tibial tunnel to the over-the-top position. The orientation of the tibial tunnel affects the ability to place the femoral aimer correctly. The guide allows a 1- to 2-mm thin posterior cortical rim after reaming. The pin is reamed to a depth 5 to 8 mm longer than the length of the femoral bone plug to allow possible recessing of the bone plug (Fig. 61-8). The femoral tunnel is smoothed, and the arthroscope is placed in the femoral tunnel and rotated

360 degrees to ensure that the posterior wall is intact (Fig. 61-9).

5. Graft Insertion and Fixation

A Beath pin is placed through the tibial tunnel and into the femoral tunnel and advanced out the anterior thigh. The sutures from the femoral bone plug are passed through the eyelet of the Beath pin, and by pulling the Beath pin out of the thigh, the sutures are retrieved. The graft is pulled in a retrograde fashion, seating the femoral bone plug into the femoral tunnel, with use of the arthroscope to confirm placement. The bone plug is pushed nearly flush with the femoral surface entrance. The graft is left 3 to 5 mm in the joint to act as a skid for placement of the interference screw guide pin. An accessory anteromedial portal is made to facilitate placement of the nitinol guide pin (see Fig. 61-2). The nitinol pin is placed through the accessory portal and slid into the femoral tunnel, anterior to the graft and bone plug. The bone plug is then seated flush with the femoral tunnel entrance. A 7 × 20-mm cannulated metal interference screw is advanced over the guide wire while the knee is kept flexed 110 to 120 degrees. The guide pin should be removed before the screw is fully seated; otherwise it may be difficult to remove. Advance the screw until its base is flush with the base of the femoral plug, taking care not to lacerate the soft tissue of the graft while placing the screw (Fig. 61-10).

The knee is cycled through a full range of motion, noting the movement of the tibial bone plug within its tunnel. While the knee is cycled 90 degrees to full extension, the graft should shorten 1 to 2 mm during the final 20 to 30 degrees of full extension ("gross isometry test"). The graft is rotated 180 degrees, which places the tibial bone plug cortical surface anterior. The screw is placed on the cortex for better fixation. By placement of the screw

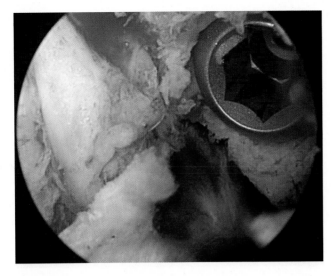

Figure 61-10 Femoral fixation of graft.

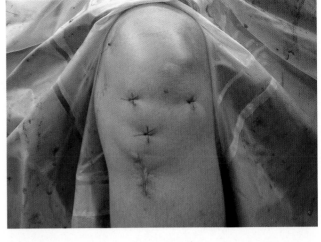

Figure 61-12 Skin incisions at completion of procedure.

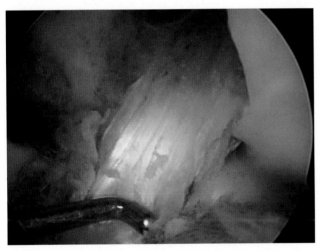

Figure 61-11 Final arthroscopic view of graft.

anterior to the graft, it is less likely to injure the graft if it extends beyond the tendo-osseous junction proximally. With the knee extended and axially loaded, an 8 × 20-mm cannulated metal interference screw is used to secure the tibial bone plug. A final arthroscopic evaluation is performed to confirm graft placement and to irrigate the knee of any loose debris (Fig 61-11).

6. Closure

The periosteal flap over the tibial tunnel and hardware is loosely approximated with No. 0 Vicryl. The subcutaneous layer is closed with No. 2 Vicryl. The skin is closed with a running 4-0 Monocryl suture. The portals are closed with a simple 3-0 Prolene suture (Fig. 61-12). The incisions, the deep tissues, and the knee joint are injected with bupivacaine. Steri-Strips, gauze pads, and a loose single-layer of

Kerlix are placed over the wounds. A cryotherapy device and drop-lock brace in full extension are placed on the knee.

Postoperative Considerations

Follow-up

- The first postoperative visit is scheduled within 5 days for an incision check and suture removal.
- The patient is again encouraged and instructed (as done preoperatively and in the post-anesthesia care unit) in patellar mobilization, isometric quadriceps exercises, and knee flexion exercises.

Rehabilitation

- Immediate weight bearing is permitted as tolerated with the knee in full extension for 2 weeks in a hinged knee brace.
- The patient should be weaned off crutches within the first postoperative week.
- Physical therapy is initiated 5 to 7 days postoperatively with emphasis on achieving full extension and beginning flexion exercises.
- The patient may begin bicycling at 3 to 4 weeks, stair-climbing machines at 8 weeks, light jogging at 12 weeks, and a gradual return to sports at 9 months (longer for allograft because of graft incorporation).

Table 61-2 Clinical Results of Bone–Patellar Tendon–Bone Allograft ACL Reconstruction

Author	Follow-up	Outcome
Harner et al[7] (1996)	3-5 years	No significant difference in laxity, functional testing, or failure rate compared with autograft Decreased loss of extension with allograft vs. autograft ($P=.009$)
Peterson et al[9] (2001)	5 years	No significant difference in laxity, functional testing, or failure rate compared with autograft Decreased loss of extension with allograft vs. autograft ($P=.027$)
Chang et al[4] (2003)	2-year minimum	91% good–excellent results vs. 97% good–excellent results with autograft No significant difference
Poehling et al[10] (2005)	5 years	Decreased pain postoperatively with allograft vs. autograft at 1 week, 6 weeks, and 3 months ($P=.0006$, $P=.0007$, $P=.0270$) Fewer activity limitations at 3 and 6 months with allograft ($P=.0431$, $P=.0014$) Increased laxity by KT-1000 in allograft ($P=.0520$)
Gorschewsky et al[6] (2005)	2 and 6 years	Increased rupture rate of allograft vs. autograft at 2 and 6 years ($P=.004$) with use of irradiated grafts
Bach et al[1] (2005)	2-year minimum	94% primary allograft reconstructions mostly or completely satisfied

61

Complications

- Graft failure at fixation or intrasubstance tear
- Infection (case reports of infection with *Clostridium septicum*[3])
- Arthrofibrosis
- Neurovascular injury
- Disease transmission (risk estimated to be 1:1,600,000,[2] no documented cases with current screening standards)

Results

Most studies that have compared outcomes of ACL reconstruction by bone–patellar tendon–bone allograft versus autograft have shown no significant difference in laxity, functional testing, or failure rate. Significantly decreased postoperative pain and smaller incisions have been shown with the use of allograft. The one study that showed significant difference in failure rates used only irradiated allografts, which have been shown to be weaker (Table 61-2).

PEARLS AND PITFALLS

- Have informed consent from the patient to use an allograft.
- Know your allograft supplier's track record and tissue-processing techniques.
- Double-check the allograft label before bringing the patient to the operating room.
- Have a second allograft available in case something is wrong with the first specimen (labeling error, tissue quality, technical error) or discuss use of the patient's own tissue if something is wrong with the allograft.
- Estimate the length of the patellar tendon allograft on the basis of the patient's height (see Table 61-1).
- Treat all associated intra-articular pathologic changes.
- Tunnel placement is the key; whether you use autograft or allograft, be vigilant.
- Be sure to have stable aperture femoral fixation without compromise of the bone-tendon junction.
- If graft mismatch is encountered, be sure to obtain stable fixation at the tibia. Options include trough and staple, graft rotation to shorten it, soft tissue bioabsorbable fixation, and a combination.
- The ultimate return to sports with allograft reconstruction may be delayed because of longer graft incorporation compared with an autograft.

References

1. Bach B, Aadalen K, Dennis M, et al. Primary anterior cruciate ligament reconstruction using fresh-frozen nonirradiated patellar tendon allograft. Am J Sports Med 2005;33:284-292.

2. Bach B, Tradonsky S, Bojchuk J, et al. Arthroscopically assisted anterior cruciate ligament reconstruction using patellar tendon autograft: five- to nine-year follow-up evaluation. Am J Sports Med 1998;26:20-29.

3. Barbour S, King W. The safe and effective use of allograft tissue—an update. Am J Sports Med 2003;31:791-797.

4. Chang S, Egami D, Shaieb M, et al. Anterior cruciate ligament reconstruction: allograft versus autograft. Arthroscopy 2003;19:453-462.

5. Creighton R, Bach B. Revision anterior cruciate ligament reconstruction with patellar tendon allograft. Sports Med Arthrosc Rev 2005;13:38-45.

6. Gorschewsky O, Klakow A, Riechert K, et al. Clinical comparison of the Tutoplast allograft and autologous patellar tendon (bone–patellar tendon–bone) for the reconstruction of the anterior cruciate ligament. Am J Sports Med 2005;33:1202-1209.

7. Harner C, Olson E, Irrgang J, et al. Allograft versus autograft anterior cruciate ligament reconstruction. Clin Orthop 1996;324:134-144.

8. Miller S, Gladstone J. Graft selection in anterior cruciate ligament reconstruction. Orthop Clin North Am 2002;33:675-683.

9. Peterson R, Shelton W, Bomboy A. Allograft versus autograft patellar tendon anterior cruciate ligament reconstruction: a 5-year follow-up. Arthroscopy 2001;17:9-13.

10. Poehling G, Curl W, Lee C, et al. Analysis of outcomes of anterior cruciate ligament repair with 5-year follow-up: allograft versus autograft. Arthroscopy 2005;21:774-785.

11. Strickland S, MacGillivray J, Warren R. Anterior cruciate ligament reconstruction with allograft tendons. Orthop Clin North Am 2003;34:41-47.

CHAPTER 62

Hamstring Tendon Autograft for Anterior Cruciate Ligament Reconstruction

Charles H. Brown, Jr., MD

Neal Chen, MD

Nader Darwich, MD

The success of anterior cruciate ligament (ACL) reconstruction is influenced by many factors, such as the initial tensile properties of the graft tissue, the initial fixation of the graft, the healing at the graft fixation sites, the biologic remodeling of the graft, and the type of postoperative rehabilitation program used. Owing to its high initial tensile strength and stiffness, ability to be rigidly fixed to bone, rapid healing of bone to bone at the graft fixation sites, and outcome studies documenting predictable success in restoration of anterior knee laxity and elimination of the pivot shift phenomenon, the central-third patellar tendon autograft is considered by many surgeons to be the "gold standard" for ACL reconstruction. However, because of the well-documented donor site morbidity associated with the harvest of patellar tendon autografts, improvements in soft tissue graft fixation techniques, and clinical outcome studies demonstrating no significant difference between patellar tendon and hamstring tendon ACL reconstructions, four-stranded hamstring tendon autografts have become an increasingly popular graft choice for ACL reconstruction.* In this chapter, we describe our current surgical technique for performing ACL reconstruction with autogenous doubled gracilis and semitendinosus tendon (DGST) grafts.

*References 1, 2, 4, 5, 7, 12, 13, 15, 18, 22, 26, 28, 30.

Preoperative Considerations

History and Physical Examination

Patients thought to have an ACL tear should provide detailed history of the initial injury and any subsequent injuries and their treatment. The diagnosis is confirmed by the Lachman and pivot shift tests or by magnetic resonance imaging if needed. It is particularly important to recognize associated injuries to the posterolateral and posteromedial structures. Failure to recognize and to treat associated patholaxity at the time of the ACL reconstruction may result in continued complaints of instability or failure of the ACL reconstruction.

Imaging

A preoperative anteroposterior radiograph of the involved knee in full extension and standing anteroposterior and posteroanterior 45-degree flexion views of both knees are important to rule out associated bone injury or joint space narrowing and to assess skeletal maturity of the patient. A true lateral radiograph of the injured knee in maximum hyperextension allows measurement of the intercondylar roof–femoral angle, which can be useful for preoperative planning of the tibial tunnel in the sagittal plane. A Merchant view of both knees is helpful in assessment of patellar alignment and tilt. Full-length standing radiographs of both lower extremities from hips to ankles are indicated in patients with joint space narrowing to allow measurement of the mechanical axis. Combined or staged tibial osteotomy and ACL reconstruction may be indicated in patients with malalignment and symptoms of pain and instability.

Indications and Contraindications

Hamstring tendon autografts are indicated for any acute or chronic ACL reconstruction. ACL reconstructions performed with hamstring tendon grafts have been shown to result in faster recovery of quadriceps muscle strength, lower incidence of donor site pain, and less interference with kneeling and crawling than after ACL reconstructions performed with patellar tendon autografts.[12,18,26] Because of less interference with kneeling and crawling, hamstring tendon grafts are the autogenous graft of choice for patients whose occupation, lifestyle, or religion requires "knee walking," crawling, or kneeling. Hamstring tendon grafts are also our preferred autogenous graft for patients with a history of extensor mechanism surgery or trauma. We also prefer hamstring tendon grafts for patients with a history of patellofemoral pain or patellar tendinopathy. Finally, hamstring tendon grafts are the autogenous graft of choice when ACL reconstruction is indicated in patients with open growth plates.

The only absolute contraindication to use of hamstring tendon grafts for ACL reconstruction is previous harvest of the hamstring tendons. In cases in which prior pes anserine transfer or open surgical procedures on the medial side of the knee have been performed, the resulting scarring and alteration of normal tissue planes may complicate harvest of hamstring tendon grafts. In these situations, the surgeon may elect to use an alternative autograft or allograft tissue. Studies demonstrating a significant loss of knee flexor strength at high flexion angles suggest caution in use of hamstring tendon grafts for athletes such as gymnasts, wrestlers, sprinters, and American football defensive backs and safeties, who require maximum flexor strength at high angles of flexion.[9,32]

Surgical Planning

Graft Fixation

Rigid initial graft fixation is critical to the success of any ACL reconstruction.[4] Attainment of rigid initial graft fixation prevents failure and minimizes elongation at the graft fixation sites during cyclic loading of the knee before

healing at the graft fixation sites has occurred.[4] Because of the longer time required for hamstring tendon grafts to heal to bone, it is important to use graft fixations that are strong and stiff and that resist slippage under cyclic loading, to prevent the development of progressive laxity in the postoperative period. However, at present, the optimal graft fixation method for hamstring tendon grafts remains controversial, and there is little consensus as to what fixation methods produce the best clinical outcomes.

Femoral Fixation Options (Fig. 62-1)

Laboratory biomechanical studies have demonstrated that the EndoButton CL and cross pins provide strong femoral fixation with minimal slippage during cyclic loading.[6,19] Although intertunnel fixation with interference screws is a popular hamstring tendon graft fixation technique, our laboratory biomechanical studies have demonstrated that this fixation method is the weakest and has the largest amount of slippage during cyclic loading.[6,19] We prefer femoral fixation with the EndoButton CL for the following reasons:

- Fixation strength is high.
- Slippage during cyclic loading is minimal.
- The fit of the tendon in the bone tunnel is tight.
- The 360 degrees of contact between the bone tunnel wall and the hamstring tendon graft enhances healing.
- The amount of graft inserted into the femoral tunnel can be customized.
- Removal of the implant is not required in revision cases.
- Fixation properties are not dependent on the bone quality of the distal femur.

Tibial Fixation Options (Fig. 62-2)

Tibial fixation is the weak link of ACL graft fixation, and tibial fixation of hamstring tendon grafts remains problematic.[4] Problems with tibial fixation result primarily from the lower bone mineral density of the proximal tibia and the fact that tibial fixation devices must resist shear forces applied parallel to the axis of the tibial bone tunnel.[4] Cortical fixation techniques can address the issue of the lower bone mineral density of the proximal tibia. However, these implants are often prominent and may cause local skin irritation and pain and require a second operation for removal.[24] Intratunnel tibial fixation with interference screws eliminates the problem of prominent hardware; however, laboratory biomechanical studies have shown that this fixation method is the weakest and demonstrates

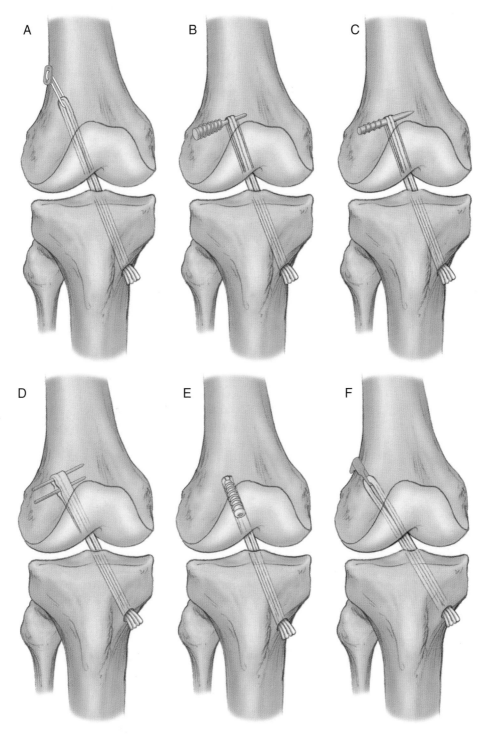

Figure 62-1 Femoral fixation options. **A,** EndoButton CL. **B,** Bone Mulch screw. **C,** TransFix. **D,** RigidFix. **E,** Bioabsorbable screw. **F,** EZLoc.

the greatest amount of slippage under cyclic loading.[20,24] On the basis of its ease of use and of biomechanical studies that demonstrate high initial fixation strength and stiffness with minimal slippage under cyclic loading conditions, we prefer intertunnel tibial fixation with the IntraFix tibial fastener (DePuy-Mitek, Norwood, Mass).[7,19]

Surgical Technique

Anesthesia and Positioning

The operation is performed as an outpatient procedure under general or regional anesthesia. A thigh-length TED

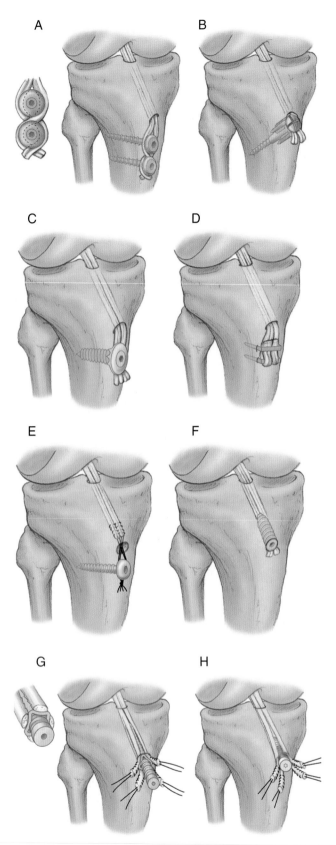

Figure 62-2 Tibial fixation options. **A,** AO ligament washers. **B,** WasherLoc. **C,** Spiked ligament washer. **D,** Staples. **E,** Suture-post fixation. **F,** Bioabsorbable screw. **G,** IntraFix tibial fastener. **H,** GTS sleeve and tapered screw.

antiembolism stocking (Kendall Company, Mansfield, Mass) and a foam rubber heel pad are applied to the well leg. A padded pneumatic tourniquet is applied high on the thigh of the operative leg but is rarely used during the operation. The patient is positioned supine on the operating room table and given 1 g of a first-generation cephalosporin intravenously followed by a continuous intravenous infusion of ketorolac at 4 mg/hr. A lead gonad shield is applied to protect the patient from radiation exposure during intraoperative fluoroscopy. Our preferred technique is to position the lower extremity so that a full, free range of motion can be performed during the procedure. Full unrestricted flexion of the knee is particularly important if the femoral tunnel is drilled by the anteromedial portal technique. We use a padded thigh post and hip positioner placed at the level of the tourniquet and a padded, L-shaped footrest that can be moved along the side rail of the operating room table, allowing the flexion angle of the knee to be changed during the procedure. The padded footrest is typically adjusted to maintain the knee at 90 degrees of flexion without manual assistance. The padded hip positioner stabilizes the patient's pelvis and the padded thigh post acts as a fulcrum to allow application of valgus force to the knee, permitting the medial compartment to be opened for performance of meniscus surgery (Fig. 62-3). Use of a standard circumferential arthroscopic leg holder and dropping the foot of the operating room table limit knee flexion and may compromise drilling of the femoral tunnel by the anteromedial portal technique.

After routine iodine skin preparation and sterile draping, a solution of 5 mg of morphine sulfate plus 20 mL of 0.25% bupivacaine (Marcaine) with 1:100,000 epinephrine is injected into the suprapatellar pouch for pre-emptive analgesia. With the use of a continuous ketorolac intravenous infusion and intra-articular administration of morphine, we have not found it necessary to use femoral nerve blocks for postoperative pain management. Use of an infusion pump improves joint distention and visualization, allowing the procedure to be performed without inflation of the tourniquet.

Specific Steps (Box 62-1)

1. Hamstring Tendon Graft Harvest

Harvest of the hamstring tendons can be performed through a vertical or oblique skin incision centered over the tibial insertion of the pes anserine tendons (Fig. 62-4). When the transtibial tunnel technique is used to drill the femoral tunnel, it is important to center the vertical skin incision midway between the anterior tibial crest and the posteromedial border of the tibia to allow the tibial tunnel to be positioned along the anterior fibers of the medial collateral ligament (MCL). If the femoral tunnel is to be drilled by the anteromedial portal technique, the vertical

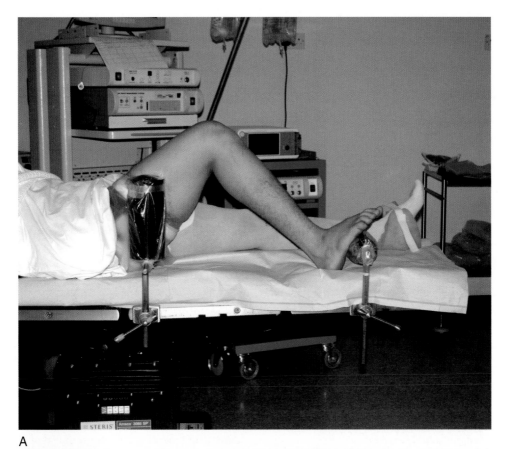

A

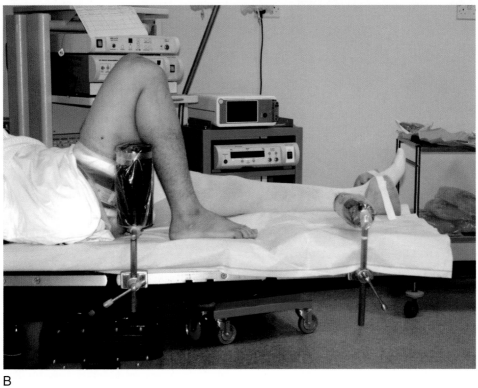

B

Figure 62-3 A, The padded thigh post and L-shaped footrest allow the knee to be positioned at 90 degrees of flexion without manual assistance. **B,** The thigh post allows full, unrestricted knee flexion during the procedure.

Box 62-1 Surgical Steps

1. Hamstring tendon graft harvest
2. Graft preparation
3. Arthroscopic portal placement
4. Preparation of the intercondylar notch
5. Femoral tunnel
6. Tibial tunnel
7. Calculation of EndoButton CL length and graft preparation
8. Graft passage and femoral fixation
9. Graft tensioning
10. Tibial fixation
11. Closure

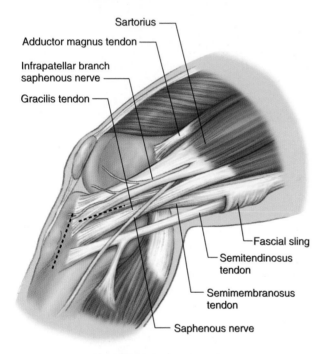

Sartorius
Adductor magnus tendon
Infrapatellar branch saphenous nerve
Gracilis tendon
Fascial sling
Semitendinosus tendon
Semimembranosus tendon
Saphenous nerve

Figure 62-4 Hamstring tendon graft harvest skin incisions and anatomic relationships on the medial side of the knee. A vertical or an oblique skin incision can be used to harvest the hamstring tendons. Important features to note are the proximity of the vertical incision to the infrapatellar branches of the saphenous nerve, the proximity of the oblique incision to the saphenous nerve, the relationship of the saphenous nerve to the gracilis tendon, the fascial connection between the medial head of the gastrocnemius, and the fascial sling that suspends the semitendinosus tendon beneath the semimembranous muscle. (From Brown CH, Sklar JH, Darwich N. Endoscopic anterior cruciate ligament reconstruction using autogenous doubled gracilis and semitendinosus tendons. Tech Knee Surg 2004;3:217.)

lines (resulting in a more cosmetic appearance), provides better proximal exposure of the tendons, and requires less skin retraction during drilling of the tibial tunnel. The anatomic course of the infrapatellar branches of the saphenous nerve also makes them less vulnerable to injury when the oblique skin incision is used.[31] However, the saphenous nerve can be injured if the oblique skin incision is positioned too close to the posteromedial corner of the tibia or sharp dissection is extended back into this region.[31] Should premature amputation of the semitendinosus tendon occur, the oblique skin incision is not extensile and an additional skin incision is required to harvest a patellar tendon autograft. We recommend against use of the oblique skin incision until experience is gained with the harvesting technique and the surgeon is able to consistently harvest hamstring tendon grafts of adequate length.

In the average-size patient, the superior border of the sartorius tendon is approximately one finger width below the tibial tubercle or three finger widths below the medial joint line (personal observation: the tendons insert more proximally in Middle Eastern patients). In revision cases involving a failed primary patellar tendon reconstruction, the distal portion of the previous patellar tendon harvest incision can be extended distally 2 to 3 cm below the tibial tubercle, allowing simultaneous harvest of the hamstring tendon grafts and removal of the tibial fixation hardware.

The skin incision and subcutaneous tissues are infiltrated with a solution of 0.25% bupivacaine with 1:100,000 epinephrine for hemostasis and pre-emptive analgesia. We routinely harvest the tendon grafts without inflation of the tourniquet. The sartorius fascia is exposed by sharp and blunt dissection. We use an inside-out technique to harvest the two tendons because this technique gives an excellent view of the internal aspect of the pes anserine and allows the surgeon to better visualize and to identify any of the associated anatomic variations or variable tendon attachments to the tibia, which are common.[21] In the inside-out technique, the conjoined tibial insertion of the two tendons is detached from the tibia by making an inverted L-shaped incision through the sartorius fascia. The sartorius fascia is grasped with an Allis clamp and lifted away from the tibia, thus protecting the underlying MCL. The fascia is incised parallel to the gracilis tendon and the tibial insertion of the two tendons is sharply released from the crest of the tibia, revealing the inner aspects of the two tendons (Fig. 62-5).

A right-angled type clamp is used to separate the two tendons from the undersurface of the sartorius fascial flap, which is preserved for later closure. The gracilis tendon is sharply divided and grasped with wide Allis-Adair tissue forceps (Codman & Shurtleff, Inc., Raynham, Mass). Blunt scissors dissection is used to free the tendon from the undersurface of the sartorius fascia. It is important to bluntly release the interconnecting fascial bands that run

skin incision can be positioned closer to the anterior crest of the tibia. This incision is more extensile and can easily be extended to harvest a patellar tendon graft should premature amputation of the semitendinosus tendon graft occur. The oblique skin incision runs parallel to Langer's

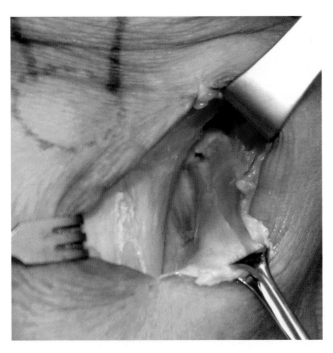

Figure 62-5 The inverted L-shaped fascial flap is reflected distally, exposing the deep aspect of the two tendons.

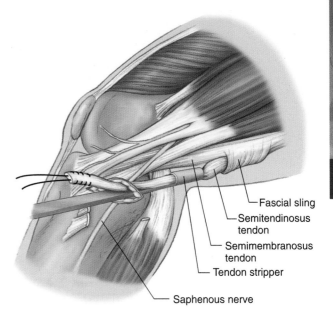

Fascial sling
Semitendinosus tendon
Semimembranosus tendon
Tendon stripper
Saphenous nerve

Figure 62-6 Passage of the tendon stripper outside of the fascial sling beneath the semimembranous muscle may result in the tendon stripper's taking an aberrant path into the thigh and causing premature amputation of the semitendinosus graft. (From Brown CH, Sklar JH. Endoscopic anterior cruciate ligament reconstruction using quadrupled hamstring tendons and EndoButton femoral fixation. Tech Orthop 1998;13:285.)

between the two tendons. Sharp or scissors dissection along the superior border of the gracilis should be avoided to prevent injury to the saphenous nerve, which leaves Hunter canal and crosses over the superior border of the gracilis tendon at the posteromedial corner of the knee.[31] Five throws of a running baseball-style whipstitch are placed in the free end of the gracilis tendon with a No. 2 nonabsorbable suture (Ti•Cron, United States Surgical, Norwalk, Conn; Ethibond special order D-5757, Ethicon, Inc., Somerville, NJ).

Depending on the surgeon's preference, the tendons can be harvested with a slotted tendon stripper, a closed Brand-type tendon stripper, or a tendon harvester (Linvatec, Largo, Fla). The gracilis tendon is harvested by flexing the knee to 90 degrees and advancing the tendon stripper parallel to the tendon by a slow, steady, rotating motion. The semitendinosus tendon is harvested in a similar fashion; however, there are more extensive fascial connections that extend from the inferior border of the semitendinosus tendon to the medial head of the gastrocnemius.[7,31] These fascial connections must be released to prevent premature amputation of the semitendinosus tendon.

More proximally in the thigh, the surgeon may encounter a second potential troublesome area at a band of thickened semimembranosus fascia that courses inferior and medial to the semimembranosus tendon.[7] This thickened band of fascia forms a sling for the semitendinosus tendon, suspending it from the inferior border of the semimembranosus muscle. Premature amputation of the semitendinosus tendon can result if the tendon strip-

per passes outside of the tendon's normal path (Fig. 62-6).[7] If excessive resistance is encountered in attempting to advance the tendon stripper through this region, it is tempting to pull harder on the semitendinosus tendon and to apply more force to the tendon stripper to advance it. However, this can cause the fascial sling beneath the semimembranosus to constrict, making it more difficult to pass the tendon stripper. Decreasing tension on the tendon and "navigating" the tendon stripper through the fascial sling will often lead to success. In a heavily muscled individual, the tendon stripper will often meet resistance at the musculotendinous junction; this can be overcome by steady pressure and rotation of the tendon stripper or by use of the larger 7.4-mm diameter stripper (Smith & Nephew Endoscopy, Andover, Mass). A successful graft harvest typically results in graft lengths of 20 to 26 cm for the gracilis and 24 to 30 cm for the semitendinosus tendon.

2. Graft Preparation

Preparation of the hamstring tendon grafts is facilitated by use of a graft preparation board (Graft Master II; Smith & Nephew Endoscopy). Residual muscle fibers on the proximal end of both tendons are removed by blunt dissection with a metal ruler, a large curet, or a Cushing-type periosteal elevator. The two tendons are cut to the same length, and the proximal end of each tendon is tubularized with a running, baseball-style whipstitch of a No. 2 nonabsorbable suture. The sutures on each end of the tendon grafts are tensioned with a "cinching" motion to remove excess slack

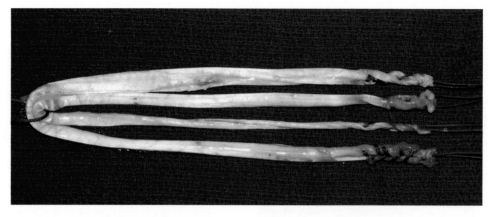

Figure 62-7 Doubled gracilis and semitendinosus tendon (DGST) graft. (From Brown CH, Sklar JH, Darwich N. Endoscopic anterior cruciate ligament reconstruction using autogenous doubled gracilis and semitendinosus tendons. Tech Knee Surg 2004;3:221.)

from the whipstitches. The two tendon grafts are looped around a No. 5 suture, making a DGST graft (Fig. 62-7). The diameter of the DGST graft is measured to the nearest 0.5 mm by use of a 0.5-mm incremental sizing block or sizing tubes. The whipstitches from the gracilis and semitendinosus tendons on each end of the graft are tied together approximately 12 cm from the end of the tendon grafts. This facilitates use of a graft-tensioning device later in the procedure. The DGST graft is looped around an EndoButton tensioning post (Smith & Nephew Endoscopy), and the DGST graft is covered with a moist laparotomy pad and pretensioned on the graft preparation board with 5 to 10 pounds for the remainder of the procedure.

3. Arthroscopic Portal Placement

As recommended by Cohen and Fu,[10] we use three portals for ACL reconstruction (Fig. 62-8). A high anterolateral portal at the level of the inferior pole of the patella adjacent to the lateral border of the patellar tendon is used for the routine viewing portal. The height of this portal places the arthroscope above the fat pad and provides an excellent "look down" view of the ACL tibial attachment site. This portal gives a frontal view of the femoral attachment site of the ACL and is most helpful in determining the clock orientation and high-low placement of the femoral tunnel. An anteromedial portal at the level of the inferior pole of the patella adjacent to the medial border of the patellar tendon is used for instrumentation and viewing of the medial wall of the lateral femoral condyle. This portal provides a more orthogonal view of the ACL femoral attachment site and allows more accurate assessment of shallow-deep femoral tunnel placement (Fig. 62-9).

An accessory medial portal located directly inferior to the anteromedial portal at the level of the medial joint line is used for drilling of the femoral tunnel.

4. Preparation of the Intercondylar Notch

Preparation of the intercondylar notch is necessary to allow visualization of the ACL femoral attachment site. A

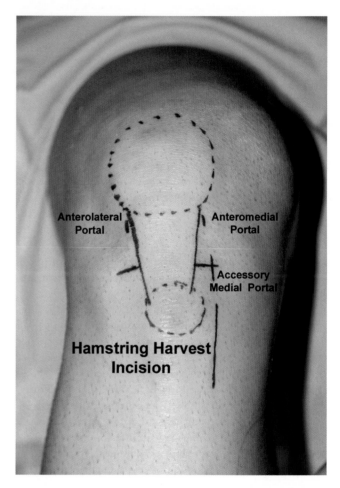

Figure 62-8 Portal location (right knee).

routine diagnostic arthroscopy is performed, and associated meniscal and chondral injuries are treated appropriately. The torn fibers of the ACL are removed from the lateral femoral condyle and the tibial attachment site by a motorized shaver, electrocautery pencil, or radiofrequency

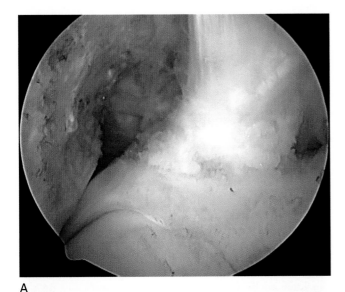

A

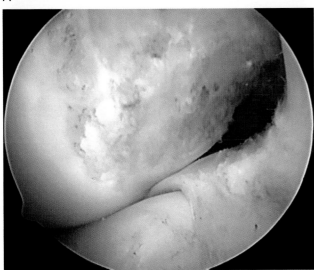

B

Figure 62-9 Arthroscopic view of femoral attachment site of the ACL from the anterolateral portal (**A**) and the anteromedial portal (**B**).

Transtibial Tunnel Technique Versus Anteromedial Portal Technique

Hamstring ACL reconstruction can be performed by the transtibial tunnel or anteromedial portal technique.[7,22,25,26,29] Regardless of the surgical technique used, the following goals must be achieved to optimize the outcome of the procedure:

- An anatomically positioned, impingement-free tibial tunnel
- A tibial tunnel with a minimum length of 40 mm
- An orientation of the femoral tunnel at a 9:30- to 10-o'clock position along the sidewall of the lateral femoral condyle
- A femoral tunnel with a minimum length of 40 mm

Achievement of these goals will eliminate roof impingement, optimize graft fixation with the EndoButton CL and IntraFix tibial fastener, and maximize the ability of a single-tunnel hamstring ACL reconstruction to control tibial rotation.[23]

Advantages of the transtibial tunnel technique are that it is familiar to most surgeons and does not require the knee to be flexed to 120 degrees during drilling of the femoral tunnel. Joint distention and the field of view in the intercondylar notch are compromised when the knee is flexed to 120 degrees or more, as required with the anteromedial technique. The transtibial tunnel technique also tends to produce longer femoral tunnels in the range of 40 to 50 mm. Femoral tunnel lengths in this range are advantageous for the EndoButton CL fixation technique because they allow a minimum of 25 mm of DGST graft to be inserted into the femoral socket. Another advantage of the transtibial tunnel technique is that the length of the femoral tunnel typically results in the EndoButton implant's resting on the stronger cortical bone of the distal femur. The major disadvantage of the transtibial tunnel technique is that free positioning of the femoral tunnel in the intercondylar notch is not possible because the femoral tunnel location is determined by the axis of the tibial tunnel.

In the transtibial tunnel technique, the angle of the tibial tunnel in the coronal plane determines femoral tunnel length and the position of the ACL graft in the intercondylar notch (Fig. 62-10).[7] Laboratory biomechanical studies have demonstrated that single-tunnel ACL grafts placed at the 10-o'clock position provide better rotational control as compared with ACL grafts at the 11-o'clock position.[23] For the femoral tunnel to be positioned at the 10-o'clock location, the tibial guide pin must be started adjacent to the anterior fibers of the MCL[7] (Fig. 62-11). However, in some cases, even when these recommendations are followed, it may not be possible to place the femoral tunnel at the desired position. When faced with this situation, we recommend switching to the anteromedial portal technique to avoid malpositioning of the

probe. We have found that use of a radiofrequency probe is faster, allows hemostasis to be achieved, and more completely removes the soft tissue along the lateral wall of the intercondylar notch, providing better visualization of the bone anatomy. Use of the anteromedial portal technique allows the femoral tunnel to be positioned lower down the sidewall of the lateral femoral condyle, resulting in a more horizontal orientation of the ACL graft. A more horizontal ACL graft avoids posterior cruciate ligament impingement and in most cases eliminates the need for notchplasty. However, a selective notchplasty may be required in the case of congenitally narrowed notches or in chronic cases with notch stenosis due to the development of notch osteophytes.

62

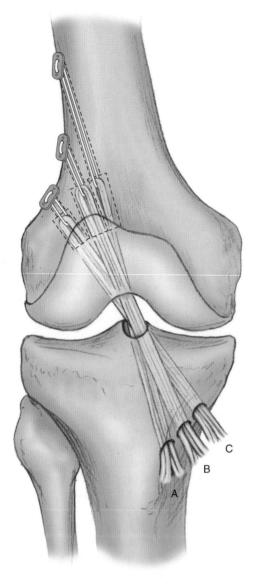

Figure 62-10 Effect of tibial tunnel starting position on femoral tunnel length. Tibial tunnel starting position close to the tibial tubercle (A) results in a long, vertically oriented femoral tunnel that requires a long continuous-loop length. A long continuous loop decreases stiffness of the femur–EndoButton CL–hamstring tendon complex. Tibial tunnel starting position midway between the tibial tubercle and the anterior fibers of the MCL (B) typically results in a femoral tunnel length of 50 to 60 mm. Tibial tunnel starting position at the anterior fibers of the MCL (C) typically results in a femoral tunnel length of 40 to 50 mm. (From Brown CH, Sklar JH. Endoscopic anterior cruciate ligament reconstruction using quadrupled hamstring tendons and EndoButton femoral fixation. Tech Orthop 1998;13:288.)

ACL graft. For a detailed description of hamstring ACL reconstruction performed by the transtibial tunnel technique, we refer the reader to our previously published technique.[7]

In the anteromedial portal technique, the femoral tunnel is drilled through the anteromedial portal or an accessory anteromedial portal.[23,29] Because the femoral tunnel is made independently of the tibial tunnel, free placement in the intercondylar notch is always possible.

Advantages of the anteromedial portal technique include the following:

- The ability to position the femoral tunnel in a more anatomic position lower down the sidewall of the lateral femoral condyle
- The freedom to locate the starting position of the tibial tunnel anywhere along the medial surface of the tibia
- The freedom to drill a steeper and therefore longer tibial tunnel
- The possibility of drilling the femoral tunnel before drilling the tibial tunnel, which helps maintain joint distention, improving joint visualization during the remainder of the procedure

However, the anteromedial portal technique requires the knee to be flexed 120 degrees or more during the drilling of the femoral tunnel, which limits joint distention and provides a more unconventional field of view in the notch that can result in spatial disorientation.[23,29] The anteromedial portal technique also tends to produce a more horizontal femoral tunnel that results in the EndoButton implant's lying on the weaker metaphyseal bone of the distal femur.[8] In our opinion, the ability of the anteromedial portal technique to allow a more anatomic placement of the femoral tunnel far outweighs its few disadvantages. For this reason, the anteromedial portal technique for femoral tunnel drilling has become our preferred surgical technique for performing ACL reconstruction.

5. Femoral Tunnel

Use of the low accessory medial portal for drilling of the femoral tunnel allows a longer femoral tunnel to be achieved than does drilling through the anteromedial portal. The resulting longer femoral tunnel is more advantageous for femoral fixation with the EndoButton CL. The location for the accessory medial portal is made by an 18-gauge spinal needle. This portal is located as low as possible just above the medial joint line. Placement of the portal too medially produces a shorter femoral tunnel and risks injury to the medial femoral condyle by the endoscopic drill bit during drilling of the femoral tunnel. The accessory medial portal is established under direct vision with a No. 11 knife blade, with care taken to avoid injury to the medial meniscus. Dilation of the portal with the blunt arthroscope obturator followed by the tips of the Metzenbaum scissors helps ease future passage of instrumentation.

A microfracture awl is passed through the accessory medial portal and used to mark the starting point for the femoral tunnel under arthroscopic guidance. Correct placement of the awl along the lateral wall of the intercondylar notch can be verified by intraoperative fluoroscopy with the radiographic quadrant method.[3] Fine tuning of

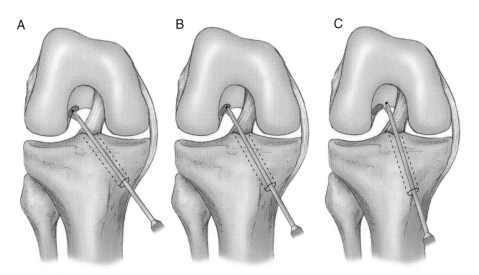

Figure 62-11 A, Tibial tunnel starting position at the anterior fibers of the MCL results in a femoral starting point at the 10-o'clock position (central portion of the ACL footprint). **B,** Tibial tunnel starting position midway between the anterior fibers of the MCL and the tibial tubercle results in a femoral starting point at the 11-o'clock position (attachment site of the anteromedial fibers). **C,** Tibial tunnel starting position close to the tibial tubercle results in a femoral starting point high in the intercondylar notch outside of the ACL footprint. (Redrawn from Brown CH, Sklar JH, Darwich N. Endoscopic anterior cruciate ligament reconstruction using autogenous doubled gracilis and semitendinosus tendons. Tech Knee Surg 2004;3:222.)

the awl's position is performed under fluoroscopic guidance. Additional confirmation of the correct starting point can be made by viewing the tip of the awl through the anteromedial portal (Fig. 62-12).

A 4- or 5-mm offset femoral aimer is passed through the accessory medial portal, and the knee is slowly flexed to 120 degrees. The blade of the femoral offset aimer is placed in the over-the-top position, and a 2.7-mm drill-tipped guide pin is positioned at the site of the microfracture awl penetration mark. Fluoroscopy can be used to check the guide pin placement. The knee is slowly brought into full flexion, and line of sight is used to verify that the guide pin will exit the lateral thigh above the intermuscular septum. The 2.7-mm drill-tipped guide wire is drilled out through the soft tissues of the lateral thigh (Fig. 62-13). Inadequate knee flexion can result in the guide pin's coming to lie inferior to the intermuscular septum, placing the peroneal nerve at risk. A 4.5-mm EndoButton drill bit (Smith & Nephew Endoscopy) is used to drill a channel through the lateral femoral cortex. A closed-end femoral socket is drilled with the appropriately sized, calibrated endoscopic 0.5-mm drill bit (Fig. 62-14). The femoral socket depth must allow for the length of the DGST graft to be inserted into the femur (usually 25 to 30 mm) plus an extra 6 mm to allow the EndoButton to clear the lateral femoral cortex and to flip. An EndoButton depth gauge (Smith & Nephew Endoscopy) inserted through the accessory medial portal is used to measure the femoral tunnel length. A loop of No. 5 nonabsorbable suture is inserted into the eyelet of the passing pin, and the ends of the suture are passed out of the lateral thigh. The loop of No. 5 suture is passed into the joint and positioned at the entrance to the femoral tunnel. This suture will be used later in the

procedure to pass the hamstring tendon graft. Because cylindric hamstring tendon grafts contact the entire edge of the femoral tunnel during cyclic motion of the knee, it is extremely important to bevel or chamfer the tunnel edges with a rasp to minimize graft abrasion.

6. Tibial Tunnel

In our surgical technique, a tibial tunnel length of 40 to 50 mm is optimal; this range will allow the 30-mm-long IntraFix sheath to be inserted flush with the tibial cortex, with no risk that the sheath will protrude into the intra-articular portion of the knee joint. Setting the adjustable tibial aimer between 50 and 55 degrees will usually allow these tunnel lengths to be achieved. The starting location of the tibial guide pin along the medial surface of the tibia is not critical when the anteromedial portal technique is used. The anterior horn of the lateral meniscus, the medial and lateral tibial spines, and the posterior cruciate ligament are used as landmarks to locate the intra-articular position of the tibial guide pin (Fig. 62-15). It is extremely helpful to use fluoroscopy to ensure correct placement of the tibial guide pin. With the knee in maximum extension, a true lateral fluoroscopic view of the knee with the femoral condyles overlapping is obtained. The tip of the guide pin should be parallel to and 2 mm posterior to Blumensaat's line (Fig. 62-16). An offset parallel drill guide can be used to reposition the guide pin if necessary. To prevent anterior drift of the tibial tunnel, a cannulated, rear-entry–style, 0.5-mm drill bit is used to drill the tibial tunnel. Half-round or angled ACL chamfering rasps are used to smooth the intra-articular edges of the tibial tunnel to minimize graft abrasion. Soft tissue around the superior edge of the

Text continued on p. 633.

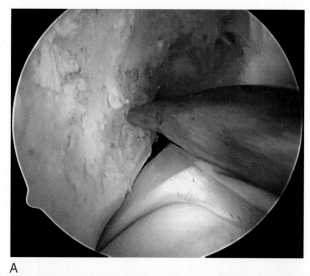

A

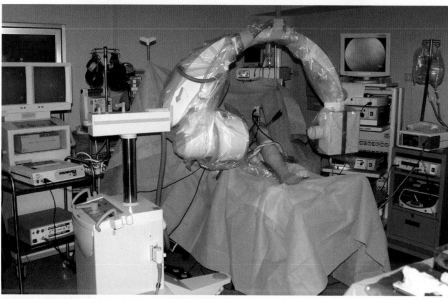

B

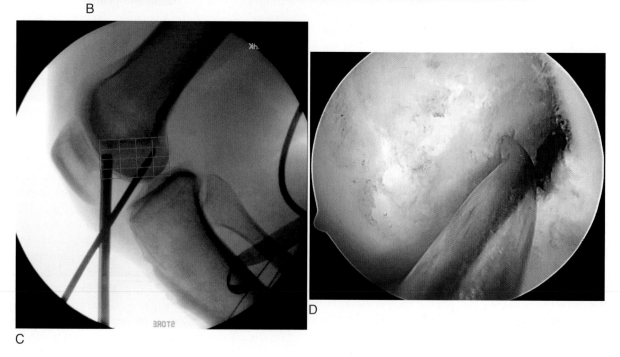

C

D

Figure 62-12 A, Microfracture awl introduced through the accessory medial portal is used to establish a starting point for the femoral tunnel (view through the anterolateral portal). **B,** Fluoroscopy is used to orient the starting point for the femoral tunnel. **C,** Digital fluoroscopic images can be captured with an Image Capture System. The radiographic quadrant of Bernard et al[3] can be used to determine the optimal starting point for the femoral tunnel. According to this method, the starting point for the femoral guide pin should be in the distal corner of the posterior superior quadrant. **D,** Fine adjustments of the starting point can be made by viewing the awl through the anteromedial portal. Viewing through this portal gives better shallow-deep spatial orientation in the notch.

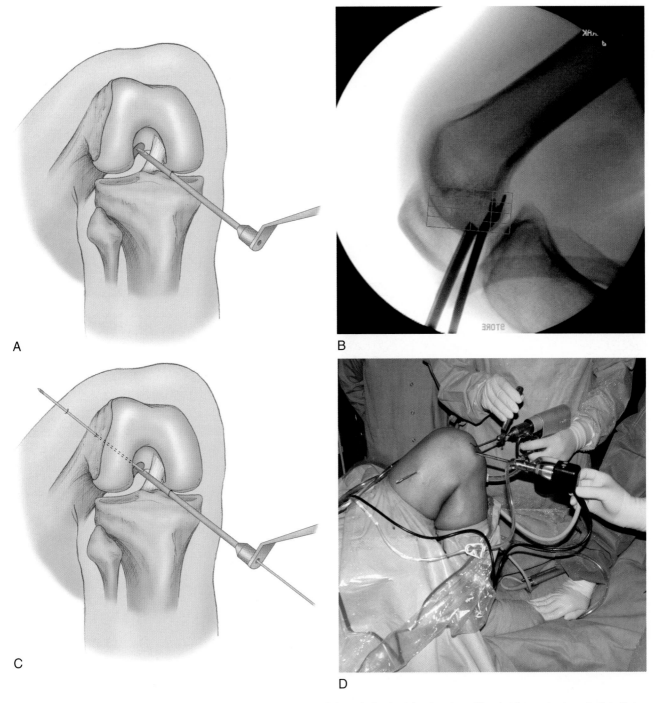

Figure 62-13 A, Femoral offset aimer is introduced through the accessory medial portal; the tip of the aimer is positioned at the previously marked starting point. **B,** Fluoroscopy can be used to confirm the starting point for the femoral guide pin. **C** and **D,** The femoral guide pin is drilled out through the lateral soft tissues with the knee in full flexion.

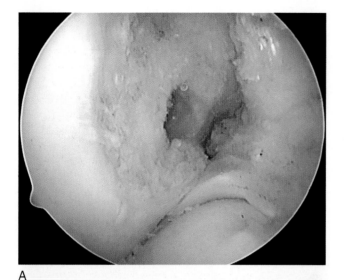

A

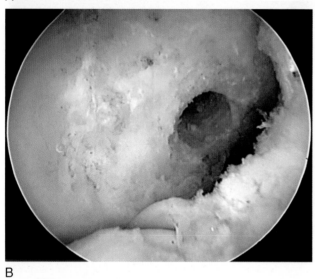

B

Figure 62-14 A, Femoral tunnel viewed through the anterolateral portal with the knee at 90 degrees of flexion. **B,** Femoral tunnel viewed through the anteromedial portal with the knee at 90 degrees of flexion.

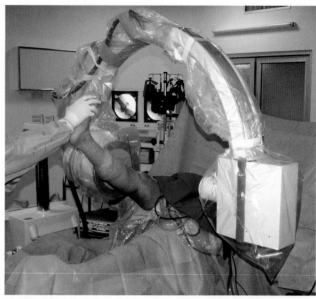

A

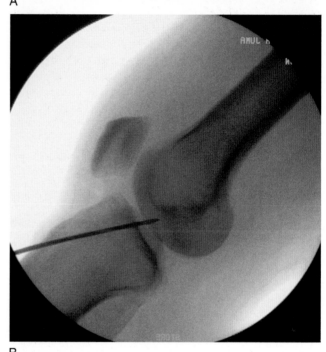

B

Figure 62-16 A, To ensure correct placement of the tibial guide pin, fluoroscopy is used to obtain a true lateral view with the knee in maximum hyperextension. **B,** The guide pin should lie 2 mm posterior to and parallel to Blumensaat's line.

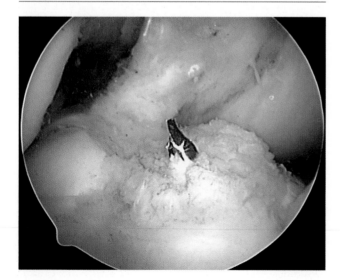

Figure 62-15 The tibial guide pin should be positioned halfway between the medial and lateral tibial spines along a line connecting the anterior horn of the lateral meniscus and the medial tibial spine.

tibial tunnel is cleared with an electrocautery pencil and a Cobb periosteal elevator in preparation for insertion of the IntraFix tibial fastener.

7. Calculation of EndoButton CL Length and Graft Preparation

The required continuous-loop length is calculated by subtracting the amount of graft to be inserted into the femoral socket from the directly measured femoral tunnel length. For example, assuming the femoral tunnel length measures 48 mm, and 30 mm of DGST graft has been chosen to be inserted into the femoral tunnel, the required continuous-loop length is calculated as follows: 48 mm − 30 mm = 18 mm. Because the continuous-loop lengths come in 5-mm increments, a 15- or 20-mm-loop comes closest to the calculated length. In general, we prefer to use the shortest possible continuous loop because this increases the stiffness of the femur–EndoButton CL–DGST graft complex. In the example cited before, we would choose a 15-mm length of loop. The appropriate length of EndoButton CL is selected and placed in the EndoButton holder (Smith & Nephew Endoscopy), and the axilla of the DGST graft is passed through the continuous loop. The two ends of the DGST graft are equalized in length and pretensioned to 10 pounds on the graft preparation board. The graft is marked with a surgical marking pen at the measured femoral tunnel length. A full-length No. 2 flipping suture and a No. 5 passing suture are passed through the end holes of the EndoButton. A second No. 5 suture can be inserted into the same hole as the No. 2 flipping suture and passed alongside the graft and out of the tibial tunnel. If necessary, this "safety suture" can be used to disengage the EndoButton from the distal femur, allowing the hamstring tendon graft to be removed from the knee.

8. Graft Passage and Femoral Fixation

The loop of No. 5 suture is retrieved from the femoral tunnel and pulled out of the tibial tunnel. The No. 2 flipping suture and No. 5 passing suture are passed through the loop of the No. 5 suture and pulled out the lateral thigh. Under arthroscopic visualization, the EndoButton and the attached hamstring tendon graft are passed across the joint and into the femoral socket by use of the No. 5 passing suture. The DGST graft must be advanced until the previously placed insertion mark is seen to pass up into the femoral socket a distance of a few millimeters. This extra distance allows the EndoButton to pass outside the lateral femoral cortex and to flip. The No. 2 flipping suture is pulled in a proximal direction, parallel to the femoral tunnel, and the EndoButton will be felt to flip against the lateral femoral cortex. Correct deployment can be verified by pulling on the No. 2 sutures and feeling the EndoButton "teeter-totter" against the lateral femoral cortex. If any doubts exist about secure deployment of the EndoButton, fluoroscopy can be used to check the position of the EndoButton.

Tension is applied to the hamstring tendon graft, and the previously placed mark at the insertion length will be seen to slide back down the femoral tunnel. If the measurements are correct, this mark should lie at the entrance of the femoral tunnel. If it should become necessary to remove the graft, the No. 5 passing suture on the EndoButton can be pulled proximally, tipping the EndoButton away from the femoral cortex. The No. 5 safety suture that exited the tibial tunnel is pulled, tipping the opposite end of the EndoButton into the 4.5-mm tunnel. The EndoButton will then disengage from the femoral cortex, and the graft can be removed by applying tension to the whipstitches on the tibial end of the graft.

9. Graft Tensioning

The opposite ends of the hamstring tendon graft are applied to a graft-tensioning device (Smith & Nephew Endoscopy), and a preload of 80 to 100 N is applied to the graft. The tensioning device is designed to apply equal tension to each end of the four-stranded hamstring tendon graft and to spread the tendons apart, allowing easier insertion of the IntraFix tibial fastener. Application of equal tension to all four limbs of the hamstring tendon graft optimizes initial fixation strength and stiffness.[16] The knee is cycled from 0 to 90 degrees for a minimum of 30 cycles, with a preload of 80 to 100 N applied to the graft by the tensioning device. Application of a preload and cycling of the knee are important steps as they allow the EndoButton CL to settle on the femoral cortex and remove creep from the polyester continuous loop, the tendon whipstitches, and the hamstring graft. At present, the optimal graft tension and knee flexion angle during tibial fixation are unknown. Depending on the graft excursion pattern detected in cycling of the knee, we tend to fix the graft with the knee positioned between 0 and 20 degrees of flexion. The usual graft excursion pattern detected with our bone tunnel placements results in pulling of the DGST graft into the tibial tunnel (tightening) during the last 20 degrees of terminal extension. When there is minimal graft excursion detected, we tend to fix the graft with the knee at 20 degrees of flexion and near full extension with greater excursions. Because of the high fixation strength and stiffness and the resistance to slippage of the IntraFix tibial fastener, we caution against applying excessive tension (>80 N) to the graft or fixing the knee at a flexion angle of more than 20 degrees. A high graft tension force in combination with the knee flexed more than 20 degrees may result in a permanent flexion contracture.

10. Tibial Fixation

Although the IntraFix tibial fastener is available as a bioabsorbable implant, we continue to prefer the original Delrin plastic version. The bioabsorbable version requires more precise sizing and a larger number of implants, increasing inventory. In addition, the bioabsorbable screw can break, leaving the surgeon with a difficult salvage situation.

Concentric placement of the IntraFix tibial fastener is critical to the success of the technique and starts with the identification of the central axis of the tibial tunnel. The central axis of the tibial tunnel is identified by passing a 1.1-mm guide wire up the center of the tensioning device and down the center of the four graft strands into the knee joint. Once the central axis of the tibial tunnel is identified, the tensioner should be held in this orientation during the subsequent steps to avoid divergent placement of the implant. The four-quadrant trial dilator is inserted down the center of the four hamstring tendon strands and oriented so that each graft strand sits in its own channel. While the desired tension is maintained on the hamstring graft, the four-quadrant trial dilator is tapped into the tibial tunnel for a distance of 30 to 35 mm. This step compresses and separates the four tendon strands and notches the bone tunnel wall to receive the 30-mm IntraFix sheath.

The 30-mm IntraFix sheath is placed on the sheath inserter with the derotational tab on the sheath oriented to match the tab on the sheath inserter. The knee is positioned at the chosen flexion angle, and a final tension of 60 to 80 N is applied to the DGST graft by use of the tensioning device. It is important to maintain the chosen flexion angle and desired graft tension during the subsequent steps. The IntraFix sheath is inserted between the four graft strands, making sure that each graft strand is positioned into a separate channel of the sheath with the derotational tab on the sheath oriented at the 3-o'clock or 9-o'clock position. Orientation of the derotational tab at these positions allows the IntraFix sheath to be inserted more deeply into the tibia, avoiding prominence. The IntraFix sheath is tapped into the bone until the derotational tab is inserted flush with the cortex (Fig. 62-17).

The sheath inserter is removed, and the 0.042-inch guide wire for the tapered screw is inserted through the center of the sheath until a loss of resistance is felt as the tip of the guide wire enters the knee joint.

An IntraFix tapered screw size of 1 mm larger than the tibial tunnel diameter is chosen. For example, we use a 7- to 9-mm tapered screw for an 8-mm tibial tunnel. Given the typical size of most DGST grafts, the 7- to 9-mm tapered screw is most commonly used. While tension is maintained on the DGST graft, the IntraFix tapered screw is inserted into the sheath until the superior aspect of the screw head is flush with or buried just below the tibial cortex (Fig. 62-18). The best bone quality is at or next to the tibial cortex, and overly deep insertion of the screw may decrease fixation strength.[5] Protruding or prominent areas of the polyethylene sheath are trimmed flush with the tibial cortex with a No. 15 blade and a small bone rongeur.

The fixation strength of any intratunnel tibial fixation device depends on the local bone mineral density.[4,20,24] If the surgeon thinks that there was inadequate torque during the insertion of the tapered screw or if the patient

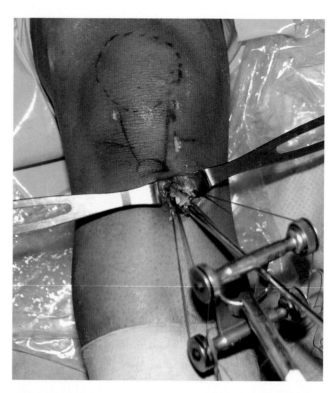

Figure 62-17 Insertion of the 30-mm IntraFix sheath. The 30-mm IntraFix sheath is inserted down the center of the DGST graft, parallel to the axis of the tibial tunnel, with each tendon graft strand positioned in its own channel.

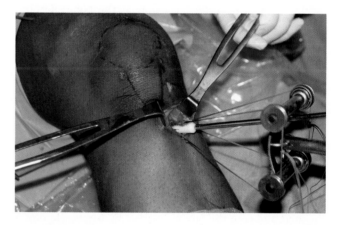

Figure 62-18 Insertion of the IntraFix tapered screw. With the knee at the chosen flexion angle, tension is maintained on the graft strands by the graft-tensioning device, and the IntraFix tapered screw is inserted along the guide wire into the IntraFix sheath.

has soft bone, we recommend that supplemental tibial fixation be used. Depending on the length of the DGST graft, the protruding tendons can be stapled below the tibial tunnel with a small barbed staple (Smith & Nephew Orthopaedics, Memphis, Tenn), or the tendon whip-stitches can be tied around an extra-small nonbarbed staple or tibial fixation post.

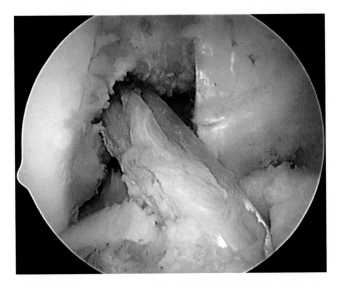

Figure 62-19 Arthroscopic appearance of the DGST graft. The femoral attachment site of the graft is located along the side wall of the lateral femoral condyle, and the graft is oriented at a 10-o'clock position in the notch.

The stability and range of motion of the knee are checked. It is important to verify that the patient has full range of motion before leaving the operating room. The arthroscope is inserted into the knee, and graft tension and impingement are assessed. Our usual graft placement and tensioning technique result in the four strands of the DGST graft being maximally tight between 0 and 20 degrees, with the graft tension decreasing slightly as the knee is flexed to 90 degrees (Fig. 62-19). After confirmation that the patient has a full range of motion and negative Lachman and pivot shift test results, the passing and flipping sutures are pulled out of the lateral thigh.

11. Closure

A closed suction drain is inserted under the sartorius fascia up into the hamstring harvest site and is helpful in preventing postoperative hematoma formation and decreasing ecchymosis along the medial side of the knee. The sartorius fascia that was preserved during the graft harvest is repaired back to the tibia with a 0 absorbable suture. The subcutaneous tissue is closed in layers with fine absorbable sutures. A running 3-0 Prolene subcuticular pullout suture produces a cosmetic closure. A second solution of 5 mg of morphine sulfate plus 20 mL of 0.25% bupivacaine with 1:100,000 epinephrine is injected into the suprapatellar pouch, and a 30-mg bolus of ketorolac is given for postoperative pain control. The continuous intravenous ketorolac infusion is continued until the patient is discharged from the day-surgery unit. A light dressing is applied over the wound, followed by a thigh-length TED antiembolism stocking, Cryo/Cuff (DJ Orthopedics, Vista, Calif), and knee immobilizer. The Hemovac drain is

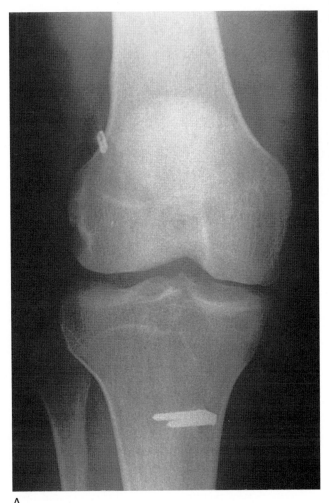

A

Figure 62-20 Postoperataive radiographs. **A,** Proper tibial tunnel placement results in placement of the EndoButton at the flare of the distal femur. A small staple was used for supplemental tibial fixation in this case.

removed when the patient is discharged from the day-surgery unit.

Postoperative Management

Follow-up

The patient is seen at 7 to 10 days for suture removal and postoperative radiographs (Fig. 62-20).

Rehabilitation

Our postoperative rehabilitation protocol is described in Table 62-1. The weight-bearing schedule is modified if a

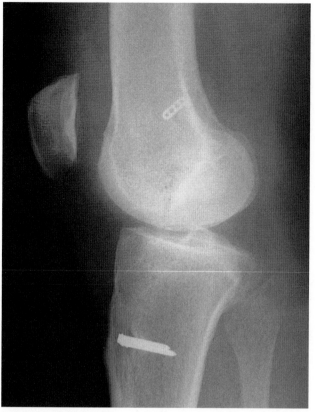

B

Figure 62-20, cont'd B, Lateral radiograph in maximum hyperextension. The tibial tunnel is parallel and posterior to Blumensaat's line.

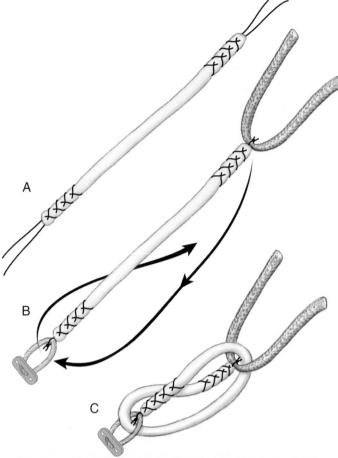

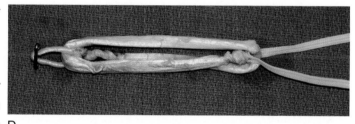

D

Figure 62-21 Technique for preparation of a triple-stranded semitendinosus graft. **A,** Semitendinosus graft with No. 2 nonabsorbable whipstitches placed at each end. **B,** The appropriate-length EndoButton CL is tied to one end of the semitendinosus graft, and the other end of the semitendinosus tendon is tied to EndoButton tape (Smith & Nephew Endoscopy). **C,** The end of the semitendinosus graft with the EndoButton tape is looped through the EndoButton CL and the EndoButton tape is passed through the resulting loop of semitendinosus graft, making a three-stranded semitendinosus graft. **D,** Final appearance of a triple-stranded semitendinosus graft. (From Brown CH, Sklar JH, Darwich N. Endoscopic anterior cruciate ligament reconstruction using autogenous doubled gracilis and semitendinosus tendons. Tech Knee Surg 2004;3:233.)

meniscus repair, microfracture, or other associated ligamentous surgery has been performed.

Complications

The risks of complications such as infection, deep venous thrombosis, and loss of motion are the same as for ACL reconstructions performed with other graft sources. However, we are unaware of reports of extensor mechanism rupture or patellar fracture after ACL reconstruction performed with hamstring tendon grafts. Complications unique to hamstring tendon grafts include premature amputation of the hamstring tendons, saphenous nerve injury, bleeding at the hamstring tendon harvest site, and hamstring muscle "pulls."

The risk of premature amputation of the tendons can be minimized by following the recommendations outlined in the section on graft harvest. If the gracilis tendon is amputated but the semitendinosus is successfully harvested, it is possible in most cases either to triple or to quadruple the semitendinosus tendon, depending on its length (Fig. 62-21). In these situations, the EndoButton CL can still be used for femoral fixation; however, because of the shorter length of the graft construct, alternative tibial fixation is obtained by tying the EndoButton tape

around a fixation post or an extra-small nonbarbed staple. If necessary, the tibial fixation can be augmented with a 25- to 30-mm bioabsorbable screw with a diameter 1 mm greater than that of the tibial tunnel. If the semitendinosus tendon is amputated, it will be necessary to use an alternative autograft, such as the patellar tendon or

Table 62-1 Postoperative Rehabilitation Protocol for Hamstring ACL Reconstruction

Goals	Exercises
Phase I: Days 0-7	
Control pain, inflammation, joint effusion, swelling	Knee Cryo/Cuff, thigh-length TED stocking, elevation
Full passive extension equal to that of the opposite knee	Heel props, pull knee into hyperextension with elastic band
Achieve 90-degree flexion	Wall slides, gravity-assisted flexion sitting on the edge of a table
Prevent quadriceps shutdown	Electrical muscle stimulation, quad isometrics, straight-leg raises, active assisted extension 90-0 degrees
Prevent heel cord contracture	Ankle pumps, calf stretches with elastic bands
Gait training	Weight bearing as tolerated with knee immobilizer and crutches; meniscus repair, revisions: ↑25% body weight/week, wean off crutches at end of week 4
Phase II: Weeks 1-2	
Control inflammation, pain, joint effusion, swelling	Continue phase I exercises
Maintain full symmetric extension	Continue phase I exercises
Achieve 100-125 degrees of flexion	Assisted flexion with use of opposite leg, wall slides, heel drags, rolling stool
Develop muscle control to be safely weaned off knee immobilizer and crutches	Continue phase I exercises, mini-squats, toe raises, active extension 90-30 degrees
Protect hamstring donor site	Prevent sudden, forceful hamstring stretching with the knee and hip in extension, such as attempting to lean forward to put on socks and shoes or leaning forward to pick up an object off the floor
Phase III: Weeks 2-4	
Maintain symmetric extension	Heel props, prone heel hangs, lock knee out, "stand at attention" Patients who fail to obtain symmetric extension should be considered for extension splinting or a "drop-out" cast
Wean off knee immobilizer	Discard immobilizer when straight-leg raises are performed without a quad lag
Wean off crutches	One crutch with ability to bear 75% of body weight; discard crutches with full weight bearing and ability to walk with normal heel-toe gait
Achieve 125-135 degrees of flexion	Heel slides, sitting back on heels
Hamstring strengthening	Hamstring isometrics 0-90 degrees, pull rolling stool backward
Quadriceps strengthening	Continue phase II exercises, mini-squats with elastic band for resistance
Hip strengthening	Side-lying hip abduction, adjustable-angle hip machine
Proprioceptive training	Balance board double-leg stance
Aerobic conditioning	Elliptical machine
Phase IV: Weeks 4-6	
Obtain full flexion	Heel slides, sitting back on heels
Continue quadriceps, hamstring, and hip strengthening	Mini-squats, leg press 50-0 degrees, front step-ups (control hip valgus), StairMaster backward, proprioceptive neuromuscular facilitation, toe raises, seated leg-curl machine 0-90 degrees
Proprioceptive training	Balance board double- and single-leg stance, add ball throws and catches
Aerobic conditioning	Stationary bike (adjust to protect patellofemoral joint), elliptical machine, pool exercises

Continued on overleaf.

62

Table 62-1 Postoperative Rehabilitation Protocol for Hamstring ACL Reconstruction—cont'd

Goals	Exercises
Phase V: Weeks 6-12	
Increase lower extremity strength and endurance	Increase intensity of phase IV exercises, high-speed (300-360 degrees/sec) isokinetics, extension (90-30 degrees), flexion (0-90 degrees), elliptical machine, StairMaster backward and forward, treadmill walking, pool exercises
Advance proprioceptive and perturbation training	Increase intensity of phase IV exercises
Phase VI: Weeks 12-16	
Increase quad and hamstring strength	Increase intensity of phase IV exercises, midrange (180-240 degrees/sec) isokinetics, extension (90-30 degrees), flexion (0-90 degrees)
Increase hamstring strength at high flexion angles	Prone leg curls with elastic tubing and leg-curl machine (90-120 degrees)
Jogging and running	Treadmill jogging and running, outdoor running on low-impact surface
Crossover drills	Lateral step-over, carioca drills
Phase VI: Weeks 16-24	
Hard cutting and sports-specific drills	Figure-of-eight, circle run, plyometrics, hopping, jumping, sprinting
Return to noncontact sports at 4-5 months	Golf, tennis, biking, hiking
Return to full sports at 6 months (revisions, 9 months)	

quadriceps tendon, or allograft tissue if preoperative consent has been obtained. The possibility of premature amputation of the tendons should be discussed during the informed consent process, and the patient and surgeon should agree on a course of action should this complication occur.

PEARLS AND PITFALLS

- Before detaching the conjoined tibial insertion of the two tendons and their dissection off the tibia, it is important to clearly identify and to bluntly separate the tendons from the underlying MCL. Failure to do so may result in the mistaken dissection of the MCL off the tibia.

- Leaving the distal 5 mm of each tendon attached to the fascial flap makes reattachment of the flap easier at the end of the procedure.

- Apply firm traction to the tendon whipstitches to release any of the remaining fascial connections before harvest of the tendon grafts.

- Complete release of the fascial connections to the medial head of the gastrocnemius can be verified by the absence of tethering of the muscle and bowing of the tendon when traction is applied to the whipstitch.

- Drilling the femoral tunnel first minimizes fluid extravasation, maintains joint distention to improve visualization, and minimizes use of the tourniquet.

- Use fluoroscopy to confirm the femoral tunnel starting point.

- Make adjustments to the femoral tunnel starting position by viewing through the anteromedial portal.

- The knee must be flexed 120 degrees or more when the anteromedial portal technique is used.

- The femoral tunnel length can be increased by drilling the femoral guide pin into the lateral femoral condyle a distance of 2 to 3 mm, then angulating the femoral offset aimer toward the midline of the knee.

- Increasing the infusion pump pressure when the knee is fully flexed can improve visualization in the notch.

- Visualization can be improved during drilling of the femoral tunnel by suctioning debris out of the joint with use of a shaver placed through the anteromedial portal.

Results

Historical perceptions of hamstring ACL reconstructions are that they produce unpredictable objective stability, tend to stretch out with time, and are not as good as reconstruction with a patellar tendon graft.

Meta-analyses of Yunes et al[33] and Freedman et al[14] concluded that patellar tendon autografts produce greater stability and result in higher postoperative activity levels. However, these studies included some series in which older hamstring fixation methods and two-stranded hamstring tendon grafts were used. Prospective randomized controlled studies comparing quadrupled hamstrings with bone–patellar tendon–bone reconstructions have demonstrated no significant differences in laxity or in clinical outcome measures at early follow-up.[1,2,13,15,22,26,30] A meta-analysis performed by Prodromos et al,[28] in which the results were stratified by graft and fixation type, demonstrated that four-stranded hamstring tendon grafts had overall stability rates equal to or higher than those of patellar tendon grafts. This study also demonstrated that the four-stranded hamstring stability rates were fixation dependent; series using Endo-Button femoral fixation and second-generation tibial fixation resulted in higher stability rates than did all other graft-fixation combinations. When the literature is carefully analyzed, four-stranded hamstring ACL reconstruction with second-generation fixation is comparable to patellar tendon autograft reconstruction, and current preconceptions regarding four-stranded hamstring ACL reconstructions may be a historical artifact (Table 62-2).

Table 62-2 Outcomes for Four-Stranded Hamstring ACL Reconstructions

Author	Year	Average Follow-up	Manual Max KT ≤2 mm	Clinical Outcome	Donor Site Morbidity
EndoButton Femoral Fixation with Second-Generation Tibial Fixation					
Cooley et al[11]	2001	5.7 years	100%	85% IKDC score normal or nearly normal	24% increased PF crepitus
Eriksson et al[12] Prospective randomized STG vs. PT	2001	33 months	STG, 43% PT, 48% NS	Lysholm score increased from 61 to 86 58% IKDC score normal or nearly normal Lysholm and Tegner scores, range of motion, laxity NS from PT	STG and PT PF pain scores NS Kneeling pain: PT>STG
Feller and Webster[13] Prospective randomized STG vs. PT	2003	3 years	85%	93% IKDC score normal or nearly normal PT greater extension deficit; quad strength, activity levels NS from PT	Kneeling pain: STG, 26%; PT, 67%
Gobbi et al[15]	2003	3 years	90%	Lysholm score, 91 72% IKDC score normal or nearly normal	Kneeling pain, 7% 10% mild PF crepitus
Gobbi ST vs. STG	2005	3 years	ST, 88% STG, 89%	Lysholm score: ST, 92; STG, 94 94% IKDC score normal or nearly normal 8% required hardware removal	Kneeling pain, 3% 10% mild PF crepitus
Prodromos et al[27]	2005	4.5 years	86%	Lysholm score, 95 72% IKDC normal or nearly normal No difference between males and females in Lysholm score or KT laxity scores No patient required hardware removal	PF crepitus: mild, 20%; moderate, 3%
Cross-Pin Femoral Fixation					
Aglietti et al[1] Prospective randomized STG vs. PT	2004	2 years	STG, 57% PT, 65% NS	IKDC score normal: STG, 57%; PT, 63% (NS) Range of motion, quad and hamstring strength, postoperative activity levels NS	PF symptoms: NS Kneeling pain: STG, 15%; PT, 62%
Harilainen et al[17] Prospective randomized STG vs. PT	2005	2 years	STG, 72% PT, 62% NS	88% negative pivot shift Lysholm score, 96 85% IKDC score normal or nearly normal Knee scores, range of motion, quad and hamstring strength NS STG: 58% required removal of tibial fixation hardware	Not reported
Fabbriciani	2005	2 years	61%	90% IKDC score normal or nearly normal	Not reported

IKDC, International Knee Documentation Committee; PF, patellofemoral; PT, patellar tendon; NS, not significant; ST, semitendinosus tendon; STG, semitendinosus tendon and gracilis construct.

62

References

1. Aglietti P, Giron F, Buzzi R, et al. Anterior cruciate ligament reconstruction: bone–patellar tendon–bone compared with double semitendinosus and gracilis tendon grafts. J Bone Joint Surg Am 2004; 86:2143-2155.

2. Aune AK, Holm I, Risberg MA, et al. Four-strand hamstring tendon autograft compared with patellar tendon–bone autograft for anterior cruciate ligament reconstruction: a randomized study with two-year follow-up. Am J Sports Med 2001;29:722-728.

3. Bernard M, Hertel P, Hornung H, Cierpinski T. Femoral insertion of the ACL. Radiographic quadrant method. Am J Knee Surg 1997; 10:14-22.

4. Brand JC, Weiler A, Caborn DNM, et al. Graft fixation in cruciate ligament reconstruction. Am J Sports Med 2000;28:761-774.

5. Brown CH, Steiner ME, Carson EW. The use of hamstring tendons for anterior cruciate ligament reconstruction. Technique and results. Clin Sports Med 1992;12:723-756.

6. Brown CH, Wilson DR, Hecker AT, Ferragamo M. Graft-bone motion and tensile properties of hamstring and patellar tendon anterior cruciate ligament femoral graft fixation under cyclic loading. Arthroscopy 2004;20:922-935.

7. Brown CH, Sklar JH, Darwich N. Endoscopic anterior cruciate ligament reconstruction using autogenous doubled gracilis and semitendinosus tendons. Tech Knee Surg 2004;3:215-237.

8. Brucker PU, Zelle BA, Fu F. Intraarticular EndoButton displacement in anatomic anterior cruciate ligament double-bundle reconstruction: a case report. Oper Tech Orthop 2005;15:154-157.

9. Carofino B, Fulkerson J. Medial hamstring tendon regeneration following harvest for anterior cruciate reconstruction: fact, myth, and clinical implication. Arthroscopy 2005;21:1257-1264.

10. Cohen SB, Fu F. Three-portal technique for anterior cruciate ligament reconstruction: use of a central medial portal. Arthroscopy 2007;23:325.e1-5.

11. Cooley VJ, Deffner KT, Rosenberg TD. Quadrupled semitendinosus anterior cruciate ligament reconstruction: 5-year results in patients without meniscus loss. Arthroscopy 2001;17:795-800.

12. Eriksson K, Anderberg P, Hamberg P, et al. There are differences in early morbidity after ACL reconstruction when comparing patellar tendon and semitendinosus tendon graft. A prospective randomized study of 107 patients. Scand J Med Sci Sports 2001;11:170-177.

13. Feller JA, Webster KE. A randomized comparison of patellar tendon and hamstring tendon anterior cruciate ligament reconstruction. Am J Sports Med 2003;31:564-573.

14. Freedman K, D'Amato M, Nedeff D, et al. Arthroscopic anterior cruciate ligament reconstruction: a meta-analysis comparing patellar tendon and hamstring tendon autograft. Am J Sports Med 2003;31:2-11.

15. Gobbi A, Mahajan S, Zanazzo M, Tuy B. Patellar tendon versus quadrupled bone-semitendinosus anterior cruciate ligament reconstruction: a prospective clinical investigation in athletes. Arthroscopy 2003;19:592-601.

16. Hamner DL, Brown CH, Steiner ME, et al. Hamstring tendon grafts for reconstruction of the anterior cruciate ligament: biomechanical evaluation of the use of multiple strands and tensioning techniques. J Bone Joint Surg Am 1999;81:549-557.

17. Harilainen A, Sandelin J, Jansson K. Cross-pin femoral fixation versus metal interference screw fixation in anterior cruciate ligament reconstruction with hamstring tendons: results of a controlled prospective randomized study with 2 year follow-up. Arthroscopy 2005; 21:25-33.

18. Kartus J, Movin T, Karlsson J. Donor-site morbidity and anterior knee problems after anterior cruciate ligament reconstruction using autografts. Arthroscopy 2001;17:971-980.

19. Kousa P, Järvinen TLN, Vihavainen M, et al. The fixation strength of six hamstring tendon graft fixation devices in anterior cruciate ligament reconstruction. Part I: femoral site. Am J Sports Med 2003;31:174-181.

20. Kousa P, Järvinen TLN, Vihavainen M, et al. The fixation strength of six hamstring tendon graft fixation devices in anterior cruciate ligament reconstruction. Part II: tibial site. Am J Sports Med 2003;31:182-188.

21. Levy M, Prud'homme J. Anatomic variations of the pes anserinus: a cadaver study. Orthopedics 1993;16:601-606.

22. Liden M, Ejerhed L, Sernert N, et al. Patellar tendon or semitendinosus tendon autografts for anterior cruciate ligament reconstruction: a prospective, randomized study with 7-year follow-up. Am J Sports Med 2007;35:740-748.

23. Loh JC, Fukuda Y, Tsuda E, et al. Knee stability and graft function following anterior cruciate ligament reconstruction: comparison between 11 o'clock and 10 o'clock femoral tunnel positions. Arthroscopy 2003;19:297-304.

24. Magen HE, Howell SM, Hull ML. Structural properties of six tibial fixation methods for anterior cruciate ligament soft tissue grafts. Am J Sports Med 1999;27:35-43.

25. O'Donnell JB, Scerpella TA. Endoscopic anterior cruciate ligament reconstruction: modified technique and radiographic view. Arthroscopy 1995;11:577-584.

26. Pinczewski LA, Lyman J, Salmon LJ, et al. A 10-year comparison of anterior reconstruction with hamstring tendon and patellar tendon autograft: a controlled, prospective trial. Am J Sports Med 2007; 35:564-574.

27. Prodromos CC, Han YS, Keller BL, Bolyard RJ. Stability results of hamstring anterior cruciate ligament reconstruction at 2- to 8-year follow-up. Arthroscopy 2005;21:138-146.

28. Prodromos CC, Joyce BT, Shi K, Keller BL. A meta-analysis of stability after anterior cruciate ligament reconstruction as a function of hamstring versus patellar tendon graft and fixation type. Arthroscopy 2005;21:1202-1208.

29. Radowski CA, Harner CD. Medial portal technique for anterior cruciate ligament reconstruction. In El Attrache NS, Harner CD, Mirzayan R, Sekiya JK, eds. Surgical Technique in Sports Medicine. Philadelphia, Lippincott Williams & Wilkins, 2007: 359-367.

30. Shaieb MD, Kan DM, Chang SK, et al. A prospective randomized comparison of patellar tendon versus semitendinosus and gracilis tendon autografts for anterior cruciate ligament reconstruction. Am J Sports Med 2002;30:214-220.

31. Soloman CG, Pagnani MJ. Hamstring tendon harvesting: reviewing anatomic relationships and avoiding pitfalls. Orthop Clin North Am 2003;34:1-8.

32. Tashiro T, Kurosawa H, Kawakami A, et al. Influence of medial hamstring tendon harvest on knee flexor strength after anterior cruciate ligament reconstruction. A detailed evaluation with comparison of single- and double-tendon harvest. Am J Sports Med 2003;31: 522-529.

33. Yunes M, Richmond JC, Engels EA, Pinczewski LA. Patellar versus hamstring tendons in anterior cruciate ligament reconstruction: a meta-analysis. Arthroscopy 2001;17:248-257.

CHAPTER 63

Central Quadriceps Free Tendon Reconstruction of the Anterior Cruciate Ligament

John P. Fulkerson, MD

Central quadriceps tendon was first used for anterior cruciate ligament (ACL) reconstruction by John Marshall in the late 1970s.[7] Marshall incorporated a portion of the retinaculum from the anterior aspect of the patella as part of this graft. Blauth, a German surgeon, then reported use of the central quadriceps tendon with bone from the proximal patella in the 1980s.[2] Hans Uli Stäubli, a Swiss orthopedic surgeon, also used the central quadriceps tendon with bone and has studied the anatomy[10] as well as the mechanical properties of the graft.[11]

In 1995, we reported use of quadriceps tendon–bone graft for ACL reconstruction as a reliable ACL graft alternative.[4] At that time, Walter Shelton was also using the quadriceps tendon with bone for ACL reconstruction. He has subsequently reported his experience.

In 1997, with the advent of improved soft tissue fixation for ACL reconstruction, we first used the central quadriceps as a free tendon graft, without bone, for ACL reconstruction, reporting this new technique in 1999.[3] Craig Morgan also used quadriceps tendon and similarly found it to be highly satisfactory as an alternative to hamstring or bone-tendon-bone reconstruction of the ACL. Peter Jokl, at Yale University, adopted the central quadriceps free tendon graft for ACL reconstruction and has reported consistently good results with it as well. We have not chosen to use any other graft type since that time, as our results have been consistently satisfactory with a very low complication rate and stability results comparable to those obtained with other graft types. We believe that the

central quadriceps free tendon provides an important alternative for ACL reconstruction, yielding results similar to those of other autografts but without some of the short- and long-term problems associated with bone-tendon-bone and hamstring reconstruction. Risk of patellar fracture[13] and anterior knee pain[9] noted after bone-tendon-bone reconstruction have been avoided with central quadriceps free tendon.[12] The long-term reports of weakness in flexion[6] and the short-term risks of hamstring spasm, bleeding, and nerve and vein injury are also obviated with use of central quadriceps free tendon.

In short, the central quadriceps free tendon is an important and desirable autograft alternative for ACL reconstruction. It is harvested from a large tendon donor site without neurovascular complication risk and without risk of patellar fracture.

Preoperative Considerations

We use central quadriceps tendon for reconstruction in virtually all patients, male and female, competitive athletes and working people. Our criteria for surgery, elicited in the history, include recurrent instability related to ACL deficiency that limits daily function or participation in desired athletic activity and an active athletic lifestyle requiring quick turning, pivoting, and cutting such that problems might be predictable without ACL reconstruction. We establish a loss of ACL function by clinical examination to detect positive Lachman and pivot shift test results. We routinely use magnetic resonance imaging for confirmation.

Contraindications include gross obesity, sedentary lifestyle in which ACL reconstruction may not be necessary, immunosuppressive therapy, and smoking on a regular basis. I find that most smokers are willing to give up smoking during the preoperative and postoperative period to allow graft healing. We have noted that small women (under 5 feet tall) may have a short quadriceps tendon. Even in such patients, an adequate graft can be harvested. No quadriceps tendon rupture has occurred in any of our patients.

Surgical Technique

The patient is placed on a standard operating room table with a tourniquet applied to the most proximal thigh; the operative leg is marked as appropriate for surgery, and an arthroscopic leg holder is placed over the tourniquet such that the leg is projecting off the end of the table with the lower table dropped (Fig. 63-1). The nonoperative leg is placed in a well-padded leg holder.

The leg is elevated and exsanguinated with an Esmarch wrap, and the tourniquet is inflated to a pressure of 250 mm Hg. The arthroscope is introduced in a standard lateral peripatellar approach, and the complete knee arthroscopy is performed before harvesting of the graft in most cases. Meniscal repair, when necessary, is performed before the ACL reconstruction.

On entering the intercondylar notch, care is taken to establish the exact nature of the ACL tear. The remnants of the ACL are probed thoroughly; a small number of patients have an intact strut of ACL plucked off the posterior intercondylar notch that may be amenable to primary repair with anchors. We have found this to be successful in the occasional appropriate patient. In such patients, the

femoral attachment site is abraded, two suture anchors are placed there, and suture ends are passed through the proximal ACL stump to secure it to the avulsion site.

If the ACL tear is not repairable, all remnants of the torn ligament are resected. A limited notchplasty is performed, primarily for visualization, and thermal cautery is used to optimize the soft tissue notchplasty, to resect some ACL remnants as needed, and to improve visualization by removal of a limited amount of fat pad in some cases.

Specific Steps (Box 63-1)

1. Graft Harvest

A short incision is made over the center of the quadriceps tendon insertion into the patella at the midpoint of the proximal pole of the patella, and this incision is extended proximally (Fig. 63-2). In most cases, a 3- to 4-cm incision is optimal (the graft has been harvested through smaller incisions on occasion when cosmetic concerns are paramount). After opening of the fascia of the quadriceps tendon, the vastus medialis is identified and the medial border of the quadriceps free tendon autograft is established approximately 5 mm from the insertion of the vastus medialis distally. This is because the thickest portion of the quadriceps tendon is medial. Because of the convergence of the quadriceps tendon proximally, it is important

Box 63-1 Surgical Steps

1. Graft harvest
   Expose quadriceps tendon.
   Define medial and lateral borders, starting at apex of vastus medialis obliquus.
   Use hemostat to define thickness of graft at 6 to 7 mm.
   Spread with hemostat to define posterior border of graft.
   Dissect graft proximally with blunt and limited sharp dissection.
   Release central quadriceps free tendon graft from harvest site at 7 cm from upper pole of patella.
   Place whipstitches of No. 5 Ethibond or FiberWire in central quadriceps free tendon graft ends.

2. Tunnels and graft passage
   Place tibial guide pin.
   Drill tibial tunnel.
   Débride and irrigate.
   Establish femoral socket and drill to 35 mm.
   Measure femoral tunnel length to anterolateral cortex for EndoButton.
   Thread and tie sutures through EndoButton.
   Adjust suture lengths in EndoButton to allow 2 cm of graft in socket.
   Tie knot adjacent to graft.
   Place lead and trailing sutures in end holes of EndoButton.

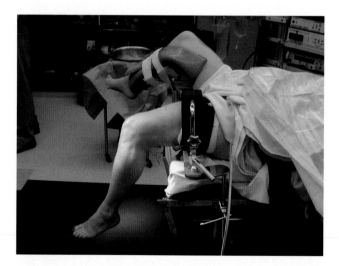

Figure 63-1 Knee in leg holder for central quadriceps free tendon reconstruction of the ACL.

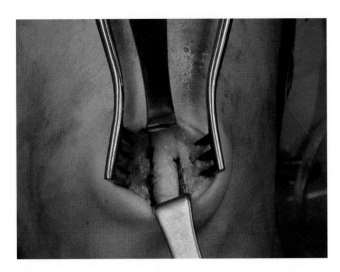

Figure 63-2 Exposure of the quadriceps tendon.

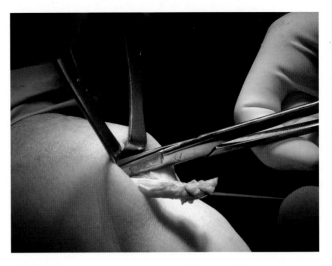

Figure 63-3 Release of the central quadriceps free tendon from the harvest site.

63

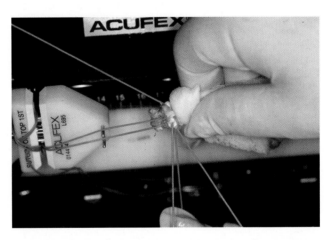

Figure 63-4 Placement of whipstitches in the central quadriceps free tendon graft.

to be not immediately at the medialis insertion but just slightly lateral of it. One may wish to establish medial and lateral borders of the graft by visualizing the apex of the quadriceps tendon with use of an Army-Navy retractor, then centering the graft proximally at the quadriceps tendon apex.

A standard No. 10 scalpel is used to incise the quadriceps tendon for a depth of only 7 mm. This is slightly less than the breadth of a No. 10 scalpel blade. This depth is incised from the proximal pole of the patella to the apex of the quadriceps tendon, which is visualized by retraction. A second incision is then made from the proximal pole of the patella 10 to 11 mm lateral to the first incision and precisely parallel to it. This incision is also made to a depth of 7 mm. The length of the incision proximally is generally 8 to 9 cm from the top of the patella.

At this point, a hemostat is placed between the two incisions to elevate the desired autograft portion of the quadriceps at a depth of 7 mm. This is generally just anterior to the suprapatellar pouch, leaving a few fibers (about 1 to 2 mm) of quadriceps tendon posterior to the desired autograft. The depth and amount of graft for harvest can be adjusted as desired by the surgeon.

Once it is clear that the desired amount of tendon is established by the hemostat, the hemostat is spread widely to release the posterior border of the quadriceps from the autograft.

At this point, a uterine T clamp is placed on the distal end of the quadriceps autograft, and No. 5 whipstitches are placed at the distal end of the graft. Only two or three whipstitches on each side of the graft are necessary. A second set of whipstitches is placed at 180 degrees to the first set so that four strands of No. 5 suture (or No. 2 FiberWire) extend from the free tendon end.

By use of blunt dissection and limited Metzenbaum scissors release proximally, the extent of the quadriceps free tendon (central quadriceps free tendon) graft is estab-

lished, and the free tendon graft is released at 7 to 9 cm from the top of the patella (Fig. 63-3). The graft is then taken to a back table, where No. 5 whipstitches are placed in the other end of the graft (Figs. 63-4 and 63-5), the graft length is confirmed, and the size of the graft is established for tibial and femoral tunnels (Fig. 63-6). The goal is to establish a tunnel size that will allow a snug fit of the autograft. In most cases, an 8-mm tunnel on each end is appropriate.

2. Tunnels and Graft Passage

Principles of central quadriceps free tendon reconstruction of the ACL are the same as those of other free tendon reconstructions of the ACL.

A tibial guide is placed through a low medial, slightly enlarged arthroscopy portal, and the angle of the guide is placed at 55 degrees. The guide pin is placed through a small incision midway between the tibial tubercle and the medial collateral ligament. The guide pin is placed to exit

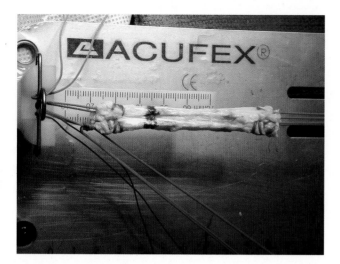

Figure 63-5 No. 5 whipstitches in both ends of the central quadriceps free tendon graft.

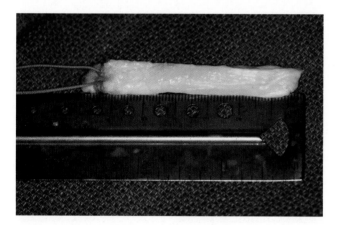

Figure 63-6 Measurement of the central quadriceps free tendon graft.

at the midpoint of the ACL stump, generally about 8 to 9 mm anterior to the posterior cruciate ligament and at a level just posterior to the anterior horn of the lateral meniscus in most cases. The knee is taken through a full range of motion to be certain that the tunnel is free of impingement in all planes. The tibial pin is generally placed at the center of the tibial ACL insertion halfway up the intercondylar spine. It is particularly important that it not be too far lateral. A pin at the top of the tibial spine is too lateral.

The tibial tunnel is then drilled with a fully threaded drill of an appropriate size, determined by measuring the graft size with cannulas. The tibial tunnel must always be the same size as or slightly larger than the appropriate femoral tunnel size. A débridement is done after drilling of the tibial tunnel to remove ligament remnants and bone fragments that may be in the joint. A thorough irrigation is also done.

We establish the femoral tunnel with use of a guide in most cases. The goal is to be at a point consistent with the conjunction of the anteromedial and posterolateral bands of the native ACL. It is particularly important that it not be too anterior (to avoid undue tightness and stretching of the graft in flexion). Our preference, if there is any question, is to be more posterior rather than too anterior. Having said this, we establish the point for the femoral socket 6 to 7 mm anterior to the over-the-top point as determined by the blade of the guide. The guide is then rotated slightly to permit the pin to pass into the posterolateral notch at a 10:30- (right knee) or 1:30- o'clock (left knee) orientation, based on the perceived "clock face" within the notch, from the top of the notch to the articular surface of the lateral condyle. The femoral socket orientation is established with the knee at 90 degrees of flexion in all cases. Orientation of the pin is examined with a hook probe after the pin is drilled out the lateral cortex through the skin. If the orientation is thought to be appropriate and consistent with the anteromedial-posterolateral band junction, it is then drilled with an acorn-type reamer to a depth of 35 to 40 mm. Margins of the tunnel are then rasped gently. A hemostat is kept on the proximal end of the pin where it exits laterally. After this, an EndoButton drill is used to drill through the lateral cortex, and a No. 5 suture, doubled over with the loop left distally, is drawn up through tibial and femoral tunnels with a hemostat on either end.

After thorough irrigation of the joint again, the EndoButton depth gauge is used to establish distance from the lateral cortex edge to the intercondylar notch entrance of the femoral tunnel. This then determines the length of the sutures from the desired quadriceps autograft femoral intercondylar notch point to the EndoButton itself.

Sutures of the quadriceps autograft are threaded through the EndoButton on a Graft Master, and we prefer to place one of each suture through one central eye of the EndoButton and then back down through the other central eye of the EndoButton such that there are two No. 5 strands going in and out through the other central eye. These are then tied to the other ends of the No. 5 sutures immediately adjacent to the quadriceps tendon graft. After a secure knot is tied with at least four throws, the suture ends are cut. The distance from the EndoButton to a point marked at approximately 2 cm from the tip of the quadriceps graft should be exactly the same as the distance measured with the EndoButton depth gauge from the lateral cortex to the femoral socket entry point.

After this, a No. 5 suture is placed through one side of the EndoButton, a No. 2 suture through the other, and the graft is drawn up through the tibia into the femoral socket. The EndoButton is flipped after it is through the proximal femoral cortex hole.

Interference screw fixation with poly-L-lactic acid (PLLA) screws has been a successful alternative,[14] giving the option of an anchor such as an EndoPearl (Linvatec, Largo, Fla) or a bone disk[15] (Fig. 63-7) on the femoral side. We prefer EndoButton fixation alone on the femoral side.

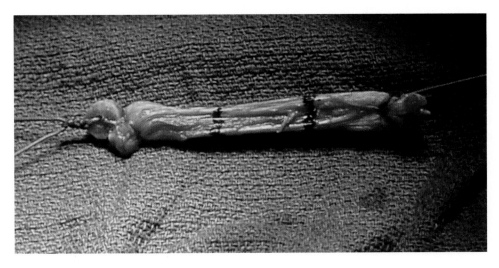

Figure 63-7 Bone disks on both ends of the graft for additional fixation.

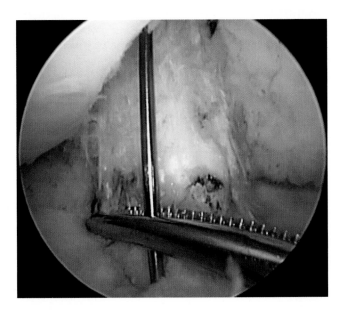

Figure 63-8 Guide pin for tibial screw fixation.

PEARLS AND PITFALLS

- Take time to be sure you have exactly the amount of tendon you want. With the quadriceps tendon, you can customize the graft's size, bulk, and length.

- Once the dimensions of the graft are defined, dissect carefully to preserve every fiber of the graft with blunt and careful sharp dissection.

- Tie the knot for FiberWires through the EndoButton such that the knot is immediately adjacent to the tendon end, not next to the EndoButton.

- Make the femoral socket deep enough to allow easy deployment of the EndoButton.

- Trim fat from the graft to maximize incorporation of bone in the bone sockets.

- Be sure to maintain tension on the graft when the tibial screw is placed so that the graft is kept at full length and tension when it is engaged by the screw.

For tibial side fixation, I prefer a polylactate bioabsorbable screw, 5 to 10 mm from the joint space (near but not *at* the tunnel opening into the joint). On the basis of studies by Nagarkatti,[8] we use a PLLA screw one size larger than the tibial tunnel size and place it carefully through the tibial tunnel, over a guide pin (Fig. 63-8), while holding the knee at 20 degrees of flexion and at tension equivalent to a 30- to 40-pound pull after thoroughly cycling the graft after femoral fixation. We are sure to insert the screw by turning (not pushing) the screw so that there is no risk of pushing the graft back. We prefer two sets of No. 5 whipstitches (FiberWire is a desirable alternative) coming off the tibial end of the graft (four strands). Although it is not necessary to achieve a stable knee, these suture ends may be tied over a button at the tunnel entrance for added security.

Postoperative Considerations

Patients are placed in a knee immobilizer after surgery but encouraged to bear full weight and to start immediate range of motion. A home program of closed-chain exercises has worked well, and loss of range of motion is extremely uncommon. Most patients achieve motion quickly as pain is less than with other autografts. Closed-chain physical therapy may be started after 10 days to 2 weeks (we generally use subcuticular closure). Most patients are off crutches with supportive quadriceps function by 2 weeks from the time of surgery. Patients do closed-chain exercises for 3 months and then progress to running. Most patients return to competitive sports at 6 months. The cosmetic results have been excellent (Fig. 63-9).

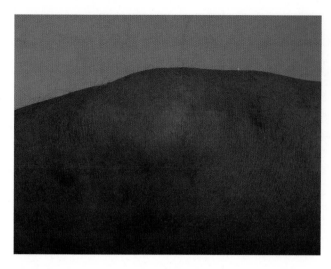

Figure 63-9 Cosmesis after central quadriceps free tendon reconstruction of the ACL.

Results

In a long-term follow-up study (all patients more than 2 years after surgery; average, 66 months) of the central

quadriceps free tendon for ACL reconstruction (DeAngelis, Cote, and Fulkerson, unpublished), the median International Knee Documentation Committee score at follow-up was 90, the average side-to-side KT-1000 difference (20-pound pull) was 1.2 mm, and the single-leg hop quotient was 0.96. There were five graft failures in the group of 124 patients. Most important, no patient had anterior knee pain or loss of knee range of motion.

Short-term pain has been less than with alternative autografts, and satisfaction of patients has been consistently high. In a short-term follow-up study by Joseph,[5] patients undergoing central quadriceps free tendon ACL reconstruction reported pain medication use for 6 days, versus 19 days in a matched group of patients receiving hamstring autografts and 22 days in a comparable group of patients with bone-tendon-bone ACL reconstruction. The patients undergoing central quadriceps free tendon reconstruction also reached rehabilitation landmarks sooner.

Finally, Adams et al[1] have demonstrated by mechanical testing that the quadriceps tendon is stronger, in general, after graft harvest than the patellar tendon is before a bone-tendon-bone graft is harvested.

References

1. Adams D, Mazzocca A, Fulkerson J. Residual strength of the quadriceps versus patellar tendon after harvesting a central free tendon graft. Arthroscopy 2006;22:76-79.
2. Blauth W. Die zweizugelige Ersatzplastik des Vorderen Kreuzband der Quadricepssehne. Unfallheilkunde 1984;87:45-51.
3. Fulkerson J. Central quadriceps free tendon for anterior cruciate ligament reconstruction. Oper Tech Sports Med 1999;7:195-200.
4. Fulkerson JP, Langeland R. An alternative cruciate reconstruction graft: the central quadriceps tendon. Arthroscopy 1995;11:252-254.
5. Joseph M, Fulkerson J, Nissen C, Sheehan TJ. Short-term recovery after anterior cruciate ligament reconstruction: a prospective comparison of three autografts. Orthopedics 2006;29:243-248.
6. Marder RA, Raskind JR, Carroll M. Prospective evaluation of arthroscopically assisted anterior cruciate ligament reconstruction. Patellar tendon versus semitendinosus and gracilis tendons. Am J Sports Med 1991;19:478-484.
7. Marshall JL, Warren RF, Wickiewicz TL, Reider B. The anterior cruciate ligament: a technique of repair and reconstruction. Clin Orthop 1979;143:97-106.
8. Nagarkatti DG, McKeon BP, Donahue BS, Fulkerson JP. Mechanical evaluation of a soft tissue interference screw in free tendon anterior cruciate ligament graft fixation. Am J Sports Med 2001;29:67-71.
9. Sachs RA, Daniel DM, Stone ML, Garfein RF. Patellofemoral problems after anterior cruciate ligament reconstruction. Am J Sports Med 1989;17:760-765.
10. Stäubli HU, Schatzmann L, Brunner P, et al. Quadriceps tendon and patellar ligament: cryosectional anatomy and structural properties in young adults. Knee Surg Sports Traumatol Arthrosc 1996;4:100-110.
11. Stäubli HU, Schatzmann L, Brunner P, et al., Mechanical tensile properties of the quadriceps tendon and patellar ligament in young adults. Am J Sports Med 1999;27:27-34.
12. Theut P, Fulkerson J. Anterior cruciate ligament reconstruction utilizing central quadriceps free tendon: a retrospective functional outcome study. Presented at the annual meeting of the American Academy of Orthopaedic Surgeons, San Francisco, 2001.
13. Viola R, Vianello R. Three cases of patella fracture in 1,320 anterior cruciate ligament reconstructions with bone–patellar tendon–bone autograft. Arthroscopy 1999;15:93-97.
14. Weiler A, Hoffmann RF, Bail HJ, et al. Tendon healing in a bone tunnel. Histological analysis after biodegradable interference fit fixation in a model of anterior cruciate ligament reconstruction in sheep. Arthroscopy 2002;18:124-135.
15. Weiler A, Richter M, Schmidmaier G, et al. The EndoPearl device increases fixation strength and eliminates construct slippage of hamstring tendon grafts with interference screw fixation. Arthroscopy 2001;17:353-359.

CHAPTER 64

Revision Anterior Cruciate Ligament Reconstruction

Ammar Anbari, MD
Bernard R. Bach, Jr., MD

Reconstruction of the anterior cruciate ligament (ACL) is one of the most common surgical procedures performed by orthopedic surgeons. More than 100,000 ACL reconstructions are performed annually. Despite its overwhelming success, 10% to 15% of patients may experience a failure of their reconstruction. In the majority of such failures, technical errors can be identified, most frequently femoral tunnel malposition. Some of these patients may require revision surgery for restoration of knee stability.

This chapter discusses the surgical planning and technique of revision ACL reconstruction.

Preoperative Considerations

Classification of ACL Failures

Although results of ACL surgery are clearly adversely affected by pain, extensor mechanism dysfunction, and arthrofibrosis, graft failure is the most obvious complication with a negative impact on clinical outcomes. This chapter focuses on graft failure with recurrent symptomatic instability. The mechanism of failure can be difficult to determine. If the failure occurs in the first 6 months, it is most likely due to a technical error, although failure of graft incorporation (especially with allografts), excessive rehabilitation, and premature return to full activities also play a role. On the other hand, failures occurring after 1 year are most likely due to a traumatic event.

Errors in surgical technique, especially with tunnel positioning, are considered the most common causes of recurrent instability. The typical mistakes seen with tunnel malpositioning have evolved during the early years. The early two-incision arthroscopic procedures were commonly associated with anteriorly placed femoral or tibial tunnels (Fig. 64-1); the single-incision endoscopic technique, at least in its early years, was associated mainly with anteriorly placed femoral tunnels. During the past 5 years, the most common patterns of tunnel malpositioning have been a combination of vertically oriented femoral tunnels and posteriorly positioned tibial tunnels (Fig. 64-2). Although commercially available femoral aiming devices have resulted in more accurately positioned femoral tunnels in the anteroposterior plane, these tools do not protect against a vertical orientation, which does not adequately restore rotational stability. On clinical examination, patients may demonstrate a normal Lachman test result but have a demonstrable pivot shift phenomenon. This problem of improper femoral tunnel position has led some surgeons to contend either that primary ACL surgery should be performed with a two-incision technique or, more recently, that double-bundle femoral and tibial tunnels be used.

History

Patients who experience recurrent instability may benefit from a revision reconstruction to stabilize the knee and to

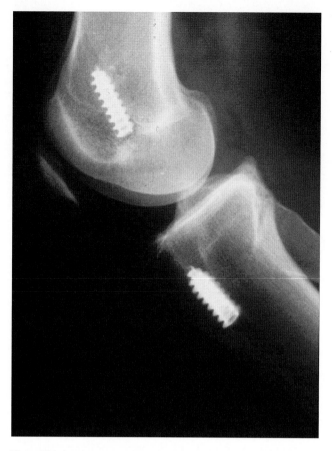

Figure 64-1 Anteriorly placed femoral tunnel.

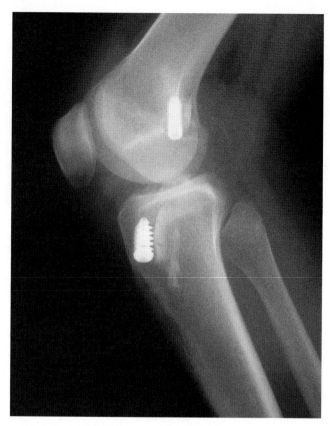

Figure 64-2 Vertical femoral tunnel and posteriorized tibial tunnel.

restore function. Preoperative data collection and planning are important to ensure the success of the reconstruction. If they are available, previous operative notes, arthroscopic images, and radiographs are reviewed to determine previous surgical tunnels and graft location. In the setting of a previous meniscectomy, staged or concomitant meniscal transplantation may be required.

Physical Examination

A thorough physical examination is performed to assess the stability of the knee not only anteriorly but also posteriorly, medially, and laterally. It is critical to exclude a subtle posterolateral or posteromedial laxity that may be contributing to graft attenuation. All test results should be compared with the opposite knee. The affected knee's range of motion should be recorded. Patellofemoral crepitation and mobility should be assessed. If it is available, a KT-1000 measurement should be performed on both knees.

A staged procedure should be considered in the following circumstances:

- Tunnel expansion of more than 1.5 cm
- Loss of extension of more than 5 degrees
- Loss of flexion of more than 20 degrees
- Significant varus or valgus malalignment requiring an osteotomy

Imaging

If no previous radiographs are available, we recommend obtaining at least two views to determine tunnel orientation and to help decide whether hardware will need to be removed during revision surgery. Standing radiographs including 45-degree posterior-to-anterior views may also provide important information about tibiofemoral arthrosis. Magnetic resonance imaging can help evaluate concomitant pathologic changes, such as meniscal tears and posterior cruciate ligament (PCL) or posterolateral corner injuries. If there is any suggestion of tunnel widening on conventional radiographs, we routinely obtain a computed tomographic scan to better delineate tunnel expansion.

Graft Choice

Several graft options are available for revision ACL reconstruction. Autografts include iliotibial band, hamstring tendon, quadriceps tendon, and patellar tendon from the ipsilateral or contralateral knee. Allograft options include Achilles tendon graft in addition to these grafts. Our preference is to use allograft tissue if a patellar tendon autograft has been harvested previously. Although some surgeons prefer the use of a contralateral patellar tendon graft, we have noted that most patients do not want to have their "normal" knee surgically violated. Although biomechanical characteristics of quadrupled hamstring grafts are more than adequate for revision reconstruction, secure fixation in the often expanded tunnels can be difficult, especially when soft tissue grafts had been used primarily. Patellar tendon allograft provides bone for supplemental grafting, and extra-large bone blocks can be customized to provide improved tunnel fill for primary interference fixation. In our institution, we have historically used non-irradiated patellar tendon allograft for revision cases, with excellent results. In a study by Harner,[4] patients who received allograft tissue had better knee scores as compared with the patients who received autograft tissue. Moreover, Noyes[6] reported 89% good to excellent results with use of allograft tissue.

Indications and Contraindications

Revision ACL reconstruction is indicated after a failed primary reconstruction, defined as a symptomatic, unstable knee that interferes with the activity level desired by the individual patient. Contraindications include significant medical comorbidities and current or recent infection. Uncorrected malalignment, decreased range of motion, and degenerative changes are relative contraindications that can frequently be addressed in staged or concomitant procedures.

Surgical Technique

Anesthesia and Positioning

Most patients undergo general anesthesia. If the patient's medical condition does not allow general anesthesia, regional spinal anesthesia can be performed instead. In some cases, a femoral nerve block can be useful in controlling postoperative pain.

Patients are positioned supine on the operating room table. The foot of the bed is flexed all the way down; a tourniquet is applied to the operative leg, which is then secured in a thigh holder. We routinely use the tourniquet only if intraoperative bleeding interferes with visualization. The contralateral leg rests in a leg holder with both hip and knee flexed no more than approximately 60 degrees to prevent traction on the femoral or peroneal nerves. To prevent lumbar spine extension and traction on the femoral nerve, we reflex the operating bed slightly and place it in

Trendelenburg position. It is important to be able to position the operative knee in approximately 110 degrees of flexion to allow proper placement of the femoral tunnel and screw if a single-incision endoscopic technique is to be used.

Surgical Landmarks, Incisions, and Portals

Landmarks
- Patella
- Patellar tendon
- Tibial plateau
- Fibular head

Portals and Approaches
- Inferomedial portal
- Inferolateral portal
- Superomedial outflow portal
- Accessory portal distal to the standard inferomedial portal for improved placement of the tibial aiming device

Examination Under Anesthesia and Diagnostic Arthroscopy

A thorough examination under anesthesia is performed to reassess ACL incompetency as well as to rule out any other injuries to the PCL, medial collateral ligament, and posterolateral corner complex.

Subsequently, a systematic diagnostic inspection of the knee is performed. The patellofemoral joint, the medial and lateral compartments and gutters, and the menisci are carefully evaluated. All necessary repairs or débridement is performed before the ACL revision. One should be particularly attentive of partial-thickness meniscal tears, which appear more commonly on the undersurface medially and on the superior surface laterally. Any arthritic changes or articular surface wear should be well documented.

Specific Steps (Box 64-1)

1. Notch Preparation

The general principles of ACL reconstruction apply to revision surgery. Before removal of the ACL remnant, inspect the footprints of the torn ACL on both the tibia and femur and mark their location with an arthroscopic electrocautery. With use of a combination of electrocautery, an arthroscopic curet, and a full-radius shaver, the

64

1. Notch preparation

2. Notchplasty

3. Removal of old hardware

4. Tibial tunnel

5. Femoral tunnel

6. Bone grafting procedures for tunnel widening

7. Graft preparation and placement

8. Femoral fixation

9. Tibial fixation

10. Wound closure

remnant of the ACL is removed from the lateral wall of the notch all the way back to the over-the-top position and from the tibial insertion. If bleeding is encountered, it can be controlled by electrocautery, increase of the inflow pressure, reduction of the systolic pressure, or inflation of the tourniquet.

2. Notchplasty

Intercondylar notch impingement and roof impingement are two common causes of ACL failure. At least 20 mm of notch width is necessary in the midtunnel region to avoid graft impingement. If a notchplasty is necessary, it can be performed with either a quarter-inch osteotome or a spherical bur. Alternatively, a curet can also be used. The notchplasty is performed from anterior to posterior and from apex to inferior. One should avoid elevating the apex of the notch (except if there are apical notch osteophytes) as the patella contacts this region in the extremes of flexion. A rasp can be used to smooth the wall of the intercondylar notch. After the notchplasty is performed, a probe is placed to palpate the over-the-top position. One should be able to hook this area easily with a probe; if the probe slides off the back edge, it is advisable to re-evaluate and to débride this area further.

3. Removal of Old Hardware

It is critical to consider whether former hardware will require removal or whether it may be bypassed at revision surgery. A variety of interference screws are commercially available with differing morphologic appearances radiographically. Most can be removed with a standard 3.5-mm screwdriver, although a screw manufactured by Instrument Makar (Okemos, Mich) requires a threaded extractor. If previous tunnels are nonanatomic and non-overlapping, the hardware can generally be left in place (Figs. 64-3 and 64-4). If the tunnels will overlap, the hardware may require initial removal for the new tunnel to be made, but it may have to be subsequently reinserted to provide construct fixation stability. In our experience, bioabsorbable screws are generally not resorbed at the time of revision surgery and frequently fracture on attempted removal secondary to softening. The surgeon may therefore have to ream through these screws to properly position the new tunnel.

If a metallic screw was used previously for femoral fixation, it may require removal. The surgeon may consider deferment of femoral screw removal until after the new tibial tunnel is made. The bone overgrowth around the screw along with any remaining soft tissue (Fig. 64-5) has to be débrided to prevent stripping of the screw. A flexible nitinol pin is placed through the screw, and an appropriate screwdriver is used to remove the old screw. This "technical pearl" may facilitate alignment of the screwdriver more easily within the femoral screw hexagonal recess and reduce the possibility of stripping the screw. If the screw is stripped, commercially available screw extractors may need to be used. Alternatively, when the femoral tunnel is placed too vertically, the screw can be advanced forward and not removed, which creates a medial wall support for the new graft.

If the tibial tunnel is in an acceptable position and a metallic screw was used, it needs to be removed as well. On the other hand, the old screw can be left in place if it is bioabsorbable or if it does not interfere with the new tunnel. It is critical to identify the location of the screw before a cortical window is made. If the screw edge is not easily detectable, the surgeon should consider use of radiographic imaging to minimize cortical violation, which could subsequently compromise tibial bone plug fixation if it is improperly positioned. One technical pearl that we routinely use during primary ACL reconstruction is to cut the tibial bone plug sutures long, leaving a tail that facilitates location of the screw for later removal if it is needed. Because we routinely place our screw on the cortical surface of the bone plug and anterior to the bone plug, these sutures will lead us to the tunnel, which frequently has been covered with new bone formation.

There are several commercially available revision screwdriver sets. They generally include reverse extractors and a variety of different-sized screwdrivers. It is critically important to be prepared for unforeseen events regarding hardware removal.

4. Tibial Tunnel

The previous tibial incision is used when possible, and it can be extended proximally or distally if necessary. A medially based rectangular periosteal flap is developed medial to the tibial tubercle and proximal to the pes. A tibial aiming device is placed through an accessory inferomedial or transpatellar portal with the angle set between 50 and 55 degrees. The higher the angle, the longer the tibial tunnel. The entry point of the guide pin should be at least 25 mm below the joint line. We choose the angle of entry

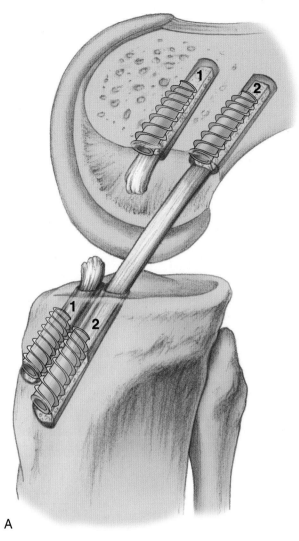

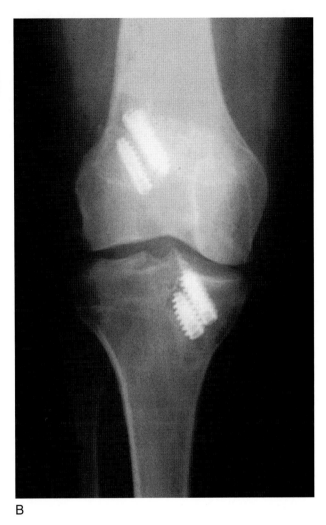

A   B

Figure 64-3 A and **B,** Nonanatomic tunnels.

by the N+10 rule, where N is the length of the soft tissue component of the graft. For example, if the length of the soft tissue of the graft is 40 mm, the angle of entry should be 40+10=50 degrees. A technical pearl is to establish an accessory inferomedial portal or transpatellar portal that facilitates proper orientation of the tibial aiming device. In the endoscopic technique, the position of the femoral tunnel is affected by the orientation of the tibial tunnel if it is drilled in a transtibial fashion. If this tunnel is angled too close to the sagittal plane, the resultant femoral tunnel is likely to be positioned too vertically (Fig. 64-6). An entrance point on the tibial cortex midway between the tibial tubercle and the posteromedial border of the tibia will allow proper tunnel orientation.

Intra-articularly, tibial tunnel orientation aims to avoid intercondylar notch impingement. In general, two types of aiming devices are available. One device creates a "point-to-point" placement of the preliminary drill pin; the other type of aimer drills the pin to the "elbow" of the

aiming device (Fig. 64-7). As a general reference point, the pin entry should be at the level of the posterior edge of the anterior horn of the lateral meniscus. Alternatively, some surgeons advocate an entrance point 7 mm anterior to the PCL. In the coronal plane, the device is placed in a central location to allow clearance of the graft between the PCL and notch wall. The knee should be extended to visualize the placement of the tibial pin, which should not impinge on the apex of the intercondylar notch with the knee in full extension. The pin will frequently be unstable and visibly mobile within the previous tibial tunnel and will therefore need to be stabilized before overreaming. After correct pin placement has been verified, the guide pin is tapped into the femoral roof to improve stability during reaming. It can also be further secured with a hemostat or Kocher clamp (Fig. 64-8). A cannulated acorn or solid fluted reamer is used to make the new tibial tunnel. A 10- or 11-mm reamer is generally used. If tunnel widening is suspected, some surgeons recommend use of a smaller

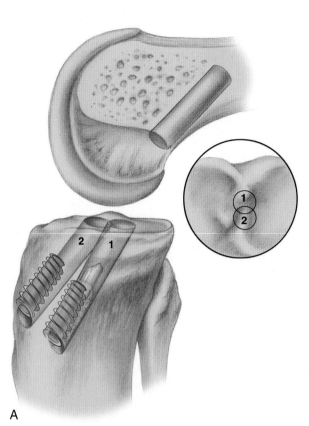

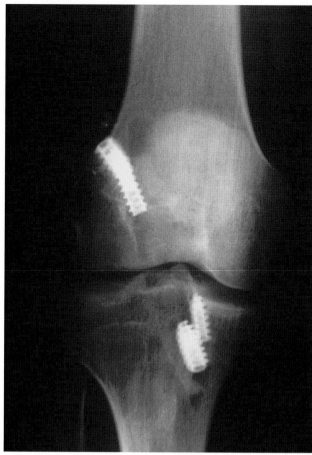

Figure 64-4 **A** and **B**, Nonoverlapping tunnels.

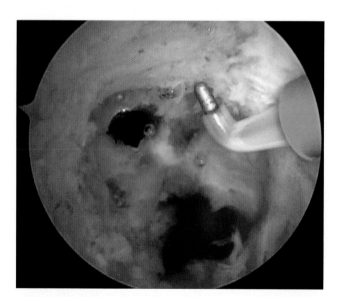

Figure 64-5 Débridement of bone and soft tissue overgrowth around the old femoral screw.

reamer first, then placement of the arthroscope through the tunnel to examine the quality of the tunnel before it is sequentially enlarged to the desired width. Once the tunnel is made, the arthroscope can be passed up the tibial tunnel to assess for residual soft tissue (Fig. 64-9), which can then be débrided with a shaver or rasp.

5. Femoral Tunnel

The ideal location for the femoral tunnel is in the 1-o'clock (left knees) or 11-o'clock (right knees) position with 1 to 2 mm of intact posterior wall. Careful inspection of the previous tunnel is performed; if it is in the correct location, it can be reused. However, if it is positioned too anterior, a new tunnel is drilled behind it (see Fig. 64-3A). In this case, we recommend keeping the old hardware in place to act as an anterior buttress. On occasion, a deficient posterior wall precludes interference screw fixation with the endoscopic technique, in which case a two-incision technique can be used to secure the ACL on the anterior femur instead.

We generally use a 7-mm offset guide, which is placed transtibially and therefore is sensitive to correct

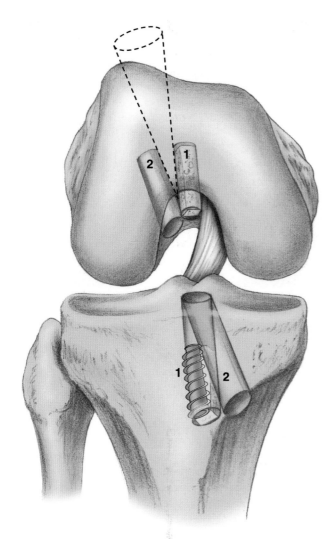

Figure 64-6 The position of the femoral tunnel is affected by the orientation of the tibial tunnel.

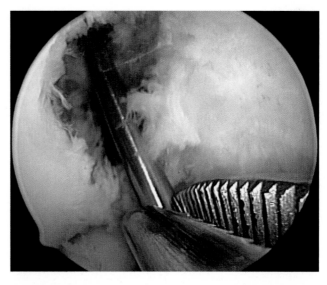

Figure 64-8 The guide pin is tapped into the femur and further stabilized with a Kocher clamp during reaming.

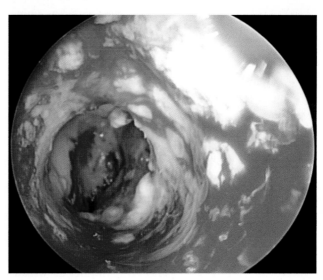

Figure 64-9 Some soft tissue remnant from the old ACL graft is still seen within the tibial tunnel.

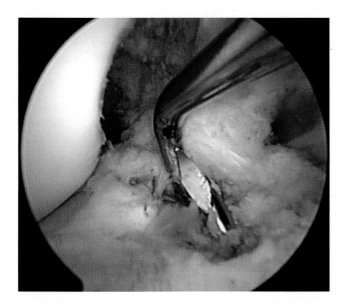

Figure 64-7 An "elbow" aiming device. Note how the guide pin touches the corner or elbow of the aiming device.

tibial tunnel orientation (Fig. 64-10). If an ideal femoral starting point cannot be achieved with this technique, the femoral tunnel should instead be drilled by use of an accessory inferomedial portal and hyperflexion of the knee to 130 degrees. A provisional guide pin is then drilled to a depth of approximately 3 to 4 cm. The surgeon may feel more resistance as this pin is drilled if it contacts the cortical bone plug from the previous reconstruction.

With a probe used to retract and to protect the PCL, reaming is performed initially to a depth of 6 to 8 mm to make the footprint. The reamer is withdrawn to allow visualization of the preliminary starting point, and a probe is used to verify the integrity of the posterior wall. A 10-mm reamer is routinely used, although one could begin

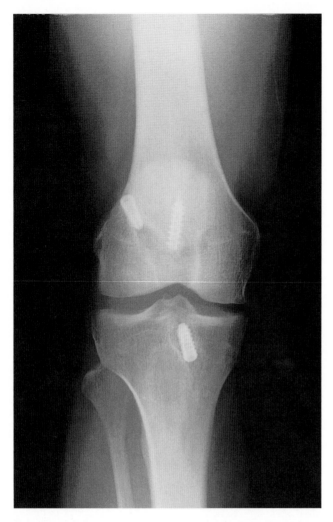

Figure 64-10 Tibial tunnel widening. Secure fixation cannot be achieved in the same procedure.

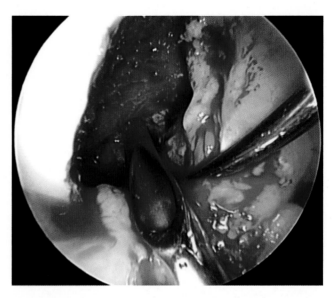

Figure 64-11 A 7-mm offset guide placed through the tibial tunnel. A probe is used to protect the PCL.

6. Bone Grafting Procedures for Tunnel Widening

After preparation of both tibial and femoral tunnels, bone grafting may be performed in either a concomitant or staged fashion to address overlapping or widened tunnels (Fig. 64-11). Graft choices include autograft and, more commonly, allograft to avoid the morbidity associated with iliac crest graft harvesting. Allograft bone chips or struts and bone left over from preparation of the tendon graft are commonly used. In the case of overlapping tibial tunnels, either bone graft or a larger tibial bone plug can be used to fill the defect and still allow interference screw fixation. Similarly, if the old and new femoral tunnels overlap, bone graft can be used to fill the defect left by the previous tunnel. To minimize extravasation of bone graft material into the joint, we found it helpful to use a clear shoulder-arthroscopy cannula or, alternatively, a 3-mL syringe with the front end cut off. The syringe is filled with morcellized bone graft, introduced through a slightly enlarged arthroscopy portal, and directed into the defect, and the bone graft is delivered by advancing the plunger. Other options include placing cortical allograft "matchsticks" into the defect and leaving the graft bone plugs sufficiently large to fill the tunnel defects. Alternatively, screws may be "stacked" to enhance bone plug fixation in overlapping or widened tunnels. Supplemental fixation (EndoButton, staples, post, suture button) on both the femoral and tibial sides should be strongly considered whenever secure graft fixation may be compromised by enlarged or bone grafted tunnels.

If bone stock is severely compromised because of extensive tunnel widening, primary bone grafting is advisable. All hardware is removed, and both tibial and femoral tunnels are filled with morcellized bone graft. After 4 months, the patient returns for staged ligament reconstruction.

with a smaller-diameter reamer (e.g., 8 mm) and then convert to the 10-mm reamer. The reamer is usually advanced to a 35-mm depth as a 25-mm bone plug is generally prepared on the graft. This allows for some space to potentially recess the graft if there is a graft-tunnel mismatch. As the reamer is advanced, the surgeon may feel more resistance than in a primary procedure in case of a previously placed cortical bone plug. Once reaming is completed, cancellous bone debris is removed with the shaver. A rasp or a shaver is used to smooth the anterior ledge of the femoral tunnel. The arthroscope is placed transtibially to inspect the femoral tunnel and to rule out posterior wall insufficiency or intratunnel "blowout." An intratunnel blowout could occur if the knee is extended too much during femoral reaming. In general, the knee should be in 70 to 80 degrees of knee flexion to position the femoral aimer. If the knee has to be extended farther to position the femoral aimer, the tibial tunnel may have been placed too far anteriorly, or a posterior ledge at the tibial tunnel entrance may be pushing the aimer anteriorly.

7. Graft Preparation and Placement

In revision cases, it may be advisable to defer graft preparation until the tunnels are made. This optimizes the potential of making custom-sized bone plugs if needed in situations in which there may be tunnel expansion or overlap. However, if one makes tunnels without knowing the length of the soft tissue construct, the likelihood of graft-construct mismatch may be increased. As a generalization, if the osseous tunnels do not appear expanded, we will make our tunnels while the graft is being prepared. An advantage of a patellar tendon allograft is that there is additional bone that can be used for grafting if necessary.

The bone plugs are shaped, contoured, and sized to fit 10-mm sizing tubes. The femoral plug bone-tendon interface is marked with a sterile marking pen. This helps determine the depth of entry of the plug in the femoral tunnel. Two or three 2-mm holes are drilled through the tibial plug, and No. 5 braided sutures are placed through them. Some surgeons prefer to do the same for the femoral plug; however, we prefer the "push-in" technique instead. In this method, the femoral bone plug is initially oriented with the cancellous bone facing anteriorly and the tendon facing posteriorly. The plug is pushed through the tibial tunnel by a two-pronged pusher (Fig. 64-12). Once it is inside the joint, a small curved hemostat is used to grasp the bone plug in its midportion and to guide the plug into the femoral tunnel. Once the plug is almost seated, the tibial plug is inspected with respect to the tibial tunnel to assess for graft-tunnel mismatch. Before seating of the bone plug is completed, a 14-inch hyperflex nitinol pin is inserted at the 11- to 12-o'clock position of the femoral tunnel, the knee is further flexed, and the pin is advanced until it meets resistance within the depth of the socket. At this point, the bone plug can be advanced until it is flush with the articular margin, and the construct is assessed again for mismatch. If the tibial bone plug resides within the tibial tunnel, one can continue with standard femoral and tibial fixation.

However, if the graft protrudes significantly because of graft-tunnel mismatch, potentially compromising tibial fixation, several treatment options exist: further recessing of the graft into the femoral tunnel; use of staple fixation or screw-post fixation on the tibial side; rotation of the graft up to 540 degrees, which can shorten the graft by up to 6 mm; performance of a free bone block modification (Fig. 64-13); and combination of these modifications (e.g., recession of the femoral bone plug and rotation of the graft). The disadvantage of recessing the graft is that there is an increased chance of tendon laceration during femoral bone plug fixation; staple or screw-post fixation has a lower strength of fixation and increased likelihood of painful hardware. Graft rotation is controversial; although the ultimate failure strength in vitro is similar to that of a nonrotated graft, cyclic loading studies suggest that the graft may be negatively affected with hyperrotation. Our

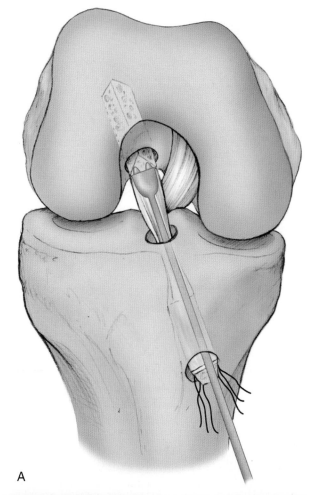

A

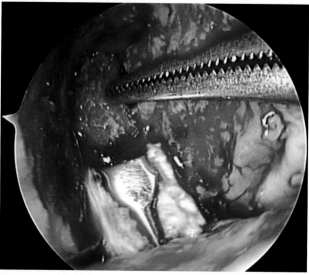

B

Figure 64-12 A and **B**, Push-in technique. The graft is advanced by a two-pronged pusher.

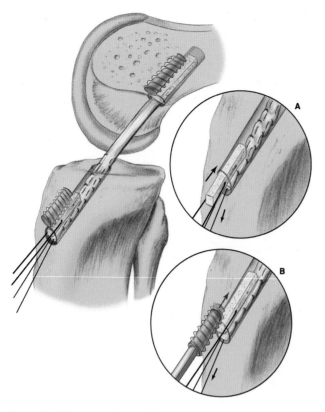

Figure 64-13 Free bone block technique.

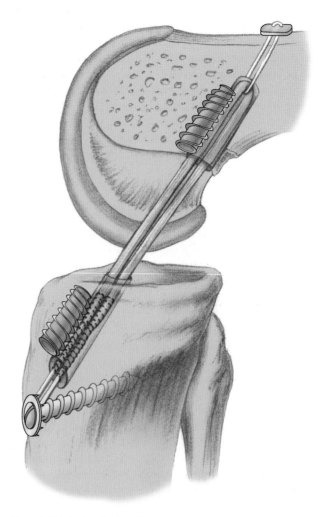

Figure 64-14 Backup fixation with a post.

general preference with more than 50% bone plug extrusion on the tibia is to remove the graft, to excise the tibial bone plug (thus making a "pseudo–quad tendon" graft), and to reinsert the graft with standard femoral fixation followed by tibial fixation by insertion of the "free" bone block into the tibial tunnel and sandwiching the plug with an interference screw. This can be supplemented by a whipstitch through the tendinous portion of the graft, which is then tied over a tibial staple or post.

8. Femoral Fixation

Once the femoral bone plug has been positioned and the hyperflex nitinol pin inserted, a 7- ×25-mm metallic cannulated interference screw is placed over the wire and advanced into the femoral tunnel. It is critical to flex the knee at least 100 degrees to ensure parallel screw placement. One should carefully inspect the graft as the screw is inserted to avoid graft laceration. Ideally, we attempt to place the screw anterior on the plug; the plug can effectively function as a skid, allowing parallel placement of the screw. If the screw is placed on the side of the plug, the likelihood of screw divergence is increased.

9. Tibial Fixation

The knee is cycled several times and isometry is inspected. In general, the graft should shorten only 1 to 2 mm in the terminal 30 degrees of extension. The graft is rotated 180

degrees so that the screw is placed against cortical rather than cancellous bone, since cortical fixation is preferable to cancellous apposition of the interference screw.[9] The interference screw is placed anterior to the graft with a cannulated metallic screw (9×20 mm). In addition, the screw pushes the graft farther posterior so that it is less likely to impinge in extension. Posteriorly placed screws carry a higher risk of screw divergence. Finally, if the screw is placed anteriorly, one can extend beyond the tendo-osseous junction without the screw's violating the soft tissue aspect of the graft, whereas if the screw is placed posteriorly, the screw tip could abrade the soft tissue. If the bone is osteopenic, one should consider supplemental fixation (Fig. 64-14). If any excess bone is protruding after placement of the tibial screw, it is cut flush with the tibia by use of a bur or a saw. In situations in which the bone plug is recessed within the tibia, we will use a longer interference screw to avoid burying the screw intraosseously. If a soft tissue graft, such as an Achilles allograft, is used on the tibial side, the size of the screw should be equal to or slightly larger than the tunnel width. Alternatively, other devices, such as a Richards staple, can be used to secure the soft tissue graft.

Once the graft is secured, it is critical to confirm the integrity of the construct fixation. The knee is multiply cycled and serially examined to confirm that Lachman and pivot shift test results are normal.

10. Wound Closure

The portal sites along with the joint are injected with 0.5% bupivacaine (Marcaine). The portal sites are closed with simple 3-0 Prolene sutures. The periosteal flap is approximated with No. 1 Vicryl sutures. The subcutaneous layer is closed with 2-0 Vicryl, and the skin is closed with a running 3-0 Prolene suture.

PEARLS AND PITFALLS

- To ensure the success of a revision, previous operative notes, arthroscopic images, and radiographs should be reviewed for information on the condition of the articular surface, previous surgical tunnels and graft location, and fixation.

- It is important to position the patient to allow flexion to approximately 110 degrees to facilitate placement of the femoral tunnel and screw and removal of previous hardware.

- Consider deferment of femoral screw removal until after the new tibial tunnel has been drilled. This may facilitate alignment of the screwdriver more easily and reduce the possibility of stripping the screw.

- Establishment of an accessory inferomedial portal or transpatellar portal can facilitate proper orientation of the tibial aiming device in a medial to lateral direction.

- After the tibial guide pin is placed, the knee should be extended to visualize the placement of the pin relative to the intercondylar apex in knee extension. If it is placed in a proper position, the guide pin should not impinge on the roof of the intercondylar notch. In flexion, the pin should cross the lower third of the PCL.

- In cases of tibial tunnel expansion, we recommend use of bone graft to fill it. This can be done on a staged basis if the tunnel is so wide that secure fixation of the graft would be compromised.

- In cases of femoral tunnel expansion, one can use cancellous bone from the allograft patella and introduce it with a 3-mL syringe with its tip removed.

- During the reaming process of both tunnels, as the reamer is advanced, the surgeon may feel more resistance than in a primary procedure because of previously placed cortical bone plugs.

- After reaming of the tunnels, the arthroscope is placed antegrade through the tibial tunnel to take a close look at both tibial and femoral tunnels.

- Defer graft preparation until the tunnels are made. This optimizes the potential of making custom-sized bone plugs if needed in situations in which there may be tunnel expansion or overlap.

- Before the tibial screw is placed, the graft is rotated 180 degrees so that the screw is placed against cortical rather than cancellous bone.

- If there is any question about the integrity of tibial fixation, one should consider "backup" fixation.

Postoperative Considerations

Rehabilitation

In most cases, the patients are allowed to progress to full weight bearing with the knee locked in extension in the brace. If secure fixation is achieved on both sides of the graft, rehabilitation follows the same protocol as for a primary ACL reconstruction.

Straight-leg raises and quadriceps sets are initiated immediately after surgery. Crutches are generally used for the first 2 weeks, and physical therapy initially concentrates on achievement of full extension and progressive flexion. Full flexion should be reached within 6 weeks. Bicycling (stationary) can be started 1 week after surgery, StairMaster-type exercises at 4 to 6 weeks, and light jogging without cutting or pivoting in 12 weeks. Gradual return to full activities is achieved 6 months after surgery.

Complications

Complications of revision ACL surgery are similar to those seen in primary ACL reconstruction. They include infection, arthrofibrosis, neurovascular injury, and failure of the revision graft to be incorporated or macrotraumatic retear.

Results

Most studies have demonstrated good results with revision ACL reconstruction, which, however, are inferior to those of primary reconstructions (Table 64-1). These findings stress that revision ACL reconstruction should be considered a salvage procedure, and patients should be carefully counseled about their expectations before the revision is performed.

Table 64-1 Results of Studies of Anterior Cruciate Ligament Reconstruction

Author	Follow-up	Outcome	Notes
Fox et al[3] (2004)	32 patients for 4.8 years	87% had grade 0/1+ Lachman and 0/1+ pivot shift test results 84% of patients had side-to-side difference of 3 mm or less on KT-1000 testing 87% of patients were satisfied with their surgery	With nonirradiated fresh-frozen bone–patellar tendon–bone allograft
O'Neill[8] (2004)	48 patients for 90 months	73% of patients had normal or nearly normal evaluation by IKDC scale 67% of patients had KT-2000 side-to-side difference of 3 mm or less 21% of patients had KT-2000 side-to-side difference of 3 to 5 mm 6% failure	With previously unharvested autograft
Siebold et al[10] (2002)	38 months	67% normal IKDC score 2.3-mm side-to-side difference on KT-1000 testing 15% failure	With allograft
Labs et al[5] (2002)	82 patients for 35 months	Tegner score improved from 2.4 to 4.6 Lysholm score improved from 54 to 76	
Texier et al[11] (2001)	32 patients for 48 months	18 of 23 athletes returned to their sports Residual laxity in 3 of 32 patients	
Colosimo et al[1] (2001)	13 patients for 39 months	11 of 13 had good to excellent results 1.9-mm side-to-side difference on KT-1000 testing No patients had loss of range of motion One patient with moderate patellofemoral problems	With reharvested ipsilateral patellar tendon
Noyes and Barber-Westin[7] (2001)	54 patients for at least 24 months	Significant improvement in pain, activities of daily living, sports participation, satisfaction 60% of revisions were fully functional, 16% were partially functional, and 24% failed	With bone–patellar tendon–bone autograft
Woods et al[12] (2001)	10 patients for 42.9 months	2.4-mm side-to-side difference on KT-1000 testing All had a negative pivot shift result All returned to previous activities Extension within 5 degrees and flexion within 15 degrees of contralateral side	With lateral third of ipsilateral patellar tendon after failure of central third
Eberhardt et al[2] (2000)	44 patients for 41.2 months	3.5-mm side-to-side difference on KT-1000 testing 75% rated knee as normal or nearly normal	With bone–patellar tendon–bone autograft

IKDC, International Knee Documentation Committee.

References

1. Colosimo AJ, Heidt RS Jr, Traub JA, Carlonas RL. Revision anterior cruciate ligament reconstruction with a reharvested ipsilateral patellar tendon. Am J Sports Med 2001;29:746-750.
2. Eberhardt C, Kurth AH, Hailer N, Jager A. Revision ACL reconstruction using autogenous patellar tendon graft. Knee Surg Sports Traumatol Arthrosc 2000;8:290-295.
3. Fox JA, Pierce M, Bojchuk J, et al. Revision anterior cruciate ligament reconstruction with nonirradiated fresh-frozen patellar tendon allograft. Arthroscopy 2004;20:787-794.
4. Harner CD, Olson E, Irrgang JJ, et al. Allograft versus autograft anterior cruciate ligament reconstruction: 3- to 5-year outcome. Clin Orthop 1996;324:134-144.

5. Labs K, Hasart O, Perka C. Results after anterior cruciate ligament revision surgery. Zentralbl Chir 2002;127:861-867.

6. Noyes FR, Barber-Westin SD, Butler DL, Wilkins RM. The role of allografts in repair and reconstruction of knee joint ligaments and menisci. Instr Course Lect 1998;47:379-396.

7. Noyes FR, Barber-Westin SD. Revision anterior cruciate surgery with use of bone–patellar tendon–bone autogenous grafts. J Bone Joint Surg Am 2001;83:1131-1143.

8. O'Neill DB. Revision arthroscopically assisted anterior cruciate ligament reconstruction with previously unharvested ipsilateral autografts. Am J Sports Med 2004;32:1833-1841.

9. Rupp S, Seil R, Krauss PW, Kohn DM. Cortical versus cancellous interference fixation for bone–patellar tendon–bone grafts. Arthroscopy 1998;14:484-488.

10. Siebold R, Buelow JU, Boes L, Ellermann A. Primary and revision reconstruction of the anterior cruciate ligament with allografts: a retrospective study including 325 patients. Zentralbl Chir 2002;127:850-854.

11. Texier A, Hulet C, Acquitter Y, et al. Arthroscopy-assisted revision in failed reconstruction of anterior cruciate ligament: 32 cases. Rev Chir Orthop Reparatrice Appar Mot 2001;87:653-660.

12. Woods GW, Fincher AL, O'Connor DP, Bacon SA. Revision anterior cruciate ligament reconstruction using the lateral third of the ipsilateral patellar tendon after failure of a central third graft: a preliminary report on 10 patients. Am J Knee Surg 2001;14:23-31.

64

CHAPTER 65

Anatomic Double-Bundle Anterior Cruciate Ligament Reconstruction

Anthony M. Buoncristiani, MD

James S. Starman, BS

Freddie H. Fu, MD, DSc (Hon), DPs (Hon)

Anterior cruciate ligament (ACL) reconstruction remains one of the most common procedures performed by orthopedic surgeons in the United States, with approximately 100,000 reconstructions performed per year.[9] ACL surgery has evolved tremendously from the original open techniques to modern procedures focusing on endoscopic reconstruction of the anteromedial bundle with use of a variety of graft choices and fixation techniques. However, the success of single-bundle ACL reconstruction ranges from 69% to 90%.[6,22]

Single-bundle ACL reconstruction is the "gold standard," but some authors have noted persistent instability with functional testing of single-bundle ACL reconstruction.[18,19] Thus, there is a growing trend toward a more anatomic ACL reconstruction that re-creates both the anteromedial and the posterolateral bundles. The double-bundle anatomy of the ACL was first described in 1938.[17] The terminology of the anteromedial and posterolateral bundles is chosen according to their tibial insertions. The tibial and femoral insertion sites of both the anteromedial and posterolateral bundles have been well described.[11,16] Although the two bundles are intertwined, their functional tensioning pattern is independent throughout knee range of motion.[8]

The idea of reconstructing both bundles of the ACL was originated by Mott and Zaricznyj in the 1980s.[14,23] They independently described a double-bundle technique with use of a single femoral tunnel and two tibial tunnels. Despite publication of their results, the technique did not become mainstream. There is recent biomechanical evidence to support that anatomic double-bundle ACL reconstruction more accurately re-creates the natural anatomy.[20] We present the senior author's (F. H. F.) technique of anatomic double-bundle ACL reconstruction with two femoral and two tibial tunnels using two tibialis anterior allografts.

Preoperative Considerations

History

Signs and Symptoms

ACL injuries occur frequently in sports that involve running, jumping, and cutting movements. They can occur without contact when the foot is anchored to the playing surface—usually by way of cleats or a rubber sole—and the body rotates beyond the tolerance of the ligament as the knee buckles. Thus, it is important to ask how the injury occurred and the position of the knee during the injury, which may also allude to the ACL bundle injury pattern. This may be associated with an audible "pop." Asking whether the athlete was able to continue to play will give you an idea of the severity of the injury. Knee pain and a hemarthrosis are usually present acutely. A complaint of instability is also common, especially when walking downhill or down stairs.

Physical Examination

Inspect and palpate for an effusion. If a large effusion is present, consider aspiration for pain relief and inspection of the aspirate for any fat globules, which would suggest a fracture. Check the range of motion; if it is limited, a magnetic resonance imaging evaluation should be obtained to ensure that no displaced meniscal tear is present. The physical examination of an isolated ACL tear is usually significant for a side-to-side difference with regard to Lachman and pivot shift maneuvers. If a discrepancy between the Lachman and pivot shift maneuvers exists, this may signify a partial tear involving either the anteromedial or posterolateral bundle. The posterolateral bundle is mainly responsible for rotational stability, and a large pivot shift will be evident if it is torn. Similarly, the anteromedial bundle is mainly responsible for translational stability when the knee is flexed, and a large Lachman maneuver will be present if it is torn. KT-1000 testing can also confirm a side-to-side difference in anterior translation. A more prominent anterior drawer compared with a Lachman test result should clue the examiner to consider a concomitant posteromedial or posterior horn medial meniscal injury. Varus or valgus instability testing should be performed to ensure that no collateral injury is present. Dial testing and posterolateral drawer testing at 30 degrees should be performed to assess for a posterolateral knee injury. Gait analysis should be performed to inspect for any underlying varus laxity. Tests for possible meniscal disease should also be performed (i.e., joint line tenderness and McMurray maneuver), but it may be difficult to distinguish between a lateral meniscal tear and a bone contusion acutely. Thus, appropriate imaging is important.

Imaging

A complete knee series consisting of weight-bearing anteroposterior and notch, lateral, and patellofemoral sunrise views should be obtained. The soft tissues can be inspected for an effusion. The bone anatomy should be inspected for any fractures or subtle signs of a rotational injury (i.e., Segond or reverse Segond capsular lesion). In addition, the status of the physes and any arthritic changes should be noted. Long-cassette films should be obtained for any patient with varus alignment on examination or if any arthritic changes are noted on the knee series obtained. This will help determine whether an osteotomy should be performed. Magnetic resonance imaging is essential not only to confirm an ACL tear but, more important, to assess for any concomitant ligamentous or cartilaginous injuries that will affect the operative plan. The posterolateral bundle is more easily visualized on coronal sectioning. Specifically, it may be seen at the level of the first cut that includes the posterior cruciate ligament.

Indications and Contraindications

The absolute indications for double-bundle ACL reconstruction are in evolution. Even though single-bundle ACL reconstruction is considered the gold standard, the technique can be improved. Gait analysis after single-bundle reconstruction has demonstrated that rotatory instability persists.[18] Furthermore, biomechanical cadaver studies have shown that even lowering of the femoral insertion site to the 3- or 9-o'clock position does not fully prevent rotatory instability.[4] Clinically, up to one fifth of the patients do not resume preinjury activities and usually complain of vague instability symptoms that objectively correspond to a mild persistent pivot shift.[2] In comparison, double-bundle ACL reconstruction does restore the rotational component in a cadaver model.[20] It has been suggested that a positive pivot shift result after ACL reconstruction is correlated with the development of later osteoarthrosis.[13]

In the young athlete with open physes, the double-bundle technique is contraindicated. Two tunnels would risk physeal arrest with subsequent malalignment and possible leg length discrepancy.

Surgical Technique

Anesthesia and Positioning

The operative extremity is identified by the patient and initialed by a member of the surgical team. All patients undergo a preoperative femoral nerve block in the holding area by our anesthesia colleagues. The patient is then placed in a supine position and given intravenous conscious sedation. A careful examination under anesthesia is performed and recorded to document the Lachman and pivot shift maneuvers. Once again, the senior author is interested in correlating the examination findings with the tear pattern of the individual bundles of the ACL. A tourniquet is applied to the proximal thigh. The extremity is then secured within a circumferential leg holder placed at the level of the tourniquet. The foot of the operating table is completely retracted to permit hyperflexion of the knee, which is crucial for later placement of the posterolateral femoral tunnel. The contralateral extremity is placed within a well-padded leg holder with the hip flexed approximately 90 degrees and abducted and externally rotated away from the surgical field to allow unobstructed access to the operative knee (Fig. 65-1). The leg is elevated for 5 minutes, and the tourniquet is then inflated. The knee is then prepared and sterilely draped.

ACL Graft Preparation

Two tibialis anterior allografts are individually fashioned as a double loop. The folded length of each graft should be

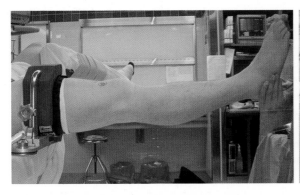
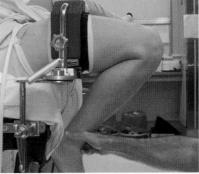

Figure 65-1 Leg positioned to allow range of motion between full extension and 120 degrees of flexion.

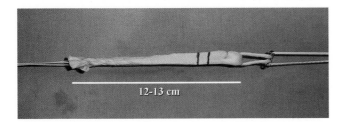

Figure 65-2 Doubled over tibialis anterior allograft with whipstitch; 8-mm diameter for anteromedial bundle, 7-mm diameter for posterolateral bundle. EndoButton CL is pictured at right.

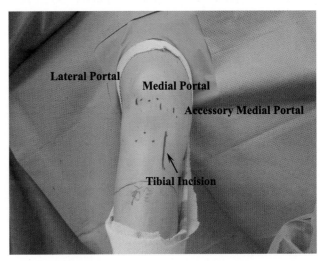

Figure 65-3 Arthroscopic portal placement and skin incisions.

approximately 12 cm for sufficient graft tissue. The grafts are trimmed to a folded diameter of 7 mm for the postero-lateral bundle and 8 mm for the anteromedial bundle. A No. 2 braided suture is whipstitched up and down both ends of the graft for 3 cm. The stitch depth is alternated, and care is taken to avoid penetrating the suture and risking weakening or breaking. The graft is then passed through the closed-loop EndoButton (Smith & Nephew, Inc., Andover, Mass). Two FiberWire (Arthrex, Naples, Fla) sutures (one stripped and one nonstripped for later identification) are placed within the buttonholes. A 2-0 absorbable suture is tied through both strands of the folded graft to secure them once the graft is passed within the closed-loop EndoButton. Each graft is marked to alert the surgeon when to engage or to "flip" the EndoButton (Fig. 65-2).

Surgical Landmarks

With the knee flexed approximately 45 degrees, the inferior pole of the patella is marked. The inferior extent of the lateral parapatellar portal begins at the level of the inferior pole of the patella and extends proximally for approximately 2 cm. The medial parapatellar portal begins at the level of the inferior pole of the patella and extends distally along the medial aspect of the patellar tendon for approximately 2 cm. The high placement of the portals

will allow the arthroscopic instruments to enter the knee above the level of the fat pad. The No. 11 blade scalpel is angled approximately 45 degrees to the skin and distally toward the notch to safely enter the knee without harming the articular cartilage. A low anteromedial accessory portal will be placed with the assistance of a spinal needle to ensure proper trajectory for the posterolateral femoral tunnel (Fig. 65-3). The knee is flexed 90 degrees, and the No. 11 scalpel blade is angled upward as it enters the skin at the level of the spinal needle marking. The portal is extended proximally approximately 1 cm, avoiding injury to both the underlying meniscus and the articular cartilage.

Diagnostic Examination

The knee is flexed approximately 25 degrees, and the arthroscopic trocar is placed in the lateral parapatellar portal angled toward the notch and then redirected beneath the patella. The patellofemoral joint is visualized. Any cartilage defects are addressed as needed. The arthroscope is then dropped down over the trochlea and into the notch to view the ACL grossly. The knee is then extended, and a valgus stress is applied to open the medial compartment. The entire meniscus is visualized and probed for stability. Medial meniscal tears are usually seen with chronic ACL tears. Any meniscal disease is addressed with either repair or débridement. The knee is brought through a range of motion to inspect the femoral condylar articular surface for any defects. The tibial plateau articular cartilage is also inspected for any defects.

The knee is then placed in a figure-four position to view the lateral compartment. The posterolateral bundle is best visualized in this position. The entire meniscus is once again observed and probed for stability. Lateral meniscal longitudinal tears are commonly seen with acute ACL tears at the junction of the middle and posterior thirds. The posterior third of the lateral meniscus is more easily viewed with the knee flexed to 90 degrees; the middle third, with the knee flexed to 60 degrees; and the anterior third, with the knee flexed to 30 degrees. Medial meniscal tears are usually seen with chronic ACL tears. Any meniscal disease is addressed with either repair or débridement. The lateral femoral condylar articular surface is inspected for any defects as the knee is brought through an entire range of motion.

Specific Steps (Box 65-1)

Attention is then redirected to the notch. Any obstructing fat pad or ligamentum mucosum is removed with the shaver or ArthroCare Coblation device. The bundles of the ACL are carefully dissected with a small ArthroCare Coblation device to fully appreciate the injury tear pattern. Because the two bundles are differentially tensioned according to the position of the knee at the time of injury, the tear patterns can be quite different for each bundle (Fig. 65-4).[7] The remnant of the ACL bundles is then débrided from both their femoral and tibial insertions. The ArthroCare Coblation device is used to mark the anteromedial and posterolateral femoral and tibial footprints (Fig. 65-5). No notchplasty is performed.

An 18-gauge spinal needle is directly visualized as it passes from the location of the low anteromedial portal onto the medial face of the lateral femoral condylar notch in the region of the previously marked posterolateral bundle (Fig. 65-6). Once satisfactory trajectory for the posterolateral bundle with the spinal needle is determined, the spinal needle is removed and the low anteromedial portal is made with a No. 11 scalpel blade angled upward to avoid cutting the anterior horn of the medial meniscus. A ³⁄₃₂-inch Steinmann pin is then passed through the low anteromedial portal onto the medial face of the lateral

Box 65-1 Surgical Steps

1. Patient positioning
2. Graft preparation
3. Medial and lateral parapatellar tendon portal placement above the fat pad
4. Injury pattern assessment
5. Insertion site marking
6. Accessory medial portal placement
7. Posterolateral femoral tunnel placement
8. Tibial posterolateral and anteromedial tunnel placement
9. Anteromedial femoral tunnel placement
10. Posterolateral graft is passed first
11. Anteromedial graft is passed second while tension is maintained on the posterolateral graft
12. Final graft fixation
13. Closure

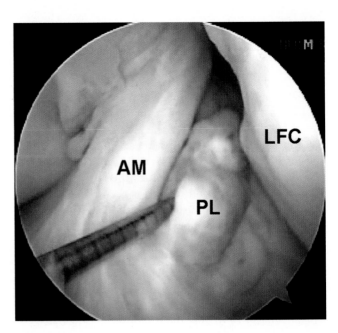

Figure 65-4 ACL tear of anteromedial and posterolateral bundles, each from femoral insertion. Preoperative examination demonstrated 2+ Lachman test score and 3+ pivot shift test score.

femoral condylar notch. The pin is placed approximately 7 or 8 mm posterior to the anterior articular margin and approximately 3 to 5 mm superior to the inferior articular margin of the lateral femoral condyle. Once correct placement of the pin is obtained, the knee is brought into approximately 110 degrees of hyperflexion and the pin is tapped into place with a mallet (Fig. 65-7). Ensure that the

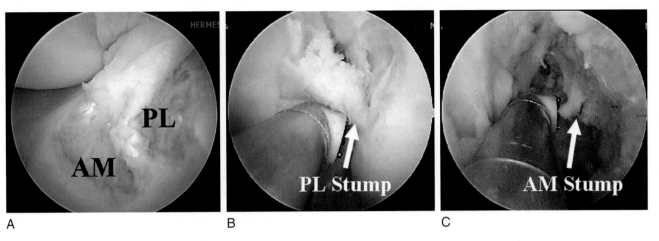

Figure 65-5 Anteromedial (AM) and posterolateral (PL) tibial (**A**) and femoral (**B** and **C**) footprints marked.

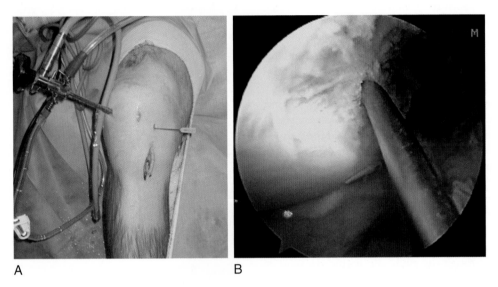

Figure 65-6 A and **B,** Accessory medial portal visualization with 18-gauge needle.

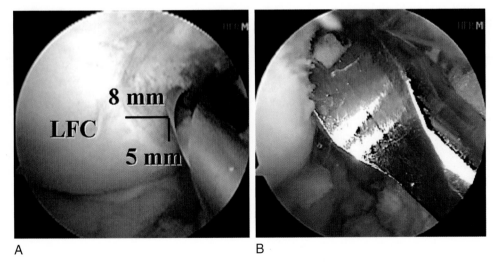

Figure 65-7 A, Guide pin placement for posterolateral femoral tunnel. **B,** A 7-mm acorn reamer, inserted from accessory medial portal.

pin did not penetrate the medial meniscus. Then slide the 7-mm acorn reamer over the Steinmann pin and have it rest against the medial face of the lateral femoral condylar notch. Ream to a depth of 25 mm. Then place the Endo-Button drill within the previously reamed canal and drop your hand before starting the drill, which will maximize the posterolateral tunnel length. With the knee still flexed 110 degrees, have your assistant place a hand on the lateral aspect of the knee and push the biceps tendon inferiorly, which will deflect the common peroneal nerve away from the drill trajectory. Barely perforate the lateral femoral cortex with the EndoButton drill and quickly retract it backward to minimize the risk of injury to the common peroneal nerve. Measure the transcondylar length and choose the appropriately sized continuously looped Endo-Button. If the length is greater than 35 mm, replace the 7-mm acorn reamer within the posterolateral tunnel and dilate the tunnel depth to 30 mm by hand. There should be at least 15 mm of graft tissue within the tunnel (Fig. 65-8).

A 3- to 4-cm incision is made over the anteromedial surface of the tibia to drill the tibial tunnels and to pass the grafts. This is in a location midway between the tibial tubercle and the posteromedial border of the tibia. Dissect the soft tissues both medially and laterally for easy access to the future tibial anteromedial and posterolateral tunnels. Identify the tibial posterolateral footprint, which is just medial to the posterior horn of the lateral meniscus and anterior to the posterior cruciate ligament. The footprint should have been previously marked with the ArthroCare Coblation device. Place the ACL Director guide (Smith & Nephew) at 55 degrees with the tip centered within the posterolateral tibial footprint (Fig. 65-9). Drill a ³⁄₃₂-inch Steinmann pin through the guide and within the joint so that a few millimeters are visible. With the ArthroCare Coblation device, identify the anteromedial tibial footprint, which is a couple of millimeters anterior to the ideal

single-bundle reconstruction location—the posterior aspect of the anterior horn of the lateral meniscus, downward sloping side of the medial tibial eminence, and approximately 7 mm anterior to the posterior cruciate ligament. Reset the ACL Director guide to 45 degrees and place it within the previously marked anteromedial tibial footprint (Fig. 65-10). Drill a second ³⁄₃₂-inch Steinmann pin through the guide and into the joint so that a few millimeters are visible. Note that the posterolateral tibial guide pin is quite vertical in comparison to the anteromedial tibial guide pin, which is quite horizontal. This pin attitude also prevents impingement within the notch because the posterolateral tunnel is centered within the knee and the anteromedial tunnel is horizontal. Once

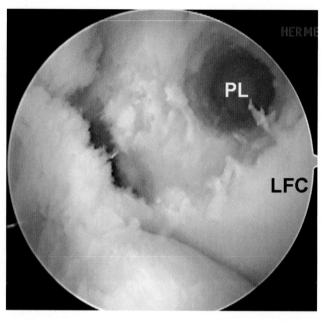

Figure 65-8 Posterolateral femoral tunnel.

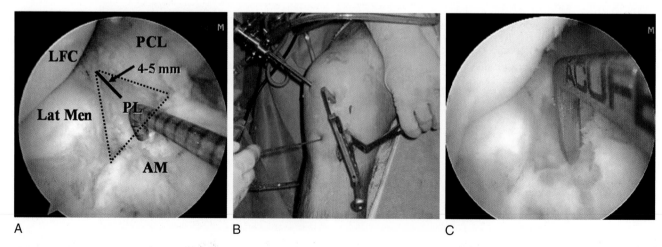

Figure 65-9 A, Posterolateral tibial insertion landmarks—centered approximately 4 to 5 mm anteromedial from the posterior horn of the lateral meniscus. **B,** ACL Director guide set at 55 degrees. **C,** Guide pin drilling.

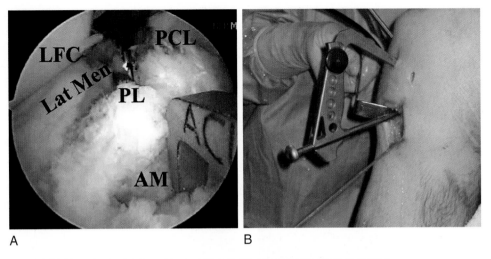

Figure 65-10 A, Anteromedial tibial insertion landmarks, guide pin drilling. **B,** ACL Director guide set at 45 degrees.

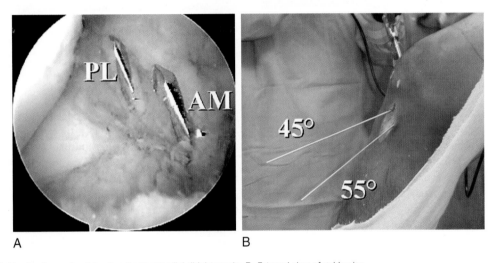

Figure 65-11 A, Guide pins for posterolateral and anteromedial tibial tunnels. **B,** External view of guide pins.

again, no notchplasty is necessary. The posterolateral tibial guide pin also enters the anteromedial surface of the tibia more posteromedially than the anteromedial tibial guide pin, which is more lateral and centered (Fig. 65-11). The skin on the tibia is retracted to allow placement of a 7-mm reamer over the posterolateral tibial guide pin, and a curet is placed within the joint overlying the posterolateral pin to protect the articular surfaces. The posterolateral tunnel is reamed, and debris is removed with a shaver. The 8-mm reamer is then placed over the anteromedial tibial guide pin, and a curet is once again placed overlying the pin to protect the articular surfaces. The anteromedial tunnel is then reamed, and debris is removed with a shaver. There should be an approximately 1-cm bone bridge between the two tibial tunnels.

Attention is then directed to the anteromedial femoral footprint. The anteromedial femoral tunnel is guided off the previously made femoral posterolateral tunnel and not off the back wall of the notch, which is traditionally done with over-the-top femoral tunnel drill guides. The ³⁄₃₂-inch Steinmann pin is placed 3 mm posterior and slightly superior to the previously drilled femoral posterolateral tunnel. The Steinmann pin can be placed transtibially through the previously drilled anteromedial tunnel or through the low anteromedial portal, whichever one will allow the proper trajectory low enough within the notch (Fig. 65-12). The knee is hyperflexed as the Steinmann pin is then tapped into place. An 8-mm acorn reamer is then placed over the pin and passed within the joint to rest against the notch wall. The anteromedial femoral tunnel is then reamed to a depth of 40 mm. The EndoButton drill is then placed within the anteromedial tunnel. Your hand should be dropped as the knee is maintained in the hyperflexed position to maximize tunnel length and to ensure that the anterolateral femoral cortex will be perforated to allow passage of the Beath pin distal to the

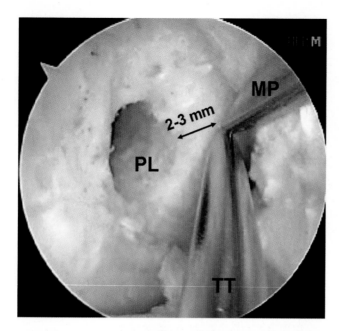

Figure 65-12 Anteromedial femoral guide pin landmarks. TT, transtibial; MP, medial portal.

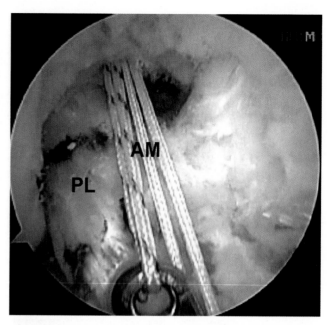

Figure 65-13 Posterolateral graft in place; anteromedial graft position is represented by FiberWire sutures in tunnel. Note that the position of the two bundles is parallel with the knee in full extension.

tourniquet. The transfemoral diameter is then measured, and the appropriately sized closed-loop EndoButton is chosen. Ideally, there should be at least 15 to 20 mm of graft tissue within the canal.

With the knee hyperflexed, place a Beath pin through the low anteromedial portal, through the posterolateral femoral tunnel, and out through the skin on the lateral aspect of the knee. Once again, you want to drop your hand and push the biceps tendon inferiorly as you pass the pin, to protect the common peroneal nerve from injury. A long looped suture is tied through the eyelet of the Beath pin, which is pulled intra-articularly and through the tibial posterolateral tunnel with arthroscopic suture retrievers. The 7-mm prepared posterolateral allograft is placed within the long looped suture attached to the Beath pin and pulled through the respective tibial and femoral tunnels. The EndoButton is flipped, and the graft is pulled to ensure proper engagement. The Beath pin is then passed through the tibial and femoral anteromedial tunnels with the knee hyperflexed to ensure that the pin exits the thigh distal to the tourniquet and remains sterile. Depending on the trajectory of the tunnels, the Beath pin may first need to be passed via the low anteromedial portal through the anteromedial femoral tunnel, and the long looped suture is pulled out through the anteromedial tibial tunnel with arthroscopic suture retrievers. The 8-mm prepared anteromedial allograft is placed within the long looped suture attached to the Beath pin and pulled through the respective tibial and femoral tunnels. The EndoButton is flipped, and the graft is pulled to ensure proper engagement (Fig. 65-13).

The knee is then cycled through a full range of motion from approximately 0 to 120 degrees for 20 to 30 times while tension is maintained on both graft ends to remove any slack and to check the isometry. The posterolateral bundle is tensioned first between 0 and 10 degrees of flexion. The anteromedial bundle is then tensioned with the knee in approximately 60 degrees of flexion. Tibial fixation is achieved with bioabsorbable interference screws that are the same diameter as the corresponding tunnel. One staple is used as adjunctive fixation for each graft on the tibial side (Fig. 65-14).

Postoperative Considerations

Rehabilitation

Postoperatively, the patient is placed in a hinged knee brace. Full weight bearing is allowed with the knee locked in extension. Continuous passive motion is started immediately from 0 to 45 degrees of flexion and increased by 10 degrees per day until maximum obtainable flexion permitted by the continuous passive motion machine is achieved for 2 consecutive days. This is usually after 1 to 2 weeks. The brace is unlocked at 1 week, and crutches are maintained until quadriceps control is re-established, typically 4 to 6 weeks. The accelerated rehabilitation protocol described by Irrgang[12] is implemented with return to contact sport at 6 months with a brace after successful function testing.

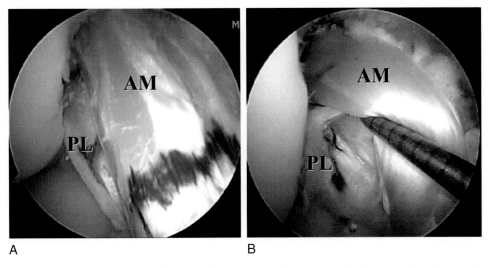

A   B

Figure 65-14 Anteromedial (AM) and posterolateral (PL) grafts in situ. The posterolateral bundle is partially obscured by the anteromedial bundle (**A**) and becomes visible with retraction of the anteromedial bundle (**B**).

Complications

We have had three graft failures, all occurring after return to sport. Two were sustained during contact injuries in playing collegiate football. The third occurred in a non-compliant patient 3 months after reconstruction when she returned to playing high-school basketball without a brace. Four patients have undergone staple removal for symptomatic hardware. To date, after 186 double-bundle ACL reconstructions, we have had no fractures and no radiographic signs of femoral condylar avascular necrosis or tunnel widening.

PEARLS AND PITFALLS

- Proper portal placement is essential for good visualization of the ACL insertion sites. Take care to place the anteromedial and anterolateral portals superior to the fat pad of the knee.

- The accessory medial portal should be placed under direct visualization, with use of a spinal needle as a guide, to ensure proper trajectory for future femoral tunnel placement.

- In removing the damaged ligament, it is useful to mark the individual anteromedial and posterolateral insertion sites with a thermal device to provide landmarks for tunnel drilling locations later in the procedure.

- In identifying tunnel locations, be aware of the flexion angle of the knee, because the insertion site alignment changes as the knee moves from extension to flexion.

- In some cases, the desired anteromedial femoral tunnel location is not accessible by the transtibial approach. In these cases, it may be necessary to drill the anteromedial femoral tunnel through the accessory medial portal. This should be done with care, as it leads to more parallel tunnels.

- Graft fixation should be done independently for the anteromedial and posterolateral grafts to reflect the normal tensioning pattern of the ACL. The posterolateral bundle should be tensioned with the knee in full extension; the anteromedial bundle should be tensioned with the knee in 60 degrees of flexion.

Results

According to Fithian et al,[5] 95% of patients who underwent single-bundle ACL reconstruction developed medial compartment degenerative radiographic changes after 7 years, and only 47% were able to return to their previous activity level. In addition, several in vivo functional biomechanical studies demonstrate that the kinematics are not completely restored with single-bundle reconstruction.[18,19] Amis[4] has shown that even if the femoral tunnel is placed in a lower position than the traditionally described location (more "anatomic") the kinematics are still not normal with regard to rotational stability. In contrast, Yagi et al[20] published their results of double-bundle ACL reconstruction in a cadaver model, showing that both translation and coupled rotation-translation were significantly less in the specimens with double-bundle ACL reconstruction. Clinical results of double-bundle ACL reconstruction surgery are still in evolution (Table 65-1).[1,3,10,15,21,23]

Conclusion

ACL reconstruction is one of the most common orthopedic procedures performed in the United States. Single-bundle ACL reconstruction, which focuses mainly on the anteromedial bundle, remains the gold standard that has enjoyed great success and returned many athletes to their sport. However, several authors have demonstrated that rotational instability persists. The goal of anatomic double-bundle ACL reconstruction is to address this issue and better restore kinematics to normal. It is hoped that this will decrease the rate of degenerative changes, but long-term clinical outcome studies are imperative. Regardless of

Table 65-1 Clinical Results of Anatomic Double-Bundle ACL Reconstruction

Author	Patients	Postoperative Anterior-Posterior Translation	Postoperative Pivot	Functional Outcome
Adachi et al[1] (2004)	105	KT: all <3 mm side-to-side difference	Not reported	100% normal
Hamada et al[10] (2001)	106	KT: all <3 mm side-to-side difference	Not reported	IKDC score: 96% normal–nearly normal
Muneta et al[15] (1999)	54	KT: 2 patients >5 mm	Not reported	Lysholm score: 94.5±5.3
Yasuda et al[21] (2004)	57	KT: 49<3 mm 8, 3-5 mm	0: 56 patients 1+: 1 patient	Noyes score: 47.5
Zaricznyj[23] (1987)	14	Negative Lachman test result: 11 patients 1+ Lachman score: 3 patients	0: 14 patients	Marshall score: 12 good–excellent, 2 fair
Aglietti (unpublished)	50	KT: all <3 mm side-to-side difference	0: 40 patients	IKDC score: 96% normal–nearly normal
Fu (unpublished)	192	KT: average 1.2-mm side-to-side difference	0: 105 patients 1+: 6 patients	93% normal, 6% nearly normal, 1% fair

IKDC, International Knee Documentation Committee.

whether a double-bundle reconstruction technique is chosen, knowledge of the underlying anatomy of the individual bundles will make one a better ACL reconstruction surgeon.

References

1. Adachi N, Ochi M, Uchio Y, et al. Reconstruction of the anterior cruciate ligament. Single- versus double-bundle multistranded hamstring tendons. J Bone Joint Surg Br 2004;86:515-520.
2. Aglietti P, Giron F, Buzzi R, et al. Anterior cruciate ligament reconstruction: bone–patellar tendon–bone compared with double semitendinosus and gracilis tendon grafts. A prospective, randomized clinical trial. J Bone Joint Surg Am 2004;86:2143-2155.
3. Aglietti P. Double-bundle ACL reconstruction: single versus double incision. Personal communication.
4. Amis AA. Persistence of the mini pivot-shift after anatomically placed ACL reconstruction. Personal communication.
5. Fithian DC, Paxton EW, Stone ML, et al. Prospective trial of a treatment algorithm for the management of the anterior cruciate ligament–injured knee. Am J Sports Med 2005;33:335-346.
6. Freedman KB, D'Amato MJ, Nedeff DD, et al. Arthroscopic anterior cruciate ligament reconstruction: a metaanalysis comparing patellar tendon and hamstring tendon autografts. Am J Sports Med 2003;31:2-11.
7. Fu FH. Rupture pattern of the anteromedial and the posterolateral bundle of the anterior cruciate ligament. Personal communication.
8. Gabriel MT, Wong EK, Woo SL, et al. Distribution of in situ forces in the anterior cruciate ligament in response to rotatory loads. J Orthop Res 2004;22:85-89.
9. Griffin LY, Agel J, Albohm MJ, et al. Non-contact anterior cruciate ligament injuries: risk factors and prevention strategies. J Am Acad Orthop Surg 2000;8:141-150.
10. Hamada M, Shino K, Horibe S, et al. Single- versus bi-socket anterior cruciate ligament reconstruction using autogenous multiple-stranded hamstring tendons with EndoButton femoral fixation: a prospective study. Arthroscopy 2001;17:801-807.
11. Harner CD, Baek GH, Vogrin TM, et al. Quantitative analysis of human cruciate ligament insertions. Arthroscopy 1999;15:741-749.
12. Irrgang JJ. Modern trends in anterior cruciate ligament rehabilitation: nonoperative and postoperative management. Clin Sports Med 1993;12:797-813.
13. Jonsson H, Riklund-Ahlstrom K, Lind J. Positive pivot shift after ACL reconstruction predicts later osteoarthrosis: 63 patients followed 5-9 years after surgery. Acta Orthop Scand 2004;75:594-599.
14. Mott HW. Semitendinosus anatomic reconstruction for cruciate ligament insufficiency. Clin Orthop Relat Res 1983;172:90-92.
15. Muneta T, Sekiya I, Yagishita K, et al. Two-bundle reconstruction of the anterior cruciate ligament using semitendinosus tendon with EndoButtons: operative technique and preliminary results. Arthroscopy 1999;15:618-624.
16. Odensten M, Gillquist J. Functional anatomy of the anterior cruciate ligament and a rationale for reconstruction. J Bone Joint Surg Am 1985;67:257-262.
17. Palmer I. On the injuries to the ligaments of the knee joint. Acta Chir Scand 1938;91:282.
18. Ristanis S, Stergiou N, Patras K, et al. Excessive tibial rotation during high-demand activities is not restored by anterior cruciate ligament reconstruction. Arthroscopy 2005;21:1323-1329.
19. Tashman S, Collon D, Anderson K, et al. Abnormal rotational knee motion during running after anterior cruciate ligament reconstruction. Am J Sports Med 2004;32:975-983.

65

20. Yagi M, Wong EK, Kanamori A, et al. Biomechanical analysis of an anatomic anterior cruciate ligament reconstruction. Am J Sports Med 2002;30:660-666.

21. Yasuda K, Kondo E, Ichiyama H, et al. Anatomic reconstruction of the anteromedial and posterolateral bundles of the anterior cruciate ligament using hamstring tendon grafts. Arthroscopy 2004;20:1015-1025.

22. Yunes M, Richmond JC, Engels EA, Pinczewski LA. Patellar versus hamstring tendons in anterior cruciate ligament reconstruction—a meta-analysis. Arthroscopy 2001;17:248-257.

23. Zaricznyj B. Reconstruction of the anterior cruciate ligament of the knee using a doubled tendon graft. Clin Orthop Relat Res 1987;220:162-175.

Transtibial Tunnel Posterior Cruciate Ligament Reconstruction

Gregory C. Fanelli, MD
Craig J. Edson, MS, PT, ATC
Kristin N. Reinheimer, PAC
Raffaele Garofalo, MD

The incidence of posterior cruciate ligament (PCL) injuries is reported to be 1% to 40% of acute knee injuries. This range depends on the population of patients described, and the incidence is approximately 3% in the general population and 38% in reports from regional trauma centers.[2,3,8] Our practice at a regional trauma center has a 38.3% incidence of PCL tears in acute knee injuries, and 56.5% of these PCL injuries occur in patients with multiple trauma. Of these PCL injuries, 45.9% are combined anterior cruciate ligament (ACL) and PCL tears; 41.2% are PCL–posterolateral corner tears. Only 3% of acute PCL injuries seen in the trauma center are isolated.

This chapter illustrates my (G. C. F.) surgical techniques for the arthroscopic single-bundle/single femoral tunnel and double-bundle/double femoral tunnel transtibial PCL reconstruction. We also present the Fanelli Sports Injury Clinic 2- to 10-year results of PCL reconstruction by this surgical technique. The information presented in this chapter has also been presented elsewhere, and the reader is referred to these sources for additional information about this topic.[1,4-7,9-20]

The single-bundle/single femoral tunnel transtibial PCL reconstruction is an anatomic reconstruction of the anterolateral bundle of the PCL. The anterolateral bundle tightens in flexion, and this reconstruction reproduces that biomechanical function. Whereas the single-bundle/single femoral tunnel transtibial PCL reconstruction does not

reproduce the broad anatomic insertion site of the normal PCL, there are certain factors that lead to success with this surgical technique:

- Identification and treatment of all pathologic changes (especially posterolateral instability)
- Accurate tunnel placement
- Anatomic graft insertion sites
- Strong graft material
- Minimal graft bending
- Final tensioning at 70 to 90 degrees of knee flexion
- Graft tensioning (Arthrotek mechanical tensioning device)
- Primary and backup fixation
- Appropriate rehabilitation program

Preoperative Considerations

History and Physical Examination

The typical history of a patient with a PCL injury includes a direct blow to the proximal tibia with the knee in 90 degrees of flexion. Hyperflexion, hyperextension, and a direct blow to the proximal medial or lateral tibia in varying degrees of knee flexion as well as a varus or valgus force will induce PCL-based multiple ligament knee injuries.

Physical examination of the injured knee compared with the noninjured knee reveals a decreased tibial step-off and a positive result of the posterior drawer test. Because concomitant collateral ligament injury is common (posterolateral and posteromedial corner injuries), posterolateral and posteromedial drawer tests, dial tests, and external rotation recurvatum tests may elicit abnormal results; varus and valgus laxity and even anterior laxity may be present.

Diagnostic Features

Isolated PCL Injury

- Abnormal posterior laxity of less than 5 mm
- Abnormal posterior laxity decreases with tibial internal rotation
- No abnormal varus
- Abnormal external rotation of the tibia on the femur of less than 5 degrees compared with the uninvolved side tested with the knee at 30 degrees and 90 degrees of knee flexion

PCL–Posterolateral Corner Injury

- Abnormal posterior laxity of more than 10 mm with a negative tibial step-off
- Abnormal varus rotation at 30 degrees of knee flexion is variable and depends on the posterolateral instability grade
- Abnormal external rotation thigh-foot angle of more than 10 degrees compared with the normal lower extremity tested at 30 degrees and 90 degrees of knee flexion (If you can see the difference, then posterolateral ligament injury exists.)
- Posterolateral drawer test result positive

Combined ACL-PCL Injuries

- Grossly abnormal anterior-posterior tibial-femoral laxity at both 25 degrees and 90 degrees of knee flexion
- Positive Lachman and pseudo-Lachman test results
- Positive pivot shifting phenomenon
- Negative tibial step-off (posterior sag)
- Increased varus-valgus laxity in full extension

Imaging

Radiography

Plain radiographs to evaluate PCL injuries include the following views:

- Anteroposterior weight-bearing view of both knees
- 30-degree flexion lateral view
- Intercondylar notch view
- 30-degree axial view of the patella
- Stress views at 90 degrees of knee flexion of both knees

Other Modalities

Magnetic resonance imaging is helpful in acute cases, but we have found it to be less beneficial in chronic PCL injuries. Bone scan is used in chronic cases of PCL instability presenting with pain to define early degenerative joint disease.

Indications

Our indications for surgical treatment of acute PCL injuries include insertion site avulsions, tibial step-off decreased 6 to 10 mm or more, and PCL tears combined with other structural injuries. Surgical treatment of chronic PCL injuries is indicated when an isolated PCL tear becomes symptomatic as demonstrated by progressive functional instability.

Surgical Technique

Anesthesia and Positioning

The patient is positioned on the operating table in the supine position, and the surgical and nonsurgical knees are examined under general or regional anesthesia. A tourniquet is applied to the operative extremity, and the surgical leg is prepared and draped in a sterile fashion. Allograft tissue is prepared before the surgical procedure is begun, and autograft tissue is harvested before the arthroscopic portion of the procedure. The arthroscopic instruments are inserted with the inflow through the superior lateral patellar portal, the arthroscope in the inferior lateral patellar portal, and the instruments in the inferior medial patellar portal. The portals are interchanged as necessary. The joint is thoroughly evaluated arthroscopically, and the PCL is evaluated by the three-zone arthroscopic technique.[13] The PCL tear is identified, and the residual stump of the PCL is débrided with hand tools and the synovial shaver.

Specific Steps (Box 66-1)

1. Initial Incision

An extracapsular posteromedial safety incision approximately 1.5 to 2.0 cm long is made (Fig. 66-1). The crural

Box 66-1 Surgical Steps

1. Initial incision
2. Elevation of the posterior capsule
3. Drill guide positioning
4. Tibial tunnel drilling
5. Drilling of the femoral tunnel
6. Tunnel preparation and graft passage
7. Graft tensioning and fixation
8. Additional surgery

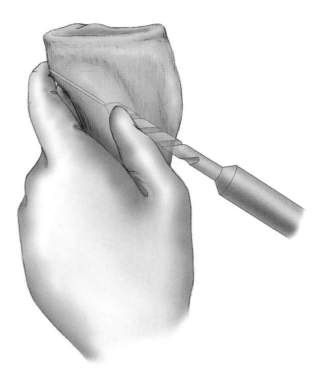

Figure 66-2 The surgeon is able to palpate the posterior aspect of the tibia through the extracapsular extra-articular posteromedial safety incision. This enables the surgeon to accurately position guide wires, to drill the tibial tunnel, and to protect the neurovascular structures. (Redrawn with permission of Arthrotek, Inc., Warsaw, Ind.)

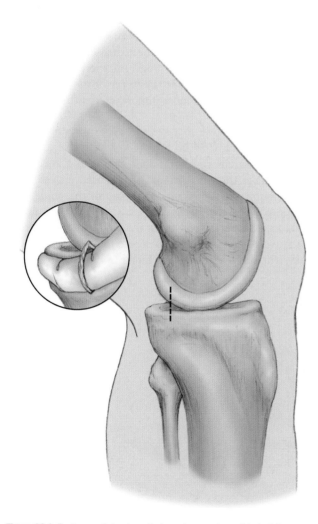

Figure 66-1 Posteromedial extra-articular extracapsular safety incision. (Redrawn with permission of Arthrotek, Inc., Warsaw, Ind.)

neurovascular structures are posterior to the finger and the posterior aspect of the joint capsule is anterior to the surgeon's finger. This technique enables the surgeon to monitor surgical instruments, such as the over-the-top PCL instruments and the PCL-ACL drill guide, as they are positioned in the posterior aspect of the knee. The surgeon's finger in the posteromedial safety incision also confirms accurate placement of the guide wire before tibial tunnel drilling in the medial-lateral and proximal-distal directions (Fig. 66-2). This is the same anatomic surgical interval that is used in the tibial inlay posterior approach.

2. Elevation of the Posterior Capsule

The curved over-the-top PCL instruments are used to carefully lyse adhesions in the posterior aspect of the knee and to elevate the posterior knee joint capsule away from the tibial ridge on the posterior aspect of the tibia. This capsular elevation enhances correct drill guide and tibial tunnel placement (Fig. 66-3).

3. Drill Guide Positioning

The arm of the Arthrotek Fanelli PCL-ACL drill guide is inserted into the knee through the inferior medial patellar portal and positioned in the PCL fossa on the posterior tibia (Fig. 66-4). The bullet portion of the drill guide contacts the anterior medial aspect of the proximal tibia

fascia is incised longitudinally, with precautions taken to protect the neurovascular structures. The interval is developed between the medial head of the gastrocnemius muscle and the posterior capsule of the knee joint, which is anterior. The surgeon's gloved finger is positioned so that the

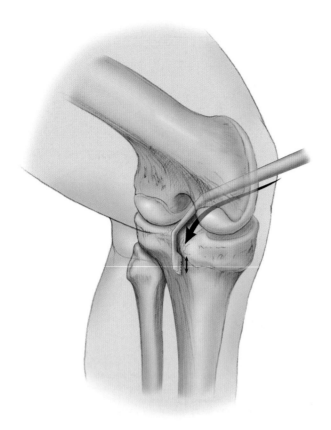

Figure 66-3 Posterior capsular elevation with the Arthrotek PCL instruments. (Redrawn with permission of Arthrotek, Inc., Warsaw, Ind.)

approximately 1 cm below the tibial tubercle, at a point midway between the tibial crest anteriorly and the posterior medial border of the tibia. This drill guide positioning creates a tibial tunnel that is relatively vertically oriented and has its posterior exit point in the inferior and lateral aspect of the PCL tibial anatomic insertion site. This positioning creates an angle of graft orientation such that the graft will make two smooth 45-degree angle turns on the posterior aspect of the tibia, eliminating a 90-degree graft angle referred to as the "killer turn" (Fig. 66-5).

The tip of the guide in the posterior aspect of the tibia is confirmed with the surgeon's finger through the extracapsular posteromedial safety incision (see Fig. 66-2). Intraoperative anteroposterior and lateral radiographs may also be obtained, as well as arthroscopic visualization to confirm drill guide and guide pin placement. A blunt spade-tipped guide wire is drilled from anterior to posterior and can be visualized with the arthroscope, in addition to being palpated with the finger in the posteromedial safety incision. We consider the finger in the posteromedial safety incision the most important step for accuracy and safety.

4. Tibial Tunnel Drilling

The appropriately sized standard cannulated reamer is used to make the tibial tunnel. The closed curved PCL curet may be positioned to cup the tip of the guide wire (Fig. 66-6). The arthroscope, when it is positioned in the posteromedial portal, visualizes the guide wire being captured by the curet and ensures protection of the neurovascular structures. The surgeon's finger in the posteromedial

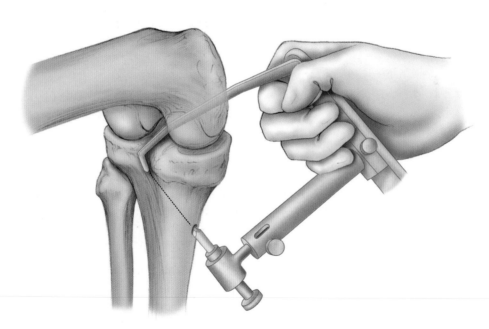

Figure 66-4 Arthrotek Fanelli PCL-ACL drill guide positioned to place guide wire in preparation for drilling of the transtibial PCL tibial tunnel. (Redrawn with permission of Arthrotek, Inc., Warsaw, Ind.)

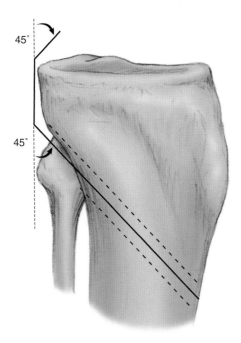

Figure 66-5 Drawing demonstrates the desired turning angles that the PCL graft will make after the tibial tunnel is made. (Redrawn with permission of Arthrotek, Inc., Warsaw, Ind.)

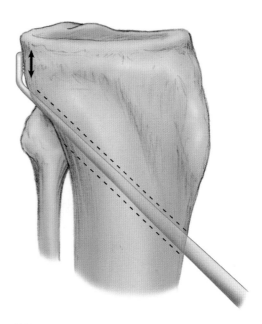

Figure 66-7 The tunnel edges are chamfered after drilling to smooth any rough edges. (Redrawn with permission of Arthrotek, Inc., Warsaw, Ind.)

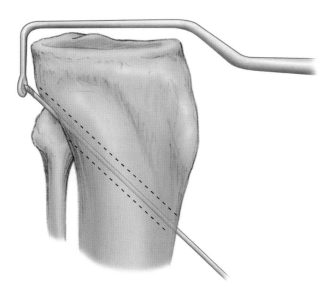

Figure 66-6 The Arthrotek PCL closed curet is used to cap the guide wire during tibial tunnel drilling. (Redrawn with permission of Arthrotek, Inc., Warsaw, Ind.)

safety incision is monitoring the position of the guide wire. The standard cannulated drill is advanced to the posterior cortex of the tibia. The drill chuck is then disengaged from the drill, and completion of the tibial tunnel reaming is performed by hand. This gives an additional margin of safety for completion of the tibial tunnel. The tunnel edges are chamfered and rasped with the PCL-ACL system rasp (Fig. 66-7).

5. Drilling of the Femoral Tunnel

The Arthrotek Fanelli PCL-ACL drill guide is positioned to drill the femoral tunnel (Fig. 66-8). The arm of the guide is introduced into the knee through the inferior medial patellar portal and positioned such that the guide wire will exit through the center of the stump of the anterolateral bundle of the PCL. The blunt spade-tipped guide wire is drilled through the guide, and just as it begins to emerge through the center of the stump of the anterolateral bundle of the PCL, the drill guide is disengaged. The accuracy of the guide wire position is confirmed arthroscopically by probing and direct visualization. Care must be taken to ensure that the patellofemoral joint has not been violated by arthroscopic examination of the patellofemoral joint before drilling of the femoral tunnel.

The appropriately sized standard cannulated reamer is used to make the femoral tunnel over a guide wire from outside in or from inside out per the surgeon's preference (Fig. 66-9). When the double-bundle/double femoral tunnel surgical technique is performed, the two tunnels are placed at the anatomic insertion sites of the anterolateral and posteromedial bundles to approximate the anatomic footprint of the PCL femoral insertion site (Fig. 66-10). The reaming debris is evacuated with a synovial shaver to minimize fat pad inflammatory response with subsequent risk of arthrofibrosis. The tunnel edges are chamfered and rasped.

6. Tunnel Preparation and Graft Passage

The Arthrotek Magellan suture-passing device is introduced through the tibial tunnel and into the knee joint; it

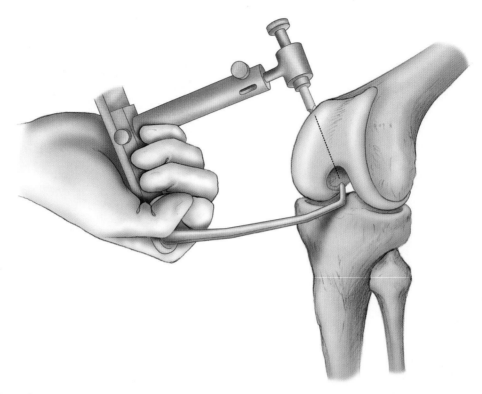

Figure 66-8 The Arthrotek Fanelli PCL-ACL drill guide is positioned to drill the guide wire from outside in. The guide wire begins at a point halfway between the medial femoral epicondyle and the medial femoral condyle trochlea articular margin, approximately 2 to 3 cm proximal to the medial femoral condyle distal articular margin, and exits through the center of the stump of the anterolateral bundle of the PCL stump. (Redrawn with permission of Arthrotek, Inc., Warsaw, Ind.)

is retrieved through the femoral tunnel with an arthroscopic grasping tool (Fig. 66-11). The traction sutures of the graft material are attached to the loop of the Arthrotek Magellan suture-passing device, and the PCL graft material is pulled into position.

7. Graft Tensioning and Fixation

Fixation of the PCL substitute is accomplished with primary and backup fixation on both the femoral and tibial sides. Our preferred graft source for PCL reconstruction is the Achilles tendon allograft alone for single-bundle reconstructions and Achilles tendon and tibialis anterior allografts for double-bundle reconstructions. Femoral fixation is accomplished by cortical suspensory backup fixation with polyethelene ligament fixation buttons, and aperture opening fixation is achieved with the Arthrotek Bio-Core bioabsorbable interference screws. The Arthrotek graft tensioning boot is applied to the traction sutures of the graft material on its distal end, set for 20 pounds, and the knee is cycled through 25 full flexion-extension cycles for graft pretensioning and settling (Fig. 66-12). During single-bundle PCL reconstructions, the graft is tensioned in approximately 70 degrees of knee flexion. During double-bundle reconstructions, the anterolateral bundle is tensioned at approximately 70 degrees of knee flexion, and the posteromedial bundle is tensioned at approximately 30

degrees of knee flexion. Tibial graft fixation is achieved with primary aperture opening fixation with the Arthrotek Bio-Core bioabsorbable interference screw; backup fixation is performed with a ligament fixation button or screw and post or screw and spiked ligament washer assembly (Fig. 66-13).

8. Additional Surgery

When multiple ligament surgeries are scheduled at the same operative session, the PCL reconstruction is performed first, followed by the ACL reconstruction, followed by the collateral ligament surgery. The reader is referred to other sections of this textbook for descriptions of multiple ligament surgeries of the knee. At the completion of the procedure, the tourniquet is deflated, and the wounds are irrigated. The incisions are closed in the standard fashion.

Postoperative Considerations

Rehabilitation

The knee is immobilized in a long leg brace in full extension for 6 weeks, with non—weight bearing with use of crutches. Progressive range of motion occurs during weeks

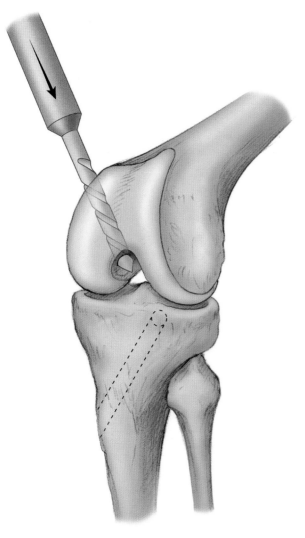

Figure 66-9 Completion of femoral tunnel reaming by hand for an additional margin of safety. (Redrawn with permission of Arthrotek, Inc., Warsaw, Ind.)

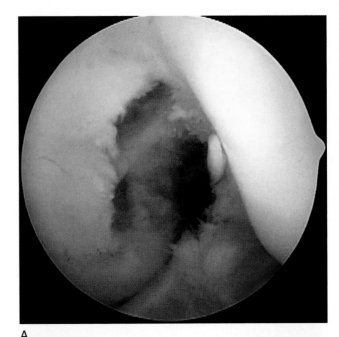

A

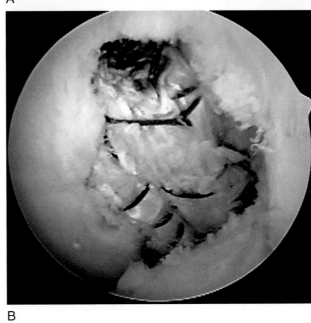

B

Figure 66-10 A, Tunnel placement for double-bundle PCL reconstruction. **B,** Double-bundle PCL reconstruction with Achilles tendon allograft for the anterolateral bundle and tibialis anterior allograft for the posteromedial bundle.

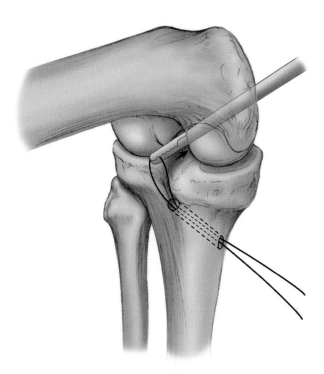

Figure 66-11 Arthrotek Magellan suture-passing device. (Redrawn with permission of Arthrotek, Inc., Warsaw, Ind.)

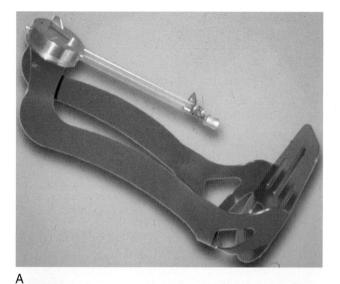

A

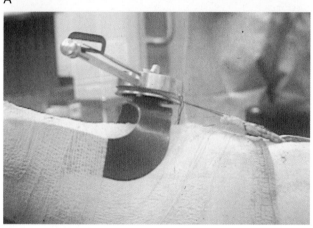

B

Figure 66-12 A, A picture of the Arthrotek knee ligament graft tensioning boot. This mechanical tensioning device uses a ratcheted torque wrench device to assist the surgeon during graft tensioning. **B,** The Arthrotek graft tensioning boot attached to the traction sutures on the PCL graft. (Redrawn with permission of Arthrotek, Inc., Warsaw, Ind.)

4 through 6. The brace is unlocked between 3 and 6 weeks, and progressive weight bearing at 25% body weight per week is instituted during postoperative weeks 7 through 10. The crutches are discontinued at the end of postoperative week 10. Progressive strength training and range-of-motion exercises are performed. Return to sports and heavy labor occurs after the sixth to ninth postoperative month, when sufficient strength, range of motion, and proprioceptive skills have returned.

Complications

PCL reconstruction is technically demanding surgery. Complications encountered with this surgical procedure include failure to recognize associated ligament injuries, neurovascular complications, persistent posterior sag,

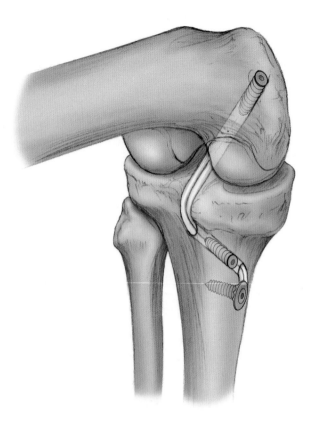

Figure 66-13 Final graft fixation with primary and backup fixation. (Redrawn with permission of Arthrotek, Inc., Warsaw, Ind.)

osteonecrosis, knee motion loss, anterior knee pain, and fractures. A comprehensive preoperative evaluation, including an accurate diagnosis, a well-planned and carefully executed surgical procedure, and a supervised postoperative rehabilitation program, will help reduce the incidence of these complications.

PEARLS AND PITFALLS

- Identify and treat all pathologic changes (especially posterolateral instability).
- Ensure accurate tunnel placement.
- Place strong graft material at anatomic graft insertion sites.
- Minimize graft bending.
- Perform final tensioning at 70 to 90 degrees of knee flexion.
- Use a mechanical tensioning device for graft tensioning (Arthrotek mechanical tensioning device).
- Use primary and backup fixation.
- Institute an appropriate program of rehabilitation.

Fanelli Sports Injury Clinic Results

After PCL reconstruction by the single-bundle surgical technique tensioned with the Arthrotek graft tensioning boot, both a normal posterior drawer test result and a

Table 66-1 Fanelli Sports Injury Clinic Results

Author	Follow-up	Outcome
Fanelli and Edson[10] (2002)	2 to 10 years	46.0% normal posterior drawer test results and tibial step-offs, and 54.0% grade 1 posterior drawer and tibial step-offs in combined ACL-PCL reconstructions; no Arthrotek graft tensioning boot was used
Fanelli and Edson[11] (2004)	2 to 10 years	70% normal posterior drawer test results and tibial step-offs for the overall study group, and 91.7% normal posterior drawer test results and tibial step-offs in the subgroup with the Arthrotek graft tensioning boot in combined PCL-posterolateral reconstructions
Fanelli et al[12] (2005)	2 years	86.6% normal posterior drawer test results and tibial step-offs in combined ACL-PCL reconstructions with the Arthrotek graft tensioning boot

normal tibial step-off are restored in 86.6% of the combined ACL-PCL reconstruction group[12] and in 91.7% of the PCL–posterolateral reconstruction group.[11] These results are outlined in Table 66-1.

Conclusions

The arthroscopically assisted single-bundle transtibial PCL reconstruction technique is a reproducible surgical procedure. There are documented results demonstrating statistically significant improvements from preoperative to postoperative status evaluated by physical examination, knee ligament rating scales, arthrometer measurements, and stress radiography. Factors contributing to the success of this surgical technique include identification and treatment of all pathologic changes (especially posterolateral instability), accurate tunnel placement, placement of strong graft material at anatomic graft insertion sites, minimization of graft bending, performance of final graft tensioning at 70 to 90 degrees of knee flexion with the Arthrotek graft tensioning boot, use of primary and backup fixation, and appropriate postoperative rehabilitation program. Because of a more anatomic reconstruction, double-bundle reconstruction may provide better results. This will need to be demonstrated in long-term clinical studies.

References

1. Arthrotek PCL Reconstruction Surgical Technique Guide. Fanelli PCL-ACL Drill Guide System. Arthrotek, Inc., Warsaw, Ind, 1998.
2. Daniel DM, Akeson W, O'Conner J, eds. Knee Ligaments: Structure, Function, Injury, and Repair. New York, Raven Press, 1990.
3. Fanelli GC. Posterior cruciate ligament injuries in trauma patients. Arthroscopy 1993;9:291-294.
4. Fanelli GC. Arthroscopic posterior cruciate ligament reconstruction: single bundle/single femoral tunnel. Arthroscopy 2000;16:725-731.
5. Fanelli GC. Arthroscopic evaluation of the PCL. In Fanelli GC, ed. Posterior Cruciate Ligament Injuries. A Guide to Practical Management. New York, Springer-Verlag, 2001.
6. Fanelli GC. Arthroscopic PCL reconstruction: transtibial technique. In Fanelli GC, ed. Posterior Cruciate Ligament Injuries. A Guide to Practical Management. New York, Springer-Verlag, 2001.
7. Fanelli GC. Complications in PCL surgery. In Fanelli GC, ed. Posterior Cruciate Ligament Injuries. A Guide to Practical Management. New York, Springer-Verlag, 2001.
8. Fanelli GC, Edson CJ. Posterior cruciate ligament injuries in trauma patients. Part II. Arthroscopy 1995;11:526-529.
9. Fanelli GC, Edson CJ. Management of posterior cruciate ligament and posterolateral instability of the knee. In Chow J, ed. Advanced Arthroplasty. New York, Springer-Verlag, 2001.
10. Fanelli GC, Edson CJ. Arthroscopically assisted combined anterior and posterior cruciate ligament reconstruction: 2- to 10-year follow-up. Arthroscopy 2002;18:703-714.
11. Fanelli GC, Edson CJ. Combined posterior cruciate ligament–posterolateral reconstruction with Achilles tendon allograft and biceps femoris tendon tenodesis: 2- to 10-year follow-up. Arthroscopy 2004;20:339-345.
12. Fanelli GC, Edson CJ, Orcutt DR, et al. Treatment of combined anterior cruciate–posterior cruciate ligament–medial-lateral side knee injuries. J Knee Surg 2005;28:240-248.
13. Fanelli GC, Giannotti B, Edson C. The posterior cruciate ligament: arthroscopic evaluation and treatment. Arthroscopy 1994;10:673-688.
14. Fanelli GC, Giannotti BF, Edson CJ. Arthroscopically assisted combined anterior and posterior cruciate ligament reconstruction. Arthroscopy 1996;12:5-14.
15. Fanelli GC, Giannotti B, Edson CJ. Arthroscopically assisted posterior cruciate ligament/posterior lateral complex reconstruction. Arthroscopy 1996;12:703-714.
16. Fanelli GC, Monahan TJ. Complications of posterior cruciate ligament reconstruction. Sports Med Arthrosc Rev 1999;7:296-302.
17. Fanelli GC, Monaghan TJ. Complications and pitfalls in posterior cruciate ligament reconstruction. In Malek MM, ed; Fanelli GC, Johnson D, Johnson D, section eds. Knee Surgery: Complications, Pitfalls, and Salvage. New York, Springer-Verlag, 2001.
18. Fanelli GC, Monaghan TJ. Complications in posterior cruciate ligament and posterolateral complex surgery. Oper Tech Sports Med 2001;9:96-99.
19. Malek MM, Fanelli GC. Technique of arthroscopically assisted PCL reconstruction. Orthopedics 1993;16:961-966.
20. Miller MD, Cooper DE, Fanelli GC, et al. Posterior cruciate ligament: current concepts. Instr Course Lect 2002;51:347-351.

CHAPTER 67

Double-Bundle Posterior Cruciate Ligament Reconstruction

Anthony M. Buoncristiani, MD

Jon K. Sekiya, MD

Posterior cruciate ligament (PCL) injuries are rare and infrequently occur in isolation. Despite our increased knowledge of the anatomy and mechanism of injury, PCL reconstruction has not obtained the success of ACL reconstruction.[1] Frustrating to the surgeon is the lack of consensus regarding the optimal management of PCL injuries. Even when surgical intervention is determined, the confusion does not cease—graft type, single versus double bundle, acute versus chronic reconstruction, and transtibial versus inlay technique are issues that are difficult to resolve.

The clinical outcome of PCL deficiency has not been uniformly poor.[16] Thus, indications for surgical intervention of isolated PCL tears are disputed. The majority of PCL reconstructions occur in conjunction with other ligamentous reconstructions or repairs. Therefore, the timing of PCL reconstruction may depend on the concomitant ligamentous repairs or reconstructions, which risks jeopardizing stability or stiffness. In addition, the chronicity of the injury has been shown to affect the clinical results.[15]

In this chapter, we discuss indications, physical examination findings, and three different techniques of double-bundle PCL reconstruction with a bifid bone–patellar tendon–bone allograft: transtibial, open tibial inlay, and arthroscopic tibial inlay. Previously, the senior author (J. K. S.) reported our technique for a bifid bone–patellar tendon–bone allograft for reconstruction of the PCL.[14] This graft closely re-creates the anatomic configuration and size of the native PCL

Preoperative Considerations

History

Acutely, there is usually a history of a direct blow to the anterior lower leg or a hyperextension injury associated with concomitant mild swelling. A PCL injury may also occur in the setting of a knee dislocation in conjunction with other ligamentous injuries. In trauma, 95% of patients with a PCL injury have an associated ligamentous injury, with the posterolateral structures being most common (approximately 60%).[2] Chronically, instability may be the only complaint.

Physical Examination

On physical examination, it is important to assess the neurovascular status of the injured limb. This is especially important if there is a history of a knee dislocation, which has a higher risk of such an injury. Inspection and palpation for an effusion is followed by assessment of the range of motion. With the knee in a flexed position, palpate for the natural tibial step-off and evaluate the anterior border of the tibial plateau in relation to the femoral condyles. In addition, a Godfrey test can be performed, whereby the lower leg is elevated with the knee flexed approximately 90 degrees to assess for the presence of a "sag." A posterior

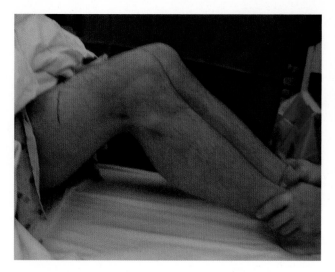

Figure 67-1 In 90 degrees of flexion, an obvious posterior subluxation of the right knee is observed. This is consistent with a PCL injury.

drawer test with the knee in 90 degrees of flexion is also performed to evaluate the amount of posterior tibial translation (Fig. 67-1). It is important to recognize the presence of a posterolateral corner knee injury, which is commonly associated with a PCL injury and will accentuate the posterior drawer.[13] The gait pattern is inspected for any varus thrust. If a posterolateral corner injury is suspected, the physical examination should include a reverse pivot shift test, a dial test, a posterolateral drawer test, and varus stress testing at both 30 degrees and 90 degrees.

Imaging

Radiography

Radiographs of the knee are obtained to inspect for any fracture in the acute setting or for any medial or patellofemoral compartmental arthrosis in the chronic setting. Long-cassette films should be obtained if any fixed or dynamic instability is suspected. Posterior tibial subluxation can sometimes be seen on the lateral radiograph. Otherwise, a comparative stress lateral radiograph can also be obtained (Fig. 67-2).

Other Modalities

A bone scan may be useful in chronic PCL insufficiency to identify degenerative changes. A magnetic resonance imaging evaluation is essential, not only to confirm a PCL injury but, more important, to assess for any concomitant posterolateral corner injury that will affect the operative plan (Fig. 67-3).

Indications and Contraindications

Isolated PCL injuries (grades I and II) can be treated nonoperatively with protected weight bearing and

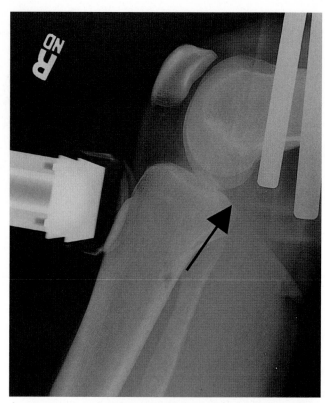

A

B

Figure 67-2 Stress views of the uninjured (**A**) and injured (**B**) knees. Note the amount of posterior tibial subluxation of the injured knee (**B**) consistent with a significant PCL injury (demonstrated by the arrows).

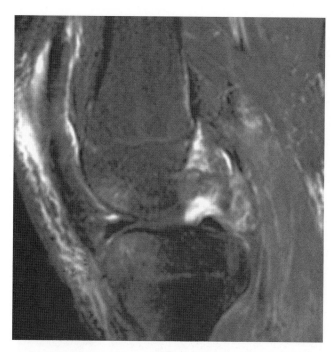

Figure 67-3 Magnetic resonance image of the same patient as in Figure 67-2 demonstrates an acute complete tear of the PCL off the tibia. There is an associated posterolateral corner injury.

quadriceps muscle rehabilitation. The absolute indications for reconstruction of an isolated PCL tear are persistent instability (grade III) and bone avulsion, although some authors dispute the existence of an isolated grade III PCL injury.[13,15] Regardless, most PCL reconstructions occur in conjunction with a knee dislocation or multiligamentous injury. The timing of PCL reconstruction is controversial, but an acute reconstruction is generally accepted for bone avulsion injuries or for addressing combined ligamentous injuries—especially a posterolateral corner injury. Acute PCL reconstruction is contraindicated in the setting of a traumatic open knee injury or a significantly stiff knee.

Surgical Technique

Graft Preparation

A whole, nonirradiated, frozen patellar tendon allograft is thawed at room temperature in antibiotic saline. To improve efficiency, the graft may be prepared during induction of anesthesia or by a trained assistant during the diagnostic arthroscopy. If uncertainty exists as to whether the PCL reconstruction should be performed, the graft is thawed after the diagnostic arthroscopy.

The required minimum dimensions of the patellar tendon allograft are 45 mm of tendon length and 22 mm of tendon width. For patients taller than 6 feet, we prefer

a minimum tendon length of 50 mm, particularly if an open inlay technique is chosen for tibial fixation. The central 20-mm segment of the graft is identified and incised with a scalpel to form two bundles. Both an 11-mm and a 9-mm graft are fashioned to re-create the anterolateral and posteromedial bundles, respectively. For a right knee, the 11-mm anterolateral bundle is lateral with the cancellous side facing anterior, and the 9-mm posteromedial bundle is medial. This most closely mimics the normal PCL morphologic appearance as described by Harner et al[6] and reproduces the PCL "twist." The patellar bone segment is used for the femoral attachments and is split with an oscillating saw along the line of the tendon fibers between the two bundles. Each patellar bone block is then cut to a length of approximately 20 mm. A rongeur is used to fashion the bone blocks to fit the respective femoral tunnel sizes of 11 mm and 9 mm corresponding to the size of the tendon. It is important to "bullet-tip" the ends of each plug to facilitate later passage within the femoral tunnels. Each femoral bone plug is then drilled with two separate 2.0-mm holes, and passing sutures of No. 2 FiberWire (Arthrex, Naples, Fla) are then placed through them. One additional No. 2 FiberWire suture is placed at the bone-tendon interface for additional fixation. The prepared femoral bone plugs are suitable for use with either the tibial inlay or the arthroscopic transtibial tunnel technique. However, preparation of the tibial bone plug is different for the arthroscopic and open inlay procedures. For the tibial inlay reconstruction, the tibial bone plug is sized to approximately 20 mm long, 13 mm wide, and 12 mm thick. A single 4.5-mm gliding hole is placed in the center of the plug for later placement of a 4.5-mm fully threaded cortical screw (Synthes, Paoli, Pa) for fixation of the graft within the tibial trough.

The arthroscopic transtibial graft dimensions differ from the inlay with regard to the tibial bone plug. The transtibial bone plug is approximately 30 mm long and 12 mm in diameter. Two 2.0-mm drill holes are drilled in the bone plug and threaded with No. 2 FiberWire. An additional FiberWire suture is sewn to the tendon-graft interface. The graft tip is "bulleted" to facilitate later passage within the tibial tunnel (Fig. 67-4).

Anesthesia and Positioning

The anesthesia team places both femoral and sciatic peripheral nerve catheters in the preoperative holding area (but they are not dosed) for postoperative pain management. No anesthetic is introduced until neurologic assessment has occurred on completion of the case. The patient is then brought to the operating room and placed supine on a radiolucent table. The patient then undergoes endotracheal intubation, but no long-acting paralytics are given to hide neurologic stimulation. An examination under anesthesia is performed to document PCL

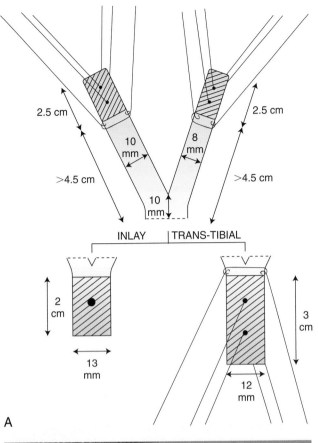

A

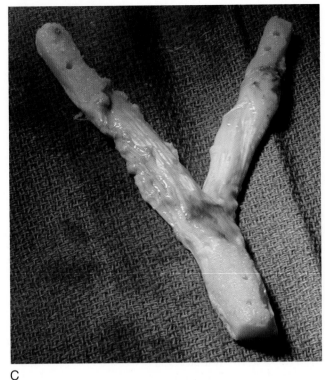

C

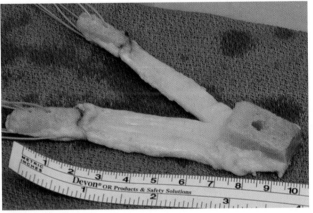

B

Figure 67-4 **A,** Diagram representation of the tibial inlay and transtibial graft preparation. Note the differences between the tibial inlay (**B**) and transtibial allograft (**C**) preparation. The inlay graft has a 4.5-mm gliding hole for tibial fixation; the transtibial graft is smaller and bulleted to facilitate tibial tunnel passage. (**A** reprinted with permission from Sekiya JK, Kurtz CA, Carr DR. Transtibial and tibial inlay double-bundle posterior cruciate ligament reconstruction: surgical technique using a bifid bone–patellar tendon–bone allograft. Arthroscopy 2004;20:1095-1100.)

deficiency. A tourniquet is applied to the thigh but is usually not used. A post is attached to the operating room table at the level of the tourniquet. For the open inlay technique, a gel pad bump is placed under the contralateral hip to facilitate later exposure to the posteromedial knee of the operative extremity in the figure-four position. A 5-pound beanbag is secured to the operating room table at a location that will maintain the knee in approximately 90 degrees of flexion. The leg is prepared with both alcohol and DuraPrep, and an extremity drape is applied to the lower leg. A preoperative time-out is performed to identify the patient, the extremity, and the procedure (Fig. 67-5).

Open Tibial Inlay

Surgical Landmarks, Incisions, and Portals

A bump is placed between the post and the leg to help stabilize the knee in a flexed position while the foot rests on the prepositioned sandbag. With the knee flexed approximately 90 degrees, standard anteromedial and anterolateral portal incisions are made and diagnostic arthroscopy is performed initially to address and to document additional injuries. The PCL stump is arthroscopi-

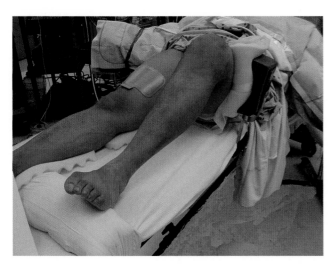

Figure 67-5 A gel pad is placed under the contralateral hip, and a beanbag keeps the operative knee flexed in approximately 90 degrees. This allows access to and exposure of the posteromedial knee.

cally débrided from the femoral origin, and any anatomic variations in bundle location are noted. An attempt is made to preserve any intact meniscofemoral ligaments, but they are often sacrificed because they hinder passage of the large PCL graft. The center of the medial femoral condyle is identified, and a 4-cm incision is placed along the posterior border of the vastus medialis. This incision will be used later for femoral tunnel placement.

Exposure

The leg is then flexed to 90 degrees and brought into a figure-four position while the bump is repositioned under the lateral ankle. This accentuates the external rotation of the hip and facilitates access to the posteromedial lower leg. A 5- to 7-cm incision is made starting in the crease of the popliteal fossa and curving distally along the posteromedial border of the tibia (Fig. 67-6). The dissection is continued through the subcutaneous fat down to the level of the sartorius fascia and the fascia overlying the medial head of the gastrocnemius. The fascia is incised along the palpable posteromedial tibial border. The semimembranosus and pes anserinus tendons are retracted anteriorly and proximally while the medial head of the gastrocnemius is elevated from the tibial cortex and retracted posteriorly. The medial border of the gastrocnemius is followed distally along the posterior tibia, and the proximal border of the popliteus muscle is identified (Fig. 67-7). The popliteus muscle is elevated subperiosteally off the posteromedial surface of the tibia and mobilized laterally and distally.

Specific Steps (Box 67-1)

Femoral Tunnels

An outside-in femoral target PCL guide is used to place the two ³⁄₃₂-inch Steinmann pins by arthroscopic guidance.

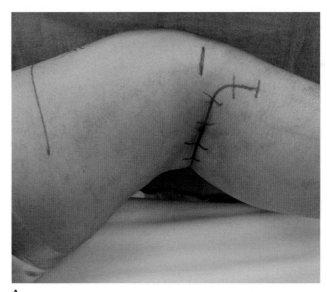

A

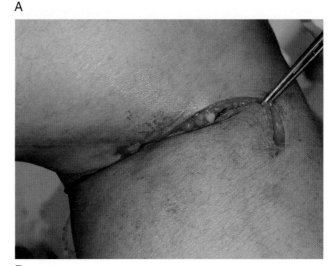

B

Figure 67-6 A 5- to 7-cm incision is made starting in the crease of the popliteal fossa and curving distally along the posteromedial border of the tibia.

One pin is placed at each center of the anatomic locations of the anterolateral and posteromedial bundles. We prefer to drill the two femoral tunnels from outside in for three reasons: (1) a study by Handy et al[4] suggested that the femoral tunnel–to-graft angle is less severe with this technique; (2) we can more easily tension the grafts and fix them outside-in as opposed to inside-out; and (3) we can supplement metal interference screw fixation by tying the sutures over the bone bridge for the two tunnels or over a plastic button. On the basis of anatomic studies of the PCL origin, for the right knee the Beath pin for the anterolateral bundle is placed at the 12:30-o'clock position approximately 5.5 mm from the articular margin, and the smaller posteromedial bundle is placed at the 3-o'clock position approximately 6 to 7 mm from the articular margin.[6,10] Cannulated reamers are drilled over the guide

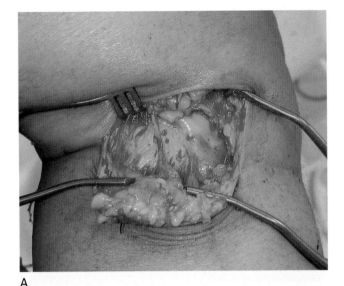

A

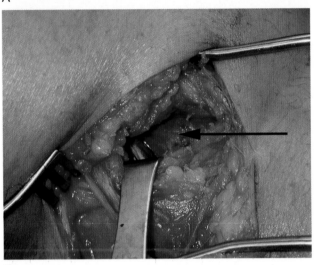

B

Figure 67-7 A, The fascia overlying the semimembranosus and pes anserinus tendons (anteriorly) and the medial head of the gastrocnemius (posteriorly) is exposed. **B,** This plane is then entered, which exposes the underlying popliteus muscle (identified by the arrow).

Box 67-1 Surgical Steps

1. Positioning
2. Examination under anesthesia
3. Graft preparation
4. Tibial attachment
5. Femoral tunnel drilling
6. Graft passage
7. Graft fixation
8. Closure

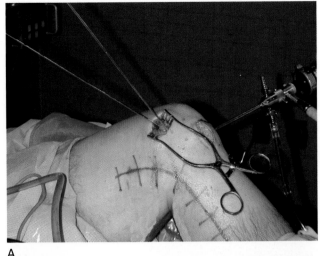

A

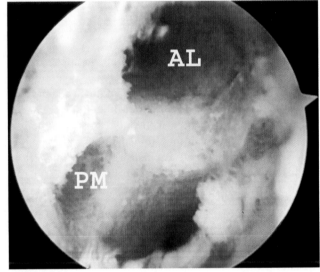

B

Figure 67-8 A, An outside-in femoral target PCL guide is used to place the Beath pin for the anterolateral bundle at the 12:30-o'clock position approximately 5.5 mm from the articular margin. The smaller posteromedial bundle is placed at the 3-o'clock position approximately 6 to 7 mm from the articular margin. **B,** An arthroscopic view of the anterolateral (AL) and posteromedial (PM) tunnels is shown.

pins to make an 11-mm anterolateral and a 9-mm posteromedial tunnel (Fig. 67-8).

Tibial Trough Preparation

The knee is placed into the figure-four position, and attention is redirected to the posteromedial exposure of the tibia. The superior tibial insertion site of the PCL begins in a fossa between the two palpable prominences of the medial and lateral plateaus of the tibia.[17] The fossa serves as a guide to the location of the trough (Fig. 67-9). A vertical arthrotomy is made with a scalpel between the two prominences. The remaining PCL insertion is identified and débrided. A quarter-inch curved osteotome or bur is used to make a trough 13 mm wide, 12 mm deep, and

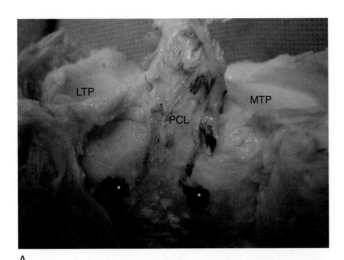

A

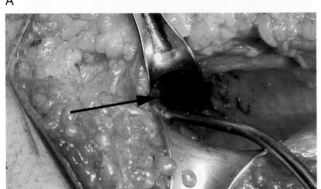

B

Figure 67-9 A, The superior tibial insertion site of the PCL begins in a fossa between the two palpable prominences of the posterior medial and lateral plateaus of the tibia *(asterisks)*. MTP, medial tibial plateau; LTP, lateral tibial plateau. (From Whiddon DR, Sekiya JK. Double-bundle PCL reconstruction with a bifid bone-patellar tendon-bone allograft. Oper Tech Sports Med 2006;13(4):233–240.) **B,** A trough for the tibial inlay is made *(arrow)* with a curved osteotome or bur. It is important to keep a shelf of bone superiorly in the trough to help stabilize the graft when it is later recessed into place.

extending distally 2 cm. It is important to keep a shelf of bone superiorly in the trough to help stabilize the graft when later it is recessed into place.

Tibial Inlay Graft Passage and Fixation

A 3.2-mm transtibial drill hole is placed in the center of the trough corresponding to the 4.5-mm gliding hole in the graft's tibial bone plug. The transtibial depth is measured, and a 3.2-mm tap is then placed. The graft is more easily passed in an anterior to posterior direction from inside the joint into the trough. The anteromedial parapatellar portal is slightly extended to accommodate the graft's passage. The sutures are kept separated for each respective graft bundle for later identification and passage. A 4.5-mm fully threaded cortical screw corresponding to the measured length plus 10 mm is used to lag the bone block into the trough (Fig. 67-10). We use intraoperative fluoroscopy to verify the location of the graft. The lateral view is easily obtained with the knee in the figure-four position, and the leg is extended for the anteroposterior view.

Femoral Graft Passage and Fixation

The anterolateral and posteromedial bundle grafts are then passed through the femoral tunnels by use of a suture passer. The extended medial parapatellar arthrotomy is often useful for passage and manipulation of the bone plugs into their respective tunnels. After the graft is fully seated in the femoral tunnels, the natural PCL twist is observed (Fig. 67-11).[6] Several cycles of flexion and extension are recommended to pre-tension each graft. On the basis of biomechanical evidence, both the anterolateral and posteromedial bundles of the PCL graft are fixed at 90 degrees of knee flexion with a metal interference screw placed from outside in.[3] A gentle anterior drawer force is applied during screw insertion to re-create the natural tibial step-off.

The knee is then placed through a range of motion, with any limitation of full extension or flexion noted. Anterior and posterior laxity is carefully examined. If any problems exist, the femoral fixation is released, the problem is rectified, and the grafts are retensioned. Any remaining bone plug protruding from the femoral tunnels is removed with a rongeur before skin closure. The sutures are tied together over the tunnel bone bridge or over a plastic button for additional fixation. Dorsalis pedis and posterior tibial artery pulses are checked. Anteroposterior and lateral radiographs are obtained before leaving the operating room (Fig. 67-12).

Transtibial Tunnel

Technical Steps

A bump is placed between the post and the leg to help stabilize the knee in a flexed position while the foot rests on the pre-positioned sandbag. The previously mentioned medial and lateral parapatellar tendon portals are used for the diagnostic arthroscopy. The 70-degree arthroscope is placed through the notch to facilitate placement of an accessory posteromedial portal. The PCL insertion is identified, and the majority of the remaining PCL is débrided. However, the PCL footprint is preserved to properly identify the placement of the transtibial tunnel.

Tibial Tunneling

An arthroscopic tibial PCL guide is placed in the center of the PCL footprint approximately 1.5 cm distal to the articular edge of the posterior plateau (Fig. 67-13). This corresponds to the junction of the middle and distal thirds of the posterior tibial slope. The PCL guide is set at 60 degrees (a more vertical position) to decrease the acuity of the turn as the graft enters the joint. The centering bullet device is then used to mark the anteromedial tibial skin for incision placement. The guide pin is drilled under direct visualization. Again, we use intraoperative

67

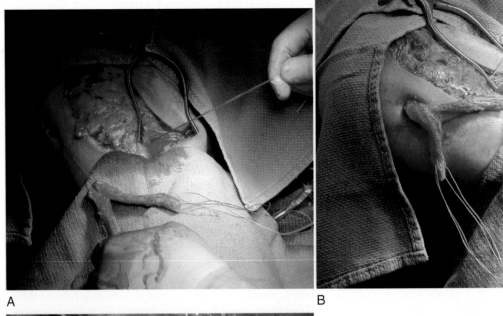

A

B

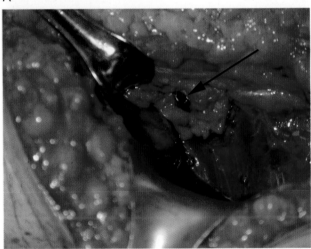

C

Figure 67-10 A, The graft is more easily passed in an anterior to posterior direction. **B,** The anteromedial parapatellar portal is slightly extended to accommodate the graft and to facilitate passage from inside the joint into the trough. **C,** A 4.5-mm, fully threaded cortical screw *(arrow)* corresponding to the measured length plus 10 mm is used to lag the bone block into the trough. Note that a concomitant medial collateral ligament reconstruction is being performed. Thus, the pictured incision is much larger than required for a routine double-bundle tibial inlay procedure to accommodate exposure of both the femoral and tibial insertion sites of the medial collateral ligament.

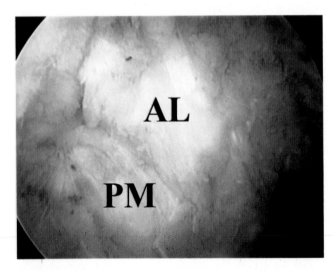

Figure 67-11 An arthroscopic view of the anterolateral (AL) and posteromedial (PM) bundles of the PCL after graft passage.

fluoroscopy to verify the position of the guide wire on a lateral projection to ensure that the pin just penetrates the posterior cortex and is not driven into any neurovascular structures posteriorly. The guide wire is then overdrilled with a 12-mm reamer under fluoroscopic guidance to ensure that the integrity of the posterior tibial cortex remains intact (Fig. 67-14). The tunnel is dilated with a 12-mm dilator, and the anterior edge of the tunnel is chamfered to decrease possible graft abrasion.

Transtibial Graft Passage and Fixation

The medial parapatellar portal is extended to accommodate the graft. A No. 2 braided suture is placed into the posterior knee through the transtibial tunnel with an arthroscopic grasper. It is visualized and grasped out the medial parapatellar arthrotomy and used as a suture shuttle to pull the tibial bone plug anterograde down the tunnel. The knee may need to be cycled to facilitate seating

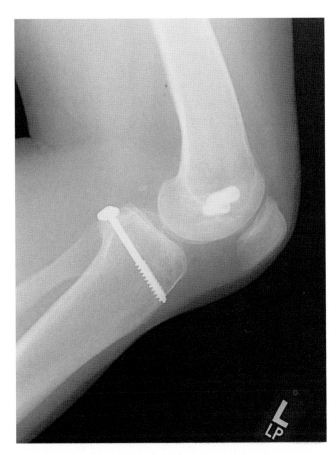

Figure 67-12 A postoperative lateral radiograph demonstrating graft location and reduction. The 4.5-mm cortical screw securing the tibial bone plug and the two metal interference screws corresponding to the anterolateral and posteromedial femoral tunnels are demonstrated.

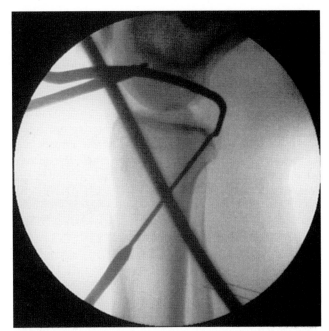

A

B

Figure 67-14 A, Intraoperative fluoroscopy is used to verify the position of the guide wire on a lateral projection to ensure that the pin just penetrates the posterior cortex and is not driven into any neurovascular structures posteriorly. **B,** The guide wire is then overdrilled with a 12-mm reamer under fluoroscopic guidance to ensure that the integrity of the posterior tibial cortex remains intact.

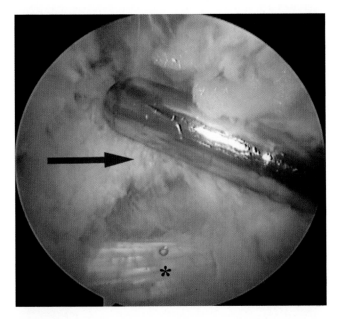

Figure 67-13 The PCL footprint is approximately 1.0 cm distal to the articular edge of the posterior plateau. The arrow points to the PCL stump, which is being débrided by an arthroscopic shaver. The asterisk marks the location of the transverse fibers of the posterior horn of the medial meniscus. This is an excellent landmark for PCL reconstruction.

of the graft within the transtibial tunnel. The posteromedial and anterolateral limbs of the graft are then placed into their respective femoral tunnels. The tibial bone plug is pulled distally in the tunnel so that the posteromedial bundle is set approximately 10 mm from the outer femoral cortex. This will ensure that no graft protrudes from the outer femoral cortex. The tibial bone plug is tensioned and then fixed with a 10-×30-mm metal interference screw. The tibial fixation is augmented by tying the sutures over a button at the entrance of the tibial tunnel. The anterolateral and posteromedial bundles are then tensioned and secured as previously described.

Arthroscopic Tibial Inlay

Technical Steps

Brick Campbell and the senior author (J. K. S.) have developed an arthroscopic PCL inlay technique that has undergone successful in vitro preliminary testing.[20] Similar anterolateral, anteromedial, and posteromedial portals are made as previously described. The PCL footprint is prepared. Custom arthroscopic instrumentation is used to make two overlapping circular defects 12 mm in diameter and totaling 18 mm in length (Smith & Nephew, Inc, Andover, Mass). By use of a modified PCL tibial pin guide, two parallel pins are drilled from the anterior tibial cortex into the PCL footprint (Fig. 67-15). Again, we use intraoperative fluoroscopy to observe advancement of the pins posteriorly. The Beath pins are observed exiting at the appropriate location, with overpenetration prevented by the guide. A centering sleeve from the guide is removed, and each pin is overreamed with an EndoButton reamer (Smith & Nephew, Inc.). An end-threaded rod is passed

into each drill site, emerging from the footprint. The 12-mm retrograde reamer blade is then placed onto the threads through the posteromedial portal and tightened as the rod rotates clockwise (Fig. 67-16). The tibial PCL footprint is then engaged by the reamer and cut retrograde to a depth of approximately 10 mm. The rod is then advanced and the reamer blade removed. The rod is then moved to the second hole and the reaming process repeated, making a figure-of-eight defect 12 mm wide by 18 mm long. A correspondingly shaped tibial bone block is fashioned with two 2.0-mm drill holes. A jig has been fabricated to check the bone block fit in the tibial defect. Once good bone block–defect match is obtained, one No. 2 FiberWire suture is looped through each of the two bone block drill holes. The FiberWire suture is passed down the tibial drill holes with a suture passer and tied over the anteromedial tibial cortex (Fig. 67-17). The graft is passed anterograde through the extended anteromedial portal arthrotomy and secured as previously described.

Postoperative Considerations

Rehabilitation

A hinged knee brace locked in full extension is applied to the operative extremity. Cryotherapy is used to assist with management of postoperative pain and swelling. Extension bracing is continued for 4 weeks, providing support to the tibia to prevent posterior translation and excessive stress on the graft. Partial weight bearing (30%) and quadriceps exercises are started on the first postoperative day. Sym-

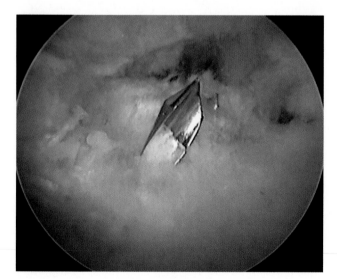

Figure 67-15 Arthroscopic view of the PCL footprint demonstrating two parallel pins that are drilled by use of a modified PCL tibial pin guide.

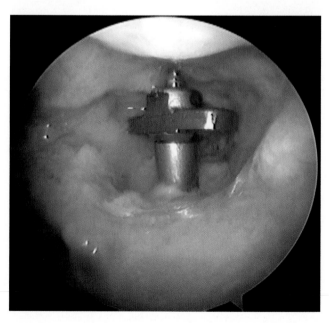

Figure 67-16 A customized arthroscopic 12-mm retrograde reamer blade is used to cut a 10-mm-deep trough in the tibial PCL footprint.

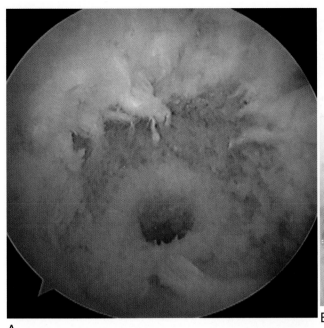

A

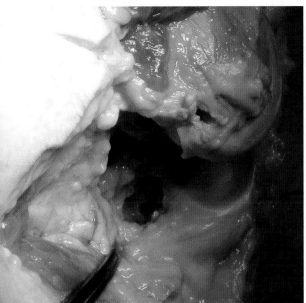

B

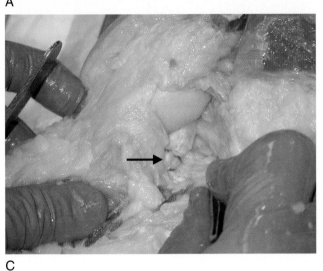

C

Figure 67-17 A, Arthroscopic view of the tibial inlay trough made by the retrograde reamer blade. **B,** Open dissection of the same cadaver knee demonstrating the tibial inlay trough. **C,** Once the trough is prepared, the graft is passed and secured into place with one No. 2 FiberWire suture looped through two bone block drill holes *(arrow)*. The FiberWire suture is passed down the tibial drill holes with a suture passer and tied over the anteromedial tibial cortex.

metric full hyperextension is achieved, and passive prone knee flexion, quadriceps sets, and patellar mobilization exercises are performed with the assistance of a physical therapist for the first month. A continuous passive motion machine is used with a maximum flexion of 90 degrees. In the second month, a stationary bicycle is begun, and full flexion is achieved by 3 months. At 4 months, focused rehabilitation with closed-chain exercises and many repetitions are begun—leg presses, step-ups, mini-squats, hamstring curls, elliptical trainer. At 6 months, slow running without cutting is initiated. At 9 to 12 months, sport-specific functional training exercises are begun with gradual return to previous sport. The criteria for return to sport are as follows: quadriceps and hamstring strength at least 90% of opposite leg; one-leg hop test and vertical jump at least 90% of opposite leg; full-speed run, shuttle run, and figure-of-eight running without a limp; squat and rise from a full

squat; and no effusion or quadriceps atrophy in conjunction with a satisfactory clinical examination.

Complications

Complications are rare but can happen. Failure to carefully position the extremity with adequate padding can lead to neurapraxia. Loss of motion (usually decreased flexion) can result from errors in graft positioning and excessive tensioning during graft fixation or from inadequate range-of-motion exercises during postoperative rehabilitation. Residual laxity can also occur.

Injury to the popliteal vessels is an infrequent but serious complication. With the transtibial technique, great care must be taken to ensure that overpenetration of the posterior tibial cortex does not occur. With the inlay technique, the vessels need to be retracted laterally, and the surgeon should always be aware of their location while drilling. In addition, the thigh and calf should be routinely palpated to ensure that no compartment syndrome develops from fluid extravasation into the soft tissues.

Avascular necrosis of the medial femoral condyle can be avoided by placing the femoral tunnel entry and exit points proximal enough to allow preservation of the subchondral bone.

PEARLS AND PITFALLS

- The required minimum dimensions of the patellar tendon allograft are 45 mm of tendon length and 22 mm of tendon width.

- It is important to bullet-tip the ends of each plug to facilitate later passage within the femoral tunnels.

- Regardless of the technique used for reconstruction, always be cognizant of the location of the neurovascular bundle. Advance the guide pin and reamer under direct fluoroscopic guidance (arthroscopic technique).

- Know the anatomic landmarks for proper placement of the tibial and femoral tunnels.

- On the basis of biomechanical evidence, both the anterolateral and posteromedial bundles of the PCL graft are fixed at 90 degrees of knee

flexion with a metal interference screw placed from outside in with a gentle anterior drawer force applied to re-create the natural tibial step-off.

- Loss of motion can result from errors in graft positioning and excessive tensioning during graft fixation or from inadequate range-of-motion exercises during postoperative rehabilitation.

- Avascular necrosis of the medial femoral condyle can be avoided by placing the femoral tunnel entry-exit points proximal enough to allow preservation of the subchondral bone.

- Routinely palpate the thigh and calf to ensure that no compartment syndrome develops from fluid extravasation into the soft tissues.

- After fixation of all reconstructive grafts, check for full hyperextension and flexion to make sure that the knee is not being overconstrained.

Results

Biomechanical in vitro cadaver studies have documented the advantage of a double-bundle PCL construct.[5,8,12,22] Race and Amis[12] demonstrated that anatomic double-bundle PCL reconstruction with a bone–patellar tendon–bone graft more closely approximates normal knee kinematics in a cadaver model compared with single-bundle reconstruction. Harner et al[5] published a paper supporting double-bundle PCL reconstruction with a

transtibial Achilles allograft. However, a biomechanical cadaver study noted no difference between a transtibial and a tibial inlay technique for PCL reconstruction.[9] In addition, Sekiya et al[22] demonstrated that an open double-bundle PCL reconstruction with a bifid bone–patellar tendon–bone tibial inlay allograft was significantly more stable than a single-bundle construct as compared with intact knees by stress radiography measurements. Furthermore, Sekiya et al,[20] in a separate study, noted that arthroscopic tibial inlay double-bundle PCL

Table 67-1 Clinical Results of Double-Bundle PCL Reconstruction

Author	Patients	Follow-up	Graft	Postoperative Anterior-Posterior Translation	Functional Outcome
Yoon et al[21] (2005)	27	25 months	Transtibial; Achilles allograft	2.4-mm side-side (average)	Lysholm score: 91.8 (average)
Noyes and Barber-Westin[11] (2005)	19	35 months	Tibial inlay; quadriceps tendon autograft	2.3-mm side-side (average)	IKDC score: 14 A, B; 5 C, D
Stannard et al[18] (2003)	30	25 months	Tibial inlay; Achilles allograft	0.2-mm side-side (average)	Lysholm score: 89.4 (average)
Houe and Jorgensen[7] (2004)	10 double-bundle	35 months	Transtibial; hamstring autograft	3-mm side-side (average)	Lysholm score: 95 (average)
	6 single-bundle	35 months	Transtibial; bone-tendon-bone autograft	2-mm side-side (average)	Lysholm score: 100
Wang et al[19] (2004)	16 double-bundle	41 months	Transtibial; hamstring autograft	3.1-mm side-side (average)	Lysholm score: 89 (average)
	19 single-bundle	28.2 months	Transtibial; hamstring autograft	2.3-mm side-side (average)	Lysholm score: 88 (average)

IKDC, International Knee Documentation Committee.

reconstruction with a bifid bone–patellar tendon–bone construct was comparable to an open technique by stress radiography measurements and physical examination.

Clinical double-bundle PCL reconstruction studies are in evolution (Table 67-1).[7,11,18,19,21] The report of Wang et al[19] is the only published randomized prospective study. Thirty-five patients underwent either single- or double-bundle transtibial PCL reconstruction with autogenous hamstring autograft. No statistically significant clinical or radiographic differences were demonstrated. However, the two hamstring tendons were separated during the double-bundle technique, with the smaller gracilis tendon being used as the posteromedial bundle. Thus, the laxity testing may have been different if a larger, more anatomic graft had been used instead.

67

References

1. Bach BR. Graft selection for posterior cruciate ligament surgery. Oper Tech Sports Med 1993;1:104-109.
2. Fanelli GC, Edson CJ. Posterior cruciate ligament injuries in trauma patients. Part II. Arthroscopy 1995;11:526-529.
3. Fox RJ, Harner CD, Sakane M, et al. Determination of the in situ forces in the human posterior cruciate ligament using robotic technology: a cadaveric study. Am J Sports Med 1998;26:395-401.
4. Handy MH, Blessey PB, Miller MD. Measurement of the tibial tunnel/graft angle and the graft/femoral tunnel angle in posterior cruciate ligament reconstruction: a cadaveric study comparing two techniques for femoral tunnel placement. Arthroscopy 2003;19(suppl):36.
5. Harner CD, Janaushek MA, Kanamori A, et al. Biomechanical analysis of a double-bundle posterior cruciate ligament reconstruction. Am J Sports Med 2000;28:144-151.
6. Harner CD, Xerogeanes JW, Livesay GA, et al. The human posterior cruciate ligament complex: an interdisciplinary study: ligament morphology and biomechanical evaluation. Am J Sports Med 1995;23:736-745.
7. Houe T, Jorgensen U. Arthroscopic posterior cruciate ligament reconstruction: one- vs. two-tunnel technique. Scand J Med Sci Sports 2004;14:107-111.
8. Mannor DA, Shearn JT, Grood ES, et al. Two-bundle posterior cruciate ligament reconstruction: an in vitro analysis of graft placement and tension. Am J Sports Med 2000;28:833-845.
9. Margheritini F, Mauro CS, Rihn JA, et al. Biomechanical comparison of tibial inlay versus transtibial techniques for posterior cruciate ligament reconstruction: analysis of knee kinematics and graft in situ forces. Am J Sports Med 2004;32:587-593.
10. Mejia EA, Noyes FR, Grood ES. Posterior cruciate ligament femoral insertion site characteristics: importance for reconstructive procedures. Am J Sports Med 2002;30:643-651.
11. Noyes FR, Barber-Westin S. Posterior cruciate ligament replacement with a two-strand quadriceps tendon–patellar bone autograft and a tibial inlay technique. J Bone Joint Surg Am 2005;87:1241-1252.
12. Race A, Amis AA. PCL reconstruction: in vitro biomechanical comparison of "isometric" versus single and double-bundle "anatomic" grafts. J Bone Joint Surg Br 1998;80:173-179.
13. Sekiya JK, Haemmerle MJ, Stabile KJ, et al. Biomechanical analysis of a combined double bundle posterior cruciate ligament and posterolateral corner knee reconstruction. Am J Sports Med 2005;33:360-369.
14. Sekiya JK, Kurtz CA, Carr DR. Transtibial and tibial inlay double-bundle posterior cruciate ligament reconstruction: surgical technique using a bifid bone–patellar tendon–bone allograft. Arthroscopy 2004;20:1095-1100.
15. Sekiya JK, West RV, Ong BC, et al. Clinical outcomes after isolated arthroscopic single-bundle posterior cruciate ligament reconstruction. Arthroscopy 2005;21:1042-1050.
16. Shelbourne KD, Rubinstein RA. Methodist Sports Medicine Center's experience with acute and chronic isolated posterior cruciate ligament injuries. Clin Sports Med 1994;13:531-543.
17. Sheps DM, Otto D, Fernhout M. The anatomic characteristics of the tibial insertion of the posterior cruciate ligament. Arthroscopy 2005;21:820-825.
18. Stannard JP, Riley RS, Sheils TM, et al. Anatomic reconstruction of the posterior cruciate ligament after multiligament knee injuries: a combination of the tibial-inlay and two-femoral-tunnel techniques. Am J Sports Med 2003;31:196-202.
19. Wang CJ, Weng LH, Hsu CC, Chan YS. Arthroscopic single- versus double-bundle posterior cruciate ligament reconstructions using hamstring autograft. Injury 2004;35:1293-1299.
20. Whiddon DR, Miller MD, Sekiya JK, et al. Double-bundle PCL reconstruction: an open versus a new arthroscopic inlay technique. The American Orthopaedic Society for Sports Medicine, Hershey, Pa, 2006. Unpublished data.
21. Yoon KH, Bae DK, Song SJ, Lim CT. Arthroscopic double-bundle augmentation of posterior cruciate ligament using split Achilles allograft. Arthroscopy 2005;21:1436-1442.
22. Zehm CT, Miller MD, Sekiya JK, et al. Single bundle versus open double bundle inlay. The American Orthopaedic Society for Sports Medicine, Hershey, Pa, 2006. Unpublished data.

CHAPTER 68

Posterior Cruciate Ligament Tibial Inlay

L. Joseph Rubino, MD

Mark D. Miller, MD

Injuries to the posterior cruciate ligament (PCL) are much rarer than those to the anterior cruciate ligament (ACL). Knowledge of and experience in evaluation and management of the PCL still lag behind those of the ACL. Recently, more emphasis has been placed on accurate evaluation and treatment of PCL injuries, either in isolation or in combined ligament injury patterns. The PCL serves as the primary restraint to posterior tibial translation at 90 degrees. Classically, the posterior drawer examination has been the standard for evaluation of PCL stability (Fig. 68-1). More recently, emphasis has been placed on objective measurement of posterior tibial subluxation (Fig. 68-2).[10,11] Other components of the physical examination include the reverse pivot shift, quadriceps sag, quadriceps active test, and dial test. As always, comparison with the contralateral extremity should be performed. Radiologic evaluation should include anteroposterior and lateral radiographs and magnetic resonance imaging of the knee.

Preoperative Considerations

Anatomy

The PCL is attached to the posterolateral portion of the medial femoral condyle and passes posteriorly and laterally to attach into a depression on the posterior aspect of the tibia, bordered by a medial and lateral prominence. The attachment on the posterior tibia is approximately 1 cm distal to the joint line. The average length is 38 mm, and the average width is 13 mm; the midpoint of the ligament is the narrowest point—an average of 11 mm.[8,9] The two

bundles of the PCL are the anterolateral and posteromedial. Traditionally, attention has been focused on the reconstruction of the anterolateral bundle. More recent research has verified the importance of the posteromedial bundle as well as of the meniscofemoral ligaments of Humphrey and Wrisberg. The anterolateral and posteromedial bundles appear to function in a reciprocal pattern, with the anterolateral bundle tight in flexion and the posteromedial bundle tight in extension.

History

PCL injuries occur with a posteriorly directed blow to the proximal tibia, often from a dashboard or hyperextension injury to the knee. When the mechanism of injury involves a direct blow to the anterior tibia, the foot position at the time of contact plays a role in the injury pattern; ankle plantar flexion is associated with PCL injury, and ankle dorsiflexion is associated with patellofemoral injury (Fig. 68-3). Patients often suspect an injury to the knee, although the presentation is much less dramatic than with ACL injuries. Most isolated PCL injuries are grade I or grade II and may be treated nonoperatively with emphasis on regaining of full range of motion and quadriceps rehabilitation to counteract the tendency toward posterior tibial subluxation. In many circumstances, the PCL may actually "heal" as seen on magnetic resonance imaging (Fig. 68-4). Debate continues about persistent objective laxity in these "healed" PCL tears; however, lower grade, isolated PCL injuries are still treated nonoperatively.[17,18] Grade III PCL injuries are rare in isolation and are most frequently seen with loss of secondary restraints and concomitant

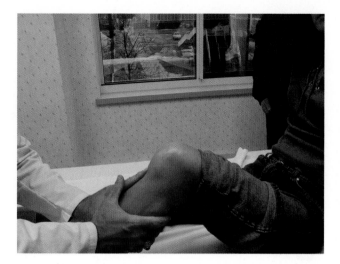

Figure 68-1 Posterior drawer examination indicating grade III PCL laxity.

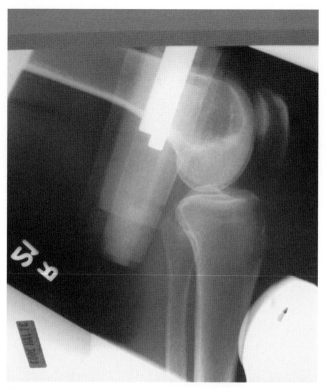

A

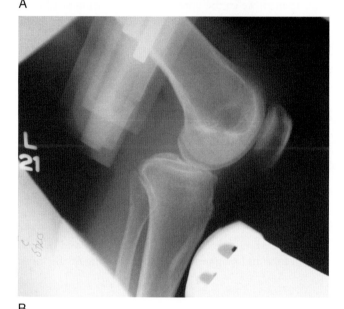

B

Figure 68-2 A, Normal knee examination finding with Telos testing. **B,** Abnormal Telos test result.

posterolateral knee injury. It is extremely important that PCL injuries associated with lateral side injuries are identified because this will affect both the treatment and results of PCL injury and reconstruction (Fig. 68-5). The grade III and the symptomatic isolated grade II PCL injury should be surgically reconstructed.

Surgical Technique

There are multiple techniques for PCL reconstruction. This chapter deals with operative treatment of the PCL by a single-bundle tibial inlay technique with bone–patellar tendon–bone autograft. This technique is called the inlay because the bone from the graft is placed into a trough made in the posterior aspect of the tibia (inlaid), at the footprint of the PCL. This posterior approach for fixation of the tibia avoids the "killer turn" associated with transtibial PCL reconstructions, reducing the stress placed across the graft.[2] This single-bundle technique reliably reconstructs the anterolateral bundle of the PCL.

It is our preference to use bone–patellar tendon–bone autograft because of the bone to bone fixation possible with this graft and because of problems with allograft, including delayed incorporation, infection risk, late laxity, and cost. If autograft is not available, an allograft with a bone block is another option (i.e., Achilles tendon, bone–patellar tendon–bone, or quadriceps tendon).

Examination Under Anesthesia, Positioning, and Diagnostic Arthroscopy

The surgical procedure starts with a thorough examination under anesthesia to confirm the preoperative examination findings. It is imperative at this time to ensure that the posterolateral structures are intact. A tourniquet is placed high on the thigh, and it is deflated before closure of the posterior wound to ensure that there is no injury to the posterior vascular structures.

The patient can be positioned either supine or in the lateral decubitus position. Arthroscopy can be performed in the lateral decubitus position, alleviating the need for intraoperative repositioning, or the patient can be repositioned after arthroscopy to facilitate the approach to the

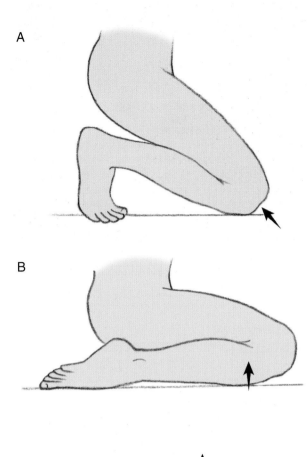

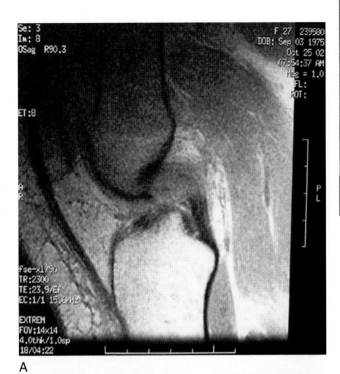

A

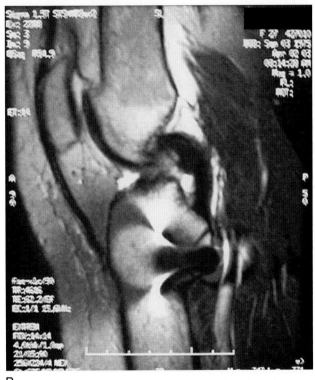

B

Figure 68-4 Magnetic resonance images of a PCL tear off of the femur (**A**) and 6 months later (**B**) showing healing of the PCL fibers.

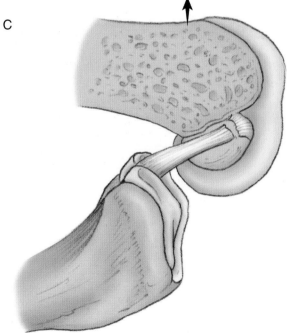

Figure 68-3 The sagittal plane of the foot at the time of a direct blow to the anterior tibia determines the injury pattern. **A,** Dorsiflexion at impact imparts force to the patella. **B,** Plantar flexion causes a posteriorly directed force to the tibia and places the PCL at risk for injury. **C,** Hyperflexion injuries are also associated with PCL tears.

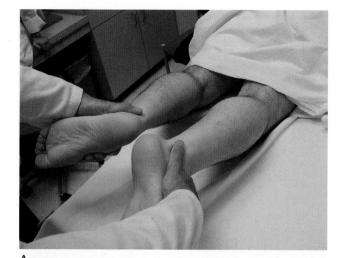

A

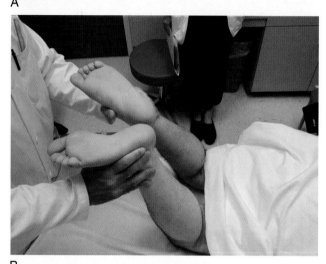

B

Figure 68-5 Dial test showing asymmetric external rotation at 30 degrees (**A**) and symmetric rotation at 90 degrees (**B**).

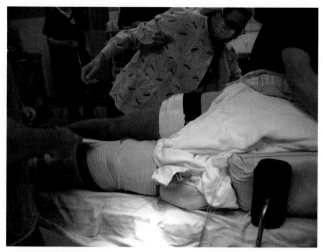

Figure 68-6 The sloppy lateral position is used for both arthroscopy and PCL reconstruction. Note the well-padded contralateral knee and the use of a beanbag and post for support.

Box 68-1 Surgical Steps

1. Graft harvest

2. Femoral tunnel placement

3. Posterior approach

4. Graft passage and fixation

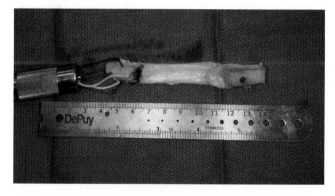

Figure 68-7 The autograft before passage. Note the bullet-shaped bone plug for the femoral side to facilitate passage.

posterior tibia. The authors' preference is to use the lateral decubitus position for both arthroscopy and PCL reconstruction (Fig. 68-6). Care must be taken to adequately pad the contralateral leg to avoid pressure necrosis. The operative extremity can be abducted and externally rotated to facilitate the arthroscopy as well as the exposure of the medial side of the knee.

All intra-articular pathology is addressed at this time. The torn PCL may be difficult to recognize until it is viewed completely. An indication of a PCL tear is a "sloppy ACL sign" or ACL pseudolaxity.[6] Once the torn PCL is identified, the PCL stump is débrided, with preservation of any fibers in continuity.

Specific Steps (Box 68-1)

1. Graft Harvest

While the extremity is abducted and externally rotated, the bone–patellar tendon–bone autograft is harvested from the ipsilateral knee in standard fashion. The graft is harvested and prepared to be rectangular on the tibial inlay side and bullet shaped on the femoral side to allow smooth passage into the femoral tunnel (Fig. 68-7).

2. Femoral Tunnel Placement

An incision is made in Langer's lines at the medial knee slightly anterior and superior to the medial femoral epicondyle (Fig. 68-8). Dissection is carried down in line with the vastus medialis muscle to the level of the condyle. It is important to visualize the bone at this stage for protection

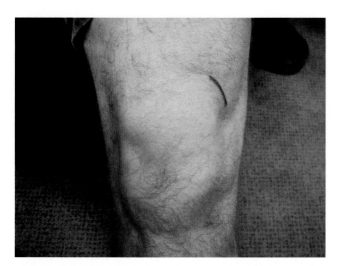

Figure 68-8 The skin incision on the medial side of the knee used for exposure of the medial condyle for drilling of the femoral tunnel. The incision is oblique and over the distal portion of the vastus medialis.

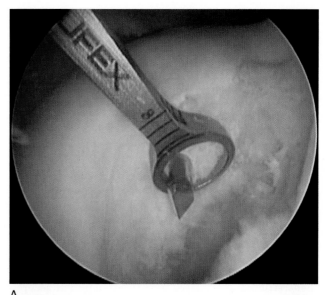

A

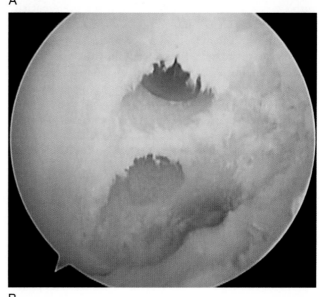

B

Figure 68-9 A, Arthroscopic view of the PCL guide in place for single-bundle PCL reconstruction with the guide pin drilled from outside in. B, Femoral tunnels for a two-bundle PCL reconstruction. The blue plug is positioned in the tunnel for the anterolateral bundle.

of the soft tissues and for accurate placement of the PCL guide. In addition, good visualization allows easy identification of the tunnel when you are ready to perform femoral tunnel fixation. The guide is placed with arthroscopic assistance at the 1-o'clock position (on the right knee) or the 11-o'clock position (on the left knee) and 8 mm deep (away from the articular surface) (Fig. 68-9). The guide pin is drilled from outside in by use of the PCL guide, with the ideal placement in the medial femoral notch confirmed arthroscopically. The starting point of the guide pin must be proximal (farther from subchondral bone) enough to avoid subchondral collapse, insufficiency fractures, or avascular necrosis of the condyle from drilling of the femoral tunnel.[1] The tunnel is then drilled over the guide wire, and the edges are débrided to facilitate graft passage at a later stage. A looped smooth 18-gauge wire is placed retrograde through the tunnel into the joint and used to pass the autograft from the back of the knee into the joint and femoral tunnel at a later stage.

3. Posterior Approach

The extremity is then placed back in the lateral decubitus position. A posterior approach is made in line with the flexion crease of the knee, providing for excellent exposure and cosmesis (Fig. 68-10). The fascial incision is made in a hockey stick fashion, perpendicular to the skin incision at the most lateral part of the skin incision and curving distally between the medial gastrocnemius and the semimembranosus muscle belly. The most important landmark to identify at this time is the medial head of the gastrocnemius muscle. Once the plane between the medial gastrocnemius and the semimembranosus is identified, blunt dissection is used and the gastrocnemius muscle is mobilized and retracted laterally. It is useful at this point to place a series of smooth Steinmann pins from posterior to

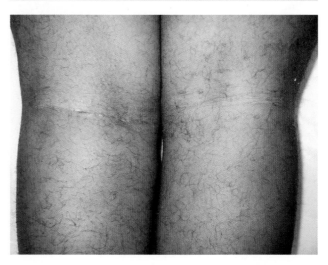

Figure 68-10 The posterior skin incision heals with few cosmetic problems. The operative side is on the left.

anterior and to bend them to serve as a self-retainer.[13] Staying in this interval protects the neurovascular bundle, and it is not necessary to visualize the posterior neurovascular structures with this technique. Once the gastrocnemius and neurovascular bundle are retracted and protected, the posterior tibia and capsule are identified. The medial and lateral prominences of the posterior tibia mark the PCL footprint. The lateral prominence is smaller and often more difficult to palpate; however, the medial prominence should be readily apparent at this point. Therefore, the trough is prepared lateral to the medial prominence. Preparation of the bone trough for the inlay is fashioned by hand, with either osteotomes or a high-speed bur. The trough should be closely size matched to the bone plug from the graft, as this is an inlay graft. A generous, vertical, posterior arthrotomy is made to form the trough proximally. Once the trough is completed, the prepared graft is then retrieved and inlayed into the trough and secured with two pins from a cannulated screw set, preferentially for a screw size of 4.5 mm (Fig. 68-11). The graft is then passed into the joint with the previously placed looped smooth 18-gauge wire. Screw fixation is then performed with two bicortical screws securing the bone plug into the posterior trough. Alternatively, the bone plug can be fixed with one 6.5-mm cancellous screw or with a staple. It is our preference to fix this graft with two bicortical 4.5-mm screws.

4. Graft Passage and Fixation

The graft is passed from posterior into the joint. The bullet-shaped bone plug is passed into the previously drilled and prepared femoral tunnel. Once the graft is positioned in the femoral tunnel, a guide pin is placed on the anterior side of the graft from outside in. While maximum manual tension is applied to the graft, the knee is cycled to remove any kinks in the graft. While tension is continued on the graft, an anterior drawer force is applied with the knee at 90 degrees. An interference screw is then placed over the guide pin, and it should be removed when the interference screw is about halfway seated to avoid having the guide pin bound up in the fixation. The interference screw is then seated the remainder of the way, and the graft is visualized arthroscopically to ensure that the interference screw is not proud at the joint level. Tension on the graft is constant until the interference screw is fully seated. Depending on the choice of grafts and the stability of the reconstruction, double fixation can be obtained with a post and washer, with staples, or over a button on the medial femoral cortex (Figs. 68-12 and 68-13). A Hemovac drain may be placed in the posterior wound if there is a concern of postoperative hematoma. Routine dressings are applied, and ice to the knee is recommended.

PEARLS AND PITFALLS

Pearls

- Fully mobilize the medial head of the gastrocnemius with aggressive blunt dissection.
- Use a long retractor that is "toed in" to hold the gastrocnemius while you are drilling the Steinmann pins that will be used for retraction.
- Palpate the posterior prominences. Stay lateral to the more prominent medial prominence.
- Make a generous arthrotomy by extending the initial incision for the trough proximally.
- Make sure that the graft does not spin or get wrapped up during fixation.
- If the graft does not go right up into the femoral tunnel, pass it anteriorly and then up the tunnel. This is performed in two separate steps.
- Cycle the knee and palpate the graft to ensure that there is good tension before final fixation.
- Look down the femoral tunnel during and after interference screw placement with the arthroscope.

Pitfalls

- Do not forget to fix the posterolateral corner if there is a combined injury (most common).
- Do not use a tourniquet or leg holder for more than 120 minutes. This requires a well-planned operation, particularly if a multiple ligament reconstruction is performed.
- Pad the extremities and opposite leg well to prevent pressure injuries.
- Failure to make a generous posterior arthrotomy can make graft passage difficult.
- Do not hesitate to back up graft fixation.
- Do not leave the operating room unhappy.

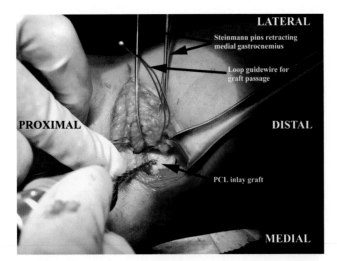

Figure 68-11 Photograph of the posterior knee incision with Steinmann pins for retraction of the gastrocnemius muscle in a lateral direction, a looped guide wire for graft passage, and the inlay graft ready for fixation.

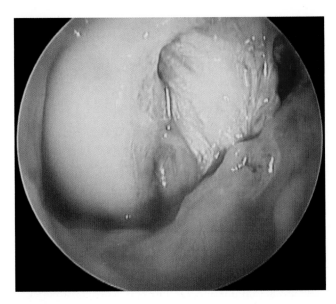

Figure 68-12 Arthroscopic view of the PCL graft in a two-bundle reconstruction. Note the position of the larger, anterolateral bundle.

Postoperative Considerations

Follow-up and Rehabilitation

Postoperative extension bracing may help prevent tibial subluxation for the first 1 to 2 weeks. Postoperative care of the PCL reconstruction focuses on regaining full range of motion. We prefer to stress prone extension modalities to allow gravity both to help obtain extension and to protect against posterior sag. Active quadriceps activity is allowed, with no active hamstring motion or strengthening. Hamstring exercises can be started actively at 3 to 4 months. It is important to be aware and to counsel the patient that PCL rehabilitation is more difficult than ACL rehabilitation, and full recovery including full range of motion can often take up to a year.

Complications

PCL reconstructions are not common in the routine practice setting. The operation can be lengthier than other more common surgical procedures, and thus certain precautions need to be taken. Careful positioning and padding of the contralateral extremity need to be performed preoperatively to prevent neurapraxia or pressure sores. Loss of motion is not uncommon and is often related to excessive graft tension, tensioning in extension, and inadequate postoperative rehabilitation. Neurovascular injuries are rare; however, the posterior approach to the tibia places the surgeon close to the popliteal artery and tibial nerve. Finally, patients may continue to have postoperative laxity in the knee by instrumented and objective testing measures. Fortunately, this laxity is rarely associated with func-

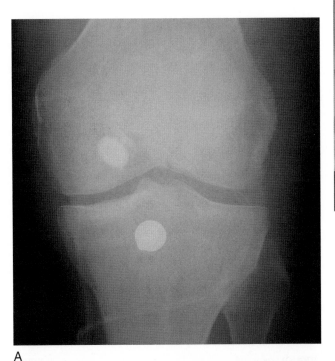

A

B

Figure 68-13 A and **B,** Anteroposterior and lateral radiographs of the PCL graft fixation.

tional instability, and patients are routinely unaware of this subtle asymmetry. Accurate tunnel placement and proper graft tensioning may reduce the incidence of laxity after surgical reconstruction of the PCL.

Results

Patients with chronic PCL insufficiency tend to have increased knee pain, effusions, and late chondrosis of the

68

Table 68-1 Summary of Results for Single-Bundle Inlay PCL Reconstruction

Author	Follow-up	Results
Cooper and Stewart[5] (2004)	Minimum 2 years	34 of 41 grade I or better on posterior drawer examination; average Telos side-to-side difference of 4.11 mm
Seon and Song[16] (2006)	Minimum 2 years	20 of 22 grade I or better on posterior drawer examination
Berg[2] (1995)	Minimum 2 years	KT-1000 quadriceps active drawer at 70 degrees improved in all patients (4/4)
Jung et al[19] (2004)	Minimum 2 years	Telos improved from 10.8 to 3.4 mm; KT-1000 improved from 9.0 to 1.8 mm

medial and patellofemoral compartment.[3,7] The PCL-deficient knee also increases stress across both the medial and lateral meniscus,[15] possibly accounting for the recurrent effusions and late chondrosis. Although these patients often report good subjective results, they have functional deficits and late changes as described.[17] The long-term outcome of the PCL-injured knee remains highly variable.

The results of PCL reconstruction are generally good (Table 68-1).[4,12,14] The patient can expect return to grade I laxity or better. Many studies have confirmed varying degrees of residual laxity after reconstruction by objective and clinical examination. Despite this laxity, most patients have minimal or no symptoms. The functional results of PCL reconstruction are not necessarily correlated with the objective laxity observed.

References

1. Athanasian EA, Wickiewicz TL, Warren RF. Osteonecrosis of the femoral condyle after arthroscopic reconstruction of a cruciate ligament. Report of two cases. J Bone Joint Surg Am 1995;77:1418-1422.
2. Berg EE. Posterior cruciate ligament tibial inlay reconstruction. Arthroscopy 1995;11:69-76.
3. Boynton MD, Tietjens MB. Long-term followup of the untreated isolated posterior cruciate ligament–deficient knee. Am J Sports Med 1996;24:306-310.
4. Clancy WG, Shelbourne KD, Zoellner GB. Treatment of knee joint instability secondary to rupture of the posterior cruciate ligament. J Bone Joint Surg Am 1983;65:310-332.
5. Cooper DE, Stewart D. Posterior cruciate ligament reconstruction using single-bundle patella tendon graft with tibial inlay fixation: 2- to 10-year follow-up. Am J Sports Med 2004;32:346-360.
6. Fanelli GC, Giannotti BF, Edson CJ. The posterior cruciate ligament: arthroscopic evaluation and treatment. Arthroscopy 1994;10:673-688.
7. Gill TJ, DeFrate LE, Wang C, et al. The effect of posterior cruciate ligament reconstruction on patellofemoral contact pressures in the knee joint under simulated muscle loads. Am J Sports Med 2004;32:109-115.
8. Girgis FG, Marshall JL, Monajem A. The cruciate ligaments of the knee joint. Anatomical, functional and experimental analysis. Clin Orthop 1975;106:216-231.
9. Harner CD, Livesay GA, Kashiwaguchi S. Comparative study of the size and shape of human anterior and posterior cruciate ligaments. J Orthop Res 1995;13:429-434.
10. Hewett TE, Noyes FR, Lee MD. Diagnosis of complete and partial posterior cruciate ligament ruptures: stress radiography compared with KT-1000 arthrometer and posterior drawer testing. Am J Sports Med 1997;25:648-655.
11. Margheritini F, Mancini L, Mauro CS, Mariani PP. Stress radiography for quantifying posterior cruciate ligament deficiency. Arthroscopy 2003;19:706-711.
12. Miller MD, Bergfeld JA, Fowler PJ, et al. The posterior cruciate ligament injured knee: principles of evaluation and treatment. Instr Course Lect 1999;48:199-207.
13. Miller MD, Olszewski AD. Posterior cruciate ligament injuries. New treatment options. Am J Knee Surg 1995;8:145-154.
14. Noyes FR, Barber-Westin SD. Treatment of complex injuries involving the posterior cruciate and posterolateral ligaments of the knee. Am J Knee Surg 1996;9:200-214.
15. Pearsall AW, Hollis JM. The effect of posterior cruciate ligament injury and reconstruction on meniscal strain. Am J Sports Med 2004;32:1675-8160.
16. Seon JK, Song EK. Reconstruction of isolated posterior cruciate ligament injuries: a clinical comparison of the transtibial and tibial inlay techniques. Arthroscopy 2006;22:27-32.
17. Shelbourne KD, Davis TJ, Patel DV. The natural history of acute, isolated, nonoperatively treated posterior cruciate ligament injuries. Am J Sports Med 1999;27:276-283.
18. Shelbourne KD, Muthukaruppan Y. Subjective results of nonoperatively treated, acute, isolated posterior cruciate ligament injuries. Arthroscopy 2005;21:457-461.
19. Young-Bok Jung, Suk-Kee Tae, Ho-Joong Jung, Kee-Hyun Lee. Replacement of the torn posterior cruciate ligament with a mid-third patellar tendon graft with use of a modified tibial inlay method. J Bone Joint Surg Am 2004;86:1878-1883.

CHAPTER 69

Posterolateral Corner Reconstruction

Warren Ross Kadrmas, MD
Russell F. Warren, MD

Injury to the posterolateral corner of the knee is a rare but often debilitating entity. Posterolateral corner injury is usually associated with additional ligament injury and can be missed on initial physical examination.[2,3,6,7] If it is identified early (within 3 weeks), many authors recommend acute repair of the posterolateral corner. However, recent data suggest that the results of reconstruction may be equivalent to those of acute repair.[11] Reconstruction of the posterolateral corner is indicated for those who present after 3 weeks of injury or who have inadequate soft tissue for successful repair. Biomechanical data have shown that reconstruction of the posterolateral corner must restore function of the lateral collateral ligament and popliteofibular ligament to resist posterior translation, varus opening, and external rotation of the tibia on the femur.[4,5,12]

Preoperative Considerations

History

It is essential to obtain a complete history of the injury at the time of the initial evaluation. Injuries to the posterolateral corner of the knee are rarely isolated and are usually associated with significant trauma to the knee. A detailed account of previous treatments, as well as operative reports, if they are available, should be obtained before consideration of additional surgical intervention.

Typical History

- Acute, traumatic knee injury
- Activity-related instability
- Previous ligament reconstruction (anterior or posterior cruciate ligament) may have failed

Physical Examination

Examination of the cruciate and collateral ligaments as well as of the neurovascular status of the patient should be well documented. A significant percentage of posterolateral corner injuries occur in the setting of knee dislocation. Examination of the acute injury may be limited by pain.

Acute

- Tenderness over posterolateral aspect of the knee with ecchymosis (Fig. 69-1)
- Positive varus instability at 30 degrees (and 0 degrees with combined injury)
- Associated ligamentous instability may be present (anterior cruciate ligament, posterior cruciate ligament)
- Positive result of posterolateral drawer test
- Positive result of external rotation (dial) test: increased only at 30 degrees, isolated posterolateral corner injury; increased at 30 degrees and 90 degrees, posterior cruciate ligament and posterolateral corner injuries
- Positive result of external rotation recurvatum test (with combined injury) (Fig. 69-2)
- Positive result of reverse pivot shift test
- Examination findings may be consistent with peroneal nerve injury

Chronic

- Similar to acute, although a varus thrust during gait may develop
- Lateral joint line pain

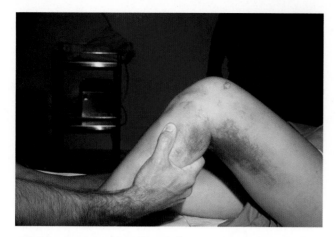

Figure 69-1 Clinical appearance of the knee after posterolateral corner injury.

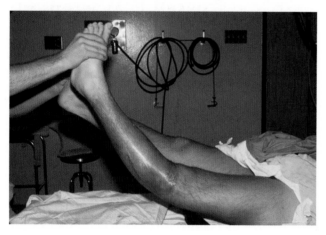

Figure 69-2 Positive result of external rotation recurvatum test.

Imaging

Radiography

- Weight-bearing anteroposterior radiograph in full extension
- Weight-bearing posteroanterior 45-degree flexion radiograph
- Non–weight-bearing 45-degree flexion lateral radiograph
- Patella Merchant radiograph
- Long-cassette mechanical axis radiograph if varus deformity suspected (chronic cases)

Other Modalities

Magnetic resonance imaging is performed to assess meniscus and ligamentous structures. Magnetic resonance arteriography may be considered, in conjunction with magnetic resonance imaging, for evaluation of acute or subacute posterolateral corner injuries in the setting of suspected knee dislocation.

Electromyelography is performed at 3 weeks if peroneal nerve injury is present.

Indications and Contraindications

Reconstruction of the posterolateral corner of the knee is generally indicated for complete disruptions (grade III) or grade II injuries with symptomatic instability. Associated ligamentous injuries may need to be addressed at the time of posterolateral corner reconstruction. A relative contraindication for posterolateral corner reconstruction is varus knee alignment. High tibial osteotomy, before or in conjunction with the posterolateral corner reconstruction, should be considered in chronic cases.

Surgical Planning

Concomitant Procedures

Significant limb malalignment, chondral injury, or associated ligament injuries may need to be addressed before or in conjunction with the posterolateral corner reconstruction in chronic cases.

Graft Selection

Graft selection should be discussed with the patient at the preoperative visit. Graft options include hamstring autograft, Achilles tendon allograft, and anterior tibial tendon allograft tissue.

Surgical Technique

Anesthesia and Positioning

Reconstruction of the posterolateral corner of the knee can be performed under general, combined spinal and epidural, or regional anesthesia on the basis of the patient's, anesthesiologist's, and surgeon's preferences. The patient is placed supine on a standard operating room table, and a tourniquet is applied to the upper thigh. The knee is flexed 20 to 30 degrees over a bump.

Surgical Landmarks

- Fibular head
- Gerdy tubercle
- Lateral epicondyle of the femur

Examination Under Anesthesia and Diagnostic Arthroscopy

Examination under anesthesia is performed to test the ligamentous structures of the knee. Diagnostic arthroscopy may be performed to further evaluate the lateral compartment and intra-articular structures. If combined ligamentous reconstruction, cartilage restoration procedures, and tibial osteotomy are to be considered, they may be done under arthroscopic assistance before the posterolateral corner is addressed.

Specific Steps (Box 69-1)

1. Exposure

An incision is made in the skin from a point just proximal and posterior to the lateral epicondyle and extended in line with the iliotibial band to a point just distal to Gerdy tubercle, midway between Gerdy tubercle and the fibular head. The incision is carried sharply down to the level of the iliotibial band with a scalpel or electrocautery. Anterior and posterior soft tissue flaps are raised to expose the lateral epicondyle, the Gerdy tubercle, and the fibular head.

2. Fibular Tunnel Preparation

The posterior border of the long head of the biceps femoris is identified and incised sharply. The peroneal nerve is identified at the posterior border of the muscle belly and dissected from proximal to distal as it passes across the fibular head. The fascia overlying the peroneal muscles should be released to allow adequate decompression of the nerve. A vessel loop is placed around the nerve for identification and protection throughout the remainder of the case. After identification and protection of the peroneal nerve, anterior and posterior subperiosteal dissection of the fibular head is performed. A guide wire is placed from anterior to posterior, inclined distally, approximately 2 cm from the tip of the fibula, and overreamed with a 7- to 8-

mm acorn reamer (Fig. 69-3). A No. 5 Ethibond (Ethicon, Inc., Somerville, NJ) suture is placed through the fibular hole and tagged for later graft passage (Fig. 69-4).

3. Femoral Tunnel Preparation

Attention is turned to the lateral epicondyle of the femur, which is easily palpated. A 3- to 4-cm incision is made in the iliotibial band at the level of the lateral epicondyle and extended distally. Blunt dissection is performed deep to the iliotibial band, and the lateral collateral ligament remnant and popliteus insertion are visualized. The isometric point on the femur is generally located midway between the lateral collateral ligament origin and the popliteus insertion. The most isometric point on the femur is determined by placing a suture from the fibular head to a pin on the lateral epicondyle at the center of rotation and cycling the knee from flexion to extension (Fig. 69-5). The isometric point on the femur should not allow more than 2 mm of excursion of the suture when the knee is taken through a full range of motion. Subperiosteal dissection is performed at the isometric point, and a slotted guide pin is drilled across the femur (Fig. 69-6). Placement of the

Box 69-1 Surgical Steps

1. Exposure
2. Fibular tunnel preparation
3. Femoral tunnel preparation
4. Graft preparation
5. Graft passage
6. Graft fixation
7. Compartment release
8. Closure

69

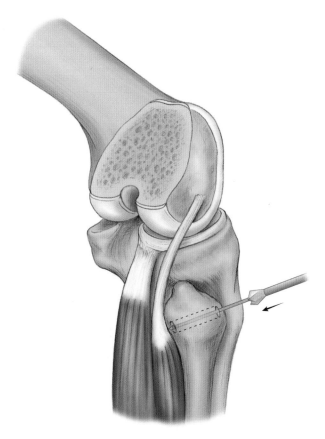

Figure 69-3 A guide wire is placed from anterior to posterior, angled distally, approximately 1 cm from the tip of the fibula, and overreamed with a 7- or 8-mm acorn reamer. (Redrawn with modification from Verma NN, Mithofer K, Battaglia M, MacGillivray J. The docking technique for posterolateral corner reconstruction. Arthroscopy 2005;21:238-242.)

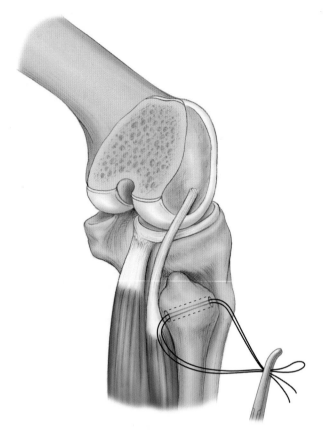

Figure 69-4 A No. 5 Ethibond suture is placed through the fibular tunnel and tagged for later graft passage. (Redrawn with modification from Verma NN, Mithofer K, Battaglia M, MacGillivray J. The docking technique for posterolateral corner reconstruction. Arthroscopy 2005;21:238-242.)

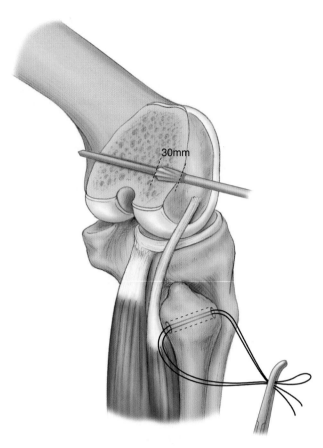

Figure 69-6 A slotted guide pin is placed at the isometric point on the femur and overdrilled with an 8-mm reamer to a depth of 30 mm. (Redrawn with modification from Verma NN, Mithofer K, Battaglia M, MacGillivray J. The docking technique for posterolateral corner reconstruction. Arthroscopy 2005;21:238-242.)

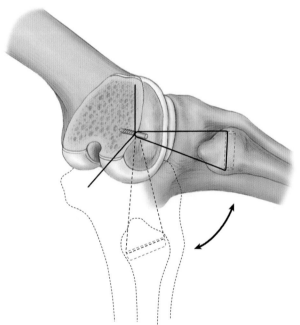

Figure 69-5 The isometric point on the femur is determined by placing a suture from the fibular tunnel to a pin on the lateral epicondyle at the center of rotation and cycling the knee from flexion to extension. The suture should maintain less than 2 mm of excursion throughout a full range of motion. (Redrawn with modification from Verma NN, Mithofer K, Battaglia M, MacGillivray J. The docking technique for posterolateral corner reconstruction. Arthroscopy 2005;21:238-242.)

guide pin is made parallel to the joint line and may be confirmed with fluoroscopy. The guide pin is overdrilled with an 8-mm reamer to a depth of 30 mm. Two No. 2 FiberWire (Arthrex, Naples, Fla) sutures are placed in the slot of the guide pin, and the free ends are brought out the medial side of the knee (Fig. 69-7).

4. Graft Preparation

The selected graft is subsequently prepared. A No. 2 FiberWire suture is placed in one end of the graft in a Krakow-type fashion; the other end is left free for future measurement and division.

5. Graft Passage

The graft is brought through the fibular tunnel by the previously placed No. 5 Ethibond passing suture (Fig. 69-8). Dissection under the iliotibial band is performed with a large clamp, and both ends of the graft are passed beneath it. The end of the graft with the Krakow suture is docked into the femoral tunnel by use of one of the passing sutures and manual traction applied from the medial aspect

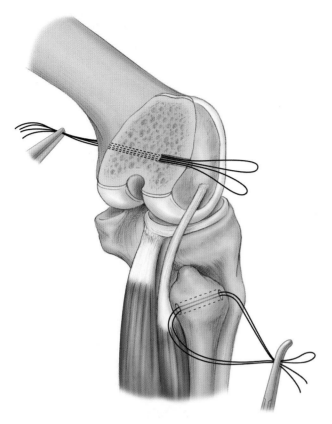

Figure 69-7 Two No. 2 FiberWire sutures are placed in the slot of the guide pin, and the free ends are brought out the medial side of the knee. (Redrawn with modification from Verma NN, Mithofer K, Battaglia M, MacGillivray J. The docking technique for posterolateral corner reconstruction. Arthroscopy 2005;21:238-242.)

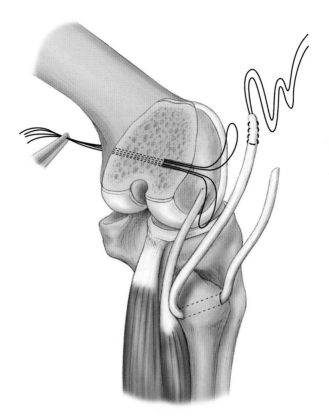

Figure 69-8 Graft passed through fibular tunnel. (Redrawn with modification from Verma NN, Mithofer K, Battaglia M, MacGillivray J. The docking technique for posterolateral corner reconstruction. Arthroscopy 2005;21:238-242.)

of the knee (Fig. 69-9). The knee is subsequently reduced and taken through a full range of motion with the tibia held in internal rotation and a valgus stress applied. The free end of the graft is tensioned and brought to the aperture of the femoral tunnel for measurement. A No. 2 FiberWire suture is placed in a Krakow-type fashion from the point marked at the femoral tunnel and extended 20 mm distally. The free end of the graft is then divided immediately distal to the Krakow-type stitch. The suture ends in the graft are then shuttled into the tunnel and brought out the medial side of the knee with the remaining passing suture.

6. Graft Fixation

A soft tissue interference screw is placed from anterior to posterior in the fibular tunnel to secure the graft distally. The ends of the graft are firmly docked into the femoral tunnel, and the knee is again taken through a gentle range of motion to eliminate creep within the graft and to confirm isometry. The knee is brought to 20 degrees of flexion, and the tibia is maintained in internal rotation with a valgus stress. The graft ends are secured within the femoral tunnel with an interference screw. In the setting of osteoporotic bone or poor primary fixation, supplemental fixation with a soft tissue button may be performed on

the medial cortex of the femur through a separate small incision (Fig. 69-10).

7. Compartment Release

The anterior and lateral compartments of the leg are released distally with a long-handled Metzenbaum scissors before wound closure.

8. Closure

The incisions are closed in layers, and a drain is placed within the wound. Care should be taken to ensure that the peroneal nerve is not under tension during the closure.

Combined Procedures

Tibial Osteotomy and Posterolateral Corner Reconstruction

- High tibial osteotomy should be performed before or in conjunction with the posterolateral corner reconstruction.
- If they are performed in conjunction, the tibial osteotomy should be done before the posterolateral corner reconstruction.

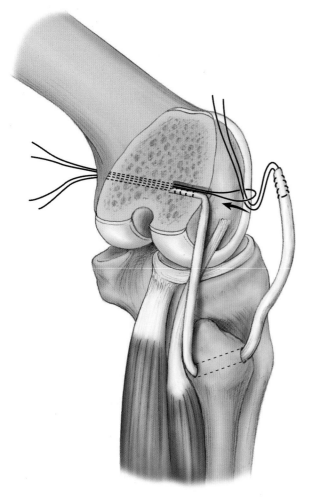

Figure 69-9 Single end of graft docked in femoral tunnel. (Redrawn with modification from Verma NN, Mithofer K, Battaglia M, MacGillivray J. The docking technique for posterolateral corner reconstruction. Arthroscopy 2005;21:238-242.)

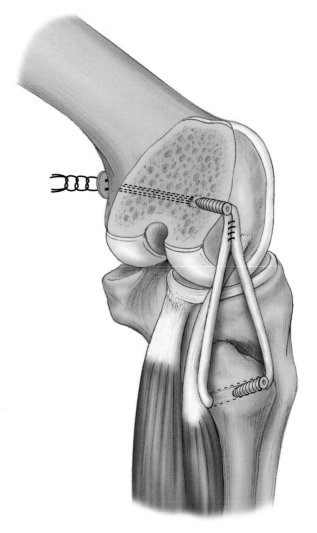

Figure 69-10 Final graft fixation. (Redrawn with modification from Verma NN, Mithofer K, Battaglia M, MacGillivray J. The docking technique for posterolateral corner reconstruction. Arthroscopy 2005;21:238-242.)

- Medial opening wedge osteotomy is indicated for patients with medial laxity and varus deformity.
- Consider medial opening wedge osteotomy for patients with varus deformity and grade I or grade II varus instability.
- Lateral closing wedge osteotomy is performed in patients with varus deformity without medial laxity or with grade III varus instability.

Combined Cruciate Ligament and Posterolateral Corner Reconstruction

Posterior and anterior cruciate ligaments should be secured within the tibial and femoral tunnels, respectively, before completion of posterolateral corner reconstruction. The knee is held in a reduced position during subsequent fixation of the posterolateral corner. The final posterior or anterior cruciate ligament fixation should be performed after completion of the posterolateral corner reconstruction.

Postoperative Considerations

Follow-up

- At 7 to 10 days for suture removal and postoperative radiographs

Rehabilitation

- The patient is initially maintained non–weight bearing in a hinged knee brace; range of motion is limited to 0 to 90 degrees of flexion (continuous passive motion may be used).
- Gentle strengthening exercises are initiated at 4 weeks.
- Progression of weight bearing to full begins 6 to 8 weeks postoperatively.
- In-line running is permitted after 16 weeks.

Table 69-1 Results of Posterolateral Corner Reconstruction

Author	Follow-up	Outcome
Noyes et al[9] (1996)	42 months	16/21 (76%) good–excellent
Albright and Brown[1] (1998)	4 years	26/30 (87%) clinical improvement
Latimer et al[8] (1998)	28 months	10/10 (100%) resolution of subjective instability
Stannard et al[11] (2005)	2 years	20/22 (91%) successful
Yoon et al[13] (2006)	Minimum 1 year	Anatomic reconstruction: 20/21 (95%) good–excellent Posterolateral corner sling: 21/25 (84%) good–excellent

69

- Return to full activities is allowed after 6 months (if strength is within 80% of contralateral side).

Complications

- Peroneal nerve injury
- Infection
- Arthrofibrosis
- Recurrent instability

Results

After posterolateral corner reconstruction, good to excellent results can be expected in 85% to 90% of cases (Table 69-1). Patients will generally have resolution of instability but may continue to have some degree of pain, depending on the cartilage injury at the time of the initial trauma. Recent data suggest that results of anatomic reconstructions may be better than those of procedures that do not attempt to restore the normal anatomy.[13]

PEARLS AND PITFALLS

- Avoid soft tissue reconstruction. If a varus alignment is present with chronic instability, an osteotomy is required.
- Peroneal nerve injury needs exploration. If hematoma is present, epineurolysis may be required. This marks the most dangerous area for future exploration.
- Acute lateral collateral ligament injuries have some potential to heal as they are extra-articular. Popliteal injuries will not heal as well.
- Isometry for the reconstruction is important to avoid stretching of the graft.
- Screw fixation with the graft in the femur is risky if the bone quality is poor. Pull the sutures medially if in doubt.
- Avoid reconstruction in a smoker until smoking is stopped.
- It is easy to break the fibular tunnel if the drill hole is larger than 8 mm.
- Use screw fixation within the fibula to remove excess laxity from the system.
- Prescribe a long leg brace for 6 weeks.
- No weight bearing is permitted for 6 to 7 weeks.

References

1. Albright JP, Brown AW. Management of chronic posterolateral rotatory instability of the knee: surgical technique for the posterolateral corner sling procedure. Instr Course Lect 1998;47:369-378.
2. Baker CL Jr, Norwood LA, Hughston JC. Acute posterolateral rotatory instability of the knee. J Bone Joint Surg Am 1983;65:614-618.
3. DeLee JC, Riley MB, Rockwood CA Jr. Acute posterolateral rotatory instability of the knee. Am J Sports Med 1983;11:199-207.
4. Gollehon DL, Torzilli PA, Warren RF. The role of the posterolateral and cruciate ligaments in the stability of the human knee: a biomechanical study. J Bone Joint Surg Am 1987;69:233-242.
5. Grood ES, Stowers SF, Noyes FR. Limits of movement in the human knee: effect of sectioning the posterior cruciate ligament and posterolateral structures. J Bone Joint Surg Am 1988;70:88-97.
6. Hughston JC, Andrews JR, Cross MJ, Moschi A. Classification of knee ligament instabilities. Part II. The lateral compartment. J Bone Joint Surg Am 1976;58:173-179.
7. Hughston JC, Jacobson KE. Chronic posterolateral rotatory instability of the knee. J Bone Joint Surg Am 1985;67:351-359.
8. Latimer HA, Tibone JE, ElAttrache NS, McMahon PJ. Reconstruction of the lateral collateral ligament of the knee with patellar tendon allograft: report of a new technique in combined ligament injuries. Am J Sports Med 1998;26:656-662.
9. Noyes FR, Barber-Westin SD. Surgical restoration to treat chronic deficiency of the posterolateral complex and cruciate ligaments of the knee joint. Am J Sports Med 1996;24:415-426.
10. Noyes FR, Stowers SF, Grood ES, et al. Posterior subluxations of the medial and lateral tibiofemoral compartments: an in vitro ligament sectioning study in cadaveric knees. Am J Sports Med 1993;21:407-414.
11. Stannard JP, Brown SL, Farris RC, et al. The posterolateral corner of the knee: repair versus reconstruction. Am J Sports Med 2005;33:881-888.
12. Veltri DM, Warren RF. Anatomy, biomechanics, and physical findings in posterolateral knee instability. Clin Sports Med 1994;13:599-614.
13. Yoon KH, Bae DK, Ha JH, Park SW. Anatomic reconstructive surgery for posterolateral instability of the knee. Arthroscopy 2006;22:159-165.

Medial Collateral Ligament Repair and Reconstruction

David R. McAllister, MD
Timothy J. Henderson, MD

Injury to the medial ligamentous structures of the knee is one of the most common ligament injuries involving the knee.[1,9] The treatment of medial-sided knee injuries has evolved from aggressive surgical treatment in the past to nonoperative treatment of most of these injuries currently. Although the majority of isolated medial-sided knee injuries can be treated nonoperatively, with full return to function expected,[3,4,6] many complex medial-sided knee injuries or injuries combined with other ligament disease may require surgical intervention.

Preoperative Considerations

History

The common mechanism of injury to the medial structures of the knee is secondary to the knee's being subjected to a valgus force either from a direct lateral blow or from the foot's being planted and the body's imparting a valgus force to the knee.[6] With increased force, additional injuries to the cruciates may occur.

Physical Examination

The severity of injury to the medial collateral ligament (MCL) may be graded according to its stability in resisting a valgus stress at 30 degrees of knee flexion. A grade I injury, which is described as a partial tear to the MCL, exhibits tenderness over the course of the ligament and pain with valgus stress as well as abnormal laxity limited to 5 mm or less with valgus stress.[5] A grade II injury exhibits tenderness to palpation and to valgus stress, no laxity at 0 degrees, and 5 to 9 mm of opening at 30 degrees of flexion (in comparison with the unaffected side).[5] Grade I and grade II injuries have definite endpoints to valgus stress on physical examination. A grade III injury represents complete rupture of the medial ligaments with tearing of the deep capsular structures. Examination of a grade III injury allows opening at 0 degrees (variable, depending on the presence or degree of injury to the cruciates) and at 30 degrees of flexion. A grade III injury indicates medial opening of 10 mm or more.[5] There is no firm endpoint to valgus stress at 30 degrees of flexion. Opening of more than 5 to 10 mm in full extension should suggest other associated ligament and capsular injuries.

Anatomy

Common to medial-sided knee injuries are injuries to the posteromedial corner. The posterior medial corner consists of the posterior horn of the medial meniscus, the posterior oblique ligament (POL), and the semimembranosus muscle and its expansions.[2,4,11] It is believed by many authors that the posteromedial corner operates in a coordinated fashion throughout normal range of motion as both a static and a dynamic restraint to anteromedial rotary instability.[4]

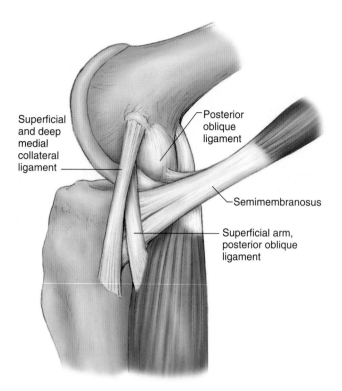

Figure 70-1 Normal anatomy of the medial side of the knee. The superficial and deep portions of the medial collateral ligament as well as the posterior oblique ligament are seen.

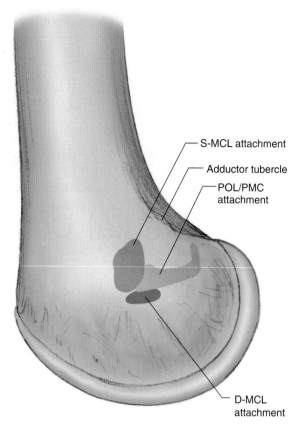

Figure 70-2 Bone anatomy of the medial femoral condyle. The adductor tubercle as well as the attachment sites of the posterior oblique ligament/posterior medial capsule (POL/PMC), superficial medial collateral ligament (S-MCL), and deep medial collateral ligament (D-MCL) can be seen.

The medial complex of the knee has been described as a sleeve of tissue extending from the midline anteriorly to the midline posteriorly. The important static structures (Fig. 70-1) responsible for valgus stability are the superficial MCL, the deep MCL, and the POL.[2,12] Dynamic support is provided by the aforementioned posterior medial corner structures. The superficial MCL runs from the medial femoral epicondyle proximally, anterior to the adductor tubercle (Fig. 70-2), and inserts on the anteromedial tibia 4 to 7 cm distal to the joint line, beneath the insertion of the pes anserinus. It is between 9 and 11 cm long and 1 to 2 cm wide.[2] The anterior parallel fibers of the superficial MCL are in constant tension throughout flexion, whereas the posterior fibers are oblique and lax in flexion.[1,2] The deep MCL is a short structure deep to the superficial MCL; it attaches to the medial meniscus.[11] Whereas the deep MCL can be separated from the superficial MCL distally, the fibers of both structures fuse proximally. The POL (also referred to as the posterior medial capsule) is a triangular capsular ligament originating posterior to the superficial MCL at the adductor tubercle and inserting just below the joint line at the flare of the proximal medial tibia.[2] It is approximately 5 cm long and 0.5 cm wide.[10] Approximately one third of the POL fibers are attached to the posterior horn of the medial meniscus; two thirds pass directly from the femur to the tibia.[4] The POL becomes lax in flexion, and it is theorized that to function, it must be dynamized by the pull of the attached semimembranosus.[2]

Imaging

Radiography

Radiographs to evaluate the injured knee include the standard anteroposterior, lateral, and patellofemoral views. Films should be evaluated for fractures, ligament avulsions, and lateral capsular signs such as the Segond fracture, loose bodies, and Pellegrini-Stieda lesions. Stress radiographs are important in adolescents to rule out potential epiphyseal lesions.

Magnetic Resonance Imaging

Magnetic resonance imaging is a valuable tool to identify not only meniscal and cruciate pathologic changes but also the location of the MCL injury (Fig. 70-3).[9,10] This can aid greatly at the time of surgery by helping to locate the zone of injury and the area in need of repair.[8] If a magnetic resonance imaging evaluation of an MCL tear demonstrates a type I lesion (located at the femoral origin), the likelihood of nonoperative treatment being effective is high. If a type III lesion is encountered (a tear from the femoral origin that extends distally across the joint line),

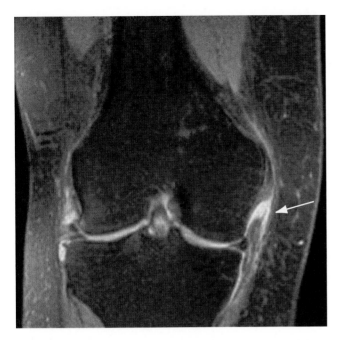

Figure 70-3 Coronal magnetic resonance imaging sequence showing full-thickness injury to the MCL at its femoral attachment site.

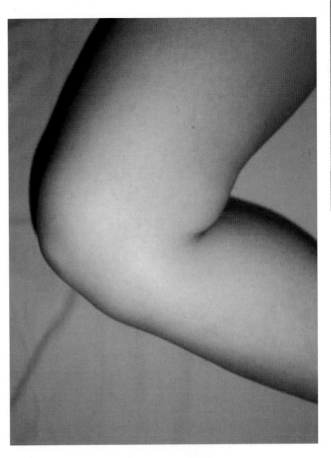

Figure 70-4 Figure-four position of the knee during surgical repair.

the chance of successful nonoperative treatment is low, and the possibility that residual chronic laxity will remain is significant.[9]

Surgical Planning

Although it is commonly accepted that isolated tears of the MCL, regardless of grade, can be treated with early functional rehabilitation and bracing, the treatment of torn medial ligaments associated with other ligamentous injuries is still controversial.[1,2,3,6] Some authors advocate reconstruction of the anterior cruciate ligament with nonoperative treatment of the medial structures; others report satisfying results with combined medial ligament repair and anterior cruciate ligament reconstruction. Nevertheless, combined grade III MCL and cruciate ligament injuries can lead to complex symptomatic instability because the functional deficiency of one ligament may affect the healing of the other.[3,9] Less commonly, isolated grade III injuries, after a trial of nonoperative treatment, may heal with residual symptomatic medial instability.

Surgical repair or reconstruction of the medial ligamentous complex may be recommended if there is a chronic grade III MCL injury with symptoms of instability with excessive medial joint line opening to valgus stress.[3]

Surgical Technique

Examination Under Anesthesia and Positioning

At the time of surgery, a knee examination under anesthesia is performed to help confirm the suspected diagnosis and to rule out other ligament deficiencies. The patient is positioned supine on the operating table, and a tourniquet is placed as high as possible on the operative leg. Suture anchors, interference screws, a tendon harvester, and an allograft (on standby) should be available before the procedure is started. Care should be taken to ensure that the operative leg may be easily placed in a figure-four position to allow medial exposure (Fig. 70-4).

Specific Steps (Box 70-1)

Repair

We agree with Muller[7] and have found that there is often sufficient local tissue for repair and that a graft is not usually necessary. We avoid arthroscopy before repair of MCL injuries. We have found that arthroscopy may cause

Box 70-1 Surgical Steps

Repair

- The superficial and deep MCLs are detached from their proximal attachments on the femur and reflected inferiorly (attached to sutures at bottom).
- The POL is detached from its femoral attachment and reflected posteriorly (attached to sutures on right).
- The posteromedial portion of the medial femoral condyle is exposed.
- The superficial and deep MCLs are advanced and reattached to the medial femoral condyle with suture anchors.
- The POL is advanced proximally and anteriorly (attached to sutures on left).

Reconstruction

- The femoral side is fixed with an interference screw, and the tibial side is secured with suture anchors.

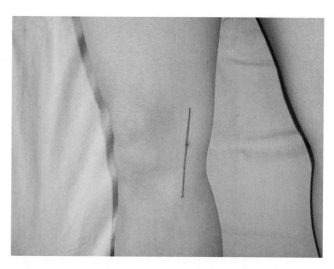

Figure 70-5 Line of medial incision coursing over the medial epicondyle (marked with a dot).

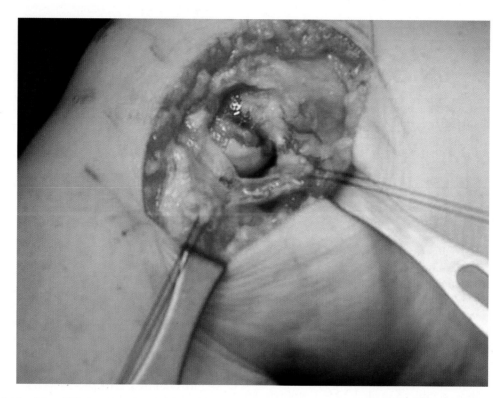

Figure 70-6 The superficial and deep MCLs have been detached from their proximal attachments on the femur and reflected inferiorly (attached to sutures at bottom). The POL has been detached from its femoral attachment and is reflected posteriorly (attached to sutures on right). The posteromedial portion of the medial femoral condyle is exposed.

significant fluid extravasation into the soft tissues, making dissection more difficult. The leg is exsanguinated with the use of an Esmarch bandage, and the tourniquet is inflated to 300 mm Hg. The leg is placed in the figure-four position, which should allow excellent exposure to the medial aspect of the knee. An 8-cm incision is made on the medial aspect of the knee coursing over the medial epicondyle (Fig. 70-5). The saphenous vein and nerve should be identified and protected when possible during the approach.[12] The sartorius fascia is incised and retracted anteriorly and posteriorly. The superficial MCL as well as the POL can normally be easily identified (Fig. 70-6).

The site of injury to the MCL will dictate the operative technique. Ligaments torn from their bone attachments should be reattached to their anatomic origins. If the MCL is torn proximally, it should be advanced to the medial epicondyle and repaired with the knee flexed to 30 degrees, under a varus-directed force, and with moderate tension (Fig. 70-7). Staples, suture anchors, or nonabsorbable sutures placed through drill holes can be used. If the MCL is torn at its distal insertion, it should be advanced to its distal insertion beneath the pes anserinus and fixed in a similar fashion. Similarly, fixation can be performed with ligament screws and washers, suture anchors, or No. 5 nonabsorbable sutures placed through drill holes in the bone. Once the superficial MCL is repaired, the POL is advanced and repaired to the adductor tubercle proximally and to the posterior edge of the repaired MCL (Fig. 70-8). Posterior to and confluent with the POL will be the posterior medial capsule and its connection to the semimembranosus. If these structures are disrupted or lax, they should be advanced to the POL and included in the repair. Acute midsubstance ruptures of the superficial MCL or the POL can be repaired primarily with suture.

Reconstruction

Autograft

If the tissue quality of the superficial MCL is poor or the ligament tear is such that it cannot be repaired anatomically, consideration should be given to use of a tendon graft, although we have rarely found this to be necessary. If additional ligamentous injury and reconstruction are needed on the affected knee, we may recommend an allograft to limit additional operative morbidity. If the medial injury is the only ligamentous reconstruction to be performed, an autograft may be an acceptable choice.

Autogenous reconstruction can be accomplished with the use of a harvested semitendinosus or a gracilis tendon.[3] The hamstring tendons are harvested in the standard fashion[3] and are fashioned into double-bundle tendon grafts. The graft should be positioned proximally at the medial epicondyle and may be fixed with an EndoButton or with an interference screw technique. If interference screw fixation is preferred, the diameter of the graft is measured, and an appropriately sized tunnel is reamed to a depth of 25 to 30 mm. The graft sutures from the looped end are placed in the eyelet of the guide pin and pulled through the lateral cortex. A 25-mm soft tissue interference screw, the same size as the graft tunnel diameter, is placed in the tunnel to fix the graft. The position of the distal end of the graft is approximated with the use of the remaining fibers of the distal insertion of the MCL. The knee is put through range of motion with the graft tentatively held at the presumptive distal fixation site to test for isometry. A change in graft length of 3 to 4 mm is considered an acceptable amount of excursion.[3] The distal end of the graft is then fixed to the distal insertion site

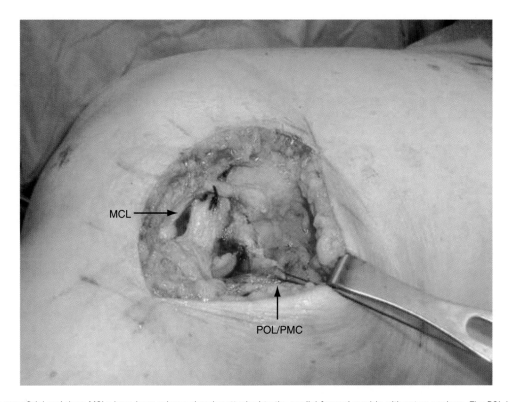

Figure 70-7 The superficial and deep MCLs have been advanced and reattached to the medial femoral condyle with suture anchors. The POL is reflected posteriorly (attached to sutures on right).

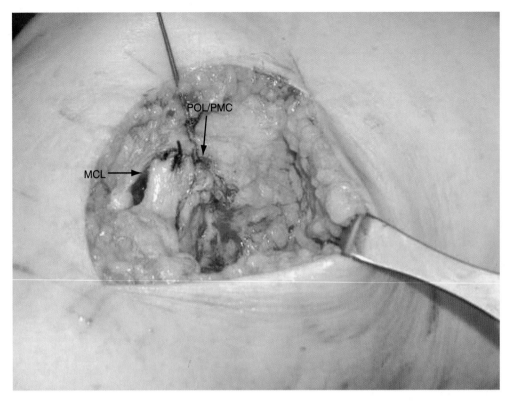

Figure 70-8 The superficial and deep MCLs have been advanced and reattached to the medial femoral condyle with suture anchors. The POL is advanced proximally and anteriorly (attached to sutures on left).

with suture anchors or nonabsorbable sutures placed through drill holes in the bone. Take care to fix the tibial side with the knee held in 30 degrees of flexion[3] as described previously in the repair section (Fig. 70-9). The POL can then be advanced anteriorly and proximally and sutured to the reconstructed MCL. It is rarely necessary to reconstruct the POL because there is almost always suitable POL/posterior medial capsular tissue to be advanced and repaired.

Allograft

The decision to use an allograft for reconstruction can be made to limit morbidity, particularly in the multiple ligament–injured knee. Semitendinosus or tibialis anterior grafts are attractive choices because they are of sufficient size and length to reconstruct the superficial MCL. The allograft reconstruction is performed in a way similar to the autograft reconstruction.

PEARLS AND PITFALLS

Pearls

- It may be difficult to visualize the injury to the MCL intraoperatively in chronic cases. A preoperative magnetic resonance imaging evaluation is useful to clearly identify the zone of injury.

- The medial epicondyle is located in the posterior third of the medial condyle when it is viewed on a lateral radiograph. It is essential to recognize the location of the epicondyle for appropriate proximal repair or fixation.

Pitfalls

- The saphenous nerve and vein are vulnerable during this surgical approach. Care should be taken to identify and to protect these structures.

- In placing the guide wire for the interference screw at the medial epicondyle, care should be taken to ensure that the wire is drilled slightly anterior and proximal. The peroneal nerve is potentially at risk if the guide pin is placed in a posterior and distal direction.

- During rehabilitation, care should be taken to prevent unprotected weight bearing that might allow the knee to drift into valgus, which may result in residual valgus instability.

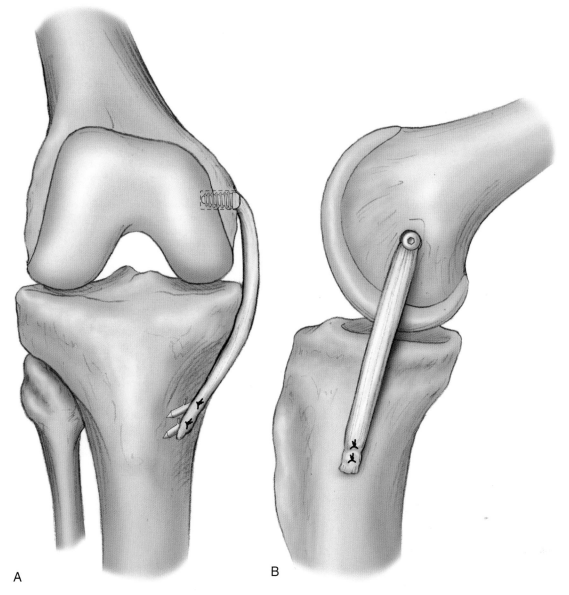

A   B

Figure 70-9 MCL reconstruction with a free soft tissue graft. The femoral side is fixed with an interference screw, and the tibial side is secured with suture anchors.

Postoperative Considerations

Rehabilitation

Postoperatively, the leg is placed in a hinged knee brace locked in 30 degrees of flexion. The patient is initially non–weight bearing with crutches. The patient may be allowed to undergo protected range of motion from 0 to 90 degrees and protected weight bearing in a hinged knee brace locked in extension at 14 days postoperatively. Our goal is for patients to regain full range of motion at 6 weeks after surgery. The patient may return to full weight bearing at 6 to 8 weeks with the hinged knee brace unlocked, and

the physical therapy program may advance to bicycling and closed-chain kinetic exercises. If the medial ligament repair is performed in combination with a cruciate reconstruction, the postoperative protocol should be geared toward the cruciate rehabilitation.

Complications

Knee stiffness and the formation of heterotopic bone are complications of acute medial ligament repair.[1] Arthrofibrosis or a knee flexion contracture is minimal if the patient adheres to a regimented rehabilitation program, however.

References

1. Beltran J. The distal semimembranosus complex: normal MR anatomy, variants, biomechanics and pathology. Skeletal Radiol 2003;32:435-445.

2. Bosworth D. Transplantation of the semitendinosus for repair of laceration of medial collateral ligament of the knee. J Bone Joint Surg Am 1952;34:196-202.

3. Haimes J, Wroble R, Grood E, Noyes F. Role of the medial structures in the intact and anterior cruciate ligament–deficient knee. Am J Sports Med 1994;22:402-409.

4. Hughston J. The importance of the posterior oblique ligament in repair of acute tears of the medial ligaments in knees with and without an associated rupture of the anterior cruciate ligament. J Bone Joint Surg Am 1994;76:1328-1344.

5. Hughston J, Eilers A. The role of the posterior oblique ligament in repairs of acute medial (collateral) ligament tears of the knee. J Bone Joint Surg 1973;55:923-955.

6. Loredo R, Hodler J, Pedowitz R, et al. Posteromedial corner of the knee: MR imaging with gross anatomic correlation. Skeletal Radiol 1999;28:305-311.

7. Muller W, ed. The Knee: Form, Function, and Ligament Reconstruction. New York, Springer-Verlag, 1983:241-246.

8. Nakamura N, Horibe S, Toritsuka, et al. Acute grade III medial collateral ligament injury of the knee associated with anterior cruciate ligament tear. The usefulness of magnetic resonance imaging in determining a treatment regimen. Am J Sports Med 2003;31:261-267.

9. Pressman A, Johnson D. A review of ski injuries resulting in combined injury to the anterior cruciate ligament and medial collateral ligaments. Arthroscopy 2003;19:194-202.

10. Robinson J, Bull A, Amis A. Structural properties of the medial collateral ligament complex of the human knee. J Biomech 2005;38:1067-1074.

11. Robinson J, Sanchez-Ballester J, Bull A, et al. The posteromedial corner revisited. An anatomical description of the passive restraining structures of the medial aspect of the human knee. J Bone Joint Surg Br 2004;86:674-681.

12. Sims W, Jacobson K. The posteromedial corner of the knee: medial-sided injury patterns revisited. Am J Sports Med 2004;32:337-345.

CHAPTER 71

Multiligament Knee Reconstruction

Christopher A. Radkowski, MD
Christopher D. Harner, MD

Knee dislocations are rare but severe injuries. The diagnosis and management of multiligament knee injuries remain challenging and complex. Knee dislocations can occur from trauma of relatively high or low energy and can be overlooked in the setting of polytrauma with a spontaneous reduction of the knee before the time of presentation. These injuries usually result in damage to at least three of the four major ligaments of the knee, commonly involving both the anterior (ACL) and posterior cruciate ligaments (PCL) and either the medial collateral ligament (MCL) or the lateral collateral ligament (LCL) and the posterolateral corner (PLC).[6]

Knee dislocations are also associated with neurologic and vascular insults. The incidence of popliteal artery injury after knee dislocation is estimated to be between 32% and 45%.[7,17] Neurologic damage may occur in 16% to 40% of all knee dislocations.[10,17] Classification of these injuries is based on the direction of tibial translation in relation to the femur: anterior, posterior, medial, lateral, or rotatory.[6]

Historically, multiligament knee injuries have been treated with cast immobilization. Advances in imaging, clinical awareness, and surgical techniques have led to improved diagnosis and management of these injuries. Results of existing studies are difficult to compare, given the different populations of patients (including the severity of injuries), the different techniques used for treatment of cruciate and collateral ligament injuries, and the various outcome measurements and rating scales. Some controversy still exists concerning the timing of surgery, the decision of ligament repair versus reconstruction, and the

surgical technique in the management of multiligament knee injuries.

Preoperative Considerations

History

A complete history can be difficult to obtain from an obtunded or sedated polytrauma patient, but it is important nonetheless. The mechanism of injury can provide insight into the direction of dislocation and focus attention to other potentially injured structures in the knee. High- or low-energy trauma may cause a knee dislocation, and this aspect should be noted. The time of injury and the time at onset of symptoms of neurologic or vascular compromise are vital to obtain and to document. Previous knee injuries and treatments should also be recorded.

Physical Examination

After the evaluation and treatment of the trauma patient, a thorough examination of the uninvolved and involved knees is performed. For an unreduced dislocated knee, a neurovascular examination is conducted and documented. If there is no apparent vascular compromise, anteroposterior and lateral radiographs are obtained to note the direction of dislocation and to exclude periarticular or intra-articular fractures. Conscious sedation is administered, and a gentle closed reduction is performed.

Several components of the physical examination are crucial in determining whether emergent arteriography or surgery is required. All aspects of the examination should be compared with the contralateral knee. A deteriorating neurovascular status may represent ongoing leg ischemia or compartment syndrome; therefore, serial examinations are imperative.

Inspection of Skin

- Note open wounds, abrasions, and soft tissue injuries.
- Dimpling of skin (may be present in irreducible knee dislocations)
- Previous incisions

Vascular Examination

- Assess dorsalis pedis and posterior tibialis pulses with palpation, Doppler study, and ankle-brachial indices.
- Assess capillary refill, color, and temperature of affected extremity.

Neurologic Examination

- Test motor and sensory function in lower extremity.

Ligamentous Examination

- Anterior tibial translation at 30 and 90 degrees
- Posterior tibial translation at 90 degrees
- Varus and valgus stress at 0 and 30 degrees
- Posteromedial and posterolateral rotatory instability

Other Associated Injuries

- Bone injuries: bone contusion, avulsion fractures, peri-articular or intra-articular fractures
- Meniscal injury
- Articular cartilage injury

Imaging

Radiographs

- Acute cases: anteroposterior and lateral radiographs
- Chronic cases: anteroposterior, lateral, and 45-degree flexion, weight-bearing radiographs

Other Modalities

- Magnetic resonance imaging to evaluate ligament and capsular injuries, meniscal tears, and occult fractures
- Arteriography for any concerns with the vascular supply to the extremity

Indications and Contraindications

Absolute indications for surgery include open knee dislocations, open fracture-dislocations, and irreducible knee dislocations. Compartment syndrome may occur after the initial injury or after revascularization and should be treated emergently. Vascular injuries warrant a consultation with a vascular surgeon and require immediate intervention. For nonemergent cases, surgery is generally recommended for most patients with multiligament knee injuries.

Surgery for multiligament knee injuries is contraindicated for patients with an active infection, sedentary lifestyle, advanced osteoarthritis of the knee, severe medical comorbidities, and intra-articular or periarticular fractures of the involved knee.

Other Preoperative Considerations

Ligamentous Repair Versus Reconstruction

The majority of multiligament knee injuries involve disruption of both cruciate ligaments and either medial- or lateral-sided injuries. Tibial avulsions of the cruciate ligaments are treated with repair; however, most cruciate ligament injuries are intrasubstance tears and are best managed with ligament reconstruction. If any bundles of the ACL or PCL remain intact, these are preserved, and a single-bundle cruciate ligament augmentation is performed.

For MCL, LCL, and PLC tears, primary repair may be attempted within 3 weeks of injury. For femoral- or tibial-sided MCL ruptures, repair can be performed with a screw and spiked soft tissue washer or suture anchors. Acute LCL and PLC intrasubstance tears may be repaired primarily with nonabsorbable suture, whereas avulsions from the fibular head may be treated with suture anchors or sutures tied through transosseous tunnels.

More chronic medial or lateral ruptures are less amenable to repair secondary to muscle contracture and scar formation. In these cases, repair with graft augmentation or ligament reconstruction is performed.

Timing of Surgery

The timing of multiligament knee surgery is debated. Factors affecting this decision include the vascular status of the lower extremity, the condition of the skin and soft tissues, the presence of other intra-articular injuries, the associated traumatic or systemic injuries, the capsuloligamentous structures injured, and the extent of these injuries.[5]

In general, multiligament knee surgeries are performed 2 to 3 weeks after injury. This interval is chosen to allow time for soft tissue and capsular injuries to heal and to decrease the likelihood of fluid extravasation with arthroscopy, yet to operate before significant scar formation and soft tissue contractures occur.[9] Some combined cruciate and medial ligamentous injuries can be managed with initial bracing of the MCL and later reconstruction of the ACL and PCL. With so many variables to consider, the timing of surgery must be tailored to the individual patient.

Surgical Technique

Anesthesia and Positioning

Multiligament reconstruction procedures may be performed under general epidural or regular anesthesia with intravenous sedation, depending on the preferences of the surgeon, the anesthesiologist, and the patient. Preoperative femoral and sciatic blocks are routinely performed to assist in postoperative pain relief. The patient is positioned supine on the operating room table. A Foley catheter is passed, and all extremities are well padded. A gel pad is placed under the ipsilateral hip. A padded bump is taped to the foot of the table to hold the knee flexed at 90 degrees without manual assistance. A side post with bump is placed lateral at the proximal thigh to support the leg in flexion. A tourniquet is placed on the proximal thigh but not routinely used.

Surface Anatomy and Skin Incisions

The following are surgical landmarks for multiligament knee reconstruction (Fig. 71-1):

- Patella and patellar tendon
- Medial and lateral femoral epicondyles
- Medial and lateral joint lines
- Fibular head
- Path of common peroneal nerve
- Tibial tubercle and Gerdy tubercle

The knee is flexed to 90 degrees, and the vertical arthroscopy portals are delineated. If patellar height is considered normal, the anterolateral portal is placed just lateral to the lateral border of the patellar tendon at the level of the inferior pole of the patella. The anteromedial portal for outflow is positioned approximately 1 cm medial to the medial border of the superior aspect of the patellar tendon. An outflow portal may be used superolaterally. For PCL reconstruction, an accessory posteromedial portal is established just proximal to the joint line and posterior to the MCL under spinal needle localization. The incision for the cruciate ligament tibial tunnels is positioned approximately 2 cm distal and medial to the superior portion of the tibial tubercle. The femoral tunnel incision for the PCL graft is marked over the proximal anteromedial knee. If an MCL repair or reconstruction is to be performed, a curvilinear incision is planned from the tibial tunnel incision extending proximally above the medial epicondyle. If a posterolateral dissection is required, a curvilinear incision is made from the lateral aspect of the lateral femoral condyle to just anterior to the fibular head. The proposed

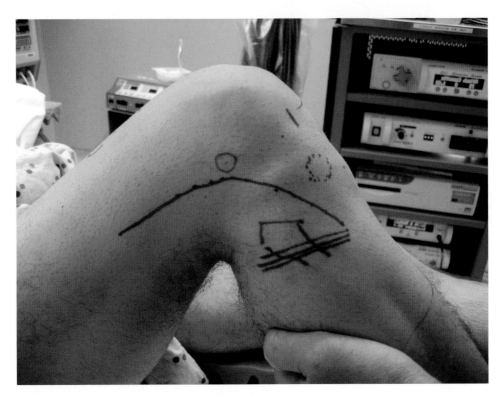

Figure 71-1 A lateral view shows the surgical landmarks drawn on a right knee.

incisions are then cleaned with sterile povidone iodine (Betadine) paint and then injected with a 0.25% bupivacaine with 1:100,000 diluted epinephrine.

Examination Under Anesthesia and Diagnostic Arthroscopy

An examination under anesthesia is then performed. The nonoperative knee is examined, followed by the operative knee. The alignment and range of motion are assessed with specific attention to terminal extension and flexion. A thorough ligamentous examination is conducted to determine the patterns of laxity. Once the leg is prepared and draped, the dorsalis pedis artery is palpated and marked, and a hole is cut in the stockinette for access to the pulse throughout the case (Fig. 71-2).

The arthroscopic equipment is prepared, and the fluoroscopy machine is later draped. A complete diagnostic arthroscopy is performed to assess for intra-articular pathologic changes, including inspection of the menisci and articular surfaces. The intercondylar notch is exam-

ined for any remaining intact bundles of the cruciate ligaments, which are preserved for augmentation.

Specific Steps (Box 71-1)

1. Graft Selection and Preparation

Findings from the history, physical examination, imaging studies, examination under anesthesia, and arthroscopic

Box 71-1 Surgical Steps

1. Graft selection and preparation
2. Cruciate ligament tunnel preparation
3. Cruciate graft passage and proximal fixation
4. Lateral-sided injuries
5. Medial-sided injuries
6. Graft tensioning and distal fixation
7. Closure

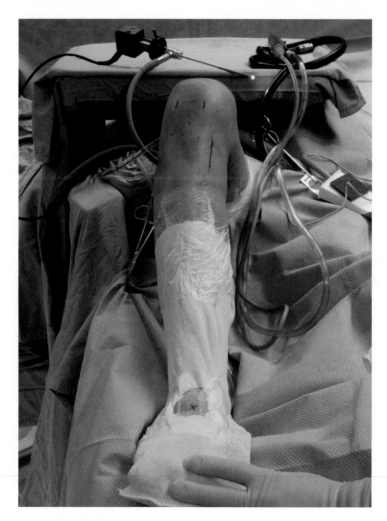

Figure 71-2 A right knee is prepared and draped. The dorsalis pedis pulse is marked and accessible throughout the case.

examination are combined to determine which structures require repair or reconstruction. Options for graft selection include allograft and autograft (Fig. 71-3). Whereas autograft offers potentially more rapid incorporation, decreased infection risk, and decreased cost, use of allograft tissue has no donor site morbidity, offers a variety of graft sizes, and decreases operative time. At our institution, allograft tissue is preferred in multiligament knee reconstruction surgery. In general, hamstring autograft is not harvested in the setting of a medial ligament injury.

For ACL reconstruction, bone–patellar tendon–bone allograft provides sufficient strength with good osseous fixation. The bone plugs are usually fashioned to 11×25 mm; the graft width is 11 mm. Smaller-diameter grafts may be used in augmentation cases. Drill holes are placed in both bone plugs for passage of No. 5 nonabsorbable sutures. Alternatively, soft tissue allograft may also be used. Soft tissue grafts are doubled on themselves over a closed endoloop with the EndoButton (Smith & Nephew, Inc., Andover, Mass) removed. This is done to maximize the amount of graft within the tunnel, which has been shown in a dog model to improve pullout strength.[8] All grafts are placed on the tensiometer and kept moist in a damp sponge.

For PCL reconstruction, Achilles tendon or tibialis anterior allograft is preferred. Achilles tendon grafts offer a bone plug for rigid femoral fixation, which is fashioned to 11×25 mm. A No. 5 nonabsorbable suture is passed through bone plug drill holes, and another suture is used to whipstitch the tendinous portion of the graft. For augmentation of the anterolateral or posteromedial bundles, tibialis anterior allograft or hamstring autograft may also be used.

Reconstruction of the LCL is performed with Achilles tendon allograft or remaining graft from the bone–patellar tendon–bone allograft initially used for the ACL reconstruction. The bone plug is sized to 7 to 8 mm in diameter. The PLC is reconstructed with tibialis anterior allograft or hamstring autograft.

2. Cruciate Ligament Tunnel Preparation

The tibial tunnel of the PCL reconstruction is addressed first. A 70-degree arthroscope is placed through the anterolateral portal and used to visualize the PCL tibial footprint. A spinal needle is used for establishment of the posteromedial portal. A transseptal portal is established as described by Ahn et al.[1,2] The PCL footprint is exposed by débridement of the surrounding synovial tissue with a PCL curet and arthroscopic shaver (Fig. 71-4). Care is taken to avoid injury to the neurovascular bundle posteriorly. The 30- and 70-degree arthroscopes are frequently exchanged in the posteromedial and anterolateral portals, respectively, for adequate visualization. A PCL drill guide is set to 50 to 55 degrees, and its placement posteriorly is confirmed with fluoroscopy and arthroscopy. A vertical incision is made over the anteromedial aspect of the proximal tibia (or the anterolateral aspect if an ACL reconstruction is not required and a lateral incision will be performed).

The guide wire is passed under fluoroscopic guidance to the posterior tibial cortex and then through the cortex under arthroscopic visualization. The wire exits the tibia along the sloped face of the posterior tibial fossa, in the distal and lateral aspects of the PCL footprint. A parallel drill guide may be used to optimize placement of the guide wire.

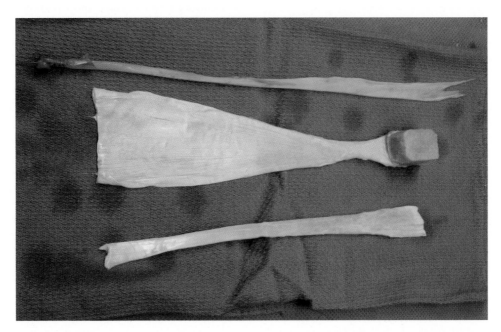

Figure 71-3 Graft choices for multiligament reconstruction include hamstring autograft, Achilles tendon allograft, and soft tissue allograft.

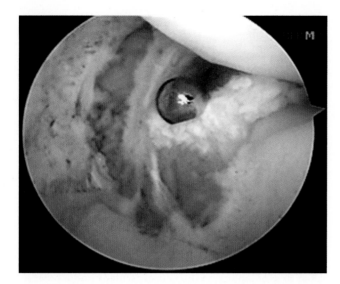

Figure 71-4 An arthroscopic view through the posteromedial portal shows the shaver being used to débride the PCL tibial origin in a left knee. The medial femoral condyle is seen on the top right, and just below it is the posterior horn of the medial meniscus.

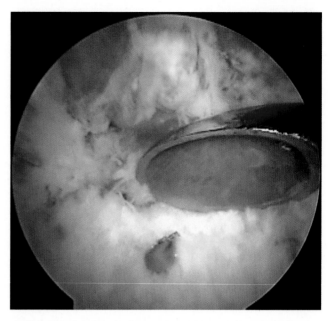

Figure 71-5 An anterolateral portal arthroscopic view of the posterior right knee shows the guide wire of the PCL tibial tunnel protruding from the posterior tibia. The curet is passed from the posteromedial portal to protect the posterior neurovascular structures.

Both ACL and PCL guide wires are placed before drilling of the tibial tunnels. To prepare the ACL tibial tunnel, the ACL stump is débrided and any intact bundles are preserved. An ACL guide is set to 45 degrees, and a guide wire is drilled into the center of the ACL footprint. A lateral fluoroscopic image is obtained to confirm correct placement of both wires.

A cannulated compaction drill is passed over the wire to drill the PCL tibial tunnel; a curet is placed over the guide wire posteriorly for protection from neurovascular injury (Fig. 71-5). Final drilling of the posterior cortex is done by hand. Serial tunnel dilators are passed to match the size of the graft. The tibial tunnel for the ACL is drilled in similar fashion. The tibial tunnels between the ACL and PCL are at least 1 to 2 cm apart.

Femoral tunnel preparation for PCL reconstruction involves identification and débridement of the PCL femoral insertion. For single-bundle PCL reconstruction, a guide wire is inserted through the anterolateral portal in the center of the PCL insertion site. A cannulated compaction drill is inserted by hand to avoid injury to the patellar chondral surface and to confirm tunnel location in relation to the articular cartilage of the medial femoral condyle. The drill is passed to a depth of 25 to 30 mm, and sequential dilators are passed up to the graft diameter. A smaller drill is used to drill through the cortex for graft passage. Separate tunnels are drilled and smaller grafts are used if double-bundle PCL reconstruction is to be performed.

For placement of the ACL femoral tunnel, a notch-plasty is performed, and the over-the-top position is identified with a curet. An anteromedial portal technique with the knee flexed to 120 degrees is preferred for placement of the femoral ACL tunnel (Fig. 71-6). An angled awl is

placed in the 10-o'clock or 2-o'clock position for the right or left knee, respectively, to make a starting hole 5 to 6 mm anterior to the posterior wall. A guide wire is then advanced into the medial wall of the lateral femoral condyle through the starting hole. The compaction drill is again used to make a hole 25 to 30 mm in depth, the cortex is broached with a smaller drill, and serial dilators are passed (Fig. 71-7).

3. Cruciate Graft Passage and Proximal Fixation

The compartments of the leg should be checked regularly during the arthroscopic portion of the procedure. Graft passage may be performed arthroscopically "dry" if there is concern about fluid extravasation. An 18-gauge bent wire loop is passed through the PCL tibial tunnel and retrieved through the anterolateral portal with a pituitary rongeur. The leading No. 5 suture is then pulled antero-grade through the tibial tunnel as the wire loop is removed. A Beath pin is inserted through the anterolateral portal into the PCL femoral tunnel. The leading sutures for the femoral side of the PCL graft are passed through the eye of the Beath pin and pulled proximally with the pin into the tunnel. For the ACL, the graft is passed in retrograde fashion through the tibial tunnel. The leading femoral-sided suture limbs are passed through the tibial tunnel with a pituitary rongeur and grasped through the antero-medial portal with another pituitary rongeur. A Beath pin is passed through the ACL femoral tunnel with the lead sutures, and the graft is pulled into the femoral tunnel.

Femoral fixation for both grafts is performed with a post. A 4.5-mm AO cortical screw and washer are used for

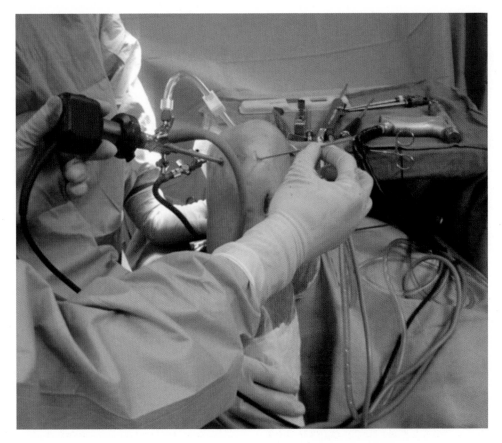

Figure 71-6 The ACL femoral tunnel guide wire is being passed by the medial portal ACL reconstruction technique.

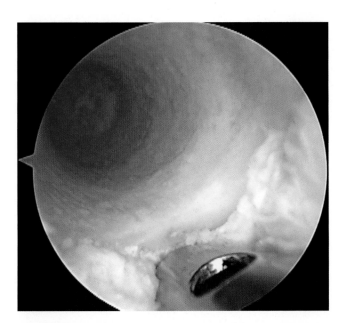

Figure 71-7 An arthroscopic view shows the ACL femoral tunnel after drilling and dilation. The posterior wall is visible between the tunnel and the suction instrument.

the ACL, and a 6.5-mm cancellous screw and washer are used for PCL fixation. The lead sutures may be tied over the post, or the screw may be passed through a closed endoloop attached to the graft. Careful planning should ensure that these screws are placed at different levels within the distal femur. Alternatively, interference screws may be used.

4. Lateral-Sided Injuries

A hockey stick lateral incision is made to address injuries to the PLC. The iliotibial band is retracted anteriorly, and the biceps femoris muscle and tendon are retracted posteriorly. The common peroneal nerve is identified and protected throughout the procedure. Acute bone avulsion injuries of the LCL, popliteus, iliotibial band, or biceps tendon are generally repaired to bone with suture anchors. For irreparable, intrasubstance, or chronic PLC ruptures, reconstruction is recommended.

LCL reconstructions are performed with allograft passed through a bone tunnel in the fibular head (Fig. 71-8) and into a blind femoral tunnel measuring 7 to 8 mm in diameter. No. 2 nonabsorbable suture may be placed in whipstitch fashion in the native popliteus and LCL for advancement with the graft into the femoral tunnel (Fig. 71-9). A small drill is used to penetrate the medial femoral

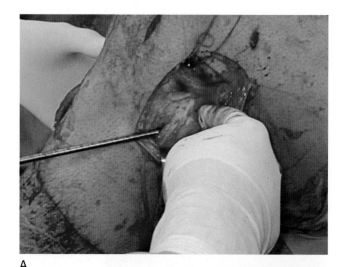

A

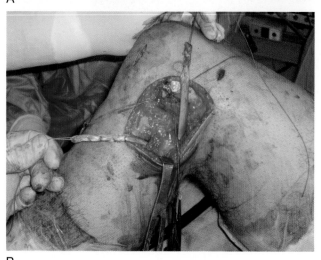

B

Figure 71-8 A, For posterolateral reconstructions, the fibula is drilled from anterior and inferior to posterior and superior. **B,** The graft is passed through the fibular tunnel and may be tied over a post or placed into a blind femoral tunnel.

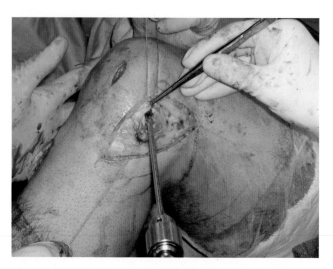

Figure 71-9 An acorn reamer is used to make a blind femoral tunnel laterally for PLC reconstruction. The native LCL and popliteus have been whipstitched and will be advanced into the femoral tunnel.

cortex, and a Beath pin may be used to pass the leading sutures to the medial side. The graft and native tissue are pulled into the femoral tunnel, and the sutures are tied over a post on the medial femur (or the post from the femoral PCL fixation). Native tissue is sutured to graft tissue to augment the reconstruction.

5. Medial-Sided Injuries

If a medial-sided injury is to be addressed, a curvilinear incision is extended from the anteromedial proximal tibial incision. Peripheral medial meniscal tears may be repaired through this incision. The MCL is usually repaired in grade III injuries. For femoral or tibial avulsion injuries, the ligament is repaired to a prepared bone bed with suture anchors or a screw and spiked soft tissue washer or both for deep and superficial layers (Fig. 71-10). Intrasubstance tears may be primarily repaired in acute cases or reconstructed with augmentation of native tissue in chronic cases. The posterior oblique ligament (POL) may be injured in cases of posteromedial rotatory instability. The POL is separated from the posterior MCL and the underlying meniscus. The peripheral meniscus is rasped, and a suture repair is performed through the anteriorly advanced POL. The anterior flap of the POL is advanced and imbricated deep to the posterior MCL with cottony Dacron sutures (Fig. 71-11).

6. Graft Tensioning and Distal Fixation

The order of distal fixation is as follows:

- PCL
- ACL
- Lateral structures
- Medial structures

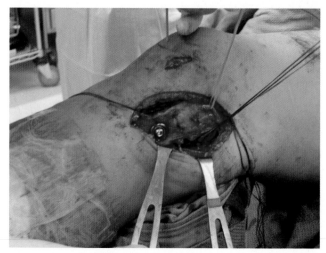

Figure 71-10 A spiked soft tissue washer and screw may be used for MCL repair. The deep layer was repaired with use of suture anchors and tied over the superficial MCL.

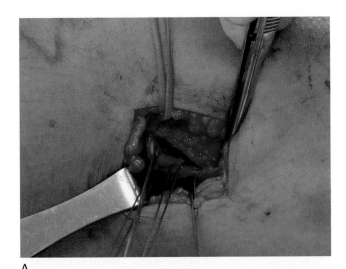

A

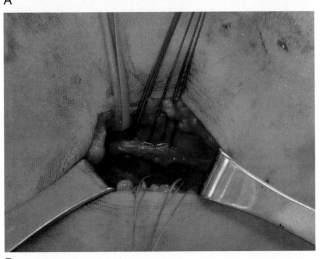

B

Figure 71-11 A, For posteromedial repairs, tagging sutures are placed in the medial meniscus and POL. The posterior border of the MCL is seen just anterior to the POL. **B,** The POL is then advanced underneath the posterior MCL in a pants-over-vest fashion.

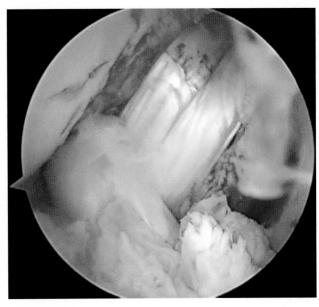

Figure 71-12 An arthroscopic notch view of a right knee shows the reconstructed ACL and PCL grafts.

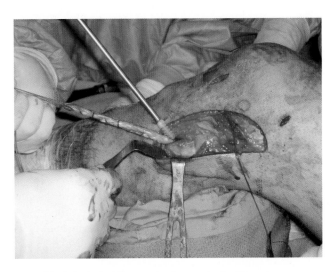

Figure 71-13 Grafts for LCL reconstruction may be fixed through a transosseous fibular tunnel with a bioabsorbable interference screw.

Single-bundle PCL reconstructions are tensioned at 90 degrees of flexion to approximate the anterolateral bundle. An anterior tibial force is applied to reduce the tibia on the femur. The lead sutures of the graft may be tied over a 4.5-mm AO screw and washer, or an interference screw may be used. Tension and tibial fixation of the ACL graft are performed in full extension. Fixation may be achieved with a screw and washer post or an interference screw. The position of the graft and the fixation are checked arthroscopically (Fig. 71-12) and clinically.

The PLC graft is tensioned at 30 degrees of knee flexion with internal rotation of the tibia. Fibular fixation of reconstructed LCL or popliteofibular ligament may be performed with an interference screw (Fig. 71-13). The reconstructed MCL is also tensioned at 15 to 30 degrees and may be fixed with a screw and washer or an interference screw. The POL advancement is tensioned at full extension. After final fixation, the knee's range of motion is assessed, and final fluoroscopic images are obtained.

7. Closure

All incisions are irrigated with antibiotic solution. Deep layers are closed with 0 nonabsorbable suture, subcutaneous tissues are approximated with 2-0 nonabsorbable suture, and skin is closed with staples. The arthroscopic portals are closed with 3-0 nylon suture. The dorsalis pedis pulse is palpated or assessed by sterile Doppler study if necessary, and the leg is palpated to assess the compartments. A standard surgical dressing is placed with a bias stockinette wrap. A hinged knee brace is applied and locked in extension.

Postoperative Considerations

The patient is discharged from the hospital on the following day and returns in 7 to 10 days for staple or suture removal and radiographs (Fig. 71-14). Dressing changes are performed with posterior tibial support to avoid stress to the reconstructed PCL.

Rehabilitation

The rehabilitation program for multiple ligament knee reconstruction is as follows.[3,9]

- Immediate partial weight bearing is allowed with the brace locked in extension.
- Quad sets, straight-leg raises, and calf pumps are done while the patient is in the brace.
- Closed-chain exercises (mini-squats) are performed with the brace unlocked, with a goal of 90 degrees of flexion by 4 weeks. The brace is locked in extension with ambulation.
- Unlock the hinged knee brace at 4 weeks and advance to full weight bearing.
- Avoid active knee flexion with hamstrings for 6 weeks to prevent posterior tibial translation; avoid open-chain hamstring exercises for 12 weeks.
- Quadriceps strengthening, including limited arc open-chain knee extension exercises, begins after 4 weeks.
- Active-assisted range of motion and stretching begin at 6 weeks.
- Discontinue the brace at 6 weeks.
- The goals are full extension and 100 degrees of flexion by 12 weeks. If progress is unsatisfactory, manipulation under anesthesia may be performed.
- Low-impact aerobic activities are permitted at 8 to 12 weeks; running is permitted at 6 months if quadriceps strength is 80% of the contralateral side.
- Return is allowed to heavy labor in 6 to 9 months and to sports in 9 to 12 months.

Complications

- Neurovascular injury, including popliteal vessels, peroneal and saphenous nerves (missed and iatrogenic injuries)
- Compartment syndrome (missed and iatrogenic injuries)
- Tibial plateau fracture (missed and iatrogenic injuries)
- Infection
- Arthrofibrosis
- Residual laxity due to failure to recognize or to treat all injured components, failure of graft incorporation, or recurrent rupture of graft

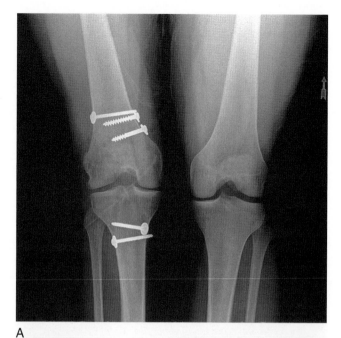

Figure 71-14 Flexion weight-bearing 30-degree posteroanterior (**A**) and lateral (**B**) postoperative radiographs show tunnel position and fixation of ACL and PCL grafts. The additional medial femoral screw was used to tie PCL reconstruction sutures pulled through a femoral tunnel.

PEARLS AND PITFALLS

- Intraoperative compartment syndrome should be avoided and calf pressures should be monitored manually before, during, and after the procedure. Significant fluid extravasation can lead to increased compartment pressures. This risk can be minimized by using gravity inflow instead of a pump, completing a quick but thorough diagnostic arthroscopy, and performing parts (such as graft passage) of the procedure "dry." If there is growing concern for a developing compartment syndrome, the compartment pressures may be checked, and the deep and superficial posterior compartments should be released.

- Neurovascular injuries should be avoided. The pulses should be evaluated before, during, and after surgery. Routine use of the tourniquet can be avoided. Multiligament reconstruction procedures are complicated and should be performed in a facility with immediate vascular surgical support; this is not always readily available at outpatient surgical centers.

- Carefully plan skin incisions with large skin bridges between parallel incisions to avoid skin necrosis, infection, and problems with exposure.

Results

Management of the dislocated knee has changed with the advancement of arthroscopic techniques. Some authors have shown improved clinical results in comparing operative with nonoperative treatment of multiligament injuries.[16,21] However, comparison of studies involving multiligament reconstruction is difficult for a number of reasons. There are variations in the populations of patients in these studies; some include or exclude patients with neurovascular injuries, many include both acute and chronic ligament injuries, and the different ligament injury combinations in each study are widely varied. In addition, different surgical techniques have been used in different studies. These variables include ligament repair or reconstruction, open or arthroscopic techniques, choice of graft tissue, single- or double-bundle cruciate reconstruction,[19] and method of PCL reconstruction. Finally, use of different clinical outcomes also limits comparisons between studies. Postoperative knee stability has been evaluated with physical examination, side-to-side differences with KT-1000 arthrometer measurements, and stress radiography. Functional results are reported in different rating scales. The Meyers scoring system was developed for knee dislocations and is based on subjective ratings.[12,13] However, it does not account for functional or objective scores and is less strict than other knee-scoring systems.[20] A list of studies involving surgical treatment, including bicruciate ligament injuries and their results, is shown in Table 71-1.[4,9,11,14,15,18,20]

71

Table 71-1 Results of Studies

Author	Number of Knees	Mean Follow-up	Clinical Results
Harner et al[9] (2004)	31	44 months	Meyers: 23/31 (74%) good–excellent IKDC: 0 normal, 11 (35%) nearly normal, 12 (39%) abnormal, 8 (26%) severely abnormal
Fanelli and Edson[4] (2002)	35	2-10 years	Significant improvement over Tegner, HSS, and Lysholm preoperative scores
Ohkoshi et al[15] (2002)	9	40 months	IKDC: 0 normal, 7/9 (78%) nearly normal, 2/9 (22%) abnormal
Mariani et al[11] (2001)	14	36 months	IKDC: 3 (20%) normal, 7 (47%) nearly normal, 3 (20%) abnormal, 1 (7%) grossly abnormal HSS: 12/14 (86%) good–excellent
Wascher et al[20] (1999)	13	38 months	Meyers: 11/13 (85%) good–excellent IKDC: 6 (50%) nearly normal, 5 (42%) abnormal, 1 (8%) grossly abnormal
Noyes and Barber-Westin[14] (1997)	11	58 months	3/7 (43%) good–excellent (acute only rated)
Shapiro and Freedman[18] (1995)	7	51 months	Meyers: 6/7 (86%) good–excellent

Meyers, Meyers knee dislocation rating system; IKDC, International Knee Documentation Committee form; HSS, Hospital for Special Surgery knee ligament rating scale.

References

1. Ahn JH, Chung YS, Oh I. Arthroscopic posterior cruciate ligament reconstruction using the posterior trans-septal portal. Arthroscopy 2003;19:101-107.

2. Ahn JH, Ha CW. Posterior trans-septal portal for arthroscopic surgery of the knee joint. Arthroscopy 2000;16:774-779.

3. Chhabra A, Cha PS, Rihn JA, et al. Surgical management of knee dislocations. Surgical technique. J Bone Joint Surg Am 2005;87(suppl 1, pt 1):1-21.

4. Fanelli GC, Edson CJ. Arthroscopically assisted combined anterior and posterior cruciate ligament reconstruction in the multiple ligament injured knee: 2- to 10-year follow-up. Arthroscopy 2002;18:703-714.

5. Fanelli GC, Edson CJ, Orcutt DR, et al. Treatment of combined anterior cruciate–posterior cruciate ligament–medial-lateral side knee injuries. J Knee Surg 2005;18:240-248.

6. Fanelli GC, Orcutt DR, Edson CJ. The multiple-ligament injured knee: evaluation, treatment, and results. Arthroscopy 2005;21: 471-486.

7. Good L, Johnson RJ. The dislocated knee. J Am Acad Orthop Surg 1995;3:284-292.

8. Greis PE, Burks RT, Bachus K, Luker MG. The influence of tendon length and fit on the strength of a tendon-bone tunnel complex: a biomechanical and histologic study in the dog. Am J Sports Med 2001;29:493-497.

9. Harner CD, Waltrip RL, Bennett CH, et al. Surgical management of knee dislocations. J Bone Joint Surg Am 2004;86:262-273.

10. Helgeson MD, Lehman RA Jr, Murphy KP. Initial evaluation of the acute and chronic multiple ligament injured knee. J Knee Surg 2005;18:213-219.

11. Mariani PP, Margheritini F, Camillieri G. One-stage arthroscopically assisted anterior and posterior cruciate ligament reconstruction. Arthroscopy 2001;17:700-707.

12. Meyers MH, Harvey JP Jr. Traumatic dislocation of the knee joint. A study of eighteen cases. J Bone Joint Surg Am 1971;53:16-29.

13. Meyers MH, Moore TM, Harvey JP Jr. Traumatic dislocation of the knee joint. J Bone Joint Surg Am 1975;57:430-433.

14. Noyes FR, Barber-Westin SD. Reconstruction of the anterior and posterior cruciate ligaments after knee dislocation. Use of early protected postoperative motion to decrease arthrofibrosis. Am J Sport Med 1997;25:769-778.

15. Ohkoshi Y, Nagasaki S, Shibata N, et al. Two-stage reconstruction with autografts for knee dislocations. Clin Orthop Rel Res 2002;398:169-175.

16. Richter M, Bosch U, Wippermann B, et al. Comparison of surgical repair or reconstruction of the cruciate ligaments versus nonsurgical treatment in patients with traumatic knee dislocations. Am J Sports Med 2002;30:718-727.

17. Rihn JA, Cha PS, Groff YJ, Harner CD. The acutely dislocated knee: evaluation and management. J Am Acad Orthop Surg 2004;12: 334-346.

18. Shapiro MS, Freedman EL. Allograft reconstruction of the anterior and posterior cruciate ligaments after traumatic knee dislocation. Am J Sports Med 1995;23:580-587.

19. Stannard JP, Riley RS, Sheils TM, et al. Anatomic reconstruction of the posterior cruciate ligament after multiligament knee injuries. A combination of the tibial-inlay and two-femoral-tunnel techniques. Am J Sports Med 2003;31:196-202.

20. Wascher DC, Becker JR, Dexter JG, Blevins FT. Reconstruction of the anterior and posterior cruciate ligaments after knee dislocation. Results using fresh-frozen nonirradiated allografts. Am J Sports Med 1999;27:189-196.

21. Wong CH, Tan JL, Chang HC, et al. Knee dislocations—a retrospective study comparing operative versus closed immobilization treatment outcomes. Knee Surg Sports Traumatol Arthrosc 2004;12:540-544.

CHAPTER 72

Medial Patellofemoral Ligament Reconstruction and Repair for Patellar Instability

Andrew J. Cosgarea, MD

Numerous surgical procedures have been described for treatment of patellar instability, most with generally favorable success rates. The medial patellofemoral ligament (MPFL) is the primary soft tissue passive restraint to pathologic lateral patellar displacement[4,7,17] and is torn when the patella dislocates.[15,19,23] There has been a great deal of interest recently in soft tissue procedures that address the MPFL. Techniques have been described to repair[5,13,15,23] or to reconstruct[8,18,24] the MPFL in an attempt to restore its function as a checkrein. Regardless of which approach is taken, successful surgical treatment requires that the surgeon have a thorough understanding of the relevant anatomy and a working knowledge of patellofemoral biomechanics.

Preoperative Considerations

History

Patellofemoral complaints are among the most common problems encountered by physicians treating knee disorders, and instability represents a distinct subset that is usually amenable to surgical treatment. Instability represents a continuum ranging from minor incidental subluxation episodes to traumatic dislocation events. Patients with frequent subluxation episodes and patients who dislocate usually experience substantial knee pain, swelling, and stiffness, resulting in interruption of their normal occupational and recreational activities.

Patellar dislocations can occur from an indirect twisting mechanism as the upper body rotates while the foot remains planted on the ground. Less commonly, a direct blow to the medial aspect of the patella from contact sport or motor vehicle accident drives the patella laterally. The patella may be spontaneously reduced as the knee is extended, or a formal reduction maneuver may be necessary. With initial dislocation episodes, significant pain and swelling are caused by soft tissue and articular surface damage. The resulting hemarthrosis and quadriceps weakness may take several weeks to resolve. The degree of morbidity tends to decrease in patients who sustain multiple recurrent episodes.

Subluxation episodes are usually less dramatic and manifest as a feeling of instability and pain. Patients often describe the sense that the knee may "give out." These episodes usually occur with trunk rotation during physical activity and result in a variable degree of pain and swelling. The pain is usually anterior and may be bilateral, especially in patients with malalignment or diffuse ligamentous laxity. The most important clinical determination to be made is whether the pain described by the patient is associated with patellar instability, as the common clinical entity of isolated anterior knee pain (patellofemoral pain syndrome) is nearly universally treated nonoperatively.

Physical Examination

Tibiofemoral alignment is evaluated with the patient standing. The knee is then observed for intra-articular and extra-articular swelling, and the knee's range of motion is formally measured and compared with the contralateral leg. The soft tissues are palpated for areas of tenderness. The examiner should try to identify the area of greatest tenderness along the course of the MPFL; this usually identifies the location of the tear.

A thorough ligamentous examination is necessary to rule out concomitant cruciate or collateral ligament tears. It is not uncommon to confuse the symptoms of a torn anterior cruciate ligament with patellar instability. Medial collateral ligament injuries occur commonly at the time of patellar dislocation. Measurement of the quadriceps angle (Q angle) can be used as a gross assessment of the lateral force vector. Patellar tracking is observed during active knee extension. The patella is observed for a tendency to slip laterally as the knee approaches the last 20 degrees of extension and the patella is no longer constrained by the lateral trochlear ridge (J sign). Patellar translation is estimated by applying a laterally directed force to the medial side of the patella with the knee in extension. The examiner attempts to quantify the amount of translation in quadrants and the consistency of the endpoint. An indistinct or "soft" endpoint suggests MPFL incompetence. A sense of apprehension with this maneuver (apprehension sign) supports the diagnosis of instability. Conversely, apprehension with medial translation may suggest medial instability. Lateral retinacular tightness is assessed by attempting to lift the lateral edge of the patella (tilt test). The retinaculum is considered tight if the patella will not correct to a neutral or horizontal position.

Imaging

Radiography

The standard radiographic series includes anteroposterior, lateral (30 degrees of flexion), tunnel, and sunrise (30 to 45 degrees of flexion) views. The tunnel view is useful to demonstrate osteochondral lesions or loose bodies in the notch. The lateral view gives information about patellar height and trochlear morphologic features. The tangential view shows the degree of subluxation and tilt as well as any osteochondral lesions.

Other Imaging Modalities

Computed tomographic axial images (20 degrees of flexion) are helpful in some cases to quantify subluxation and tilt. Magnetic resonance imaging will demonstrate a characteristic bone bruise pattern affecting the medial facet of the patella and the lateral femoral condyle in patients who have recently sustained a traumatic dislocation. Chondral and osteochondral injuries are clearly localized by magnetic resonance imaging.

Indications and Contraindications

MPFL reconstruction is indicated in skeletally mature patients with symptomatic recurrent lateral subluxation or dislocation episodes. Attempts at nonoperative treatment, including activity modification, physical therapy, and bracing, have failed in most patients. Femoral fixation can be modified in skeletally immature patients so that the distal femoral growth plate is not at risk. Tibial tuberosity osteotomy procedures like the Elmslie-Trillat, which directly decrease the Q angle, have a theoretical advantage in patients with greater degrees of malalignment. The Fulkerson anteromedialization osteotomy is preferred in patients with malalignment and degenerative changes.[14] MPFL reconstruction or repair can be combined with distal osteotomy if neither alone is sufficient to provide adequate stability. Lateral retinacular release is reserved for patients with excessive lateral patellofemoral pressure and is ineffective as an isolated procedure in patients with instability.

Some authors recommend MPFL repair after first-time patellar dislocation.[23] I usually treat an initial subluxation or dislocation episode nonoperatively but will repair an acute MPFL tear when surgery is indicated for concomitant intra-articular disease (such as a large loose body or meniscus tear). MPFL repair may also be used to treat recurrent instability. With repeated instability episodes, the MPFL becomes attenuated and functionally incompetent. To re-establish the normal checkrein effect, the MPFL is tightened by cutting, shortening, and reattaching it at the patellar or femoral insertion or by midsubstance imbrication.

MPFL repair or reconstruction is contraindicated in patients with medial instability or isolated anterior knee pain. In patients with significant medial patellofemoral degenerative changes, great care should be taken not to overtighten the MPFL as this will result in excessive medial joint pressures and is likely to exacerbate patellofemoral pain.

Surgical Technique

Anesthesia and Positioning

Surgery is performed with the patient supine on a standard operating room table. A vertical thigh post is used to facilitate arthroscopic evaluation and is removed before the reconstruction is started. A tourniquet is placed around the proximal thigh on the operative side. A compressive thigh-high stocking is placed on the contralateral leg. The procedure is performed on an outpatient basis with use of general or regional anesthesia techniques. Prophylactic intravenous antibiotics are administered before incision.

Examination Under Anesthesia

Once adequate anesthesia has been established, a comprehensive examination is performed. It is usually easier to characterize patellar stability, translation, and tilt when the patient is anesthetized. With the knee in extension, the position of the patella is determined at rest and with a lateral translation force applied (Fig. 72-1). Even an unstable patella will not stay dislocated unless the knee is maintained in a flexed position (Fig. 72-2). It is important to compare the amount of translation on the symptomatic side with the normal lateral patellar translation in the contralateral knee. The examiner should use his or her thumb to push the patella laterally and assess the amount of translation as well as the consistency of the endpoint (Fig. 72-3). It is also important to assess the patient for lateral retinacular tightness. If the examiner is unable to evert the lateral edge of the patella to the neutral or horizontal position, and if the patient's symptoms and preoperative radiographs are consistent with excessive lateral pressure, consideration should be given to a concomitant arthroscopic lateral retinacular release.

Arthroscopic Examination

Diagnostic arthroscopy is performed by standard superolateral, inferomedial, and inferolateral portals. The suprapatellar pouch, the medial and lateral parapatellar gutters, and the posteromedial and posterolateral compartments are carefully assessed for loose bodies. The articular surfaces of the patella and trochlea are thoroughly visualized for chondral lesions. Most often, the medial facet of the patella and the proximal portion of the lateral femoral condyle are injured after traumatic patellar dislocation. Hemorrhage in the soft tissue and a capsular defect along the medial edge of the patella suggest a recent traumatic avulsion of the MPFL insertion. Patellar tracking in the trochlear groove is visualized as the knee is flexed and extended. The menisci and cruciate ligaments are assessed for concomitant pathologic changes. Any significant chondral lesions are addressed surgically with débridement, marrow stimulation, or repair techniques as indicated. Careful consideration should be given to whether large defects should be unloaded by tibial tuberosity osteotomy techniques, such as anteromedialization. If there is excessive tightness of the lateral

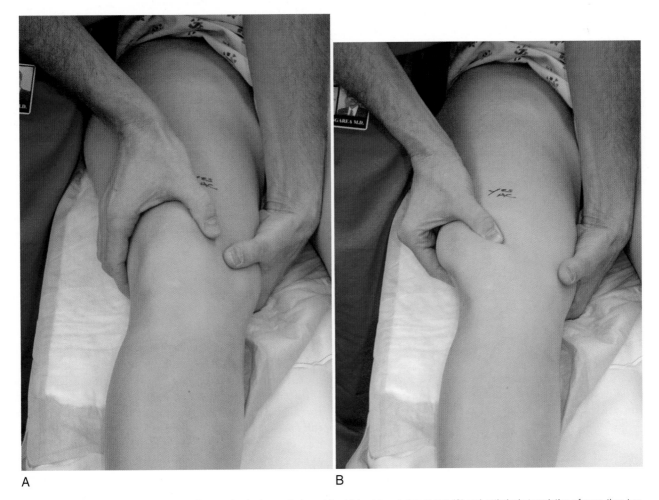

A
B

Figure 72-1 Examination of the right knee under anesthesia demonstrates minimal lateral translation at rest (**A**) and pathologic translation of more than two quadrants with lateral force applied (**B**).

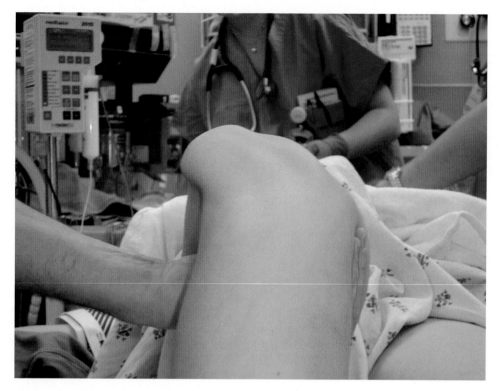

Figure 72-2 Lateral dislocation of the right patella.

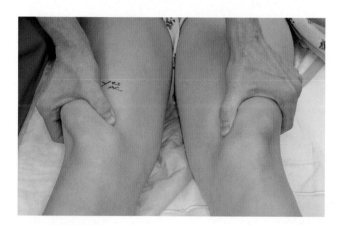

Figure 72-3 Comparison of patellar translation between symptomatic right knee and asymptomatic left knee with equal lateral forces applied under general anesthesia.

retinaculum, an arthroscopic release may be performed at this point, although we have not found that to be routinely necessary.

Surgical Landmarks and Incisions

A marking pen is used to identify the location of the patella and tibial tuberosity (Fig. 72-4). Marks are also made over the adductor tubercle and just distally over the medial

femoral epicondyle. The pes anserine tendon insertion site is localized by palpation. A 3- to 4-cm oblique mark is made for the harvest incision directly over the sartorial fascia insertion on the proximal medial tibia. A second 3- to 4-cm line is drawn directly over the midportion of the MPFL, halfway between the medial border of the patella and the medial femoral epicondyle. The position of this incision is modified if the location of the MPFL tear has been ascertained from the preoperative examination or magnetic resonance imaging and an MPFL repair rather than reconstruction is planned.

Specific Steps (Box 72-1)

1. MPFL Exposure

The leg is exsanguinated with an Esmarch bandage, and the tourniquet is raised while the knee is in an extended position. A longitudinal incision is made directly over the MPFL midway between the medial edge of the patella and the medial epicondyle. Blunt dissection is used to expose the thick medial retinacular layer contiguous with the inferior border of the vastus medialis obliquus (Fig. 72-5). With gentle dissection, the MPFL is usually identifiable (Fig. 72-6). In the case of a recent dislocation, it may be possible to identify the site of failure at the medial border of the patella, at the medial femoral epicondyle, or less commonly in midsubstance.

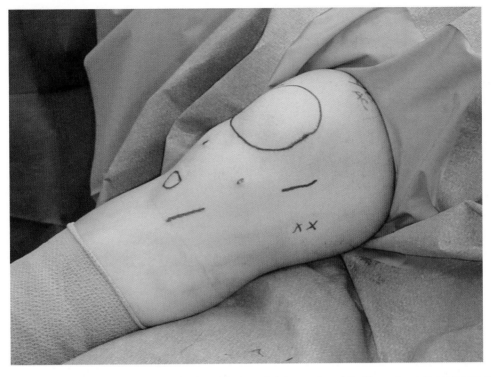

Figure 72-4 Surface landmarks, right knee, after diagnostic arthroscopy. The large circle is over the patella; the smaller circle overlies the tibial tuberosity. The proximal X is over the adductor tubercle; the distal X overlies the medial epicondyle. The proximal line is over the midportion of the MPFL and is where the incision is made to expose the medial border of the patella and medial femoral epicondyle. The distal line overlies the pes anserine insertion and is where the incision is made to harvest the gracilis tendon.

Box 72-1 Surgical Steps

1. MPFL exposure

2. MPFL repair

3. Graft harvest for MPFL reconstruction

4. Patellar tunnel

5. Femoral tunnel

6. Graft tensioning and fixation

7. Closure

2. MPFL Repair

With a medially directed force applied to the lateral edge of the patella, the medial border of the patella is brought into the operative field. If the MPFL is avulsed at this location, a direct repair can be performed with bone tunnels or suture anchors. With retraction of the posterior edge of the wound, the adductor tubercle and medial femoral epicondyle can be exposed through the same incision. Some authors believe that the most common site of failure is off of the femur.[23] In this location, the torn MPFL can be repaired to a stump of remaining tissue with No. 2 nonabsorbable sutures or reattached directly to a freshened bone surface by two or three suture anchors. Repair of a midsubstance rupture is more challenging. It is not always possible to identify the location of tissue failure, and especially in chronic cases, it can be difficult to determine how much to shorten the attenuated ligament. Overtightening of the ligament will result in subsequent repair failure or overconstrain the patella. I generally reserve MPFL repair techniques for patients who have experienced recent instability episodes when acute surgical intervention is indicated for concomitant intra-articular disease.

3. Graft Harvest for MPFL Reconstruction

A variety of different autologous or allogeneic graft sources are available for reconstruction of the MPFL. I prefer to use the gracilis tendon, which is immediately adjacent to the reconstruction site and relatively easy to harvest. An incision is made directly over the pes anserine insertion, and blunt dissection is used to expose the sartorial fascia. The superior edge of the sartorial fascia is identified anterior to the superficial medial collateral ligament. The sartorial fascia is then incised and everted to expose the underlying gracilis and semitendinosus tendons. A combination of blunt and sharp dissection is used to separate the gracilis tendon from the sartorial fascia. The free end of the tendon is tagged, and a tendon stripper is then used to harvest the gracilis tendon. Although the gracilis is smaller and shorter than the semitendinosus tendon, it is still significantly stronger than the native MPFL[1,3,4,16] and is almost

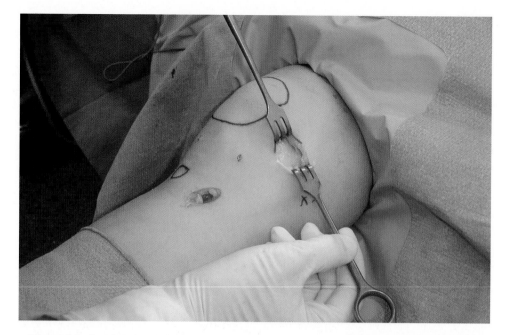

Figure 72-5 Exposure of the medial retinaculum just inferior to the vastus medialis obliquus. The gracilis tendon has been harvested.

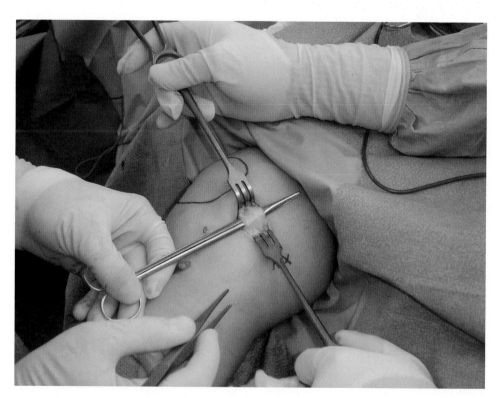

Figure 72-6 Exposure of the midsubstance of the MPFL.

always long enough to construct an adequate graft. After harvesting of the gracilis tendon, the sartorial fascia is sutured back to its insertion on the proximal medial tibia.

The gracilis tendon is then prepared for implantation by removal of muscle and other debris from the surface. The tendon is then folded over so that double-looped length can be measured. The diameter is also measured with a tunnel sizer. A double-looped graft length of 9 to 10 cm is sufficient and will be increased as necessary once the graft construct has been completed.

4. Patellar Tunnel

Soft tissue is cleared from the medial edge of the patella with a rongeur. The proximal and distal poles of the patella are localized digitally. A small transverse incision is made at the MPFL insertion on the medial edge of the patella (Fig. 72-7). A 2.5-mm drill bit is drilled from medial to lateral in the midportion of the MPFL insertion on the medial border of the patella (Fig. 72-8), which is usually just above the equator of the patella. The surgeon must carefully advance the drill bit so that it exits the lateral edge of the patella without violating either the anterior bone cortex or posterior articular surface. The drill bit is then removed from the drill, and lateral fluoroscopy can confirm appropriate positioning (Fig. 72-9). The 2.5-mm drill bit is then replaced by a 2.0-mm eyelet K-wire, which is then overdrilled with a 4.5-mm cannulated drill bit. A depth gauge is then used to measure the length of the tunnel. On the basis of the length of the graft and the

amount of graft that the surgeon wants in the patellar tunnel, the appropriate length Endobutton CL fixation device (Acufex; Smith & Nephew Endoscopy, Andover, Mass) is chosen. The graft construct is completed at the back table by passing the gracilis tendon tissue through the loop of the EndoButton and suturing it to itself with a No. 2 nonabsorbable woven suture. Sutures are also woven through the femoral end of the graft and will be used later to pull the graft into the femoral tunnel (Fig. 72-10). Two different-sized sutures are then passed through the two holes in the metal EndoButton. If the graft diameter is more than 4.5 mm, the patellar tunnel is enlarged with the appropriately sized cannulated drill bit to a depth of approximately 1 cm longer than the length of gracilis tissue that is intended to remain in the tunnel.

The 2.0-mm eyelet K-wire is passed from medial to lateral across the patellar tunnel and directed to exit the superolateral inflow portal. The four suture ends from the EndoButton are loaded through the eyelet of the K-wire, and the K-wire is pulled out through the superolateral portal site. With the EndoButton positioned lengthwise, the graft is pulled through the patellar tunnel until it clears the lateral edge of the patella (Fig. 72-11). Once it clears the patellar tunnel, tension is placed on the femoral end of the graft so that the EndoButton sits flush along the lateral edge of the patella. The position of the EndoButton can be confirmed fluoroscopically, and it can be manually manipulated so that it lies flush and lengthwise along the lateral edge of the patella.

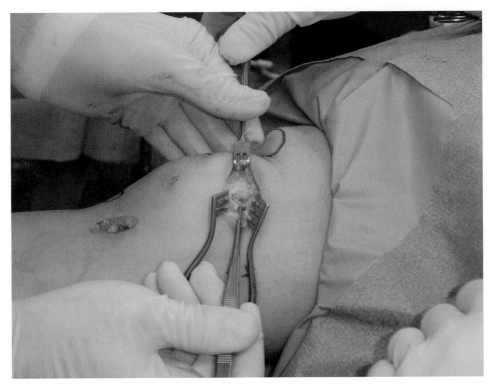

Figure 72-7 Exposure of the medial edge of the patella in preparation for drilling of the patellar tunnel.

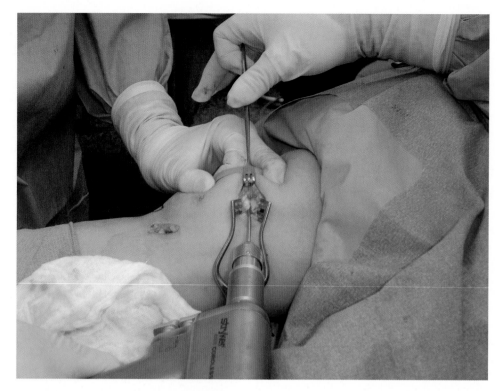

Figure 72-8 The 2.5-mm drill bit is passed transversely from medial to lateral.

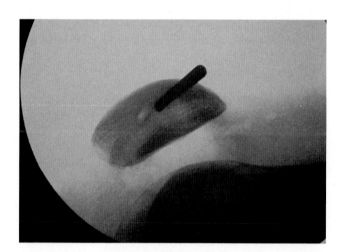

Figure 72-9 Fluoroscopic image confirming appropriate position of the drill bit in the patella, proximal to the equator.

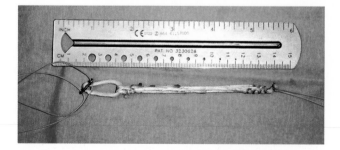

Figure 72-10 Double-looped gracilis tendon autograft with Endobutton CL used for patellar fixation.

5. Femoral Tunnel

A common technical error that occurs during MPFL reconstruction surgery is to place the femoral tunnel adjacent to the adductor tubercle rather than the medial femoral epicondyle; therefore, it is crucial to distinguish between these two bone prominences. Several anatomic studies have demonstrated that the femoral attachment site of the MPFL is at the medial epicondyle, which is approximately 1 cm distal to the adductor tubercle.[20,21,25] Others report the femoral attachment to be just anterior to the medial femoral epicondyle.[12,26] A biomechanical study suggests that malpositioning of the femoral tunnel even 5 mm too far proximal can result in increased graft force and pressure applied to the cartilage of the medial facet of the patella.[11]

Once the anatomy is defined, a 2.5-mm drill bit is placed just anterior to the medial femoral epicondyle. This position can be confirmed fluoroscopically (Fig. 72-12). The graft is then passed through a soft tissue tunnel underneath the medial retinaculum and the remnant of the MPFL. The graft can then be wrapped around the drill bit, allowing assessment of graft isometry as the knee is flexed and extended. Minor changes in the position of the drill bit will allow fine-tuning of tunnel positioning. Once the optimal position for the femoral tunnel has been determined, the drill bit is replaced with a 2.0-mm eyelet K-wire. The K-wire is then overdrilled with a 6.0-mm cannulated drill bit to the appropriate depth based on the remaining length of the graft (Fig. 72-13). The suture ends

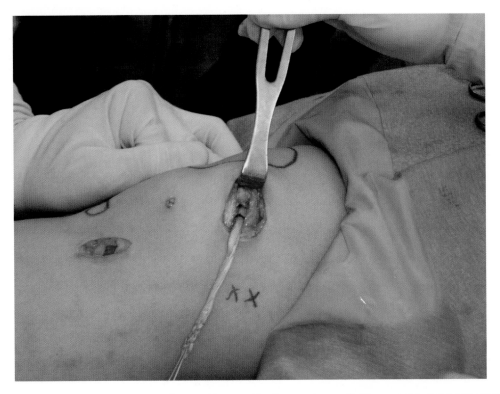

Figure 72-11 The gracilis graft is being pulled into the patellar tunnel by manual traction on sutures exiting the superolateral portal. The EndoButton passes the lateral border of the patella and is rotated to lie flush.

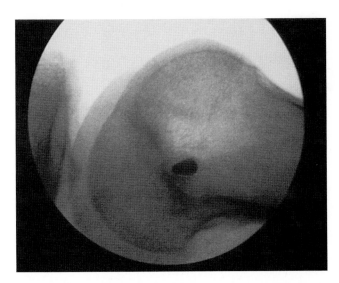

Figure 72-12 Fluoroscopic image confirming appropriate position of the 2.5-mm drill bit at the femoral tunnel location just anterior to the medial epicondyle.

are then passed through the eyelet of the K-wire, and the graft is pulled into the femoral tunnel as the K-wire is pulled out the lateral side of the knee (Fig. 72-14).

6. Graft Tensioning and Fixation

Tension is placed on the free suture ends on the lateral aspect of the knee as the surgeon moves the knee several times through a full range of motion. As the knee flexes and extends, the amount of tension in the graft can be ascertained by the amount of traction felt on the free suture ends (Fig. 72-15). In addition, the graft tension is directly palpated and visualized through the medial incision. It is extremely important not to overconstrain the graft. The knee is placed in full extension, and the patella is translated laterally. An attempt is made to identify the graft length that reproduces the same amount of normal lateral translation noted on the contralateral side. Once the appropriate graft length is identified, graft fixation is obtained by a 7.0-mm bioabsorbable cannulated femoral interference screw (Fig. 72-16). The screw is countersunk below the surface of the bone, and fixation can be augmented by sewing the graft to the adjacent soft tissue at the tunnel opening (Fig. 72-17). It should then be confirmed that the knee has full range of motion, the patella is no longer dislocatable, and the graft provides a firm checkrein preventing pathologic lateral translation.

7. Closure

Subcuticular wound closure offers excellent cosmesis (Fig. 72-18). Cryotherapy devices are routinely used to help control pain and swelling. A compressive dressing is then applied, followed by a thigh-high compression stocking and a postoperative brace locked in full extension.

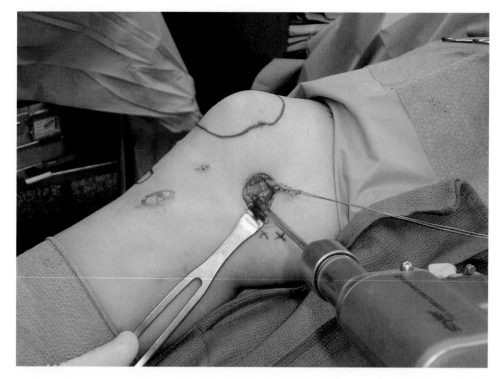

Figure 72-13 Femoral tunnel drilled with 6.0-mm drill bit.

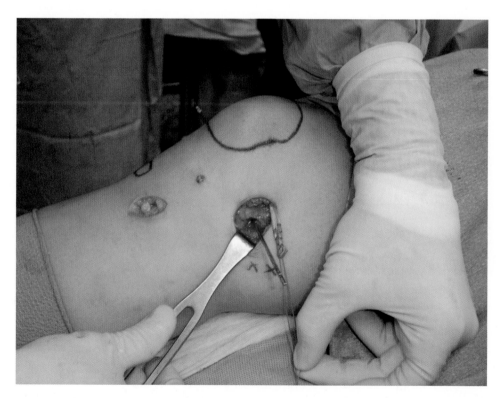

Figure 72-14 The 2.0-mm eyelet K-wire is used to pull the femoral end of the graft into the femoral tunnel.

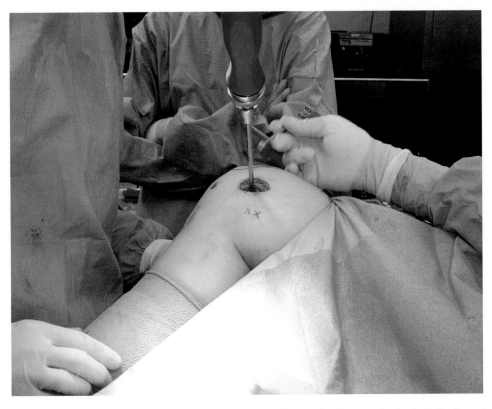

Figure 72-15 The knee is ranged through a full flexion arc several times. Graft isometry is determined by assessing tension in the femoral sutures, which are held where they exit the skin on the lateral side of the knee.

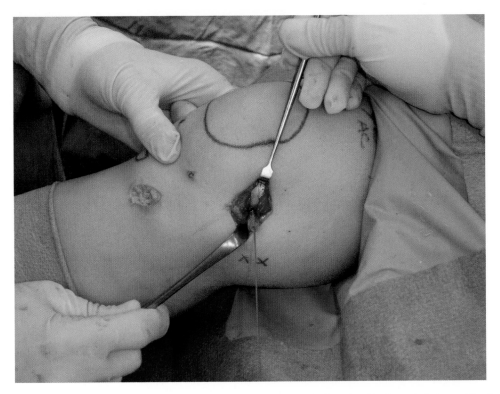

Figure 72-16 Femoral fixation is obtained by a 7.0-mm bioabsorbable interference screw with the knee flexed to the angle that was determined to cause the greatest amount of tension in the MPFL graft. An attempt is made to replicate the passive lateral translation of the patella in the normal contralateral knee.

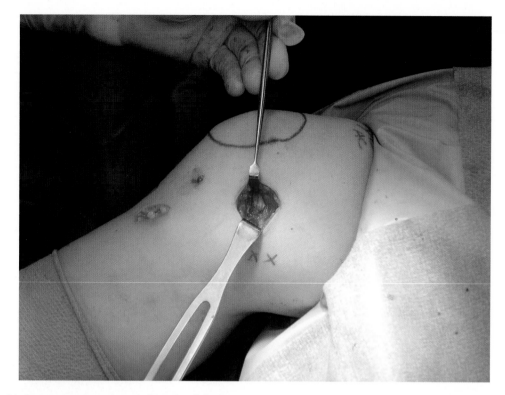

Figure 72-17 The interference screw is countersunk. Femoral graft fixation may be augmented with sutures.

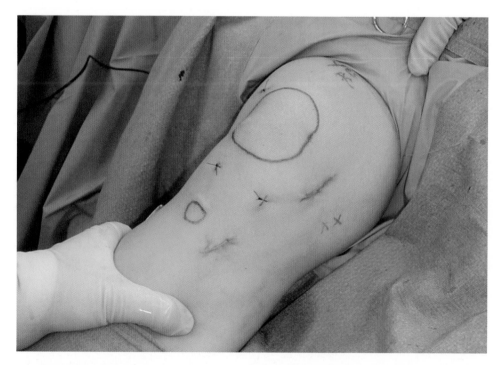

Figure 72-18 Subcuticular wound closure allows excellent cosmesis.

Postoperative Considerations

Rehabilitation (Box 72-2)

Immediately postoperatively, patients are instructed in quadriceps sets and straight-leg raises. Patients are instructed in crutch ambulation and are allowed touch-down weight bearing. The brace remains locked in full extension for 1 week, at which point patients are encouraged to begin knee range of motion and to progress as tolerated. Weight bearing is also allowed to progress as tolerated. Patients are encouraged to attend formal physical therapy three times per week, where knee range of motion and quadriceps-strengthening exercises are emphasized. The brace is unlocked for ambulation as soon as quadriceps strength is sufficient. Patients are given the goal of achieving 120 degrees of knee flexion by 4 weeks postoperatively, and the brace is generally discontinued by 6 weeks. Patients are encouraged to achieve full knee range of motion by 8 weeks and allowed to progress to jogging and sports-specific drills by 12 weeks. Most patients are able to return to sports by 4 to 5 months.

Box 72-2 Postoperative Rehabilitation Protocol

Discharge
- Touch-down weight bearing with brace locked in extension
- Quadriceps sets, straight-leg raises, ankle pumps
- Cryotherapy device

Week 1
- Advance to full weight bearing as tolerated with brace locked in extension
- Unlock brace for active and active-assisted range-of-motion exercises
- Physical therapy referral three times per week for 12 weeks

Week 2
- Straight-leg raises with 1-pound weight
- Begin stationary bicycle for range of motion

Week 4
- Straight-leg raises: 100 reps daily
- Should have 120 degrees of flexion

Week 6
- Discontinue hinged brace when quadriceps strength allows

Week 8
- StairStepper, treadmill
- Should have normal range of motion

Month 3
- Initiate progressive jogging program

Month 4-5
- Advance to cutting and sport-specific drills
- Return to regular sports

Complications

As with many knee reconstruction procedures, the most common postoperative complication is loss of motion. Flexion and extension deficits may be secondary to inadequate postoperative rehabilitation. This risk can be minimized by early weight bearing and motion exercises. Flexion deficits may also be secondary to intraoperative technical errors (malpositioning or overtensioning of the graft). These errors could also overload the medial patellofemoral joint, resulting in pain and arthrosis, especially in the setting of a traumatic medial patellar chondral lesion. Other complications include recurrent instability, painful hardware, and patellar fracture.

PEARLS AND PITFALLS

- The most important clinical determination is whether the patient's symptoms are caused by patellar instability or the common entity of isolated anterior knee pain (patellofemoral pain syndrome), which is nearly universally treated nonoperatively.
- Patellofemoral instability represents a distinct subset of the spectrum of patellofemoral disorders and is usually amenable to surgical treatment.
- Successful surgical treatment requires that the surgeon have a thorough understanding of the relevant anatomy and a working knowledge of patellofemoral biomechanics.
- The MPFL is the primary soft tissue restraint to pathologic lateral patellar displacement and is torn when the patella dislocates.
- MPFL repair and reconstruction are contraindicated in patients with medial instability.
- The position of the incision is modified if the location of the MPFL tear has been ascertained from the preoperative examination or magnetic resonance imaging and if an MPFL repair rather than reconstruction is planned.
- It is not always possible to identify the location of the MPFL tear, especially in chronic cases, and it can be difficult to determine how much to shorten the attenuated ligament.
- An attempt is made to identify the graft length that reproduces the same amount of normal lateral translation noted on the contralateral side.
- A common technical error is to place the femoral tunnel adjacent to the adductor tubercle rather than the medial femoral epicondyle. Malpositioning of the femoral tunnel by as little as 5 mm too far proximal can result in significantly increased graft force and pressure applied to the patellofemoral cartilage.
- In drilling of the patellar tunnel, the surgeon must carefully advance the drill bit across the patella so that it exits the lateral edge without violating either the anterior bone cortex or posterior articular surface.
- MPFL reconstruction or repair can be combined with tibial tuberosity osteotomy if neither alone is sufficient to provide adequate stability.
- If the patient's symptoms and preoperative radiographs are consistent with excessive lateral pressure, a concomitant arthroscopic lateral retinacular release should be considered.
- Femoral fixation can be modified in skeletally immature patients so that the distal femoral growth plate is not placed at risk.
- The most common postoperative complication is loss of motion. Whereas motion deficits may be secondary to inadequate postoperative rehabilitation, they can also be secondary to intraoperative technical errors like malpositioning of the tunnels or overtensioning of the graft.

72

Table 72-1 Results of Surgical Treatment

Author	No. of Patients	Follow-up	Results
MPFL Reconstruction			
Deie et al[6] (2003)	4	7.4 years	Dislocation, 0; Kujala score: 96.3
Drez et al[8] (2001)	15	2.6 years	Dislocation, 0; Kujala score: 88
Ellera Gomes[9] (1992)	30	3.25 years	83% good–excellent
Ellera Gomes et al[10] (2004)	15	5.0 years	87% satisfied
MPFL Repair			
Avikainen et al[2] (1993)	14	6.9 years	Dislocation, 1; 86% good–excellent
Garth et al[15] (2003)	20	2.7 years	95% good–excellent
Nomura et al[22] (2004)	5	5.9 years	Kujala score: 97.6; 80% good–excellent
Sallay et al[23] (1996)	12	3 years	Dislocation, 0; 58% good–excellent

Results

Published studies reporting outcome after MPFL repair or reconstruction have been limited by small numbers of patients, retrospective design, and lack of control groups but have been generally favorable.[2,6,8,9,10,15,22,23] Most authors report satisfactory outcomes (good and excellent) in the range of 83% to 96% (Table 72-1).[1,8,9,10,15,22] Because a variety of different outcome parameters have been used, it is difficult to compare results, indicating the need for larger, multicenter controlled studies.

References

1. Amis AA, Firer P, Mountney J, et al. Anatomy and biomechanics of the medial patellofemoral ligament. Knee 2003;10:215-220.
2. Avikainen VJ, Nikku RK, Seppanen-Lehmonen TK. Adductor magnus tenodesis for patellar dislocation. Technique and preliminary results. Clin Orthop Relat Res 1993;297:12-16.
3. Ciccone WJ, Bratton DR, Weinstein DM, Elias JJ. Viscoelasticity and temperature variations decrease tension and stiffness of hamstring tendon grafts following anterior cruciate ligament reconstruction. J Bone Joint Surg Am 2006;88:1071-1078.
4. Conlan T, Garth WP Jr, Lemons JE. Evaluation of the medial soft-tissue restraints of the extensor mechanism of the knee. J Bone Joint Surg Am 1993;75:682-693.
5. Davis DK, Fithian DC. Techniques of medial retinacular repair and reconstruction. Clin Orthop Relat Res 2002;402:38-52.
6. Deie M, Ochi M, Sumen Y, et al. Reconstruction of the medial patellofemoral ligament for the treatment of habitual or recurrent dislocation of the patella in children. J Bone Joint Surg Br 2003;85:887-890.
7. Desio SM, Burks RT, Bachus KN. Soft tissue restraints to lateral patellar translation in the human knee. Am J Sports Med 1998;26:59-65.
8. Drez D Jr, Edwards TB, Williams CS. Results of medial patellofemoral ligament reconstruction in the treatment of patellar dislocation. Arthroscopy 2001;17:298-306.
9. Ellera Gomes JL. Medial patellofemoral ligament reconstruction for recurrent dislocation of the patella: a preliminary report. Arthroscopy 1992;8:335-340.
10. Ellera Gomes JL, Stigler Marczyk LR, Cesar de Cesar P, Jungblut CF. Medial patellofemoral ligament reconstruction with semitendinosus autograft for chronic patellar instability: a follow-up study. Arthroscopy 2004;20:147-151.
11. Elias JJ, Cosgarea AJ. Technical errors during medial patellofemoral ligament reconstruction could overload medial patellofemoral cartilage: a computational analysis. Am J Sports Med 2006;34:1478-1485.
12. Feller JA, Feagin JA Jr, Garrett WE Jr. The medial patellofemoral ligament revisited: an anatomical study. Knee Surg Sports Traumatol Arthrosc 1993;1:184-186.
13. Fithian DC, Meier SW. The case for advancement and repair of the medial patellofemoral ligament in patients with recurrent patellar instability. Oper Tech Sports Med 1999;7:81-89.
14. Fulkerson JP, Becker GJ, Meaney JA, et al. Anteromedial tibial tubercle transfer without bone graft. Am J Sports Med 1990;18:490-496.
15. Garth WP Jr, DiChristina DG, Holt G. Delayed proximal repair and distal realignment after patellar dislocation. Clin Orthop Relat Res 2000;377:132-144.
16. Hamner DL, Brown CH Jr, Steiner ME, et al. Hamstring tendon grafts for reconstruction of the anterior cruciate ligament: biomechanical evaluation of the use of multiple strands and tensioning techniques. J Bone Joint Surg Am 1999;81:549-557.
17. Huberti HH, Hayes WC, Stone JL, Shybut GT. Force ratios in the quadriceps tendon and ligamentum patellae. J Orthop Res 1984;2:49-54.
18. Muneta T, Sekiya I, Tsuchiya M, Shinomiya K. A technique for reconstruction of the medial patellofemoral ligament. Clin Orthop Relat Res 1999;359:151-155.
19. Nomura E. Classification of lesions of the medial patello-femoral ligament in patellar dislocation. Int Orthop 1999;23:260-263.
20. Nomura E, Horiuchi Y, Kihara M. Medial patellofemoral ligament restraint in lateral patellar translation and reconstruction. Knee 2000;7:121-127.

21. Nomura E, Inoue M. Surgical technique and rationale for medial patellofemoral ligament reconstruction for recurrent patellar dislocation. Arthroscopy 2003;19:E47.
22. Nomura E, Inoue M, Osada N. Augmented repair of avulsion-tear type medial patellofemoral ligament injury in acute patellar dislocation. Knee Surg Sports Traumatol Arthrosc 2005;13:346-351. Epub Nov 27, 2004.
23. Sallay PI, Poggi J, Speer KP, Garrett WE. Acute dislocation of the patella. A correlative pathoanatomic study. Am J Sports Med 1996;24:52-60.
24. Schock E, Burks R. Medial patellofemoral ligament reconstruction using a hamstring graft. Oper Tech Sports Med 2001;9:169-175.
25. Smirk C, Morris H. The anatomy and reconstruction of the medial patellofemoral ligament. Knee 2003;10:221-227.
26. Steensen RN, Dopirak RM, McDonald WG 3rd. The anatomy and isometry of the medial patellofemoral ligament: implications for reconstruction. Am J Sports Med 2004;32:1509-1513.

72

CHAPTER 73

Management of Arthrofibrosis of the Knee

Kevin Doulens, MD

Kurt Spindler, MD

Decreased range of motion is a primary concern after virtually any type of injury or surgery about the knee. Arthrofibrosis is generally defined as a loss in range of motion secondary to the buildup of dense intra-articular scar tissue. This complication can be difficult to prevent and even more difficult to predict. Extra-articular lesions, such as capsule and muscle contractures, can also contribute to the patient's motion deficit. The motion loss can be in the direction of flexion, extension, or both and varies in severity. Most patients will tolerate a loss of flexion better than a loss of extension, as extension loss makes ambulation both more difficult and energy intensive by altering gait mechanics and placing increased strain on structures around the knee.

Although arthrofibrosis is most commonly seen after surgery or injury to the knee, it can also occur in the face of sepsis, neurologic deficits that compromise motion, complex regional pain syndrome, and other inflammatory processes. Nonoperative treatment, including supervised physical therapy, anti-inflammatory medications, oral or intra-articular steroids, and narcotic pain relievers, are the mainstay of treatment and are successful in resolving the majority of cases. Unfortunately, a significant number of patients will be refractory to conservative treatment and require operative intervention.

Historically, the operative procedures used were open techniques that allowed the débridement of intra-articular scar tissue and the release of tight capsular structures. Arthroscopy is now the mainstay of treatment, allowing both débridement and releases with minimal additional morbidity. The surgical procedures most commonly associated with arthrofibrosis are intra-articular ligament reconstruction and total knee arthroplasty. Several published articles have addressed possible causes or predisposing factors leading to postoperative decreased range of motion. Contributing factors include surgery performed acutely after injury, injury that involves the proximal aspect of the medial collateral ligament, poor preoperative motion, and improper placement of reconstruction grafts. There is, however, no clear consensus on causation.

The incidence of stiffness after knee surgery as reported by various authors varies from as low as 4% to as high as 57% and represents a heterogeneous mix of injury caused versus postoperative patients, making it difficult to fully assess the extent of this condition. Studies have shown a correlation between the development of arthrofibrosis postoperatively and the presence of preoperative irritation and limited range of motion, along with poorly controlled perioperative pain. It has also been suggested that early postoperative rehabilitation and timely intervention, when necessary, can minimize the risk for development of arthrofibrosis.

Preoperative Considerations

The timing of operative intervention for arthrofibrosis is a factor that has a large impact on the ultimate success or failure of treatment. Early intervention has been shown to have better outcomes than those of procedures undertaken later. In general, after the first 3 months following injury or surgery with use of an early and aggressive physical therapy program, any remaining flexion or extension deficit should be approached surgically. This time frame allows a reasonable attempt at nonoperative resolution of knee stiffness but does not give the proliferating scar tissue adequate time to mature. After 9 months to a year, surgical procedures will have a lower chance to regain and, just as important, to maintain an increase in range of motion because of scar maturation and extra-articular contracture of the capsule and surrounding musculature.

The range of motion of the knee preoperatively can provide insight into the likely areas of pathologic change. If the knee lacks extension, the pathologic process is often in the intercondylar notch region. A lack of flexion usually indicates exuberant tissue in the suprapatellar pouch or the medial and lateral gutters. In the case of arthrofibrosis that follows total knee arthroplasty, the scar tissue often encompasses the entire intra-articular space.

Physical Examination

Physical examination of a knee with arthrofibrosis often reveals more than just a loss of motion. Swelling, effusion, and warmth about the joint, typical of an inflammatory process, are common. Because the majority of these cases follow trauma or surgery to the knee, pain is often a presenting factor. Atrophy of the musculature and an antalgic gait are seen in more progressed instances. It is important to accurately assess the amount of flexion and extension that the joint exhibits, along with a history of the inciting events and their time line. A joint that demonstrates progressive and worsening loss of motion is typical of a global process of inflammation and scarring. Loss of motion that reaches a limit and then stabilizes is more indicative of a focal process, such as the "cyclops" lesion that can develop in the anterior knee after anterior cruciate ligament reconstruction.

Imaging

Preoperative imaging is of marginal value in arthrofibrosis, especially in postoperative patients well known to the surgeon. Plain radiographs may demonstrate a distal position of the kneecap, known as patella infra, and may show evidence of soft tissue calcification, especially in long-standing cases. Post-reconstruction bone scans are not routinely obtained as they will continue to show increased uptake as a result of the previous surgical intervention. Magnetic resonance imaging adds little to the preoperative assessment of arthrofibrosis. The proliferative soft tissues may be visualized in various compartments of the joint, including the cyclops lesion in the anterior aspect of the knee, but these are of little value for preoperative planning and usually do little to alter decision-making.

Contraindications

Extrinsic factors that might influence knee function also need to be considered. Neurologic impairment that causes weakness about the knee will not be altered by removal of intra-articular scar tissue. Furthermore, surgical insult to a knee that does not function normally may lead to additional scarring. The same holds for a knee joint showing signs of an inflammatory process. Without proper prior medical treatment of the underlying pathologic process, surgical intervention may worsen the situation. Sepsis of the knee poses an interesting situation in that the operative intervention to clear the pathologic process, arthroscopic lavage and débridement, can also be used to remove proliferative scar tissue. If scar tissue recurs after resolution of the infection, repeated arthroscopy can remove this tissue easily.

A firm contraindication to operative intervention for arthrofibrosis is complex regional pain syndrome. This difficult and multifactorial entity is often made worse by surgical procedures. Standard treatment of complex regional pain syndrome should be undertaken and the condition improved or stabilized before an attempt at arthroscopic treatment of stiffness is undertaken. Softer contraindications to surgery include concomitant medical problems and a patient who is not motivated (or able) to cooperate with postoperative therapy.

Surgical Technique

Anesthesia and Positioning

With the decline in need for open procedures, the patient is positioned in the usual manner for knee arthroscopy. A thigh tourniquet is applied, and the knee is prepared and draped in a flexed position with the table end at 90 degrees. The tourniquet is inflated only if bleeding is encountered during the case that cannot be controlled with arthroscopic cautery. A straight post, rather than a standard knee holder, is positioned along the outside of the thigh at the level of the tourniquet to allow full manipulation of the knee after removal of the scar tissue while the patient is still anesthetized.

Specific Steps (Box 73-1)

1. Establish Portals

The first step in the procedure is to establish the portals. With decreased motion of the knee and swelling secondary to proliferative intra-articular soft tissue, finding the joint line as a surgical landmark can be difficult. When possible, a mark is made to indicate the medial and lateral joint

Box 73-1 Surgical Steps

1. Establish portals

2. Establish initial working space

3. Complete débridement throughout knee

4. Inspection

5. Manipulation under anesthesia

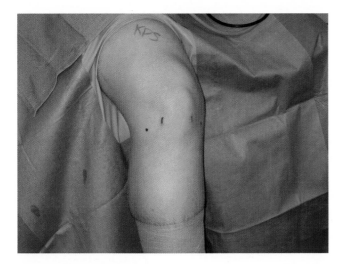

Figure 73-1 Portal placement.

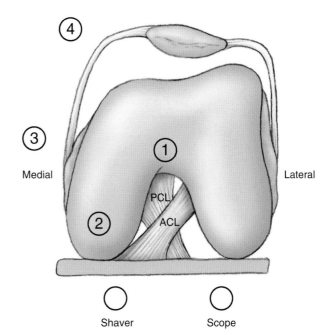

Figure 73-2 Medial débridement pattern.

lines, and the portals are then established on the basis of the markings (Fig. 73-1). An anterolateral portal is made just above the joint line and a few millimeters lateral to the edge of the patellar tendon. If the joint line is not discernible, the inferior border of the patella can serve as a reference. By drawing a horizontal line across the knee at this level, the initial portal can be made one fingerbreadth (i.e., approximately 2 cm) lateral to midline so that it bisects this line.

2. Establish Initial Working Space

If the knee has some motion preoperatively, indicating preservation of some of the normal intra-articular spaces, the cannula and trocar are advanced into the suprapatellar pouch through the anterolateral portal in the standard fashion. An inspection of the knee, with appropriate picture documentation, is completed as much as allowed by the intra-articular scar tissue. With use of the arthroscope to visualize the anterior medial compartment, a spinal needle is placed to localize the anteromedial portal, and this portal is then established. Once again, if there is insufficient space to visualize the spinal needle, the inferior patellar line can serve as a reference for this portal, placing it 2 cm medial to midline and bisecting the horizontal mark.

In a knee with minimal motion due to abundant scar tissue or, more commonly, after a total knee arthroplasty, it is not possible to insert the camera and tools in the usual fashion. Débridement of a knee with extensive scarring requires diligence. The previously described landmarks are made on the patient's skin. The anterolateral portal is made, and the cannula and trocar are inserted into the notch. The anteromedial portal is then made, and a shaver is inserted through this portal directed at the notch. In the intercondylar area behind the patellar tendon and fat pad, the shaver is located and visualized. With care taken not to engage the fat pad for avoidance of excessive bleeding, the scar tissue in the notch is then carefully débrided to establish a working space. Once a working area has been established, the camera and tools can be advanced outward toward the medial and lateral gutters (Fig. 73-2).

3. Complete Débridement Throughout Knee

On the basis of the amount and location of the pathologic process as identified by arthroscopy, a 4.5- or 5.5-mm shaver is inserted into the medial portal to begin débridement of the scar tissue in the medial compartment. An arthroscopic punch tool or the cautery is often needed to establish an edge in the fibrous tissue for the shaver effectively to take hold and to begin débridement of the scar. It is generally possible to work through the scar tissue until a plane appears between the scar and the more normal appearing capsular tissue. Development of this plane with the shaver or punch will allow sufficient removal of tissue in the various compartments of the knee. The medial gutter is débrided of its scar tissue burden. With the intercondylar notch and gutter cleaned out, débridement can

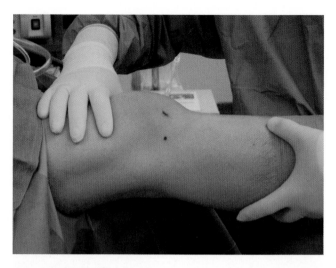

Figure 73-4 Extension manipulation.

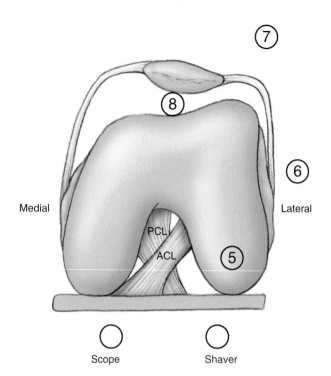

Figure 73-3 Lateral débridement pattern.

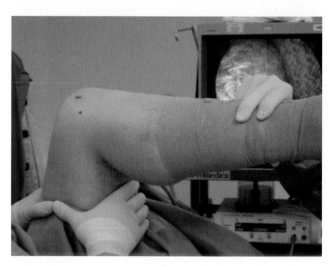

Figure 73-5 Flexion manipulation.

proceed up into the suprapatellar pouch. This pattern is then reversed and repeated for the lateral compartments (Fig. 73-3).

4. Inspection

Once the fibrous soft tissues have been removed from the compartments of the knee, an inspection can now be completed. A full inspection of the medial and lateral gutters, the suprapatellar pouch, and the intercondylar notch is required to ensure that adequate tissue has been removed. In general, this is a slow and time-consuming process, and patience is required to correctly establish the planes of dissection and to remove sufficient scar.

5. Manipulation Under Anesthesia

After débridement of the intra-articular scar tissue, a gentle manipulation can be performed on the knee. If there is an extension deficit, the knee can be supported by the heel and gentle downward pressure applied in a constant manner to the anterior knee, attempting to stretch and to release any tissue that might be preventing extension (Fig. 73-4). Similarly, manipulation can be used for lack of flexion. The hip is flexed to 90 degrees and the back of the knee supported while a gentle, steady two-finger pressure is applied to the lower leg in an attempt to release any tissue hindering flexion (Fig. 73-5). Care must be taken to use gentle pressure in both these maneuvers; excessive force or bouncing might cause unwanted damage, such as fracture. Once the manipulation has been completed,

the range of motion should again be assessed and documented.

Postoperative Considerations

Follow-up

The patient is seen 5 to 7 days postoperatively for inspection of the surgical site and evaluation of motion. Sutures can be removed from portals if they are well healed. Range of motion should be documented.

Rehabilitation

The patient is placed into a straight knee immobilizer and allowed immediate weight bearing as tolerated. Physical therapy begins on postoperative day 1, with range-of-motion exercises, quadriceps strengthening, and patellar mobilization. Therapy is ideally conducted every day for the first 2 weeks and then at least three times per week thereafter. An emphasis is placed on increasing range of motion steadily with the goal of achieving the same measurements gained in the operating room, although this is often difficult to achieve fully. On occasion, patients will be unable to regain full or nearly full extension, despite therapy and intra-articular débridement, and open posterior capsular release will be required. The description of this procedure is beyond the scope of this chapter but is covered in several of the provided references.

Complications

Typical problems to watch for include hematoma, compartment syndrome from fluid extravasation, infection, and loss of motion.

Table 73-1 Clinical Results of Treatment for Arthrofibrosis

Author	No. of Patients	Outcome
Mayr et al[3] (2004)	223	96.8% improved
Noyes et al[5] (2000)	23	All full extension
Millett et al[4] (1999)	8	All satisfactory (open)
Shelbourne et al[7] (1996)	16	1 unsuccessful, 5 not full extension
Cosgarea et al[1] (1994)	37	36 satisfactory
Steadman et al[8] (1993)	44	33 excellent, 8 good, 1 fair, 2 poor
Noyes et al[6] (1992)	207	205 satisfactory
Harner et al[2] (1992)	27	All satisfactory, 6 required open procedures

73

PEARLS AND PITFALLS

Pearls

- Most loss of motion will respond to proper therapy and anti-inflammatory medications, steroids, and pain medications as needed.
- Early rehabilitation and timely intervention can decrease scarring after surgery or injury.
- After injury or surgery, 3 months is a reasonable period in which to try nonoperative treatment before surgery for any remaining deficit.
- For extension loss, look for scarring and lesions in the notch. For flexion loss, look in the suprapatellar pouch and the medial and lateral gutters.
- A progressive loss of motion indicates a scarring process; a stable block to motion indicates a discrete lesion.

- Patients must be willing and able to participate in physical therapy postoperatively.

Pitfalls

- Mature scar tissue, usually encountered 12 months or longer after injury or surgery, is more difficult to remove and produces poorer results in the long term.
- In dealing with total knee arthroplasty, care must be taken not to damage the components. A shaver can easily remove portions of the polyethylene spacer, and any tool or camera can scratch or abrade the metal. Either of these can lead to accelerated wear of the components and premature failure of the arthroplasty.
- Extension loss that does not respond to débridement may come from posterior capsular tightness. Unresolved flexion loss may result from quadriceps tightness.
- Complex regional pain syndrome is an absolute contraindication to operative intervention.

Results

The best treatment for arthrofibrosis of the knee is prevention. Through the use of anti-inflammatory medications, cryotherapy, adequate pain control, and early rehabilitation programs, postoperative patients can achieve their maximal range of motion and avoid this potentially debilitating complication.

With early recognition and timely intervention, arthrofibrosis can often be treated successfully. In patients with discrete lesions or less dense scarring, better results have been reported than in patients with extensive scarring. Through diligent postoperative physical therapy, many patients will experience a significant recovery of motion and maintain the gains achieved in the operating room (Table 73-1).

References

1. Cosgarea AJ, DeHaven KE, Lovelock JE. The surgical treatment of arthrofibrosis of the knee. Am J Sports Med 1994;22:184-191.
2. Harner CD, Irrgang JJ, Paul J, et al. Loss of motion after anterior cruciate ligament reconstruction. Am J Sports Med 1992;20:499-506.
3. Mayr HO, Weig TG, Plitz W. Arthrofibrosis following ACL reconstruction—reasons and outcome. Arch Orthop Trauma Surg 2004;124:518-522.
4. Millett PJ, Williams RJ, Wickiewicz TL. Open débridement and soft tissue release as a salvage procedure for the severely arthrofibrotic knee. Am J Sports Med 1999;27:552-561.

5. Noyes FR, Berrios-Torres S, Barber-Westin SD, Heckmann TP. Prevention of permanent arthrofibrosis after anterior cruciate ligament reconstruction alone or combined with associated procedures: a prospective study in 443 knees. Knee Surg Sports Traumatol Arthrosc 2000;8:196-206.

6. Noyes FR, Mangine RE, Barber SD. The early treatment of motion complications after reconstruction of the anterior cruciate ligament. Clin Orthop 1992;277:217-228.

7. Shelbourne KD, Patel DV, Martini DJ. Classification and management of arthrofibrosis of the knee after anterior cruciate ligament reconstruction. Am J Sports Med 1996;24:857-862.

8. Steadman JR, Burns TP, Peloza J, et al. Surgical treatment of arthrofibrosis of the knee. J Orthop Tech 1993;1:119-127.

Suggested Reading

DeHaven KE, Cosgarea AJ, Sebastianelli WJ. Arthrofibrosis of the knee following ligament surgery. Instr Course Lect 2003;52:369-381.

Kim DH, Gill TJ, Millett PJ. Arthroscopic treatment of the arthrofibrotic knee. Arthroscopy 2004;20:187-194.

Lidenfeld TN, Wojtys EM, Husain A. Surgical treatment of arthrofibrosis of the knee. Instr Course Lect 2000;49:211-221.

Petsche TS, Hutchinson MR. Loss of extension after reconstruction of the anterior cruciate ligament. J Am Acad Orthop Surg 1999;7:119-127.

Shelbourne KD, Patel DV. Treatment of limited motion after anterior cruciate ligament reconstruction. Knee Surg Sports Traumatol Arthrosc 1999;7:85-92.

CHAPTER 74

Distal Realignment for Patellofemoral Disease

Jack Farr, MD

Although the emphasis of this chapter is on tibial tuberosity surgery for patellofemoral disease, the multifactorial nature of patellofemoral dysfunction requires an acknowledgement that a patellofemoral problem is rarely addressed by a single surgical treatment. Tibial tuberosity repositioning must be examined with a full appreciation of proximal soft tissue balance, limb rotation, and articular cartilage disease (grade, site, and extent). Although positive outcomes were initially reported for many distal realignment patellofemoral surgeries, early positive results often deteriorated markedly over time. In the case of the Hauser posterior medial tuberosity transfer, although stability was maintained, patellofemoral cartilage degeneration predictably occurred over time. Thus, in general, patellofemoral surgery not only must address the acute problem but do so without causing intermediate and long-term problems, such as chondrosis and arthrosis. Application of a more scientific approach to patellofemoral dysfunction has led to the identification of the importance of the medial patellofemoral ligament (MPFL) in restraint to lateral patellar instability, and it has refined and focused the limited role of lateral release to isolated, documented patellar tilt rather than global patellofemoral pain or instability. Likewise, the role of tibial tuberosity surgery for patellofemoral dysfunction continues to evolve both as an isolated procedure and in conjunction with proximal patellofemoral surgery.

Indications espoused for tuberosity surgery (often in combination with proximal soft tissue surgery) at one point included patellofemoral pain, instability, chondrosis, and arthrosis. Straight tibial tuberosity medialization

(TTM) was initially associated with the names of specific surgeons, including Roux, Elmslie, and Trillat; anteriorization, with Maquet; and anteromedialization (AMZ), with Fulkerson. These tuberosity surgeries have, at times, been used to treat static patellar subluxation, recurrent lateral patellar instability, patellar pain, and patellofemoral chondrosis. Tuberosity surgery for treatment of recurrent or chronic patellofemoral dislocation or subluxation was based on the assumption that the primary pathologic process was an increased Q (quadriceps) angle; for pain and chondrosis, elevation was promoted as the preferred procedure to dramatically decrease patellofemoral stress. Whereas it is obvious that repositioning of the distal point of the Q angle (tibial tuberosity) surgically does modify the Q angle, today the MPFL is accepted as the main restraint to lateral patellar instability. In fact, the Q angle, which formed the rational basis for planning of a TTM, is being questioned as a benchmark in light of the poor intraobserver and interobserver reproducibility of the measurement as reviewed by Post. In addition, Fithian is questioning the role of TTM for lateral patellar instability. At the annual meeting of the American Orthopaedic Society for Sports Medicine in 2005, he presented a case series of recurrent lateral patellar instability treated by MPFL reconstruction with or without TTM. The results were the same in both groups. On the other hand, it must be acknowledged that Cox has reported excellent long-term results in prevention of recurrent patellar instability with TTM, although critics note that his report is a clinical outcome series without radiographs that might have demonstrated arthrosis (as predicted to occur with excessive medialization of the tuberosity in biomechanical studies by Andrish and Kuroda). Furthermore, as the extent of medialization with TTM has been variably defined, critics could imply that (1) some of the patients with instability successfully treated by TTM had spontaneous healing of the MPFL, (2) the MPFL lesion was marginally injured, or (3) the TTM "overmedialized" the tuberosity and constrained the patella into stability.

From a basic science approach, the initial tuberosity surgery focused on the action of the various force vectors on patellar position and motion and on the effect of tuberosity position on those vectors. However, the equation is more complicated, as Teitge, Powers, Heino, and others have emphasized the importance of the "other half" of the joint in motion: the trochlea and associated tibiofemoral torsion. Furthermore, Dejour has brought to attention the importance of trochlear morphologic features (dysplasia) in patients with lateral patellar instability. In an attempt to objectify tuberosity surgery, we must define normal and abnormal positions of the tuberosity. We must additionally consider the extent of femoral internal torsion and tibial external torsion as per Teitge and Heino.

This objective approach to limb coronal and axial alignment from hip to ankle also measures (at the knee) an objective alternative to the Q angle, that is, the tibial tuberosity to trochlear groove (TT-TG) distance (Fig. 74-1). The TT-TG distance, as popularized by Dejour, quantitates the concept of tibial tuberosity malalignment locally at the knee. Studies suggest that a TT-TG distance of more than 15 to 20 mm is abnormal; most asymptomatic patients have distances that are less than 15 mm. Likewise, anteriorization was first shown mathematically to reduce patellofemoral stress, but direct measurements with pressure-sensitive film, real-time pressure transducer arrays, and finite element analysis modeling such as by Cohen and Ateshian show that although stresses are typically reduced with anteriorization, there is a unique response for each knee, and a global "50%" force reduction cannot be assumed. Thus, load transfer should play an important role in surgical planning, rather than assuming that there will be an absolute decrease in stress. By use of these and other objective parameters, future studies may objectively quantify the preoperative pathologic process to aid in planning of tuberosity surgery.

Preoperative Considerations

History

Subgroups considered for tuberosity surgery are those with static subluxation of the patella, those with patellofemoral chondrosis that requires load optimization, and those with recurrent lateral instability with or without static subluxation. The history will be highly variable for each subgroup, from insidious onset of patellofemoral pain to pain that began after a patellar instability episode. The standard patellofemoral history as outlined by Post should be elicited. Functional aspects need to be documented, including the amount of energy needed to cause instability and the degree of stress necessary to cause pain. Prior surgical operative notes are useful, as are intraoperative photographs.

Typical History

- Failure of prolonged appropriate physical therapy and bracing
- Patellofemoral area pain with prolonged flexed knee position, stairs, or squats
- Giving way with either pain or patellar instability
- Patellofemoral crepitation and intermittent effusion and occasional loose bodies
- Often prior chondroplasty and lateral release

Signs and Symptoms

Patellofemoral symptoms are ubiquitous but nonetheless must be documented as to functional impairments with respect to pain, crepitation, swelling, giving way, and frank patellar instability and loose body sensations. Clinical signs overlap with the physical examination findings and include documentation of crepitation during the specific arc of motion, effusion, and loose body appearance.

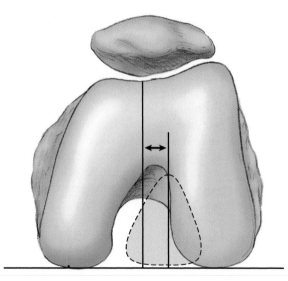

Figure 74-1 Tibial tuberosity to trochlear (femoral) groove distance is measured between perpendicular lines drawn from posterior condyles through the deepest aspect of the trochlea and the midpoint of the patellar tendon attachment of the proximal tibial tuberosity.

Physical Examination

As for all patients with patellofemoral dysfunction, a standard examination is performed of the knee and the entire functional kinetic chain from the pelvis to the foot. A standard patellofemoral examination as detailed by Post pays particular attention to the following:

- Focal site or sites of maximal pain (especially at prior scars) or diffuse pain with any touch (to suggest chronic regional pain syndrome; see contraindications)
- Patellar displacement (measured in trochlear quadrants)
- Patellar height (normal, infera, alta)
- Tuberosity position relative to center of trochlea (Q angle less reliable)
- Limb rotation (femoral and tibial internal and external rotation)
- Muscle bulk and strength, with attention to vastus medialis obliquus
- Patellar tracking through active and passive range of motion
- Individual variations of adequacy of the MPFL
- Patellar tilt or extent of eversion, especially with prior lateral release
- Patellar crepitation (document angle of flexion at which this occurs)
- Apprehension: classic lateral versus global versus medial
- Fulkerson medial instability test

Imaging

Radiography

- Standard weight-bearing anteroposterior and true lateral views
- Shallow flexion angle axial view (i.e., Merchant view)
- Long limb alignment to evaluate coronal limb malalignment
- Rosenberg (skier's) weight-bearing posteroanterior view

Other Modalities

Magnetic resonance imaging with or without contrast enhancement will add information about the extent and position of articular cartilage disease. Magnetic resonance imaging or computed tomography delineates patellofemoral morphologic features (extent of dysplasia), evaluates congruity of the patella in the trochlea, and provides objective measurement of the TT-TG distance and patellar height—with the understanding that cartilage contour does not always match bone contour.

Technetium bone scan may indicate areas of overload and arthrosis or suggest complex regional pain syndrome (sympathetically mediated pain).

Indications and Contraindications

Indications for Tibial Tuberosity Medialization

- Objective measurement of an increased TT-TG distance and symptoms, which can be directly related to abnormal stress secondary to resultant force vectors. The joint has normal or nearly normal articular surfaces of the patellofemoral compartment.
- Objective measurement of a markedly increased TT-TG distance in patients undergoing MPFL reconstruction or repair in an effort to decrease abnormal stress to the MPFL
- Potentially, those patients with the diagnosis of static chronic patellar subluxation, in addition to recurrent patellofemoral instability, who are undergoing MPFL surgery. In this case, TTM is performed in an effort to improve patellofemoral joint congruity, thus improving contact area, which may decrease stress.
- Objective measurement of an increased TT-TG distance in a patient who has undergone patellofemoral arthroplasty that demonstrates chronic patellar subluxation after correct implantation and adequate lateral release and MPFL repair or reconstruction

Indications for Anteromedialization

- As for TTM, but with chondrosis in the distal lateral region of the patella with an intact trochlea or minimal trochlear chondrosis. (Restated, this includes excessive lateral compression with tilt, chronic static patellar subluxation, and a combination as described originally by Fulkerson.)
- As in the preceding, but with more extensive chondrosis (grade, distribution, and trochlear condrosis). AMZ may be combined with cartilage restoration procedures, when AMZ can decrease stress to the restored regions.

Contraindications to Tibial Tuberosity Medialization

- Normal TT-TG distance
- Abnormal femoral anteversion or tibial torsion as per Teitge
- Problem not explained by an increased TT-TG distance
- Medial patellofemoral chondrosis that would be subjected to increased loading after TTM
- Grade III or higher (Outerbridge or International Cartilage Repair Society) chondrosis of the patella or trochlea

- Standard contraindications to knee osteotomy, such as nicotine use, nonspecific pain, infection, inflammatory arthropathy, marked osteoporosis (which would compromise fixation), complex regional pain syndrome, patella infera, and arthrofibrosis
- Relative contraindication in the markedly varus knee that could have increased stress to the medial tibiofemoral compartment after TTM as per Andrish

Contraindications to Anteromedialization (without cartilage restoration)

- As for contraindications to TTM and when AMZ would be expected to increase the stress in areas of damaged cartilage (e.g., proximal patellar pole after impact chondrosis, diffuse mid-waist patellar chondrosis, or medial facet chondrosis)
- Trochlear chondrosis of grade II or higher

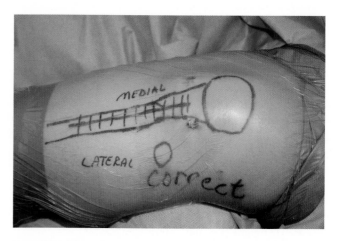

Figure 74-2 Skin landmarks for AMZ incision include patella, patellar tendon, tibial crest, and Gerdy tuberosity.

Surgical Planning

The goal of medialization is normalization of the tuberosity position rather than overmedialization, so preoperative radiographic or clinical assessment of TT-TG distance is useful in planning.

Concomitant Procedures

If lateral release and MPFL repair (or reconstruction) are performed in conjunction with TTM or AMZ, the procedure order is lateral release, then tuberosity surgery, and finally MPFL surgery. If cartilage restoration is planned, in addition to the TTM or AMZ, these procedures can be performed concomitantly to reduce total knee exposure to surgery and to ease the patient's rehabilitation.

Surgical Techniques

Anesthesia and Positioning

The less invasive TTM can be performed under local anesthetic with sedation. TTM as well as AMZ may be performed by use of regional blocks (femoral and sciatic), with postoperative femoral nerve block for prolonged pain control. Alternatively, epidural, spinal, or general anesthetics may be used according to the surgeon's preference. Both AMZ and TTM are performed with the patient in the supine position, often with a roll under the ipsilateral pelvis to decrease external rotation. In light of bone surgery, they are often performed with the foot of the operating

table elevated and a side post used for the arthroscopic portion of the procedure rather than with the foot in a dependent position.

Surgical Landmarks, Incisions, and Portals (Fig. 74-2)

Landmarks

- Patella
- Trochlear margins
- Patellar tendon attachment to tibial tuberosity
- Gerdy tuberosity
- Crest of tibia

Portals and Approaches

- The arthroscopic portion of the procedure is performed through standard anteromedial and anterolateral portals with the option of an additional proximal portal to view patellar tracking in the trochlea.
- For the isolated TTM, a longitudinal 5-cm incision is made lateral to the tibial tuberosity.
- AMZ is performed either through an oblique 12-cm incision from the anterolateral portal to the midline distally or directly in the midline beginning 2 cm proximal to the patellar tendon attachment to the tibial tuberosity and continuing distally.

Structures at Risk

- Anterior tibial artery
- Deep peroneal nerve
- Patellar tendon
- Sites of long-term overload (leading to chondrosis).

Examination Under Anesthesia and Diagnostic Arthroscopy

Under anesthesia, range of motion (comparison of passive patellar tracking to known preoperative active) and the full extent of patellar displacement and tilt are documented. Diagnostic arthroscopy allows mapping and grading of all areas of chondrosis. These findings enter into final planning and in some instances suggest cancellation of the tuberosity surgery in light of discovery of a contraindication.

The arthroscopic examination documents the associated tibiofemoral and patellofemoral chondral (grade and region of lesions) and morphologic features of the pathologic process. This information allows fine-tuning of the tuberosity surgery for the indications listed before. Arthroscopic chondral treatment may be performed as indicated, followed by titration of the lateral release, if necessary. For those patients with reversible patellar tilt and significant medial patellar displacement (two trochlear quadrants), a lateral release will not be performed; for patients with patellar tilt and minimal medial patellar dis-

placement (one trochlear quadrant or less), a limited lateral release or stepcut lateral lengthening will be titrated to allow reversal of tilt and to achieve two quadrants of medial patellar displacement.

Specific Steps (Box 74-1)

Tibial Tuberosity Medialization (Fig. 74-3A and B)

1. Exposure

The skin incision is based on whether the TTM is an isolated or combined surgery. The standard longitudinal

Box 74-1 Surgical Steps

1. Exposure
2. Planning of the osteotomy
3. Performance of the osteotomy
4. Tubercle fixation

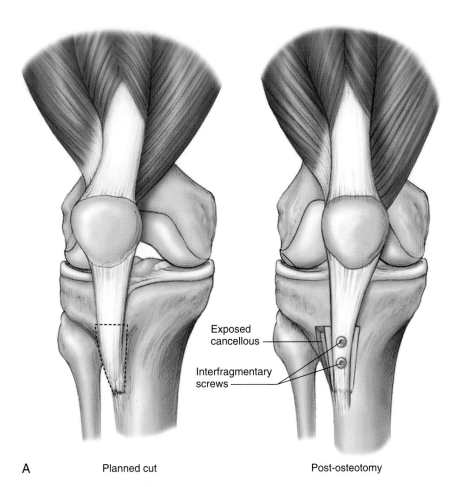

Exposed cancellous

Interfragmentary screws

A   Planned cut   Post-osteotomy

Figure 74-3 A, Overview of tibial tuberosity medialization.

74

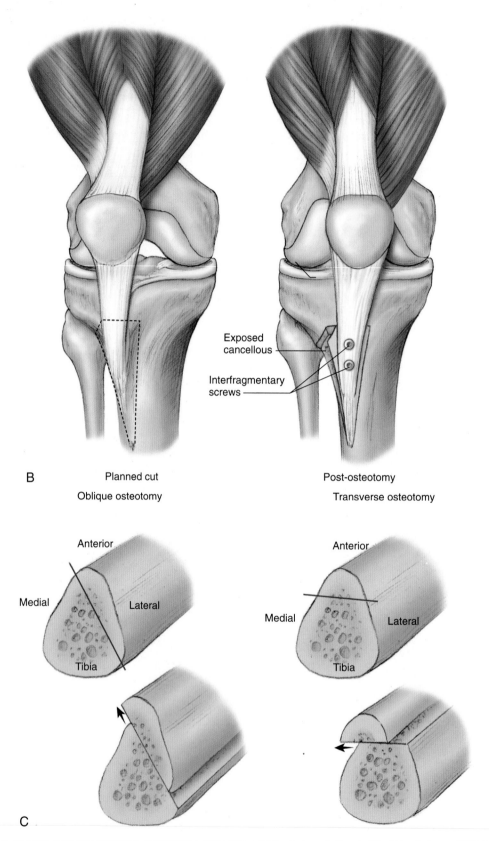

Exposed cancellous

Interfragmentary screws

B — Planned cut
Oblique osteotomy

Post-osteotomy
Transverse osteotomy

Anterior

Medial — Lateral

Tibia

Anterior

Medial — Lateral

Tibia

C

Figure 74-3, cont'd B, Overview of anteromedialization. **C,** Orientation of the oblique AMZ osteotomy *(left)* and of the flat osteotomy of TTM *(right)*.

incision is made lateral to the tibial tuberosity, with approximately 2 cm of the incision above the tuberosity and 3 cm of the incision below the tuberosity. It may be modified to a more universal direct anterior longitudinal approach as dictated by concomitant surgery. The patellar tendon is identified, and the lateral release (if it is performed) is extended along the lateral border of the patellar tendon with emphasis on hemostasis. A 1.5-cm subperiosteal exposure of the lateral aspect of the tibial tuberosity is performed.

2. Planning of the Osteotomy

The coronal plane cut is referenced from the anterior joint lines to be flat in the coronal plane. If there is a desire to unload the distal lateral patella, the cut is made with a mild anteriorly directed slope (Fig. 74-3C, *right*).

3. Performance of the Osteotomy

A 1.5-cm-deep cut in the axial plane is performed just proximal to the protected patellar tendon proximal attachment to the tibial tuberosity. A second bone cut begins at the posterior aspect of this cut and extends distally for approximately 5 cm while remaining 1.5 cm posterior to the crest of the tibial tuberosity. With the distal anterior tibial crest kept intact, the tuberosity is rotated medially, making a greenstick fracture at the distal portion of the osteotomy. The tuberosity is medialized to the extent that the TT-TG distance is normalized, but not overmedialized.

4. Tuberosity Fixation

The tuberosity is temporarily fixed with a Kirschner wire. Patellar tracking is viewed, and if it is acceptable, the tuberosity is fixed with interfragmentary screws (the screws are aimed medially, with care taken to avoid vascular injury).

Anteromedialization

1. Exposure

If the AMZ is an isolated procedure, begin the midline longitudinal incision midway between the patella and tuberosity and extend it distally 10 to 15 cm. Alternatively, the incision can course from the anterolateral portal to the same point on the tibial crest distally. Proximal extension may be performed to allow concomitant patellofemoral cartilage restoration. The patellar tendon is exposed subcutaneously. The lateral aspect of the patellar tendon is released, isolated, and protected. This lateral peripatellar tendon incision is extended proximally to the lateral release (noting the specific lateral release indications discussed earlier) and then distally along the anterior tibial crest to begin elevation of the anterior compartment musculature (Fig. 74-4). To allow anteriorization, a release is also performed immediately adjacent to the patellar tendon medially. The freed patellar tendon is protected with a retractor

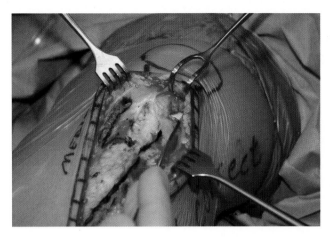

Figure 74-4 The pointer is at the distal extent of the arthroscopically performed lateral release. The peripatellar tendon and lateral tibial crest incision sites are marked. Note that a tourniquet was not used during this procedure.

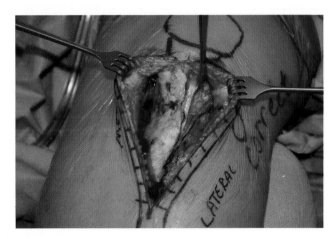

Figure 74-5 An Army-Navy retractor demonstrates that both margins of the patellar tendon have been released.

(Fig. 74-5). The anterior compartment musculature is subperiosteally dissected, and a retractor is positioned at the posterior extent of the lateral tibial wall to protect the posterior neurovascular structures (Fig. 74-6).

2. Planning of the Osteotomy

With use of a commercially available AMZ osteotomy system (Tracker by Mitek, Raynham, Mass), the osteotomy starting entrance position is planned by placing the cutting block jig medial to the patellar tendon attachment to the tibial tuberosity (Fig. 74-7). The planned osteotomy begins adjacent to the medial patellar tendon and courses laterally as it runs distally to allow the osteotomy to exit distally and laterally (a triangle shape). A drill guide–like arm is inserted into the cutting block. The tip of the slope selector arm predicts the lateral wall exit of the oblique osteotomy (Fig. 74-8). The tip (osteotomy exit) should be on the lateral wall of the tibia, always anterior to the

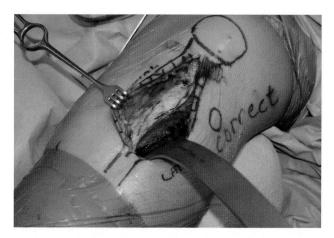

Figure 74-6 The anterior compartment musculature has been subperiosteally elevated from the lateral wall of the tibia and held with a custom retractor.

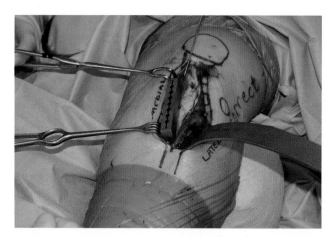

Figure 74-7 The cutting block is angled laterally as it extends distally from the medial aspect of the patellar tendon attachment to the tuberosity, which makes a thin shingle of bone distally to allow the necessary repositioning of the tuberosity. The nerve hook is retracting the medial edge of the patellar tendon.

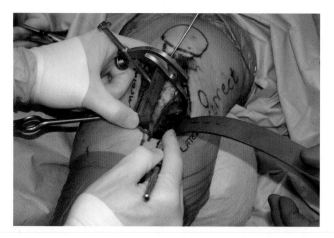

Figure 74-8 The tip of the slope selector guide (highlighted by the probe) shows where the osteotomy will exit. By moving the cutting block more medial and the tip of the slope selector more anterior up the wall of the tibia, the angle of the slope is decreased. With the osteotomy exiting just anterior to the posterior wall, the steepest slope (approximately 60 degrees) is obtained.

posterior wall. With the cutting block immediately adjacent to the patellar tendon attachment medially and the slope selector tip just anterior to the posterior wall, the slope is approximately 60 degrees (Fig. 74-3C, *left*). By moving the cutting block medially and the slope selector anteriorly, the slope can be decreased, for example, to 45 degrees. A smaller angle provides increased medialization relative to anteriorization. That is, the suggested anteriorization of 1.2 to 1.5 cm is "constant," and thus with a steep slope (60 degrees), the medial displacement would be 0.6 to 0.75 cm; for a 45-degree slope, the same elevation would allow 1.2 to 1.5 cm of medialization.

3. Performance of the Osteotomy

With the desired slope selected, the cutting block is temporarily fixed to the tibia with pins through drill holes (Fig. 74-9). The oblique cut is made with an oscillating saw cooled with saline. The saw is directly observed as it exits on the lateral wall of the tibia anterior to the retractor (Fig. 74-10). The cutting block is removed. The oblique cut is

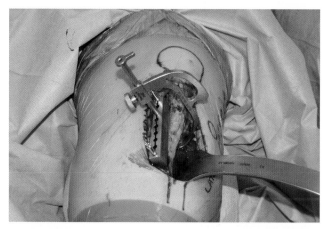

Figure 74-9 After the desired slope and cutting block position are selected, the cutting block is temporarily fixed to the tibia with pins through drill holes. Note that the cutting block is positioned more laterally at the distal aspect.

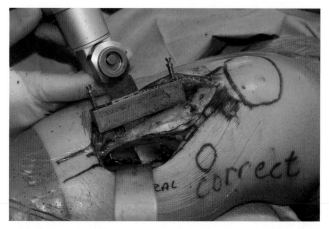

Figure 74-10 The saw is observed at all times as it exits the posterior aspect of the lateral wall. The retractor helps protect underlying tissues.

finished proximally and distally with use of the original bone cut as a captured saw guide (Fig. 74-11). To finish the proximal osteotomy, an osteotome connects the posterolateral wall saw exit site to the lateral aspect of the patellar tendon attachment to the tibial tuberosity (Fig. 74-12). Changing the angle of the osteotome, the last bone cut connects the previous cuts that have extended just proximal to the patellar tendon attachment to the tibial tuberosity medially and laterally. At this point, the tuberosity pedicle is free to rotate up the inclined slope.

4. Tuberosity Fixation

The completed oblique cut allows movement of the tuberosity pedicle up the inclined plane, affecting the desired anteromedialization. The tuberosity is temporarily fixed with a Kirschner wire, and the anteriorization and medialization are measured (Fig. 74-13). The tuberosity is fixed with interfragmentary technique, with avoidance of vascular structures as discussed by Miller (Fig. 74-14).

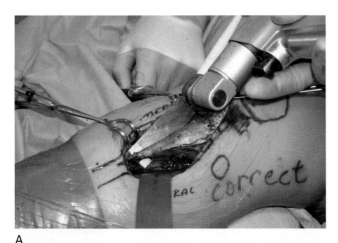

A

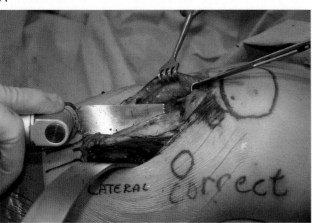

B

Figure 74-11 After the main portion of the oblique cut is made through the jig, the cutting block is removed and the osteotomy is used as a captured guide to finish the distal (**A**) and proximal (**B**) aspects of the oblique cut.

Postoperative Considerations

Follow-up

- Standard knee management includes a protective brace locked at or near extension initially, compression, cryotherapy, elevation, and possible continuation of the femoral nerve block (Fig. 74-15). The limb is observed for compartment syndrome and any problems with skin healing.
- Sutures and staples are removed at 7 to 10 days.
- Radiographs are typically obtained perioperatively and then at 6 weeks postoperatively. For comparison of preoperative and postoperative radiographs, see Figure 74-16.

Rehabilitation

- The less extensive osteotomy of the TTM allows the patient to begin weight bearing with crutches as tolerated. AMZ requires limited weight bearing with two crutches for 6 weeks to minimize fracture. The initial protective brace may be discontinued when the patient is safe and has excellent quadriceps control.
- Early postoperative exercises serve to improve venous flow, to maintain quadriceps function, and to maintain

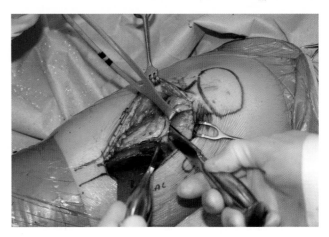

Figure 74-12 The two osteotomes represent the final proximal cuts. The more posterior osteotome courses from the proximal extent of the posterior oblique cut to the lateral attachment of the patellar tendon to the tuberosity. The second osteotome connects the lateral cut just made to the cut already present on the medial aspect of the patellar tendon attachment to the tuberosity. Note the retractor protecting the patellar tendon. Also note that the angles of the cuts are quite different.

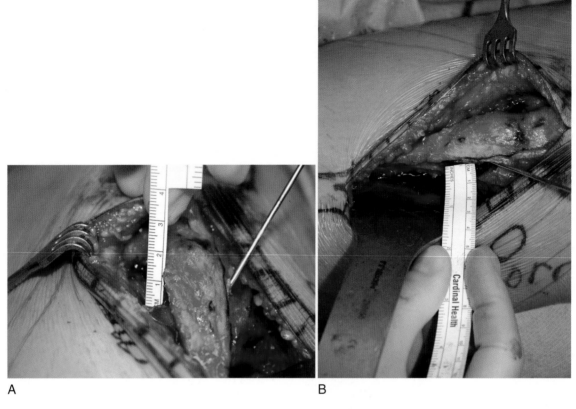

A   B

Figure 74-13 After the tuberosity is repositioned up the slope of the osteotomy, it is fixed temporarily with a K-wire, and the anteriorization (**A**) and medialization (**B**) are checked.

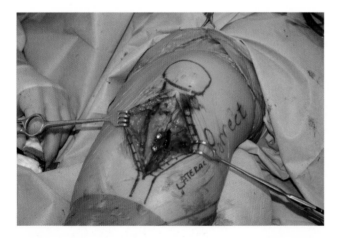

Figure 74-14 The tibial tuberosity is fixed with two 4.5-mm interfragmentary screws in the new position.

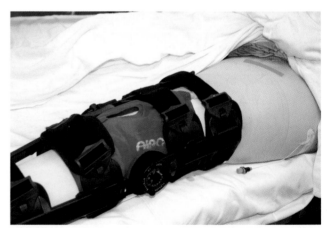

Figure 74-15 Postoperative management with antithrombotic hose, a cryotherapy device, and a hinged brace locked in extension or 0 to 30 degrees. Note the two catheters proximally for the femoral and sciatic regional nerve blocks. The sciatic catheter is removed immediately after surgery; the femoral catheter may be used for added pain control.

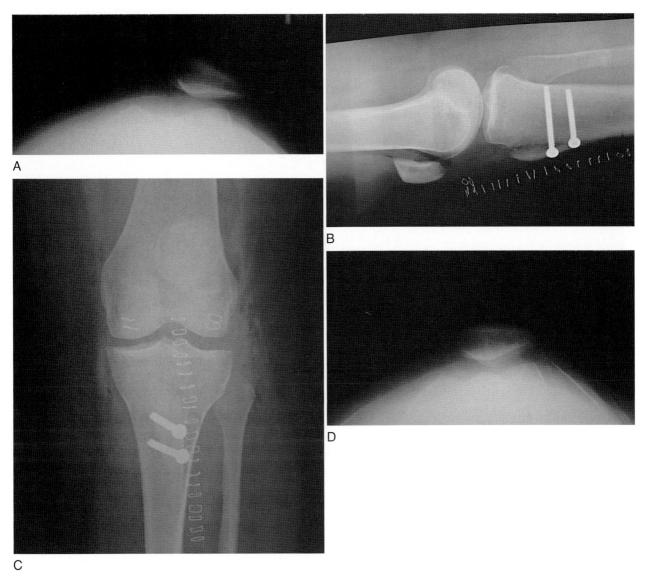

Figure 74-16 Radiographs of the case described here. **A,** Preoperative Merchant view with chronic static subluxation (no instability). **B,** Lateral view showing tuberosity elevation and fixation. **C,** Anteroposterior view showing medialization. **D,** Postoperative Merchant view with improved centralization of the patella.

patellar mobility. The patient is rapidly progressed to a comprehensive core proximal muscle strengthening program and range-of-motion exercises. Depth, grade, and region of chondral lesions and restoration will dictate the type and flexion angle of patellofemoral loading exercises.

- The AMZ is protected with a brace locked in full extension or 0 to 30 degrees for ambulation; the brace is removed for supine heel slides. The stationary bicycle is started early for range of motion.

Complications

Complications are similar to those of any open bone procedure of the knee. These include fracture, malunion, loss of fixation, nonunion, infection, thromboembolic phenomenon, compartment syndrome, sympathetically mediated pain, arthrofibrosis, patella infera, and long-term progression of patellofemoral chondrosis. Additionally, failure to address preoperative surgical indications may lead to postoperative complications.

PEARLS AND PITFALLS

Pearls

- The goal for all tuberosity surgeries is "normalization" of the tuberosity position, that is, the surgery in not just to medialize or to anteriorize.

- Although computed tomographic scans are not obtained routinely, most patients have undergone a magnetic resonance imaging evaluation, which is useful for defining the regions of any chondrosis. This will aid in the planning of tubercle surgery (e.g., AMZ to unload a distal lateral area of chondrosis).

- The magnetic resonance imaging evaluation may have been performed at another facility, but it is still possible for the radiologist to go back to the images and to measure the TT-TG distance and the Caton-Deschamps ratio.

- The mean TT-TG distance of asymptomatic patients is 13 mm.

- The TT-TG distance is abnormal above 20 mm.

- The steepest AMZ angle is 60 degrees. For the typical 15 mm of elevation, this results in medialization of approximately 8 mm, which would normalize the elevated TT-TG distances in the majority of patients.

- An elevated Caton-Deschamps ratio (patella alta) would suggest that a component of distalization be added to normalize the position of the tibial tuberosity.

- Always measure hip internal and external rotation in the prone position. If there is excessive internal hip rotation, this implicates an increase in femoral anteversion, which should then be evaluated with computed tomography (hip, knee, and ankle) that will also detect excessive tibial external rotation.

- Preoperative rehabilitation prepares the limb and patient for recovery.

- Rehabilitation must emphasize proximal and core musculature and not just local muscles.

- The combination of cartilage restoration with AMZ (when specific chondral lesions are noted) may allow improved outcomes compared with either procedure alone.

- Be alert for pain that is disproportionate to the surgery. Early intervention (including sympathetic blocks) may avoid progression to classic complex regional pain syndrome.

Pitfalls

- Tibial tuberosity overmedialization increases medial patellofemoral forces and may lead to patellofemoral chondrosis and arthrosis.

- Medial tibiofemoral forces also increase with tuberosity medialization, so be very careful in considering the procedure in a varus knee to avoid acceleration of medial compartment wear.

- Warn patients of hardware pain and the potential need for removal.

- AMZ significantly weakens the tibia until healing. Early weight bearing will lead to an increased tibial fracture rate.

- Whereas a "little" medialization may be beneficial, more is not better. The goal is to normalize the TT-TG distance.

- Tibial tuberosity surgery cannot substitute for patholaxity of the MPFL causing patellar dislocations.

- The lateral release with tibial tuberosity surgery is only to balance the soft tissue. Overzealous lateral release may cause both medial iatrogenic dislocations and paradoxically an increase in lateral patholaxity.

- Tibial tuberosity surgery is contraindicated when the apparent lateral position is from a combination of excessive femoral anteversion and tibial external rotation.

- In patients with extreme trochlear dysplasia, the "bump" at the entrance to the trochlea will continue to interfere with tracking unless it is directly addressed.

- Too much anteriorization can cause problems with skin healing and may significantly rotate the patella, causing abnormal contact areas.

- AMZ outcomes are poor with proximal pole, panpatellar chondrosis or if there is trochlear chondrosis.

- Patella infera is a complicated problem and should be treated with a continuum of care; tuberosity surgery must have a thorough, scientifically based role if it is contemplated in that situation.

Results

Both short- and long-term case series for TTM and AMZ demonstrate high percentages of good and excellent results (Table 74-1). However, these are case series and need interpretation within the ranking of evidence-based medicine. In addition, these results need to be reviewed with biomechanical studies (i.e., Cohen and Kuroda) in mind.

Table 74-1 Results

Investigator	Surgery Type	Follow-up (average)	Outcomes
Bellemans et al[2] (1997)	AMZ	32 months	Lysholm scores: preoperative, 62; postoperative, 92
Buuck and Fulkerson[3] (2000)	AMZ	8.2 years	86% good and excellent
Cameron et al[4] (1986)	AMZ	2 years	82% good and excellent
Carney et al[5] (2005)	TTM	26 years	54% good and excellent
Fulkerson[11] (1983)	AMZ		All patients received substantial relief of pain
Fulkerson et al[12] (1990)	AMZ	35 months	89% good and excellent
Naranja et al[17] (1996)	TTM+Ant	74.2 months	53% good and excellent
Pidoriano et al[18] (1997)	AMZ	46.8 months	72% improvement
Sakai et al[20] (1996)	AMZ	5 years	20/21 satisfactory

AMZ, anteromedialization; Ant, anteriorization; TTM, tibial tuberosity medialization.

References

1. Beck PR, Thomas AL, Farr J, et al. Trochlear contact pressures following anteromedialization of the tibial tubercle. Am J Sports Med 2005;33:1710-1715.
2. Bellemans J, Cauwenberghs F, Witvrouw E, et al. Anteromedial tibial tubercle transfer in patients with chronic anterior knee pain and a subluxation-type patellar malalignment. Am J Sports Med 1997; 25:375-381.
3. Buuck D, Fulkerson J. Anteromedialization of the tibial tubercle: a 4- to 12-year follow-up. Oper Tech Sports Med 2000;8:131-137.
4. Cameron HU, Huffer B, Cameron GM. Anteromedial displacement of the tibial tubercle for patellofemoral arthralgia. Can J Surg 1986;29:456-458.
5. Carney JR, Mologne TS, Muldoon M, Cox JS. Long-term evaluation of the Roux-Elmslie-Trillat procedure for patellar instability. Am J Sports Med 2005;33:1220-1223.
6. Cohen ZA, Henry JH, McCarthy DM. Computer simulations of patellofemoral joint surgery. Patient-specific models for tuberosity transfer. Am J Sports Med 2003;31:87-98.
7. Cosgarea AJ, Schatzke MD, Seth A, Litsky AS. Biomechanical analysis of flat and oblique tibial tubercle osteotomy for recurrent patellar instability. Am J Sports Med 1999;27:507-512.
8. Dejour H, Walch G, Nove-Josserand L, Guier C. Factors of patellar instability: an anatomic radiographic study. Knee Surg Sports Traumatol Arthrosc 1994;2:19-26.
9. Farr J. Anteromedialization of the tibial tubercle for treatment of patellofemoral malpositioning and concomitant isolated patellofemoral arthrosis. Tech Orthop 1997;12:151-164.
10. Ferrandez L, Usabiaga J, Yubero J, et al. An experimental study of the redistribution of patellofemoral pressures by the anterior displacement of the anterior tuberosity of the tibia. Clin Orthop 1989;238:183-189.
11. Fulkerson JP. Anteromedialization of the tibial tuberosity for patellofemoral malalignment. Clin Orthop 1983;177:176-181.
12. Fulkerson JP, Becker GJ, Meaney JA, et al. Anteromedial tibial tubercle transfer without bone graft. Am J Sports Med 1990;18:490-497.
13. Heino Brechter J, Powers CM, Terk MR, et al. Quantification of patellofemoral joint contact area using magnetic resonance imaging. Magn Reson Imaging 2003;21:955-959.
14. Kline AJ, Gonzales J, Beach WR, Miller MD. Vascular risk associated with bicortical tibial drilling during anteromedial tibial tubercle transfer. Am J Orthop 2006;34:30-32.
15. Kuroda R, Kambic H, Valdevit A, Andrish JT. Articular cartilage contact pressure after tibial tuberosity transfer. Am J Sports Med 2001;29:403-409.
16. Morshuis WJ, Pavlov PW, de Rooy KP. Anteromedialization of the tibial tuberosity in the treatment of patellofemoral pain and malalignment. Clin Orthop 1990;255:242-250.
17. Naranja RJ, Reilly PJ, Kuhlman JR, et al. Long-term evaluation of the Elmslie-Trillat-Maquet procedure for patellofemoral dysfunction. Am J Sports Med 1996;24:779-784.
18. Pidoriano AJ, Weinstein RN, Buuck DA, et al. Correlation of patellar articular lesions with results from anteromedial tibial tubercle transfer. Am J Sports Med 1997;25:533-537.
19. Post WR. Clinical evaluation of patients with patellofemoral disorders. Arthroscopy 1999;15:841-851.
20. Sakai N, Koshino T, Okamoto R. Pain reduction after anteromedial displacement of the tibial tuberosity: 5-year follow-up in 21 knees with patellofemoral arthrosis. Acta Orthop Scand 1996;67:13-15.

74

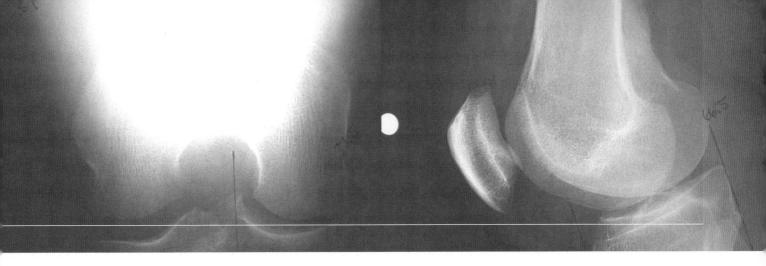

Index

Note: Pages numbers followed by the letter b refer to boxed material; those followed by f refer to figures, and those followed by t refer to tables.

Selected 2013 ed dm 2/11/14